Feline soft tissue and general surgery

There is no such thing as "Just a cat."
Robert A. Heinlein

Content Strategist: Robert Edwards
Content Development Specialist: Catherine Jackson
Project Manager: Sukanthi Sukumar
Designer: Miles Hitchen
Illustration Manager: Jennifer Rose
Illustrator: Antbits Ltd

Feline soft tissue and general surgery

Edited by

Sorrel J. Langley-Hobbs MA, BVetMed, DSAS(O), DipECVS, MRCVS

European Specialist in Small Animal Surgery, University Surgeon, Head of Small Animal Surgery, Department of Veterinary Medicine, University of Cambridge, Cambridge, UK

Jackie L. Demetriou BVetMed, CertSAS, DipECVS, MRCVS

European Specialist in Small Animal Surgery, Hon. Assoc. Professor of Small Animal Surgery, University of Nottingham, Dick White Referrals, Suffolk, UK

Jane F. Ladlow MA, VetMB, DipECVS, MRCVS

European Specialist in Small Animal Surgery, Lecturer, Soft Tissue Surgery, University of Cambridge, Cambridge, UK

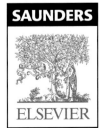

Edinburgh   London   New York   Oxford   Philadelphia   St Louis   Sydney   Toronto   2014

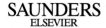

SAUNDERS
ELSEVIER

ISBN 978 0 7020 4336 9

British Library Cataloguing in Publication Data
A catalogue record for this book is available from the British Library

Library of Congress Cataloging in Publication Data
A catalog record for this book is available from the Library of Congress

Notices
Knowledge and best practice in this field are constantly changing. As new research and experience broaden our understanding, changes in research methods, professional practices, or medical treatment may become necessary.

Practitioners and researchers must always rely on their own experience and knowledge in evaluating and using any information, methods, compounds, or experiments described herein. In using such information or methods they should be mindful of their own safety and the safety of others, including parties for whom they have a professional responsibility.

With respect to any drug or pharmaceutical products identified, readers are advised to check the most current information provided (i) on procedures featured or (ii) by the manufacturer of each product to be administered, to verify the recommended dose or formula, the method and duration of administration, and contraindications. It is the responsibility of practitioners, relying on their own experience and knowledge of their patients, to make diagnoses, to determine dosages and the best treatment for each individual patient, and to take all appropriate safety precautions.

To the fullest extent of the law, neither the Publisher nor the authors, contributors, or editors, assume any liability for any injury and/or damage to persons or property as a matter of products liability, negligence or otherwise, or from any use or operation of any methods, products, instructions, or ideas contained in the material herein.

ELSEVIER your source for books, journals and multimedia in the health sciences
www.elsevierhealth.com

Working together to grow libraries in developing countries

www.elsevier.com • www.bookaid.org

The publisher's policy is to use paper manufactured from sustainable forests

Printed in China

Contents

Contents

Preface

There are many general and oncologic soft tissue surgical conditions that are unique to the cat, which more than justifies the need for a book dedicated to the subject. Examples of such conditions include feline injection site sarcomas, hyperthyroidism, axillary wounds, megacolon and feline lower urinary tract disease. There are significant anatomic differences between cats and dogs, which affect and influence surgical approaches and management of specific conditions.

Cats are popular pets, and are growing in popularity, with 33% of Americans owning a cat, and more than half of those owning more than one cat. Cats are also living longer, therefore conditions that are associated with older patients, such as neoplasia, are being recognized with increasing frequency in this species. Hyperthyroidism is also becoming more common, possibly due to the felines' increased longevity and also due to an increased awareness of this illness by both owners and veterinarians. Curative treatment options such as thyroidectomy become especially appealing when this condition is diagnosed at a younger age. Owners' expectations are also increasing, perhaps due to improved and more widespread access to information from the media, and as a result owners are also aware of the requirement to treat cats as a separate species. This book will enable the veterinarian to be fully informed and up-to-date on the management of all soft tissue surgical conditions in this species, so as to be able to offer the client and animal the best possible treatment advice.

The book should appeal to veterinarians in general practice, specialist veterinarians and veterinary students. Its aim is to provide a useful description of how to perform many surgical procedures in the cat, from straightforward procedures, which a general practitioner may feel competent to perform, to more specialized surgery. The book covers in detail surgical procedures specific to the cat that are either not described in detail in other textbooks or are described for the dog; such as total ear canal ablation, mandibulectomy, perineal urethrostomy, colectomy, adrenalectomy or hypophysectomy. This textbook is intended to be a partner to *Feline Orthopedic Surgery and Musculoskeletal Disease*. Together they will form a comprehensive pair of textbooks that cover the management of most surgical diseases in the cat.

There are many excellent books on feline diseases and their medical management available on the market and this book is not designed to replace such textbooks. For more information on the pathogenesis and medical management of such diseases the reader should refer to such texts. Additionally, there are excellent and thorough texts on both feline dentistry and feline ophthalmology, so no attempt was made to replicate these subjects. Periorbital and eyelid surgery is included as it was felt that this type of surgery is often attempted by general and specialist surgeons but intraocular surgery would usually be performed by an ophthalmologist and similarly advanced dentistry techniques by a specialist dentist.

The book is divided into seven parts. The first part deals with pre, intra and postoperative assessment and care of the surgical patient with separate chapters included on nutrition and blood transfusion.

The second part covers diagnostics including radiology, magnetic resonance imaging, scintigraphy and endoscopy from the nose to the bladder. A separate chapter is included on the cat ward. Further chapters cover instruments, sutures, implants, drains and feeding tubes. The third part in the book is the final introductory topics that covers some principles of diagnosis and surgery for oncology cases. In order to recognize the importance of multimodal cancer treatment, chapters are included on radiotherapy and chemotherapy.

The final four parts of the book cover surgical disease of the skin and adnexa, abdominal cavity, thoracic cavity and finally the head and neck. The general format of each chapter follows a similar pattern. A brief description of the anatomy of the organ or part of the body is followed by sections on general considerations such as specific concerns or imaging that is recommended for investigation of relevant diseases. Then all the most common surgical diseases from congenital, acquired to neoplastic are described. This section is followed by the surgical techniques performed on the organ or part of the body with specific descriptions included in textboxes so the reader is guided as to how to perform the surgery. The end of the chapter highlights the relevant aspects of specific postoperative care, complications that can occur and the prognosis for the specific diseases. The emphasis on the sections of the chapters varies according to the organs and diseases being covered.

S.J. Langley-Hobbs
J.L. Demetriou
J.F. Ladlow

Acknowledgments

We would like to acknowledge the following colleagues for their generous contributions to this book, including reading chapters, taking photographs, and other contributions:

Hayley Carne BSc(Hons), RVN
Rob Foale BSc, BVetMed, DSAM, DipECVIM-Ca, MRCVS
Jon Hall MA, VetMB, CertSAS, MRCVS
Karen Harris BVetMed, MRCVS

Graham Hayes MA, VetMB, CertSAS, DipECVS, MRCVS
Christina Knudsen DVM, MRCVS
Liz Leece BVSc, CVA, DipECVAA, MRCVS
Sam McMillan VTS(Anaesthesia), DipAVN(Medical), RVN
Nic Rousset BSc, BVSc, MRCVS
Julie Sales DCR
Silke Stein DVM, DipECVS
Chrissie Willers

Contributors

Kimberly A. Agnello DVM, MS, DipACVS
Consultant in Surgery,
Faculty Surgeon,
School of Veterinary Medicine,
University of Pennsylvania,
Philadelphia, Pennsylvania, USA

Davina M. Anderson MA, VetMB, PhD, DSAS(ST), DipECVS, MRCVS
RCVS Recognised Specialist in Small Animal Surgery (Soft Tissue),
European Specialist in Small Animal Surgery,
Anderson Moores Veterinary Specialists Ltd,
Winchester, UK

Lillian R. Aronson VMD, DipACVS
Associate Professor of Surgery,
University of Pennsylvania,
School of Veterinary Medicine,
Philadelphia, Pennysylvania, USA

Nicholas J. Bacon MA, VetMB, CertVR, CertSAS, DipECVS, DipACVS, MRCVS
ACVS Founding Fellow, Surgical Oncology,
Imparato Clinical Associate Professor, Surgical Oncology,
Oncology Service Chief,
Department of Small Animal Clinical Sciences,
College of Veterinary Medicine,
University of Florida,
Gainesville, Florida, USA

Stephen J. Baines MA, VetMB, PhD, CertVR, CertSAS, DipECVS, DipClinOnc, MRCVS
European Specialist in Small Animal Surgery,
RCVS Specialist in Small Animal Surgery,
RCVS Specialist in Veterinary Oncology,
Willows Referral Service,
Solihull, UK

Vanessa R. Barrs BVSc(Hons), MVetClinStud, MACVSc(Small Animal), FANZCVSc(Feline), GradCertEd(Higher Ed)
Registered Feline Medicine Specialist,
Director of the University Veterinary Teaching Hospital,
Associate Professor and Head of Small Animal Medicine,
Faculty of Veterinary Science,
The University of Sydney,
NSW, Australia

Julia A. Beatty BSc(Hons), BVetMed, PhD, FANZCVSc(Feline Medicine), GradCertEd(HigherEd), MRCVS
RCVS Recognised Specialist in Feline Medicine,
Associate Professor of Small Animal Medicine,
Faculty of Veterinary Science,
The University of Sydney,
NSW, Australia

Mark W. Bohling DVM, PhD, DipACVS
Assistant Professor of Surgery,
Department of Small Animal Clinical Science,
College of Veterinary Medicine,
University of Tennessee,
Knoxville, Tennessee, USA

Malcolm J. Brearley MA, VetMB, MSc(Clin Onc), DipECVIM-CA(Oncology), FRCVS
RCVS Emeritus Specialist in Veterinary Oncology,
Frostenden,
Suffolk, UK

Paolo Buracco DVM, DipECVS
Full Professor of Veterinary Surgery,
Department of Animal Science,
University of Turin,
Grugliasco (Turin), Italy

Contributors

Rachel Burrow BVetMed, CertSAS, CertVR, DipECVS, MRCVS
Lecturer in Small Animal Soft Tissue Surgery,
Small Animal Teaching Hospital,
Wirral, UK

Nicole J. Buote DVM, DipACVS
Veterinary Specialist,
Surgeon,
VCA West Los Angeles,
Los Angeles, California, USA

Marge Chandler DVM, MS, MANZCVSc, DACVN, DACVIM,
DipECVIM-CA, MRCVS
Small Animal Nutrition Service,
University of Edinburgh,
Roslin, UK

Jackie L. Demetriou BVetMed, CertSAS, DipECVS, MRCVS
European Specialist in Small Animal Surgery,
Hon. Assoc. Professor of Small Animal Surgery,
University of Nottingham,
Dick White Referrals,
Suffolk, UK

Jane M. Dobson MA, DVetMed, DipECIVM-CA(Int Med & Onc),
MRCVS
University Reader in Veterinary Oncology,
Department of Veterinary Medicine,
University of Cambridge,
Cambridge, UK

Gary W. Ellison DVM, MS, DipACVS
Professor and Service Chief,
Small Animal Surgery,
Department of Small Animal Clinical Sciences,
University of Florida,
Gainesville, Florida, USA

Edward J. Friend BVetMed, CertSAS, DipECVS, MRCVS
Teaching Associate in Small Animal Surgery,
School of Veterinary Science,
University of Bristol,
Bristol, UK

Gabriele Gradner DVM, DipECVS
Clinical Department of Small Animal Surgery,
University of Veterinary Medicine,
Vienna, Austria

Zoe Halfacree MA, VetMB, CertVDI, CertSAS, FHEA,
DipECVS, MRCVS
Senior Lecturer in Small Animal Surgery,
Clinical Sciences and Services,
Small Animal Medicine and Surgery Group,
The Royal Veterinary College,
Hatfield, UK

Elizabeth Hardie DVM, PhD, DipACVS
Department Head, Clinical Sciences,
College of Veterinary Medicine,
Raleigh, North Carolina, USA

Robert J. Hardie DVM, DipACVS, DipECVS
Clinical Associate Professor,
Small Animal General Surgery,
University of Wisconsin,
School of Veterinary Medicine,
Department of Surgical Sciences,
Madison, Wisconsin, USA

Andrea Harvey BVSc, DSAM(Feline), DipECVIM-CA, MRCVS
RCVS Recognised Specialist in Feline Medicine,
European Veterinary Specialist in Internal Medicine,
Feline Medicine Clinician,
Small Animal Specialist Hospital,
Sydney, Australia

David Holt BVSc, DipACVS
Professor of Surgery,
University of Pennsylvania,
School of Veterinary Medicine,
Philadelphia, Pennysylvania, USA

Mark W. Jackson BSc, DVM, PhD, DipACVIM
Senior Lecturer,
Small Animal Internal Medicine,
University of Glasgow,
Glasgow, UK

Debra A. Kamstock DVM, PhD, DipACVP
Chief Pathologist/Director,
KamPath Diagnostics and Investigation;
Faculty Affiliate,
College of Veterinary Medicine and Biomedical Sciences,
Colorado State University;
President,
Oncology Pathology Working Group,
A joint venture of the Veterinary Cancer Society and the American
College of Veterinary Pathologists,
Colorado, USA

Sabine B.R. Kästner Prof Dr med vet, MVetSci, DipECVAA
Professor in Veterinary Anaesthesiology,
University of Veterinary Medicine,
Hannover, Germany

Barbara Kirby BS, RN, DVM, MS, DipACVS, DipECVS
Associate Professor and Discipline Leader Small Animal Surgery,
Section of Veterinary Clinical Sciences,
University College Dublin,
Dublin, Ireland

Patrick R. Kircher Prof Dr med vet, PhD, DipECVDI
Head of Division for Diagnostic Imaging,
Vetsuisse-Faculty,
University of Zurich,
Zurich, Switzerland

Jolle Kirpensteijn DVM, PhD, DipACVS, DipECVS
Professor in Surgery,
Department of Clinical Sciences of Companion Animals,
Faculty of Veterinary Medicine,
Utrecht University,
Utrecht, The Netherlands

Clare Knottenbelt BVSc, MSc, DSAM, MRCVS
Professor of Small Animal Medicine and Oncology,
University of Glasgow,
Glasgow, UK

Jane F. Ladlow MA, VetMB, DipECVS, MRCVS
European Specialist in Small Animal Surgery,
Lecturer, Soft Tissue Surgery,
University of Cambridge,
Cambridge, UK

Sorrel J. Langley-Hobbs MA, BVetMed, DSAS(O), DipECVS,
MRCVS
European Specialist in Small Animal Surgery,
University Surgeon,
Head of Small Animal Surgery,
Department of Veterinary Medicine,
University of Cambridge,
Cambridge, UK

John Lapish BSc, BVetMed, MRCVS
Chairman,
Veterinary Instrumentation,
Sheffield, UK

Philip Lhermette BSc(Hons), CBiol, MSB, BVetMed, MRCVS
Principal Veterinary Surgeon,
Elands Veterinary Clinic,
Sevenoaks, Kent;
Special Lecturer in Veterinary Endoscopy and Endosurgery,
The University of Nottingham School of Veterinary Medicine and Science,
Nottingham, UK

Lea M. Liehmann DipECVS
European Specialist in Small Animal Surgery,
Department for Companion Animals and Horses,
Clinic for Small Animals: Small Animal Surgery,
University for Veterinary Medicine,
Vienna

Victoria Lipscomb MA, VetB, CertSAS, FHEA, DipECVS
European Specialist in Small Animal Surgery,
Senior Lecturer in Small Animal Surgery,
Head of Soft Tissue Surgery,
Department of Veterinary Clinical Sciences,
Royal Veterinary College,
University of London,
Hatfield, UK

Jeffrey P. Little DVM
Small Animal Surgeon,
Department of Surgical Sciences,
School of Veterinary Medicine,
University of Wisconsin,
Madison, Wisconsin, USA

Janet K. McClaran DVM, DipACVS
Staff Surgeon,
The Animal Medical Center,
New York, New York, USA

Björn P. Meij DVM, PhD, DipECVS
Associate Professor,
Department of Clinical Sciences of Companion Animals,
Faculty of Veterinary Medicine,
Utrecht University, The Netherlands

Alison L. Moores BVSc(Hons), CertSAS, DipECVS, MRCVS
RCVS Specialist in Small Animal Surgery,
European Specialist in Small Animal Surgery,
Anderson Moores Veterinary Specialists,
Winchester, UK

Pieter Nelissen DVM, CertSAS, MRCVS
Consultant in Small Animal Surgery,
Dick White Referrals,
Suffolk, UK

Mauria O'Brien DVM, DACVECC
Clinical Assistant Professor,
Small Animal Emergency and Critical Care,
College of Veterinary Medicine,
University of Illinois,
Urbana, Illinois, USA

Stefanie Ohlerth PD, Dr med vet, DipECVDI
Senior Lecturer,
Diagnostic Imaging,
Vetsuisse Faculty,
University of Zurich,
Zurich, Switzerland

Laura J. Owen BVSc, CertSAS, DipECVS, MRCVS
European Specialist in Small Animal Surgery,
Lecturer, Soft Tissue Surgery,
University of Cambridge,
Cambridge, UK

Caryn E. Plummer DVM, DACVO
Assitant Professor and Service Chief,
Comparative Ophthalmology College of Veterinary Medicine,
University of Florida,
Gainesville, Florida, USA

Barbara Posch CertVR, DECVDI, MRCVS
Staff Radiologist,
The Queen's Veterinary School Small Animal Hospital,
University of Cambridge,
Cambridge, UK

Kathryn M. Pratschke MVB, MVM, CertSAS, DipECVS, MRCVS
RCVS Specialist in Small Animal Surgery,
European Specialist in Small Animal Surgery,
School of Veterinary Medicine,
College of Medical, Veterinary and Life Sciences,
University of Glasgow,
Glasgow, UK

Suzanne Rudd DipAVN(Medical), RVN
Senior Feline Veterinary Nurse,
Langford Veterinary Services/University of Bristol,
Bristol, UK

Bernard Séguin DVM, MS, DipACVS
ACVS Founding Fellow (Surgical Oncology),
Associate Professor,
Department of Clinical Sciences,
College of Veterinary Medicine,
Oregon State University,
Corvallis, Oregon, USA

Chris Shales MA, VetMB, CertSAS, DipECVS, MRCVS
European Specialist in Small Animal Surgery,
RCVS Specialist in Small Animal Surgery,
Willows Veterinary Referral Service,
Solihull, UK

Thomas Sissener MS, DVM, CertSAS, DipECVS, MRCVS
Surgeon and European Specialist in Small Animal Surgery,
Oslo, Norway

Contributors

Ramesh K. Sivacolundhu BSc, BVMS, MVS, FANZCVS
Specialist in Small Animal Surgery,
Director of Surgery and Oncology,
Balcatta Veterinary Hospital,
Perth, Australia

Kinley D. Smith MA, VetMB, PhD, CertSAS, MRCVS
Clinician in Small Animal Surgery,
Small Animal Hospital,
Faculty of Veterinary Medicine,
University of Glasgow,
Glasgow, UK

Andrew Sparkes BVetMed, PhD, DipECVIM, MRCVS
Veterinary Director,
International Society of Feline Medicine and International Cat Care,
Wilts, UK

Michael S. Tivers BVSc, PhD, CertSAS, DipECVS, MRCVS
RCVS and European Specialist in Small Animal Surgery,
Cave Veterinary Specialists,
West Buckland, UK

S.A. van Nimwegen DVM, PhD, DipECVS
Specialist in Small Animal Surgery,
Assistant Professor,
Department of Clinical Sciences of Companion Animals,
Faculty of Veterinary Medicine,
University Utrecht,
The Netherlands

Robert N. White BSc(Hons), BVetMed, CertVA, DSAS(Soft Tissue), DipECVS, MRCVS
European Specialist in Small Animal Surgery,
RCVS Specialist in Small Animal Soft Tissue Surgery,
Willows Veterinary Referral Service,
Solihull, UK

Dick White BVetMed, PhD, DSAS, DVR, FRCVS, DipACVS, DipECVS
ACVS, European and RCVS Specialist in Small Animal Surgery,
RCVS Specialist in Veterinary Oncology,
ACVS Founding Fellow (Surgical Oncology),
Director, Dick White Referrals,
Suffolk, UK

John M. Williams MA, VetMB, LLB, CertVR, DipECVS, FRCVS
Honorary Visiting Professor,
University of Liverpool;
Soft Tissue Surgeon,
Northwest Surgeons,
Cheshire, UK

Donald A. Yool BVMS, PhD, DipECVS, CertSAS, MRCVS
Senior Lecturer,
Head of Small Animal Soft Tissue Surgery,
Royal (Dick) School of Veterinary Studies,
University of Edinburgh,
Edinburgh, UK

Section | 1 |

S.J. Langley-Hobbs, J.L. Demetriou, J.F. Ladlow

The perioperative period

The success of a surgical procedure is reliant on thorough preoperative preparation and good postoperative nursing and nutrition, in addition to surgical technique. In recent years there has been an increased awareness of pain assessment and treatment in cats and also the development of cat friendly environments.

Initially, a thorough preoperative assessment of the patient is required and this is covered in detail in the first chapter in the book. Cats need a calm approach to assessment, and there are many aspects of both the physical examination and the environment in which the cat is examined that can be adapted to suit the nature of the cat.

The second chapter on anesthesia and analgesia focuses on cats with surgical diseases of the various organ systems including the thorax, abdomen, and head and neck. Analgesia of the cat should continue throughout the perioperative period. There have been big advances and progress made in the assessment of pain in the cat. Pain in cats is not always easy to detect, particularly as cats are often anxious and stressed due to their visit to the veterinarian. Pain scoring of cats should be something that is done routinely in both the preoperative and postoperative period. A cat that has had surgery performed should always be given the benefit of the doubt and given analgesia even if the signs of pain are not obvious. The subsequent two chapters are also focused on postoperative care. During the postoperative period the cat needs regular assessment to ensure it has a smooth recovery from surgery so complications are avoided, or recognized and treated promptly when they do occur. Thoughtful postoperative nursing can improve the recovery for the cat, and decrease the stress of hospitalization.

Surgical patients may require blood or blood products and the mechanisms and practicalities associated with giving a cat a blood transfusion are well described. If there is pre-existing blood loss or anemia, then the transfusion can be given preoperatively. If it is anticipated that there may be significant blood loss intraoperatively, then blood should be readily available in case it is needed. In either case the cat should be blood typed and cross-matched in preparation for a safe transfusion.

Cats that are unwell and hospitalized are not always keen to eat, and inappetent cats, particularly if overweight, are at risk of hepatic lipidosis. The importance of adequate nutrition and encouraging oral feeding cannot be overlooked and this topic is discussed in detail in the final chapter of this part of the book. Cats that eat postoperatively can usually be discharged more quickly and recover more swiftly.

Chapter | **1** |

Preoperative assessment for surgery

V.R. Barrs, J.A. Beatty

Pre-operative assessment of the patient provides a solid foundation for a safe and successful surgical procedure. The assessment relies heavily on information obtained from a thorough history and physical examination. It establishes the baseline physiologic data for the individual, facilitates assessment of intercurrent disease and its potential relevance, identifies current medications that may need adjustment in the perioperative period and directs appropriate preoperative testing.

ARRIVAL AND HISTORY TAKING

Evaluation of the patient begins at reception. Sick cats often present for lethargy and inappetence regardless of their underlying disease. Cats should be observed in their carriers by staff on arrival to identify injured or dyspneic patients that require immediate stabilization.

History taking

Regardless of the surgical procedure planned, the clinician should familiarize themselves fully with the medical history. The history can be considered in two parts; the general history and the specific history. The general history involves collection of background epidemiological information for the patient (Box 1-1). Signalment should be confirmed. Owners may, unwittingly, provide inaccurate information on their cat's age, breed or sex. It should be ascertained whether the cat was acquired as a kitten or as an adult of unknown background. A reasonable estimate of age can be made in cats that are still growing (up to 18–24 months) and in geriatric cats if there is iris discoloration or age-associated disease, e.g., most cats with hyperthyroidism are over 10 years old. Information regarding the cats' living circumstances is important. Owners of cats living in apartments can usually provide detailed information on toileting, appetite and activity levels that owners of cats that roam will be unable to provide. Owners should be questioned about current medications with the drug, dose, frequency and time of last dosing being recorded. In presurgical patients, special attention should be given to medications that may affect coagulation (e.g., heparins, warfarin, aspirin, and clopidogrel) and wound healing (e.g., prednisolone).

The specific history relates to the presenting complaint (Box 1-2). This establishes what abnormalities the owner has noticed, their duration and the pattern of disease. It is the responsibility of the clinician to find a way of communicating with each owner that best facilitates information flow. Although the problem might not be exactly what the owner perceives it to be, if a problem is reported, there almost certainly is one.

PHYSICAL EXAMINATION

A complete preoperative physical examination is essential to identify factors that may affect surgical outcome. Most cats will allow a thorough examination and respond best to minimal restraint. Special care should be taken with cats that are particularly timid or aggressive. Maintaining a quiet environment and avoiding sudden movement is helpful. Doors and windows should be closed. Further information on providing an appropriate environment for examining cats and the most cat friendly consulting room is provided in Chapter 9.

Handling and acclimatization

The demeanor of the cat and its resting respiratory rate and effort should be observed while it is in its carrier. If the cat appears relaxed, it should be stroked and talked to before lifting it onto the floor or table. If the cat appears aggressive (e.g., ears back and flattened) it is prudent to remove the cat from the top of its carrier swiftly by scruffing the back of the neck with one hand and supporting the cat's body under its chest with the other hand (Fig. 1-1). Some cats feel threatened when approached to be removed from their cage. Hesitating to remove these cats can precipitate aggressive swiping or biting. A non-aggressive cat can be removed from its carry cage at the start of the consultation and given time to acclimatize while the history is taken. The cat can sit on the consulting table while being gently held or stroked by the owner, or if the cat is not injured or dyspneic, it can explore the room. This can reduce anxiety in an unfamiliar environment before the physical examination begins and permits observation of the cat's mentation and gait. The 'window of opportunity' for examination of the cat can be small and the examination should

Box 1-1 **General history: An outline of questions to assist in obtaining background information**

Confirm signalment (age, sex, breed)
Determine origin of cat
    shelter/breeding cattery/pet-shop/stray?
    geographic origin/travel history?
    age when acquired?
Present environment
    outdoor access? (free roaming/restricted?)
    rural/urban?
    other pets? (number/species/health status)
    exposure to other animals?
    toxin exposure?
Diet
    amount and type including supplements and treats
    ingestion of prey? (e.g., rodents, reptiles, birds)
Previous medical problems
    type of illness, management, outcome
    current medications (prescription, over-the-counter, holistic)
Vaccination and parasite control status

Box 1-2 **Specific history: An outline of questions to assist in characterizing the presenting complaint**

What is the presenting complaint?
Is this a recurrence of a previously investigated problem?
What were the first signs?
What is the duration of these signs?
Are signs intermittent or continuous?
Are signs static, progressive or resolving?
Present status
    weight loss/gain?
    activity level, demeanor?
    appetite, water intake?
    urination and defecation characteristics?
    any gastrointestinal or respiratory signs?

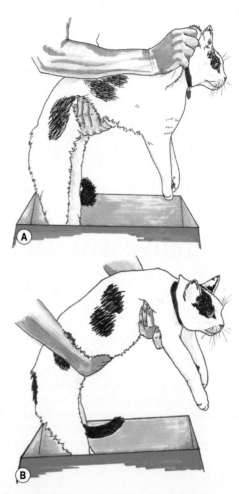

Figure 1-1 Removing cat from a top-loading box. **(A)** An anxious or aggressive cat can be held at the scruff and under the abdomen and swiftly removed. **(B)** A friendly cat can be supported under the chest and abdomen for removal.

the physical examination, after acclimatization. This avoids artefactual, anxiety-induced increases or decreases in blood pressure, known as the 'white-coat' effect (Fig. 1-2, Box 1-3). Doppler techniques are preferred over oscillometric techniques for measurement of SBP in conscious cats as they are more accurate and faster to measure.[2,3]

Head-to-tail examination

The physical examination can be completed by starting at the head and working caudally. The cat should first be weighed using accurate scales and its body condition score assessed using established 5-point or 9-point scoring systems (see Chapter 6):

Head
    Assess the shape and symmetry of the head
    Look/feel for muscle atrophy
Eyes
    Check pupil shape and symmetry
    Examine for discharge or blepharospasm
    Retract upper and lower eyelids to examine conjunctiva and sclera (Fig. 1-3)
    Examine cornea, iris and anterior chamber
    Prolapse nictitating membrane by placing thumb over upper eyelid and retropulsing globe with lower lid retracted (Fig. 1-4).

proceed from least invasive to most invasive procedures, with abdominal palpation, rectal temperature and manipulation of an area suspected to be painful generally performed last.

BLOOD PRESSURE MEASUREMENT

Measurement of systolic blood pressure (SBP) is indicated in any cat with evidence of target organ damage, including cats with chronic kidney disease (CKD), retinopathy or choriodopathy, intracranial signs, cardiovascular signs (murmur, gallop, arrhythmia) or epistaxis. SBP pressure should also be measured in obese cats and where thyroid or adrenal disease is suspected. Given that CKD and hyperthyroidism are the most common causes of hypertension in cats, it is prudent to measure blood pressure routinely in any cat that is 10 years of age or older.[1] Measurement of SBP should be carried out at the beginning of

Box 1-3 Systolic blood pressure measurement using Doppler sphygmomanometry

1. To minimize the 'white-coat' effect bring the cat, with the owner, into a quiet consultation room away from extraneous noises such as barking dogs. Allow five to ten minutes for the cat to acclimatize to these conditions.
2. With the cat in sternal recumbency or sitting, use an alcohol soaked swab to wet the hair on the palmar aspect of one forelimb adjacent to the metacarpal pad and just proximal to the first phalanx (Fig. 1.2A). Clipping the hair is NOT necessary in most cats. A hindlimb or the tail can also be used.
3. Measure the circumference of the forelimb mid-way between the carpus and the elbow, where the cuff will be placed. The cuff width should be >30% and closest to 40% of the circumference. An undersized cuff overestimates, and an oversized cuff underestimates blood pressure. Place the cuff.

4. Apply coupling gel to the Doppler probe and place the probe on the area prepared, level with the first phalanx and directly over the median artery to obtain a pulse signal. The cuff should be positioned level with the heart. Inflate the cuff to 20–30 mmHg beyond where the pulse is no longer audible. Slowly deflate the cuff. The point at which the pulse is again first audible is the systolic blood pressure (Figs 1.2B, 1.2C).
5. Leaving 30 to 60 seconds between each reading, take five consecutive readings, discard the first, and then calculate the mean systolic blood pressure. Record the cuff size used.
6. Perform fundoscopy to look for evidence of hypertensive choriodopathy or retinopathy (Fig. 1.2D).

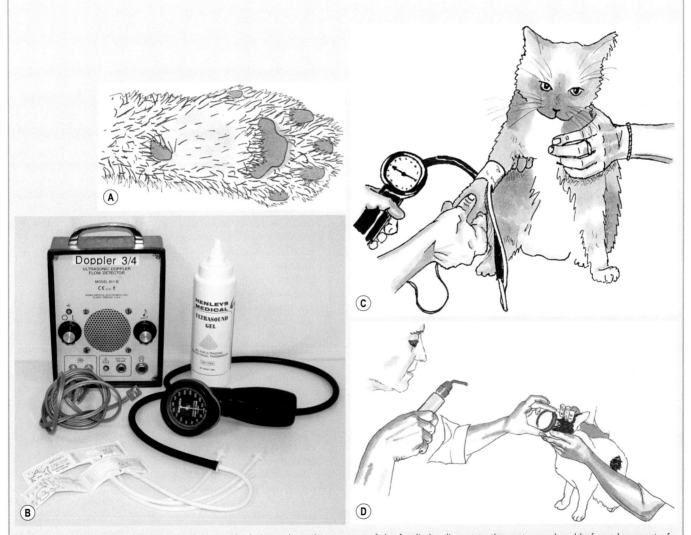

Figure 1-2 **(A)** An alcohol swab is used to wet the hair on the palmar aspect of the forelimb adjacent to the metacarpal pad before placement of the Doppler ultrasound probe. Clipping of the hair is not necessary and could contribute to "white-coat" hypertension. **(B)** Equipment for indirect blood pressure measurement in the cat: ultrasonic Doppler flow detector, sphygmomanometer, blood pressure cuff and coupling gel. **(C)** Technique for blood pressure measurement with cat gently restrained. The cuff is placed mid-way between the carpus and elbow. The Doppler probe is held lightly over the median artery on the palmar aspect of the forelimb adjacent to the metacarpal pad. **(D)** Indirect ophthalmoscopy using a Finnoff transilluminator and a 20–30 diopter lens. The examination can usually be completed in low ambient light without topical mydriatics. Otherwise, 1% tropicamide can be used. ([B] With thanks to Henleys Medical Supplies Ltd.).

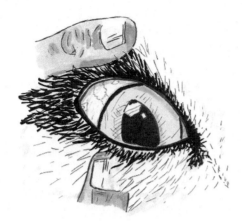

Figure 1-3 Examination of the sclera.

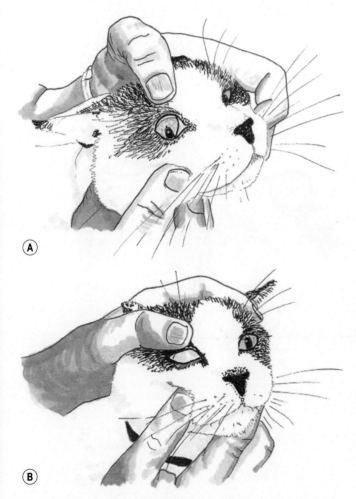

Figure 1-4 Examination of the nictitating membrane. **(A)** The lower lid is retracted downwards while **(B)** placing gentle pressure on the globe.

Fundic examination is essential when there is suspicion for chorioretinal disease (e.g., toxoplasmosis, feline infectious peritonitis (FIP)) or whenever blood pressure is measured (Fig. 1-2D)

Ears
  Examine pinnae
  Inspect and smell external ear canal for evidence of infection

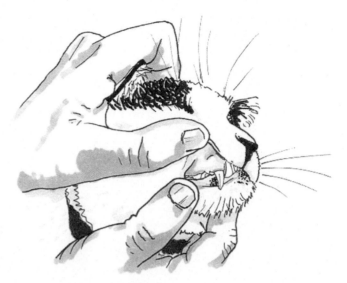

Figure 1-5 Examination of the gums.

Otoscopic examination to the level of the tympanic membranes, if permitted by the cat. Sedation or anesthesia is required for complete visualization if the cat has sensitive or painful ears

Mouth and hydration status
  Examine lips/commissures
  Elevate upper lip to assess mucous membrane color, moistness, capillary refill time (CRT) (Fig. 1-5). In comparison to the dog, the normal mucous membrane color for cats is paler. Assess the cat's hydration status (Table 1-1). Signs of dehydration include dry or tacky mucous membranes, a loss of skin turgor (skin tenting between the shoulder blades), prolonged CRT and enophthalmos. Skin tenting as a measure of hydration can be unreliable in geriatric or emaciated cats and the moistness of mucous membranes is more difficult to assess in cats than in dogs
  Assess teeth and gingiva
  The mouth should be opened (Fig. 1-6). The fauces, tongue and soft palate can be inspected. Subtle jaundice can sometimes be detected first on the soft palate
  The underside of the tongue is examined for masses or string foreign bodies by pressing the thumb of the second hand into the intermandibular space to elevate the tongue

Nose
  Assess nasal planum for altered pigmentation, ulceration or crusts
  Assess nares for symmetry, flare (with increased inspiratory effort), discharge and patency (microscope slide fogs on exhalation)
  Assess nasal bridge for shape and symmetry

Thyroid gland, larynx trachea, jugular vein
  With the head fully extended the thyroid lobes can be palpated by sliding the thumb and forefinger in a continuous movement from the larynx to the thoracic inlet. Enlarged thyroid lobes are palpated as a flick through the fingers (Fig. 1-7)
  The larynx can be gently palpated to elicit a swallow allowing non-invasive assessment of the gag reflex. One or two soft coughs may be elicited
  While the head is elevated the jugular vein is inspected for distension and/or pulsation. The hair may be damped down if the vein is not visible

Table 1-1 Assessment of hydration status

% Dehydration	Attitude	Eyes	Mucous membranes	Skin tent	Capillary refill time
5	Normal	Normal	Dry	Mildly prolonged <2 seconds	Normal or mildly prolonged
6–9	Mildly lethargic	Mildly sunken	Tacky/dry	Prolonged >3 seconds	Prolonged
10–12	Lethargic	Deeply sunken	Dry ± cold	Persists	Prolonged
>15%	Moribund, death impending	Deeply sunken	Dry/cold	Persists	Prolonged

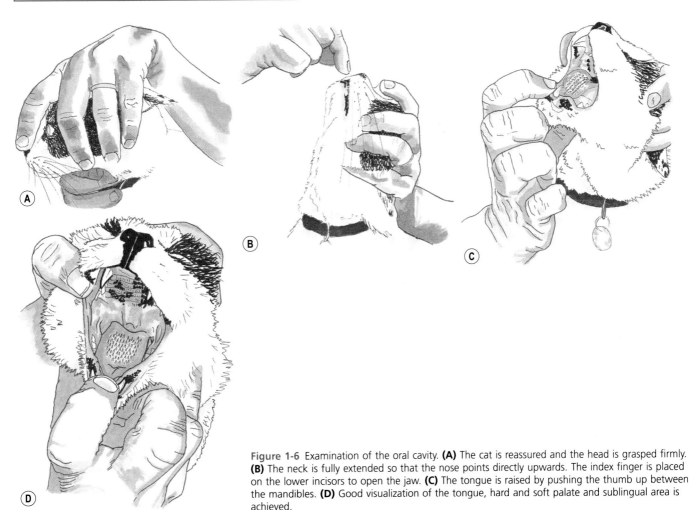

Figure 1-6 Examination of the oral cavity. **(A)** The cat is reassured and the head is grasped firmly. **(B)** The neck is fully extended so that the nose points directly upwards. The index finger is placed on the lower incisors to open the jaw. **(C)** The tongue is raised by pushing the thumb up between the mandibles. **(D)** Good visualization of the tongue, hard and soft palate and sublingual area is achieved.

Peripheral lymph nodes

Mandibular lymph nodes are located rostral and lateral to the mandibular salivary gland. They are palpated by grasping the soft tissues ventral to the vertical ramus of the mandibles and sifting through tissues until the node is felt as a small 'bean' that is harder and smoother than the lobulated salivary gland

Superficial cervical (prescapular) lymph nodes lie medial to the point of the shoulder, near the clavicle remnant

The popliteal lymph nodes lie between the gastrocnemius muscle bellies in the pelvic limbs and must be differentiated from surrounding fatty tissue

The axillary, inguinal lymph nodes and often prescapular lymph nodes, are not palpable unless enlarged

Thorax

Cardiovascular System

Palpate the cardiac apex beat noting intensity and presence of any thrills

Place the diaphragm of the stethoscope over the sternum with the cat standing or sitting and auscultate the heart in sternal and parasternal locations. In a veterinary hospital environment the normal feline heart rate ranges from 140 to 200 beats per minute

Take the heart rate and palpate the femoral pulses simultaneously, noting the pulse amplitude, pulse symmetry and any pulse deficits. Evaluation of femoral pulses is more difficult in the cat than the dog as they are more easily occluded during firm palpation, but their presence should be ascertained

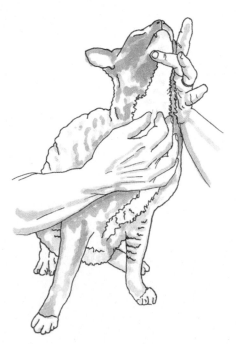

Figure 1-7 Thyroid palpation.

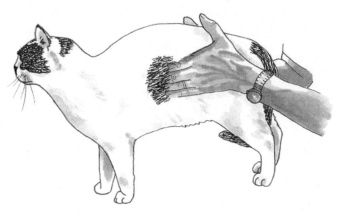

Figure 1-8 Abdominal palpation, two-handed technique.

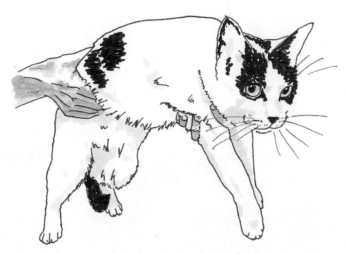

Figure 1-9 Abdominal palpation one-handed technique, R kidney palpation.

Listen for murmurs, grade them from I to VI and find the point of maximum intensity (PMI). Murmurs can be induced if the stethoscope is pressed too firmly against the chest
Listen for gallop (extra, abnormal) heart sounds. S4 is the gallop sound most often heard in cats. It arises from atrial contraction against a diastolically compromised ventricle, e.g., in hypertrophic cardiomyopathy. The S3 gallop is rare in cats. It is caused by sudden cessation of rapid ventricular filling with vibration of the walls and muscles
Assess the rhythm of the heart as regular, regular–irregular (e.g., sinus arrhythmia, rare in cats compared with dogs) or irregular–irregular (e.g., atrial fibrillation)

Respiratory System
Dyspnea is best detected by observation, not auscultation. Rate and effort should be determined while the cat is still in its carrier. The presence of a subtle increase in inspiratory effort is easier to appreciate from above. The presence of audible respiratory noise (stridor, stertor, wheeze) should be noted
Normal respiratory rate is 16 to 32 breaths per minute
In cats the cranial thoracic cage is compressible. Abnormal resistance can indicate an intrathoracic mass
Auscultation of lower respiratory tract: start mid-thorax at the 8th intercostal space (level of tracheal bifurcation). Move the stethoscope dorsally, ventrally, cranially and caudally to auscultate all areas of the lungs. Record the exact location of any abnormal lung sounds and their characteristics, e.g., crackles, wheezes
Auscultate over the trachea and larynx. Upper respiratory sounds may be referred to the lower respiratory tract. If sounds are loudest over the upper respiratory tract, it is likely that this is their origin
If the cat is purring, options are to reposition it, show the cat a running tap or tap the nose, gently palpate the larynx or auscultate through the purring until there is a gap, or try again later

Percussion of the thorax can help identify areas of decreased resonance caused by fluid, consolidation or a mass

Abdominal palpation
Examine the animal from behind. Start at the mid-abdomen pressing gently at first, and then slowly increasing the pressure in increments. If you apply too much pressure initially the patient may splint the abdomen and normal structures will not be palpable
The abdomen can be palpated using a one or two-handed technique (Figs 1-8 and 1-9). For the latter, the flat of each hand is placed against the abdominal wall in a mid-abdominal location and slowly pressed together. The kidneys are palpated first. The right kidney lies cranial to the left kidney and if not palpable with the cat standing, the forelegs are lifted off the table with the left hand under the chest. The right kidney then drops into a more caudal location and can be grasped with the right hand. The left kidney is easily palpable with the cat in a standing position. The size of the kidneys should be noted as well as any irregularities of the renal cortex
Next reach forward into the cranial abdomen. The caudal border of a normal liver can usually just be palpated as a sharp edge on the cranioventral abdomen adjacent the costal arch
A palpable spleen usually indicates splenomegaly

Small intestinal loops are palpated in the ventral third of the abdomen and should be evaluated for wall thickening

Enlarged mesenteric lymph nodes may also be palpable

The descending colon is palpable when feces are present. Feces are usually compressible, whereas intestinal masses are not

Musculoskeletal, skin and coat

Examine each forelimb from scapula to toes. Examine forelimb muscles for symmetry, palpate for masses under the hair coat

Check feet, flex carpus and elbow, check toes and nails. Cats with digital metastases have swollen, painful distal digits, this may be the only physical abnormality with some neoplasms

Palpate the muscles of the back and trunk. Apply pressure over the vertebrae to detect back pain

Palpate rear limb muscles, check toes and nails

If the animal has presented for a musculoskeletal problem a more detailed examination is required[4]

Examine the hair coat, combing the coat the wrong way. Thoroughly examine the skin color and coat consistency. Check for alopecia

Ventral abdomen

Lay the cat in lateral or dorsal recumbency and examine the ventral abdomen. Check the skin and palpate the nipples, inguinal and axillary areas carefully

Rectal temperature

Normal temperature 37.8–39.2°C

Use lubricant to insert the thermometer gently into the rectum. Cats often clamp their internal anal sphincter, preventing the thermometer from entering further. Wait for a few seconds and stroke the cat. Once the cat has relaxed then gently insert the thermometer at least 2 or 3 cm into the rectum. The thermometer must be held at an angle so that the bulb lies against the rectal wall. If the thermometer is held in the lumen of the rectum or in feces it may record an erroneously low value. Rigid thermometers are preferred to more flexible thermometers since the latter may bend away from the rectal wall

While measuring the temperature inspect the perineum and tail base

Examine the thermometer for the presence of fecal material and note color, presence of blood, mucus, and so on.

Due to their small size digital rectal examinations are only performed in cats if clinical signs of rectal, urethral or, rarely, prostatic disease are present. Some cats require sedation to perform a rectal examination.

PROBLEM-BASED PATIENT ASSESSMENT

Once the history and physical examination are complete, the next step is to determine and assess the active problems based on the information acquired. A problem is defined as anything that interferes with the patient's well-being that requires further attention or management. A problem may be a specific diagnosis, a clinical sign, a syndrome, an abnormal physical finding, an abnormal laboratory test result or an abnormal diagnostic imaging finding. It may be something requiring immediate investigation and/or treatment or something that is not of immediate concern but is potentially important. Once the problem list is defined, except for specific diagnoses, each problem is assessed in terms of:

The body systems involved
The anatomic localization of lesions
The possible pathogenetic mechanisms
The possible etiologies.

Box 1-4 **VITAMIN D acronym used to create differential diagnoses list**

Vascular: ischemia + hemorrhage
Infection/inflammation/immune-mediated: (bacterial, fungal, viral, protozoal, parasitic)
Trauma
Anomalous: congenital + inherited disease
Metabolic/toxic/nutritional
Idiopathic
Neoplastic: primary, metastatic
Degenerative

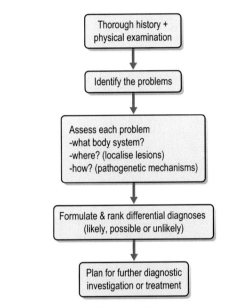

Figure 1-10 Flow diagram of problem-based patient assessment.

A list of differential diagnoses is made for each problem by following this pathway of clinical reasoning. Differential diagnoses should be ranked as likely, possible or unlikely. To assist in considering possible etiologies, acronyms such as VITAMIN D are useful (Box 1-4). Plans for the diagnostic investigation are then formulated and recorded in the medical record. The problem-based approach is summarized in Figure 1-10. For presurgical patients, where the history and physical examination reveal evidence of intercurrent disease, an assessment needs to be made as to whether these problems or their management could impact on the proposed surgical procedure and whether further investigation or treatment is required. Implications of this assessment should be fully discussed with owners prior to obtaining consent for surgery.

PREOPERATIVE LABORATORY DATABASE

The minimum database

The minimum database required prior to anesthesia and surgery will depend on the physical status of the cat and whether the surgical procedure is minor (< 60 minutes) or major. For healthy cats, or cats less than 7 years of age undergoing minor surgery (e.g., repair of a skin laceration) a packed cell volume (PCV), total plasma protein (TP) and urine specific gravity are recommended. For the same patients undergoing major surgery, and for healthy cats of 7 years or older, or cats with non-life-threatening systemic illnesses undergoing minor surgery a complete blood count (CBC), urinalysis (UA) and biochemistry panel (urea, creatinine, alkaline phosphatase (ALP), alanine aminotransferase (ALT), glucose, sodium, potassium, chloride, TP) are recommended. For cats with non-life-threatening systemic illnesses undergoing major surgery or for cats with life-threatening illness undergoing any surgery a CBC, UA and complete biochemical and electrolyte panel is recommended. These guidelines are adapted from the American Society of Anesthesiologists physical status classification system[5] (see Chapter 2).

Retrovirus testing

Serological testing for feline leukemia virus (FeLV) antigen and feline immunodeficiency virus (FIV) antibody is recommended for all cats. Cats returning a positive FeLV antigen test should have the result confirmed by virus isolation, immunofluorescence assay or polymerase chain reaction (PCR). A positive FIV antibody test in a cat older than 6 months of age that has not been vaccinated for FIV indicates that the cat is infected. Where vaccination status is unknown, a PCR test will determine whether the positive antibody test is a result of vaccination or infection. While the prognosis for FeLV infected cats is guarded, the prognosis for FIV-infected cats cannot be predicted from its infection status alone as many FIV-infected cats have a normal life-expectancy.

Coagulation testing

Abnormalities in coagulation mechanisms confer a risk of excessive bleeding or thrombosis. Acquired and heritable defects in primary and secondary coagulation are recognized in the cat.

Screening for heritable defects

Most heritable defects, other than vitamin K-dependent coagulopathy of Devon Rex cats, are clinically silent but manifest as excessive surgical or postsurgical bleeding.

Vitamin K-dependent coagulopathy of Devon Rex cats is a combined factor deficiency (II, VII, IX and X).[6] All Devon Rex cats should have activated partial thromboplastin time (APTT) measured prior to elective surgery to identify affected cats. This coagulopathy is associated with spontaneous bleeding which can be severe, and careful history taking may reveal previous episodes of lameness associated with hemarthrosis. Oral vitamin K treatment normalizes coagulation.[6] Although not associated with a bleeding tendency, erythrocyte pyruvate kinase (EPK) deficiency in Abyssinian and Somali cats can cause cyclic anemia and genetic testing is advised in these breeds prior to surgery, especially if anemia is present.

Other heritable coagulopathies in the cat differ from those in the dog in that they are rare and are often not breed related. The absence of a well-defined risk population for screening means that, except for cats related to known affected cats, heritable coagulopathies are unlikely to be diagnosed until clinical signs are evident. Inherited thrombocytopathias are exceedingly rare, with Chediak-Higashi syndrome (Persian cats) and von Willebrand disease reported.[7] Single factor deficiencies VIII (hemophilia A), IX (hemophilia B), X, XII and combined VIII/XII, IX/XII occur infrequently. The hemophilias are sex-linked but females can be affected as the trait usually does not affect survival. The activated coagulation time (ACT) and activated partial thromboplastin time (APTT) will be prolonged in these factor deficiencies.

Screening for acquired defects

Uremia and paraproteinemia (normal or abnormal plasma protein appearing in large quantities as a result of a pathological condition) can be associated with thrombocytopathias and platelet function testing is indicated. Indications for screening of secondary coagulation defects include patients with hepatic insufficiency, biliary obstruction, intestinal malabsorption, exocrine pancreatic insufficiency, hypoproteinemia and neoplasia.

Tests of primary hemostasis

Platelet function can be assessed by measurement of buccal mucosal bleeding time (BMBT) in-house (Box 1-5). Sedation may be required. Platelet function can be assessed in vitro using platelet aggregation studies and platelet function analyzers.

Tests of secondary hemostasis

If a coagulopathy is suspected, screening tests include activated coagulation time (in-house) initially, or preferably a laboratory-based coagulation profile, including prothrombin time, activated partial thromboplastin time, thrombin time and fibrinogen. Explanations of these tests are detailed in Chapter 5.

SPECIAL CONSIDERATIONS FOR PRE-EXISTING CONDITIONS

Current medications and antimicrobial prophylaxis

Adjustments or short-term discontinuation of medications may be required if they increase the anesthetic risk (e.g., induce bradycardia or hypotension), are contraindicated in fasting animals or can adversely affect coagulation or wound healing. Drugs commonly used in cats that require review include non-steroidal anti-inflammatory drugs (e.g., meloxicam), angiotensin converting enzyme-inhibitors (e.g., benazepril), calcium channel blockers (e.g., amlodipine), beta blockers (e.g., atenolol), prednisolone, antiplatelet drugs (e.g., clopidogrel) and anticoagulants (e.g., low-molecular weight heparin). For cats with diabetes mellitus receiving insulin, a reduced dose of insulin is given on the morning of surgery to avoid intra- or postoperative hypoglycemia. Depending on the morning blood glucose reading a 50% or greater, reduction in insulin is given (see Chapter 2, Table 2-3).

Antimicrobial prophylaxis may be indicated perioperatively depending on the type of wound, surgical site, operative time, use of surgical implants, level of contamination, and systemic immunocompetence

Table 1-2 A classification system for surgical incisions

Classification	Description
Clean	No entry into the respiratory, gastrointestinal or genitourinary tracts No break in asepsis No inflammation and no infection
Clean-contaminated	Entry into the gastrointestinal, respiratory or genitourinary tracts without significant spillage and in the absence of known infection Minor break in asepsis
Contaminated	Entry into the gastrointestinal tract with spillage and entry into the genitourinary or biliary tracts when infection is present
Dirty	Entry into a collection of purulent material Foreign body, devitalized tissue or old and contaminated wound debridement Fecal contamination

(From Hart D, Postlethwait R, Brown I, et al. (1968) Postoperative Wound Infections: a further report on ultraviolet irradiation with comments on the recent (1964) National Research Council Cooperative Study Report. Annals of Surgery 167(5):728–43. Reprinted with permission from Wolters Kluwer Health, www.lww.com with permission.)

of the patient. Surgical wounds can be classified as clean, clean-contaminated, contaminated or dirty (Table 1-2). Antimicrobial prophylaxis is unnecessary for clean wounds where the gastrointestinal, genitourinary, oropharyngeal or respiratory tract is not entered, unless surgical time exceeds 90 minutes. For clean-contaminated and contaminated procedures, such as gastrointestinal surgery, antimicrobial prophylaxis is usually indicated (see Gastrointestinal disease section below).

Anemia and hypoproteinemia

Consideration should be given to a preoperative blood transfusion where the hematocrit is <20% or if the clinical status of the patient suggests an uncompensated or acute anemia. Factors to consider when deciding whether to transfuse include severity and chronicity of the anemia, the degree of regeneration, presence of intercurrent cardiorespiratory disease, the anticipated blood loss during surgery and the duration of the procedure (Chapter 5).

Serum albumin concentrations should be maintained above 20 g/L preoperatively. Fresh frozen feline plasma can be administered at 4–6 mL/minute in acute crises such as hypovolemic shock, or for normovolemic patients at 6–22 mL/kg in a 24-hour period. However, plasma transfusion alone is ineffective in increasing intravascular protein levels, especially if losses are ongoing, since large volumes of plasma are required to increase the albumin by only small increments (22 mL/kg of plasma is estimated to increase the albumin by 5 g/L). Further, the availability of fresh frozen feline plasma is limited in some countries. Colloid oncotic pressure (COP) can be provided instead with synthetic colloids such as hydroxyethyl starch (hetastarch). In general it is recommended that the dose of hetastarch in cats not exceed 20 mL/kg/day administered as a 1 mL/kg/hour constant rate infusion (CRI).[8] When using synthetic colloids for ongoing management of critically ill hypoproteinemic patients, measurement of colloid osmotic pressure is recommended.

Iso-oncotic (5%) human serum albumin (HSA) can be given as a CRI in cats with albumin of <20 g/L administered through a peripheral vein at 2 mL/kg/hour for ten hours per day (total volume 20 mL/kg/day) until albumin reaches 20 g/L;[9] however, this should be administered with caution. In a study of 170 hypoalbuminemic cats treated with HSA the median number of days of HSA infusion required for serum albumin to reach 20 g/L was three days. The albumin solution was made from 25% commercial HSA (Albital, Hardis S.P.A, Naples, Italy) diluted to 5% in 0.9% saline. While hypersensitivity reactions were not noted in any patients, diarrhea, hyperthermia or tremors occurred in 36.5% and perivascular inflammation at catheter sites occurred in 34% of cats treated with HSA. Once cats have been exposed to HSA, antibodies develop such that re-administration of HSA risks life-threatening anaphylaxis.

SPECIFIC CONSIDERATIONS FOR ORGANS SYSTEMS

Skin and adnexa

There are not many specific preoperative considerations for conditions of the skin and adnexa, which include superficial wounds, mammary masses and vaccine associated sarcomas. However, affected cats may be elderly and therefore have intercurrent disease, such as hyperthyroidism or diabetes mellitus, which may need preoperative treatment. Cats that have suffered wounds may have trauma to other organs and systems. Wounds may be contaminated or infected so preoperative antibiotics should be given unless a sample is going to be submitted for culture and sensitivity, in which case the administration of the antibiotic is delayed until after the sample is obtained.

Gastrointestinal disease

Intestinal obstruction

Preoperative considerations for cats with obstructive small intestinal disease (e.g., foreign bodies) include fluid and electrolyte imbalances, anemia, hypoproteinemia and sepsis. Intestinal obstruction results in fluid losses into the intestinal lumen through increased secretion while absorption of intraluminal fluid and electrolytes is decreased. Dehydration may be severe. The most common electrolyte abnormalities are hypokalemia, hyponatremia, and hypochloridemia. High duodenal obstructions can result in metabolic alkalosis subsequent to loss of hydrochloric acid containing gastric secretions in vomitus. However, metabolic acidosis can also occur in association with fluid depletion from vomiting, insensible water losses, lack of intake or catabolism of body stores. More distal small intestinal obstructions also result in metabolic acidosis from loss of sodium, water and bicarbonate-rich duodenal secretions. Fluid and electrolyte abnormalities should be corrected before anesthetic induction if possible. Preoperative fresh whole blood or fresh frozen plasma transfusion may be indicated in anemic and/or hypoalbuminemic cats, especially where there is concurrent hypovolemia.

Antimicrobial therapy in intestinal surgery

Perioperative antimicrobial therapy is indicated in patients with obstructive intestinal disease, for non-obstructive intestinal disease where ileus is present and for patients undergoing intestinal biopsies. Cefazolin (20 mg/kg IV) is considered an appropriate prophylactic antimicrobial to prevent surgical site infections of the upper small intestine of cats and dogs,[10] while for distal small intestinal and colonic surgery second generation cephalosporins (e.g., cefoxitin 15–30 mg/kg IV or cefmetazole 15 mg/kg IV) are recommended.[10,11]

These recommendations are based on the conception that Gram positive cocci and enteric Gram negative bacilli are prevalent in the upper gastrointestinal tract, while the distal small intestine contains large numbers of aerobic and anaerobic bacteria and in the colon anaerobes predominate over aerobic organisms.[10] However, it should be noted that even in the upper small intestine of healthy cats, large numbers of Gram positive cocci, enteric Gram negative bacilli and anaerobic organisms are typically present.[12] Prophylactic antimicrobial agents should be administered 30 to 60 minutes before surgery, repeated every one to three hours during surgery, and discontinued at the conclusion of surgery. Where infection is identified intra-operatively, therapeutic antimicrobials should be continued post-operatively until resolution of infection (see Chapters 27 to 30).

Hepatobiliary disease

Surgical treatment of portosystemic shunts should generally be delayed until the patient can be medically stabilized. Presurgical considerations include poor wound healing, hypoalbuminemia, hypoglycemia, coagulopathies, hepatic encephalopathy and seizures. The goals of medical management include decreasing bacterial ammonia production (e.g., cleansing enemas, oral lactulose, lactulose retention enemas, antibiotics), maintaining hydration and electrolyte balance, preventing gastrointestinal ulceration (H2 blockers, proton pump inhibitors), seizure control (e.g., phenobarbitone, levatiracetam) and nutritional support. Parenteral or partial parenteral nutrition may be considered in cats with poor body condition, and parenteral glucose administration is indicated in hypoglycemic patients. Serum albumin concentrations should be maintained above 20 g/L preoperatively. Fresh frozen feline plasma can be administered, if available. Otherwise synthetic colloids can be used to raise COP. For patients with prolonged APTT, preoperative whole blood or fresh frozen plasma transfusion and vitamin K1 treatment are indicated. Blood typing should be performed in case intraoperative blood transfusion is required, particularly for cats with intrahepatic shunts. For more information on general considerations for patients with hepatobiliary disease see Chapters 31 and 32.

Genitourinary disease

Chronic kidney disease

Presurgical considerations for patients with intercurrent CKD include hydration status, SBP, electrolyte/acid-base abnormalities and the potential for primary hemostatic dysfunction. It is prudent to admit cats with CKD to hospital 24 hours prior to surgery to evaluate and correct electrolyte/acid–base disorders and fluid deficits. Maintaining these cats on IV fluids during the nil per os period prevents excessive dehydration in patients with an obligatory polyuria. Azotemia can interfere with platelet function, increasing the risk of surgical bleeding. A BMBT is recommended preoperatively.

Urethral obstruction/urinary tract rupture

In cases of urethral obstruction or urinary tract rupture, medical stabilization is required prior to surgery. The metabolic consequences of urethral obstruction / urinary tract rupture include electrolyte abnormalities (hyperkalemia, hyperphosphatemia, hypocalcemia), metabolic acidosis, central nervous system and cardiovascular depression and hypovolemia, which are progressive and life threatening. IV

fluid support is essential. A crystalloid replacement IV fluid, 0.9% NaCl or Hartmann solution, should be used initially. Maintenance solutions such as 0.45% NaCl/2.5 % glucose are hypotonic, contain less sodium to hold water in the intravascular space and are not suitable for fluid resuscitation. In collapsed cats, fluid resuscitation with an initial bolus of 20–30 mL/kg (100 mL/cat) may be required. The fluid rate can then be reassessed based on improvement in cardiovascular function and the degree of azotemia. Ability to measure central venous pressure is useful, especially in cats with pre-existing cardiovascular disease. Ideally, azotemia prior to anesthesia should be addressed by urethral catheterization and IV fluid diuresis or by peritoneal dialysis.

Hyperkalemia is the most common electrolyte abnormality in cats with urethral obstruction. The clinical consequences of hyperkalemia reflect altered muscle and cardiac conduction fiber function. Weakness and bradyarrhythmias may be seen. Classic ECG changes in hyperkalemia include bradycardia, peaked T waves, flattened P waves, increased duration of QRS, ST segment depression and shortened QT interval, progressing to sine wave. Hyperkalemia can be treated in bradycardic or arrhythmic patients using 10% calcium gluconate with simultaneous ECG monitoring (1 mL/kg by slow IV infusion over five to ten minutes). It antagonizes the effects of hyperkalemia on cell membranes (and therefore does not affect serum potassium level). Calcium gluconate works immediately and its effect lasts for 20–30 minutes. It also corrects ionized hypocalcemia, which is common in urethral obstruction and often subclinical until acidosis is reversed. Soluble (regular) insulin, which works by driving potassium ions intracellularly, can be used as an alternative (0.1–0.25 U/kg IV + glucose bolus 0.5 g/kg IV). Administration of a glucose bolus alone, with the intention of stimulating endogenous insulin secretion, is often ineffective as most cats will have stress hyperglycemia on admission.

Specific treatment for metabolic acidosis should be considered when the cat is obtunded and the venous pH is <7 or bicarbonate <12 mmol/L. Treatment with bicarbonate carries potential risks including CSF acidosis, decreased release of oxygen from hemoglobin, increased osmolality and precipitation of hypocalcemic tetany. Appropriate patient selection and careful administration are required. The following formula is used to calculate the required dose of bicarbonate:

$$\text{dose of bicarbonate (mmol)} = 0.3 \times \text{body weight (kg)} \times (\text{desired-actual bicarbonate mmol/L})$$

The desired bicarbonate level should be set at approximately 15 mmol i.e., not too high. One-third of the calculated dose is given IV over 15 minutes. If bicarbonate is still low the remainder of the calculated dose is given. Otherwise the remainder is administered over 12 hours with IV fluids.

Cardiorespiratory conditions

Cardiac murmurs may be detected on physical examination when other cardiovascular parameters are normal. Such incidental murmurs are common in cats, and may be physiologic (e.g., due to dynamic right ventricular outflow tract obstruction) or pathologic, and hemodynamically significant or otherwise. A decision must to be made as to whether to investigate incidental murmurs further. The grade of murmur does not differentiate pathologic from physiologic murmurs or correlate well with the severity of any underlying cardiovascular disease. For cats older than 8 years of age with cardiac murmurs and no signs of congestive heart failure (CHF) on physical examination, a serum T4 and SBP measurement are recommended initially. Cardiac biomarkers may assist in differentiating cats with asymptomatic heart disease from healthy cats and from cats with CHF.[13,14] For example, elevations in the natriuretic peptide NT-pro-BNP are an indication for further investigation including thoracic radiographs and echocardiography.

The absence of a murmur should not be taken as evidence of a normal cardiovascular system. Cats may have compensated cardiac disease with no physical abnormalities. An S4 gallop sound is not uncommon in cats and usually indicates underlying structural cardiac disease. If a gallop sound is auscultated, electrocardiography, SBP, thoracic radiographs and echocardiography are indicated. Where a cardiac murmur is detected on physical examination the potential for iatrogenic relative volume overload should be recognized. It is prudent not to exceed 1.5–2 × maintenance rates for IV fluids preoperatively in cats with systemic hypertension or cardiac murmurs. Measurement of central venous pressures is also useful in these patients. Cats with symptomatic cardiorespiratory disease such as congestive heart failure or pleural effusion must be stabilized prior to anesthesia. For example, in cases of pyothorax, drainage of effusion by needle thoracocentesis before anesthetic induction to place thoracostomy tubes decreases perioperative mortality.[15]

Thoracic trauma

Pulmonary contusions have been reported in up to 50% of animals with thoracic trauma and are a potential indication for limited fluid volume resuscitation. Limited fluid volume resuscitation is defined as the smallest volume of fluid possible to restore the intravascular compartment and resolve shock while minimizing fluid extravasation into the brain or lungs and the risk of disrupting an incipient blood clot. The mean arterial blood pressure should be maintained between 60–70 mmHg to keep the brain and kidneys perfused. Hypertonic saline 7.2–7.5% can be given at a dose of 3–8 mL/kg but should not be given faster than 1 mL/kg/minute. It can be mixed with colloids that increase volume expansion over 30 minutes to 2-3 hours. Hydroxyethyl starch can be used at a dose of 5 ml/kg over 10 to 15 minutes with a maximum dose of 20 ml/kg/day.[8] These treatment regimens should be followed by slow rate crystalloids to avoid dehydration.[16]

Head and neck

Hyperthyroidism

Important preoperative considerations in hyperthyroid cats are renal function, cardiac function and SBP. Ideally euthyroidism should be induced before thyroidectomy is performed, to minimize anesthetic complications associated with hyperthyroid heart disease and postoperative complications such as thyroid storm (the acute exacerbation of clinical signs of thyrotoxicosis).[17] Treatment with thioureylene antithyroid drugs (e.g., carbimazole, methimazole) is effective in reducing heart rate when euthyroidism is achieved, usually after two or more weeks. An alternative treatment for tachycardia or tachycardia-based arrhythmias for cats that are not in congestive heart failure is a beta-adrenergic drug (atenolol 6.25–12.5 mg once or twice daily, or propranolol 2.5–5 mg two to three times daily) commencing two to five days preoperatively.[18] These drugs can also be used manage tachypnea, hypertension and hyperexcitability preoperatively in cats not being treated with antithyroid drugs. Atenolol confers an advantage over propranolol because of its once daily dosing regimen, and as a selective beta-1 adrenergic blocker can be given to cats with asthma.

Although hyperthyroidism increases glomerular filtration rate, decreases serum creatinine concentration and can mask underlying CKD, there is no significant difference between the survival times of cats that develop azotemia post-treatment and those without azotemia.[19] Thus induction of euthyroidism to determine which cats will become azotemic prior to thyroidectomy confers no survival advantage. A reversible thiourylene trial is recommended for cats that are azotemic at presentation to determine the extent of underlying CKD before thyroidectomy as this may affect their suitability for surgery.

A cardiac evaluation is recommended to assess for the presence and significance of thyrotoxic cardiomyopathy. Thoracic radiographs are recommended and echocardiography and ECG may be indicated, especially in cats with gallop sounds or arrhythmias. SBP should be measured in all cases and if hypertension does not resolve after induction of euthyroidism preoperatively, treatment with the calcium channel blocker amlodipine (0.13–0.3 mg/kg once daily) is indicated. For in depth information on feline hyperthyroidism see Chapter 53.

REFERENCES

1. Brown S, Atkins C, Bagley R, et al. Guidelines for the identification, evaluation and management of systemic hypertension in cats. J Vet Intern Med 2007;21:542–58.

2. Jepson RE, Hartley V, Mendl M, et al. A comparison of CAT Doppler and oscillometric memoprint machines for non-invasive blood pressure measurement in conscious cats. J Fel Med Surg 2005;7:147–52.

3. Acierno MJ, Seaton D, Mitchell MA, da Cunha A. Agreement between directly measured blood pressure and pressures obtained with three veterinary-specific oscillometric units in cats. J Am Vet Med Assoc 2010;237:402–6.

4. Voss K. Chapter 1 Patient Assessment. In: Montavon PM, Voss K, Langley-Hobbs SJ, editors. Feline orthopedic surgery and musculoskeletal disease. Elsevier; 2009. p. 8–10.

5. Dyson DH. Pre operative assessment. In: Hall LW, Taylor PM, editors. Anesthesia of the cat. London: Bailliere Tindall; 1994. p. 105.

6. Maddison JE, Watson AD, Eade IG, Exner T. Vitamin K-dependent multifactor coagulopathy in Devon Rex cats. J Am Vet Med Assoc 1990;197:1495–7.

7. Parker MT, Collier LL, Kier AB, Johnson GS. Oral mucosa bleeding times of normal cats and cats with Chediak-Higashi syndrome or Hageman trait. Vet Clin Pathol 1988;17:9–12.

8. Chan D. Colloids: current recommendations. Vet Clin North Am Small Anim 2008;38:587–93.

9. Viganó F, Perissinotto L, Bosco VR. Administration of 5% serum albumin in critically ill small animal patients with hypoalbuminaemia: 418 dogs and 170 cats (1994-2008). J Vet Emerg Crit Care 2010;20:237–43.

10. Howe LM, Boothe, HW. Antimicrobial use in the surgical patient. Vet Clin Small Anim 2006;36:1049–60.

11. Fossum TW, Hedlund CS. Gastric and intestinal surgery. Vet Clin Small Anim 2003;33:1117–45.

12. Sparkes AH, Papasouliotis K, Sunvold G, et al. Bacterial flora in the duodenum of healthy cats and effect of dietary supplementation with fructo-oligosaccharides. Am J Vet Res 1998;59:431–5.

13. Connolly DJ, Magalhaes RJ, Syme HM, et al. Circulating natriuretic peptides in cats with heart disease. J Vet Intern Med 2008;22:96–105.

14. Ettinger SJ, Yee K, Beardow, et al. Diagnostic test parameters in cats with heart disease and their correlation with NT-proANP, NT-proBNP and troponin I measurements. J Vet Intern Med 2010;24:671 (abstract).

15. Barrs VR, Allan GS, Martin P, et al. Feline pyothorax: a retrospective study of 27 cases in Australia. J Fel Med Surg 2005;7: 211–22.

16. Hammond TN, Holm JL. Limited fluid volume resuscitation. Compend Contin Ed 2009;7:309–26.

17. Ward CR. Feline thyroid storm. Vet Clin Small Anim 2007;37:745–54.

18. Flanders JA. Surgical options for the treatment of hyperthyroidism. J Fel Med Surg 1999;1:127–34.

19. Williams TL, Elliott J, Syme HM. Association of iatrogenic hypothyroidism with azotaemia and reduced survival time in cats treated for hyperthyroidism. J Vet Int Med 2010;24:1086–92.

Chapter | 2 |

Anesthesia and analgesia for general surgery

S.B.R. Kästner

Choosing an anesthetic protocol for a specific patient depends on the pre-anesthetic examination, the presence of systemic disease, and type and duration of the intended procedure. When anesthetizing a diseased cat it is important to take the disease process and its pathophysiology into consideration. A young healthy cat might be able to compensate for the effects of drugs, whereas a compromised animal might not be able to compensate. For a more detailed description of general anesthesia techniques, drugs, and equipment the reader is referred to Chapters 17 and 18 of *Feline Orthopedic Surgery and Musculoskeletal Disease*.[1,2] This chapter is designed to augment the previously mentioned chapters. To avoid repetition this chapter will concentrate specifically on anesthesia and analgesia of cats with intercurrent systemic disease that might have implications for anesthetizing them for surgery and cats with diseases of specific organ systems and the different considerations that might arise in such situations.

GENERAL CONSIDERATIONS

Sedation

Excitement or stress caused by excessive restraint will induce high levels of circulating catecholamines, which will not be tolerated by severely compromised cats. Stress will lead to increased anesthetic requirements and consequently more severe cardiovascular depression. Pre-medication can help alleviate this stress. A full description of drugs that can be administered in cats and their indications is described in *Feline Orthopedic Surgery and Musculoskeletal Disease*.[1]

Anesthesia

Injectable anesthetics can be used for induction of anesthesia followed by inhalational anesthesia for maintenance or they can be used as the sole anesthetic agent (total intravenous anesthesia [TIVA]). Inhalation anesthesia is still the preferred technique for producing general anesthesia for prolonged and invasive surgical procedures because the depth of anesthesia can easily be adapted and drug accumulation is not a problem with modern inhalation anesthetics. Modern protocols use the principle of balanced anesthesia, with a combination of different analgesic, sedative–hypnotic and muscle-relaxing drugs, with the aim of reducing the concentration of volatile anesthetics required (Table 2-1).

New drugs

Since the recent publication of the *Feline Orthopedic Surgery and Musculoskeletal Disease* textbook,[1,2] the variety of drugs available for anesthesia and analgesia in cats has changed very little. However, the use of tramadol in small animal practice has risen dramatically. It has the advantage of oral administration. A new non-steroidal anti-inflammatory drug (robenacoxib) is licensed for use in cats, and anti-epileptic agents (gabapentin and pregabalin) are being used more commonly in small animal practice. These drugs will be described below.

Tramadol

Tramadol is an atypical opioid with weak μ-receptor binding activity in combination with serotonin and noradrenaline reuptake inhibition as its analgesic mechanism. Cats produce the active metabolite, which is responsible for the opioid analgesia, more effectively than dogs. Oral bioavailability is high in cats (93%). For cats a dose of 1–2 mg/kg IV and oral dosing of 2–4 mg/kg twice a day has been recommended clinically. In experimental animals 2–4 mg/kg was effective and dosing every six hours seemed to be necessary to maintain analgesia at a maximal effect.[3] The liquid formulation often contains peppermint oil, which induces copious salivation and is not well liked by cats.

Robenacoxib

Robenacoxib is a selective COX-2 inhibitor in the cat (ex vivo and in vivo) and is licensed for the treatment of acute musculoskeletal pain and postoperative pain after soft tissue surgery in the cat. Because of the high degree of COX-2 selectivity the gastrointestinal toxicity is low. Maximal plasma concentrations in the cat are reached after 0.5 hours and one hour after oral and subcutaneous application, respectively.[4,5]

DOI: 10.1016/B978-0-7020-4336-9.00002-0

Table 2-1 Infusions used in conjunction with inhalational or injectable anesthetics for balanced anesthesia in cats

Drug	Induction/loading dose (mg/kg)	Maintenance dose		Comment
Fentanyl	0.003–0.005 IV	0.005–0.015 mg/kg/hour	VRI to effect	IPPV Bradycardia
Alfentanil	0.0025–0.005 IV	0.03–0.3 mg/kg/hour	VRI	IPPV Bradycardia
Sufentanil	0.001–0.003 IV	0.001–0.006 mg/kg/hour	VRI	IPPV Bradycardia
Remifentanil		0.012–0.036 mg/kg/hour	VRI	IPPV Bradycardia
Ketamine	0.3–0.5 IV	0.1–1.2 mg/kg/hour (common 0.3 mg/kg/hour)	CRI	High doses lead to ketamine 'signs'
Medetomidine	0.0005–0.001 IV over ten minutes very slowly	0.001–0.002 mg/kg/hour	CRI	Bradycardia
Dexmedetomidine	0.0005–0.001 IV over ten minutes very slowly	0.0005–0.001 mg/kg/hour	CRI	Bradycardia
Morphine + ketamine (MK)	Premedication and induction doses	3.3 µg/kg/minute 10 µg/kg/minute infused at 10 mL/kg/hour postoperative 2 mL/kg/hour	CRI	5 mg morphine 15 mg ketamine in 250 mL NaCl

CRI, constant rate infusion; IPPV, intermittent positive pressure ventilation; VRI, variable rate infusion.

Anti-epileptic medication

Originally introduced as anti-epileptic drugs, gabapentin and its 'successor', pregabalin, are used as adjunctive drugs in combination with other analgesics for the control of neuropathic conditions, osteoarthritis and tumor-related pain. The exact analgesic mechanism is still not clear and they do not change nociceptive thresholds. Controlled studies for cats are not available. Dose recommendations for gabapentin range from 5–20 mg/kg orally two to three times a day. Initial treatment can induce sedation and sleepiness, long-term treatment leads to weight gain.

Fluid administration

During inhalational anesthesia a significant amount of fluids is lost via the respiratory tract, open wounds or hemorrhage. In addition, with most anesthetics vascular tone is reduced and intravascular volume has to be replaced to maintain an adequate perfusion pressure.

In a systemically healthy patient any isotonic crystalloid solution (i.e., lactated Ringer solution, saline) can be used at a rate of 5–10 mL/kg/hour depending on the expected fluid and blood loss during the planned procedure. For prolonged procedures without opening major body cavities the lower rate should be chosen in cats to avoid overzealous dilution and disturbance of colloid osmotic pressure and pulmonary edema formation. A large study on small animal perioperative mortalities found an increased anesthetic risk for cats receiving intravenous fluids.[6,7] This might be related to the fact that in practice only diseased, high-risk feline patients will be treated with infusions; however, it might also indicate overinfusion when the rate is not controlled properly which can occur when using large giving sets.

Emergency resuscitation

Cats with systemic disease may require emergency resuscitation. A list of recommended drugs and doses is included in Table 2-2.

SYSTEMIC AND METABOLIC DISORDERS

Cats presenting for general and oncological surgery may have concurrent disease that needs treating prior to anesthesia or that influences the choice of anesthetic agents and analgesics that can be safely administered. Anemia, hypoproteinemia, diabetes and obesity will be discussed in the following sections.

Anemia

Arterial oxygen content depends on hemoglobin concentration (or packed cell volume (PCV)) and saturation with oxygen. A normal arterial oxygen content of 16–20 mL/dL is reached with 12–15 mg/dL hemoglobin. In anemia, compensatory increases in cardiac output are required to maintain adequate oxygen delivery, which increases myocardial work and in combination with low oxygen content can lead to myocardial hypoxia and death. Therefore, anemia should be treated before anesthesia and 100% oxygen given during anesthesia.

There are no standard, clear cut transfusion triggers available for cats. However, transfusion is recommended with a PCV of less than 13% in chronic anemia and 20% in acute anemia. Signs of hemorrhagic shock can become evident when 20% of the circulating blood volume (in cats approximately 7% of bodyweight) is lost. In cats with concomitant anemia and reduced cardiac performance a careful individual decision for transfusion has to be made and volume overload needs to be avoided.

Whole blood is recommended with acute hemorrhage and erythrocyte concentrate for treatment of chronic normovolemic anemia, to avoid volume overload. If stored blood is used in planned procedures the transfusion should be scheduled the day before surgery to allow for compensation for the changes in oxygen-carrying capacity of the stored products. In cats, blood transfusion requires blood typing or cross-matching even with the first transfusion because of preformed antibodies (Chapter 5).

Table 2-2 Drugs used in emergency situations and cardiovascular resuscitation

Drug	Dose (mg/kg)	Indication	Comments
Epinephrine (1 : 10,000 = 0.1 mg/mL)	0.01–0.1 mg/kg IV/IO, repeat every five minutes if no effect or CRI 0.001–0.01 mg/kg/minute	Asystole	Avoid high dose in sinus rhythm (electromechanical dissociation)
Norepinephrine	0.05–0.1 mg/kg IV 0.001–0.01 mg/kg/minute	Hypotension	
Dopamine	0.002–0.001 mg/kg/minute	Hypotension	
Dobutamine	0.005–0.02 mg/kg/minute	Hypotension, low cardiac output	
Vasopressin	0.4–0.8 U/kg IV one dose	Increase myocardial blood flow	
Atropine	0.02–0.05 mg/kg IV/IM	Bradycardia, AV block	
Glycopyrrolate	0.02–0.04 mg/kg IV/SC	Bradycardia, AV block	
Lidocaine	0.5–1 mg/kg IV 0.01–0.04 mg/kg/minute	Ventricular premature contractions, ventricular tachycardia,	Contraindicated if bradycardia
Calcium gluconate (10%)	0.5 mL/kg slow IV	Hyperkalemia, hypocalcemia, electromechanical dissociation	Tachycardia possible
Fluids Isotonic saline Lactated Ringer Hypertonic saline Hydroxyethyl starch	10–(50) mL/kg/hour 10–(50) mL/kg/hour 4–6 mL/kg over ten minutes 10-20 mL/kg (5–10 mL/kg/hour) daily dose should not exceed 20 mL/kg	Volume depletion, shock therapy	Can cause hypernatremia
Furosemide	2–5 mg/kg IV repeat after ten minutes	Pulmonary edema, brain edema, oliguria	
Methylprednisolone dexamethasone	10–30 mg/kg IV 0.5–2 mg/kg IV	Post resuscitation	
Esmolol	0.1–0.5 mg/kg IV CRI: 0.01–0.05mg/kg/minute IV	Sinus tachycardia	

AV, artrioventricular; CRI, constant infusion rate; IM, intramuscular; IO, intraocular; IV, intravenous; SC, subcutaneous.

Hypoproteinemia

Many drugs used for anesthesia are reversibly bound to transport proteins in the albumin fraction of blood. Only the unbound amount of drug is pharmacologically active. If the plasma protein (albumin) bound fraction in blood is decreased, then more unbound drug is available, resulting in an increased (anesthetic) effect. Therefore, there is the potential for an increased anesthesia effect in hypoproteinemic animals and the principle of giving anesthesia to effect and incremental dosing should be followed.

Decreased albumin concentrations lower plasma oncotic pressure and high amounts of crystalloid fluids are not well tolerated as they increase the risk of pulmonary edema. If the plasma protein concentration is below 35 g/L (3.5 g/dL) then giving colloidal fluids like hydroxyethyl starch or plasma transfusion should be considered.

Diabetes

Diabetic patients may present for a variety of diabetes-related or unrelated procedures. There are no specific indications or contraindications for a special type of anesthetic agent in diabetic cats. Whenever possible, anesthesia should be undertaken when the diabetes is adequately controlled; if this is not possible then short-acting agents with short recovery times allow early return to eating.

In diabetic animals the management of blood glucose levels in the perioperative period is the major consideration for the veterinary surgeon. Fasting times should be kept short; surgery should be scheduled for the morning to avoid long periods of fasting. In animals being admitted on the morning of surgery owners should be advised to feed the animal for the last time late at night instead of the early evening.

Insulin administration after fasting increases the risk of hypoglycemia. However, insulin activity is necessary to enable metabolism and uptake of nutrients by the tissues. In addition, preoperative stress with the release of catecholamines and corticosteroids increases glucose levels and insulin requirements. Therefore, insulin should not be withheld in the preoperative period. The usual recommendation on the proportion of the animal's usual insulin dose varies from one half to one quarter of the usual dose. Ideally this is adapted according to the glucose levels on the morning of surgery (Table 2-3).

If the cat is on a twice-daily insulin regime it can often be returned to its usual feeding and insulin regime in the evening after surgery. If the animal is inappetent it can be maintained on a dextrose infusion and given regular/soluble insulin every six hours.

Table 2-3 Blood glucose management during anesthesia in diabetic patients

Blood glucose in the morning (pre insulin)	Insulin	Dextrose (2.5–5%) infusion
<5.5 mmol/L	No	Start 2–4 mL/kg/hour
5.5–11 mmol/L	One-quarter of the usual dose	Start 2–4 mL/kg/hour
>11 mmol/L	Half the usual dose	No infusion necessary until glucose <8 mmol/L

Box 2-1 **Goals for anesthesia of the obese cat**

Avoid SC administration of drugs and be aware of respiratory depression/obstruction—monitor the patient closely

Pre-oxygenate as long as stress-free

Rapid induction (IV) is preferred for rapid control of airways

Anesthesia maintenance—preferably with an inhalational agent

Patients usually benefit from intermittent positive pressure ventilation (± positive end expiratory pressure)

Calculate ventilation parameters like tidal volume for intermittent positive pressure ventilation based on lean body mass

Continue monitoring into recovery and after tracheal extubation

Return to feeding as soon as possible as obese patients don't tolerate acute starvation due to the risk of hyperlipemia

Ideally, 'managed weight loss' preoperatively would help improve risk

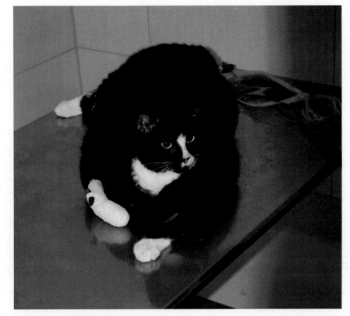

Figure 2-1 Morbidly obese cat.

The glucose target range during surgery lies between 8.3 and 14 mmol/L; glucose monitoring during surgery is recommended every 30 to 60 minutes. A 2.5–5% dextrose infusion is given according to the cat's systemic glucose concentrations (Table 2-3).

If the cat is on oral hypoglycemic agents, e.g., glipizide, then these should be withheld on the day of surgery; instead, the glucose concentration is monitored and stabilized with short-acting soluble insulin and dextrose infusion if necessary.

Obesity

There is an increasing incidence of obesity in domestic cats[8] (Fig. 2-1). In obese animals the veterinarian is faced with a variety of general problems as well as specific anesthesia-related problems. Venous access as well as palpation of arterial pulses is impaired. Increased fat in the throat region may make endotracheal intubation more difficult and may also increase the risk of airway obstruction. Increased superficial fat obtunds thoracic auscultation and obscures landmarks for locoregional techniques and may act as a thermal insulator and increase the risk of heat stress.

Increased total body fat is accompanied by decreased total body water (on a mL/kg basis) resulting in decreased volume of distribution for water-soluble drugs and increased volume of distribution for lipid-soluble drugs. Most anesthetic agents are fat soluble. Excessive body fat in/on the chest and abdomen leads to reduced chest wall and lung compliance, reduced total lung capacity, reduced expiratory reserve volume, reduced functional reserve capacity (FRC) and increased work of breathing. Reduced FRC means reduced oxygen reserves and the patient can desaturate rapidly if it becomes apneic or intubation fails. The FRC may decrease below closing capacity and atelectasis and hypoxemia may occur during normal tidal breathing.

The goals of the anesthetic protocol in obese cats are listed in Box 2-1.

SKIN AND ADNEXA

Patients with skin and adnexal problems (Chapters 17 to 22) may not have any specific anesthetic requirements related directly to the lesions. However tumors are often seen in older cats who are prone to problems such as hyperthryroidism, diabetes and obesity. Wounds or masses may be infected or ulcerated and therefore cause systemic illness and require preoperative stabilization prior to anesthesia (Chapter 1).

If lesions are on the distal limbs then appendicular nerve blocks like the femoral. sciatic or brachial may be useful for giving specific analgesia of the area and reducing the requirement for systemic anesthetic drugs.

If masses are large then analgesia after resection is essential. Consideration can be given to using wound infusion catheters (Chapter 11) in addition to multimodal analgesia with non-steroidal anti-inflammatory drugs, opioids and other adjuncts such as ketamine and the alpha-2 agonists.

Brachial plexus block

A brachial plexus block in the cat is performed under general anesthesia. A brachial plexus block at the height of the shoulder is suitable for operations on the front limb within or distal to the elbow. A 22G 5 cm needle is inserted medial to the shoulder joint and advanced parallel with the spine directed towards the costochondral junction of the ribs. If no blood can be aspirated, lidocaine or bupivacaine diluted to a volume of 5 mL to facilitate spread is injected during withdrawal to reach the radial, ulnar, median and musculocutaneous nerves (RUMM block). The use of a nerve stimulator to locate the nerves and set specific depots improves the results (Fig. 2-2).

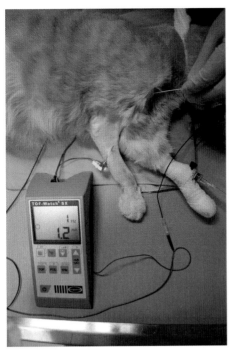

Figure 2-2 Use of a nerve stimulator allows a more specific block of the brachial plexus.

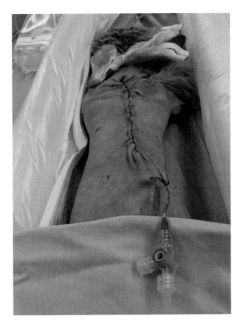

Figure 2-3 Self-made wound catheter placed after removal of a large fibrosarcoma.

Femoral nerve block

Anesthetizing the femoral nerve desensitizes the medial part of the thigh, tibia and tarsus and achieves motor blockade of the quadriceps femoris muscle. After aseptic preparation of the inguinal area, a 22G needle is inserted 1–2 cm in a craniodorsal direction immediately cranial to the femoral artery, below the inguinal ligament.

Use of a nerve stimulator induces a twitch distal (extension of the knee) to the stimulating site and helps to verify appropriate needle placement. Ultrasound-guided nerve infiltration will also improve results.

Sciatic nerve block

The sciatic nerve block gives motor block to the caudal muscles of the thigh and desensitizes the surrounding tissue and skin. Landmarks for needle insertion in the laterally recumbent animal are the greater trochanter of the femur and the ischiatic tuberosity. At the level of one-third of the distance between the two points, a 22G needle is inserted in a cranial direction. Using a nerve stimulator will result in dorsal flexion of the foot.

Wound catheter infusion systems

Fenestrated wound catheters (Chapter 11), can be used for analgesia of defined wound regions, for example after ear canal ablation or large tumor excisions like fibrosarcoma removal (Chapter 17). Commercial systems come in different lengths with bacterial filters, a flow restrictor and a balloon pump (i.e., ON-Q PainBuster, Kimberly Clark or Diffusion/Wound catheter, MILA International Inc. Erlanger, KY, USA), but it is also possible to purchase the catheter and filter without the pump. The catheter can also be constructed from red rubber or polyethylene tubing (Fig. 2-3). The elastomeric reservoir (pump) delivers fluid at a rate of 0.5–5 mL/hour; alternatively, a syringe pump can be used in non-ambulatory patients. The catheter

is usually placed subcutaneously during surgery in the desired area and can either be continuously perfused with a local anesthetic (lidocaine (1%) 0.2–0.4 mg/kg/hour) or repeated boluses of a long-acting local anesthetic can be given intermittently (1 mg/kg bupivacaine [0.25%] first dose followed by 0.5 mg/kg every six hours for one to two days).[9]

ABDOMINAL SURGERY

Multimodal analgesia should be provided where possible in patients undergoing a laparotomy. Non-steroidal anti-inflammatory medication is contraindicated in patients that may be suffering from gastrointestinal ulceration and patients that are hypovolemic. Pure μ agonist opioids such as morphine and methadone are excellent analgesic drugs, but they can cause nausea, constipation and urine retention, particularly after prolonged usage. Pethidine, unlike morphine, relaxes intestinal spasms. Butorphanol is a moderate analgesic for visceral pain but poor for somatic pain, therefore it is good for abdominal procedures, although its duration of action is quite short lived. Another good analgesic agent for abdominal surgery is buprenorphine, which has the benefit of a longer duration of action, good efficacy and fewer side effects than pure μ agonist opioids.

Epidural anesthesia

This provides useful adjunctive analgesia for both abdominal and thoracic procedures. Contraindications for epidural anesthesia are septicemia, coagulation disorders, hypovolemia, shock, skin infections at the puncture site and deformity, dislocations or fractures of the spine or pelvis. Possible complications include local skin infection, meningitis and trauma to the spinal cord, but these are rare. The procedure is described in Chapter 18 of *Feline Orthopedic Surgery and Musculoskeletal Disease*.[2]

GASTROINTESTINAL DISEASE

Pre-medication with systemic gastroprotectant medication (cimetidine or ranitidine) may be indicated in cats with a high risk of gastroesophageal reflux or regurgitation; elevation of the pH of gastric fluid ameliorates the potential effects upon the esophagus or lungs should regurgitation and/or aspiration occur.

If there is megaesophagus, gastric fluid retention, or proximal small intestinal obstruction there is a risk of regurgitation and therefore aspiration at the time of induction. It is important to achieve a smooth induction and intubate the patient promptly; stomach tubes and suction apparatus should be made available.

HEPATOBILIARY DISEASE

As many drugs are metabolized by the liver, care should be taken when using them in patients with hepatobiliary disease. It may still be possible to use such drugs but lower doses should be used and they should be administered less frequently. Intravenous anesthesia can be used for induction and then the cat should be maintained on inhalational gases such as isoflurane or sevoflurane: halothane should be avoided as it can cause hepatotoxicity. Non-steroidal anti-inflammatory drugs are contraindicated in cats with hepatic disease.

UROGENITAL DISEASE

In general, almost all anesthetics decrease glomerular filtration by either directly altering renal blood flow (RBF) or indirectly by changing cardiovascular conditions or neuroendocrine activity. Inhalation anesthetics decrease RBF and glomerular filtration rate (GFR) in a dose-dependent manner directly related to systemic blood pressure. Renal autoregulation is preserved at low end-tidal concentrations of volatile anesthetics, whereas high concentrations depress renal autoregulation and decrease RBF. If disease such as renal or postrenal failure and azotemia is present, then the cat's response to the anesthetic drugs administered may be altered in this situation. Acidosis might increase the fraction of unbound drugs in the blood and lower doses of highly protein bound anesthetic drugs are needed. Acidosis also contributes to the development of hyperkalemia. In hyperkalemia the resting potential of cardiac muscle cells is changed and bradycardia can occur due to decreased conductivity, contractility and excitability. Changes associated with hyperkalemia in the ECG trace are illustrated in Figure 2-4 and listed in Box 2-2.

Chronic renal failure

Patients with chronic renal failure might present with hypokalemia and anemia because of bone marrow suppression, chronic blood loss via the gastrointestinal tract, reduced erythrocyte life span and suppressed erythropoietin production. If the packed cell volume is decreased, then administration of a blood transfusion before anesthesia may be recommended (see Chapter 5 for further information). Chronic renal disease can also be associated with hypertension and compensatory high cardiac output but reduced cardiac reserve. Arterial blood pressure should be estimated preoperatively by Doppler or oscillometric techniques and hypertension be controlled by amlodipine or calcium channel blockers. However, calcium channel blockers have to be used with caution as they can promote hypotension during anesthesia.

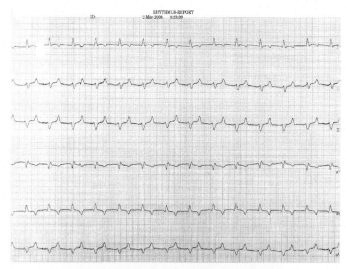

Figure 2-4 ECG trace of a cat with hyperkalemia (8.91 mmol/L). Note the loss of the P wave and wide QRS complexes.

Box 2-2 Changes seen with hyperkalemia

Peaked T wave
Prolonged PR interval, wide QRS complexes
Small or loss of P wave (atrial standstill)
Shortened Q-T interval

Box 2-3 Stabilization and treatment of hyperkalemia and atrial standstill

Restoration of myocardial contractility and conductivity

0.1 mg/kg 10% calcium chloride (0.5 ml/kg calcium gluconate) over 20 minutes IV re-establishes normal gradient between resting and threshold potential
NB: does not change potassium concentrations

Lowering plasma potassium concentration

50% glucose (1–2 mL/kg IV) induces endogenous insulin release
Insulin 0.25 IU/kg in 2 g/IU glucose IV followed by glucose containing and potassium free fluids (e.g., 5% glucose in 0.9% NaCl); monitor for hypoglycemia
Treat acidosis (H+/K+ shift)
Sodium bicarbonate 1–2 mmol/kg IV
Intermittent positive pressure ventilation (prevents respiratory acidosis)

Principles of anesthesia for cats in renal or postrenal failure are listed in Box 2-3.

Urethral obstruction or bladder rupture

Urethral obstruction or a ruptured bladder are often associated with hyponatremia, hypochloremia, hypocalemia, hyperphosphatemia, or hyperkalemia. If possible, correction of electrolyte disturbances is recommended before general anesthesia. If plasma potassium is increased above 5.5 mmol/L then this should be corrected (Box 2-4) before induction of anesthesia because of the possible interference with cardiac performance by the hyperphosphatemia.

Postoperative oliguria

Postoperative oliguria (<0.5 mL/kg/hour urine production) requires immediate attention. In the absence of congestive heart failure a fluid bolus of isotonic NaCl or a balanced electrolyte solution can be given at 5 mL/kg. Furosemide at 1–2 mg/kg or as a constant rate infusion at 0.6–1 mg/kg/hour promotes diuresis. However, furosemide in the presence of hypovolemia can increase nephrotoxicity of other drugs.

Box 2-4 Goals for anesthesia of a cat with renal or post renal failure

Assess fluid balance
Control electrolyte disturbances
Control acidosis
Control blood pressure (preoperative hypertension)
Avoid **nephrotoxic substances** like aminoglycoside antibiotics, NSAIDs, free hemoglobin, iodinated radiographic contrast agents
Avoid intraoperative hypotension and prevent renal hypoperfusion:
   avoid alpha-2 agonists
   analgesia with μ-agonistic opioids
   low doses of volatiles
   IV fluids
   promote cardiac contractility with dobutamine or dopamine
Measure and control urine production (>0.5 mL/kg/hour)

The use of dopamine to promote renal perfusion, diuresis and natriuresis is questionable in cats. Dopamine (DA1) receptors present in the kidney of cats might be different from other species and an increase in renal perfusion might be more related to cardiovascular stimulation. Even low doses of dopamine carry the risk of alpha adrenergic related vasoconstriction with decreased renal blood flow (RBF). Therefore, dobutamine (1–10 μg/kg/minute) might be a better choice as it has little effect on α-adrenergic receptors and increase in RBF is obtained by increasing cardiac output.

Prepubertal neutering

Kittens, particularly if less than 12 weeks of age, have an increased sensitivity to drugs, suffer a prolongation of their effects, and have a limited capacity for cardiovascular compensation. This has important implications in terms of anesthesia, and the choice of what to use for early or prepubertal neutering. Table 2-4 lists a number of protocols that have been used successfully for early age neutering,[10] including a protocol known as the 'quad' protocol[10] whereby kittens are given equal volumes of drugs dependent on their surface area rather than body weight.

Younger animals have a large body surface area, a reduced ability to thermoregulate and limited subcutaneous fat reserves so they are at greater risk of hypothermia both intraoperatively and postoperatively so surgical times should be kept as short as possible, wetting of hair kept to a minimum and adequate warming used intraoperatively and postoperatively.

Cesarean section

In animals being prepared for cesarean section, there are additional considerations. Oxygen should be administered by mask or flow by pre-induction. It is recommended to use rapidly metabolized or reversible agents so the fetuses are not unduly affected by

---

Table 2-4 Useful protocols for general anesthesia in kittens undergoing early age neutering

Agent(s)	Dose and route	Analgesia	Comments
Medetomidine + Ketamine	30–40 μg/kg IM 7–10 mg/kg IM	Reasonable	Good depth of anesthesia in kittens >1.5 kg
Quad:[a] Medetomidine + Ketamine + Midazolam + Buprenorphine	600 μg/m² IM 60 mg/m² IM 3 mg/m² IM 180 μg/m² IM	Very good, six to 12 hours postoperatively	Good depth of anesthesia Quick induction and recovery Multimodal analgesia Reversal agent can be used[b]
Propofol	Unpremedicated: 8.0 mg/kg IV Premedicated: 6.0 mg/kg IV	Dependent on premedication	IV route may be difficult in kittens
Isoflurane	Mask Induction	None	Strong, unpleasant odor
Sevoflurane	Mask Induction	None	Mild, inoffensive odor Expensive Rapid uptake and elimination compared to isoflurane

[a]The dosing protocol for the quad protocol, whereby equal volumes of each drug are administered IM, BSA = (K X BW $^{0.67}$) / 100; K = 10.4 (cats), body weight (BW) measured in kg, body surface area (BSA) is measured in m².

[b]Atipamezole (Antisedan: Pfizer) is recommended as a reversal agent, at 10–50% volume of the previously administered medetomidine (Domitor; Pfizer), no sooner than 20 minutes after initial intramuscular injection. Note that its use at 10% volume is unlicensed in cats.

IV, intravenous; IM, intramuscular.

(Modified from Joyce A & Yates D. Help stop teenage pregnancy. Early-age neutering in cats. J Fel Med Surg 2011;13:3–10, with permission from Elsevier.)

the anesthetic agents. Almost all drugs will cross the placenta so it is difficult to avoid any transplacental transfer. Alpha-2 agonists result in lower puppy survival and therefore should also be avoided in cats. Then the cat should be induced with a short-acting intravenous anesthetic agent such as propofol or alfaxalone. Nitrous oxide should be avoided if possible until the fetuses are removed. A midline lidocaine block or epidural/spinal anesthesia should be considered to reduce the amount of intravenous or gaseous anesthesia required, although performing an epidural will result in an inevitable delay in starting surgery due to the time taken to perform the procedure. The author has had good results with gaseous anesthetic agents when performing cesareans.

When positioning for surgery the head can be elevated slightly to reduce pressure on the diaphragm by the enlarged abdominal contents. In addition, a slight rotation to the side avoids the full weight of the uterus compressing the caval vein. In debilitated cats, anesthesia time should be kept as short as possible and clipping of the surgical site can also be performed before anesthesia induction.

THORACIC SURGERY

Despite the development of minimally invasive techniques (Chapter 42), which lower surgical morbidity, opening the thoracic cavity is still necessary for a variety of procedures (Chapter 41). The goals for anesthesia of cats with specific thoracic conditions are listed in Box 2-5.

> ### Box 2-5 Goals for anesthesia for cats with specific thoracic conditions
>
> #### Thoracic trauma and flail chest (Chapter 43)
>
> Pre-oxygenate
> Rapid induction to gain rapid airway control
> Monitor for pneumothorax
>
> #### Diaphragmatic rupture (Chapter 45)
>
> Pre-oxygenate
> Fluid resuscitation
> Preparation of the surgical field in an 'upright position' if severe dyspnea is present
> Tilt table (cat) so that head and thorax are higher than abdomen
> Rapid induction
> Immediate controlled ventilation, but with low to moderate inflation to avoid immediate re-expansion and reperfusion injury, ventilate enough to prevent hypoxemia (SpO_2 <95%, PaO_2 <60 mmHg) and severe hypercapnia ($PaCO_2$ >60 mmHg)
> NB: capnography will underestimate $PaCO_2$ because of lung atelectasis und uneven lung emptying
>
> #### Pulmonary lesions
>
> Pre-oxygenate
> If major lung leak expected use a TIVA technique
> Animals with pulmonary contusions should be ventilated very carefully with low tidal volumes and high frequencies (i.e., 20 breaths per minute, 7–10 mL/kg) to avoid stretching of affected blood vessels. If the procedure allows, maintain spontaneous ventilation

Thoracotomy

Thoracotomy can be associated with a high degree of pain, with the sternal approach being more invasive than the lateral, intercostal, approach. Before performing such a major surgical intervention a thorough evaluation of the cardiopulmonary function of the patient is necessary. Stabilization procedures should be performed as far as possible and the risk of intraoperative blood loss should be assessed and necessary preparations made.

Opening of the thoracic wall will lead to retraction of the lung and atelectasis formation with reduction of the alveolar area for gas exchange and consecutive hypoxemia. Therefore, controlled ventilation should be established before opening the chest. A combination of intermittent positive pressure ventilation (IPPV) with peak pressures of 10–20 cm H_2O and positive end expiratory pressure (PEEP) of 5 cm H_2O and 100% oxygen will help to avoid lung collapse and hypoxemia in cats. If the lung tissue is very stiff (low compliance) higher pressures might be necessary. Close cooperation of the surgeon and the anesthetist is necessary to adapt lung inflation. Particularly with a lateral approach, too much lung inflation can hinder the surgical procedure. Ventilators that are suitable for use in cats (human pediatric, small animal ventilators) come in different designs depending on the cycling and controlling mechanism and the mechanism producing the inspiratory phase (pressure or flow generator). For cats the ventilator should be able to deliver small tidal volumes (20–200 mL) at a safe working pressure (10–60 cm H_2O) to avoid barotrauma to the lungs. Ventilator settings (Table 2-5) have to be adapted to the individual animal's needs to maintain eucapnia (30–35 mmHg).

Volatile anesthetics as well as TIVA techniques can be used for cats undergoing thoracotomy. Nitrous oxide should be avoided because to be useful it has to be given at high percentage concentrations, making high inspired oxygen fractions impossible. In addition, nitrous oxide diffuses down the concentration gradient very rapidly into closed air spaces, increasing their volume.

Monitoring during thoracotomy

Continuous monitoring should be done to assess for arrhythmias, ventilation, and oxygenation status of the animal. The ventilation and lung inflation need to be adapted to the animal's needs. With an open chest the information provided by capnography is not representative of arterial CO_2 tensions. End-tidal CO_2 is lower than the arterial values indicating ventilation perfusion mismatch due to lung collapse. A decreasing end-tidal CO_2 is not necessarily an indication to reduce ventilation in these circumstances. Arterial or free-flow lingual samples are necessary (which can be difficult to obtain in cats) for information on the adequacy of minute ventilation. Pulse oximetry will indicate desaturation with severe alterations in ventilation perfusion matching

Table 2-5 Suggested ventilator settings in cats[1]

Ventilator	Settings
Tidal volume	15–20 mL/kg
Respiratory rate	12–20/minute
Minute volume	400–600 mL
Peak inspiratory pressure	20 cm H_2O
Inspiratory to expiratory time ratio	1 : 2 to 1 : 3

or shunting. Information on less severe changes in gas exchange is limited with pulse oximetry. Obstruction of the endotracheal tube can occur with secretions from the respiratory tract, for example pus from a pulmonary abscess.

Analgesia

A thoracotomy is a painful procedure, particularly when performed through a sternotomy. It requires effective analgesia and close attention for several days in the postoperative period. Analgesia needs to be well planned and should start before the operation (Box 2-6).

Intercostal nerve block

The intercostal nerves lie adjacent to the caudal border of each rib. Two or three nerves on either side of the incision site need to be blocked. The needle is inserted distal to the angle of the rib close to the epaxial muscles and is directed dorsally along the caudal border of the rib. It is common for the surgeon to perform this block once the pleural cavity has been entered to allow direct visualization of the nerve and minimize the risk of hemorrhage, which can occur to a catastrophic degree when done blind. Additionally, the pleural cavity is punctured very easily and the cat has to be watched closely for signs of pneumothorax if the procedure is not followed by thoracotomy. If multiple nerves are infiltrated care has to be taken not to reach toxic doses of the local anesthetic.

Interpleural anesthesia

Interpleural infusion of bupivacaine or lidocaine diluted in 5 mL saline infused into the interpleural space via a chest tube every eight to 12 hours provides anesthesia of intercostal nerves and analgesia after thoracotomy. A wound diffusion catheter placed after a sternotomy could also be considered, as it provides an effective route for delivering local anesthesia and for longer than the duration that the thoracic drain may stay in place.

Box 2-6 **Analgesia considerations for thoracic surgery**
Systemic analgesia with an opioid, ideally with a constant rate infusion or a multimodal approach with a combination of an opioid and ketamine with or without lidocaine. NB: cats can develop hypotension with lidocaine
An epidural with a local anesthetic and morphine at a total volume of 1 mL/3.5 kg can provide analgesia for thoracotomy. An epidural catheter can be used for repeated injections and postoperative treatment
An intercostal nerve block rostral and caudal to the incision site can be used. When performed before thoracic surgery analgesia is often not complete; specific local injection, after opening the thorax, close to the vertebrae will improve the results
An interpleural block is given with the aim that the anesthetic diffuses through the thoracic wall to the intercostal nerves. The anesthetic can be injected through a chest drain with the animal in a sternal or a standing position after sternotomy and in a lateral position (lying on the affected side) after lateral thoracotomy. The first infusion should be performed after the thorax is closed and the animal is still anesthetized. The infusion can then be repeated every eight to 12 hours

---

CARDIOVASCULAR DISEASE

Cardiovascular disease comprises a variety of congenital and acquired conditions. In general, uncontrolled cardiac failure is a contraindication for immediate general anesthesia and patients must be stabilized (Box 2-7) and cardiac function improved pre-anesthesia if feasible. If cardiac failure is related to non-cardiac conditions like hyperthyroidism (Chapter 53) then the primary condition should be treated.

There is no 'gold standard' anesthetic protocol for animals with cardiovascular disease and the technique has to be adapted to the intended procedure und underlying condition. The goals of a chosen protocol should be stress-free induction and analgesia to avoid catecholamine release, minimal depression of myocardial contractility, maintenance of blood pressure, maintenance of adequate ventilation and minimal interaction with the effects of the medical treatment of the heart condition. Catecholamines contribute to arrhythmia formation in combination with certain anesthetics (i.e., thiopentone, halothane), so these should be avoided in cats with cardiovascular disease.

In the following section principles of anesthesia management for the most commonly encountered cardiac diseases in the cat are described.

Hypertrophic cardiomyopathy (HCM)

In cats, HCM is a common disease that can occur in young to middle aged animals. Any breed can be affected but the Maine Coon is predisposed.

The main pathology is muscular hypertrophy with restricted ventricular volume. One special form of HCM involves systolic anterior motion of the septal mitral valve leaflet (SAM), which momentarily restricts ventricular outflow and induces mitral regurgitation. On physical examination and auscultation it cannot be distinguished from dynamic right ventricular outflow tract obstruction (DR VOTO), which represents a more benign heart murmur; echocardiography is necessary for a definitive diagnosis. Outflow tract obstruction is exacerbated by tachycardia, increased myocardial contractility and increased afterload.

Cats with pulmonary edema and heart failure should be stabilized before elective surgery. Acute therapy includes cage rest, oxygen therapy, vasodilators (i.e., benazepril, enalapril), and furosemide. Heart rate and contractility can be reduced with atenolol (β1-blocker) and diltiazem (calcium-channel blocker).

Stress before anesthesia should be avoided and effective analgesia should be used, including an opioid to reduce heart rate and the use of regional anesthesia techniques, dependent on the planned procedure. The aims during anesthesia are listed in Box 2-8. Ketamine as an induction agent or for maintenance of anesthesia should be avoided because it increases myocardial contractility, myocardial

---

Box 2-7 **Stabilization procedures for cats in cardiac failure**
Reduction of retained fluids (diuretics, thoracocentesis, pericardiocentesis)
Reduction of cardiac work by afterload reduction (i.e., angiotensin-converting enzyme inhibitors, nitroprusside, hydralazine, prazosin) cage rest, oxygen therapy and anxiolytic drugs
Improvement of cardiac contractility, where indicated, with pimobendan, dobutamine, digoxin
Control of arrhythmias

> **Box 2-8 Goals for anesthesia of the cat with hypertrophic cardiomyopathy**
>
> Avoid heart rate increases
> Lower contractility
> Maintain or mildly increase afterload (systemic vascular resistance)
> Maintain filling pressures

> **Box 2-9 Analgesia considerations for aural surgery**
>
> The aural area is very well innervated and surgical procedures in this region are often very painful and irritating for the animal
> Start gabapentin treatment before surgery 10 mg/kg two to three times a day
> Opioid or opioid/ketamine infusion during surgery
> Wound catheter placement and intermittent bupivacaine (0.5%)
> Continue opioid/ketamine infusion post-surgery
> Use non-steroidal anti-inflammatory drugs to reduce wound swelling

> **Box 2-10 Analgesia considerations for mandibulectomy or maxillectomy**
>
> Start gabapentin treatment before surgery 10 mg/kg two to three times a day
> Opioid or opioid/ketamine infusion during surgery
> Deep infraorbital (maxillary) block with bupivacaine 0.5%
> Continue opioid/ketamine infusion post surgery in combination with a NSAID over three days, re-evaluate pain and possibly change to non-steroidal anti-inflammatory drugs only

work and myocardial oxygen consumption. The author prefers a fentanyl, midazolam, etomidate protocol.[1] Etomidate is known for minimal cardiovascular effects and maintenance of vascular tone. If the vagotonic effect of the opioid (i.e., fentanyl, morphine) is insufficient to control heart rate, a short-acting beta-blocker like esmolol can be added. Supported by an echocardiographic study, the alpha-2 agonist medetomidine has been used as part of an anesthetic protocol in cats with HCM to successfully prevent mitral regurgitation. Medetomidine has been shown to be able to reduce SAM by its peripheral effects on vascular alpha-2 receptors and increases in afterload.[11]

If HCM is associated with hyperthyroidism, preoperative euthyroidism should be restored if possible (Chapter 58) and special attention should be paid to the occurrence of ventricular arrhythmias.

Traumatic myocarditis (myocardial contusion)

Blunt thoracic trauma with contusion of the myocardium can result in ventricular arrhythmias 24 to 48 hours after the event. In combination with pain, anxiety, electrolyte disturbances and hypovolemia the risk of the development of life-threatening arrhythmias is increased. Every animal with thoracic trauma should have an ECG examination before surgery. After correction of hypovolemia and electrolyte disturbances, anxiolysis and pain control are important to prevent further catecholamine release. In the absence of hypovolemia a low dose of acepromazine (0.01–0.02 mg/kg) can be beneficial because of its antiarrhythmogenic and anxiolytic effects. Treatment of ventricular arrhythmias with lidocaine infusions[1] can be maintained throughout anesthesia with due consideration that in cats lidocaine can induce low blood pressure and cardiovascular depression.[12]

Congenital cardiac diseases

In cases of congenital cardiac diseases like persistent ductus arteriosus (PDA) and ventricular septal defect (VSD) undergoing surgical correction, the animals are often quite young and the thoracic cavity has to be opened. All anesthetic principles for these conditions have to be followed, including consideration of the cat's age and therefore its ability to metabolize drugs and maintain normothermia and the surgical approach, such as a thoracotomy (Chapter 41).

A common feature of several congenital disorders is an abnormal blood flow between the left, systemic circulation, and the right, pulmonary circulation. As long as the blood shunts from left to right, oxygenation of the blood is not a problem. Oxygenated blood re-circulates through the lung. Cyanosis develops with right to left shunts, when deoxygenated blood enters the systemic circulation. Therefore, the goal in anesthesia is to maintain left to right shunting by maintaining cardiac output, avoiding a massive decrease in systemic vascular resistance (extreme vasodilation) and avoiding an increase in pulmonary vascular resistance. Cardiac output is maintained by fluids and dobutamine, avoiding high doses of volatiles. Acepromazine will reduce vasodilation and an increase in pulmonary

vascular resistance is prevented by using low inflation pressures for ventilation.

HEAD AND NECK SURGERY

When operating in the region of the head and neck, and in particular the larynx and pharynx, it is important to maintain a patent airway and also to monitor the cat carefully following surgery for any upper respiratory distress due to swelling. It is imperative to provide adequate analgesia both preoperatively and postoperatively when operating around the cat's head. Aural surgery can be particularly painful and consideration of how to provide appropriate analgesia is listed in Box 2-9. Postoperative pain may result in difficulty or reluctance to eat, particularly after surgery of the mandible and maxillectomy (Box 2-10). If the surgery or disease is likely to result in the animal being inappetent postoperatively then consideration should be made to place a feeding tube (Chapter 12). Local anesthetics provide good specific local analgesia and are relatively easy to administer for surgery of the head.

Local anesthetics and nerve blocks

Local anesthetics are useful adjuncts for providing analgesia during surgery; their usage enables reduced doses of anesthesia to be used and the analgesia provided by the block is often continued postoperatively. Nerve blocks that are of specific use for procedures of the head include the infraorbital nerve block, the mental nerve block and the mandibular nerve block.

Infraorbital nerve block

The nerves of the head can be desensitized by infiltrating 0.1–0.3 mL of 1–2% lidocaine or mepivacaine, 0.5% ropivacaine or 0.25–0.5% bupivacaine.

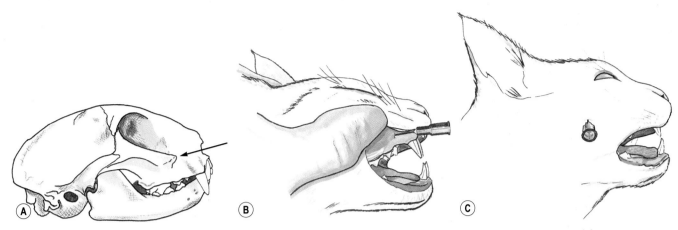

Figure 2-5 Infraorbital nerve block. **(A)** The infraorbital canal is just cranial to the palpable ridge (arrow). **(B)** Intraoral approach. **(C)** Cutaneous approach.

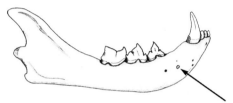

Figure 2-6 The middle mental foramen on a cat's mandible (arrow), site of the mental nerve block.

The infraorbital canal starts at the rostral floor of the orbit and opens rostral to the zygomatic arch at the infraorbital foramen. In the cat the canal is very short and the infraorbital foramen is recessed and cannot be palpated directly but the ridge is obvious above the premolars. The canal contains the infraorbital nerve as well as the infraorbital artery and vein. The needle is inserted into the opening of the canal by either an oral or transcutaneous access (Fig. 2-5). Anesthesia will affect the ipsilateral premolar, canine and incisor teeth as well as the bone and soft tissue buccal to the teeth. If the needle is inserted about 0.5 cm into the 'canal' and pressure is placed over the foramen the agent will flow distally and block the caudal maxillary alveolar nerve which anesthetizes the maxillary molars, the roof of the nasal cavity, the upper lip and muzzle and the soft and hard palate.

Mental nerve block

In cats, the middle mental foramen is located midway between the mandibular canine tooth and the third premolar tooth (cats have no first or second mandibular premolar teeth) at the dorsoventral midpoint of the mandible. From an intraoral approach, the needle enters the mucosa rostral to the mandibular frenulum and is advanced into the opening of the foramen (Fig. 2-6). This block anesthetizes the buccal mucosa and lip rostral to the foramen. If the needle is advanced deeper into the mandibular canal, the canine and incisor teeth will also be anesthetized. However, due to the small opening in cats and the potential to cause trauma to the nerve and vessels, it is preferable to place the needle tip just inside the foramen and then apply digital pressure to force the agent deeper into the canal.

Mandibular nerve block

The inferior alveolar nerve is located within the mandibular canal; therefore, to block this nerve it must be accessed before it enters the

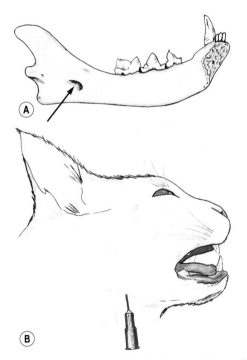

Figure 2-7 Mandibular nerve block. **(A)** The foramen is situated on the medial aspect of the mandible (arrow). **(B)** The nerve can be blocked by a cutaneous approach or intraoral.

body of the mandible. The site at which the nerve is accessible is just before it enters the inferior alveolar foramen on the medial side of the ramus of the mandible. This block may be achieved with either an intraoral or an extraoral approach (Fig. 2-7). In cats, the foramen lies ventral to the midpoint of the zygomatic arch. The author prefers the intraoral approach to the inferior alveolar foramen. The needle is inserted through the oral mucosa just behind the last molar and then walked off the medial side of the mandible. With the tip of the needle pointing in the direction of the angular process it is advanced halfway between the last molar and the angular process. The ipsilateral mandibular teeth and bone as well as all of the soft tissue lingual to the mandible are blocked. Care has to be taken to keep the needle close to the mandible and foramen to avoid also blocking the lingual nerve, which might paralyze the tongue and risk the cat biting its tongue on recovery.

BRAIN SURGERY

The primary goal in anesthesia for cats undergoing brain surgery is to maintain cerebral blood flow (CBF), which depends on cerebral perfusion pressure (CPP) and cerebral vascular resistance (CVR). Cerebral perfusion pressure results from mean arterial pressure (MAP) opposed by intracranial pressure (ICP). This shows that perfusion is directly related to MAP and maintenance of cardiac output and MAP above a certain level is crucial for animals with intracranial lesions; CPP should be maintained above 70 mmHg, which translates to a MAP of 70–80 mmHg.

In the healthy brain, blood flow is autoregulated and remains constant over a wide range of CPP (50–150 mmHg); outside this range it depends on MAP. The CBF is also matched to the metabolic requirements of the brain. Brain injury or certain anesthetics can interfere with the metabolic coupling. Ventilation and oxygenation also play an important role in the regulation of cerebral vascular tone. Hypercapnia or hypoxia result in cerebral vasodilation; hypocapnia leads to increasing vasoconstriction in a linear manner with decreasing $PaCO_2$. Therefore hypoxemia as well as hypoventilation or extreme hyperventilation has to be prevented in animals with brain injury.

Intracranial pressure

Management of ICP (Box 2-11) is a major issue in head trauma patients as well as patients with space-occupying intracranial lesions that undergo craniotomy.

Signs of raised ICP are depression, pupillary changes (from miosis to anisocoria and bilateral mydriasis) and changes in respiratory pattern. In severely increased ICP, the Cushing triad can occur with hypertension, reflex bradycardia and respiratory alterations.

There is a major difference in the indication for preoperative use of steroids in head trauma patients and cats with intracranial tumors. In tumor patients, perioperative use of steroids reduces peritumor edema and can significantly improve clinical signs. In head trauma patients that may require anesthesia, steroids are contraindicated as they induce hyperglycemia. Hyperglycemia is part of the stress response after head injury. However, hyperglycemia increases brain damage when traumatic brain injury is complicated by secondary ischemia.

Anesthesia

The choice of what premedication to use is dependent on the mental status and cooperation of the individual patient (Box 2-12).

Anesthetic induction should be smooth and extensive coughing during intubation prevented. Pre-oxygenation can help to minimize hypoxia during induction. Propofol and thiopental are suitable for induction of anesthesia in patients with raised ICP. Mechanical ventilation should be started immediately after intubation and normocapnia or mild hypocapnia maintained (30–35 mmHg).

For maintenance of anesthesia for neurosurgery a propofol TIVA is often used in humans. However, in cats prolonged infusion times of propofol can lead to cumulation and prolonged recoveries due to the cats' limited ability to metabolize phenolic compounds.[13] When using volatile agents, sevoflurane is the best choice as it maintains blood flow metabolism coupling, causes less vasodilation than isoflurane and anesthetic depth is easily altered. Halothane should be avoided as it disturbs flow–metabolism coupling. Nitrous oxide should be avoided as it increases cerebral blood flow and oxygen demand and increases the potential for air embolism.

Box 2-11 General measures to reduce intracranial pressure

Position of the head slightly elevated

Avoid increase in central venous pressure

Avoid jugular compression or occlusion with tight bandages or venous catheters – use peripherally inserted central venous lines

Avoid coughing during intubation

Avoid high inspiratory pressures with IPPV

Mannitol 0.5 g/kg IV over 20 minutes can be repeated as a bolus; a constant rate infusion is less effective

Furosemide 1 mg/kg IV followed by constant rate infusion with 1 mg/kg/hour (loop diuretics reduce CSF production and brain fluid)

Intermittent positive pressure ventilation to maintain eucapnia or mild hyperventilation

Systemic lidocaine reduces intracranial pressure

Box 2-12 Premedication considerations for craniotomy

Opioids have no direct effect on intracranial pressure, but high doses cause hypoventilation

Morphine may induce vomiting

Ketamine might increase intracranial pressure at the high end of the dose range because of muscle rigidity. However, it can be used in the low dose range (3–5 mg/kg IM) in combination with benzodiazepines for uncooperative cats. Avoid in seizuring animals or those with a history of seizures

Medetomidine can induce vomiting, but it is helpful for sedation of fractious animals at 1–5 μg/kg IM. It causes systemic vasoconstriction and cardiovascular depression

---

A combination of an infusion of fentanyl, alfentanil or remifentanil is suitable to reduce the anesthetic requirements and avoid sudden changes in MAP. Fentanyl can cumulate after long infusions. Remifentanil and alfentanil do not cumulate but require introduction of another analgesic before the infusion is stopped (Table 2-1).

For good surgical access the brain should be relaxed, which can be obtained by mannitol infusion at the rate given for ICP control before opening the cranium.

The removal of meningiomas (Chapter 58) in cats can be associated with extensive bleeding, therefore cats should be blood typed before surgery and preparations for potential blood transfusion made (Chapter 5).

Postoperative anesthesia

Craniotomy patients require intensive postoperative care (Chapters 4 and 58). In general a smooth rapid recovery is desirable to allow early neurologic assessment. However, in cases that had intraoperative hemorrhage or unstable patients it can be advantageous to maintain anesthesia or deep sedation and ventilation for prolonged periods.

Analgesia for brain surgery

Analgesia is best given based on a multimodal approach. Adequate analgesia is important to avoid postoperative hypertension and excitement. Non-steroidal anti-inflammatory drugs should only be used in cats without previous or concurrent steroid treatment. In severely depressed patients care has to be taken not to overdose with opioids; they should be titrated to effect. High doses of opioids can induce central excitation in cats, and opioids can alter pupil reactivity in cats.

Seizure activity has to be controlled. Many brain tumor patients present with seizures and they are often already on anti-epileptic treatment before surgery. If the patient is not on long-term anti-epileptic medication, phenobarbital or gabapentin given before surgery might help to reduce the risk of seizures and will give some 'background' sedation after surgery. The type of postoperative nutritional support needs to be planned (Chapter 6) and placement of a percutaneous endoscopic gastrostomy (PEG) tube should be considered (Chapter 12).

REFERENCES

1. Kästner S. Anesthesia. In: Montavon PM, Voss K, Langley-Hobbs SJ, editors. Feline orthopedic surgery and musculoskeletal disease. Elsevier Edinburgh; 2009. p. 177–98.

2. Kästner S. Analgesia. In: Montavon PM, Voss K, Langley-Hobbs SJ, editors. Feline orthopedic surgery and musculoskeletal disease. Elsevier Edinburgh; 2009. p. 199–205.

3. Pypendop BH, Siao KT, Ilkiw JE. Effects of tramadol hydrochloride on the thermal threshold in cats. Am J Vet Res 2009;70: 1465–70.

4. Pelligand L, King JN, Toutain PL, et al. In vivo COX-2 selectivity of robenacoxib in a feline tissue cage model of inflammation. J Vet Pharmacol Ther 2009;32(Suppl. 1): 103–4.

5. Giraudel JM, Toutain PL, King JN, Lees P. Differential inhibition of cyclooxygenase isoenzymes in the cat by the NSAID robenacoxib. J Vet Pharmacol Ther 2009;32:31–40.

6. Brodbelt DC, Pfeiffer DU, Young LE, Wood JL. Risk factors for anaesthetic-related death in cats: results from the confidential enquiry into perioperative small animal fatalities (CEPSAF). Br J Anaesth 2007;99:617–23.

7. Brodbelt D. Feline anesthetic deaths in veterinary practice. Top Companion Anim Med 2010;25:189–94. Review.

8. German AJ. The growing problem of obesity in dogs and cats. The Journal of Nutrition 2006;136:1940S–6S.

9. Abelson AL, McCobb EC, Shaw S, et al. Use of wound soaker catheters for the administration of local anesthetic for post-operative analgesia: 56 cases. Vet Anaesth Analg 2009;36: 597–602.

10. Joyce A, Yates D. Help stop teenage pregnancy. Early-age neutering in cats. J Fel Med Surg 2011;13:3–10.

11. Lamont LA, Bulmer BJ, Sisson DD, et al. Doppler echocardiographic effects of medetomidine on dynamic left ventricular outflow tract obstruction in cat. J Am Vet Med Assoc 2002;221:1276–81.

12. Pypendop B, Ilkiw J. Assessment of the hemodynamic effects of lidocaine administered IV in isoflurane anesthetized cats. Am J Vet Res 2005;66:661–8.

13. Pascoe PJ, Ilkiw JE, Frischmeyer KJ. The effect of the duration of propofol administration on recovery from anaesthesia in cats. Vet Anaesth Analg 2006;33:2–7.

Chapter | **3** |

Postoperative monitoring and management of complications

J.A. Beatty, V.R. Barrs

The postoperative period from anesthetic recovery to discharge from hospital is a crucial period for initial healing and return to function. Success relies on an integrated, team approach to optimizing the patient environment, hydration status, electrolyte balance, nutritional and analgesic needs. Despite best efforts, complications can occur during the postoperative period. Having routine monitoring procedures in place to identify complications at the earliest opportunity, facilitating timely interventions, will achieve the best outcome. This chapter will cover general aspects of postoperative monitoring and management; specific information will be included in the individual chapters on separate organs.

DAILY INPATIENT MONITORING

A cornerstone of excellent patient care is careful, appropriate monitoring. Staff should be aware of the importance of the procedures that they perform and the data that they record. For example, essential information will be lost if the litter tray, bedding and cage are cleaned without noting and recording urination. Where urine output is inappropriately low, an opportunity will have been lost for early intervention to prevent acute renal failure (ARF). Minimum monitoring for the postoperative inpatient is a twice-daily examination. A useful approach to direct this examination and to record its findings is the SOAP (subjective, objective, assessment, plan) protocol (Box 3-1).

Using the SOAP protocol

The SOAP protocol facilitates consistent, comprehensive medical evaluation that can be clearly communicated in a standardized, concise format. The subjective and objective components involve data collection and are followed by a succinct assessment and a plan. The SOAP directs the frequency and the nature of additional individual monitoring, avoiding excessive handling and sampling. For practical reasons, the order in which data is collected does not correspond with the order in which it is recorded.

Data collection

Observing the cat undisturbed in its cage allows assessment of its demeanor and resting respiratory rate and effort, all of which may change upon handling. Unless there are specific indications otherwise, physical examination is best completed on the examination table. Physical examination has been described in Chapter 1. For patients with reduced mobility or where handling causes discomfort, the bedding can be used to support the patient during transfer from the cage (Fig. 3-1). Cats should be weighed using scales that are accurate for small patients, such as pediatric scales (Fig. 3-2). A fall in body weight can accompany dehydration or catabolism, whereas a rapid increase can signal occult effusion. Surgical wounds, drains and feeding tube sites and intravenous (IV) catheter sites should be inspected for discharge, redness, swelling, or evidence of self-trauma. Gentle palpation of surgical sites can assist with pain scoring. The cage should be checked for evidence of urination (estimated volume, color), defecation (amount, color, consistency, presence of mucus, blood), vomitus or hemorrhage. Food and water intake should be recorded. For cats on IV fluids, the rate and type of fluid being administered should be confirmed. Patients receiving IV fluids typically have hematocrit, total plasma protein (TP), electrolytes and, where available, blood gases monitored every 24 hours. Judicious sampling minimizes handling and restraint and avoids exacerbating anemia. Using an insulin syringe for venipuncture is well tolerated, minimally traumatic and provides sufficient sample for microhematocrit, TP, electrolytes, blood glucose and blood film preparation.

Assessment

Subjective and objective data form the basis of the patient assessment. All problems identified should be ranked and assessed (Chapter 1) and an overall assessment of the cat's status as stable, improving or deteriorating made. Consideration should be given to the pain score, hydration/nutritional status, changes in body weight, new problems, or problems that cannot be accounted for.

Plan

The plan schedules investigations, treatments and ongoing monitoring, including adjustments to fluid therapy, nutrition, the analgesia

© 2014 Elsevier Ltd
DOI: 10.1016/B978-0-7020-4336-9.00003-2

Box 3-1 SOAP protocol for recording clinical information

Subjective data	Electrolytes
Objective data	Fluids
Weight	Food intake
Temperature	Urination
Heart rate	Defecation
Pulse rate	Water consumption
Pulse quality	Additional notes
Respiratory rate	Medications given
MM	Procedures performed
Capillary refill time	**A**ssessment
Packed cell volume	**P**lan
Total plasma protein	

MM, mucous membrane colour.

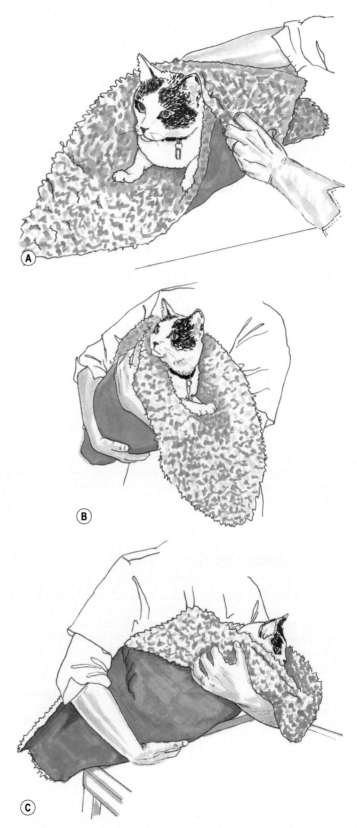

Figure 3-1 Using the bedding to transport a weak, immobile or painful patient.

plan, other medications (type, dose, route and frequency) and care of surgical drains, feeding tubes, venous access or closed urine collection systems. Environmental adjustments, such as a litter tray with low sides or a privacy area (a sleeping box or a curtain over part of the cage door) for timid cats undergoing less intensive monitoring, are included.

FLUID THERAPY

The goals of fluid therapy are to maintain hydration and effective circulating volume and to contribute to acid–base and electrolyte balance. Evidence on which to base recommendations for fluid therapy in the postoperative feline patient is limited, mainly comprising extrapolation of data relating to other species and pathophysiological justification. The volume, composition and rate of IV fluids should be tailored to the individual based on serial monitoring of physical and laboratory parameters.

Route of fluid administration

A pump should be used to deliver IV fluids and a peripheral catheter is suitable for most purposes. Where a fluid pump is not available, a pediatric burette (Fig. 3-3) is preferable to a standard giving set to avoid fluid overload. The required rate is converted to the number of drips/minute for the giving set:

$$\text{Drops per minute} = \frac{\text{required rate (mL/hour)} \times \text{drops/mL (check individual set)}}{60}$$

Subcutaneous (SC) administration is not suitable for irritant solutions and an unpredictable rate of absorption can precipitate congestive heart failure or hypokalemia. Administration via a feeding tube or the intraosseous route may be indicated.

Volume of fluid administration

The volume of fluid required for a 24 hour period is the sum of current deficits, maintenance requirements, and ongoing losses (Box 3-2). Losses during surgery include hemorrhage, evaporation from serous surfaces, transudation from traumatized tissues, and gastrointestinal sequestration. The maintenance requirement for an adult

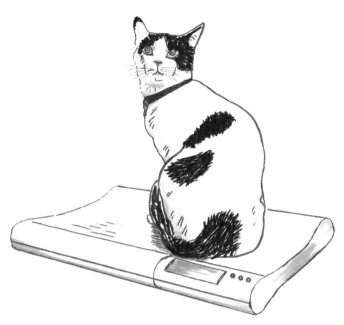

Figure 3-2 Pediatric scales for accurate weighing.

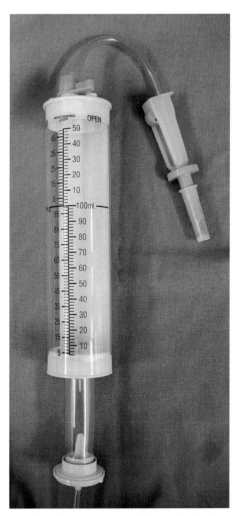

Figure 3-3 A pediatric burette prevents fluid overload when a fluid pump is not available.

Box 3-2 **Example of a fluid replacement calculation**

A 5 kg cat is estimated to be 5% dehydrated. The cat is vomiting four times per day, approximately 10 mL per vomit
  Maintenance requirement (60 mL/kg/day) for this cat is 60 × 5 = 300 mL in 24 hours, or **150 mL** in 12 hours
  Fluids deficit (in mL) is body weight (kg) × % dehydration (as a decimal) × 1000
    This cat's fluid deficit is (5 × 0.05 × 1000) = **250 mL**
    The *ongoing losses* are 40 mL in 24 hours, or **20 mL** in 12 hours
    So, if the fluid deficit is replaced over 12 hours, the total volume of fluid to be delivered in 12 hours is 150 + 250 + 20 = 420 mL, or (420/12) = **35 mL/hour**

cat is approximately 60 mL/kg/day.[1] Ongoing losses include those associated with vomiting, diarrhea, polyuria, surgical drains, and transudation into body cavities or externally. Hydration status is estimated based on the patient's history, physical findings and laboratory data. Changes from objective baseline data such as weight, hematocrit, TP and creatinine are particularly useful.

Rate of fluid administration

The rate at which fluid is administered depends on the severity and clinical consequences of the deficit, taking into account pre-existing conditions, which may predispose to fluid overload. Deficits are usually replaced over six to 12 hours.

The maximum rate of infusion for cats, 60 mL/kg/hour (90 mL/kg/hour in the dog), is reserved for patients with non-cardiogenic shock, and even then, is given as smaller boluses, repeated as necessary (see below, Management considerations for the septic cat). Care should be taken to avoid interstitial fluid overload, the consequences of which include pulmonary edema, pleural effusion and delayed healing due to prolonged ileus, edema and poor tissue oxygenation. Compensated cardiac and renal disease, chronic anemia, and colloid administration all increase the risk of fluid overload. Urine output should be monitored and maintained above 1–2 mL/kg/hour (or higher where there is obligatory polyuria). Compensated cardiac disease is difficult to detect without echocardiography. Detection of a murmur is neither sensitive nor specific for this purpose.[2] Assessment of vertebral heart score, atrial size, and pulmonary vasculature on thoracic radiographs can assist. However, in contrast to dogs, hypertrophic cardiomyopathies are common in cats and significant structural changes can produce minimal change in the cardiac silhouette. Where an increased risk of fluid overload is identified, for example in a cat with advanced hyperthyroidism where significant structural cardiac disease might be predicted despite medical stabilization, conservative fluid rates and additional monitoring should be instituted. Resting respiratory rate and effort can be recorded cage-side, hourly. Increased rate and effort from baseline should prompt assessment for jugular distension or pulsation, thorough auscultation for signs of pulmonary edema or pleural effusion and, if necessary, thoracic radiographs. Serial central venous pressure (CVP) monitoring is useful for avoiding volume overload (normal CVP 0–10 cmH$_2$O).[3] As maintenance needs are gradually met from other sources, such as enteral feeding or voluntary food intake, fluid rates should be reduced and then ceased.

Fluid composition

The exact composition of the fluid administered will depend on individual requirements. In humans and dogs, anesthesia and surgery are associated with a transient increase in antidiuretic hormone (ADH)

31

secretion lasting from one to four days.[4] ADH promotes fluid retention and natriuresis. The administration of hypotonic, maintenance solutions in the immediate postsurgical period has been associated with dilutional hyponatremia and fluid overload, which can be severe.[5] Assuming that the same is true in cats, then even in a well-hydrated patient, a rehydration solution, such as 0.9% saline or Hartmann solution, is recommended in the initial postsurgical period. Since high rates of potassium-free crystalloids are often administered during surgery, prompt supplementation of fluids after surgery with potassium is necessary to prevent iatrogenic hypokalemia.

ELECTROLYTE ABNORMALITIES

It is essential to monitor for postoperative electrolyte abnormalities. Hypokalemia is common after surgery, particularly in cats that have been inappetent preoperatively.

Hypokalemia

Hypokalemia results from reduced intake, increased losses or redistribution in alkalosis. In the postsurgical patient, reduced food intake, inadequate supplementation of fluids, solute diuresis, diarrhea, chronic vomiting and diuretic use (loop and thiazide diuretics) can contribute. Other causes of hypokalemia, including primary hyperaldosteronism (Conn syndrome) (Chapter 35), a condition likely underdiagnosed in the cat,[6] and breed-associated hypokalemia of Burmese cats, will be identified preoperatively. Intracellular potassium concentrations are actively maintained at much higher levels than extracellular levels and this potassium gradient contributes to the resting membrane potential of excitable cells. When IV fluids are delivered at maintenance rates, supplementation with potassium chloride at 20 mmol/L usually maintains normokalemia. The clinical consequences of severe hypokalemia (<3 mmol/L) include generalized weakness, cervical ventroflexion and reduced gastrointestinal motility. Where the potassium deficit is mild, oral or enteral supplementation can be used (4–10 mmol of potassium gluconate/cat/day divided) or the concentration of potassium in the fluids can be increased up to 40 mmol/L. Where potassium is added to a bag of fluids in use, the fluids must be turned 'off' to the patient while adding concentrated potassium solution to prevent infusion until the solution is adequately mixed. The maximum rate of potassium supplementation, 0.5 mmol/kg/hour, should not be exceeded or life-threatening cardiotoxicity can result. If plasma potassium is <3.0 mmol/L, a maximum-rate potassium infusion can be delivered using a syringe driver (Fig. 3-4), or as a secondary infusion on a pump, for one hour, after which electrolytes should be retested and the infusion repeated if necessary (Box 3-3).

Hyperkalemia

Hyperkalemia can occur with reduced renal excretion, translocation in acidosis, over-supplementation of fluids and massive tissue necrosis. In the postsurgical period, hyperkalemia should prompt immediate assessment for ARF. Adequate urine output (1–2 mL/kg/hour) should be confirmed without delay and renal parameters determined (plasma creatinine, urea and phosphate). If azotemia is confirmed the contribution of prerenal, renal and postrenal causes should be investigated. Where loss of integrity of the urinary tract is a possibility, e.g., after urinary tract surgery, abdominal ultrasonography is indicated. If an abdominal effusion is identified, simultaneous comparison of creatinine concentration in the plasma and the effusion confirms uroperitoneum, if the creatinine level is higher in the effusion (urea

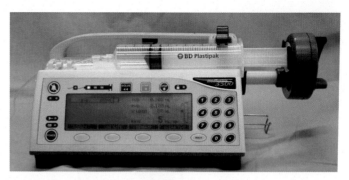

Figure 3-4 A syringe driver can be used to deliver a supplementary potassium infusion.

Box 3-3 **Preparing a maximum-rate potassium infusion**

A 10 mL quantity of a 1 mmol/mL solution of potassium chloride is added to 10 mL of 0.9% sodium chloride. The resulting 0.5 mmol/mL solution is delivered using a syringe driver (Fig. 3-4) at 1 mL/kg/hour for one hour only. Plasma potassium is re-measured. The infusion can be repeated until normokalemia is achieved, but this rate should not be exceeded.

equilibrates quickly and is less useful for diagnosing uroperitoneum). Hyperkalemia in the face of normal renal function can accompany excessive supplementation, acidosis and drug administration (e.g., spironolactone, angiotensin-converting enzyme inhibitors). The most significant clinical consequence of hyperkalemia is cardiotoxicity, manifesting as bradycardia or arrhythmias, and specific treatment with calcium gluconate may be indicated (see Chapter 1 for consequences and treatment of hyperkalemia).

Hyponatremia

Fluctuations in plasma sodium concentration affect the volume and osmolality of the extracellular and intracellular fluid compartments. Where hyponatremia is identified, artefact due to hyperglobulinemia or hyperlipidemia or dilution of plasma sodium by solute accumulation, such as glucose or mannitol, can be quickly ruled out. Hyponatremia with concurrent hypovolemia can occur with renal, gastrointestinal and third space losses, severe burns, post-obstructive diuresis, hypotonic fluid administration, certain drugs (e.g., barbiturates) and severe hepatic, renal or cardiac failure.[7] The clinical significance of hyponatremia depends on the magnitude and speed of change; a rapid or severe fall in sodium concentration can cause cerebral edema manifesting as obtundation and seizures. Treatment should address the underlying cause. Where this fails to resolve the problem, or where hyponatremia is severe (<125 mmol/L), specific therapy is indicated. Rapid reversal of cerebral edema can cause cerebral dehydration and hemorrhage if the deficit was acquired gradually. Volume deficits are replaced first, using a rehydrating crystalloid (e.g., 0.9% saline). The patient should be monitored every 1 to 2 hours to ensure that the maximum rate of sodium replacement, 0.5–0.7 mmol/L/hour, is not exceeded. Normovolemic hyponatremia can be addressed by restricting fluid intake to less than urine output.

Hypernatremia

Hypernatremia follows pure water or hypotonic fluid loss, or excess sodium administration. Clinical signs due to central nervous system (CNS) cellular dehydration and hemorrhage (e.g., vomiting, muscle fasciculations, seizure and coma) are seen when the plasma sodium concentration exceeds 170 mmol/L. Again, the speed and severity of the sodium elevation are important. Patients tolerate gradual sodium elevations better because of idiogenic osmole generation within CNS cells. If the patient is concurrently hypovolemic, then hypotonic losses such as gastrointestinal, third space and renal losses are the most likely cause of the hypernatremia. Normovolemic hypernatremia is less common and results from pure water loss, including loss from body cavities during surgery or reduced water intake. Sodium gain can accompany primary hyperaldosteronism or administration of sodium bicarbonate, and is associated with hypervolemia. The underlying cause should be addressed. The rate of sodium reduction should not exceed 0.5–0.7 mmol/L/hour or cerebral edema can result. Any volume deficit should be replaced first using 0.9% saline because its sodium concentration (154 mmol/L) is usually less than that of the plasma in hypernatremic animals. Free water is then replaced with hypotonic crystalloids such as 0.45% saline over 2 to 4 days. Sodium gain can be treated with furosemide (1 mg/kg every 12 hours PO).

Hypocalcemia

Total serum calcium comprises protein bound, complexed and ionized (iCa) fractions which represent 40%, 8% and 52% of the total, respectively, in the cat.[8] Serum iCa, the physiologically active fraction, has numerous roles and is essential for normal neurological, muscular and gastrointestinal function. Close monitoring of calcium is indicated in a subset of postoperative patients at risk from hypocalcemia. Failure to preserve parathyroid function during thyroidectomy is a common cause of postoperative hypocalcemia. Less commonly, removal of a parathyroid hormone-related peptide-secreting tumor may reveal a parathyroid response blunted by chronic humoral hypercalcemia of malignancy (HHM). HHM is less common in the cat than the dog, but has been reported with lymphoma, squamous cell carcinoma, multiple myeloma, osteosarcoma, and thyroid and bronchogenic carcinoma.[9]

Other patients at risk of hypocalcemia include those undergoing parathyroidectomy (Chapter 56) (although primary hyperparathyroidism is rare in the cat), cesarian section, patients with urethral obstruction or urinary tract rupture, or any cat that becomes acutely ill. Following iatrogenic loss of parathyroid function, clinical signs can develop within 12 hours. Early signs are subtle, such as pawing or rubbing of the face and behavioral change. Weakness, muscle fasciculations, tetany and seizures can develop. A fall in total serum calcium below 1.5 mmol/L or iCa below 0.8 mmol/L can be associated with clinical signs. iCa should be monitored every six hours after surgery in patients at risk. If iCa measurement is not available, total serum calcium is used.

Formulae to correct total calcium values for hypoalbuminemia have not been validated in the cat. Adherence to the appropriate sample collection protocol, including anaerobic collection unless correction for an aerobic sample is to be made, is essential to avoid errors in iCa measurement. In cats with clinical signs, 1 mL/kg of 10% calcium gluconate can be given IV over ten to 20 minutes with electrocardiographic monitoring or constant auscultation. The infusion should be stopped if arrhythmias occur, or repeated if clinical signs persist. SC administration of 1 mL/kg 10% calcium gluconate, diluted 1:1 with 0.9% saline, can be given after IV supplementation or when mild hypocalcemia is detected in patients at risk with no clinical signs. Calcium chloride is irritant and not suitable for SC use. Calcium salts should not be mixed with bicarbonate-containing solutions (e.g. Hartmann solution) as precipitation can occur. In patients that develop hypocalcemia, oral supplementation with calcium (e.g., calcium carbonate 200 mg/cat/day divided and administered with food) and calcitriol, or a synthetic analog, is commenced and may be required

indefinitely. Calcitriol treatment can be initiated at 20–30 ng/kg/day for three to four days then gradually reduced.[10]

Hypophosphatemia

Phosphate is the major intracellular anion and is required for energy generation. Hypophosphatemia occurs with increased renal loss, decreased intestinal absorption or transcellular shifts. Intravascular hemolysis may occur when plasma phosphate falls below 0.5 mmol/L. Phosphate should be monitored in the postoperative patient at risk of diabetic ketoacidosis or re-feeding syndrome. Hypophosphatemia can be treated by supplementation of IV fluids with a 50:50 mixture of potassium chloride:potassium phosphate. Alternatively, 0.01–0.03 mmol/kg potassium phosphate can be given IV in 0.9% saline over six hours.

POSTOPERATIVE ANEMIA

Anemia is readily identified from daily hematocrit monitoring. Even where anemia is mild, consideration should be given to the cause/s in the assessment, and appropriate plans made. Cats are relatively predisposed to anemia compared with dogs because they have a lower blood volume (66 mL/kg compared to 90 mL/kg in the dog) and feline red blood cells have a shorter life span (approximately 70 days compared to 120 days in the dog). Clinical consequences of anemia include pale mucous membranes, weakness and, if severe, a hemic murmur. Anemia in the cat is often multifactorial. Major mechanisms in the surgical patient are hemorrhage and hemolysis and these should be ruled out first. In this acute setting, a reduced bone marrow response will not cause anemia, but can contribute to its degree and duration. Examination of a blood film can provide very useful information (Fig. 3-5). The absence of features of regeneration on a blood film (Fig. 3-6) should not be interpreted as necessarily indicating a non-regenerative cause as they take three to five days to appear. Anemia can be exacerbated by the dilutional effect of IV fluids.

Consideration should be given to potential causes and sites of occult hemorrhage. Disruption of tissue architecture with loss of vascular integrity (e.g., surgery-associated, ulceration, neoplasia, inflammatory disease) and coagulopathies should be considered. Inherited coagulopathies are uncommon in the cat, but postsurgical hemorrhage may be the first clinical manifestation of these disorders (Chapter 1). Excessive blood sampling and internal and external parasitism may also contribute. Major sites for occult hemorrhage are the peritoneal cavity, the pleural space, the gastrointestinal tract and the urinary tract. Black/brown vomit, resembling coffee grounds, or tarry feces suggest gastrointestinal hemorrhage. Pleural and peritoneal cavities can be rapidly screened for free fluid using ultrasonography, although hemorrhage can be reabsorbed rapidly. Reduced plasma TP increases suspicion of occult hemorrhage, especially where other causes of reduced protein are unlikely, but a normal value does not rule out hemorrhage.

The platelet count and morphology should be determined from a blood film. A simple platelet estimate can be performed by counting the number of platelets in a high-power, oil-immersion monolayer field. This is repeated ten times and average number/high-power field obtained. This figure is multiplied by 20 to give the number of platelets $\times 10^9$/L.[11] Automated counts should not be relied on in the cat because of the large size of feline platelets and their propensity to clump (Fig. 3-7). Where true thrombocytopenia is identified, consumption, destruction and sequestration should be considered. Reduced production of platelets in isolation is rare. Immune-mediated thrombocytopenia in cats is usually secondary to

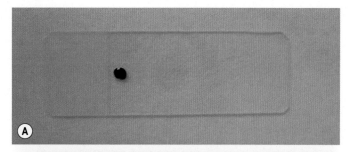

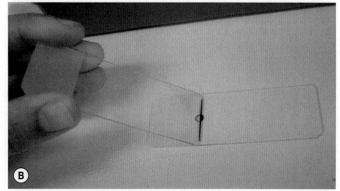

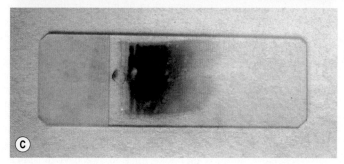

Figure 3-5 Preparation of a blood film. **(A)** A tiny drop of freshly collected EDTA blood is placed on a slide. **(B)** The angle of the second slide is adjusted so that the feathered edge of the film is well within the limit of the bottom slide **(C)**.

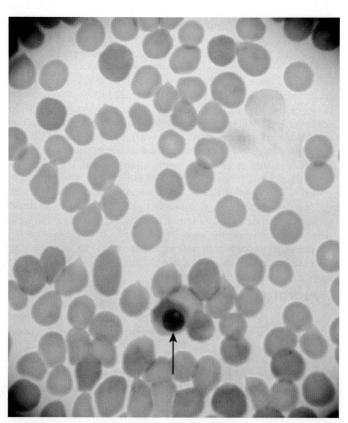

Figure 3-6 Features of erythrocyte regeneration on a blood film. Note anisocytosis (cells of unequal size) and a normoblast (arrow). Diff Quik, × 100, oil immersion.

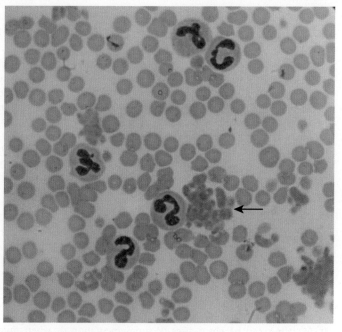

Figure 3-7 Platelet clumping on a blood film (arrow).

infection, neoplasia or drug administration (e.g., griseofulvin) and can occur concurrently with immune-mediated hemolytic anemia (IMHA).[12]

The absolute platelet count is useful to help determine if thrombocytopenia is a consequence or cause of hemorrhage; spontaneous bleeding occurs with platelet counts less than 50×10^9/L. A buccal mucosal bleeding time can assist in assessing for thrombocytopathies (Chapter 1). If a disorder of secondary hemostasis is suspected, the activated coagulation time (ACT) and activated partial thromboplastin time (aPTT) are useful screening tests. Samples for coagulation testing are collected into citrate using atraumatic jugular venipuncture to minimize tissue factor release, which can activate clotting factors and/or platelets. If prolonged, a coagulation profile, including prothrombin time, aPTT, thrombin time and fibrinogen can be submitted to characterize the defect (Box 3-4).

Inherited factor deficiencies VIII (hemophilia A), IX (hemophilia B), X, XI and fibrinogen, either alone or in combination, should be considered.[13,14] Even though hereditary deficiencies are uncommon, their first manifestation is often excessive bleeding after surgical intervention. Factor XII deficiency is associated with a prolonged aPTT but no bleeding tendency. Individual factor assays are required to diagnose these problems. A hereditary, vitamin K-responsive coagulopathy occurs in Devon Rex cats and an ACT or aPTT should be evaluated in

this breed prior to surgery. Acquired disorders of secondary hemostasis result from reduced absorption of vitamin K (hepatobiliary disease, gastrointestinal disease), reduced factor synthesis (hepatic disease) and loss or consumption of factors (hemorrhage, hypoproteinemia, disseminated intravascular coagulation [DIC]).[3,5]

Primary immune-mediated hemolytic anemia (IMHA) is less common in the cat than the dog. In the cat, IMHA can occur secondary to infection, neoplasia, inflammatory disease and certain drugs, including methimazole. Serology for FeLV and FIV PCR and PCR for occult *Mycoplasma haemofelis* may be indicated. A slide (in saline) agglutination test can be performed in-house (Fig. 3-8) and a direct Coombs test (at 4°C and 37°C) should be requested.[15]

Box 3-4 Coagulation testing

Activated coagulation time (ACT)

Useful for rapid in-house evaluation of the intrinsic and common pathways of coagulation. Reference ranges in cats vary depending on the type of activator used:

Becton Dickinson ACT tube 366522 (BD, Franklin Lakes, NJ, USA) contains inert siliceous earth to activate factor XII from 2 mL blood sample. Reference range 55 to 185 seconds.[25]

MAX-ACT tube (Helena Laboratories, Beaumont, TX, USA) containing celine, kaolin and glass beads to activate factor XII from 0.5 mL sample. Reference range 55 to 85 seconds.[26]

Prothrombin time (PT)

Identifies abnormalities in the extrinsic pathway (factor VII) and common pathways (fibrinogen, II, V and X). PT prolongation occurs in congenital and acquired vitamin K deficiency, hepatobiliary disease, specific factor deficiencies and DIC. In acquired vitamin K deficiency, the short half-life of factor VII means that PT may be prolonged while APTT is normal in early stage deficiency.

Activated partial thromboplastin time (aPTT)

Identifies abnormalities in the intrinsic (kininogen, prekallekrein, XII, XI, IX and VIII) and common pathways (fibrinogen, II, V and X). APTT prolongation occurs in later-stage vitamin K deficiency, liver disease, specific factor deficiencies and DIC.

Note: mild prolongation of the PT or APTT can occur with handling or analyzer error.

Thrombin time (TT)

TT is the time required for thrombin to convert fibrinogen to a fibrin clot. TT is inversely proportional to the fibrinogen concentration.

Fibrin/fibrinogen degradation products (FDP)

Plasmin cleaves fibrin/fibrinogen to yield FDPs. D-Dimers are produced from fibrin breakdown and their presence demonstrates that coagulation and fibrinolysis have been activated. Information on assays validated for feline samples is limited.

DISSEMINATED INTRAVASCULAR COAGULATION

Disseminated intravascular coagulation (DIC) occurs when a predisposing condition triggers widespread activation of the coagulation and fibrinolytic systems concurrently. Inhibitors of these systems are consumed and microthrombus formation causes end organ damage. Hemorrhage is less common in DIC in cats (5–15% of cases) than in dogs (26%). DIC in the cat has been associated with neoplasia, pancreatitis and infection, with or without sepsis, and it carries a poor prognosis, with only 7% of cats surviving in one study (16). Diagnosis requires three or more of the following coagulation abnormalities; prolonged prothrombin time (PT) or aPTT, elevated fibrin degradation products (FDP), thrombocytopenia, low fibrinogen concentration and identification of a predisposing condition.

A better understanding of coagulation abnormalities in the cat awaits the availability of robust assays validated for use in this species. Treatment of the underlying disease should be initiated. The efficacy of heparin to reduce thrombus formation is controversial, even in human medicine. Heparin should not be used in cats with evidence of hemorrhage. The appropriate dose of low molecular weight heparin in the cat is unknown and its effect cannot be monitored because anti-Xa activity assay is not routinely available. Unfractionated heparin at 200–250 IU/kg SC every six to eight hours, monitored with a daily coagulation panel, has been recommended.[17] Whole blood or, where available, component therapy may be indicated where there is hemorrhage (Chapter 5).

INFECTION

Factors which increase the risk for postoperative wound infection in small animals include age >8 years, clipping of surgical sites before anesthetic induction, duration of anesthesia >60 minutes, duration of surgery >90 minutes, use of the anesthetic agent propofol, intraoperative bacterial contamination of the wound (>10^5 organisms/g of tissue), local wound factors, and use of braided or multifilament suture material. Selection of therapeutic antimicrobials should be based on antimicrobial culture and susceptibility testing results. Pending results, factors that influence empiric choice include identifying the most likely genera of bacteria to be causing the infection in light of the clinical history, known bacterial resistance patterns for the suspected isolate, ability of the antimicrobial agent to penetrate into

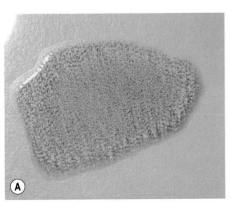
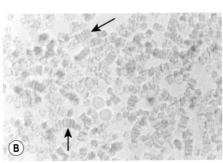
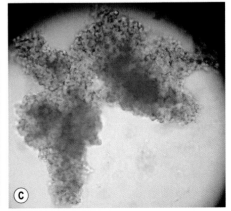

Figure 3-8 Slide (in saline) agglutination test. Light microscopy can be used to differentiate **(A)** macroscopic clumping of red cells due to **(B)** rouleaux formation (arrows) from **(C)** genuine agglutination.

the target tissue and toxicity of the drug.[18] Bactericidal drugs are preferred over bacteriostatic agents and only synergistic drug combinations should be used.

SHOCK

Shock is a clinical syndrome that occurs when the circulatory system fails to meet tissue needs. It is characterized by poor perfusion, hypotension and reduced tissue oxygenation. There are some major differences in presentation and management of shock in cats compared with dogs. Cats are often bradycardic and hypothermic, especially with septic shock, and balancing fluid resuscitation against the risk of fluid overload can be challenging. The major categories of shock are cardiogenic, hypovolemic and distributive (anaphylactic and septic) shock. Where shock develops in the postoperative period, septic or hypovolemic etiologies are most likely.

Systemic inflammatory response syndrome, sepsis and septic shock

Where infection, which is usually bacterial, is accompanied by a systemic inflammatory response syndrome (SIRS), the patient is said to be septic. SIRS is the clinical syndrome resulting from a systemic inflammatory response to an infectious or non-infectious (e.g., pancreatitis), process. It is distinct from, but can be accompanied by, bacteremia. Local inflammation at the site of infection can progress to become a systemic process where pro-inflammatory mediators, such as TNF-α and IL-6, predominate.[19] NF-kB plays a central role in the progression of inflammation in Gram negative sepsis. SIRS is associated with cardiovascular dysfunction, increased vascular permeability, aberrant coagulation and dysfunction of other organs including gastrointestinal, renal, hepatic, and respiratory systems. Severe sepsis can progress to septic shock, characterized by cardiovascular compromise, reduced effective circulating volume, inadequate tissue oxygenation, and organ dysfunction. Even in human medicine, consensus is evolving regarding the exact definitions of these terms which reflect, partly, that the pathogenesis of these syndromes is incompletely understood. Since far less is understood about SIRS and septic shock in cats, attempting firm definitions is less important than a broad grasp of the concepts required to recognize the unique clinical signs of sepsis in the cat and to institute appropriate treatment.

Clinical features of SIRS and sepsis in cats

Based on a study of 29 cats with sepsis, confirmed at necropsy, it has been proposed that a clinical diagnosis of SIRS can be made when cats fulfill three of the four objective criteria listed in Box 3-5.[20] Concurrent evidence of infection is required to make a diagnosis of sepsis. The cat is unusual in that bradycardia, a response that seems detrimental in a poorly perfused animal, is common in SIRS and septic shock. Bradycardia occurs independently of hypothermia and may be

relative; for example, a heart rate of 160 beats/minute is inappropriate for a hypotensive, hypoperfused animal. In contrast, in the dog tachycardia, fever and hyperemic mucous membranes are noted, at least in the initial, hyperdynamic phase of sepsis. Other physical findings in cats with sepsis include pale mucous membranes, weak pulses, hypotension, hypothermia, diffuse abdominal pain (unrelated to peritonitis) and tachypnea. When assessing perfusion, peripheral sites, such as the metatarsus, are more useful than femoral pulses because the former are lost first. Laboratory abnormalities in sepsis include hypoalbuminemia, hypoglycemia, icterus, anemia, thrombocytopenia, and neutrophilia with a left shift. Infections most often associated with sepsis in cats include pyothorax, pneumonia, peritonitis and bacteremia secondary to gastrointestinal disease (Figs 3-9 and 3-10).

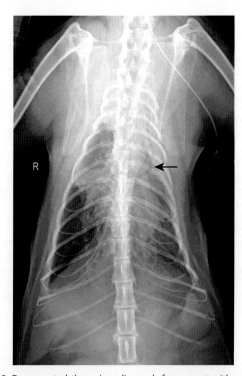

Figure 3-9 Dorsoventral thoracic radiograph from a cat with aspiration pneumonia. Changes include loss of aeration of the right middle and left cranial lung lobes and an air bronchogram (arrow). An absence of radiographic changes does not rule our pneumonia.

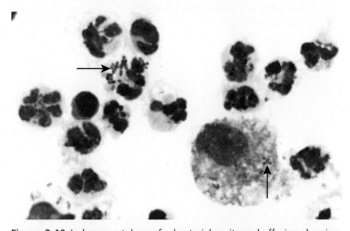

Figure 3-10 In-house cytology of a bacterial peritoneal effusion showing intracellular bacteria (arrows). Cytology is often diagnostic for septic effusions and should be performed while fluid analysis and culture are pending.

Box 3-5 **Objective criteria for SIRS**
Abnormal values are indicative of SIRS if cats have at least three abnormal parameters:[19]
Rectal temperature: >39.7 or <37.8°C (>103.5 or <100°F)
Heart rate: >225 bpm or <140 bpm
Respiratory rate: >40 breaths/minute
White cell count: >19.5 × 10^9 /L, or <5 × 10^9 /L, or bands >5%

Physical abnormalities in cats with peritonitis can be subtle; pain is often not a feature and an abdominal fluid wave can be difficult to appreciate in cats. Thoracic radiographs and abdominal ultrasonography are indicated where sepsis is suspected. Bacterial infection should be confirmed by culture of appropriate samples, such as blood, urine, pleural, peritoneal, or bronchoalveolar fluid.

Management considerations for the septic cat

Management can be considered in two parts: treating the infection and hemodynamic stabilization. Broad-spectrum, parenteral, preferably IV, bactericidal antibiotics should be used until the results of sensitivity testing are available to guide the choice of a reduced spectrum agent. *Escherichia coli* was the most common bacterial isolate in 12 septic cats, with beta-hemolytic *Streptococcus* spp and *Pseudomonas* spp also being detected.[20] However, in feline pyothorax specifically, *E. coli* is an uncommon isolate. Empirical therapy using penicillin G or an aminopenicillin, either alone, or in combination with metronidazole, or monotherapy with a potentiated penicillin, e.g., amoxicillin-clavulanic acid or ticarcillin-clavulanic acid, is recommended for pyothorax.[21] Other treatment for infection, such as drainage or debridement, may be indicated.

Fluid resuscitation should be initiated to address hypotension and poor perfusion. A bolus of 10–20 mL/kg of warmed, isotonic crystalloid can be given IV over ten to 20 minutes. This dose can be repeated, with the total dose not exceeding 50–60 mL/kg. Crystalloids distribute to all fluid compartments rapidly. Pulmonary edema and pleural effusion can result from relative fluid excess in the face of cardiovascular compromise, increased vascular permeability, and reduced plasma oncotic pressure. If perfusion does not improve after one to three crystalloid boluses, then one or two boluses of 2–3 mL/kg of colloid, e.g., hetastarch (hydroxyethyl starch, HES), can be given IV over 15–20 minutes. Warming can be initiated after the first bolus of fluids. Active warming without fluid replacement can cause peripheral vasodilation, further reducing effective circulating volume and making perfusion worse. Options include forced air temperature management units (Fig. 3-11), and circulating water blankets. Microwaveable heat pads and hot water bottles should be avoided as they can cause burns (Fig. 3-12). Also hot water bottles can promote cooling, as their temperature drops below that of the patient.

Monitoring of an individual's response guides ongoing treatment. Improved tissue oxygenation and cardiovascular function can be detected by serial monitoring of peripheral pulse quality, SBP, heart rate, rectal temperature, capillary refill time, mentation, and CVP where available. A continuous rectal temperature probe causes minimal disturbance to the patient. Serial lactate readings will fall as perfusion improves. Urine output should be closely monitored in a closed collection system or by weighing absorbent pads. Where SBP remains below 90 mmHg despite fluid resuscitation, inotropic support can be provided with a constant rate infusion (CRI) of dobutamine (1–5 µg/kg/minute). Cats being treated with dobutamine for more than 24 hours can develop seizures that cease on withdrawal of the medication. A dopamine CRI, (5 µg/kg/minute) has positive inotropic and chronotropic effects. At >10 µg/kg/minute, dopamine promotes vasoconstriction which may be counterproductive. Other vasopressors can be tried sequentially (noradrenaline CRI 0.1–3 µg/kg/minute; adrenaline 0.1–2 µg/kg/minute; vasopressin 0.5–2 mU/kg/minute).[22]

Other treatments include supplemental oxygen delivered by nasal catheter to improve tissue oxygenation. Hypoalbuminemia can affect plasma oncotic pressure, coagulation parameters, and wound healing. Plasma therapy, or colloid support, may be required. Hypoglycemia should be treated with an IV glucose bolus (1 mL/kg of a 20%

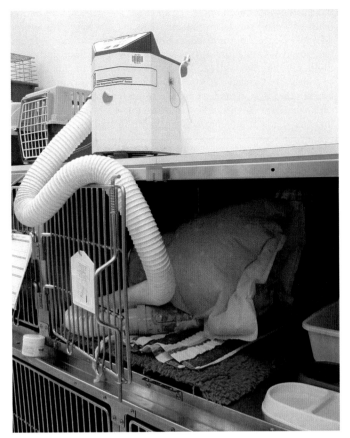

Figure 3-11 Active warming using a forced air temperature management unit (Bair Hugger).

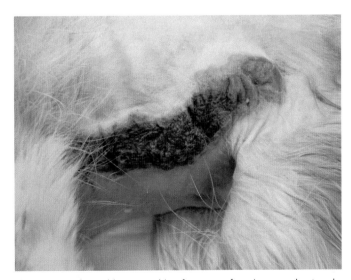

Figure 3-12 Thermal burns resulting from use of a microwave heat pad in a recumbent cat with poor mobility.

solution). If there is marked, sustained hyperglycemia, soluble insulin should be considered. Nutritional needs can be met with enteral or total parenteral nutritional support. Combined with gastrointestinal protectants, such as omeprazole and famotidine, this will help maintain gastrointestinal integrity, preventing bacterial translocation. Analgesia requirements should be considered, although monitoring analgesic effectiveness in a critical patient can be difficult. In anemic patients or those with abnormal coagulation parameters, whole blood transfusion may be indicated (Chapter 5). The plan should address management of wounds, urine and feces elimination, turning every two hours if sternal positioning cannot be maintained and intermittent positive stimulation, such as grooming, while maximizing opportunities for rest. Low-dose corticosteroid therapy for the management of critical illness-related corticosteroid insufficiency is controversial.[23] Where other treatments have failed, 0.5 mg/kg prednisolone sodium succinate IV can be considered. Research into specific therapies targeting endotoxins or inflammatory mediators is ongoing.[19,24]

Other types of shock

Hypovolemic shock follows major hemorrhage, gastrointestinal losses, or third space losses. Clinical signs are referable to poor perfusion and tachycardia or bradycardia may be present. The diagnosis can usually be made on the basis of history and clinical findings.

Treatment involves restoring circulating volume and improving perfusion, as above. Where hemorrhage is the cause, then rapid infusion of whole blood is ideal.

Cardiogenic shock occurs when the cardiac output is not maintained because of systolic or diastolic dysfunction or obstruction (e.g., aortic thromboembolism). The spectrum of cardiac diseases affecting cats is different to that seen in dogs. In cats, systolic dysfunction is less common and pericardial effusion is rare and does not typically cause tamponade. In addition to poor perfusion, there may be clinical signs referable to a cardiac problem such as an arrhythmia, murmur, gallop or pulse deficits, and/or to congestive heart failure (e.g., pulmonary edema, pleural effusion). It can sometimes be difficult to know whether bradycardia (or tachycardia) in a poorly perfused cat is a cause or consequence of shock. Echocardiography is the most useful diagnostic tool here. Treatment will depend on the underlying problem, but fluids are contraindicated in cardiogenic shock.

REFERENCES

1. Wellman M, Dibartola S, Kohn C. Applied physiology of body fluid in dogs and cats. In: Fluid, electrolyte, and acid-base disorders in small animal practice. 3rd ed. St. Louis, Mo: Saunders Elsevier; 2006. p. 3–26.

2. Paige CF, Abbott JA, Elvinger F, Pyle RL. Prevalence of cardiomyopathy in apparently healthy cats. J Am Vet Med Assoc 2009;234:1398–403.

3. Kudnig ST, Mama K. Guidelines for perioperative fluid therapy. Compend Contin Educ Vet 2003;25:102–11.

4. Ishihara H, Ishida K, Oyama T, et al. Effects of general anaesthesia and surgery on renal function and plasma ADH levels. Can Anaesth Soc J 1978;25:312–18.

5. Kruegener GH, Kerin MJ, MacFie J. Post-operative fluid therapy–put not thy faith in dextrose saline: discussion paper. J R Soc Med 1991;84:611–12.

6. Ash RA, Harvey AM, Tasker S. Primary hyperaldosteronism in the cat: a series of 13 cases. J Feline Med Surg 2005;7:173–82.

7. Martin LG, Veatch AE. Electrolyte disorders. In: Drobatz KJ, Costello M, editors. Feline emergency and critical care medicine. 2010. p. 439–65.

8. Schenck P, Chew D, Behrend E. Updates on hypercalcemic disorders. In: August JR, editor. Consultations in feline internal medicine, vol. 5. St Louis: Saunders; 2006. p. 157–68.

9. Savary KC, Price GS, Vaden SL. Hypercalcemia in cats: A retrospective study of 71 cases (1991–1997). J Vet Intern Med 2000;14:184–9.

10. Chew DJ, Nagode LA: Treatment of hypoparathyroidism. In: Bonagura JD, editor. Kirk's current veterinary therapy: Small animal practice XIII. Philadelphia: WB Saunders Co; 2000. p. 340–5.

11. Séverine T, Cripps PJ, Mackin AJ. Estimation of platelet counts on feline blood smears, Vet Clin Pathol 1999;28:42–5.

12. Wondratschek C, Weingart C, Kohn B. Primary immune-mediated thrombocytopenia in cats. J Am Anim Hosp Assoc 2010;46:12–19.

13. Baldwin CJ, Cowell RL. Inherited coagulopathies. In: August JR, editor. Consultations in feline internal medicine, vol. 3. 1997. p. 488–98.

14. Gookin JL, Brooks MB, Catalfamo JL, et al. Factor X deficiency in a cat. J Am Vet Med Assoc 1997;211:576–9.

15. Tasker S, Murray JK, Knowles TG, Day MJ. Coombs', haemoplasma and retrovirus testing in feline anemia. J Small Anim Pract 2010;51:192–9.

16. Estrin MA, Wehausen CE, Jessen CR, Lee JA. Disseminated intravascular coagulation in cats. J Vet Intern Med 2006;20:1334–9.

17. Estrin MA, Spangler EA. Disseminated intravascular coagulation. In: August JR, editor. Consultations in feline internal medicine. Chapter 62, Volume 6. Elsevier Saunders; 2010. p. 639–51.

18. Boothe DM. Principles of antimicrobial therapy. Vet Clin Small Anim 2006;36:1003–47.

19. DeClue AE, Williams KJ, Sharp C, et al. Systemic response to low-dose endotoxin infusion in cats. Vet Immunol Immunopathol 2009;132:167–74.

20. Brady CA, Otto CM, Van Winkle TJ, King LG. Severe sepsis in cats: 29 cases (1986-1998). J Am Vet Med Assoc 2000;217:531–5.

21. Barrs VR, Beatty JA. Feline pyothorax – new insights into an old problem: Part II. Treatment recommendations and prophylaxis. The Vet J 2009;179:171–8.

22. Costello M. Shock. In: Drobatz KJ, Costello M, editors. Feline emergency and critical care medicine. 2010. p. 23–9.

23. Marik PE, Pastores SM, Annane D, et al. Recommendations for the diagnosis and management of corticosteroid insufficiency in critically ill adult patients: consensus statements from an international task force by the American College of Critical Care Medicine. Crit Care Med 2008;36:1937–49.

24. Sharp CR, DeClue AE, Haak CE, et al. Evaluation of the anti-endotoxin effects of polymyxin B in a feline model of endotoxemia. J Feline Med Surg 2010;12:278–85.

25. Bay JD, Scott MA, Hans JE. Reference values for activated coagulation time in cats. Am J Vet Res 2000;61:750–3.

26. See AM, Swindells KL Sharman MJ, et al. Activated coagulation times in normal cats and dogs using MAX-ACTTM tubes. Aust Vet J 2009;87:292–5.

Chapter | 4 |

Postoperative nursing care

S. Rudd, J.L. Demetriou, S.J. Langley-Hobbs

Nursing care is defined by the American Association of Feline Medicine (AAFM) and the International Society of Feline Medicine (ISFM) as any interaction between the cat and the veterinary team (veterinarian, technician or nurse, receptionist or support staff) in the clinic, or between the cat and its owner at home, that promotes wellness or recovery from illness or injury and addresses the patient's physical and emotional well-being.[1] Nursing care also helps the sick or convalescing cat engage in activities that it would be unable to perform without help. To provide optimal support to a sick, injured or recovering cat, the art of nursing care is as important as the medical science.[1]

The postoperative care of a cat should not be neglected; attention to this aspect of the cat's treatment can make a big difference to the nature of the recovery and well-being of the patient. In some cases the provision and quality of postoperative care can mean the difference between a successful and unsuccessful outcome. This chapter will focus on the provision of nursing care for the postoperative period up until and including discharge of the recovering cat to the owner (for other aspects of postoperative management and monitoring see Chapter 3). Short sections are included on the pertinent points on provision of nursing care of cats, which have undergone skin and adnexal surgery, abdominal surgery, thoracic surgery, and head surgery.

RECOVERY FROM ANESTHESIA

The recovery period can be the most critical stage of anesthesia for a cat. Current estimates indicate that approximately 0.11% (1 in 895 anesthetics) of healthy cats die of an anesthetic-related death, which is more than twice as frequent as has been recently reported in dogs (0.05% or 1 in 1849). Most of these deaths occur in the postoperative period.[2] Greater attention to patient monitoring during and after anesthesia could reduce perioperative complications in cats;[2] the recovery area should be appropriately equipped and have trained personnel monitoring recovery of patients after anesthesia and surgery.

Emergency anesthesia equipment

It may be necessary or advisable to continue to administer oxygen to the postoperative cat and re-intubation is occasionally required in a cat that is having severe breathing difficulties or in one that undergoes cardiac arrest and requires resuscitation. It is therefore essential that there is easy access to anesthetic equipment in the recovery area.

An anesthetic machine with an Ayres T-piece should be readily accessible. A range of different-sized face masks should also be available. Clear Perspex masks are usually tolerated better by cats than opaque ones such as black rubber ones. Many cats, however, will not tolerate a mask and an oxygen tent may be preferred. Oxygen tents are available commercially or they can be made by covering the front of a kennel with a polymethyl methacrylate sheet (e.g., Perspex) or plastic such as food wrap.

In the event of the cat requiring re-intubation, laryngoscope blades of a suitable small size and a range of endotracheal tubes (both cuffed and uncuffed) are required. A cuffed endotracheal tube is essential for intermittent positive pressure ventilation (IPPV). Even when intubating a cat in an emergency, local anesthetic should still be applied to the larynx to avoid laryngospasm. In anticipation of a difficult intubation, a 6FG dog urinary catheter should be included in the emergency box. This can either be used as a guide for insertion of the endotracheal tube or used alone to intubate the cat if it is not possible to insert anything larger in diameter. A 3.5 mm blue Portex tube connector can be placed on the end to allow connection to an anesthetic circuit so oxygen can be given as a temporary measure until the airway is established further. For resuscitation, when oxygen and an Ayres T-piece are not available, an Ambu bag can be used. Pediatric or neonatal Ambu bags (small sizes suitable for cats) can be connected to oxygen and as they are self-filling and have no valve to turn, they may even be more advantageous than an Ayres T-piece in an emergency.

Obstruction of the airway due to fluid or mucus is a common cause of acute hypoxia during the recovery phase.[3] If obstruction is suspected the airway should be carefully aspirated. A suction device is an essential piece of equipment for the ICU. In cases where an airway cannot be established, due to an obstruction for example, an emergency tracheostomy may need to be performed (Chapter 46). Alternatively,

© 2014 Elsevier Ltd
DOI: 10.1016/B978-0-7020-4336-9.00004-4

a large gauge needle can be inserted directly into the trachea to allow immediate oxygenation until a tracheotomy can be performed.

Emergency box

A fully stocked emergency box should be kept in the recovery area. This should be checked weekly and replenished after every use. It is important to ensure all members of staff know where the emergency box is kept and that it is kept within easy access. The contents of the box should be set out clearly and the box should not be overcrowded with drugs and equipment, so that anyone using it can locate what they need quickly and efficiently. To avoid overloading the general emergency box, it can be helpful to have smaller kits for specific procedures made up ready for use, for example for thoracocentesis (Chapter 41) or tracheotomy (Chapter 46). To minimize preparation time, commonly used emergency drugs e.g., adrenaline (epinephrine) and atropine, can be kept drawn up in syringes ready for immediate use. However, this is not appropriate for all emergency drugs, as not all drugs contain preservatives and so will lose effectiveness once the vial is opened. It is therefore important that expiry dates are checked and adhered to. Having some syringes with suitable sized needles already attached in the emergency box can save time when drawing up drugs. An easy-to-follow emergency 'drugs and dosage' chart is also invaluable to ensure there is minimal delay in administering the correct drug and dose in an emergency situation.

Essential recommended items for a feline emergency box are listed (Table 4-1).

Personnel

As well as ensuring all emergency equipment is available, it is equally important to make sure that all the staff involved in postoperative care are aware of what action to take in an emergency situation. Regular staff refreshment training should be scheduled to ensure a smooth, fast and effective operation for times of real emergency.

PRINCIPLES OF POSTOPERATIVE NURSING CARE

Thorough and attentive patient assessment and monitoring with effective communication of the findings can facilitate excellent patient care and an optimal recovery (Fig. 4-1). After any surgery the cat should be assessed for certain signs, parameters, behavior and functions (Box 4-1), the relevance and importance of each being dependent on the surgery performed.

Basic parameters

In the immediate postoperative stage the cat's temperature, pulse, mucous membrane color, capillary refill time, and respiration should be monitored at least hourly, reducing down gradually to every four hours and then twice daily if the patient is stable. Patients with abnormal parameters or unstable patients will need to be monitored more frequently or constantly when critically ill or after extensive surgery.

A cat's vital signs should be interpreted in conjunction with environmental factors and the temperament of the individual cat. The presence of pain can result in elevations in pulse and temperature. The significance of a high pulse count and respiratory rate should be evaluated along with the cat's other parameters (temperature, pulse quality, mucous membrane color, capillary refill time, respiratory pattern etc.), as well as assessing if the cat is stressed or fearful (Chapter 7). Stress and fear will give falsely high pulse and respiration rates so

Table 4-1 Essential recommended items for a feline emergency box

	Cat crash kit stock contents
Drugs	10 × Adrenaline 1:1000 vials (2 × 1 mL drawn up ready for use) 10 × Atropine vials (2 × 1 mL drawn up ready for use) 5 × Terbutaline vials 3 × Lidocaine 2% vials 3 × Lidocaine 1% vials 2 × Potassium chloride 1.5 g in 10 mL vials 1 × bottle Dopram 1 × bottle Propofol 1 × bottle local anesthetic spray
Consumables	10 × 1 mL, 2 mL, 5 mL, 10 mL and 20 mL syringes 10 × 25G, 23G and 21G × ⅝" needles 4 × 21G × 1.5" needles 5 × 22G and 24G IV catheters Tape – Durapore (3M) 4 × T-Ports 4 × bungs 2 × 3-way taps 1 × 500 mL Hartmanns 1 × extension set 1 × giving set 1 × white open weave (WOW) bandage 1 × Soffban (Smith and Nephew) 1 × Co-flex (Andover Healthcare Group) Gauze swabs Surgical spirit 2 × size 11 scalpel blades 1 × 6FG dog urinary catheter
Other	Laryngoscope Endotracheal tubes – size 3, 3.5, 4, 4.5, 5, 5.5 cuffed and uncuffed 1 × cuff inflator 1 × 3.5 mm endotracheal tube connector Stethoscope Ambu bag Quick reference drug dosage chart

Box 4-1 Basic parameters to measure or monitor postoperatively in the feline surgical patient

Vital signs: temperature, pulse, respiration and mucous membranes
Pain
Appetite and hydration
Weight
Urination/defecation
Infection
Movement/well-being

it is important that the cat's environment should be evaluated to determine, for example, whether the proximity of a dog or another cat is causing these elevations.

Once the cat has recovered from anesthesia, the frequency of monitoring and which vital signs are important to monitor will depend on the surgery that has been performed, how well the cat recovered from the procedure, how it is progressing clinically and how tolerant the patient is (Chapter 7).

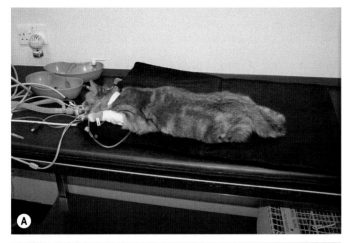

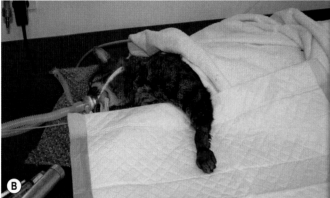

Figure 4-1 Heat loss should be minimized during anesthesia. **(A)** The cat is on a heat pad in the operating theatre. **(B)** This cat is being kept warm in the radiology room by use of bubble wrap and a towel.

Temperature

A low body temperature may both increase the chance of postoperative infection through immune function suppression and delay recovery from anesthesia. Most postoperative cats will be hypothermic to a degree, and therefore it is of utmost importance to monitor the temperature during the recovery phase and quickly implement methods of restoring normothermia before further temperature reductions occur. To prevent or minimize postoperative hypothermia in the recovery room provision should be made first to keep cats warm while under anesthesia (Fig. 4-1). Cats in the recovery area can then be warmed by warm air blankets (Bair Huggers), a warming mat, bubble wrap, blankets, warm gloves, warm bean or rice bags.

While being warmed the cat's temperature should be monitored regularly to avoid hyperthermia. In addition to excessive warming, hyperthermia in cats in the postoperative phase is also seen with opioid administration, including hydromorphone, morphine, butorphanol and buprenorphine.[4] The increase of temperature seen is usually mild to moderate (<40.1°C [104.2°F]) and self-limiting.[4] If the cat is hyperthermic due to overheating, infection or opioid administration and this is of concern, the cat should be judiciously cooled by removing all warming aids in the first instance. If hyperthermia still does not resolve then other methods of cooling can be considered such as the use of fans, or the application of surgical spirit to the foot pads in combination with continued temperature monitoring. Reversal of the opioid can be achieved by administering naloxone, but this will also remove the analgesic effect of the drug, so alternative pain therapy will be required.

Box 4-2 **Behavioral and physical signs that may be exhibited in painful and fearful cats**

Quiet and withdrawn
Tense and hunched posture – body low to the ground, limbs tightly kept towards the body, often pressed up against the back of the kennel or in their litter tray
An unwillingness to interact with people
Eyelids pointing down (like the cat is frowning)
Dilated pupils
Ear position starting to turn then flatten
Whiskers flattening then coming forward immediately before aggression
Trembling
Tachypnea
Hypersalivation
Hissing
Vocalizing
Aggression
Tachycardia
Anorexia
Reduced urine and fecal output
Reduced/no self-grooming

Cats that have undergone colonic, rectal, perineal, or urethral surgery should not have their rectal temperature recorded in the first stages of postoperative recovery unless absolutely necessary. Skin and ear thermometers and identichips with thermal indicators have been shown to be variable in their accuracy, but these methods may still be useful in cats who do not need such accurate temperature recording or where rectal thermometers are not advised or not tolerated.

Pain recognition

The assessment of pain is an essential skill that should be acquired by all personnel involved with the postoperative recovery of cats. Recognition of pain in cats is challenging as the signs are often more subtle than in dogs.[5] Cats show mainly postural signs, without vocalization.[6]

To make things even more difficult, many of the signs of pain that cats show are also displayed when they are fearful and so it can be very challenging to differentiate between the two (Box 4-2). An initial assessment should begin by observing the cat in its cage from a distance. Cats that are happy and pain free will be alert, responsive and move freely around the cage with no signs of distress. Cats that are in pain will be quiet and withdrawn and may well be hunched up at the back of their cage. They will not usually move around freely or respond when called or spoken to. The environment should also be taken into consideration; if the cat is in a ward with barking dogs or if the cat has a nervous disposition it may display similar signs to that of a cat in pain. After the initial assessment of observing the patient from a distance has been completed, the cage door can then be opened. The cat can be talked to and gently stroked. Pain-free cats tend to respond well to this interaction. Some cats will get up and approach the assessor and even nervous cats will sometimes raise their hind quarters when being tickled at the base of their tail. Very fearful cats may growl or show aggression and not allow any physical contact, but this behavior is not necessarily related to pain. The area peripheral to but in close vicinity to the surgical site, should then be gently palpated. In any assessment of pain mere observation is insufficient and interactive means such as palpation must also be used.[7] Changes in wound sensitivity have correlated well with visual analog pain scores in cats, suggesting that palpation, which is a simple clinically applicable technique, is a valuable tool and should be incorporated into an overall assessment protocol.[8] A painful cat will become tense, look uncomfortable and may flinch or vocalize during palpation. Some cats will also hypersalivate in response to pain. If these signs are shown palpation should be stopped immediately until more analgesia has been administered.

Purring is thought to be always associated with cats being happy but in some circumstances cats that are really sick will still purr. Most commonly, however, cats that are in pain will not purr and if stroked they may squint or flinch.

Isolated physiological measures such as heart rate, respiratory rate, and rectal temperature are generally poor indicators of postoperative pain in cats.[5,9] However, these parameters should not be ignored but monitored in conjunction with pain scoring because in some painful cats the respiratory rate, pulse, and temperature may increase; measurements should be made every four to 12 hours, the frequency being dependent on the patient's temperament, type of surgery, recovery and progress.

Reducing fear in hospitalized cats will help to eliminate fear behavior and therefore make pain assessment more accurate as both share common features. There should be an understanding of the signs of fear behavior (Box 4-2). Additionally, there should be a general expectation on the degree of pain anticipated depending on the cat's history and on what surgical procedure has been performed. It should be assumed, however, that all cats that have undergone any type of surgery need some form of analgesia so it is important that this aspect is not overlooked, particularly in fearful cats. If it is uncertain whether a cat is painful it is better to provide some analgesia and then reassess the patient once that has had a chance to take effect rather than potentially leave a painful cat with no or inappropriate analgesia. Excitement can occur after opioid administration in some cats and it is important to appreciate the signs of this, which include dilated pupils (Fig. 4-2) and dysphoria, so this is not misinterpreted as pain.

Simple descriptive (SDS) and numerical rating scales (NRS) and visual analog scales (VAS) have all been used in cats to quantify pain.[9,10] Recent research has been concerned with how to assess pain more accurately in cats, including assessing posture and facial expressions (Fig. 4-3). Colorado State University has a feline acute pain scale for use in cats which encompasses psychological and behavioral elements, response to wound palpation and body tension and this can be downloaded (Fig. 4-4).[11]

Movement and well-being

As soon as it is safe to do so after surgery the cat should be encouraged to move. Physiotherapy is often indicated and the potential benefits include an increase in blood flow to the surgical site and an improvement of muscle tone, which in turn should enable and encourage movement. In cases of nerve damage, physiotherapy is very useful in nerve stimulation, encouraging neural regeneration and the return of sensation.

The benefit and need for physiotherapy will depend on the type of surgery the cat has undergone and whether it has any pre-existing conditions such as osteoarthritis which may slow down recovery, for example after amputation. A full description of rehabilitation of the cat and the modalities that can be used is given in Chapter 21 of *Feline Orthopedic surgery and Musculoskeletal Disease*.[12] Physiotherapeutic manipulation should be initially performed over a short time period with a gradual increase in duration over time, depending partly on how well the cat is tolerating the treatment and the response to the therapy. It is vital that the cat has sufficient analgesia when starting physiotherapy because initially manipulation can be painful and inadequate analgesia could cause the cat to develop aversion to future treatments.

Cats that are hospitalized will not be able to carry out normal feline behavior. An important aspect that is often overlooked is that they will be unable to move around freely as they would do at home, which could cause adverse physical effects such as muscle atrophy, gut stasis and also may result in a depressed mental state. In particular, a cat that has to wear a rigid Elizabethan collar will be unable to groom and sometimes have difficulty in eating and drinking. All cats should be given a 'time out' period each day, whether this is by removing the Elizabethan collar to allow grooming, letting the cat out of the cage so it can stretch (Fig. 4-5) or taking it out in a carrier to allow the cat to get some fresh air. This will not only provide great stimulation but may aid in a quicker recovery. All time out periods should be observed, especially when a surgical site is being left without protection of an Elizabethan collar. Soft Elizabethan collars are better suited for cats as they can adopt normal sleeping positions and reach their food and water bowls more easily (Fig. 4-6). However, these collars are not suitable for all cats as some may be able to reach around the collar to the surgical site.

NURSING CARE AFTER SKIN AND ADNEXAL SURGERY

Cats that have had large tumor excisions, wound closure, and skin grafts will often be painful after surgery. This should be anticipated early so the cat is given pre-emptive analgesia[13] and a plan should be in place, with drug doses and frequency of administration, in case there is additional unexpected pain and excitement on recovery. Recovery excitement could result in premature bandage removal or wound breakdown if this is not anticipated and dealt with. Analgesic considerations would generally be multimodal and include local blocks, constant rate infusions, and wound infusion catheters (see Chapters 2 and 11).

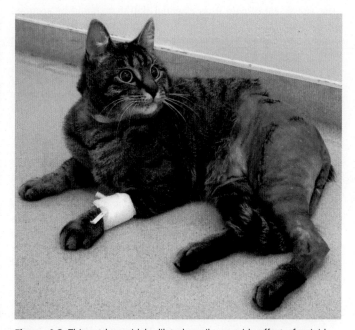

Figure 4-2 This cat has widely dilated pupils as a side effect of opioid administration. Methadone was stopped and the cat given the partial agonist buprenorphine and the side effects abated.

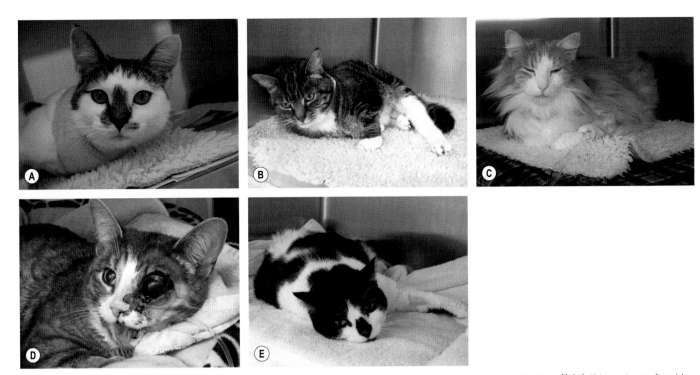

Figure 4-3 Cats exhibiting different degrees of pain, scored according to the Colorado State University Acute Pain Score.[11] **(A)** This cat is comfortable and interested in its surroundings and was not bothered by wound palpation (pain score =0). **(B)** This cat is slightly unsettled in the hospital and less interested in its surroundings, mild or no reaction to palpation of incision (pain score = 1). **(C)** This cat is quiet, lays curled up, tail tucked in and eyes partially closed, decreased appetite – untouched food can be seen near the cat that is reluctant to move around its cage (pain score = 2). **(D)** This cat was yowling when unattended. It was very reluctant to move and responded to palpation around its proptosed eye (pain score = 3). **(E)** This cat is recumbent and unresponsive of its surroundings. The cat's response to palpation was to tense up (pain score = 4).

Bandages and dressings

Cats can be very adept and determined to remove even the most carefully placed bandage. It is therefore important that the cat is adequately supervised on recovery ensuring it remains comfortable (Fig. 4-7) and relaxed and that the cat is not given the opportunity to interfere with external coaptation. Bandages should be regularly monitored to ensure that they are not too tight and that they remain dry. If there is strike through of wound discharge or the dressing becomes soiled or wet, then the dressing should be removed and replaced as necessary. If the cat seems unduly distressed, is biting or scratching at the bandage and seems determined to remove it then the necessity for the bandage should be reassessed as there may be a better option than bandaging that is equally effective and more comfortable for the cat. It is important to differentiate between a cat that is in pain and a cat that is determined to remove its bandage. Bandages alone cause stress, a 200% increase in urine cortisol was recorded in a study on onchyectomy in cats.[14] If the digits appear swollen or cold then the bandage should be removed immediately and replaced as necessary (Fig. 4-8). It is not an uncommon occurrence for a bandage that is too tight to rapidly lead to ischemia of the distal limb (which effectively acts as a tourniquet) causing pressure sores and necessitating intensive and often prolonged wound management (Fig. 4-9) or in the worst instance, if the damage is severe, amputation.[15]

Incisions and wounds

Wounds and incisions should be inspected twice a day unless covered with a dressing or bandage. The wound should be assessed firstly visually and then, if appropriate, gently palpated with gloved hands.

If the wound is infected it will be painful, swollen, hot and it may also secrete discharge. It is important to note color, consistency and smell of any discharge seen and a sample should be taken from the wound (after flushing with sterile isotonic saline solution), which can then be sent for Gram stain and culture to identify the organism(s) responsible and determine the appropriate antibiotic sensitivity (see Chapter 18).

Drains

Open and closed suction drains may be placed after tumor resections, wound or abscess debridement or in other instances of skin and adnexal surgery where the surgeon anticipates the formation of excess fluid postoperatively. The management of these drains is discussed in Chapter 11.

NURSING CARE AFTER THORACIC SURGERY

Cats that have undergone thoracic surgery (see Chapters 41 to 48) will need very close monitoring during the recovery and in the early postoperative stage. Basic parameters (temperature, pulse, respiration) should be monitored regularly initially, with particular attention to the cat's respiratory rate, pattern, SpO_2 levels and pain. After extubation the cat should be placed in an oxygen enriched environment such as an oxygen tent, or in an incubator with piped oxygen if the cat is also hypothermic. The cat will initially need constant monitoring after thoracic surgery. The basic considerations for postoperative nursing care of cats after thoracic surgery are listed in Box 4-3.

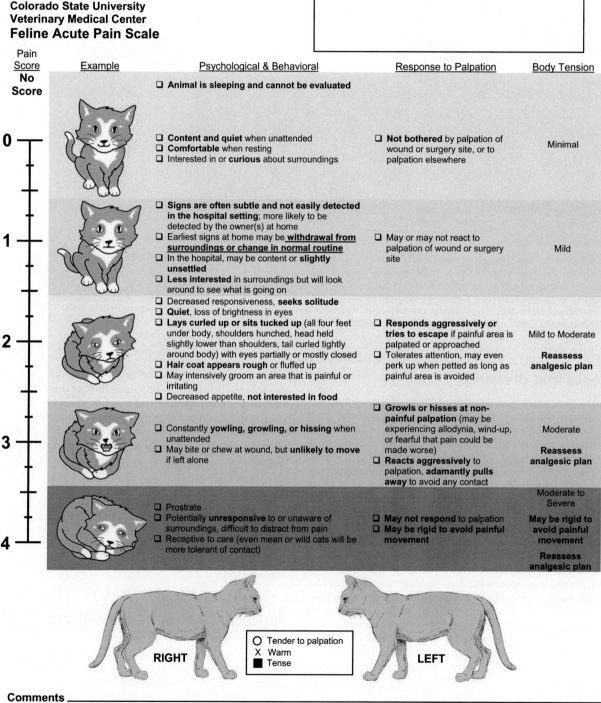

Colorado State University
Veterinary Medical Center
Feline Acute Pain Scale

Pain Score	Example	Psychological & Behavioral	Response to Palpation	Body Tension
No Score		☐ Animal is sleeping and cannot be evaluated		
0		☐ **Content and quiet** when unattended ☐ **Comfortable** when resting ☐ Interested in or **curious** about surroundings	☐ **Not bothered** by palpation of wound or surgery site, or to palpation elsewhere	Minimal
1		☐ **Signs are often subtle and not easily detected in the hospital setting**; more likely to be detected by the owner(s) at home ☐ Earliest signs at home may be **withdrawal from surroundings or change in normal routine** ☐ In the hospital, may be content or **slightly unsettled** ☐ **Less interested** in surroundings but will look around to see what is going on	☐ May or may not react to palpation of wound or surgery site	Mild
2		☐ Decreased responsiveness, **seeks solitude** ☐ **Quiet**, loss of brightness in eyes ☐ **Lays curled up or sits tucked up** (all four feet under body, shoulders hunched, head held slightly lower than shoulders, tail curled tightly around body) with eyes partially or mostly closed ☐ **Hair coat appears rough** or fluffed up ☐ May intensively groom an area that is painful or irritating ☐ Decreased appetite, **not interested in food**	☐ **Responds aggressively or tries to escape** if painful area is palpated or approached ☐ Tolerates attention, may even perk up when petted as long as painful area is avoided	Mild to Moderate **Reassess analgesic plan**
3		☐ Constantly **yowling, growling, or hissing** when unattended ☐ May bite or chew at wound, but **unlikely to move** if left alone	☐ **Growls or hisses at non-painful palpation** (may be experiencing allodynia, wind-up, or fearful that pain could be made worse) ☐ **Reacts aggressively** to palpation, **adamantly pulls away** to avoid any contact	Moderate **Reassess analgesic plan**
4		☐ Prostrate ☐ Potentially **unresponsive** to or unaware of surroundings, difficult to distract from pain ☐ Receptive to care (even mean or wild cats will be more tolerant of contact)	☐ **May not respond** to palpation ☐ **May be rigid to avoid painful movement**	Moderate to Severe **May be rigid to avoid painful movement** **Reassess analgesic plan**

RIGHT   LEFT

○ Tender to palpation
X Warm
■ Tense

Comments _____

© 2006/PW Hellyer, SR Uhrig, NG Robinson

Figure 4-4 Colorado Acute Pain Score sheet. *(Reproduced with kind permission of Peter W Hellyer, Colorado State University.)*

Management of the thoracic drain

Chest drains are managed by placing a small dry adhesive dressing at the entry site into the thorax to protect the insertion site from infection and to absorb any serous discharge, which may be produced in the first 24–48 hours (Fig. 4-10). To prevent patient interference and to support the weight of the chest drain an elasticated string vest (Surgifix, FRA Production S.p.A) can be used. These dressings are very useful to cover any thoracic or abdominal tubes; however, a large enough size (size 6) should be used to ensure that the elastic does not compress the thorax or abdomen. Holes need to be made in the vest to place the limbs through and these holes should be large enough so that the elastic does not cut into the axillary area of the limbs. The use of a soft Elizabethan collar is also advisable to ensure the patient does not lick at the site or bite the tube. The tube insertion site should be undressed, checked and cleansed with a dilute chlorhexidine solution and redressed every 12–24 hours. Gloves must be worn when examining and cleaning any wounds both from the drain and the

thoracic surgical incision, to reduce the chance of iatrogenic infection. If either wound begins to look inflamed or is producing any purulent discharge the site should be swabbed and sent for culture and the cat monitored carefully for development of sepsis (see Chapter 2). For information on wounds and dressing materials see Chapter 18. After drain removal the stoma is covered with a small sterile dressing and the site is left to heal by secondary intention.

NURSING CARE AFTER ABDOMINAL SURGERY

Nursing care after abdominal surgery will consist of regular monitoring of basic parameters including pulse, temperature, respiration, pain, and urine and fecal production (Fig. 4-12). Monitoring peripheral pulse quality, respiration, mucous membrane color and particularly temperature is essential in detecting the first signs of any postoperative complications such as hemorrhage, shock or peritonitis (see Chapter 26). The basic considerations for postoperative nursing care of cats after abdominal surgery are listed in Box 4-4. Cats with

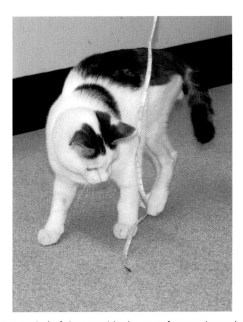

Figure 4-5 A period of time outside the cage for exercise and play can be very beneficial to the cat's recovery and demeanour.

Box 4-3 **Postoperative nursing care considerations after thoracic surgery**

Oxygen: All patients having thoracic surgery will benefit from oxygen supplementation in recovery

Monitoring: Cardiovascular parameters should be closely monitored via respiratory rate and effort, capnography, pulse oximetry and electrocardiography

Analgesia: A multimodal approach using systemic opioids, intrapleural block with local anesthetic agents, non-steroidal anti-inflammatories (unless contraindicated). The cat should be regularly reassessed for the presence of pain and analgesia continued for as long a period as necessary (see Chapters 2 and 41)

Thoracostomy drain: A plan with timing intervals for thoracostomy tube drainage should be put in place (see Chapter 41). The drain should be protected from patient interference by use of bandaging and a buster collar

Nutrition: Cats should be encouraged to eat once recovered from anesthesia and there is no risk of aspiration (see Chapter 6)

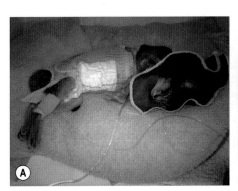
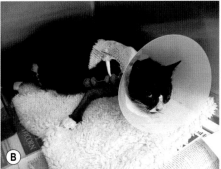
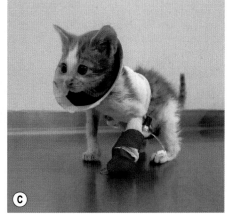

Figure 4-6 **(A)** A cat with a soft Elizabethan collar to prevent interference with its drain, catheters and surgical site. An elasticated string vest has been fitted to hold the drain against the cat's body and to minimize the risk of being inadvertently pulled out. **(B)** A large and rigid Elizabethan collar placed on a cat after enucleation, to prevent self-trauma to the surgical site. This can cause stress to the cat; a softer collar would have been functional in this cat. **(C)** A rigid Elizabethan collar has been shortened and modified in this young kitten that had urethral surgery; a less rigid collar was not feasible in this situation as it did not prevent interference with the surgical site.

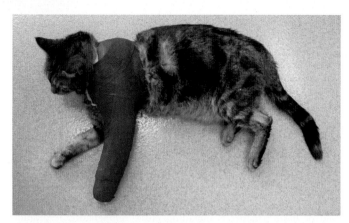

Figure 4-7 A cat with a spica splint protecting a surgical repair of a ruptured tendon. Many cats would not tolerate this type of immobilization.

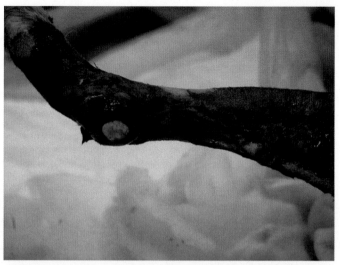

Figure 4-9 A bandage that was placed on this cat has resulted in a severe pressure sore on the caudal aspect of the distal pelvic limb and hock. The wound is shown after ten days of treatment, granulation tissue is well established but the tip of the calcaneus is still visible.

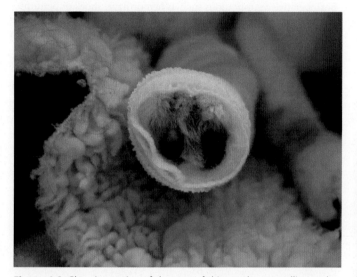

Figure 4-8 Close inspection of the toes of this cat shows swelling and divergence of the toes and protrusion of the toe nails. The bandage may have been applied too tightly and it should be removed and the foot inspected before a less restrictive bandage is reapplied, or if the bandage is not essential then consideration should be given to leaving it off.

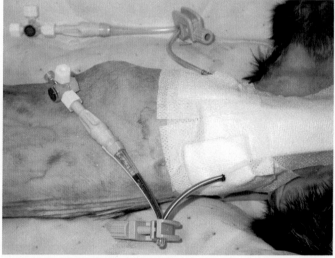

Figure 4-10 A cat with two thoracic drains. The drain insertion sites are covered by self-adherent dressings.

abdominal pain adopt a hunched sternal posture, with their head hung lower than their body, elbows drawn back, stifles forward and abdominal muscles tensed.[16]

Postoperative nutrition

Before any surgery it is important to plan ahead and anticipate the patient's expected requirements after surgery (see Chapter 6). Postoperative nutrition is essential and if the cat has been anorexic or is likely to be anorexic after surgery, then a plan for assisted feeding should be made. The type of feeding tube (see Chapter 12) to be placed will depend on the patient's requirements, the estimated time that assisted feeding will be needed and the cat's general preoperative condition and disease. Enteral feeding or total or partial parenteral nutrition (TPN or PPN) are also options for consideration. Forward planning is essential as a catheter for TPN or PPN and esophagostomy, gastrotomy and jejunostomy tubes will need to be placed at the time of surgery. It is advisable when feeding through gastrotomy or jejunostomy tubes that this should not begin until the cat is fully recovered and able to maintain a sternal position with an elevated head without

assistance. It is important to slowly introduce any new diet and gradually increase the volume of food fed to avoid overfilling the stomach and potentially risk inducing vomiting or regurgitation.

Feeding tubes are managed as described for a thoracic drain although due to the length of the external portion of tube, it may be necessary to use additional conforming bandage and a carefully placed layer of cohesive bandage around the tube in addition to the vest, ensuring the bandage is not placed too tight around the cat's abdomen.

Monitoring urination

The cat's ability to urinate and the frequency of urination should be recorded as part of the general postoperative monitoring. Some cats will be reluctant to urinate while hospitalized due to a number of factors, including stress, unwillingness to use a litter tray and unfamiliar cat litter. Bladder palpation to check on size and fullness may be necessary and gentle palpation of the bladder can initiate urination in some cats (Fig. 4-11). Surgery involving the urinary tract may

Box 4-4 **Postoperative nursing care considerations after abdominal surgery**

Monitoring: Basic parameters such as pulse respiration and temperature should be regularly monitored for changes associated with signs of shock, hemorrhage and peritonitis

Excretion: Urine and fecal production and intestinal movement by auscultation should be monitored and recorded

Analgesia: A multimodal approach is generally used using systemic opioids, local analgesic agents and non-steroidal anti-inflammatories. If a wound infusion catheter has been placed, then local anesthetics can be infused down this intermittently or continuously. The cat should be regularly reassessed for the presence of pain and analgesia continued for as long a period as necessary (see Chapter 2)

Abdominal drains: Fluid production is regularly monitored and drains emptied aseptically and volume / characteristics of fluid produced recorded. Patient interference with the drain is prevented by the use of bandaging and Elizabethan collar

Nutrition: If feeding tubes have been placed then a plan should be made when to start feeding with volume and frequency of meals. Encouragement to eat is usually indicated in cats after abdominal surgery

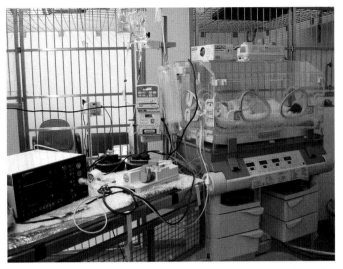

Figure 4-12 A cat recovering from abdominal surgery in an incubator in the well-equipped intensive care unit and recovery room.

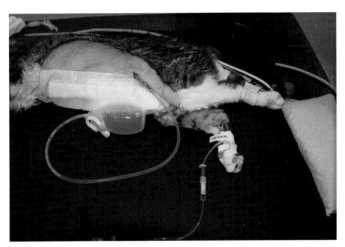

Figure 4-13 A closed suction drain has been placed in a cat with peritonitis after surgical exploration. A Primapore dressing (Smith and Nephew) provides a protective layer over the surgical incision, and can be replaced if strike through occurs due to discharge. If the incision stays dry then the dressing can be removed after 24 hours. An 'arterial' label, denoting that an arterial catheter has been placed in the left metatarsal artery, is a useful way of imparting this information to other members of the veterinary staff who may be administering intravenous fluids and drugs to the cat.

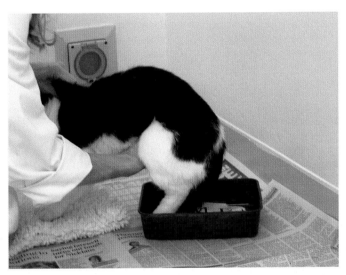

Figure 4-11 A cat having its bladder palpated for size and fullness. In a cat that is unable to urinate, for example due to neurological disease, it may be necessary to express the bladder.

require a cat to have a long-stay silicone urinary catheter placed, or a cystotomy tube. In these circumstances urine production will need to be closely monitored to check hydration status, that the kidneys are producing urine effectively and that there are no obstructions in the catheter or tube; often a closed collection system will be used for accurate monitoring. Urine production should be measured every four hours and calculated to ensure the cat is producing at least 1 mL/kg/hour. Urine color and turbidity should also be monitored and recorded. A reduction in urine output might indicate inadequate hydration, decreased urine production due to acute renal failure or a blocked catheter. Increased urine production may be due to over hydration or inability to concentrate urine due to renal failure. Urine from cats with indwelling catheters should be carefully monitored for the presence of a lower urinary tract infection and if there is any suspicion that such an infection is present the catheter itself should be submitted for bacterial culture and sensitivity.

Abdominal drain management

Abdominal drains are usually well tolerated in cats. Continuous suction drains attached to a reservoir bulb (Fig. 4-13) should be checked every two hours initially to establish how much fluid is being drained and then emptied twice a day or more often if necessary. Dressings for these tubes are managed in a similar manner as for a thoracic drain using a small, dry adhesive dressing and a string vest in combination with an Elizabethan collar.

Incisional dressings

Depending on the type of surgery performed abdominal wounds can be dressed with a small dry adhesive dressing, or for wounds where more postoperative fluid is expected surgical pads can be applied and held in place by a string vest (Fig. 4-7). Dressings should be closely monitored for the amount and color of the exudate. Gloves should always be worn when checking and replacing dressings. Dressings with little exudate should be changed daily and more often with increasing exudate. Inflammation or purulent discharge should be investigated and managed as described for thoracic wounds.

NURSING CARE AFTER HEAD AND NECK SURGERY

Upper airway surgery

If a cat has had surgery of the upper airway, such as the larynx or trachea, then careful monitoring is required postoperatively for any signs of respiratory distress or dyspnea. Mucous membranes should be assessed for normal color and respiratory rate and effort recorded. Equipment such as oxygen, a suction machine, small endotracheal tubes, a laryngoscope, local anesthetic spray and anesthetic drugs should be readily available in case emergency intubation is required (Table 4-1). In the cat that has had laryngeal surgery emergency tracheostomy surgery may occasionally be required and anticipation of this possibility should also be prepared for (see Chapter 46).

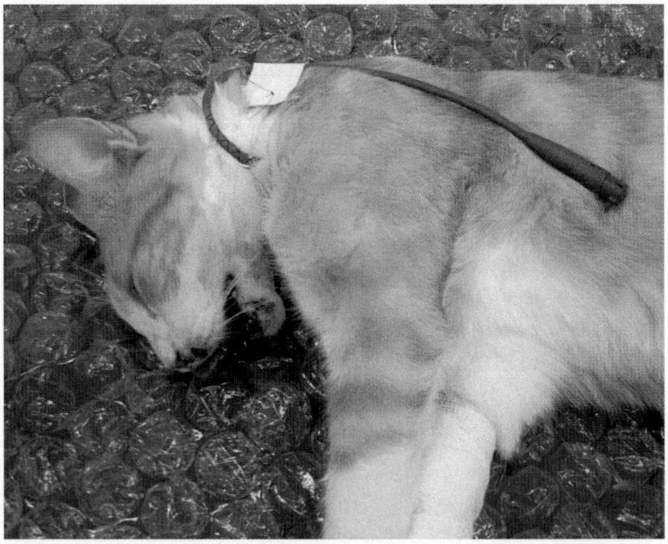

Figure 4-14 An esophagostomy tube has been placed in this cat with head trauma in anticipation that it would be reluctant to eat voluntarily on recovery from anesthesia.

Brain surgery

Careful monitoring of cats after brain surgery (see Chapter 58) is essential. Detailed aspects for intensive care postoperatively are discussed in Chapters 2 and 3. The particular emphasis on nursing care of cats after brain surgery relates to their general monitoring, seizure watch, and comfort.

Recovery after brain surgery may be slow and oxygen may be required until respiratory drive has returned. Cats are at risk of seizures after brain surgery so usually constant monitoring is required in the immediate postoperative period for this possibility. Anti-epileptic drugs and their indications and dosages should be readily available to give if required. The recovery cage should be well padded to prevent

injury if seizuring does occur. The appetite may be reduced due to central nervous system effects and possibly loss of the sense of smell. Encouraging eating by offering strong smelling food can be tried but if unsuccessful then a feeding tube may need to be placed (see Chapter 12). If it is anticipated that the cat may be reluctant to eat postoperatively after head surgery then placement of a pre-emptive feeding tube is recommended (Fig. 4-14). Central effects after brain surgery may also result in paraplegic animals that will require assistance with urination and defecation. They may require regular bathing if soiled and grooming to increase comfort levels. Physiotherapy of the limbs, to maintain muscle tone and joint mobility, will also be highly beneficial, as would coupage of the thorax in the recumbent cat.

REFERENCES

1. Carney HC, Little S, Brownlee-Tomasso D, et al. AAFP and ISFM feline friendly nursing care guidelines. J of Fel Med Surg 2012;14:337–49.

2. Brodbelt D. Feline anesthetic deaths in veterinary practice. Top Companion Anim Med 2010;25:189–94.

3. Wegner K, Pablo L. Anesthesia case of the month. Pulmonary abscess formation. J Am Vet Med Assoc 2006;228:850–3.

4. Posner LP. Effects of opioids and anesthetic drugs on body temperature in cats. Vet Anaes & Analg 2010;37: 35–43.

5. Cambridge AJ, Tobias KM, Newberry RC, et al. Subjective and objective measurements of post-operative pain in cats. J Am Vet Med Assoc 2000;217: 685–90.

6. Sanford J, and working party of the Association of Veterinary Teachers and Research Workers. Guidelines for the recognition and assessment of pain in animals. Vet Rec 1986;118:334–8.

7. Grint NJ, Murison PJ, Coe RJ, et al. Assessment of the influence of surgical technique on post-operative pain and wound tenderness in cats following ovariohysterectomy. J Fel Med Surg 2006;8:15–21.

8. Slingsby LS, Jones A, Waterman-Pearson AE, et al. Use of a new finger-mounted device to compare mechanical nociceptive thresholds in cats given pethidine or no medication after castration. Res Vet Sci 2001;70:243–6.

9. Smith JD, Allen SW, Quandt JE, et al. Changes in cortisol concentration in response to stress and post-operative pain in client-owned cats and correlation with objective clinical variables. Am J Vet Res 1999;60:432–6.

10. Holton LL, Scott EM, Nolan AM, et al. Comparison of three methods used for assessments of pain in dogs. J Am Vet Med Assoc 1998;212:61–6.

11. http://csuanimalcancercenter.org/assets/files/csu_acute_pain_scale_feline.pdf

http://www.vetclick.com/downloads/Cat%20pain%20Chart_v5.pdf.

12. Hudson S. Rehabilitation of the cat. In: Montavon PM, Voss K, Langley-Hobbs SJ, editors. Feline orthopedic surgery and musculoskeletal disease. Elsevier; 2009. p. 221–35.

13. Kästner S. Analgesia. In: Montavon PM, Voss K, Langley-Hobbs SJ, editors. Feline orthopedic surgery and musculoskeletal disease. Elsevier; 2009. p. 199–206.

14. Levy J, Lapham B, Hardie E, et al. Evaluation of laser onychectomy in the cat. In: 19th Annual Meeting of the American Society of Laser Medicine and Surgery; 1999; Lake Buena Vista, FL; 1999.

15. Anderson DM. White RAS. Ischemic bandage injuries: a case series and review of the literature. Vet Surg 2000;29: 488–98.

16. Robertson SA. Assessment and management of acute pain in cats. J Vet Emerg Crit Care 2005;15:261–72.

Chapter | 5 |

Blood transfusions in cats

C. Knottenbelt, M.W. Jackson, M. O'Brien

Blood or blood products are commonly required in surgical patients and a well-timed transfusion can be life-saving.[1-3] The presurgical and pre-anesthetic workup should identify those patients that would benefit (see Chapter 1). Pre-existing anemia, anticipated extensive blood loss during surgery and known coagulation disorders are the most common indications for transfusing fresh whole blood or blood products. However, cats must NEVER receive any blood or blood products unless they have been blood typed, and preferably cross-matched, with the donor. The risk of fatal transfusion reactions is too great, even in first transfusions, if these steps are not taken.[4] Feline blood groups are becoming increasingly complex and it is therefore impossible to safely 'guess the blood type'. Typing is technically easy to perform and commercial kits are available allowing desk-top typing in the veterinary practice. For routine surgical patients, blood typing and cross-matching can be done at admission. However, for surgical emergencies blood typing could be done at induction or during surgery if blood or blood products are required. By following the guidelines below and using standard operating procedures, cats will receive the benefits of a safe blood product supply. This will enhance the quality of life for feline surgical patients requiring transfusion while minimizing the risks to both donor and recipient cats.

ASSESSING THE NEED FOR A TRANSFUSION

Transfusion should be considered in any feline patient with a packed cell volume (PCV) of less than 20% that is due to undergo surgery or where it is indicated by the clinical condition of the patient.[5] Reasons for considering an emergency transfusion are shown in Box 5-1. Although many surgical cases would benefit from blood component therapy (e.g., platelet rich plasma, fresh plasma for clotting factors),[6,7] this is rarely available for feline patients. In general, patients with hypovolemic anemia or those expected to have substantial blood loss during surgery should receive fresh whole blood. Patients with coagulopathies, especially secondary to hepatic disorders, and/or those that are normovolemic can be given component therapy where possible.[6] Always collect any blood required for tests, such as typing, FeLV/FIV, Coomb test etc, BEFORE giving the patient a transfusion.

Unexpected blood loss during surgery

Whole blood, colloids and crystalloids are used to restore blood volume. Transfusion is only required if bleeding is severe enough to result in anemia. Healthy conscious cats can lose up to 20% of their blood volume (13 mL/kg) without adverse effects provided that circulation is supported with colloids or crystalloids. In an anesthetized patient, blood loss of greater than 10% (equivalent to 7 mL/kg) should be considered potentially life-threatening.[8] Assessment of peripheral oxygenation is an insensitive way of assessing if blood loss is significant, as most anemic patients will have an SpO_2 of 100%.[9] Similarly, during a bleeding episode the PCV may not reflect the degree of blood loss unless IV fluids are also being administered. A change in total protein can also be used to estimate blood loss. The best method of determining the need for blood is monitoring blood pressure and perfusion parameters (heart, respiration and pulse rates, pulse quality, body temperature, CRT, mentation, lactate concentration).[9] The administration of whole blood provides circulatory volume support and coagulation factors which may be beneficial in patients with bleeding disorders. Fresh whole blood also provides transient (three to four hours) benefit to patients with platelet diseases.

Expected blood loss during surgery

Where surgery is likely to result in significant blood loss, presurgical assessment and preparation for transfusion of the patient are essential. Cats can have significant anemia and show minimal clinical signs due to its chronicity. Through lifestyle adaptations they may appear normal to the owners despite an extremely low PCV. Although this chronic anemia is well tolerated, an acute blood loss can result in sudden deterioration in the patient's ability to cope with the anemia. Prior to the surgical procedure the cat's PCV and perfusion parameters (pulse quality, mucous membrane color and capillary refill time) must be assessed. Where anemia is moderate to severe (PCV <20%) it should be corrected with transfusion prior to anesthesia. In cats with mild-moderate anemia (PCV >20%), arrangements should be made to have blood available if blood loss during surgery is predicted.

© 2014 Elsevier Ltd
DOI: 10.1016/B978-0-7020-4336-9.00005-6

Stabilizing an anemic patient prior to surgery

First, the cause of the anemia must be determined. Patients with chronic blood loss or those with non-regenerative anemia may gain significant long-term benefit from transfusion. Transfusion can stabilize the patient for two to three months as transfused red blood cells can have a near normal life span (70 days). Prior to anesthesia a PCV of at least 20% should be achieved.

Cats with hemolytic anemia receive transient benefits from a transfusion and should have their hemolytic disease stabilized and under long-term control prior to surgery whenever possible.

Note that clotting factors, platelets and the anti-inflammatory/immunoregulatory properties of fresh whole blood last only two weeks in human blood units and it is likely that this is much shorter in cats.[9]

Disorders of secondary hemostasis

The most common cause of clotting problems is vitamin K deficiency, which can be caused by anorexia or hepatic disease involving the biliary tract. Vitamin K is a fat-soluble vitamin with a relatively short half-life that requires bile acids for its uptake. Cats can rapidly become deficient in the vitamin leading to coagulation disturbances similar to those seen in coumarin toxicity.[10,11] All cats with significant anorexia and those suspected of having significant biliary disease should be given vitamin K by injection 24 hours prior to surgery. Oral vitamin K will not aid those patients with compromised vitamin K uptake. In cats with disseminated intravascular coagulation, whole blood will provide clotting factors and antithrombin. However, if the patient is not anemic then fresh frozen plasma, if available, will suffice.[6,7] Further discussion on coagulopathies in cats is given in Chapter 1.

FELINE BLOOD GROUPS

Two major blood group systems have now been identified in cats. The most important is the AB system which has three types (A, B and AB).[12,13] Type A is the most common, whereas type B proportions vary both geographically and with breed.[14] Type AB cats are consistently rare and only found in breeds with type B cats (20). The prevalence of type B can be very high (approaching 50%) in some pedigree breeds, especially the British shorthair, ragdoll, Birman, and Rex breeds. Type B cats are also commonly encountered amongst Persians, Somalis, Abyssinians, Himalayans, and Scottish folds. However, notable geographic and individual variation in blood type can occur within these breeds.[14–20] It appears that feline blood types are well conserved as wild felids have the same blood groups as domesticated cats.[21]

In addition, cats have naturally occurring alloantibodies against the blood type antigen that they do not possess.[22,23] These alloantibodies result from exposure to antigenic epitopes commonly found in nature that are similar or identical to 'non-self' blood group antigens.

Therefore, when a cat with naturally formed alloantibodies encounters 'foreign' type red blood cells a transfusion reaction ensues. All type B cats have high levels of naturally occurring anti-A antibodies. Many type A cats (>70%) have low levels of naturally occurring anti-B antibodies but this varies geographically.[23] Type AB cats do not have naturally occurring alloantibodies.[13,23]

The Mik red cell antigen was recently reported. Cats whose red cells do not express the Mik cell antigen can have naturally occurring alloantibodies against the Mik antigen (approximately 4% of cats in the study).[24]

Blood typing and cross-matching techniques

Cats must receive blood of the same type as their own or significant and potentially fatal transfusion reactions can occur.[25,26] These reactions may be either immediate hemolysis or delayed (up to five days later). Compatibility can only be guaranteed if donor and recipient are the same blood type and have a negative cross-match. Cross-matching alone does not always ensure that donor and recipient are the same blood type.

A variety of desktop blood typing kits are available. In-house systems use very small volumes of blood and positive results are seen as an agglutination reaction (Rapid Vet-H), or a test line (Quick Test A+B) (Fig. 5-1). Many diagnostic laboratories will also perform these typing tests. However, blood typing will not identify incompatibilities associated with previous transfusions, which may not be AB associated. Therefore blood typing AND cross-matching (Fig. 5-2) should ideally be performed at the first transfusion and must be performed before subsequent transfusions.[27] How to perform a cross-match is summarized in Box 5-2.

SELECTING A DONOR

The ease of blood collection from the donor cat plays a large role in the success of any transfusion. Box 5-3 lists factors to consider when selecting a donor. Commercial suppliers also provide whole blood and/or blood products; however, not all commercial suppliers have ready access to rare types so a list of alternative sources is useful.

Collection of donor blood

Healthy cats can donate 10% of their total blood volume (every four to six weeks) without adverse effects. Collection of 20% of blood volume can produce short-term hypovolemia requiring therapeutic intervention. Collection of > 20% of blood volume can produce severe life-threatening hypovolemia and should not be performed.

To avoid making the donor anemic the PCV should be checked before collection and be at least 35%.[28,29] Most feline donors will be donating 20% of their blood volume (40–60 mL) and should receive crystalloids to provide circulatory support. Crystalloids should be given over 45–60 minutes with a total volume of two to three times the volume of blood collected.

The most effective anticoagulants are found in human blood collection bags (CPD-A). The amount of anticoagulant should be proportional to the volume being collected (6 mL of anticoagulant for 50 mL of blood, or 7 mL anticoagulant for 60 mL blood). If human blood bags are not available then the collection syringe can be pretreated with heparin by drawing heparin into the syringe and then flushing it out. Note that if heparin is used as an anticoagulant blood must be used immediately.

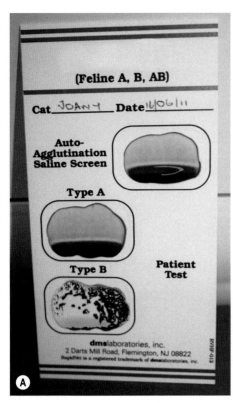

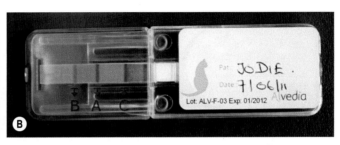

Figure 5-1 Feline blood typing systems. **(A)** Feline blood typing card that uses agglutination to indicate a positive result. **(B)** Feline blood typing gel tube which uses a test line

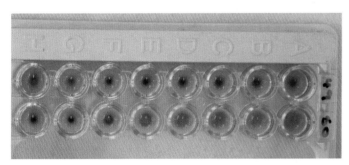

Figure 5-2 A positive cross-match.

Box 5-2 **Performing a cross-match**

1. Collect EDTA and heparin samples from both donor and recipient
2. Spin down all four samples (3000 rpm for ten minutes)
3. EDTA sample provides the cells. These need to be washed to remove all antibodies (re-suspend in saline, re-spin and remove supernatant)
4. Make 3–5% cell solution by adding saline
5. Plasma from heparin sample provides the antibodies
6. Two drops of donor cell suspension are mixed with two drops of recipient plasma (and vice versa) either on a slide or preferably in test tubes or well plates
7. The cell/plasma mixture is assessed for hemolysis (diffuse reddening of solution which fails to settle out) or agglutination (granular appearance)

   Mixing cell solution with plasma from the same animal acts as a negative control

Box 5-3 **Selecting a blood donor**

Healthy, easy to handle and friendly

Normal physical examination

Large, non-obese >4.0 kg lean body weight, ideally non-brachycephalic

Young (>1 year) to middle aged (up to 10–12 years)

Non-pregnant, not in estrus

Packed cell volume >35%

Vaccinated and de-wormed

Negative for retroviruses, *Mycoplasma haemofelis*, *Bartonella henselae* and other infectious diseases based on geographical location (e.g. ehrlichiosis, anaplasmosis, etc.)[35]

Free from external parasites, ideally without a history of foreign travel or contact with traveled pets

Known blood group

Normotensive (120–180 mmHg systolic): occult heart disease and other conditions can be associated with low blood pressure that is exacerbated by sedation and/or blood donation

Most feline donors require sedation for donation. Midazolam (0.3 mg/kg) and ketamine (2 mg/kg) given in combination intravenously, provide the required sedation without affecting blood pressure.[30] Blood is collected from the jugular veins with the cat in dorsal recumbency with support under the cat's neck (Fig. 5-3). Occlusion of both jugular veins can increase blood flow rates. Feline blood can be stored for up to 28 days in a pharmacy standard refrigerator; however, refrigeration will cause a complete loss of platelet viability after several hours.[9]

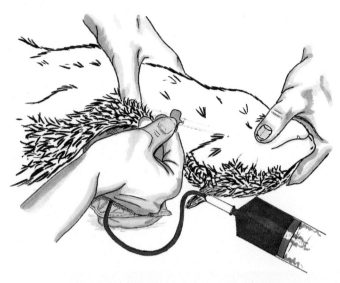

Figure 5-3 Collection of blood from a cat. The cat is placed in dorsal recumbency with support under the neck.

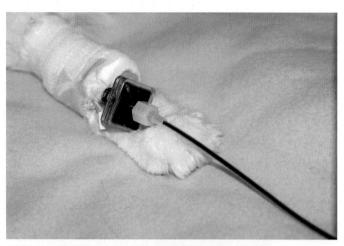

Figure 5-4 Blood administered through in-line filter.

Box 5-4 **Equation used to calculate blood volume to transfuse**

$$\text{Volume required} = \frac{66 \times \text{weight of recipient in kg} \times (\text{target PCV} - \text{patient's PCV})}{\text{PCV of donor}}$$

Permanent or semi-permanent vascular access ports (VAPs) can be employed as a more humane, labour-efficient means of repeated collections from the same donor. These devices avoid the necessity of repeated sedation, decrease the risk of infections and transfusion reactions, and allow faster, more efficient collection because only two people are required. Although these are perceived as better for feline health and welfare[31] and can be maintained for the effective 'donating' life of the donor cat they do require initial surgical placement. The benefits would only be realized in a busy hospital where multiple transfusions occur and regular donors are used.

Estimating the volume of blood needed

To raise the patient's PCV by approximately 10% you need to give 20 mL/kg of whole blood or 10 mL/kg of packed red blood cells.

The precise volume of blood to be transfused can be calculated using an equation[32] (Box 5-4).

A target PCV of 20% is usual although a higher PCV may be required if anemia is acute. It is not always possible to reach the target without giving more than one unit of blood. However, even small increases in PCV can significantly improve clinical signs and, given donor limitations, the recipient would usually get one 'unit' of blood provided by the donor (40–60 mL of whole blood depending on donor weight).

How to transfuse: practical aspects

Whole blood and packed red blood cells (PRBC) can be administered using a blood giving set that contains a filter or straight from the anticoagulated collection syringe using an in-line filter (e.g., Hemonate filter, Utah Medical Products) (Fig. 5-4). PRBC should be administered at body temperature to improve flow. Warm water should be

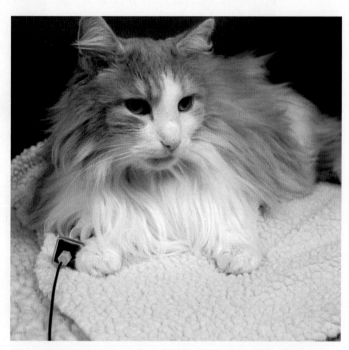

Figure 5-5 A cat receiving donor blood. This is direct from a syringe using a syringe driver and an in-line filter. This system minimizes the risk of contamination of the blood when transferring it to a blood bag.

used to heat the blood slowly. Microwave ovens should never be used as overheating the blood will result in hemolysis and coagulation of proteins.

Blood can be administered via an intravenous catheter (Fig. 5-5) or intraosseous needle/catheter as uptake into the bone marrow is very efficient (> 1 drop per minute with an infusion pump).[33]

Whole blood should be given at 5–10 mL/kg/hour (over two to four hours) in most patients. However, in hypovolemic patients the rate can be increased to 20 mL/kg/hour provided there is constant monitoring and reductions in rate as required. In patients with cardiovascular disease the rate should be reduced to 2 mL/kg/hour; however, the transfusion should not take longer than four hours in total as after this time there is a risk of bacterial contamination. Where PRBC are being used rates should be reduced by 50% to avoid volume overload.

Storage of blood products

Storage of blood results in damage to the red blood cells (known as storage lesions) and other blood components. The longer that the blood is stored the greater the risk of significant transfusion reactions associated with these storage lesions (which can look similar to an AB typing mismatch). In addition to the risk of storage lesions, the oxygen-carrying capacity of stored red cells declines over time.[9] However, this can be partially restored within hours of transfusion.[9] Current recommendations are that blood should be collected and used as soon as possible and preferably within three weeks.[9]

HEMOGLOBIN-BASED OXYGEN CARRIERS

Hemoglobin-based oxygen carriers (HBOCs) are colloid solutions containing a bovine hemoglobin glutamer (polymer) in Ringer's lactate, licensed for use in dogs. It has been used off-label in cats. It must be given at slower rates and its use and risks should be discussed with the owner as its use in cats is outside the veterinary medicine directorate (VMD) cascade.[34,35] It has a higher affinity for oxygen (both in binding and offloading) than RBCs and therefore increases the patient's oxygen-carrying potential. It is therefore used when whole blood is not available or a compatible donor cannot be found. The benefit from a single administration is short lived (half-life of 30–40 hours in dogs), compared to a blood transfusion. Oxyglobin must not be given to patients with circulatory failure or oliguric renal disease. In some cats it may be associated with acute onset respiratory distress if given too quickly. The rate should not exceed 0.5–1.0 mL/kg/hour with a maximum total dose of 5–7.5 mL/kg. The primary complication in cats is volume overload leading to pulmonary edema, pleural effusion, and cardiac impairment.[34,35]

Oxyglobin (OPK Biotech) causes a yellow-orange discoloration of tissues, notably skin, mucous membranes and sclera; red-green discoloration of feces and port wine discoloration of urine. Oxyglobin will affect refractometer readings of total solids and colorimetric measurements for some serum chemistries. Therefore, pretreatment samples MUST be taken prior to Oxyglobin administration. At the time of this writing the product is no longer available in the UK; hopefully this is not a permanent situation.

TRANSFUSION REACTIONS

Mismatched transfusions can cause a fatal reaction in some cats. Acute reactions which are commonly associated with the administration of type A or AB blood to a type B cat are very severe. Delayed reactions which are commonly seen with type B or AB blood given to a type A cat tend to be less severe but will result in a significant loss of red blood cells[26] and a return to pretransfusion PCV in a matter of days after transfusion. The speed and severity of transfusion reaction depends on the alloantibody titer and not the volume of mismatched blood given; fatal reactions to as little as 1 mL have been reported.[25] Mismatched transfusions will also cause the induction of antibody production, making subsequent reactions severe if a second mismatched transfusion is given in the future.

All cats receiving a transfusion should be monitored closely for the first 15 minutes and then monitored regularly for the signs of a transfusion reaction (Box 5-5). Mild transfusion reactions such as pyrexia and vomiting (Fig. 5-6) can usually be corrected by slowing the rate of blood administration.[36]

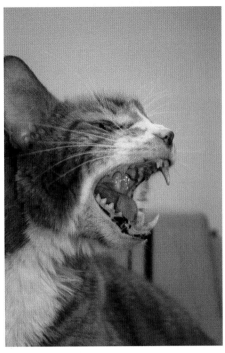

Figure 5-6 Cat showing signs of vocalization, which is a common sign of a mild or early transfusion reaction.

Box 5-5 Clinical signs associated with transfusion reactions

Mild reaction

Pyrexia
Vomiting
Vocalization
Urticaria
Erythema or pruritus

Severe reaction

Depression
Dyspnea, tachypnea or coughing
Tachycardia or bradycardia
Tremors or convulsions
Shock
Cardiopulmonary arrest
Anorexia (delayed)
Jaundice (delayed)

When a transfusion reaction is suspected, the transfusion must be stopped while the cause of the reaction is investigated. The bag should be checked for signs of hemolysis or bacterial contamination and the blood typing and cross-matching results confirmed. Some patients may require antihistamine treatment; however, the pre-emptive use of antihistamines is not recommended as it may mask the early stages of a more severe reaction. In most cases the transfusion can be restarted at a slower rate once symptoms have resolved. In more severe, potentially life-threatening reactions the patients may also require treatment for shock (intravenous fluids and corticosteroids) and close monitoring for hemoglobinemia and hemoglobinuria.

REFERENCES

1. Klaser DA, Reine NJ, Hohenhaus AE. Red blood cell transfusions in cats: 126 cases (1999). J Am Vet Med Assoc 2005;226(6): 920–3.

2. Roux FA, Deschamps JY, Blais MC, et al. Multiple red cell transfusions in 27 cats (2003–2006): indications, complications and outcomes. J Feline Med Surg 2008;(3):213–18.

3. Weingart C, Giger U, Kohn B. Whole blood transfusions in 91 cats: a clinical evaluation. J Feline Med Surg 2004;6(3): 139–48.

4. Auer L, Bell K. Transfusion reactions in cats due to AB blood group incompatibility. Res Vet Sci 1983;35: 145–52.

5. Prittie JE. Triggers for use, optimal dosing, and problems associated with red cell transfusions. Vet Clin North Am Small Anim Pract 2003;33(6):1261–75.

6. Castellanos I, Couto CG, Gray TL. Clinical use of blood products in cats: a retrospective study (1997–2000). J Vet Intern Med 2004;18:529–32.

7. Helm JR, Knottenbelt CM. Blood transfusions in the Dog and Cat – Part one – Indications for blood product transfusions. In Practice 2010;32:184–9.

8. Gaynor JS, Dunlop CI, Wagner AE, et al. Complications and mortality associated with anesthesia in dogs and cats. J Am Anim Hosp Assoc 1999;35:13–17.

9. Prittie JE. Controversies related to red blood cell transfusion in critically ill patients. J Vet Emerg Crit Care 2010;20: 167–76.

10. Lisciandro SC, Hohenhaus A, Brooks M. Coagulation abnormalities in 22 cats with naturally occurring liver disease. J Vet Intern Med 1998;12:71–5.

11. Center SA, Crawford MA, Guida L, et al. A retrospective study of 77 cats with severe hepatic lipidosis: 1975–1990. J Vet Intern Med 1993;7:349–59.

12. Auer L, Bell K. The AB blood group system of cats. An Bld Grp, Biochem Gen 1981;12:287–97.

13. Griot-Wenk M, Giger U. Cats with type AB blood in the United States. J Vet Intern Med 1991;5:139 only.

14. Knottenbelt CM. The feline AB blood group system and its importance in transfusion medicine: a review. J Feline Med Surg 2002;4:69–76.

15. Knottenbelt CM, Addie DD, Day MJ, Mackin AJ. Determination of the prevalence of feline blood types in the UK. J Small Anim Pract 1999;40:115–18.

16. Griot-Wenk M, Giger U. Feline transfusion medicine. Blood types and their clinical importance. Vet Clin N Am: Small Anim Prac 1995;25:1305–22.

17. Forcada Y, Guitian J, Gibson G. Frequencies of feline blood types at a referral hospital in the south east of England. J Small Anim Prac 2007;48(10): 570–3.

18. Malik R, Griffin DL, White JD, et al. The prevalence of feline A/B blood types in the Sydney region. Aust Vet J 2005; 83(1–2):38–44.

19. Medeiros MA, Soares AM, Alviano DS, et al. Frequencies of feline blood types in the Rio de Janeiro area of Brazil. Vet Clin Pathol 2008;37(3):272–6.

20. Arikan S, Gurkan M, Ozaytekin E, et al. Frequencies of blood type A, B and AB in non-pedigree domestic cats in Turkey. J Small Anim Prac 2006;47(1):10–13.

21. Griot-Wenk M, Giger U. The AB blood group system in wild felids. Anim Genet 1999;30:144–7.

22. Bucheler J, Giger U. Alloantibodies against A and B blood types in cats. Vet Immun Immunopath 1993;38:283–95.

23. Knottenbelt CM, Day MJ, Cripps PJ, Mackin AJ. Measurement of titres of naturally occurring alloantibodies against feline blood group antigens in the UK. J Small Anim Prac 1999;40:365–70.

24. Weinstein NM, Blais MC, Harris K, et al. A newly recognized blood group in domestic shorthair cats: the Mik red cell antigen. J Vet Int Med 2007;21:287–92.

25. Auer L, Bell K. Transfusion reactions in cats due to AB blood group incompatibility. Res Vet Sci 1983;35: 145–52.

26. Giger U, Bucheler J. Transfusion of type-A and type-B blood to cats. J Am Vet Med Assoc 1991;198:411–18.

27. Tocci LJ, Ewing PJ. Increasing patient safety in veterinary transfusion medicine: an overview of pretransfusion testing. J Vet Emerg Crit Care 2009;19(1): 66–73.

28. Wardrop KJ, Reine N, Birkenheuer A, et al. Canine and feline blood donor screening for infectious disease. J Vet Intern Med 2005;19:135–42.

29. Iazbik MC, Gómez Ochoa P, Westendorf N, et al. Effects of blood collection for transfusion on arterial blood pressure, heart rate, and PCV in cats. J Vet Intern Med 2007;21:1181–4.

30. Helm JR, Knottenbelt CM Blood transfusions in the Dog and Cat – Practicalities of giving and receiving blood. In Practice 2010;32:231–7.

31. Morrison JA, Lauer SK, Baldwin CJ, et al. Evaluation of the use of subcutaneous implantable vascular access ports in feline blood donors. J Am Vet Med Assoc 2007;230(6):855–61.

32. Pichler, ME, Turnwald GH. Blood transfusion in dogs and cats Part I. Physiology, collection, storage and indications for whole blood therapy. Comp Cont Ed Pract Vet 1985;7: 64–71.

33. Otto C, Crowe D. Intraosseous resuscitation techniques and applications. In: Kirk RW, Bonagura JD, editors. Kirk's current veterinary therapy XI. Philadelphia, PA: WB Saunders Co; 1992. p. 107–12.

34. Gibson GR, Callan MB, Hoffman V, Giger U. Use of a hemoglobin-based oxygen-carrying solution in cats: 72 cases (1998–2000). J Am Vet Med Assoc 2002;221:96–102.

35. Weingart C, Kohn B. Clinical use of a hemoglobin-based oxygen carrying solution (Oxyglobin) in 48 cats (2002–2006). J Feline Med Surg 2008;10(5):431–8.

36. Turnwald GH, Pichler ME. Blood transfusion in dogs and cats Part II. Administration, adverse effects and component therapy. Comp Cont Ed 1985;7(2):115–22.

Chapter | 6 |

Nutrition for the surgical patient

M. Chandler

Appropriate nutrition is critical for optimal preparation for and recovery from surgery, as morbidity and mortality are affected by nutritional status. Nutritional assessment and calculation of nutritional requirements of the cat provides guidance as to the appropriate feeding protocol. Virtually all hospitalized cats may be fed by oral, enteral or parenteral nutritional supplementation.

PREOPERATIVE ASSESSMENT

Preoperative nutritional status in people predicts the occurrence of postoperative complications and the severity of the inflammatory response.[1-4] Deterioration of nutritional status in patients undergoing major surgery is associated with poor wound healing and decreased immune function.[4] Other consequences of malnutrition include fatigue, decreased thermoregulation, respiratory, pancreatic, gastrointestinal, mental, endocrine and cardiovascular functions, and impaired muscle strength.[5] Morbidity and mortality rates are increased in malnourished patients. The postoperative mortality rate in human cancer patients approaches 23% for the malnourished but is only 4% in those in better nutritional condition, unrelated to differences in disease or procedure.[6] Nutritional support in elderly patients reduces the mortality rate from 18.6% to 8.6% at six months.[7] Similarly, emaciated cats are significantly more likely to die within a year than those of optimal body condition.[8]

Conversely, obesity has been cited as increasing the potential anesthetic and surgical risks in people and dogs,[9,10] though this is less well documented in cats. Obesity influences the dosing of preanesthetic and anesthetic medications, as dosing for actual weight rather than for lean body weight may result in over-dosing. With repeated dosing of some intravenous drugs there is saturation of lean body tissue and drug distribution to fat, which may result in prolonged recovery times.[11] Further, obesity can make monitoring by auscultation during anesthesia more difficult due to the muffling of heart and lung sounds.[12]

Nutritional management starts with assessment of the nutritional status, including dietary history. Dietary history should include the cat's appetite, the food brand name, flavor and type, amount fed, number of meals, and any treats, snacks, or foods given to administer

---

Box 6-1 Indications for supplemental nutritional support

Acute weight loss of ≥5%
Chronic weight loss of ≥10%
Poor body condition (see Table 6.1; <5/9)
Anorexia or poor food intake
Malassimilation of food
Increased loss of nutrients (e.g., protein losing disorders, diabetes mellitus)
Non-healing wounds

---

medications. If present, the duration of anorexia or decreased appetite should be noted. People give unreliable estimates of their own food intake,[13] but the reliability of an owner's assessment of their pet's food intake is unknown. Any history of weight loss or gain should be noted, though assessing weight change can be difficult if the animal's previous weight is unknown. Ascites may make weight loss more difficult to assess.

Impairment of organ function occurs with starvation before significant physical changes are observed, and nutritional deprivation is especially likely to be overlooked in the obese hospitalized patient.[6] Initiation of nutritional support is indicated in patients meeting any of these criteria: acute weight loss of >5%, chronic weight loss of >10%, poor body condition, anorexia for more than three days, decreased protein intake or malabsorption, weakness, or non-healing wounds (Box 6-1).

Body assessment

Many assessment protocols for humans use the body mass index (BMI), which is weight (kg)/height(m)^2, and anthropometric measurements such as midarm muscle circumference.[6] A feline version of BMI has been developed and validated by dual energy X-ray absorptiometry (DEXA) for healthy cats weighing between 3 kg and 9 kg.[14] The feline BMI uses the rib cage circumference in cm and the leg index measurement (LIM), which is the hind leg length in cm from the middle of the patella to the dorsal tip of the calcaneal process.

© 2014 Elsevier Ltd
DOI: 10.1016/B978-0-7020-4336-9.00006-8

Box 6-2 **Equation for estimation of body fat**

Percentage body fat

$$= \frac{[\text{rib cage}/0.762 - \text{leg index measurement}]}{0.9156}.$$

The amount of body fat is estimated using the equation in Box 6-2. This calculation has not been validated in ill cats, and feline BMI is not widely used in clinical practice.

Body condition scores (BCS) provide a semi-quantitative method for evaluating fat and lean body tissue percentages.[15,16] Scoring systems have been developed using systems of 1 to 5, 6, or 9 points, with lower numbers representing thinner cats and higher numbers indicating fatter animals. A feline BCS system using a 9-point scale has shown good correlation (0.91) with percentage of body fat as determined by DEXA.[16] This BCS system, using pictures and descriptions, shows good repeatability within and between observers. A score of five out of nine is optimal (Table 6-1).

The BCS systems do not take into account muscle wasting, and many ill cats have muscle loss disproportionate to fat loss due to the metabolic changes of stress. Consequently, a 4-point feline muscle mass scoring (MSS) system has been developed based on palpation of muscles over the skull, scapulae, spine, and pelvis[17] (Table 6-2). Animals with no muscle wasting are scored as a 3, mild wasting is 2, moderate wasting is 1, and a 0 score represents severe wasting. There was a fair correlation between the feline MMS system and cats' lean body mass as determined by DEXA.[17]

Multi-frequency bioelectrical impedance has been used experimentally to assess body composition in healthy cats,[18] but is not used in the clinical setting. Disturbances of water and electrolyte metabolism in the ill patient limit the usefulness of this technique in the hospital.[6] In research settings, DEXA is used for determination of body composition. It has good accuracy but requires anesthesia and is not practical for most patients.[19]

Nutritional assessment in humans has included measurements of serum albumin and other proteins, including acute phase reactants. These parameters are affected by factors other than nutrition, including metabolic changes of illness, hydration, and vascular permeability. Serum albumin does not correlate well with other nutritional assessments or with starvation in people,[6,20] although in cats admitted to a referral practice there was a positive correlation of serum albumin with body condition score.[21] This was likely due to decreases in serum albumin and BCS both reflecting the underlying disease.[20,21] Serum insulin-like growth factor (IGF)-I concentrations are reduced by short-term dietary restriction and restored by re-feeding in cats,[22] but this parameter is not widely available for daily use in practice.

While there appear to be no reliable, widely available laboratory markers for assessment of nutritional status, the identification of specific nutrient deficiencies, such as folate, cobalamin, and iron can be useful. The most practical preoperative nutritional assessment in practice combines the history of acute or chronic weight loss, dietary intake, body condition score, and muscle mass score.

Obesity concerns

Due to the potential for obese cats to have higher risks of complications with anesthesia and surgery, it may be prudent to postpone elective procedures until the cat loses weight. For more urgent procedures, the fat cat should be provided with adequate nutritional support to decrease the loss of lean body tissue and the risk of hepatic lipidosis.

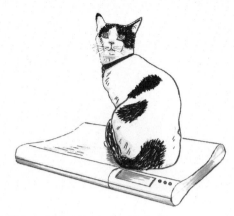

Figure 6-1 Daily weighing for the hospitalized cat.

Daily monitoring of the cat's nutritional status while hospitalized will help to ensure adequate intake. Cats should be weighed daily (Fig. 6-1), although day-to-day weight fluctuations are influenced by fluid balance.

HOW LONG TO STARVE BEFORE SURGERY?

Adult cats

Fasting has been recommended prior to general anesthesia to minimize gastric content volume and thereby decrease the risk of regurgitation and aspiration. Gastroesophageal reflux during general anesthesia is considered to be a common cause of esophagitis, and can cause esophageal strictures. The incidence of gastroesophageal reflux during anesthesia in dogs has been reported as 16.3%.[23] In another canine study, the rate of esophageal stricture caused by gastroesophageal reflux during anesthesia was 0.13%, and 30% of these cases died.[24] Studies in cats are not available.

The traditional practice in veterinary medicine has been to starve patients overnight or for at least six to 12 hours prior to anesthesia. However, canine studies have shown that prolonged fasting neither diminishes gastric volume nor decreases gastric acidity.[25] An increased duration of fasting is actually associated with an increased incidence of reflux in dogs. None of 30 dogs fasted for two to four hours refluxed during anesthesia, while 13.3% of the ones fasted for 12 to 18 hours had an episode of reflux.[23] In another study, none of 31 dogs fasted for three hours refluxed, while 16.3% of those fasted for ten hours had an episode. Dogs fasted for three hours after a canned food meal did not have a significantly increased gastric volume compared to those dogs fasted for 20 hours. Further, gastric acidity was reduced in the dogs with a three hour fast compared to those with a 20 hour fast.[26] Morphine also decreases the lower esophageal pressure; its use in combination with acetylpromazine (acepromazine) prior to anesthesia increased the incidence of gastroesophageal reflux in dogs from 27% to 60%.[27] Further, in humans, providing oral fluids and carbohydrates up to two hours before surgery attenuates postoperative insulin resistance. As dietary fat slows the rate of gastric emptying, feeding a small, low fat meal may be the best option.[28] Recent recommendations for otherwise healthy dogs undergoing elective procedures are to allow water up to two hours prior to induction, and a light meal three to four hours before induction.[29] While no feline studies are available to provide specific protocols, similar recommendations are reasonable.

Table 6-1 Body condition scores in cats

BODY CONDITION SYSTEM

TOO THIN

1 Ribs visible on shorthaired cats; no palpable fat; severe abdominal tuck; lumbar vertebrae and wings of ilia easily palpated.

2 Ribs easily visible on shorthaired cats; lumbar vertebrae obvious with minimal muscle mass; pronounced abdominal tuck; no palpable fat.

3 Ribs easily palpable with minimal fat covering; lumbar vertebrae obvious; obvious waist behind ribs; minimal abdominal fat.

4 Ribs palpable with minimal fat covering; noticeable waist behind ribs; slight abdominal tuck; abdominal fat pad absent.

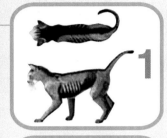

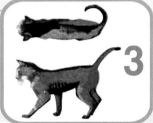

IDEAL

5 Well-proportioned; observe waist behind ribs; ribs palpable with slight fat covering; abdominal fat pad minimal.

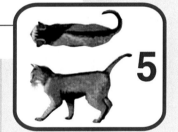

TOO HEAVY

6 Ribs palpable with slight excess fat covering; waist and abdominal fat pad distinguishable but not obvious; abdominal tuck absent.

7 Ribs not easily palpated with moderate fat covering; waist poorly discernible; obvious rounding of abdomen; moderate abdominal fat pad.

8 Ribs not palpable with excess fat covering; waist absent; obvious rounding of abdomen with prominent abdominal fat pad; fat deposits present over lumbar area.

9 Ribs not palpable under heavy fat cover; heavy fat deposits over lumbar area, face and limbs; distention of abdomen with no waist; extensive abdominal fat deposits.

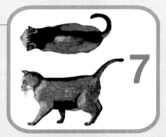

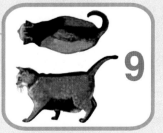

The BODY CONDITION SYSTEM was developed at the Nestlé Purina Pet Care Centre and has been validated as documented in the following publications:

Laflamme DP. **Development and Validation of a Body Condition Score System for Cats: A Clinical Tool.** *Feline Practice 1997; 25:13-17*

Laflamme DP, Hume E, Harrison J. **Evaluation of Zoometric Measures as an Assessment of Body Composition of Dogs and Cats.** *Compendium 2001; 23(Suppl 9A):88*

Body Condition Scores in cats. Image and intellectual property items are produced with the kind permission of Société des Produits Nestlé S.A.

Table 6-2 Muscle condition score

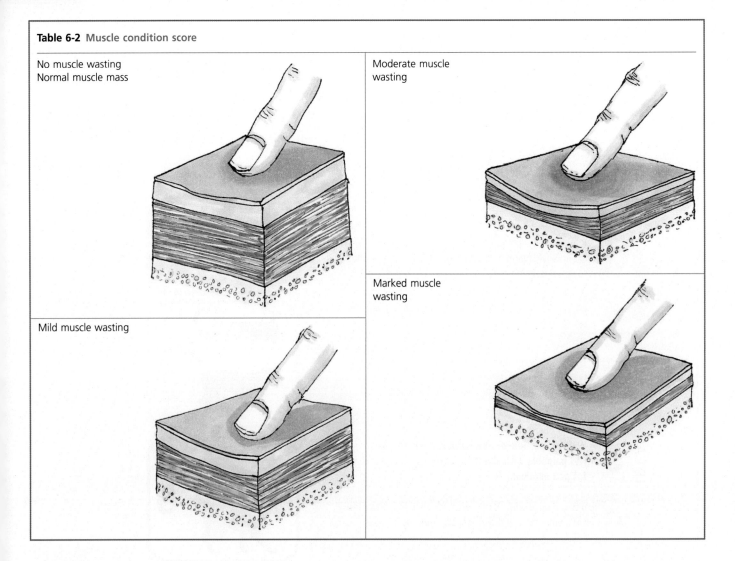

No muscle wasting
Normal muscle mass

Moderate muscle wasting

Marked muscle wasting

Mild muscle wasting

Kittens

No studies provide good evidence for the most appropriate preoperative fasting times for kittens. Similar to current recommendation for adult animals, many clinicians provide a small morning feed three to four hours prior to anesthesia to decrease the risk of hypoglycemia.[30] Checking blood glucose concentration at induction and intermittently during a procedure and treating as needed may be recommended for very young kittens, especially for longer procedures.

Diabetic cats

Where possible, surgery should be delayed until the cat's diabetic state is stable and reasonably well controlled with insulin. While surgery itself is not a greater risk for a well-controlled diabetic patient than for a healthy animal, the preoperative fast and the anesthetic drugs may cause problems, as can stresses which cause release of counter-regulatory (diabetogenic) hormones promoting insulin resistance and ketogenesis.[31] Even short hypoglycemic episodes may cause brain damage and hyperglycemia can cause an osmotic diuresis.[11]

Various different options are available for diabetic cats (Chapter 2); ultimately, careful monitoring of blood glucose is essential in all cases. One option is to provide food and insulin in the morning as normal

Table 6-3 Adjusting dextrose and insulin doses prior to anesthesia

Morning blood glucose (mmol/L) (before insulin)	2.5–3% dextrose infusion	Insulin (percentage of normal dose)
<5.5	Yes	None
5.5–11	Yes	25%
11	Not until glucose is ≤8 mmol/L	50%

and anesthetize in the afternoon. Otherwise, insulin should be administered in the morning, but if the cat will not be fed, the insulin dose should be adjusted[31] as recommended in Table 6-3.

During anesthesia the cat's blood glucose concentrations should be monitored every 30 to 60 minutes and dextrose administered to maintain a blood glucose concentration between 8.5 and 14 mmol/L. If the cat's blood glucose remains persistently above 17 mmol/L, regular crystalline insulin may be administered at 20% of the cat's normal dose. The following day, the usual schedule can be maintained unless the cat is not eating. If that occurs, it may be necessary to use intravenous dextrose and subcutaneous regular crystalline insulin (every six to eight hours) until the cat is eating regularly.

ASSESSING THE NEED FOR NUTRITION POSTOPERATIVELY

Nutritional support is essential for recovery of postoperative patients. Nutritional depletion in people increases the risk for postoperative complications[32] and is associated with reduced systemic immunity, exaggerated stress response, poor wound healing, and delayed recovery.[4] Within 24 hours of starvation changes in metabolism and function occur, including increased insulin resistance and reduced muscle function.[33] Providing nutrition in the postoperative period improves wound healing, muscle function, insulin resistance, and reduces the risk of sepsis.

When healthy animals or humans are starved (simple starvation), they primarily use fat as an energy source after glycogen stores are utilized. When ill or injured individuals are starved (stressed starvation), they catabolize more protein due to alterations in cytokines and hormones.[34] In cats, which have continuous gluconeogenesis, the mobilization of amino acids from muscles is more pronounced than in other species. Without nutritional support and adequate dietary protein, muscle catabolism is used to provide the liver with amino acids for gluconeogenesis and the acute phase protein response.[35] Cats are unable to adapt their urea cycle enzymes or amino transferase enzymes to reduced protein intake, so are less able to conserve protein than omnivorous species. These factors combine to cause rapid protein malnutrition and a negative protein balance in anorexic cats.[34-36] In healthy cats, impairment of immune function can be demonstrated by the fourth day of starvation; this would likely occur sooner in postoperative cats due to stress.[37]

What and when to feed postoperatively

The timing of feeding patients postoperatively has been controversial, especially after gastrointestinal surgery. Concerns about postoperative gastric ileus, vomiting, and intestinal incisional breakdown have meant oral feeding has been previously withheld in humans until the return of bowel function, defined as the passage of flatus or feces in the absence of vomiting or abdominal distension.[38] For most cats, offering food within 24 hours would be a reasonable recommendation even after most gastrointestinal surgeries. If the cat does not eat within two days, supplemental nutrition (e.g., feeding tube) may be advisable.

Parenteral nutrition

Because of the concerns about early enteral feeding, parenteral nutrition (PN) has been used postoperatively in people. This resulted in a high rate of septic complications and infections possibly related to bacterial translocation across the intestinal tract, especially of Gram negative coliforms.[4] Increased bacterial translocation occurs during starvation or parenteral nutrition. In humans, postoperative PN has shown benefit only in severely malnourished patients. In those with less severe malnutrition, results of PN use postoperatively have been mixed and sometimes associated with a worse outcome. Another potential complication with PN is hyperglycemia. Stressed or ill cats are at risk for hyperglycemia due to increased gluconeogenesis, depressed glycogenesis, glucose intolerance, and peripheral insulin resistance, and hyperglycemia has been associated with a poorer outcome for feline critical care patients.[39] Hyperglycemia that is caused or exacerbated by PN may be controlled by using lower rates or amounts of infusion (e.g., partial parenteral nutrition) or with insulin.[40] The lipids usually used in PN are based on n-6 fatty acids such as soybean oil. Excessive amounts of n-6 fatty acids may have a negative effect on the immune system, and replacing part of the lipid with n-3 fatty acids, monoglycerides (e.g., olive oil) or medium chain triglycerides has shown some benefits in human patients.[41]

Enteral nutrition support

When feasible, enteral nutrition is preferred to parenteral nutrition. For patients not severely malnourished and not requiring PN, withholding of enteral or oral nutrition for several days has been previously recommended; however, numerous studies in people and dogs have shown that early enteral nutrition, within 24 hours postoperatively, is beneficial for enhanced immunocompetence, reduced postoperative infections, maintenance of gut structure and function, shorter length of hospital stay, and decreased mortality rates.[42-46] Early enteral nutrition can potentially attenuate the catabolic stress responses after surgery.[45] Also, withholding nutritional support, especially in overweight cats, increases the risk of hepatic lipidosis.[36] The main complication with early postoperative feeding is an increased incidence of vomiting, likely due to gastroparesis causing ileus.[33]

Using enteral nutrition in cycles, e.g., for 6 to 12 hours, rather than continuously, has been found to improve gastric function after pancreatoduodenectomy in humans.[46] In this study, plasma cholecystokinin (CCK) concentrations stayed high in patients fed continuously, which was thought to delay the time to normal diet intake. Continuous feeding, via CCK and possibly other neurohormonal feedback mechanisms, impaired gastric emptying, prolonged postoperative gastroparesis and possibly suppressed appetite. The use of systemic opioids for analgesia also contributes to delayed gastric emptying.

Immunomodulation of enteral nutritional supplementation has been used to influence the metabolic response postoperatively. Studies in pharmaconutrition, the use of nutrients as drugs, include the use of anti-oxidants, glutamine, n-3 fatty acids, and arginine.[47-52] Major surgery induces production of reactive oxygen species, and levels of anti-oxidants such as glutathione, vitamin C, vitamin E, β-carotene, zinc, and selenium are reduced while the pro-inflammatory mediators C-reactive protein, interleukin-6, and tumor necrosis factor receptor 55 are increased.[49] In patients given enteral nutrition enriched with glutamine and anti-oxidants (vitamins C and E, β-carotene, zinc, and selenium) the immunoinflammatory response was modified.[49] Postoperative enteral nutrition enriched with the n-3 fatty acid, eicosapentenoic acid, improved maintenance of lean body mass and attenuated the stress response in humans.[52] Glutamine has been proposed to improve the tropism of enterocytes and colonocytes, enhance the immune barrier, act as a substrate for glutathione (which has anti-oxidant actions), and decrease intestinal bacterial translocation.[48] Supplementation of arginine, a conditionally essential amino acid, has been demonstrated to improve wound healing in people, and enhances lymphocyte response in postoperative patients.[47,53] It functions in the urea cycle and improves nitrogen retention. While promising, the benefits of immunomodulation have not been documented in cats, and the safety, efficacy, and dosages need to be determined before their use is recommended.

Though no studies have been done in cats to determine the optimal postoperative feeding protocol, early feeding with small amounts of easily digested foods within the first day after surgery and feeding meals rather than continuously appears to be a reasonable approach. If vomiting or nausea is present then medical treatment is recommended, and this may also improve gastric emptying.

HOW TO CALCULATE NUTRITIONAL ENERGY REQUIREMENTS

Monitoring of the patient's food intake is important, as often medical records only note that 'the patient ate', and do not describe the quantity or type of food. Basal energy requirement (BER) is the energy needed for a healthy resting animal in a postabsorptive (unfed) state in a thermoneutral environment. Resting energy requirement (RER) is BER plus the energy needed for assimilation of food. It is estimated to be about 10% greater than BER, but this difference is unlikely to have any clinical significance. The RER is the same as resting energy expenditure (REE). The most widely used and recommended allometric formula for RER in cats is shown in Box 6-3.

Maintenance energy requirement (MER) is the energy required by an animal with a moderately active life. It is usually estimated as a multiple of RER, e.g., 1.2–1.4 × RER for cats. It does not include energy needed for growth, gestation, or lactation. It has been shown that the heavier a cat is, the more likely that the energy requirements may be overestimated. An alternative equation for estimation of MER for lean cats (BCS 5/9 or less) is 100 kcal × BW0.67, and for overweight cats with a BCS of 6/9 or more, the alternative formula is 130 × BW0.4.[54] As there is considerable individual variation among cats, using any of the formulae initially and adjusting to maintain body weight and condition is appropriate.

For hospitalized patients, some clinicians previously multiplied the RER by 1.2 to 2.0 for an illness energy requirement to increase the calories thought to be necessary for the hypermetabolism of illness or injury. However, when caloric requirements were determined using indirect calorimetry in hospitalized dogs and people, most had energy requirements near RER. Similar studies have not been done in hospitalized cats, but this is a reasonable and safe approach. Human patients with energy requirements above RER include those with head trauma and severe burns. Cats with untreated hyperthyroidism would likely also have elevated energy requirements.

In a cat that has not been eating for several days, neither enteral nor parenteral supplementation should be started at full RER. It is recommended to provide one-quarter to one-third of the calories the first day, divided into several small meals or tube-fed boluses, or as a parenteral infusion. If this is well tolerated, the amount is gradually increased to full RER over several days.

Starting at full feeding is not recommended due to the risk of the 're-feeding syndrome' in cats that have been anorexic, unable to eat, or malnourished. It is characterized by weakness, cardiac disorders, hemolytic anemia, and potentially death due to respiratory or cardiac failure. In the re-feeding of a malnourished or anorexic cat, a metabolic shift from endogenous to exogenous energy sources, particularly carbohydrates, causes reductions in serum concentrations of phosphate, magnesium and potassium, which move intracellularly under the influence of insulin. The re-feeding syndrome may be seen with either parenteral or enteral nutrition. Hypophosphatemia resulting in hemolytic anemia has been described in cats during the provision of enteral nutrition.[55] Eight of these nine cats were in poor body condition prior to feeding, and the ninth, an obese cat, had a history of anorexia. In another case of feline re-feeding syndrome, the serum phosphorus, potassium, magnesium were all deficient and the cat showed concurrent cardiac abnormalities,[56] similar to human re-feeding syndrome signs.[57] Serum concentrations of phosphorus and potassium should be monitored at least daily for the first week of nutritional support in malnourished animals. As thiamine plays a role in carbohydrate metabolism and may be depleted during starvation, provision of thiamine supplementation prior to nutrient supplementation has been recommended.[55] The risk of re-feeding syndrome supports the practice of slow initiation of full nutritional support, monitoring of electrolytes and glucose, and addition of vitamins (especially thiamine) to the nutritional formula.

OPTIMAL ROUTES FOR FEEDING

Supplemental nutritional support may be provided orally, enterally via feeding tubes such as nasoesophageal/gastric, esophageal, gastrostomy or jejunostomy tubes (Fig. 6-2), or parenterally via either a central or peripheral vein. In patients that are not initially a good anesthetic risk, nasoesophageal/nasogastric (Fig. 6-3) support can be provided prior to placement of an esophageal or gastrostomy tube (see Chapter 12). Whenever possible, enteral is preferred over parenteral feeding as it stimulates the gut-associated immune system and provides nutrients such as glutamate to the intestinal mucosa.[58] Enteral nutrition is generally safer and more economical than PN. A decision tree for choosing the route for nutritional support is provided in Figure 6-4. Enteral nutrition can be combined with PN if insufficient amounts cannot be tolerated enterally (Fig. 6-5).

TEMPTING CATS TO EAT

Where possible and appropriate, persuading a cat to eat is preferred over other feeding methods. The type of food and the amount eaten must be monitored, as often the cat will be recorded as having eaten when the calories and protein consumed are still inadequate.

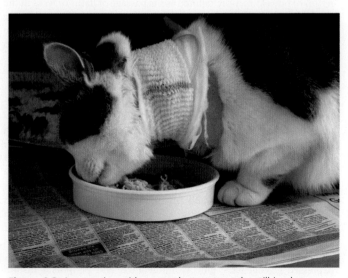

Figure 6-2 A cat eating with an esophagostomy tube still in place. *(Courtesy of SaraAnn Dickson.)*

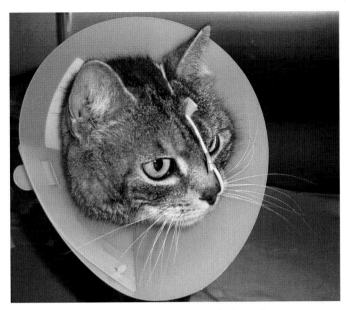

Figure 6-3 A cat with a nasoesophagostomy feeding tube.

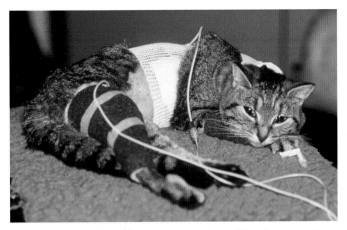

Figure 6-5 A cat with a jejunostomy tube plus peripheral parenteral nutrition via a catheter in the saphenous vein. *(Courtesy of Danielle Gunn-Moore.)*

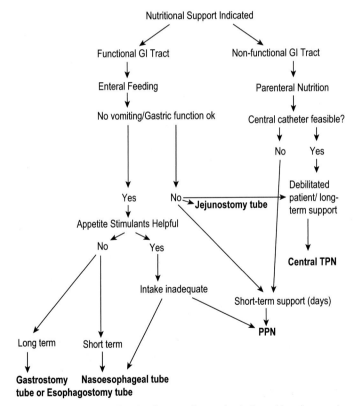

Figure 6-4 Algorithm for deciding on the method of nutritional support.

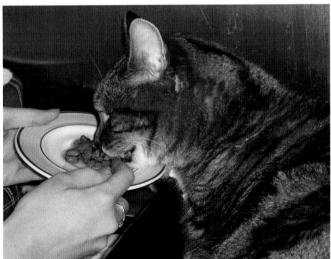

Figure 6-6 Tempting a cat to eat by hand feeding.

diet history should include the cat's preference. Warming the food to just below body temperature (e.g., the temperature of a freshly killed mouse) may help encourage intake. If this is not successful, colder foods may be tried, as cats show variation in their preferences. Some cats will eat while being petted or offered food by hand (Fig. 6-6). Placing a small amount of wet food gently in the cat's mouth or on his paws may initiate feeding. A variety of foods may be offered, but wet food should be removed if not eaten. Some cats will only eat at night when the wards are quiet. Tempting cats to eat often involves experimenting with a variety of foods and feeding patterns. Use caution with processed human foods (e.g., baby food) as some contain dried onion, which is toxic to cats.[59]

DRUGS TO STIMULATE APPETITE

Anti-emetics can be useful in cats which will not eat, as nausea may be present without vomiting. Metoclopramide promotes gastric emptying and acts centrally on the chemoreceptor trigger zone to decrease vomiting and nausea, although the effects are less potent in cats than in dogs. Ondansetron and dolasetron mesylate also act on the

Providing a safe environment for cats is important as many will not eat when stressed. The cats should be able to hide, e.g., in cardboard boxes in the kennel, and should not be exposed to barking dogs. Ideally a ward housing only cats should be used, and the cats should not be easily able to see other cats. The use of feline pheromones may help calm some cats.

Feeding frequent small meals, a normal eating pattern for cats, is beneficial. Cats generally prefer moist, high fat, high protein foods with acidic pH and strong aromas. Some cats prefer dry food and the

chemoreceptor trigger zone. While at the time of writing, maropitant has not been approved for use in cats, it has been used as a feline anti-emetic, and safety and pharmacokinetic studies for the prevention of emesis and motion sickness in cats have been performed.[60] Maropitant binds the neurokinin (NK) type 1 receptors so they cannot bind substance P. This blocks stimuli to the final common pathway in the emetic center, suppressing both central and peripheral causes of emesis.

Several drugs have been used to stimulate appetite in cats. Cyproheptadine, an antiserotoninergic, stimulates appetite in many cats, though it can cause excitability, aggression and vomiting. Benzodiazepamine derivatives such as diazepam and oxazepam have been used, but their effect is short lived, and diazepam has been associated with hepatic necrosis in cats.[61] Generally, while the cat is hospitalized, enteral or parenteral nutritional support is better than appetite stimulants, which may be more useful once the cat is recovering at home.

REFERENCES

1. Hassen TA, Pearson S, Cowled PA, Fitridge RA. Preoperative nutritional status predicts the severity of the systemic inflammatory response syndrome (SIRS) following major vascular surgery. Eur J Vasc Endovasc Surg 2007;33: 696–702.

2. D'Alegría B, Cohen C, Medeiros F, Portari Filho PE. Nutritional diagnosis obtained by subjective global assessment in surgical patients and occurrence of post-operative complications. Nutr Hosp 2008;23:619–29.

3. Smith RC, Ledgard JP, Doig G, et al. An effective automated nutrition screen for hospitalized patients. Nutrition 2009;25:309–15.

4. McClave SA, Snider HL, Spain DA. Preoperative issues in clinical nutrition. Chest 1999;115:64S–70S.

5. Allison SP. Malnutrition, disease, and outcome. Nutrition 2000;16: 590–3.

6. Pennington C. Malnutrition in hospitalised patients. In: Payne-James J, Grimble G, Silk D, editors: Artificial nutrition support in clinical practice. London: Greenwich Medical Media Ltd; 2001. p. 150–64.

7. Delmi M, Rapin CH, Bengoa JM, et al. Dietary supplementation in elderly patients with fractured neck of femur. Lancet 1990;335:1013–16.

8. Doria-rose VP, Scarlett JM. Mortality rates and causes of death among emaciated cats. J Am Vet Med Assoc 2000;216: 347–51.

9. Healy LA, Ryan AM, Sutton E, et al. Impact of obesity on surgical and oncological outcomes in the management of colorectal cancer. Int J Colorectal Dis 2010;25:1293–9.

10. Amundson DE, Djurkovic S, Matwiyoff GN. The obesity paradox. Crit Care Clin Oct 2010;26:583–96.

11. Clutton RE. The medical implications of canine obesity and their relevance to anaesthesia. Br Vet J 1988;144:21–8.

12. Self, I. Personal communication, 2011.

13. Maurer J, Taren DL, Teixeria PJ, et al. The psychosocial and behavioural characteristic related to energy misreporting. Nutr Rev 2006;62 (2 Pt 1):53–66.

14. Hawthorne AJ, Butterwick RF. The feline body mass index – a simple measure of body fat content in cats. Waltham Focus 2000;10:32–3.

15. Burkholder J. Use of body condition scores in clinical assessment of the provision of optimal nutrition. J Am Vet Med 2000;217:650–4.

16. LaFlamme D. Development and validation of a body condition score system for cats: a clinical tool. J Feline Pract 1997;25:13–18.

17. Michel K, Anderson W, Cupp C, Laflamme DP. Correlation of a feline muscle mass score with body composition determined by DEXA. Abstract. Cambridge, U.K.: The Waltham International Nutritional Sciences Symposium; September 16–18, 2010.

18. Elliott DA, Backus RC, Van Loan MD, Rogers QR. Evaluation of multifrequency bioelectrical analysis for the assessment of extracellular and total body water in healthy cats. J Nutr 2002;132:1757S–9S.

19. Toll PW, Gross KL, Berryhill SA, Jewell DE. Usefulness of dual energy x-ray absorptiometry for body composition measurement in adult dogs. J Nutr 1994;124:2601S–3S.

20. Covinsky KE, Covinsky MH, Palmer RM, Sehgal AR. Serum albumin concentration and clinical assessment of nutritional status in hospitalized older people: different sides of different coins? J Am Geriatr Soc 2002;50:631–7.

21. Chandler ML, Gunn-Moore DA. Nutritional status of canine and feline patients admitted to a referral veterinary internal medicine service. Nutr 2004;134(85):2050S–2S.

22. Maxwell A, Butterwick R, Batt RM, Camacho-Hübner C. Serum insulin-like growth factor (IGF)-I concentrations are reduced by short-term dietary restriction and restored by refeeding in domestic cats (Felis catus). J Nutr 1999;129(10):1879–84.

23. Galatos AD, Rapatopoulos D. Gastro-oesophageal reflux during anaesthesia in the dog: the effect of age positioning and type of surgical procedure. Vet Rec 1995;137:479–516.

24. Kushner LI, Shofer FS. Incidence of esophageal strictures and esophagitis after

general anesthesia. Proceedings of the 8th world congress of veterinary anaesthesia. Knoxville, Tennessee USA. 2003. p. 184.

25. Raptopoulos D, Savvas I. Preoperative fasting: 'Nil per os after midnight' – time to change? Proceedings of the world small animal veterinary association world congress. 6-9 October 2004. Rhodes, Greece.

26. Savvas I, Rallis T, Raptopoulos D, et al. The effect of pre-anesthetic fasting time and type of food on gastric content volume and acidity in dogs. Vet Anesthesia and Analgesia 2009;36: 539–46.

27. Wilson DV, Evans AT, Miller R, et al. Effects of preanesthetic administration of morphine of gastro esophageal reflux and regurgitation during anesthesia in dogs. Am J Vet Res 2005;66:386–90.

28. Fearon KCH, Luff R. The nutritional management of surgical patients: enhanced recovery after surgery. Proceedings of the Nutrition Society 2003;62:807–11.

29. Raptopoulos D. To starve or not to starve? That is the question. Proceedings of the association of veterinary anesthiologists spring conference. Cambridge, U.K.: Queens College; March 30–1, 2010.

30. Root Kustritz MV. Early spay-neuter: clinical considerations. Clin Tech Small Anim Pract 2002;17(3):124–8.

31. Feldman EC, Nelson RW. Canine diabetes mellitus. In: Canine and feline endocrinology and reproduction. 3rd ed. St Louis Missouri: Saunders; 2004. p. 486–539.

32. Ward N. Nutrition support for patients undergoing gastrointestinal surgery. Nutr J 2003;1:2–18.

33. Lewis SJ, Andersen HK, Thomas S. Early enteral nutrition within 24 h of intestinal surgery versus later commencement of feeding: a systematic review and meta-analysis. J Gastrointest Surg 2009;13:569–75.

34. Elia M. Metabolic response to starvation, injury and sepsis. In: Payne-James J, Grimble G, Silk D, editors: Artificial nutrition support in clinical practice. London: Greenwich Medical Media Ltd; 2001. p. 1–34.

35. Zoran DL. The carnivore connection to nutrition in cats. J Am Vet Med Assoc 2002;221(11):1559–67.

36. Center S. Pathophysiology of liver disease: normal and abnormal function. In: Guilford WG, Center SA, Strombeck DR, Williams DA, Meyer DJ, editors: Stombeck's small animal gastroenterology. 3rd ed. Philadelphia, PA: WB Saunders Co; 1996. p. 553–631.

37. Freitag KA, Saker KE, Thomas E, Kalnitsky J. Acute starvation and subsequent refeeding affect lymphocyte subsets and proliferation in cats. J Nutr 2000;130:2444–9.

38. Pearl ML, Valea FA, Fischer M, et al. A randomized controlled trial of early postoperative feeding in gynecologic oncology patients undergoing intra-abdominal surgery. Obstet Gynecol 1998;92:94–7.

39. Chan DL, Freeman LM, Rozanski EA, et al. Alterations in carbohydrate metabolism in critically ill cats. J Vet Emerg Crit Care 2006;16: S7–S17.

40. Thorell A, Nordenström J. Metabolic complications of parenteral nutrition. In: Payne-James J, Grimble G, Silk D, editors: Artificial nutrition support in clinical practice. London: Greenwich Medical Media Ltd; 2001. p. 445–59.

41. Calder PC. Symposium 4: hot topics in parenteral nutrition – rationale for using new lipid emulsions in parenteral nutrition and a review of the trials performed in adults. Proceedings of the Nutrition Society 2009;68: 252–60.

42. Donabedian H. Nutritional therapy and infectious diseases: a two-edged sword. Nutrition Journal 2006;5:21–30.

43. Goonetilleke KS, Siriwardena AK. Systematic review of perioperative nutritional supplementation in patients undergoing pancreaticoduodenectomy. J Parent Enteral Nutr 2006;7(1):5–13.

44. Kawasaki N, Suzuki Y, Nakayoshi T, et al. Early postoperative enteral nutrition is useful for recovering gastrointestinal motility and maintaining the nutritional status. Surg Today 2009;39:255–30.

45. Nagata S, Fukuzawa K, Iwashita Y, et al. Comparison of enteral nutrition with combined enteral and parenteral nutrition in post-pancreaticoduodenectomy patients: a pilot study. Nutrition Journal 2009;8:24–6.

46. van Berge Henegouwen MI, Akkermans LM, van Gulik TM, et al. Prospective, randomized trial on the effect of cyclic versus continuous enteral nutrition on postoperative gastric function after pylorus-preserving pancreatoduodenec-tomy. Ann Surg 1997;226:685–7.

47. Hulsewé O'Toole T, Chan DL. Nutrition support for the surgical patient. In: Payne-James J, Grimble G, Silk D, editors: Artificial nutrition support in clinical practice. London: Greenwich Medical Media Ltd; 2001. p. 605–16.

48. García-de-Lorenzo A, Zarazaga A, García-Luna PP, et al. Clinical evidence for enteral nutritional support with glutamine: a systematic review. Nutrition 2003;19:805–11.

49. van Stijn MF, Boelens PG, Richir MC, et al. Antioxidant-enriched enteral nutrition and immuno-inflammatory response after major gastrointestinal surgery. Br J Nutr 2010;103:314–28.

50. Bengmark S. Econutrition and health maintenance – a new concept to prevent GI inflammation, ulceration and sepsis. Clin Nutr 1996;16:24–8.

51. McClave SA, Chang WK, Dhaliwal R, Heyland DK. Nutrition support in acute pancreatitis: a systemic review of the literature. J Parenter Enteral Nutr 2006;30:143–56.

52. Ryan AM, Reynolds JV, Healy L, et al. Enteral nutrition enriched with eicosapentaenoic acid (EPA) preserves lean body mass following esophageal cancer surgery: results of a double-blinded randomized controlled trial. Ann Surg 2009;249:364–5.

53. Saker KE. Nutrition and immune function. Vet Clinics North Am Small Anim Pract 2006;36:1199–224.

54. National Research Council. Chapter 3. Energy. In: Nutrient requirements of dogs and cats. Washington DC: The National Academies Press; 2006. p. 28–48.

55. Justin RB, Hohenhaus AE. Hypophosphatemia associated with enteral alimentation in cats. J Vet Intern Med 1995;9:228–33.

56. Armitage-Chan EA, O'Toole T, Chan DL. Management of prolonged food deprivation, hypothermia, and refeeding syndrome in a cat. J Vet Emerg Crit Care 2006;16:S34–41.

57. Solomon SN, Kirby DS. The refeeding syndrome: a review. J Parent Enter Nutr 1990;14:90–5.

58. Saker KE, Remillard RL. Critical care nutrition and enteral assisted feeding. In: Small animal clinical nutrition. 5th ed. Topeka, Kansas, USA: Mark Morris Institute; 2010. p. 446–76.

59. Robertson JE, Christopher MM, Rogers QR. Heinz body formation in cats fed baby food containing onion powder. J Am Med Vet Assoc 1998;212:1260–6.

60. Hickman MA, Cox SR, Mahabir S, et al. Safety, pharmacokinetics and the use of the novel NK-1 Receptor antagonist maropitant (Cerenia) for the prevention of emesis and motion sickness in cats. J Vet Pharmacol Ther 2008;31: 220–9.

61. Chan DL. Nutritional support of critically ill patients. Waltham Focus 2006; 16(3):9–15.

Section | 2 |

S.J. Langley-Hobbs, J.F. Ladlow, J.L. Demetriou

Diagnostics, equipment and implants

There are many modifications that can be made to the practice, waiting room and cat ward that can ensure the cat is treated in an optimum environment and that may also minimize stress and fear that a visit to the vet may initiate. Advice and training for both owners and staff in aspects of feline behavior will help with both transporting the cat to the practice and improving owner satisfaction. Cats can be fastidious eaters, thus stress and pain following surgery can contribute to a reluctance to eat. In anticipation of postoperative anorexia, it can be sensible to place a feeding tube, and the types of tube to use and where and how to place the tube are described in a chapter on feeding tubes.

Investigating feline diseases both preoperatively and postoperatively will often require diagnostic imaging, including radiology and ultrasound or more advanced imaging such as computed tomography or magnetic resonance imaging. The more advanced imaging techniques may be particularly useful for obtaining information on metastasis and invasiveness of tumors, which can be very helpful in deciding whether surgery is indicated or planning for large surgical resections. Endoscopy is increasingly used to investigate conditions of the respiratory, gastrointestinal, and urinary tracts. The specific equipment required for this procedure, including the appropriate sizes to use in the cat, is described in a separate chapter.

The remaining chapters in Part 2 cover the indications and practical use of sutures, implants, instruments, and surgical drains that could be valuable in feline general surgery.

Chapter | 7 |

Cats in the practice

S. Rudd, J.L. Demetriou, S.J. Langley-Hobbs

For cats, a visit to a veterinary practice can be a stressful experience that begins as soon as there is a small alteration in the cat's routine. Changes such as fasting the cat in the morning, or the cat finding the cat flap locked can cause anxiety. Anything unfamiliar or threatening that the cat then sees, hears, smells, or experiences such as the sight of the cat basket, or being placed into it, followed by a journey to the clinic, is frequently stressful. This stress may then escalate into fear and a cat's natural response to fear is to run away and hide, i.e., the flight response. However, due to the physical restrictions of being in the cat basket and then the inevitable physical handling that occurs within the veterinary practice, cats are often unable to utilize the flight response and so they are only left with one option, which is to fight. This chapter, therefore, will cover all aspects of a cat's visit to the vet from home and on to the cat ward, with information provided on how to make the visit as stress free as possible.

REDUCING FELINE STRESS IN THE PRACTICE

Stress recognition

Fear and anxiety in cats may first manifest as changes in ear position, eyes and facial expression, body position, sweating from the paw pads, and tail movement (Figure 7-1).[1] Fearful cats may attempt escape, and vocalization such as hissing can indicate an escalation in stress. Overt aggressive behavior can include scratching and biting. Some fearful cats will freeze. It can sometimes be difficult to distinguish between stressed and fearful cats with those in pain. The cat-friendly practice publications and feline-friendly handling guidelines contain more information about recognition of fear and anxiety in cats.[2-4]

Management of stress

Fear aggression is commonly seen in all veterinary practices and yet it is still widely unrecognized and often misinterpreted as dominance behavior, or it is casually disregarded as a negative character trait. How a cat's behavior is interpreted will have a significant influence on how it is approached, handled, treated, and understood. Negative feelings, attitudes and poor handling techniques of a cat with fear and fear aggression will only heighten the problem. Conversely, empathy, a calm approach and careful consideration as to how to make the environment less stressful for cats will have an extremely positive impact, possibly leading to all cats receiving better treatment and more accurate and thorough monitoring. There is also the added benefit that there will be a reduction in stress for the staff as well as the cat. Stress can have a significant impact on a cat's appetite and immune system and so a reduction in stress will aid a better and more rapid recovery, which may then allow earlier discharge home.

Ideally, stress reduction should start at home and so providing accurate and concise advice to clients about getting their cat to the veterinarian is important from the very first time they contact the practice (Box 7-1).[5]

Putting measures in place to help reduce stress for cats within the practice does not mean a complete renovation of the premises. Many things can be improved, even within a small practice, to make it more cat friendly. To do this, it is necessary to 'think cat' and imagine how a cat would feel entering the clinic in its current set up. Cats have incredibly strong senses and they are very instinctive animals, so it is important to think about what a cat may see, hear, smell or experience at the practice.

WAITING ROOM

In the reception area or waiting room one of the most typical causes of stress is the sight, smell and sound of dogs. So one of the main aims is to keep these two species separate. Stress can be significantly reduced by having a separate waiting room for cats; however, this may not be possible for many mixed practices, so some alternative options are available (Table 7-1 and Fig. 7-2). If a cat-only waiting room is not possible then moving the cat out of the waiting room into the examination room as quickly as possible can be helpful, particularly if there are barking dogs in the waiting room. Wide shelves on the wall or benches, and a ledge near reception for placing the carrier on prevent the need to place the cat at ground level, which is also dog level and can be intimidating and fearful for the cat.

DOI: 10.1016/B978-0-7020-4336-9.00007-X

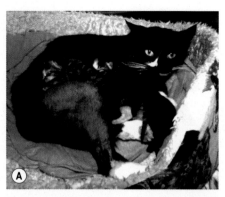
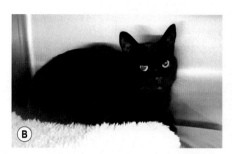
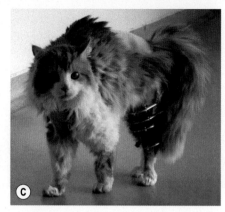

Figure 7-1 (A) A very scared feral cat with flattened ears and narrowed eyes. This cat is recovering after surgery for a hip fracture and hip dislocation and cesarean. **(B)** A cat showing mild signs of fear, seated at the rear of the cage, with dilated pupils and pricked ears. **(C)** A fearful cat with the classic 'bottlebrush' tail and arched back indicating fear escalating to aggression.

Box 7-1 Advice for owners on getting their cat to the veterinary clinic[5]

Behavior

Cats like familiar things – the cat carrier, car and veterinary clinic are unfamiliar and can cause stress

Stay calm – cats will sense changes in emotions

Reward positive behavior such as the cat sitting calmly near the carrier

Familiarize the cat with being examined, e.g., handling ears, feet, mouth, etc.

Accustomization

Leave the cat carrier in a room where the cat spends time

Put familiar used bedding inside it with the cat's scent on it

Place treats, toys, catnip inside the carrier

Be patient – accustomization may take time

If the cat still dislikes the carrier – assess the carrier itself

Getting the cat into the carrier

If accustomization has not been successful or has had insufficient time to work then:

Place the carrier in a small room with no hiding places

Stay calm and encourage the cat into carrier with treats / toys

For top opening carriers lift reluctant cats in, cradling them gently

Use familiar bedding inside the carrier

Consider use of feline pheromone spray (Feliway) inside the carrier thirty minutes prior to transport

The return

In multi-cat households a returning cat will smell differently, which may cause aggression from other cats. Minimize this by:

Leave returnee in the carrier for a few minutes to assess the other cats' reaction

If all cats appear calm and peaceful the cat can be released

If tension is present, or previous conflict has occurred then keep the cat separate for 24 hours

If there is still stress after this time, contact your veterinarian

Synthetic pheromones (e.g., Feliway) can help provide sense of familiarity

The carrier

Carriers that open from the top and front are ideal

Some cats can remain in the bottom of a top opening carrier and be examined in the base where it feels secure

Avoid carriers where the cat has to be pulled out

Choose sturdy strong carriers (cardboard ones can be fought out of by a determined fearful cat)

Consider covering the carrier with a blanket – some cats feel less anxious if they cannot see out

---

THE CONSULTATION

The consulting room

Within the consulting room, the first sources of stress that need to be considered will come from the general environment and in particularly the smell, sounds and lighting. Many of the ideas suggested in Table 7-1 can also be incorporated into the consulting room and again it is essential to try and 'see' the consulting room from a cat's point of view. The other source of stress will be the structure of the consultation and the approach of the attending clinician or nurse to the cat.

The consulting room should be suitable and secure so that the cat carrier can be placed on the ground and the door opened. It will be much less stressful for the cat if it is allowed to come out of the carrier on its own accord rather than have a pair of unfamiliar hands dragging it out. Cats that will not leave the carrier should be lifted out by removing the top of the carrier, if this is possible; it is much less confrontational to lift the cat from above than to pull the cat out from the front opening (Fig. 7-3). Top opening baskets are therefore recommended for cats.

Once out of their basket, cats frequently want to wander around the consulting room to assess their environment; and therefore they should be given this opportunity while the history is being taken. It

Table 7-1 Ways to reduce stress for the cat in the practice

Ways to reduce stress/fear	Senses it will help		
	Sight	Hearing	Smell
Have cat-only appointment/surgery times	✓	✓	✓
Section off part of the waiting room for cats only and ensure cats do not have to pass dogs to get there	✓		
Have a supply of towels/blankets for owners to cover their cats' carriers if they wish	✓		
Have ledges for people to rest their cat carriers on so that the cat is elevated from the ground	✓		
Have seat dividers between groups/pairs of seats (Fig. 7-2)	✓		
Section one end of the reception desk for cats only so owners can register and pay with no dogs around	✓		
Offer an option of the cat staying in the car until the consultation room is ready (if it is not too hot)	✓	✓	✓
Display notices asking clients to ensure their dog does not approach cats in their carriers	✓		
Use pheromone plug in/sprays			✓
Have calming music playing, e.g., classical or rainforest sounds		✓	

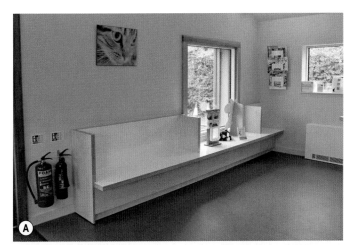

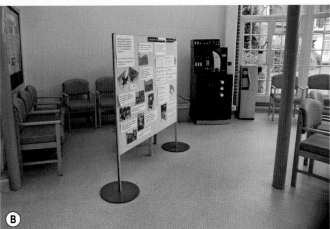

Figure 7-2 Options for feline-friendly waiting rooms. **(A)** A feline-only waiting room; the bench has been specially designed for cat carriers to be placed on them, and partitions provide the option of not placing cats adjacent to each other. **(B)** A section of this mixed cat and dog waiting room is divided by a screen to provide separate areas for cats and dogs. *([A] Courtesy of Cambridge Cat Clinic.)*

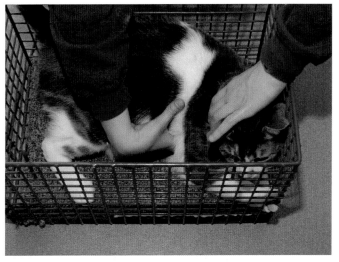

Figure 7-3 Cat basket with a top opening lid provides easy access for gently removing the cat from the basket.

is important to ensure that there are no small corners or gaps between or under the consulting room furniture that a cat may decide to hide in, which could cause a confrontational struggle to get the cat out of. Confronting a stressed cat in this way will only cause fear, which may well result in fear aggression. A cat that is stressed before the clinical examination has been conducted will inevitably be a less than ideal patient and the resulting difficulty in handling will only lead to further stress and possibly aggression.

Having a litter tray in the consulting room may be welcomed by some cats who have been kept indoors leading up to the trip to the veterinary surgery and then have had a stressful journey to the practice. Examining a cat with a full bladder may be stressful for the cat and they may be reluctant to sit still, and become agitated. Litter trays must be completely changed after every use as the smell of another cat's waste could be very threatening to the cat, as well as a potential source of infection. A set of weighing scales in the consulting room will not only be a reminder to weigh the cat at each visit but also make it a less stressful experience by not needing to take the cat back into the waiting room or ward to be weighed.

Offering guidance to owners as to how they should behave around their cat and how to interact positively with their cat to help reduce its stress levels can also help (Box 7-2), but care should be taken to present this in an empathetic manner.

The clinical examination

Some cats may find it less threatening to have the clinical examination performed at their own level, on the floor. If this is not practical or possible then lifting the cat onto the table should be done with a calm, slow and smooth approach, allowing them to sniff your hands first, then after a few strokes, scooping them up underneath their caudal thorax. If the cat is very stressed then it may exhibit fear aggression, so lifting in the same way but with one hand placed gently over the back of the neck will block the cat's view of the other hand approaching and also give more control if the cat attempts to bite. If the consulting room has a window, then it is well worth placing the examination table next to it so the cat can look outside while performing the clinical examination, as this can be a great distraction technique. Non-slip matting (e.g., a rubber mat, yoga mat or plastic table top cover) is essential for table-tops when examining cats; in addition, having a non-slip blanket on top for the cat to sit on can help them feel more at ease.

Consideration should be given to the uniform the examiner is wearing as examining a cat while wearing a scrub top rather than a white coat may be less stressful for some cats, especially if they have had a previous bad or frightening experience at a veterinary practice.

During the examination it is important to have the cat facing away from the person conducting the examination as this is less confrontational: approaching a cat face-on or staring at it can seem very threatening to them. When examining the cat's head where eye contact will be necessary, slow blinking in front of the cat conveys friendliness and trust.[6] Some components of the examination will be more stressful than others, e.g., taking the temperature, so these parts should be left until the end. Tickling the cat around the back of the ears and along the sides of the face will also often relax some cats while transferring the cat's own pheromone onto your hands. No amount of pheromones, however, will replace a good, calm handling technique. Scruffing is a very dominant and aggressive way to hold a cat, resulting in confrontation and excessive power over a cat that will lead to further stress and fear and so this technique should be avoided if

possible. For a full description of a clinical examination of the cat see Chapter 1.

The tone of voice used can make a huge difference to how a cat will respond. Nervous, fearful and especially fear aggressive cats respond to gentle, calm tones of voice, with physical contact being minimal and slow. Certain words should be avoided, particularly those which may sound like a hiss such as 'shh. …' or more blunt sounding words such as 'stop it!'. Calm reassuring words such as 'it's alright …' phrased in a sighed breath will be much more effective and also help you to keep calm if you are feeling nervous by keeping your breathing slow, steady and deep. Sometimes if the cat is getting stressed, simply stopping the examination for a short period of time can be enough to allow the cat to relax again.

Feline facial pheromones

The use of pheromones is an increasing phenomenon in veterinary practice, with the aim of reducing stress in the patient. They can be used in many environmental situations including in the waiting room, consultation room and ward as well as being directly applied to the clinician's hands while handling or examining the cat. Hospitalized cats that had synthetic feline facial pheromone (FFP) applied to a towel in their cages significantly increased both their grooming behaviors and food intake.[7] Exposing cats to synthetic FFP during premedication also made cats calmer during venous catheterization.[8] A diffuser is best for housing areas, and a spray for application to towels, cages and tables.

CAT WARD

A feline-only ward is certainly the most preferable choice when hospitalizing cats (Fig. 7-4). It is also important that a ward, whether feline-only or mixed, is used as a place of rest. Any procedure such as taking a blood sample or measuring blood pressure should be done away from the ward so that the patient having the procedure performed is not seen or heard by the other patients. It is also preferable for the patient itself that procedures are performed elsewhere, so that they associate the ward with being a place of calm and not with anxiety and stress.

Cats should be hospitalized in quiet wards with minimal traffic and away from dogs. If this is not possible, then kennels should be selected to minimize the stress, e.g., kennels furthest away from dogs, kennels that are quieter and free from traffic and kennels that are of suitable height to ensure minimal confrontation from people and dogs. It is also important to choose kennels that give consideration to the ease and safety of lifting a cat in and out of the cage. To help cats feel even more secure, the kennels can be pre-treated with a feline pheromone spray.

The ideal cat ward should be fairly small in size (housing up to 12 cats) as too many cats in the ward can be stressful. Cats are not sociable with each other unless within their own social group, and so if a cat can smell, hear or see any other cats this will cause stress. The cages should be positioned so they are on one wall and do not face other cages, or so that they are at a 90° angle to each other (Fig. 7-4). It is useful to have cages of different sizes to accommodate the patients' specific needs, e.g., larger kennels for larger cats and those who have no exercise restriction, or for use for patients who are to be hospitalized for longer periods of time. Some cages with shelving incorporated in the cage will be more desirable for cats, as sitting on an elevated shelf will help them feel more secure. If a cat is having a surgical procedure they may need to have their movement restricted postoperatively but it is important to ensure that the cat has enough room

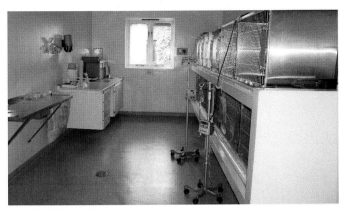

Figure 7-4 A feline-only ward with kennels facing the wall. A small ward housing no more than 12 cats is ideal. Two different-sized kennels are available for different-sized patients and differing length stays.

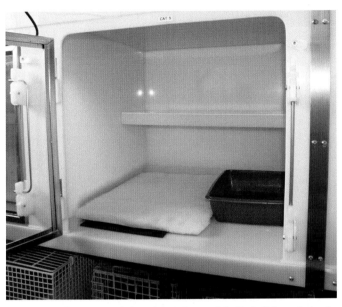

Figure 7-5 This custom designed cage has an inbuilt shelf for cats to sit on. *(Courtesy of Cambridge Cat Clinic.)*

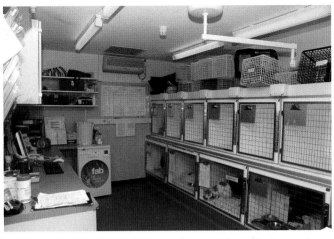

Figure 7-6 Non-stainless steel cages are warmer, less reflective and less noisy and are preferable for cats. A pheromone is shown plugged in on the far wall and cats are provided with cardboard box houses to hide or sleep in.

are used, a piece of newspaper or incontinence sheet taped to the sides of the cage may be useful to prevent this from happening.

The design of the front of the cage is also important. Perspex fronted cages have the advantage of helping to prevent aerosol-borne disease and helping in noise reduction, but they can also become quite hot and some cats do not tolerate being so enclosed. These cages are, however, useful as oxygen tents or for the nebulization of a patient. Metal open-fronted cages are therefore generally considered to be preferable and even better if they have noise reducers to lessen the sound when opening and closing the cage doors.

Bedding

Ensuring that all feline inpatients feel warm, safe and secure within their kennel is obviously essential. Putting a lining material into the kennel may not be required for cages made of fiberglass as they are not as cold as cages made from stainless steel and are easily cleaned. However, if a lining is used then it is better to use incontinence sheets rather than newspaper, as the newspaper will stain fiberglass kennels when wet and contaminate the cat with ink on contact. On top of the lining material, 'Vet Bedding' is the most appropriate bedding material for cat kennels as its soft and insulating nature makes it ideal for cats, while urine can pass through away from the patient, helping to keep them dry and reducing the risk of urine scalding.

For recumbent cats or for cats with orthopedic trauma, a mattress can be useful to give cushioning and comfort as well as helping to prevent pressure sores. Any mattress should be soft but firm and can actually provide an additional benefit for cats that are not fully ambulatory if it is the same depth as the litter tray, meaning that the cat does not have to climb into it (Fig. 7-7). The mattress should be fully covered with a waterproof layer to prevent contamination of the foam and thus becoming a fomite for infection.

Cats with diseases or injuries that cause an unsteady gait may benefit from having a non-slip surface to help them move around the kennel. Carpet tiles or a non-slip bath mat are ideal for the bottom of cages and also for when performing physiotherapy.

Hospitalization is stressful for cats and so providing them with somewhere to hide will greatly help their feeling of security. It will allow them to fulfil their natural flight response and so help to reduce the chance of fear aggression. Hiding beds such as igloos, sacks and doughnut beds are ideal in this regard (Fig. 7-8). Each cat should be

Table 7-2 Minimal suggested cage sizes for cat kennels in veterinary practices[4]			
	Height (cm)	Width (cm)	Depth (cm)
Day patient	60	60	75
Overnight patient	60	70/80	75
Longer stay	70	100	75 (or more)

for a sleeping area, litter tray, food and water bowls and that the cat is still able to stretch out and move around easily (Fig. 7-5). The minimum ideal dimension for a kennel is a width of 80 cm, depth of 75 cm and height of 56 cm (Table 7-2). Kennels made from fiberglass or plastic are preferable to stainless steel as they are warmer, less noisy and are not reflective, as some cats may find it frightening if they see a reflection of themselves (Fig. 7-6). However, if stainless steel cages

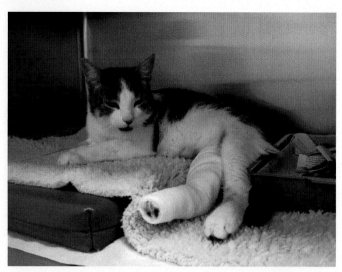

Figure 7-7 A cat recovering from surgery to its right hind limb. The cat has been provided with a mattress and vet bedding, which give a soft, comfortable and water repellent surface for resting and sleeping on.

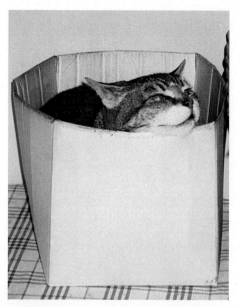

Figure 7-9 A cardboard box can provide a safe haven for a cat, and the cat can be lifted out of the cage in its box.

Bowls

Anorexia is common in hospitalized cats and so bowls for food and water should be of the correct type and size to encourage the cat to eat and drink. Most commonly, bowls are made from stainless steel, plastic or ceramic. Stainless steel autoclavable bowls are better for infection control purposes, but some cats may prefer less reflective, plastic or ceramic bowls. Ceramic bowls are good for active cats that may knock lighter bowls over and are useful for cats with limb dressings who keep knocking their water over due to poor spatial awareness and maneuverability. A clip-on bowl on the cage front is also useful for cats at risk of getting their dressing wet. Ceramic and plastic bowls are also more suitable than stainless steel for cats with magnetic collars, ensuring that the bowl does not stick to the collar. If a cat has a collar with a bell or disk on it the noise from it colliding with a stainless steel bowl as it is eating may alarm some cats and discourage them from eating. Plastic bowls are less noisy and less cold and both plastic and ceramic bowls can be easily disinfected. It is essential, however, that the disinfection is performed at the correct concentration and that the bowls are thoroughly rinsed and dried before use. Bowls for food should be shallow enough to allow a cat to eat without its whiskers touching the sides as this sensation can be off-putting for cats. The cat's muzzle size and shape should also be considered. For example, a Persian should not be given a deep bowl as they will find it difficult to reach the food. Owners may wish to bring in their own bowls to minimize the stress of unfamiliar objects but again, they must be correctly cleaned and disinfected to prevent them acting as fomites.

Cat litter

When admitting a cat into the hospital it is important to find out the cat's toileting preferences. Many cats will only toilet outside and so hospitalization can be very stressful from a toileting perspective. If a cat eliminates outside, putting soil or sand in a litter tray may be preferable to using a wood or paper based litter. However, even cats that are used to using litter trays may have a litter type preference and so it can be very helpful to check with the cat's owner on admission.

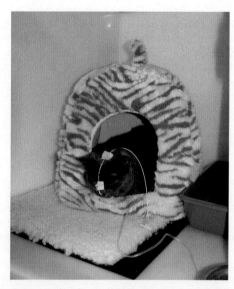

Figure 7-8 A tepee style igloo type bed provides a comfortable and safe haven for a cat while it is hospitalized for treatment. *(Courtesy of Cambridge Cat Clinic.)*

assessed to see what type of bedding is most suitable. For example, a cat who wants to hide underneath a vet bed may prefer a hiding sack to climb into rather than a tepee style igloo, whereas a slightly more confident cat may prefer a doughnut bed. The cat's temperament should also be assessed before selecting a hiding place. A bed that is difficult to get the cat out of, e.g., an igloo, will be very stressful for a fear aggressive cat. A cardboard box would be more suitable as a place to hide as it will not only provide security for the cat but make it a lot easier and less stressful for the cat as it will be simpler to remove the box (and cat) out of the cage and then lift the cat out of the top of the box (Fig. 7-9). It is important to avoid changing unsoiled bedding and cleaning marked parts of the cage as the cat will mark its territory by rubbing pheromones on parts of their cage.

Some cats may only eliminate in privacy so hooded litter trays may be helpful or, for smaller kennels, screens can be made from cardboard. The size of the litter tray should also be considered. Litter trays should be of decent size to allow the cat to get in and maneuver around comfortably (minimal size 21 cm × 31 cm). The depth of the tray is also important. Senior cats and any cat with ambulatory difficulties should have a shallow litter tray for ease of access or the access made easier still by using a mattress in the kennel the same depth as the tray. Litter trays should be cleaned out after every use as some cats will not use the litter tray again until the waste, along with any traces or smell, has been removed. To encourage normal elimination it is generally considered preferable to dispose of all of the litter and offer a fresh litter tray after every use so no trace is left. This is also a fail-safe approach to ensure no cross contamination between cats via their litter trays, which may occur if the trays are simply 'scoop cleaned;' without diligent disinfection of the scoop.

PERSONNEL

Owners will be able to detect which members of the veterinary team truly connect and offer empathy with their cats. Veterinary team members who apply both the art and science of veterinary nursing care will not only deliver optimal healthcare to the cat but earn the confidence and appreciation of the practice clients.[1] Each member of the veterinary team has a role in the cat's experience in the clinic, from the receptionist admitting the cat, to the veterinarian examining it, the veterinary nurse or technician, and ward assistants looking after the cat and nursing it when hospitalized. A team approach is therefore required to make the cat's (and owner's) visit as stress free and smooth as possible. Responsibility extends from giving advice about transporting the cat, to using feline-friendly examination techniques and recognizing feline behavior patterns.[1]

Nurses and technicians

The veterinary nurse or technician plays an important role in the practice in both caring for the cat and communicating with the owner and other members of the team. Involving the nurse can help improve efficiency and productivity in feline case management.[1] An experienced nurse should understand the basic needs of the cat, normal feline behavior, feline disease processes and subtle clinical signs that owners might overlook.[1] The nurse who is caring for the cat in the cat ward should try and develop and establish a rapport with the cat (Fig. 7-10); this will be beneficial for both the cat and the ease of nursing the cat and performing tasks such as venipuncture, catheterization, physiotherapy, dressing changes, etc. A less anxious cat will be easier to treat, making performing tasks and giving treatments easier and faster, thus saving time, and giving job satisfaction to the veterinary team, with a contented cat and tasks accomplished without aggression from the cat. Some aspects of nursing care of cats are unique: for example, cats are fastidious groomers and if unable to complete this task themselves they may need assistance. Removal of blood, tape from catheters, and antiseptic solutions by washing can decrease the amount of cleaning for the cat to do!

Time should be set aside for transfer of case responsibility to other nurses on duty, or the night staff. In addition to discussing the cat's medical problems, medication and nursing needs it is important to also discuss the cat's temperament, likes and dislikes. This information can be transferred verbally between staff or written instructions included on a sheet on the kennel, or in the animal's notes or computer record. Pertinent information would include diet, choice of food bowls, choice of bedding, and hiding place, litter tray, and any other

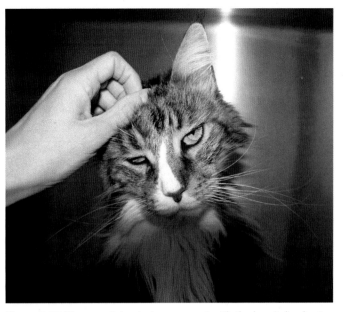

Figure 7-10 Time spent developing a rapport with the hospitalized cat, by rubbing around its head, for example, can be time well spent, reducing stress for the cat and thereby making the cat more amenable for essential procedures to be performed such as venous catheterization and venipuncture.

Box 7-3 **Nurse/technician communication with owners**
Daily communication with owners while the cat is hospitalized
Discuss and explain discharge instructions with owners
Instruct and show owners how to give medication to their cats
Petting, giving treats or stroking the cat can help
Using a bathroom sink lined with a soft towel or fleece provides an enclosed safe place for administering medication
Talk about stress reduction in the home
Discuss ways of encouraging eating in inappetent or anorexic animals
Demonstrate tube feeding
Show how to check bandages

---

special requests, such as keeping the cage covered, daily exercise, grooming, etc.

Owner communication

Many owners appreciate being able to spend time communicating with a member of the veterinary team about their cat. A significant part of this role can be delegated to the veterinary nurse or technician, particularly when the veterinarian's time may be limited; this has the benefit of increasing job satisfaction and often improving owner communication and satisfaction. There are many areas of the veterinary care and treatment on which a competent veterinary nurse or technician can communicate and demonstrate to owners very adequately (Box 7-3). Communication with the owner while the cat is hospitalized can appease the anxious owner. If an empathetic technician or nurse is talking to them on the telephone and communicating to the owner about the cat's appetite and general well-being, then that will often be more important to the owner than the veterinarian's telephone call about their cat's recovery from its illness or trauma. Often the two will go hand in hand. The nurse will also have the opportunity to ask the owner about the cat's lifestyle and preferences at home. If the cat is not urinating in the litter tray in the hospital, knowing that it always goes outside at home might prompt putting some soil in the cat's litter tray – this can often have an almost instantaneous result and prompt urination in a cat. Favourite foods, types of food bowls and bedding can also be enquired about and subsequent changes to mirror the routine at home can result in a happier and less stressed cat that is more inclined to eat while hospitalized.

It is widely held that patients remember only 80% of what they have just been told by their doctor by the time they leave the consulting room, and around 50% by the time they leave the building.[3] We should expect that pet owners would have similar powers of recall concerning their pets' health. Verbal communication with owners when discharging patients should be aided and supplemented by written instructions, with illustrations where appropriate, and demonstrations such as showing how to hold a cat for giving a tablet either on a model, their own cat, or with multimedia resources.

REFERENCES

1. Carney HC, Little S, Brownlee-Tomasso D, et al. AAFP and ISFM feline-friendly nursing care guidelines. J of Fel Med Surg 2012;14:337–49.

2. Rodan I, Sundahl E, Carney H, et al. AAFP and ISFM feline-friendly handling guidelines. J Fel Med Surg 2011;13: 364–75.

3. Riccomini F, Harvey A, Rudd S. Creating a cat friendly practice. Tisbury, UK: Feline Advisory Bureau; 2005. p. 1–41.

4. Harvey, A. Cat friendly practice 2. Tisbury, UK: Feline Advisory Bureau; 2006. p. 1–32.

5. AAFP and ISFM. Getting your cat to the veterinarian. www.fabcats.org/publications/2011_FelineFriendlyClient_Handout.pdf.

6. Natoli E, Baggio A, Pontier D. Male and female agonistic and affiliative relationships in a social group of farm cats (Felis catus L.) Behav Processes 2001;53:137–43.

7. Griffith CA, Steigerwald ES, Buffington CA. Effects of a synthetic facial pheromone on behavior of cats. J Am Vet Med Assoc 2000;217:1154–6.

8. Kronen PW, Ludders JW, Erb HN, et al. A synthetic fraction of feline facial pheromones calms but does not reduce struggling in cats before venous catheterization. Vet Anaesth Analg 2006;33:258–65.

Chapter | 8 |

Diagnostic imaging

S. Ohlerth, P. Kircher, B. Posch

Diagnostic imaging forms an essential part of the investigation for many general and oncological diseases in cats. Radiology and ultrasound remains the mainstay for initial investigations for many conditions, but with the advent of easier accessibility to advanced imaging such as computed tomography (CT) and magnetic resonance imaging (MRI) these modalities are becoming used more frequently. The indications for each imaging modality for investigation of thoracic and abdominal disease and for imaging the brain will be covered in this section. For further general information on diagnostic imaging and specifically radiography of bone diseases, the reader is referred to other specialized texts[1] and the imaging chapter in *Feline Orthopedic Surgery and Musculoskeletal Disease.*[2]

DIAGNOSTIC IMAGING MODALITIES

The present chapter focuses on the species-specific radiographic differences in the feline thorax, abdomen and neurocranium. The use of advanced imaging modalities for these areas will be briefly discussed, giving some indications where they may give additional information not provided by radiography, particularly the use of MRI for imaging the brain.

Radiology

Radiology represents the most fundamental diagnostic aid for the investigation of thoracic and abdominal soft tissue structures. It is used in conjunction with an accurate history, physical examination and other diagnostic tests. Results of the clinical, laboratory and radiographic examination may indicate the need for further diagnostic imaging. Radiographic contrast studies are routinely used to evaluate the urinary tract, the gastrointestinal tract or vascular abnormalities such as portosystemic shunts.

Ultrasound

In veterinary medicine, ultrasonography (US) is widely used for the evaluation of soft tissues in the neck, the mediastinum and, in particular, the abdomen. US is rarely specific, but it is very sensitive in depicting soft tissue disease. The size, extent, architecture, relationship to neighboring tissue and involvement of lymph nodes may be determined. For a final diagnosis, US may be used to guide fine needle aspirates or true cut biopsies.

Computed tomography

Due to an increasing availability and the advantages of multi-slice CT (fast acquisition with large anatomic coverage, thin slice thickness, increased spatial resolution), this technology has also become a highly valuable tool in veterinary medicine. As a cross-sectional imaging technique, CT avoids superimposition of adjacent structures by imaging a transverse slice. Consequently, soft tissue structures enveloped by bones e.g. the nasal cavity, brain, or pelvic organs, may be imaged well with CT whereas a radiographic image of these regions is of limited value. CT has also been increasingly used for imaging the lung, mediastinum and various abdominal organs. CT angiography is easy to perform with a peripheral intravenous injection of contrast medium (Fig. 8-1). With multi-slice CT, an arterial and venous phase, and for the liver a portal phase, can be imaged. In oncological diseases, CT angiography may indirectly help to identify and describe a neoplastic lesion on the basis of its relationship to adjacent arteries or veins (mass effect, compression and invasiveness), or the lesion itself may be outlined on the basis of its individual perfusion/contrast enhancement pattern.

Magnetic resonance imaging

MRI has long been the imaging modality of choice for neurologists and it is now also becoming a more important imaging modality for other clinical specialties. MRI has great potential for increasing use in other disease complexes, especially if soft tissue components need to be assessed, quantified and qualified. MR imaging has the potential to have a great impact in oncological and endocrinological disease in feline patients although relatively few studies exist in cats to date (Fig. 8-2).

MRI generates images without the use of X-rays. Instead it uses the magnetic properties of protons distributed in the patient's body. Two

DOI: 10.1016/B978-0-7020-4336-9.00008-1

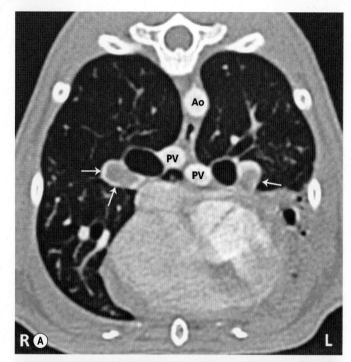

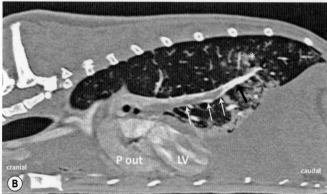

Figure 8-1 CT-angiography. **(A)** transverse plane and **(B)** left sagittal plane of a 9-year-old cat with immune-mediated hemolytic anemia and sudden onset of dyspnea and right heart failure. The pulmonary veins (PV) and the aorta (Ao) show homogeneous contrast filling; a large filling defect is seen in the right and left caudal pulmonary arteries (white arrows) consistent with thrombosis. Caudal to the thrombus, the arteries are again filled with contrast medium (black arrow). Secondary lung changes also occurred (*). P out, pulmonary outflow tract; LV, left ventricle.

MRI systems are currently in standard use in veterinary medicine, namely low-field systems (low magnetic field strength) using open scanners, and closed-bore systems with stronger magnetic fields. The open systems offer better access to the patient, the higher magnetic fields give better local resolution with slightly shorter scanning times. The higher the magnetic field, the more artefacts are possible. The high-field scanners (>1 Tesla) usually provide a large field of view (up to 50 cm) giving the possibility of performing whole-body imaging, which is excellent for tumor staging. Sequences used for staging include the fast turbo short tau inversion recovery (STIR) imaging,[3] which is widely used in human medicine nowadays.

Different sequences can be used during MRI. The recorded signal is analyzed by a computer using a complicated calculation method and eventually presented to the radiologist in the form of a section image.[4] Depending on the form, duration and intensity of the high-frequency impulses emitted into the region of interest ('pulse sequence'), the tissue contrast in the image can be determined primarily through different T1- or T2-relaxation times, but also through the proton density alone. In this context, we refer to T1-, T2- or proton density (PD)-weighted sequences. Depending on these weightings, a tissue may be visualized with different signal intensities. For example, pure water shows low signal intensity in T1-weighted sequences, and high signal intensity in T2-weighted sequences. In contrast, fat shows up with high signal intensity in both weightings, whereas muscle shows medium signal intensity in T1-weighted images, but low signal intensity in the T2-weighted ones (Fig. 8-3). The tissue contrast can be manipulated even further using special sequences. An example is the STIR sequence allowing selective suppression of the fat signal with high signal visualization of fluids in basically a T2-weighted sequence. The same can be done to extract the signal of cerebrospinal fluid (CSF) in T2-weighted images of the central nervous system. This is done with FLAIR-sequences (fluid attenuation inversion recovery) (Fig. 8-3).

Like CT and ultrasound scanning, MRI is a tomographic (slice) method for producing a two-dimensional image. For CT the two-dimensional images are formed by reconstructing the sagittal and dorsal planes from the acquired transverse slices. MRI, in contrast, is a true three-dimensional modality, which can acquire each plane by itself without the need for post-scan reconstruction.[5,6]

The high tissue contrast in MRI is a major advantage compared with X-ray techniques (radiography, computed tomography). Also, tissues can be distinguished by the different intensities created by using different sequences, allowing far better assessment of soft tissue disorders (Table 8-1). MRI is a very sensitive modality, which still lacks specificity. However, the combination of different sequences, with and without contrast enhancement, provides a great tool for depiction and description of the extent of a lesion. This modality is useful for optimal surgery planning.

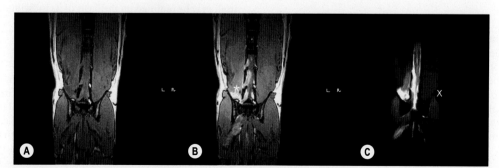

Figure 8-2 Paraspinal lymphoma invading into the spinal canal in a cat. Dorsal T1-weighted images **(A)** pre- and **(B)** post-administration of gadodiamide (gadolinium) and **(C)** dorsal STIR. In the T1-weighted image the space-occupying lesion is barely visible, whereas in the contrast enhanced image the extent of the lesion is much clearer (asterisk). Note the absence of fat signal in the STIR (x).

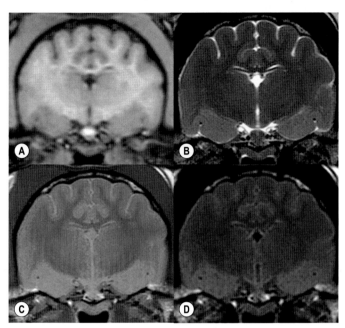

Figure 8-3 Comparison of **(A)** T1, **(B)** T2, **(C)** PD and **(D)** fluid attenuated inversion recovery (FLAIR) of the feline brain. Note the absence of fluid signal in the T1 and the FLAIR images, whereas in the T2 image the fluid is bright in signal. In the fluid-sensitive sequences (T2, FLAIR), the gray matter shows lower signal intensity than the fluid, whereas it is the opposite in T1 images. The PD, which displays the density distribution of protons, shows perfect anatomical contrast.

Table 8-1 Representative tissue types with their signal behavior in T1 and T2 images

T1 image	T2 image	Tissue
Hypointense (dark)	Hyperintense (bright)	CSF, fluid collections, edema
Hyperintense	Hypointense	Fat, some protein solutions, calcium deposits, transient blood flow
Hyperintense	Hyperintense	Paramagnetic solutions, extracellular methemoglobin, proteins
Hypointense	Hypointense	Dense calcium deposits, bone, air, rapid flow in vessels, hemosiderin, metallic artefacts

THORAX

High-quality survey radiographs can provide a lot of information on thoracic disease but there are some limitations. The use of other imaging modalities, particularly ultrasound and CT, can provide additional information, for example on heart structure and function, and earlier evidence of pulmonary metastases, respectively.

Radiology

Thoracic radiographs play an important role in the investigation of respiratory, cardiovascular and oncological diseases and in the trauma patient. They can provide a quick initial and cost-efficient general overview. However, radiographic findings are often non-specific and interpretation might be challenging, particularly of pulmonary lesions.

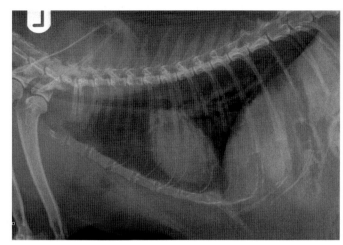

Figure 8-4 Incompletely mineralized costal cartilages in older cats can be confused with rib fractures.

Technique

A good radiographic technique is essential to maximize the usefulness of thoracic radiographs. The air-filled lungs provide a high inherent contrast. High kVp/low mAs exposure factors (long-scale contrast technique) will reduce this natural contrast and provide better lung detail. The exposure should be made at full inspiration to maximize lung contrast. The use of a fast-film screen combination reduces the exposure time and therefore motion blur. The use of a grid is not necessary in a cat. The forelimbs should be pulled forward to avoid superimposition and the head and neck are slightly extended. Rotation of the thorax should be avoided. If digital radiographic technique is used, then an appropriate algorithm should be chosen and exposure factors may need to be adapted.

Standard radiographic views

A minimum of two orthogonal views should be used for a standard thoracic examination. Right lateral and dorsoventral views are often preferred in the investigation of cardiac disease. Both lateral views (and a dorsoventral [DV] or ventrodorsal [VD]) are commonly used to screen for pulmonary metastases. Consistency and an understanding of the effect of different positioning on the radiographic appearance are important.

Atelectasis commonly occurs in the dependent lung in lateral recumbency, which can mimic or mask lung pathologies. The DV view should therefore be taken prior to lateral views. Anesthesia-induced atelectasis can be minimized by placing the patient in sternal recumbency as soon as possible after induction.[7–9]

Interpretive principles and normal anatomy

A systematic radiographic approach is important to identify pathologies and to recognize possible life-threatening conditions. The thorax can be divided into four basic anatomic regions: extra-thoracic region, pleural space, lung parenchyma, and mediastinum.

The extra-thoracic region includes the thoracic skeleton and the soft tissue of the thoracic wall and diaphragm. These structures should be included in a thorough evaluation of thoracic radiographs, in particular following trauma. Each individual rib, vertebral body and any of the included forelimbs should be scrutinized to identify skeletal lesions. Incompletely and densely mineralized costal cartilages might mimic fractures in older cats (Fig. 8-4). The thoracic surface of the diaphragm is visualized as it projects against the air-filled lung;

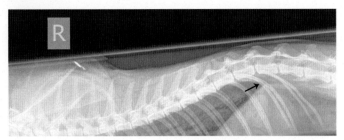

Figure 8-5 Radiograph showing the intrathoracic psoas muscles in a cat (arrow).

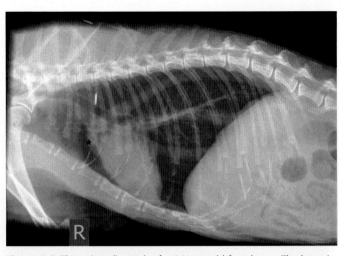

Figure 8-6 Thoracic radiograph of a 14-year-old female cat. The heart is relatively horizontal in position. The descending aorta has a meandering course and a focal aortic bulge can be seen, indicated by an asterisk. The radiopaque linear metal density object is an overlying identity chip in the cat's subcutaneous tissues.

caudally it silhouettes with the liver. In most cats, the ventral portion of the diaphragm is seen on a lateral view as a thin, soft tissue structure, outlined by mediastinal fat cranially and falciform fat caudally.

The pleural space contains only a very small quantity of fluid that is not usually visible radiographically. Space-occupying abnormalities can distend the pleural space, e.g., fluid or air accumulation, pleural masses and herniated abdominal content. In cats, unilateral pleural diseases are more common than in the dog. In contrast to dogs, the caudodorsal lung fields are separated by a triangular-shaped soft tissue opacity from the spine on a lateral view. This represents the intrathoracic psoas muscles and should not be misinterpreted as pleural effusion (Fig. 8-5).

Pulmonary vasculature, bronchi up to their secondary divisions and some interstitial markings, are usually visualized radiographically in a normal lung. Interpretation of lung parenchyma is challenging, mainly due to the wide range in appearance of normal lungs and the overlap of radiographic features between diseases of different etiology. An initial practical approach is to identify any increase or decrease in lung opacity and to determine the distribution, location and severity of the detected abnormalities. The type of pulmonary pattern (bronchial, vascular, alveolar, and interstitial) and determination of the predominant pattern are commonly used to further classify lung abnormalities. It is useful to assess whether the airways (alveolar, bronchi) are involved to determine if additional investigations are required (e.g., bronchoalveolar lavage). The presence of a mediastinal shift on the DV/VD planes is a valuable indicator of changes in volume seen in hemithorax (lung collapse, pulmonary mass).

Mediastinal structures normally seen radiographically include the heart, trachea, aorta, caudal vena cava, sometimes the esophagus, and in young animals the thymus. The normal feline heart is more consistent in shape than in dogs, with no breed-associated variations. The maximum width of the cardiac silhouette should not exceed 2–2.5 intercostal spaces on a lateral view. The apex of the heart is usually closer to the midline on a DV/VD view. In cats, the left atrium has a more cranial position, which makes it more difficult to identify on a lateral view. In older cats, the heart commonly becomes more horizontal in position and a focal aortic bulge might be noted (Fig. 8-6). In obese animals, large deposits of pericardial and mediastinal fat may mimic an enlarged cardiac silhouette. The cranial mediastinum should normally not exceed the width of the superimposed thoracic spine on a DV/VD view. Sternal and tracheobronchial lymph nodes are not visualized unless enlarged.[7-12]

Computed tomography

Computed tomography may be useful in cats with thoracic disease where other diagnostic modalities such as radiography and ultrasonography have failed to identify the cause or extent of the disease (Fig. 8-7). CT has potential for providing additional information on a variety of thoracic conditions in cats, particularly the possibility of

---

Box 8-1 **Some potential indications for thoracic CT in cats**

Pleural space

Recurrent pneumothorax
Effusion – distinguishing fluid from masses

Mediastinal disease

Thymoma
Lymphoma
Thrombosis
Heart-based tumors

Airways and lungs

Tracheal rupture
Tracheal or bronchial foreign bodies
Screening for pulmonary metastases, pulmonary thromboembolism

---

identifying pulmonary metastases that are not visible on thoracic radiographs (Box 8-1).

Magnetic resonance imaging

Imaging the thorax with MRI has been problematic due to respiratory and cardiac movement leading to distracting artefacts. With newer sequence techniques cardiac and respiratory gating is available, minimizing these artefacts and leading to useful images. Modern equipment is able to gate heart rates up to 220 beats per minute. Therefore mediastinal lesions can be imaged with all the advantages MRI provides. Also, space-occupying lesions of the pulmonary system can be examined, although CT is still a superior modality for this system.

Specific thoracic conditions

Cardiomyopathy

A variety of cardiac diseases can affect the cat, but myocardial diseases are most commonly encountered. Hypertrophic cardiomyopathy (HCM) is the most common form of myocardial disease affecting cats.

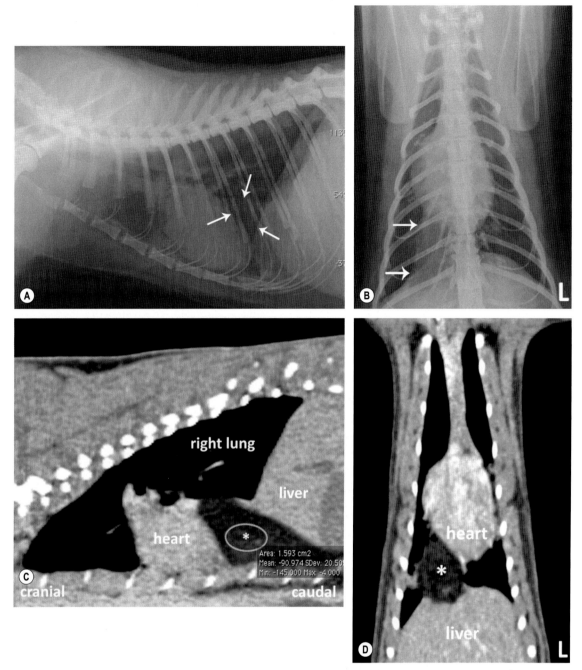

Figure 8-7 An opaque structure of fat to soft tissue density (arrows) was diagnosed radiographically in the cardiophrenic angle and on the right in a three-year-old cat with respiratory distress. The diaphragmatic contour was clearly seen in the **(A)** laterolateral view but not completely visualized on the **(B)** ventrodorsal view. It was unclear if the changes were consistent with lung pathology or a diaphragmatic hernia. With CT, a large defect was seen in the diaphragm on the right **(C)** dorsal plane and **(D)** ventrally (sagittal plane). The cardiophrenic angle was filled with fat (*, mean of −91 Hounsfield units). Findings were confirmed surgically.

Many cases of hypertrophic cardiomyopathy are clinically asymptomatic. Detection of a heart murmur and gallop rhythm should therefore warrant further investigation, even in an apparently healthy cat.

Echocardiography is the most sensitive imaging modality to diagnose and to classify cardiomyopathy. Echocardiographic changes are characterized by focal or generalized increased thickness of the left ventricular free wall and interventricular septum. Left atrial enlargement can usually be recognized in symptomatic patients. Thoracic radiographs, however, are indicated and superior to identify signs of congestive heart failure, such as pulmonary venous distension and pulmonary edema. In cats, pulmonary edema has a variable appearance and distribution (Fig. 8-8), rather than being located in the perihilar region as with dogs.[13] Pleural effusion is often present secondary to left-sided heart failure. The concentric hypertrophy of the ventricular wall is often not recognized on radiographs and only an abnormal lung pattern might be noted. Advanced left atrial enlargement is particularly obvious on the DV view, seen as a 'valentine' shaped heart.

Thoracic trauma

Patients who have suffered thoracic trauma must be stabilized prior to radiography. In dyspneic patients a DV view should be taken to avoid further respiratory compromise. Lesions that might be recognized radiographically include pulmonary contusion, pneumothorax, and rib fractures (Fig. 8-9).

Pulmonary contusion may be evident radiographically as complete lung lobe consolidation or as patchy areas of alveolar/interstitial infiltrates, commonly ipsilateral to the impact site. Radiographs taken immediately following trauma may not reveal these changes, which usually become apparent two-12 hours post-trauma.[14]

Post-traumatic rib fractures should be differentiated from older, hypertrophic non-union rib fractures, which occasionally can be seen in cats with chronic lower airway disease.

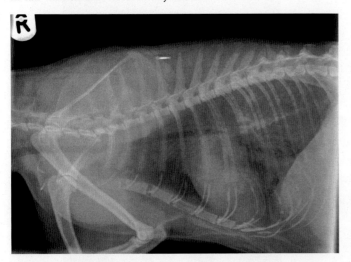

Figure 8-8 Increased opacity of the caudodorsal lung fields in an eight-year-old DSH cat with cardiogenic pulmonary edema. The cardiac silhouette is enlarged, compatible with cardiomyopathy.

Diaphragmatic rupture is a common consequence of blunt external trauma. Identification of abdominal viscera in the thoracic cavity and loss of the diaphragmatic outline are conclusive signs for diaphragmatic rupture. However, pleural effusion may be present and obscure these structures. Cranial displacement and loss of abdominal organs on an abdominal radiograph are useful, indirect signs to identify a diaphragmatic rupture. In cats, only falciform fat and omentum may herniate, which may be recognized by the loss of the diaphragmatic line ventrally and by the relatively small fat pad ventral to the liver (Fig. 8-10).[15] Positive-contrast gastrointestinal studies may aid the diagnosis.

Pulmonary metastases

Thoracic radiography is the screening tool most commonly used for detection of pulmonary metastases in cats. However, pulmonary nodules have to be at least 3–5 mm to be radiographically visible. A combination of left lateral and right lateral ± VD radiographs is recommended. Careful radiographic technique is necessary to provide high-quality films to raise the identification rate of lung nodules. Manually inflated lungs are often preferred for screening; however, anesthetic-induced atelectasis may occur. Soft tissue opacity nodules are the most common radiographic presentation of pulmonary metastatic disease (Fig. 8-11). In cats, pulmonary metastases are often poorly marginated and irregularly shaped (Fig. 8-12), in contrast to dogs. Metastasis of mammary gland tumors in cats manifests often as ill-defined nodules or as a diffuse pulmonary pattern.[16] CT is the preferred imaging modality for detecting pulmonary metastases in humans as smaller nodules (1–2 mm) can be detected.[17]

ABDOMEN

High-quality survey radiographs can provide a lot of information on abdominal disease but there are some limitations. The use of other

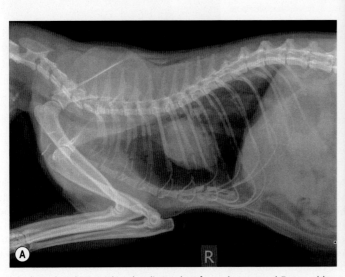
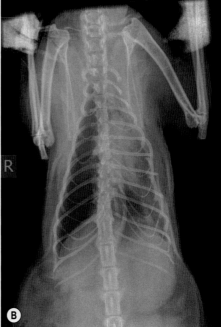

Figure 8-9 Right lateral and ventrodorsal radiographs of a male neutered 5-year-old cat that presented with dyspnea after a road traffic accident. There is pneumothorax, with elevation of the heart, lung lobe consolidation and several rib fractures.

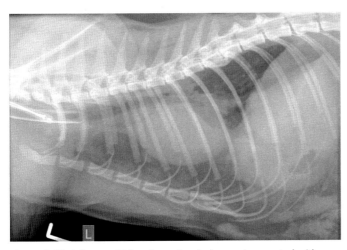

Figure 8-10 A 2-year-old female neutered obese cat presented with a pelvic fracture. Thoracic radiographs show loss of continuity of the diaphragm ventrally with elevation of the heart by a structure of fat density (suspected to be herniated falciform fat). There is also a soft tissue density structure lying ventral to the sternum, which was found to be a loop of intestine protruding through an abdominal wall rupture that was present in addition to the diaphragm rupture.

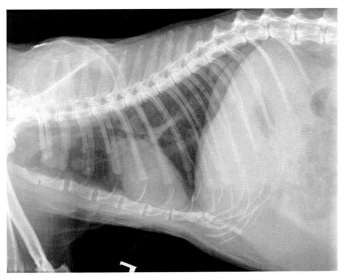

Figure 8-11 A 14-year-old male cat with multiple nodular pulmonary metastases.

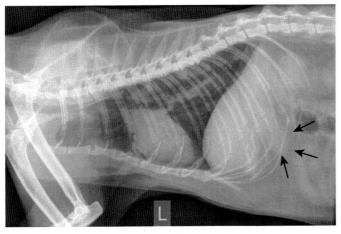

Figure 8-12 A cat with multiple ill-defined pulmonary metastases.

imaging modalities such as ultrasound, CT, or MRI can provide additional information, for example on organ structure and function and invasiveness of neoplasia.

Radiology

Technique

Abdominal radiography is best done without a grid (table top) and with a detail film-screen system. An exposure of approximately 10 mAs and 40 kVp should be used for an adult cat. For computed or digital radiography, exposures may be somewhat lower, depending on the manufacturer's recommendations. Likewise, contrast should be moderate to allow evaluation of abdominal detail and adjacent soft tissues, e.g., the abdominal wall, mammary gland or perianal region. A lateral and a ventrodorsal image should be taken during expiration and with the pelvic limbs at a 90° angle to the spine to maximize the space for the abdominal organs. Extension of the legs should be avoided. Cats should be fasted for 12 hours prior to radiography. Enemas might also be useful in some situations, such as for imaging the urinary tract, to avoid superimposition of the fecal material on the ureters and bladder.

Interpretative principles and normal anatomy

There are some important radiographic characteristics of the normal cat's abdomen. In general, due to the different radiopacities of fat, soft tissue and gas, the abdominal organs e.g., the liver, spleen, stomach, duodenum, jejunum, colon, kidneys, and urinary bladder, are well depicted in the cat. The average normal adult 'well-fed' cat has a certain amount of subcutaneous, falciform and retroperitoneal fat, which outlines the kidneys, urinary bladder and ventral border of the liver and small intestinal loops; but fat may also cause crowding of the organs in the central abdomen with a mildly reduced focal detail. In kittens and emaciated cats, the normal abdominal detail is usually reduced due to the lack of fat. In the thin or young cat, abdominal effusion may be difficult to diagnose and can sometimes only be assumed based on the fact that the abdomen appears rather large. The normal liver lobes are pointed with smooth contours; a normal size liver only just extends beyond the rib cage in the laterolateral view. A distinctive feature in the cat is the gallbladder that may protrude beyond the ventrocaudal border of the liver and this should not be misinterpreted as a liver mass. The position of the cat's stomach is normal on the lateral view if its axis is parallel with the ribs (upper limit) or perpendicular to the spine (lower limit). In contrast to the dog, the cat's stomach on the ventrodorsal view is more angled and U-shaped, with the pylorus located at or just to the right of the midline. Consequently, the duodenum does not run along the right abdominal wall but is located just right of the midline. An intramural radiolucent band (fat) in the stomach wall can be seen in some cats without concurrent clinical gastrointestinal signs. Only the head of the spleen is visible as a triangular structure just caudodorsal (lateral view) and caudolateral on the left (ventrodorsal view) of the fundus of the stomach. The spleen's tail is not normally visualized. The adrenal glands in the cat may be mineralized and, therefore, depicted craniomedial to the kidneys. This is considered an incidental finding without clinical relevance in the older cat. The normal kidneys are bean-shaped with smooth rounded contours and they are 4.0–4.5 cm long on the ventrodorsal view. The bladder neck and urethra are rather elongated. In some male cats, a very small os penis may be visible. In spayed cats, the gonadectomy sutures may mineralize and therefore become visible caudal to both kidneys and dorsal to the bladder or its neck. They may be mistaken as urinary calculi. In normal cats, the pancreas, ureters, uterus, ovaries, and abdominal lymph nodes are not visible.

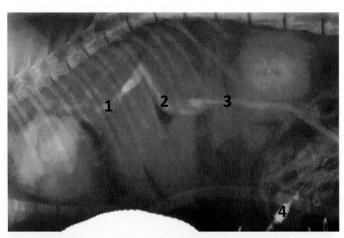

Figure 8-13 Laterolateral view of an operative mesenteric portography (4) in a cat: a large single extrahepatic anastomosis (2) is seen between the portal vein (3) and caudal vena cava (1).

Computed tomography

CT has increasingly been used for imaging various abdominal organs (Box 8-2). The cross-sectional nature of this imaging process allows greater characterization of disease processes in the abdomen. In oncological diseases, CT angiography may indirectly help to identify and describe a neoplastic lesion on the basis of its relationship to adjacent arteries or veins (mass effect, compression and invasiveness), or the lesion itself may be outlined on the basis of its individual perfusion/contrast enhancement pattern.

Magnetic resonance imaging

MRI is increasingly being used for investigation of abdominal disorders. The main focus is on liver, kidney, and adrenal disease in dogs but there is obvious potential in cats. Modern sequences use angiography for evaluation of portosystemic shunts. This technique is even less invasive than CT angiography, as it can be performed without the use of contrast media. For several years, diffusion weighted imaging (DWI) has been used in human medicine to better characterize tissues, e.g., with MR spectroscopy.[18] Its use is being investigated in veterinary medicine, with the potential for the differentiation of benign and malignant diseases.

Specific abdominal conditions

Portosystemic shunts

Diagnostic imaging plays a crucial role in the diagnosis, classification and surgical planning of portosystemic shunts. The goal is to identify an abnormal vessel or multiple vessels, determine the origin and orifice, classify a congenital intrahepatic shunt as left, central or right divisional, and assess portal hypertension.

Survey radiographs aid in assessing liver size (if the liver is small the axis of the stomach is cranial to a line perpendicular to the spine on the laterolateral view) and to search for causes of portal hypertension in acquired portosystemic shunts. In contrast to dogs, increased renal size is not a common finding in cats but it still can occur.

Selective angiography has been considered the method of choice for imaging the hepatic and portal vasculature. The techniques have been described in detail.[19,20] In general, with a portosystemic shunt, only a small or no intrahepatic portal system is outlined after the injection of iodinated contrast medium. Instead, a portosystemic anastomosis is seen (Fig. 8-13). If a shunting vessel is located cranial to the 13th thoracic vertebra, it is likely to be intrahepatic, and if it is caudal to this vertebra, it may be considered extrahepatic.[19] However, the various methods do not outline the entire portal tributary system at once and they are invasive. With operative mesenteric portography, contrast medium is injected into a jejunal vein, and the best and most complete studies of the portal venous system are usually obtained.

With cranial mesenteric arterial portography, a splenic vein shunt may not be detected and splenoportography will miss mesenteric shunts.

Ultrasound is an excellent modality for investigation of all potential hepatic, vascular and urinary lesions. However, thorough knowledge of the vascular abdominal vasculature is crucial and accuracy depends largely on the operator's experience. With B-mode, organ size can be estimated; a subjectively decreased liver volume, enlarged kidneys (>4.5 cm length) and urate urolithiasis may be found in congenital portosystemic shunts. With acquired shunts, possible findings include hepatic disease, portal vein thrombosis, or compression of the portal vein by a mass. Further, hepatic vessel morphology may be altered in portosystemic shunts, e.g., subjectively there may be a reduced size of the portal vein, low number of portal vessels, and an abnormal intra- or extrahepatic vessel or multiple extrahepatic vessels may be depicted.[21] The various tributaries of the portal vein which, in particular, are rather small in the cat, may be difficult to identify because of a lack of acoustic windows due to a small liver or intestinal gas. The drainage of an intra- or extrahepatic shunt into a hepatic vein or the caudal vena cava may be easier to look for. In a portoazygos shunt, the shunt vessel runs directly to the diaphragm without communicating with the caudal vena cava. Doppler ultrasonography may aid in the diagnosis of portosystemic shunts. In the caudal vena cava, at the site of drainage, local turbulent flow may be seen. Portal blood flow velocity (10–12 cm/second in healthy unsedated cats) measured with Doppler ultrasonography, may be increased or variable in cats with congenital portosystemic shunting, and reduced or sometimes pulsatile and hepatofugal with acquired shunts. In cats with arterioportal fistulas, multiple, large, tortuous hepatic vessels with a pulsatile flow are found.[21]

CT also represents a very sensitive tool for the diagnosis of portosystemic shunts and complete studies of the portal venous system and potential drainage vessels are obtained.[22] With multi-slice CT, dual-phase CT angiography may be performed. This technique images the liver immediately after peripheral intravenous contrast medium injection (arterial phase) and a subsequent repeat examination (portal phase) during short periods of apnea after hyperventilation. Likewise, the aorta, hepatic artery and its branches, caudal vena cava, hepatic veins, portal vein and its tributaries (e.g., cranial and caudal mesenteric veins, splenic vein, gastroduodenal vein), intrahepatic portal branches and shunt vessels are well visualized. Three-dimensional images may be reconstructed from the original data (Fig. 8-14). The anatomical information of CT angiography is of high quality and very helpful to the surgeons. It decreases surgical time and degree of dissection.

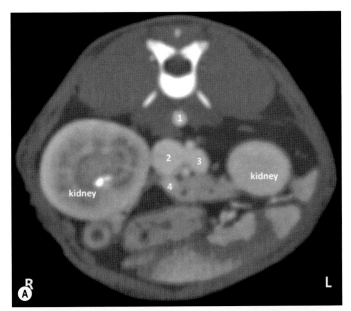

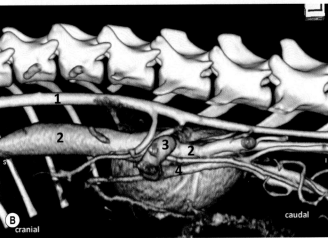

Figure 8-14 Dual CT-angiography. **(A)** Transverse image at the shunting level and **(B)** 3D-reconstruction image from the left in a cat with a single extrahepatic anastomosis (3) between the portal vein (4) and caudal vena cava (2), located in the left division (1, aorta).

Per-rectal portal scintigraphy is a reasonably sensitive, non-invasive method of detecting a portosystemic shunt. Radiolabeled technetium pertechnetate is administered by enema, and its distribution is monitored with a gamma-camera. In a normal animal, the radiopharmaceutical is absorbed into the portal circulation and subsequently enters the liver before reaching the systemic circulation. In the case of a portosystemic shunt, the majority of the radiopharmaceutical enters the systemic circulation and radioactivity appears in the heart before it appears in the liver. However, per-rectal scintigraphy provides poor anatomic shunt detail and the diagnostic quality of the studies may be poor due to inadequate rectal absorption. With trans-splenic portal scintigraphy using pertechnetate, a more consistent visualization of the portal venous system and characterization of the shunt's anatomy is achieved with a lower radionuclide dosage and improved image quality.[23]

Urogenital imaging

Diseases of the urinary tract (urolithiasis, trauma) that may require surgery are common in the cat, and diagnostic imaging plays a crucial

role in their diagnosis. Radiodense uroliths or calculi can be seen in the renal pelvis and recesses, ureters, center (deepest point) of the urinary bladder or in the urethra, e.g., the penile urethra. If radiolucent calculi are present in the urinary bladder, survey radiographs may be of limited value but typical changes include a large, rounded urinary bladder with focal loss of detail around the bladder neck due to urethral obstruction. Radiographically, the ureters cannot be seen, even if there are ureteral calculi present that are causing obstruction.

Urinary tract trauma is common in the cat. Shortly after the trauma, only little or no radiographic changes are seen. Pelvic fractures and focal bleeding/soft tissue swelling in the sublumbar or bladder neck region may be suggestive of problems. Later, retroperitoneal effusion (with renal or ureteral damage) or abdominal effusion (with urinary bladder, cranial urethral rupture or leakage from the ureters at the ureterovesical junction) may be found on the survey radiographs. Mid- or caudal-urethral rupture may lead to urinary leakage into the inguinal, perianal, and femoral soft tissues with resultant swelling.

Unilateral or bilateral regular renal enlargement may be a consequence of hydronephrosis secondary to ureteral obstruction due to calculi, pyelonephritis, ectopic ureter, ureterocele, ureteral stricture, adjacent masses or neoplasia. Other differentials relevant for a surgeon include subcapsular bleeding or perirenal pseudocyst. Irregular contours and/or focal masses may result from a hematoma, abscess, cyst, primary or metastatic neoplasia, or infarcts.

Diagnostic ultrasound represents an excellent tool to evaluate the urogenital tract. Size and content of the renal pelvis, ureters, urinary bladder and abdominal urethra may be easily examined. Normal urine is anechoic, and therefore, cellular components increase its echogenicity, and calculi show a hyperechoic surface with distal acoustic shadowing. Whereas obstructive disease may be confidently diagnosed, rupture of any segment can only be assumed. For example, a thickened and atonic urinary bladder and abdominal effusion may suggest bladder wall rupture; the leakage itself may not be detected. Ultrasound is very sensitive in detecting free fluid in the abdomen or retroperitoneal space. The abdominal or retroperitoneal fat may appear hyperechoic with inflammation. Although masses in the kidneys, retroperitoneal space and urinary bladder may be easily detected, ultrasound is not specific in their differentiation. Cystic changes of the kidneys may be easily diagnosed based on their anechoic content and thin regular hyperechoic wall. Ultrasound is also highly valuable for the diagnosis of uterine disorders, pregnancy and complications, and cryptorchidism.

Excretory urography is performed mainly to diagnose diseases of the kidneys and ureters. Food should be withheld for 24 hours, a cleansing enema performed and patients should be normally hydrated and in a stable condition for sedation or anesthesia. However, in trauma patients, the procedure may even be performed with the cat conscious. In healthy elective cases, it is advantageous to first empty and then refill the urinary bladder with 0.5–1.0 mL iodinated contrast medium and subsequently, 5–10 mL/kg body weight negative contrast medium, e.g., room air (double-contrast cystography). After abdominal survey radiographs, a bolus injection of ionic or non-ionic (in high-risk patients) iodinated contrast medium is given intravenously (dose: 800 mg iodine/kg body weight). Ventrodorsal radiographs are taken immediately. After five minutes, ventrodorsal, laterolateral, and, to investigate the ureterovesical junction, oblique views are taken. If fluoroscopy is not available, repeat radiographs may be needed to image the ureters because of the contraction waves. Late views (20, 30, and 40 minutes) are obtained to image the urinary bladder or slow leakage (extravasation) of contrast medium (Fig. 8-15). Radiolucent calculi present as filling defects within the contrast-filled structures.

If urethral or bladder rupture or radiolucent calculi are suspected, positive-contrast urethrography combined with cystography is simple and most efficient. The iodine contrast medium should be diluted

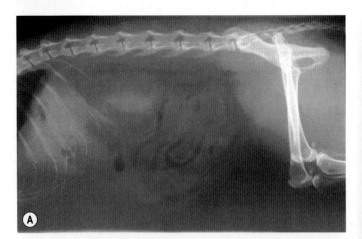

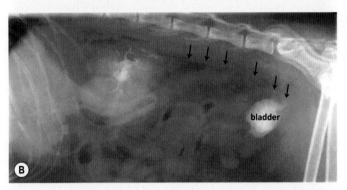

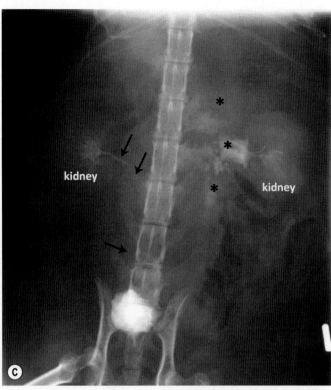

Figure 8-15 A traumatized cat with coxofemoral joint luxation. **(A)** Loss of retroperitoneal and caudal abdominal detail was found on the laterolateral radiograph; the urinary bladder was not well defined and urinary tract injury was suspected. **(B, C)** The right ureter (black arrows) appears normal during excretory urography. The left ureter cannot be depicted after five minutes. Instead, marked extravasation (*) is seen near the hilus of the left kidney. The urinary bladder is not well filled with contrast medium and therefore, appears irregular.

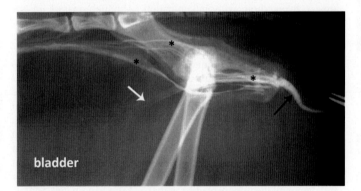

Figure 8-16 Urethral rupture at the level of the pelvic outlet: a laterolateral view of a positive contrast urethrogram shows an intact penile urethra (black arrow) and some contrast medium entering the urinary bladder (white arrow). Nevertheless, marked extravasation of contrast medium is seen within the pelvis (*).

with sterile water or saline to approximately 15% of its original concentration. Negative contrast agents should not be substituted. The urinary catheter tip is positioned in the penile urethra. Laterolateral views are usually adequate and should be taken during the injection of the last 2–3 mL of the approximately 10 mL used for imaging the urethra (Fig. 8-16). To avoid a misdiagnosis of either an intact or ruptured bladder, it is important to inject the entire calculated amount (5–10 mL/kg body weight) into the empty urinary bladder.

BRAIN

MRI is the modality of choice for imaging disorders of both the brain and spine. The main advantage of MR imaging is the high sensitivity in detection of lesions and the potential to characterize the type of lesions.[24] MRI is considered superior to CT for target delineation in brain tumors and therefore it is the modality of choice in these instances.

CT imaging continues to be widely used for radiation treatment planning because it provides necessary electron density information for accurate dosimetric calculations.[25]

Magnetic resonance imaging

Imaging the brain usually starts with T2-weighted and T1-weighted images pre-contrast and post-contrast. PD-weighted images are also often performed. In order to better assess the T2-weighted image, a FLAIR should be performed that suppresses CSF signal. In general, one can say that an MRI study without at least one inversion recovery sequence is an incomplete study. Different sequence-techniques can be used to gain information about lesion type and the use of paramagnetic contrast media such as Gadolinium (Gadodiamide) increases the possibility of differentiation of lesion type,[26] although its main value is in the increase in sensitivity in detecting lesions. Cherubini et al[24] found that signal characteristics were not useful in differentiating neoplastic from inflammatory disease, nor was the presence of perilesional edema. Imaging signs, such as mass effect or dural contact

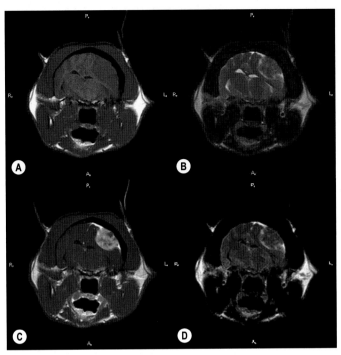

Figure 8-17 Meningioma in a cat. Transverse **(A)** T1, **(B)** T2, **(C)** T1 post-gadodiamide administration and **(D)** FLAIR images. Note the thickened calvarium under which a broad-based space-occupying lesion is seen, mildly hypointense in T1 and inhomogeneously hyperintense in T2 and FLAIR. There is marked mildly inhomogeneous contrast enhancement with the so-called dural tail. This sign is not specific for meningioma.

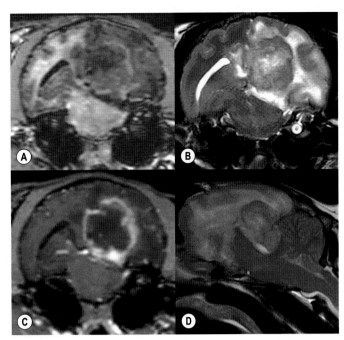

Figure 8-18 Glioma in a cat. Transverse **(A)** T1, **(B)** T2, **(C)** T1 post-gadodiamide administration and **(D)** sagittal T2. The space-occupying lesion is visible in the left hemisphere, being of low intensity in the T1-weighted image and inhomogeneously hyperintense in the T2-weighted image. The surrounding white matter is hypointense in the T1 and hyperintense in the T2-weighted images, indicating that peritumoral edema is contributing to the marked midline shift of the brain. There is a strong post-contrast rim enhancement visible. On the sagittal view the mass protrudes under the tentorium and displaces the cerebellum caudally, leading to a partial hernia of the vermis through the foramen magnum.

(dural tail sign), however, were very indicative for neoplasia, in this case meningioma. The first step in evaluating lesions in the CNS is to decide whether a lesion is extra- or intra-axial.

Specific brain conditions

Meningioma

The most common extra-axial lesion in cats is meningioma (Fig. 8-17). The tumors usually have well circumscribed distinct margins. Most of them show significant contrast enhancement, which can be homogeneous or inhomogeneous. In T2-weighted images they usually present as hyperintense compared to the surrounding tissue, whereas they can be completely isointense in T1-weighted sequences. Peritumoral edema, which appears hyperintense in both the T2-weighted and FLAIR, hypointense in T1-weighted images, is usually mild, and very inconsistent with meningioma. The dural tail sign can be identified in most of the cases and involvement of the calvarium, if present, is very indicative for this tumor type. This involvement is characterized by a thickening (sclerosis) of the overlying calvarium.

Lymphoma

Lymphoma may be classified as either an extra- or intra-axial lesion. The shape of the tumor varies from round to amorphous, usually being hyperintense on T2-weighted images with heterogeneous lesion pattern. They are iso- to hypointense in T1-weighted images and they generally show marked contrast enhancement.

Glioma

Gliomas are characterized by intra-axial origin. The tumors can be round or lobulated. They are usually hyperintense on T2-weighted images and hypointense on T1-weighted images. In one study gliomas all showed ring-enhancement, with mild to moderate peritumoral edema noted in some cases[27] (Fig. 8-18).

Pituitary neoplasia

Another important intracranial neoplasm in cats is pituitary neoplasia (see Chapter 58). As in dogs, they arise from the sella turcica, are usually well circumscribed and are hypointense and heterogeneous on T2-weighted images and isointense and heterogeneous on T1-weighted images. Contrast enhancement is usually marked. Small micro-adenomas may be missed with MRI, whereas CT can depict them in arterial phase contrast enhanced scans with a missing or displaced pituitary flush.

SCINTIGRAPHY

The physiological function of an organ or organ system is associated with its biochemical processes. These biochemical processes can be shown by the tracer principle, first described by George Hevesy, a Hungarian radiochemist (awarded the Nobel prize for chemistry in 1943). After the application of a radioactive tracer its distribution in the body can be measured from the outside. Depending on the tracer, different physiological processes can be studied. Nuclear medicine provides a non-invasive way of showing morphology, and physiological function of a targeted organ system.

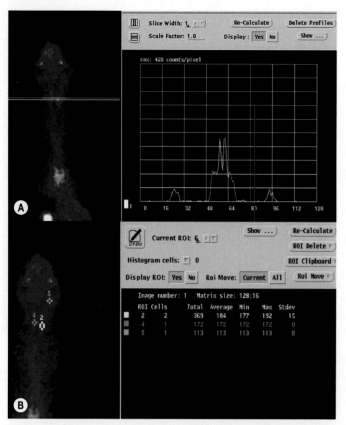

Table 8-2 The radionuclides used in thyroid nuclear medicine, their physical properties and their use

Radionuclide	Emission	Half-life	Purpose
^{99m}Technetium (Tc)	γ	6.01 hours	Morphology
^{123}Iodine (I)	γ	13.3 hours	Morphology and function
^{131}Iodine (I)	β	8.02 days	Treatment

Figure 8-19 ^{99m}Tc scan of a normal cat. Both thyroid glands accumulate the same amount of activity and the salivary:thyroid (ST-ratio) is lower than 1. **(A)** The activity is plotted over a slice line showing the same peak height over both thyroids. **(B)** The region of interest has been drawn manually over the thyroid glands (4, 2) and over one zygomatic salivary gland (5). With this, the ST-ratio can be calculated. *(Courtesy of Johann Lang, Vetsuisse-Faculty Bern)*

Equipment

The equipment consists of a gamma-camera (scintillation camera), which detects the gamma-radiation emitted from a radionuclide applied to the patient. The information collected is processed and the displayed image contains two-dimensional distribution information (equivalent to the anatomy) but also intensity per pixel (picture element). This intensity can be used to quantify the collected information. Several software solutions exist to analyze the image. Regions of interest (ROI) are drawn around the selected organ to plot the amount of accumulated radionuclide (Fig. 8-19).

This equipment is mainly limited to academic institutions, although some units exist in private clinics. The equipment is expensive and, moreover, the regulations by national nuclear regulatory commissions are very strict, making its use complicated. The most commonly used radioisotope is Technetium-99m as pertechnetate (^{99m}TcO$_4^-$). ^{99m}Tc has ideal properties for nuclear imaging as it has a short physical half-life of 6.01 hours and it does not create beta-emission but gamma-emission with a relatively low energy (140 keV) that can be measured by scintillation cameras. Another advantage is that it is readily available and relatively inexpensive.

Indications for scintigraphy in the cat

Scintigraphy is an excellent tool for diagnostic imaging of hyperthyroid cats (Box 8-3).[28] Tc-pertechnetate acts in a similar manner to iodine, being taken up and concentrated by thyroid gland tissue. As opposed to iodine it is not processed into thyroid hormone. Therefore it can locate thyroid tissue but it does not give direct information about the hormonal activity. It has to be noted that Tc-pertechnetate is also concentrated within salivary gland tissue, gastric mucosa, in the choroid plexus, and the sweat glands. As opposed to ^{99m}Tc, iodine-123 is trapped and processed in thyroid tissue. Iodine is continuously concentrated into the thyroid tissue over a period of 24 hours. Therefore it can be used to quantify the hormonal activity. Nevertheless, it is only used in selected cases as its half-life is longer and it is more expensive than ^{99m}Tc.

To summarize, ^{99m}Tc is suitable for the detection and localization of thyroid gland tissue; I-123 is used to detect, localize and quantify; and I-131 is used for therapy as it is a beta-particle emitter (Table 8-2; see Chapter 15).

Procedure for thyroid scintigraphy

The imaging protocol is well described in veterinary medicine. The patient has to remain still on the gamma-camera so sedation or general anesthesia is required.

Technetium pertechnetate

A low dose of the radioisotope (1–4 mCi/37–148 MBq for ^{99m}TcO$_4^-$) is administered intravenously. Twenty to 40 minutes after administration, orthogonal lateral and ventral views of the cervical and thoracic region are obtained.

Iodine-123

A dose of 200–400 μCi/7.4–14.8 MBq is administered intravenously. Eight hours after administration the same views are obtained for trapping and 24 hours after administration for organification.

Feline thyroid disease and nuclear imaging

The normal feline thyroid glands appear as elongated regions of radiopharmaceutical uptake either side of the trachea (see Fig. 8-19). The intensity of the thyroid glands can be measured and compared to the intensity of the zygomatic salivary glands. Therefore regions of interest are drawn over the thyroid glands and the salivary glands. A ratio is calculated (thyroid : salivary ratio). Normal cats have a ratio of 0.87 : 1 (range: 0.6–1.03 : 1). Other techniques of quantification exist but their accuracy has not been thoroughly tested yet and therefore they are not routinely used.

Hypothyroidism in cats is very rare, whereas hyperthyroidism is the most common endocrinologic disease in cats (see Chapter 53). Among the common etiologies for hyperthyroidism in cats is feline thyroid hyperplasia (adenomatous hyperplasia) affecting both thyroid glands in about 70% of the cats. Another etiology is feline thyroid adenoma, which can arise in one or both glands and can spread as ectopic thyroid tissue from the region of the tongue to the precardial region in the cranial mediastinum (Fig. 8-20). They may present as cystic and/or multifocal lesions. Adenocarcinoma of the thyroid gland is rather rare and its prevalence has been reported to be approximately 2–5%. It is to be noted that scintigraphy cannot reliably differentiate malignant from benign lesions, but certain patterns are associated with a higher probability of carcinoma.[29] Carcinomas tend to be larger, more inhomogeneous and irregularly marginated (Fig. 8-21). Uptake within the lungs is highly suspicious for metastatic lung involvement.

In thyroid scintigraphy hyperactive thyroid tissue exhibits increased uptake of the radionuclide. In unilateral cases the contralateral lobe and the surrounding thyroid tissue are classically completely suppressed by negative feedback mechanisms through the pituitary gland in cases where the lesion is hormonally active. Therefore the normal tissue does not show any uptake (Fig. 8-22).

This implies that if both lobes are visible after scintigraphy, bilateral affliction has to be considered. As thyroidectomy is one treatment possibility, bilateral excision will result in hypothyroidism, although this does not appear to be a clinical problem in cats. If affected ectopic tissue is present, which can readily be detected with nuclear scintigraphy, surgical resection of the thyroid glands alone will not be successful in treating the hyperthyroidism; radiation therapy should be considered in cases with ectopic thyroid tissue.

The use of radiation for treatment of hyperthyroidism is discussed in Chapter 15.

INTERVENTIONAL RADIOLOGY

Interventional radiology involves the use of imaging techniques such as fluoroscopy and ultrasound and specialized equipment such as catheters, guide-wires, and stents for treatment of disease or trauma (Fig. 8-23). There are many applications for its use in veterinary medicine, although it is not yet in widespread use due to the necessity for

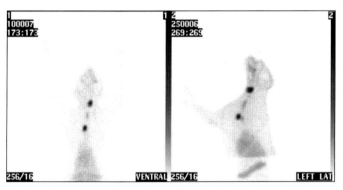

Figure 8-20 Ventral and lateral scan of a hyperthyroid cat diagnosed with a feline thyroid adenoma. Note the complete suppression of the right thyroid gland and a focus of ectopic thyroid tissue along the trachea at the level of the thoracic inlet. *(Courtesy of Johann Lang, Vetsuisse-Faculty Bern.)*

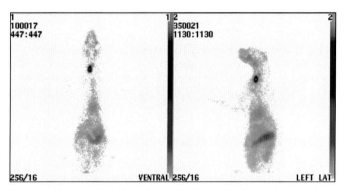

Figure 8-22 Ventral and lateral scan of a hyperthyroid cat diagnosed with a feline thyroid adenoma. A unifocal increased uptake of ^{99m}Tc in the right thyroid gland is noted, with complete suppression of the contralateral gland. No ectopic tissue is detectable. *(Courtesy of Johann Lang, Vetsuisse-Faculty Bern.)*

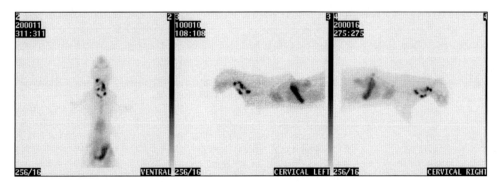

Figure 8-21 Ventral and lateral scan of a hyperthyroid cat diagnosed with a thyroid adenocarcinoma. The region of the thyroid glands shows increased uptake of ^{99m}Tc, which appears highly irregular, inhomogeneous with multiple hot spots within this area. This is considered typical for adenocarcinoma. Note the additional uptake in the stomach mucosa, which is considered normal. No ectopic tissue or metastasis can be detected in this case. *(Courtesy of Johann Lang, Vetsuisse-Faculty Bern.)*

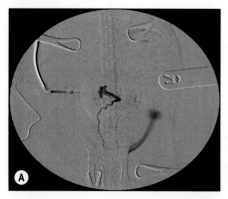 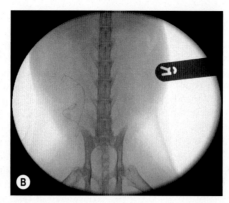 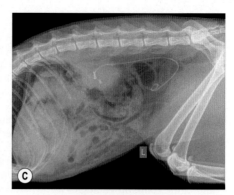

Figure 8-23 Interventional radiology was used in this cat that has had a ureteric stent placed to relieve a ureteral obstruction. **(A)** Contrast is injected into the renal pelvis under fluoroscopic guidance. **(B)** The ureteric stent is placed under fluoroscopic guidance. **(C)** A lateral radiograph confirms correct placement of the stent with the pigtails in the renal pelvis and bladder. *(Courtesy of Simon Tappin.)*

the specialized equipment and training required to become competent in its use.[30]

Indications

Interventional radiology techniques have been widely described in dogs and horses; their use in cats is less common but there are several reports in the literature of successful usage. Rheolytic thrombectomy was reported in six cats with distal aortic thromboembolism.[31] The use of the rheolytic thrombectomy system resulted in successful thrombus dissolution in five of six cats. Three of six cats survived to discharge.[31] There are several reports of stent placement in cats for a variety of reasons including nasopharyngeal stenosis, intrahepatic portosystemic shunts, ureteral obstruction and stricture, and tracheal obstruction.[32-36] Other instances of usage of interventional radiology for cats include treatment of hyperthyroidism and idiopathic chylothorax.[37-39]

Advantages and disadvantages

Patients treated by interventional radiology generally only require small incisions or implants such as stents placed through natural orifices. There is therefore low morbidity associated with the procedures, with the potential advantages of shorter hospitalization times, decreased pain, and in some cases lower cost when compared with open surgery. Some techniques such as stenting for malignant obstructions are palliative treatment options for conditions that may not be amenable to conventional treatment.[32]

The main disadvantage is associated with the costs and maintenance of the imaging equipment and the inventory of catheters, coils and stents that needs to be maintained. In addition, advanced training is required to perform these techniques.

Equipment and technique

The procedures are usually minimally invasive so do not need to be performed in the operating theatre; the necessity for imaging usually requires that the procedures are performed in the imaging area. Despite the minimally invasive nature of the techniques a high level of asepsis should still be aimed for.

A traditional fluoroscopy unit will suffice but a C-arm unit is preferable as it allows imaging of the patient in multiple planes without having to move the animal. Digital subtraction angiography and road mapping are specialized computer software imaging techniques that allow high resolution images to be gained in conjunction with minimal administration of contrast agents. This is important, particularly when performing procedures on small species such as cats. Endoscopy can be used in combination with fluoroscopy for various minimally invasive procedures and this modality is termed interventional endoscopy.[30]

REFERENCES

1. Farrow CS, Green R, Shively M. Radiology of the cat. 1st ed. St. Louis: Mosby; 1994.

2. Ohlerth S. Diagnostic imaging. In: Montavon PM, Voss K, Langley-Hobbs SJ, editors. Feline orthopedic surgery and musculoskeletal disease. Edinburgh: Elsevier; 2009. p. 21–32.

3. Mazumdar A, Siegel MJ, Narra V, Luchtman-Jones L. Whole-body fast inversion recovery MR imaging of small cell neoplasms in pediatric patients: a pilot study. AJR 2002;17:1261–6.

4. Konar M, Geissbühler U. e.hoof, eLiterature, Switzerland: Vetsuisse Faculty Zürich; 2004.

5. Bushberg JT, Seibert JA, Leidholdt EM, Boone JM. Magnetic resonance imaging MRI. In: The essential physics of medical imaging. 2nd ed. Philadelphia: Lippincott Williams and Wilkins; 2008. p. 415–46.

6. Huda W. Review of radiologic physics, textbook. 3rd ed. Philadelphia: Lippincott Williams and Wilkins; 2003.

7. Berry CR, Graham JP, Thrall DE. Interpretation paradigms for the small animal thorax. In: Thrall DE, editor. Textbook of veterinary diagnostic radiology. 5th ed. Saunders Elsevier; 2007. p. 462–85.

8. Dennis R, Kirberger, RM, Barr F, Wrigley, RH. Lower respiratory tract. In: Handbook of small animal radiology and ultrasound. 2nd ed. Saunders Elsevier; 2010. p. 145–74.

9. Schwarz T, Johnson V. BSAVA manual of canine and feline thoracic imaging. Gloucester: British Small Animal Veterinary Association; 2008.

10. Dennis R. Radiological assessment of lung disease in small animals 1. Bronchial and vascular patterns. In Practice 2008;30:182–9.

11. Dennis R. Radiological assessment of lung disease in small animals. 2. Alveolar,

interstitial and mixed lung patterns. In Practice 2008;30:262–70.

12. Thrall DE, Robertson ID. Atlas of normal radiographic anatomy and anatomic variants in the dog and cat. Saunders Elsevier; 2011.

13. Benigni L, Morgan N, Lamb CR. Radiographic appearance of cardiogenic pulmonary oedema in 23 cats. J Small Anim Prac 2009;50:9–14.

14. Parry A, Lamb C. Radiology of thoracic trauma in the dog and cat. In Practice 2010;32:238–46.

15. Lamb CR. Radiology corner: loss of diaphragmatic line as a sign of ruptured diaphragm. Veterinary Radiology and Ultrasound 2004;45:305–6.

16. Forrest LJ, Graybush CA. Radiographic patterns of pulmonary metastasis in 25 cats. Veterinary Radiology and Ultrasound 1998;39:4–8.

17. Mai W, O'Brien R, Scrivani P, et al. The lung parenchyma. In: Schwarz T, Johnson V, editors. BSAVA manual of canine and feline thoracic imaging. Gloucester: British Small Animal Veterinary Association; 2008;242–320.

18. Mullins ME. MR spectroscopy. Truly molecular imaging; past, present and future. Neuroimaging Clin N Am 2006;16:605–18.

19. Center SA. Hepatic vascular diseases. In: Guilford WG, Center SA, Strombeck DR, et al, editors. Strombeck's small animal gastroenterology. 3rd ed. Philadelphia: WB Saunders; 1996. p. 802–46.

20. Wallack ST. Mesenteric angiography. In: Wallack ST, editor. The handbook of veterinary contrast radiography. San Diego: Veterinary Imaging Inc.; 2003. p. 37–41.

21. Lamb CR. Ultrasonography of portosystemic shunts in dogs and cats. Vet Clin North Am 1998;28:725–53.

22. Zwingenberger AL, Schwarz T. Dual-phase CT angiography of the normal canine portal and hepatic vasculature. Vet Radiol Ultrasound 2004;2:117–24.

23. Daniel GB, Berry CR. Scintigraphic detection of portosystemic shunts. In: Daniel GB, Berry CR, editors. Textbook of veterinary nuclear medicine. 2nd ed. University of Tennessee; 2006. p. 231–55.

24. Cherubini GB, Mantis P, Martinez TA, et al. Utility of magnetic resonance imaging for distinguishing neoplastic from non-neoplastic brain lesions in dogs and cats. Vet Rad Ultrasound 2005;46: 384–7.

25. Prabhakar R, Julka PK, Ganesh T, et al. Feasibility of using MRI alone for 3D radiation treatment planning in brain tumors. Jpn J Clin Oncol 2007;37: 405–11.

26. Singh JB, Oevermann A, Lang J, et al. Contrast media enhancement of intracranial lesions in magnetic resonance imaging does not reflect histopathologic findings consistently. Vet Rad & Ultrasound 2011;52:619–26.

27. Troxel MT, Vite CH, Massicotte C, et al. Magnetic resonance imaging features of feline intracranial neoplasia: retrospective analysis of 46 cats. J Vet Intern Med 2004;18:176–89.

28. Daniel GB, Brawner DR. In: Daniel GB, Berry CR, editors. The handbook of veterinary nuclear medicine. Raleigh, North Carolina: North Carolina State University, College of Veterinary Medicine; 2006. p. 181–98.

29. Harvey AM. Scintigraphic findings in 120 hyperthyroid cats. J Feline Med Surg 2009;11:96–106.

30. Weisse CW, Berent AC, Todd KL, Solomon JA. Potential applications of interventional radiology in veterinary medicine. J Am Anim Med Assoc 2008;233:1564–74.

31. Reimer SB, Kittleson MD, Kyles AE. Use of rheolytic thrombectomy in the treatment of feline distal aortic thromboembolism. J Vet Intern Med 2006;20:290–6.

32. Culp WT, Weisse C, Cole SG, Solomon JA. Intraluminal tracheal stenting for treatment of tracheal narrowing in three cats. Vet Surg 2007;36:107–13.

33. Berent A, Weisse C. Balloon expandable metallic stent placement for benign nasopharyngeal stenosis in dogs and cats. J Am Anim Med Assoc 2008;233: 1432–40.

34. Weisse C, Schwartz K, Stronger R, et al. Transjugular coil embolization of an intrahepatic portosystemic shunt in a cat. J Am Vet Med Assoc 2002;221:1287–91, 1266–7.

35. Kyles AE, Hardie EM, Wooden BG, et al. Management and outcome of cats with ureteral calculi 153 cases (1984–2002). J Am Vet Med Assoc 2005;226: 937–44.

36. Zaid MS, Berent AC, Weisse C, Caceres A. Feline ureteral strictures: 10 cases (2007–2009). J Vet Intern Med 2011;25: 222–9.

37. Lafond E, Weirich WE, Salisbury SK. Omentalization of the thorax for treatment of idiopathic chylothorax with constrictive pleuritis in a cat. J Am Anim Hosp Assoc 2002;38: 74–8.

38. Wells AL, Long CD, Hornof WJ, et al. Use of percutaneous ethanol injection for treatment of bilateral hyperplastic thyroid nodules in cats. J Am Anim Hosp Assoc 2001;218:1293–7.

39. Mallery KF, Pollard RE, Nelson RW, et al. Percutaneous ultrasound-guided radiofrequency heat ablation for treatment of hyperthyroidism in cats. J Am Anim Hosp Assoc 2003;223: 1602–7.

Chapter | 9 |

Endoscopy

A. Harvey

Endoscopy can form a very useful part of the investigation of many disorders. An initial thorough assessment of any patient presenting for any form of endoscopy is of the utmost importance; the risks and benefits of endoscopy should always be carefully weighed up for the individual patient. Endoscopy is used for assessment of the upper and lower gastrointestinal tract, the respiratory tract, and the lower urinary tract. This chapter will cover diagnostic endoscopy for surgical diseases in cats.

GENERAL CONSIDERATIONS

A thorough history and physical examination is required first, and, in most instances, endoscopy should be preceded by other investigations to assess the cat for systemic disease, and to ensure that endoscopy is the most appropriate next stage in the investigation. For the majority of cases, this assessment should include hematological and biochemical analysis of blood, other appropriate laboratory investigations depending on presenting signs (e.g., total T4, fecal analysis, FeLV/FIV testing, urinalysis), blood pressure assessment, and diagnostic imaging (e.g., radiographs, ultrasound, computed tomography). The patient should be stable for anesthesia, and any concurrent diseases or complications (e.g., dehydration) should be addressed. The endoscopic examination should always be fully documented, either by completing a report or through the use of recording equipment.

Endoscopes are expensive and delicate pieces of equipment. It is therefore essential that the surgeon is familiar with how to handle the endoscopes, and how to set up and appropriately use them, in order to avoid damaging the equipment, as well as avoiding risk to the patient through inappropriate use. It is also important to be aware of the cleaning, storage and maintenance required for endoscopes to ensure that they are kept in good working order. The reader should have basic training and be familiar with the basic technique of endoscopy, particularly how to hold the flexible endoscope and use the controls correctly.

Flexible endoscopes

Flexible endoscopy is required for the gastrointestinal tract (GIT), and feline respiratory tract. Flexible endoscopes are complex pieces of equipment with channels for suction and irrigation and passage of instruments as well as light guide fibers and optical image fibers, and guide-wires for the angulation of the tip. They are composed of the insertion tube (the part that enters the patient), the hand piece (containing deflection control knobs, suction valve, air/water valve and instrument channel port) and the umbilical cord (connects hand piece to the light source and also contains the video cable connection, suction pump connection and irrigation bottle connection).

Flexible endoscopes are either fiber optic or video. Fiber optic endoscopes are cheaper, and can be smaller in size, but the image produced is pixelated and of poorer quality than that of a videoscope. Additionally, the glass fibers are very fragile and if damaged the image quality is further reduced. Video endoscopes overcome the problem of poor image quality; however, due to the size of the distal chip sensors required, video endoscopes are not widely available under 5–6 mm diameter. Therefore, many endoscopes used in feline medicine, particularly bronchoscopes, are still fiberscopes.

Rigid endoscopes

A rigid endoscope can potentially be used for tracheoscopy and anteriograde rhinoscopy. The small size of the nose in cats makes rhinoscopy challenging but often an important part of the investigation of cats with chronic nasal discharge, in combination with advanced imaging and biopsy. Rigid endoscopes consist of a fiber optic rigid telescope and a fiber optic light cable that connects to a light source which can be xenon or halogen. Xenon provides a brighter light source and is also suitable for use with flexible video endoscopes and fiberscopes.

A 2.7 mm 18 cm long rigid telescope with a 14.5Fr 17 cm length operating sheath is useful for larger cats (Hopkins II Stortz). The 1.9 mm 19 cm endoscope (cystoscope) is more suitable for most cats. The use of a 10Fr sheath with the smaller (1.9 mm) endoscope

© 2014 Elsevier Ltd
DOI: 10.1016/B978-0-7020-4336-9.00009-3

protects the delicate scope from damage and enables flushing. Both the 2.7 mm and 1.9 mm endoscopes have a 30 degree viewing angle. These endoscopes are also suitable for cystoscopy, otoscopy (and arthroscopy).

GASTROINTESTINAL ENDOSCOPY

Gastrointestinal endoscopy can be used for assessment of the stomach, upper small intestine, and the rectum and colon in the cat.[1,2]

Equipment

For gastrointestinal (GI) endoscopy, a flexible endoscope is required with four-way tip deflection (and ability to retroflex >180° in one plane), and the mechanical functions of insufflation, irrigation and suction. These functions should always be checked prior to anesthetising the cat. A single gastroscope can generally be used in all sized cats for esophagoscopy, gastroduodenoscopy and colonoscopy.

The ability to collect endoscopic biopsies is one of the major advantages and aims of performing gastroendoscopy.[3] The larger the biopsy channel, the larger the biopsies that can be collected and therefore the more likely they are to be of diagnostic quality. The compromise is that the larger the distal tip size, the more difficult pyloric intubation will be. The instrument channel should be at least 2 mm in order to be able to obtain diagnostic biopsy samples. There are several scopes on the market that can be considered (Table 9-1).

Most of these endoscopes have a 2 mm instrument channel, with the largest instrument channel being 2.8 mm. A larger instrument channel has significant advantages, but there are also disadvantages to consider with the larger size of endoscope. An experienced endoscopist will be able to intubate the pylorus of most cats with a distal tip approaching 8mm in diameter, but an inexperienced endoscopist may struggle, and it may not be possible in smaller cats. A 1.4 m length insertion tube is quite long for cats, which can make maneuvering more challenging as the insertion tube outside the patient tends to loop.

The main forceps required for feline gastrointestinal endoscopy are biopsy forceps. Grasping forceps and basket forceps are also useful for removing gastric foreign bodies, although these are less commonly encountered in cats than dogs. Basket forceps are also required for placing percutaneous endoscopic gastrostomy (PEG) tubes. There are many different types of biopsy forceps, varying in shape (oval, round), edge (smooth, serrated), fenestrated or unfenestrated, those with a central spike, and swing jaw forceps. The author prefers oval fenestrated forceps without a central spike. The fenestrated cups reduce crush artefact, and the oval cups tend to collect more tissue. Central spikes can damage the biopsy tissue. The type of edge used depends on the toughness of the tissue being sampled. The author tends to mainly use smooth edged cups, but if the tissue is tough, these can slip off, in which case switching to serrated edged cups is advisable. When taking biopsy samples of the intestine, swing jaw forceps help turn the cups into the intestinal wall, but they are much more expensive forceps.

Prior to anesthetizing the patient, ancillary equipment should be prepared (Box 9-1) and endoscopy equipment checked that it is fully functional (including air pump, suction unit and valve, air/water valve, tip deflection, light source image, biopsy forceps, recording equipment).

Uses and indications

Common reasons for performing upper GI endoscopy in cats are listed in Box 9-2.

Unless a specific esophageal disorder, e.g., a stricture that may make advancing beyond this point unnecessary, is diagnosed, full esophago-gastro-duodenoscopy should always be performed.

Colonoscopy is indicated for investigation of large intestinal diarrhea, hematochezia, tenesmus, dyschezia, constipation and investigation of a palpable rectal mass or stricture. Upper GI endoscopy should always be performed whenever colonoscopy is being performed, since lesions are rarely confined to the colon even when clinical signs are predominantly large intestinal.

GI endoscopy has the advantage of allowing examination of the mucosal surface of the GIT. It is a much less invasive way of obtaining gut biopsies compared to open surgery: the patient can be discharged the same day as the procedure, there is no convalescence or time delay due to wound healing, and immediate corticosteroid treatment can be started if indicated.

Box 9-1 Ancillary equipment required for gastrointestinal endoscopy

Protective clothing
Mouth gag
Biopsy forceps
Formalin pots
Sterile saline

Table 9-1 Examples of endoscopes suitable for gastrointestinal use in cats

Manufacturer	Type	Distal tip	Instrument channel	Working length
Olympus	Lucera video-gastroscope GIF-XP260	5 mm	2 mm	1.1 m
Olympus	Video-gastroscope EvisExera II GIF-XP180N	5.5 mm	2 mm	1.1 m
Olympus	Video-gastroscope SlimSIGHT GIF-XP160	5.9 mm	2 mm	1 m
Olympus	Video-gastroscope VET-XP20	7.9 mm	2 mm	1.4 m
Storz	Video-gastroscope 60714PKS	7.8 mm	2.8 mm	1.4 m
Storz	Video-gastroscope 13820PKS	5.9 mm	2 mm	1.1 m

Box 9-2 **Common reasons for performing upper GI endoscopy in cats**

Assessment of esophageal disease (first exclude mega-esophagus on radiographs), in cases of:
- Regurgitation
- Dysphagia
- Painful swallowing
- Excessive salivation

Dilation of esophageal strictures

Assessment of gastric and small intestinal disease in cases of:
- Chronic vomiting
- Unexplained weight loss
- Unexplained anorexia
- Hematemesis or melena
- Chronic diarrhea
- Ultrasonographically detectable thickening or loss of layering of gastric and/or intestinal wall

Per endoscopic gastrostomy (PEG) tube placement and removal

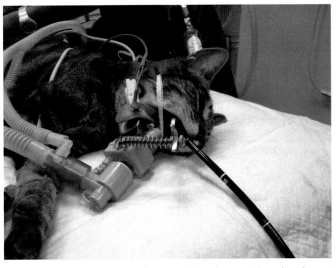

Figure 9-1 Patient positioning for upper GI endoscopy. Note that the cat is in left lateral recumbency, the ET tube is secured in place, and a gag and pulse oximeter are being used. *(Courtesy of Great Western Referrals.)*

Limitations and contraindications

There are relatively few contraindications for gastrointestinal endoscopy. The main one that is essential to consider is where systemic causes of clinical signs have not been excluded and there have been inadequate investigations performed prior to considering endoscopy. Other contraindications include patients that are a poor anesthetic risk, the presence of a bleeding disorder, any patient that has had recent GI surgery, and where food has not been withheld, or the stomach has been found to be full on imaging.

While being a very valuable way of assessing the GIT, there are limitations of endoscopy. Firstly, it does require appropriate and fully functioning equipment together with a competent endoscopist, with good biopsy technique, to allow adequate evaluation of the GIT and collection of diagnostic quality biopsies. It is also not possible to assess functional and motility disorders, hypersecretory disorders, the whole GIT, submucosal lesions, or intraperitoneal lesions. When endoscopic biopsies have failed to produce a diagnosis, where non-mucosal disease is suspected, or disease is known to be beyond the reach of an endoscope, or where there is evidence of intraperitoneal disease (e.g., mesenteric lymphadenopathy, ascites, hepatic/pancreatic abnormalities), then surgical biopsies are indicated.

Patient preparation

For upper GI endoscopy, patient preparation simply requires withdrawal of food for at least 12 hours prior to the procedure, to ensure that the stomach is empty. If any barium contrast studies have been performed, then GI endoscopy should not be performed for at least 24 hours. For colonoscopy, withdrawal of food for 24 hours is required, in addition to 'cleansing' the large intestine. There are various different laxative protocols, but the author's preference is to administer 10–15 mL/kg of polyethylene glycol laxative (Klean-Prep), via a nasoesophageal tube (just placed for each administration and then removed in between), on two or three occasions within the period approximately four to 20 hours prior to colonoscopy, and then to administer a sodium citrate rectal enema (Micralax) two to four hours prior to the procedure.

Pre-medication prior to induction of anesthesia is routine. Atropine is not used routinely, although some advocate that it can make pyloric intubation easier, and it may reduce the risk of vagally induced brady-cardia during the procedure. An intravenous catheter should be in place, and fluids administered throughout the procedure. Induction of anesthesia is routine. Nitrous oxide should not be used since insufflation of the stomach permits diffusion of nitrous oxide into it and causes gastric overdistension. Intravenous midazolam or diazepam can be useful if there is difficulty intubating the pylorus, or if the cat becomes uncomfortable (e.g., tachypneic) during this procedure, or if the GIT is particularly inflamed. For further information on anesthesia see Chapter 2.[1]

An endotracheal (ET) tube should be placed. Cuffed ET tubes are usually advised to prevent the risk of reflux, but caution needs to be used with cuffed ET tubes in cats.

Red rubber tubes with inflated cuffs should not be used, as these high pressure cuffs can cause tracheal necrosis; only the low pressure, high volume cuffed PVC tubes should be used. Presence of a cuff can, however, limit the diameter of the ET tube that can be passed and narrower tubes are more likely to become obstructed. The author prefers to use the largest possible uncuffed tube—in most average sized cats, a size 5 uncuffed ET tube can be passed. The tube should be secured in place, and a mouth gag must always be inserted to prevent damage to the endoscope. Pulse oximetry monitoring should be used, and appropriate warming equipment to ensure the cat does not become hypothermic during the procedure.

The cat should be positioned in left lateral recumbency for routine GI endoscopy (upper and lower), so that the gastric antrum is uppermost, allowing air to fill it and make the pylorus more visible, and that the descending colon lies ventrally, which aids intubation of the transverse and ascending colon (Fig. 9-1). For esophagoscopy where conditions such as mega-esophagus, esophageal strictures or esophageal foreign bodies are suspected, the cat should be kept in sternal recumbency with the head elevated in order to reduce the risk of aspiration. For PEG tube placement, the cat is positioned in right lateral recumbency. The endoscopist should be positioned in such a way that they have a good view of the video monitor, but also in a way that the insertion tube outside of the patient is kept in as straight a line as possible to prevent difficulty steering and advancing, which occurs if there is looping of the insertion tube outside the patient.

ENDOSCOPIC BIOPSY TECHNIQUE

An assistant is required to operate the biopsy forceps and it is important that they are familiar with how to operate them before starting. Instruments must always be passed through the biopsy channel in a closed position and never forced against resistance. Squeezing too hard to close the cups can break the wire of the forceps so must be avoided. Care must be taken when passing instruments through the deflected tip of the endoscope, as forceful passage can easily damage the inner lining of the instrument channel. The instrument channel also serves as a suction channel, so suction will be much reduced when an instrument is within the channel, especially if the instrument channel cap is open. When the scope has passed several intestinal flexures, the forceps can be difficult to open as the wire may be bent, and straightening the endoscope will help with this.

The quality of the biopsies obtained is determined mainly by the size of the forceps (dependent on the size of the scope), and the pressure exerted on the tissue by the operator. This is a big limitation in feline endoscopy as the patient size limits the size of endoscope, and therefore the size of biopsy forceps that can be used. Therefore, in order to obtain diagnostic quality biopsies, there is no room for poor operator technique. Exerting maximal pressure can be achieved by positioning the biopsy cups perpendicular to the tissue being sampled (Fig. 9-2). Being able to do this effectively and knowing how much pressure can safely be applied comes with experience. Deflating the viscus before biopsy also helps increase the size of the sample by reducing stretching of the mucosa.

Once the biopsy has been collected the forceps are removed from the biopsy channel, the cups opened and immersed in 10% formalin, releasing the tissue. The forceps must be rinsed in water before reintroducing into the endoscope. Alternatively, tissue samples can be laid on card or tissue cassettes prior to being placed in formalin.

GASTROINTESTINAL ENDOSCOPY TECHNIQUE

General technique

As the endoscope is inserted into a viscus, air is instilled to obtain a clear view. The rate of air insufflation needs to be adjusted to ensure adequate inflation without over inflation. The small size of cats makes it easy to over inflate the GIT and thus this needs to be monitored carefully. Using a low setting on the air pump and ensuring the airhole is not inadvertently covered leading to continuous insufflation will help avoid over inflation. The anesthetist should also observe and palpate the abdomen regularly to ensure over inflation is not occurring. This is extremely important, as over inflation not only makes the endoscopy more difficult, particularly pyloric intubation and biopsy collection, but more importantly will lead to impairment of venous return, and can quickly result in severe cardiovascular and respiratory compromise, in addition to risking perforation of a viscus. Inability to sufficiently insufflate can be the result of a faulty air pump, leaking seal, air escaping from the viscus, or may indicate significant GI pathology.

Steering is achieved through a combination of insertion and retraction of the insertion tube, longitudinal rotation of the insertion tube (torquing), up/down and left/right tip deflection, and passive movement as the endoscope follows the wall of a viscus. Attention should be paid to keeping the insertion tube as straight as possible to assist in more accurate steering.

The lens will often become obscured by blood, mucus and GI contents, and this requires flushing by depressing the air/water button. Any fluid pooling in a viscus requires suctioning to examine the underlying mucosa. Air should always be suctioned from the viscus before withdrawing the endoscope.

Upper gastrointestinal endoscopy

Delay in intubating the pylorus, combined with insufflation of air, makes pyloric intubation more difficult. Therefore it is usual to only quickly visually inspect the esophagus and stomach on the way down, leaving more complete evaluation to the end of the procedure (except where esophagoscopy is the main purpose of the procedure). The endoscope is inserted through the upper esophageal sphincter by applying only gentle pressure and insufflating small amounts of air. Once through the sphincter the tip should be adjusted so that the esophageal lumen is in the center of the view, and the endoscope gently advanced to the lower esophageal sphincter. A quick inspection of the mucosa on the way down ensures that any pathological lesions can be distinguished from iatrogenic damage when closer inspection is performed on withdrawal. In cats, the distal esophagus has distinct circular folds and the lower esophageal sphincter may be seen as a star or slit-like opening (Fig. 9-3).

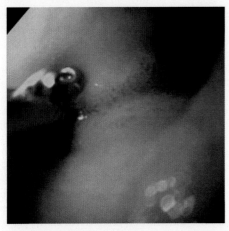

Figure 9-2 Duodenum from a cat with inflammatory bowel disease, illustrating biopsy technique, positioning the biopsy cups perpendicular to the mucosa. *(Courtesy of the University of Bristol.)*

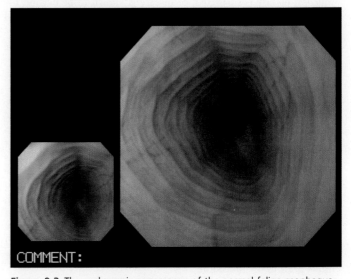

Figure 9-3 The endoscopic appearance of the normal feline esophagus. *(Courtesy of the University of Bristol.)*

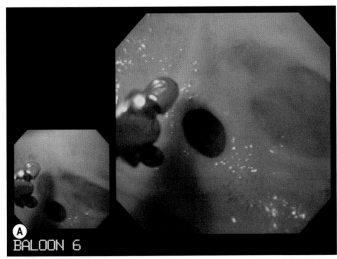

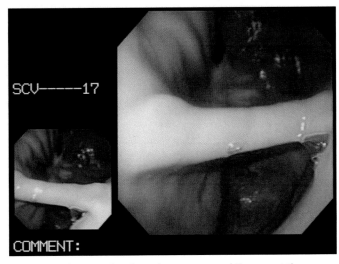

Figure 9-5 The normal endoscopic appearance of the area at the junction of the body/fundus of the stomach on the greater curvature. Note that the parallel rugal folds are running towards the pyloric antrum beneath the angularis incisura. *(Courtesy of the University of Bristol.)*

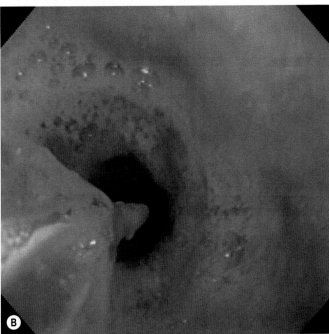

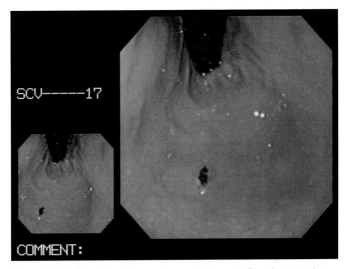

Figure 9-6 Image shows the gastroscope being retroflexed to examine the cardia. Note the small red area of hemorrhage where a biopsy has just been taken. This is a normal post-biopsy appearance. *(Courtesy of the University of Bristol.)*

Figure 9-4 Esophageal stricture. **(A)** The endoscopic biopsy forceps (oval fenestrated forceps without a central spike) give an indication of the diameter of the strictured area. **(B)** A balloon catheter is being advanced through the lumen of the oesophageal stricture to allow balloon dilation. *(Courtesy of the University of Bristol.)*

The most common pathologies observed in the feline esophagus are esophagitis, esophageal ulceration, and esophageal strictures (Fig. 9-4A). Biopsies are not routinely taken from the esophagus as the mucosa is very tough. Masses should be biopsied, but these are rare. With esophageal strictures, endoscopy can be used to guide balloon dilation, by passing a balloon catheter alongside the endoscope (Fig. 9-4B). When the stricture is very narrow it can be difficult to insert the balloon into the stricture and great care needs to be taken when directing the balloon to ensure that the tip does not cause further esophageal trauma or esophageal perforation. See Chapter 27 for more information on esophageal disease.

Once at the lower esophageal sphincter, the endoscope tip should be angled towards it with continued insufflation and gently advanced through into the stomach. As the endoscope enters the stomach the junction of the fundus and body of the stomach can be seen, with parallel rugal folds on the greater curvature running towards the

pyloric antrum (Fig. 9-5). This provides an important landmark in locating the pylorus. The other most important landmark is the angularis incisura (angle of the lesser curvature) with the cardia above, and the pyloric antrum below, and this can be located by retroflexing the endoscope tip fully to first locate the cardia (Fig. 9-6) and then slightly reducing the retroflexion to bring the lesser curvature into view. Some insufflation is required to visualize these landmarks, but over inflation will make pyloric intubation difficult, and this is the most common mistake made. In cats, the angle of the lesser curvature is quite acute, and a slide-by technique can be useful for passing the endoscope into the antrum. This involves gently advancing the endoscope along the mucosal surface of the greater curvature; the endoscope tip will be impinging on the gastric mucosa and so red-out will occur, but provided this is moving and the endoscope is not advanced against any resistance, it can continue to be advanced along the greater curvature until the pyloric antrum comes into view. Ensuring that the pylorus is in the center of the screen, and suctioning as the insertion tube is advanced towards it assists with pyloric intubation.

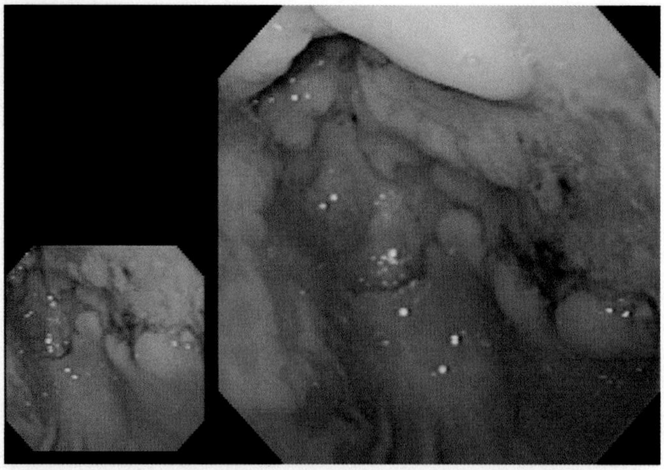

Figure 9-7 Endoscopic view of the stomach of a cat with gastric lymphoma. Note the very pale and 'lumpy' appearance. *(Courtesy of the University of Bristol.)*

Once through the pylorus the insertion tube is advanced past the cranial duodenal flexure, where red-out is likely to occur, and then with intermittent insufflation of air, and deflection of the tip, the lumen of the duodenum should come into view. The endoscope can then be gently pushed along the duodenal mucosa as far as required. With a 1 m length endoscope, the proximal jejunum may even be reached in cats. It is common for the mucosa to appear macroscopically normal even when significant microscopic disease is present. Multiple biopsies (approximately six to ten) should therefore always be taken from different regions of the small intestine.[4] The most common small intestinal disorders in cats are inflammatory bowel disease and intestinal lymphoma.

Once the duodenum has been assessed and biopsies taken, all the air should be suctioned out as the endoscope is withdrawn. The proximal duodenal flexure should be evaluated on the way out for lesions (e.g., ulcers) before withdrawing the endoscope back into the stomach for more complete evaluation. Retroflexion and rotation of the endoscope along its long axis allow full inspection of the cardia and the fundus. Multiple biopsies (total approximately six to ten) should be taken from all areas of the stomach, in addition to any macroscopic lesions. In cats, the most frequent macroscopic lesions identified are neoplastic disorders, most commonly gastric lymphoma. The mucosa is often pale, lumpy and friable; however, this is very variable and there is no pathognomonic appearance (Fig. 9-7).

Colonoscopy

Colonoscopy is more straightforward to perform than upper GI endoscopy, provided that the patient has been adequately prepared. The insertion tube should be lubricated with gel, and an assistant is required to gently pinch the anus around the insertion tube to prevent air from escaping. Once inserted into the rectum, air should be insufflated until the mucosa of the descending colon is in view, before advancing further. The junctions between the descending and transverse colon, and transverse and ascending colon can be readily detected as obvious bends, prior to reaching the ileocecocolic junction, identified by the opening into the cecum and the prominent raised appearance of the ileocolic sphincter. It is possible to pass biopsy forceps through the sphincter to biopsy the ileal mucosa. Approximately six to ten biopsies should be taken from all parts of the colon, prior to suctioning the air out and withdrawing the endoscope and examining the rectum on the way out. Ileal biopsies were found to be useful in the diagnosis of small cell lymphoma in a small

percentage of cats in one study of the utility of endoscopic biopsies in cats.[5]

Complications and aftercare

Serious complications associated with GI endoscopy are rare. The most common problem is gastric overinflation, which as well as making endoscopy more difficult, particularly pyloric intubation and biopsy collection, also leads to impairment of venous return, and can quickly result in severe cardiovascular and respiratory compromise. It is important to avoid overdistension, and to remember to remove air with suction prior to withdrawing the endoscope at the end of the procedure. Other potential complications include bradycardia, which may occur as a vagovagal reflex, usually in cats with severe GI disease, and is usually resolved with atropine, and gastrointestinal perforation, which when it occurs is usually the result of severe GI disease, accompanied by forceful use of the endoscope without adequate visualization, or poor biopsy technique. Occasionally with severe GI disease, perforation can occur with over inflation alone. Emergency laparotomy is required if perforation is evident or pneumoperitoneum develops. Significant mucosal hemorrhage associated with biopsy is rare, and it is not necessary to routinely prescribe gastrointestinal protectants following endoscopy. Most cases of routine endoscopy require no specific aftercare.

RESPIRATORY TRACT ENDOSCOPY

Equipment

For rigid rhinoscopy either a 1.9 mm or a 2.7 mm (18 cm long) rigid endoscope can be used, although the latter is only suitable for use in larger cats. Both these endoscopes have a 30° viewing angle. These endoscopes are also suitable for cystoscopy, otoscopy (and arthroscopy) (Table 9-2). Examination of the nasopharynx is also possible with the 1.9 mm rigid endoscope, which alleviates the need for flexible retrograde rhinoscopy.

The 2.7 mm telescope has a 14.5 Fr sheath containing a 5 Fr working channel and two Luer stopcocks for irrigation and suction. A range of 5 Fr flexible biopsy instruments are available which pass though the working channel. These include cup biopsy forceps and grasping forceps. The 1.9 mm 19 cm endoscope (cystoscope) is a suitable size for most cats. The use of a 10 Fr sheath with the smaller (1.9 mm) endoscope protects the delicate scope from damage and enables flushing. Use of the scope without the sheath facilitates examination of the more caudal nasal passages but risks damage to the scope. Rigid biopsy forceps are available to be used parallel to the telescope if a sheath (such as the 10 Fr) with no working channel is used.

For endoscopy of the respiratory tract in cats, a flexible endoscope is most useful. Due to the size of the distal tip sensors required for video endoscopy, video endoscopes are not widely available under 5–6 mm diameter, so the endoscopes used for feline bronchoscopy and rhinoscopy are almost always fiberscopes, which have a reduced quality of image compared to video endoscopes, but are less expensive to purchase. Bronchoscopes are simpler to use than gastroscopes, in that they just have two-way tip deflection and suction. There is no air/water channel as there is no requirement for insufflation and irrigation with respiratory tract endoscopy. The suction function is important for being able to suction any airway secretions, in addition to performing bronchoalveolar lavage (BAL), and this function should always be checked prior to anesthetising the cat. Small suction tips should also be readily available.

Table 9-2 Some suitable bronchoscopes for cats

Manufacturer	Type	Distal tip diameter	Instrument channel	Working length
Olympus OES bronchoscopes	BF 3C40	3.3 mm	1.2 mm	55 cm
Olympus OES bronchoscopes	BF-XP60	2.8 mm	1.2 mm	60 cm
Karl Storz bronchoscopes	60002 VL1	3.7 mm	1.5 mm	54 cm
Karl Storz bronchoscopes	60003 VB1	3 mm	1.2 mm	1 m

A 3–3.7 mm diameter bronchoscope should be suitable for all cats.

Box 9-3 Ancillary equipment required for feline bronchoscopy

Protective clothing
Mouth gag
Topical 1% lignocaine, 0.2 mL
Aspiration catheters
EDTA and plain collection pots for BAL fluid
Two to four 5 mL syringes containing 0.9% sterile saline for performing BALs
Biopsy forceps
Grasping forceps for foreign body retrieval
Swabs/sponges for packing the pharynx in case of nasopharyngeal hemorrhage following biopsy
Equipment for thoracocentesis in case of pneumothorax

Box 9-4 Indications for rhinoscopy

Acute onset sneezing and facial discomfort
Chronic nasal discharge
Stertorous breathing
Sneezing
Epistaxis
Gagging/retching
Facial distortion or swelling
Biopsy of nasopharyngeal masses
Retrieval of nasopharyngeal foreign bodies

One size of bronchoscope can be used in any domestic cat for both bronchoscopy and retrograde rhinoscopy (Table 9-2).

The author prefers to collect BAL samples directly through the bronchoscope, by attaching a collection tube between the bronchoscope and the suction tubing, but aspiration catheters can also be used for fluid collection, either inserted through or adjacent to the bronchoscope. It is essential that the bronchoscope is sterilized prior to use, and that scope flushes are performed for bacterial culture, to ensure there is no scope contamination. Cytology brushes, aspiration needles and small biopsy forceps can also be used for obtaining samples.

Prior to anesthetising the patient, ancillary equipment should also be ready prepared (Box 9-3) and the bronchoscopy equipment should be checked that it is fully functioning (including suction unit and valve, tip deflection, light source image, recording equipment).

Uses and indications

The most common reason for performing bronchoscopy in cats is in the assessment of chronic lower airway disease as indicated by chronic cough and/or episodic tachypnea/dyspnea (with consistent radiographic abnormalities); lung masses and focal or diffuse bronchial/bronchointerstitial/bronchoalveolar lung patterns identified on thoracic radiographs; acute cough/dyspnea, particularly for retrieval of tracheal or bronchial foreign bodies[6] and for the collection of bronchoalveolar lavage samples.[7] The indications for rhinoscopy are listed in Box 9-4; investigation of chronic nasal discharge in cats is one of the commonest indications.[8]

Limitations and contraindications

The main risk of bronchoscopy is development of hypoxemia. This can easily result in cats, given the narrowness of their airways, particularly if bronchoscopy is prolonged, if there is induction of bronchospasm, or mucus plugging of airways. Close monitoring of pulse oximetry is therefore required, and the procedure should be performed as quickly as possible while still being thorough. Contraindications to bronchoscopy include severe pre-existing hypoxemia, cardiac failure, severe dyspnea (except where likely to be resolved by the procedure e.g., foreign body retrieval), presence of a bleeding disorder, and in any patient where inadequate investigations have been performed prior to considering bronchoscopy. The limitation of bronchoscopy is that it only allows assessment of the larger airways so is not useful for evaluating interstitial pulmonary disease or the small bronchi so can miss focal disorders and foreign bodies that have migrated into distal bronchi. Sample collection is limited to samples for cytological assessment (BALs and cytology brushes) and extremely small biopsy samples.

There are few contraindications for retrograde rhinoscopy. The main contraindications are inadequate investigations being performed prior to anesthesia and patients that are a poor anesthetic risk. The limitations of retrograde rhinoscopy are that it only allows for assessment of the pharynx caudal to the choanae, and most often if any lesions are biopsied the resultant hemorrhage precludes further evaluation or additional biopsies to be taken. Furthermore, endoscopic biopsies are extremely small in size, and therefore often of limited diagnostic value.

Contraindications to rigid rhinoscopy are coagulation abnormalities, which could result in excessive hemorrhage, and if advanced imaging studies have revealed compromise of the cribriform plate that could allow excessive damage to occur on flushing of the nasal cavity.

Patient preparation

Depending on the reason for performing endoscopy of the respiratory tract, and the clinical status of the cat, pre-oxygenation is usually advisable. Pre-medication prior to induction of anesthesia is dependent on clinical status. For cats undergoing bronchoscopy, administration of terbutaline prior to the procedure reduces the risk of inducing

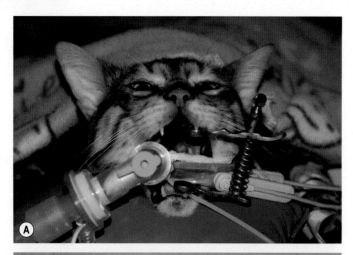

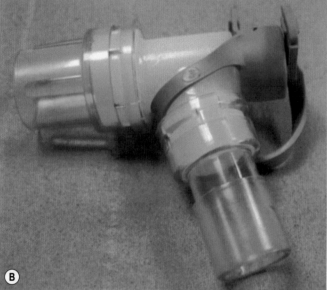

Figure 9-8 (A) Patient positioning for bronchoscopy, illustrating a **(B)** swivel tip T-adaptor to allow passage of the bronchoscope through the ET tube while allowing continuation of inhalational anesthesia.

The ET tube or catheter tubing should be secured in place, and a mouth gag used. For retrograde rhinoscopy, consideration needs to be given to reducing risk of aspiration if there are excessive secretions and/or hemorrhage. A cuffed ET tube can be used, and is often recommended; however, care does need to be taken not to traumatize the trachea with cuffed tubes in cats. The author prefers to use as large a diameter ET tube as possible (most cats can accommodate a size 5 ET tube) uncuffed, and to pack the pharynx with swabs/sponges as required. Packing the pharynx interferes with being able to introduce the endoscope over the edge of the soft palate, so the author starts off the procedure without packs but has packs and suction to hand, which are used as soon as the endoscope is withdrawn.

Pulse oximetry monitoring before, during, and after all respiratory endoscopy is vital. ECG and end-tidal capnography monitoring are also recommended. If problems are encountered the procedure should be stopped, the cat intubated, ventilated, and airway secretions suctioned if required.

RESPIRATORY ENDOSCOPY TECHNIQUE

General technique

As anesthesia is being induced, the larynx should always be fully evaluated prior to intubation for evidence of edema, hyperemia, irregularity, masses, and paralysis. Where both bronchoscopy and retrograde rhinoscopy are being performed, bronchoscopy should be performed first to avoid scope contamination. The general technique for respiratory tract endoscopy is more straightforward than for GI endoscopy, with steering being the main requirement, achieved by up/down tip deflection and longitudinal rotation of the insertion tube (torquing). Respiratory endoscopy, however, is a much higher risk procedure, and the endoscopist needs to be skilled not to cause any trauma, to ensure a thorough but quick evaluation and sample collection. Close communication should be maintained with the anesthetist at all times, so that any concerns arising can be rapidly addressed.

Bronchoscopy

Once the patient is adequately prepared, the bronchoscope is gently advanced down the trachea, observing for abnormalities such as erythema and irregularity of the mucosa, foreign material, and excessive airway secretions. Given the wide and straight nature of the trachea, it is usually straightforward to obtain a good image to the level of the carina (Fig. 9-9). Beyond this, the small size of the feline airways can make obtaining a good image quite challenging. However, it is important that the airway lumen is visualized adequately as the bronchoscope is advanced, to avoid iatrogenic airway trauma. Steering is used to direct the bronchoscope into the left or right main stem bronchi. The right main stem bronchus will be seen on the left side of the image. A standard method of systemic evaluation should be used for evaluating the airways on each side, with a map of the airways (Fig. 9-10) always borne in mind.[7,9] The airways should be evaluated for collapse, masses, compression, excessive mucus, purulent secretions, hemorrhage, mucosal erythema and irregularity, and foreign material. Both sides of the airways should be evaluated before collecting samples.

BAL samples should be routinely collected from left and right sides for cytology and culture. Once the lung lobe to be sampled has been selected, the bronchoscope should be advanced into smaller and smaller airways until it is seated in the airway and cannot be advanced any further. Sterile 0.9% saline 5 mL is then flushed either directly

bronchospasm. An intravenous catheter should be in place. The cat should be positioned in sternal recumbency with the head slightly elevated and the neck extended (Fig. 9-8A). Ideally, an ET tube is placed, and the bronchoscope passed through the lumen of the ET tube. A swivel tip T-adaptor is attached between the ET tube and the T-piece (Fig. 9-8B). This contains a rubber valve at the port allowing anesthetic gases and oxygen to be delivered while the bronchoscope is passed through the ET tube. After intravenous induction of anesthesia (e.g., with propofol) the cat is preferably maintained on inhalational anesthesia, which is possible if the endoscope can fit easily through the ET tube leaving enough space for movement of gases at the same time.

When the lumen of the ET tube is too narrow to accommodate the bronchoscope, narrow bore tubing such as a dog urinary catheter can be inserted into the trachea and used for intermittent oxygen propulsion, by connecting an ET tube connector, and a T-piece with the reservoir bag removed, to enable the anesthetist to jet propulse oxygen down the tube by intermittently covering the end of the tube with a thumb. In this situation, anesthesia needs to be maintained with total intravenous anesthesia,[1] such as small increments of propofol, as required.

down the endoscope channel or through an aspiration catheter, an assistant coupages the chest, and then suction is applied with either a syringe or using the endoscope suction system. A further 5 mL bolus may be required if inadequate fluid is retrieved. The sample should be placed in an EDTA and plain collection pot. The procedure is then repeated in a lung lobe on the opposite side.

Brush cytology can be useful, particularly of any mass type lesions, but the author does not routinely perform this. The author rarely performs airway biopsies, since the small size of samples possible with a feline bronchoscope is often of limited diagnostic value, and the risks of hemorrhage and pneumothorax are significant. The author usually reserves biopsies for airway masses, for which biopsy is useful, but risk of hemorrhage still needs to be considered.

The most common airway pathology in cats is chronic airway inflammation of varying degrees, and less commonly bronchial foreign bodies, usually associated with secondary localized broncho-pneumonia. Retrieval of bronchial foreign bodies can be difficult. The

limitations in the size of the instrument channel mean that retrieval devices generally need to be inserted alongside the endoscope, which makes directing the retrieval device into the required airway challenging even for a skilled endoscopist.

Rhinoscopy

If anteriograde rhinoscopy with a rigid endoscope and/or biopsies or nasal flushes are also going to be performed, then retrograde rhinoscopy should be performed first, as otherwise fluid/blood/discharge may obscure visualization of the nasopharynx. Retrograde rhinoscopy is performed by retroflexing the flexible endoscope over the edge of the soft palate, to look forwards towards the choanae. The endoscope can either be inserted straight into the oropharynx and then retroflexed when the tip is beyond the edge of the soft palate, or retroflexed into a 'J' shape prior to insertion. The insertion tube is then pulled rostrally, advancing the tip towards the choanae. The view on the monitor is upside down and reversed. It is normal to stimulate a strong gag reflex during this procedure, which can make it very challenging. Use of topical lidocaine spray on the soft palate can help to blunt this reflex. The nasopharynx should be evaluated for presence of discharge, hyperemic/irregular/nodular tissue, masses, polyps, nasopharyngeal stenosis and foreign bodies (e.g., a blade of grass). The most common pathology in the nasopharynx of cats is inflammatory disease. Changes seen include mild to severe erythema and mucosal irregularity; excessive secretions may obscure adequate visualization of the area. Raised nodules of benign lymphoid hyperplasia are quite commonly seen with chronic inflammatory disorders (Fig. 9-11), which may be isolated to the pharynx, or associated with inflammatory nasal disease. Other common abnormalities observed in cats are foreign bodies, polyps, and neoplastic masses, most commonly lymphoma (Fig. 9-12).

Foreign bodies such as blades of grass may be removed with endoscopic forceps. However, with the limitation in size of forceps that can be used endoscopically, it is often easier once a foreign body has been identified to remove it with grabbing forceps under direct visualization by placing the cat in dorsal recumbency and using a spay hook or Allis tissue forceps to pull the soft palate forward.

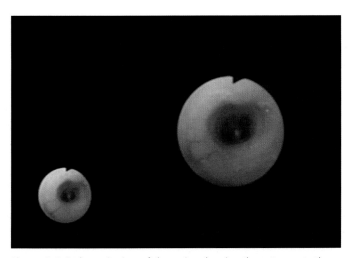

Figure 9-9 Endoscopic view of the carina showing the entrance to the left and right main stem bronchi. *(Courtesy of the University of Bristol.)*

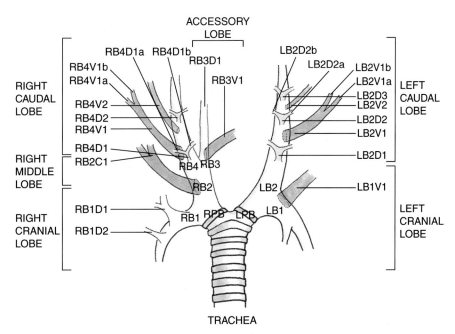

Figure 9-10 Dorsal view of the feline bronchial tree. *(Reprinted from Caccamo R. Endoscopic bronchial anatomy in the cat. J Feline Med Surg 2007;9:140–149, with permission from Sage Publications.)*

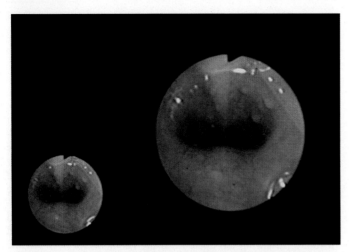

Figure 9-11 Endoscopic view of the nasopharynx by retrograde rhinoscopy. Note the multiple small raised nodules, typical of a cat with pharyngitis. *(Courtesy of the University of Bristol.)*

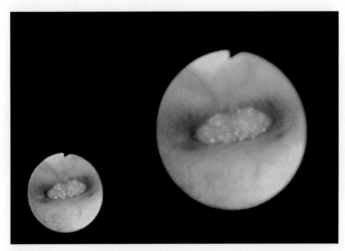

Figure 9-12 Endoscopic view of the nasopharynx by retrograde rhinoscopy of a cat with nasopharyngeal lymphoma. *(Courtesy of the University of Bristol.)*

Endoscopic guided biopsies can be useful for taking biopsy samples of masses; however, often one biopsy alone will cause significant enough hemorrhage to obscure further visualization and therefore further endoscopic guided biopsies will not be possible. When taking endoscopic biopsies, to avoid damaging the biopsy channel, it is vital that the biopsy forceps are passed through to the distal tip prior to retroflexing the tip. Depending on the reason for performing retrograde rhinoscopy, and the abnormalities identified, most cases will also require a combination of rigid rhinoscopy and/or nasal flushes and/or blindly collected anteriograde nasal biopsies to complete the investigation.

Prior to rigid rhinoscopy a coagulation profile is advisable as even minor trauma to the nasal mucosa may cause dramatic hemorrhage. A deep plane of anesthesia is required for rigid rhinoscopy due to the sensitivity of the nasal mucosa. Local anesthetic blocks such as the infraorbital nerve block are recommended (Chapter 2) and the use of a topical lidocaine spray via the external nares is helpful to numb the mucosa. The cat is placed in ventral recumbency with the head angled slightly down, with the nose over the end of the table to facilitate drainage from the nose. Before inserting the rhinoscope into the external nares, the rhinoscope is measured from the external nares to the medial canthus of the eye and a tape marker placed at this level to prevent damage to the cribriform plate.

If discharge obscures the view once the rhinoscope has been placed into the nares, flushing gently with saline or a balanced electrolyte solution either via the rhinoscope sheath or the nares can improve visualization and decrease iatrogenic damage. Both nasal cavities should be explored before taking biopsies, starting with the side least likely to be affected. Biopsies can be taken blind, through the sheath with flexible biopsy forceps, or via rigid cup forceps that are run alongside the rhinoscope so that the jaws are visible. Multiple biopsies are taken; this is particularly important if a mass is visualized. If any foreign bodies are found, alligator forceps passed parallel to the endoscope are suitable for removal in most cases. For further information on nasal disease and investigation the reader is referred to Chapter 54.

Complications and aftercare

The main potential complications associated with bronchoscopy are hypoxemia, hypercarbia, bronchospasm, trauma and hemorrhage and pneumothorax. Most of these complications are easily avoidable through good bronchoscopy technique and careful anesthesia and monitoring. Hemorrhage is a risk with rigid anteriograde rhinoscopy though this is usually controllable with ice packs and flushing with cold saline. Occasionally cotton buds are placed via the nares to obstruct blood flow and encourage clotting. These are removed after recovery from anesthesia, which should be gradual and controlled. The pharynx should be inspected prior to extubation and any blood gently removed. Patients are usually monitored overnight after rigid rhinoscopy to ensure sneezing does not cause significant hemorrhage and to protect owners' homes, as mild sneezing of hemorrhagic discharge is common. Retrograde rhinoscopy itself is relatively low risk, but it is common after pharyngeal examination for excessive mucus to be secreted, and when biopsies have been taken there can be significant hemorrhage. Care needs to be taken to prevent aspiration by use of swabs to pack the pharynx and suction to ensure clear airways.

Following all respiratory endoscopy, the cat should remain intubated and allowed to breathe 100% oxygen. Any excessive secretions should be suctioned, both from within the ET tube and the back of the pharynx. If nasopharyngeal biopsies have been taken, the pharynx should be carefully assessed for remaining hemorrhage, and any blood swabbed or suctioned to ensure a clear airway at the point that the cat is ready to be extubated. In cases of suspected bronchospasm following bronchoscopy, terbutaline administration can be continued following the procedure. It is essential that cats are closely monitored in recovery with suction equipment, ET tubes, laryngoscope, and oxygen, as it is not uncommon for airway obstruction to occur during recovery, most commonly as a result of airway secretions.

URETHROCYSTOSCOPY

P. Lhermette

The bladder and urethra in cats can be directly visualized by endoscopy. The procedure is known as cystoscopy when the bladder is examined or urethrocystography when the urethra is included in the examination. Urethrocystoscopy can be used for examining the whole of the urinary tract from the vestibule to the urinary bladder. This is a relatively easy technique in the female but the narrow urethra of the male presents more of a challenge. One of the commonest indications

Table 9-3 Some suitable urethrocystoscopes for cats

Manufacturer	Type	Outer diameter	Viewing angle	Working length	Comments
Endoscopes for urethrocystography in females					
Karl Storz	67030 BA	9 Fr (3.16 mm)	30°	14 cm	3 Fr (1 mm) instrument channel. Integral sheath therefore sturdier in construction
		2.7 mm	30°	18 cm	
		1.9 mm	30°	19 cm	Care, fragile – need protective sheath
Endoscopes for urethrocystography in males					
Karl Storz	62512	1–1.2 mm			0.3 mm infusion channel
		1 mm	0°	20 cm	Can be used without a sheath
Endoscopes need to be at least 14 cm in length to reach the bladder.					

for urethrocystography in cats is for further investigation of feline lower urinary tract disease (FLUTD).

Equipment

Female

The standard equipment for urethrocystoscopy is a rigid endoscope in a cystoscope sheath with a working channel and two additional Luer ports for flushing and irrigation. This is always used with a camera system, a monitor, and an appropriate light source, preferably a xenon 150–300W. A variety of different endoscope systems may be used for urethrocystoscopy (Table 9-3). In adult females the urethra is easily traumatized and urethral diameter varies considerably between individuals so it may be necessary to use a smaller diameter sheath such as a high flow arthroscope sheath or even a smaller endoscope and sheath. Where a smaller endoscope is used it is important to ensure it has adequate length, at least 14 cm in order to reach the bladder. Great care must be taken with the smaller scopes to avoid torsion or flexion as small endoscopes are extremely fragile. For this reason they are never used without a protective sheath of some kind. The 9 Fr operating telescope (Karl Storz 67030BA) comprises a 1.9 mm telescope and cystoscope sheath permanently fused together and is suitable for urethrocystoscopy in almost all queens.

Male

The urethra of the tom cat is extremely narrow and can only be examined with a semi-flexible 1–1.2 mm cystourethroscope. Most of these endoscopes are too small to accommodate an instrument or infusion channel, which limits their effectiveness, and they also lack directional control. A cystourethroscope with a diameter of 1.2 mm and a 0.3 mm infusion channel, that allows the infusion of saline or gas under pressure, can improve visualization. A sharp 2.1 mm 17 cm sheath (Karl Storz 26120 JX) can be used with the 1 mm Karl Storz scope as an optical veress pneumoperitoneum needle and can therefore also be used for direct percutaneous entry into the bladder if necessary.

Indications

Lower urinary tract disease is common in cats, with approximately 60% of cases being idiopathic.[10] In cats with recurrent episodes or in elderly cats it is sensible to rule out other causes of lower urinary tract disease such as urolithiasis, neoplasia or anatomical malformation. Tumors such as transitional cell carcinoma are rare but can present with similar signs to those of feline lower urinary tract disease.[11]

Investigation of FLUTD will usually include diagnostic imaging. Both ultrasound and radiography are commonly used to image the urinary tract but limitations with these techniques include relative insensitivity and the presence of the bony pelvis. They do, however, enable the clinician to visualize structures outside the urinary tract or within the bladder wall which may not be visible from within the lumen. CT and MRI may also be used but are relatively expensive and rarely available in a first opinion setting.

Other indications for urethrocystoscopy include cases of urinary tract incontinence and urinary tract trauma. The most common causes for incontinence in the cat are ectopic ureters or congenital urethral sphincter mechanism incompetence. These conditions can easily be diagnosed using urethrocystoscopy. The presence of urinary tract trauma following pelvic fracture is common. Urethrocystoscopy has been found to be a more sensitive technique for assessing bladder and urethral trauma in comparison to radiography.[12,13]

URETHROCYSTOSCOPY TECHNIQUE IN THE FEMALE

The technique for urethrocystoscopy in the queen is similar to that in the bitch.[14] It is not necessary to clip the perineal area unless it is heavily soiled. The perivulval/preputial area should be cleaned with a suitable antiseptic such as chlorhexidene. The patient is positioned in sternal recumbency on a tub table or over a gridded tray. The endoscope is placed in a matching cystoscope sheath, a camera and light guide cable are attached and the system is white balanced. A litre of saline is attached to an infusion port on the cystoscope sheath via a standard giving set. Normal (0.9%) or Hartmann's solution may be used, but it should always be warmed to body temperature to avoid hypothermia. The controls on the giving set are opened to allow adjustment of flow using the taps on the cystoscope. The cystoscope sheath is lubricated with sterile water-soluble lubricant and the tip is inserted into the vulva in a rostrodorsal direction to follow the lumen of the vestibule. The vulva is compressed by pinching around the cystoscope to form a seal and saline flow is initiated to inflate the vestibule. The vaginal os and urethral orifice are visualized (Fig. 9-13) and the cystoscope is advanced and guided into the urethra. The urethral lumen dilates with the saline irrigation and can be examined in detail for lesions or the presence of ectopic ureters as the cystoscope is advanced. Care should be taken to ensure that the lumen of the urethra is centered at the bottom of the image on the monitor. The 30° angle of the telescope is always directed opposite to the light

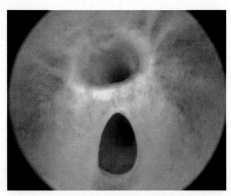

Figure 9-13 Cystoscopic view of the feline vestibule showing vaginal os above and urethral opening below.

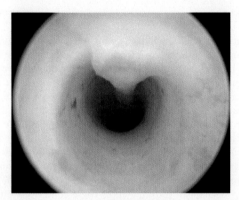

Figure 9-14 Cystoscopic view of the female feline urethra with prominent dorsal fold.

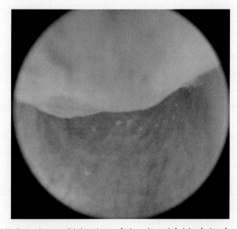

Figure 9-15 Prominent thickening of the dorsal fold of the female proximal urethra near the trigone.

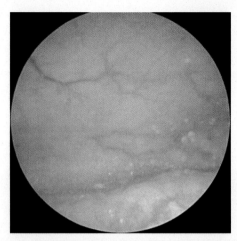

Figure 9-16 Cystoscopic view of small struvite crystals in the bladder. These can be removed by suction through the cystoscope channel.

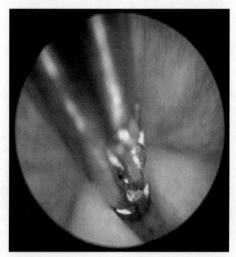

Figure 9-17 Biopsies of the bladder may be taken under direct visualization with forceps placed through the instrument channel. The bladder should be non-distended or flaccid in order to get a good sample.

guide cable so that when the light guide cable is in a ventral position the telescope's line of view will be directed up at the dorsal wall of the urethra. Attempting to maintain the lumen in the center of the image will result in trauma to the ventral wall of the urethra. The urethra of the queen has a prominent dorsal fold (Fig. 9-14), which is not present in the bitch, and there is often an obvious thickening near the trigone that must be negotiated before entering the bladder (Fig. 9-15).

The bladder is examined for calculi, polyps or masses, and hemorrhage or other abnormalities. Urine often appears cloudy and may contain cellular debris and other particulate matter (Fig. 9-16), therefore following an initial examination urine is drained from the bladder via the suction port on the cystoscope. If an arthroscope is being used with only one port, the giving set is removed and urine is drained using a 50 mL syringe. The bladder is then filled with sterile saline to improve visualization. Care should be taken not to over inflate the bladder as this may cause damage to the mucosa and hemorrhage. It will also make taking biopsies difficult. Occasionally several flushes may be required, especially if there is any hemorrhage. Insufflation with air or, preferably, carbon dioxide may be necessary if hemorrhage is severe enough to prevent adequate visualization.

The ureteral openings are visualized at approximately 10 o'clock and 2 o'clock on the dorsal wall of the trigone and these should be observed for normal function. Urine should be seen entering the bladder periodically as a clear yellow stream. Rotating the telescope around its long axis utilizes the 30° angle of view to visualize the whole of the trigone. For biopsy collection flexible biopsy forceps are introduced through the instrument channel (Fig. 9-17). If an arthroscope sheath is used then no instrument channel is available. In this case the endoscope is carefully removed, leaving the arthroscope sheath in the bladder. Biopsy forceps can then be placed through the sheath and blind biopsies taken. Biopsy samples are small and subject to artefactual damage so it is important that multiple samples are taken. The endoscope is replaced and the bladder wall inspected to ensure biopsies have been taken from a representative area. This blind technique is best for generalized bladder wall lesions where the location of the biopsy is not critical, although it is possible to get biopsies of specific lesions as long as they are not in an awkward site (e.g., the trigone) where maintaining the position of the sheath is difficult. If uroliths are present they may be grasped using forceps or a stone basket and removed individually through the urethra. If they are too large or numerous, a laparoscopic assisted cystoscopy or open cystotomy may be performed to remove them (see Chapters 24 and 37). Following sample collection the bladder is drained through the cystoscope and the instrument is carefully removed.

URETHROCYSTOSCOPY TECHNIQUE IN THE MALE

The small diameter endoscopes required for transurethral cystoscopy in the tom cat do not have an instrument channel and so biopsies of specific lesions must be collected by a laparoscopic assisted approach or open cystotomy. For generalized bladder wall lesions small 3.5 Fr biopsy forceps can be passed blindly up the urethra to obtain samples from the bladder wall. However, histological interpretation can be difficult due to the very small sample size. If a perineal urethrostomy has been performed, rigid urethrocystoscopy may be performed as for the queen. Alternatively, with the right equipment, the bladder can be entered by direct percutaneous entry.

The urethra in the tom cat has a distinct bend in it where it approaches the pelvic brim, which can impede the advancement of the endoscope. To avoid this difficulty the tip of the penis should be gently grasped with a moistened swab and pulled caudally and slightly dorsally to straighten the urethra before attempting to pass the endoscope (Fig. 9-18).

Complications and aftercare

The urethra is delicate and easily traumatized. Great care must be taken during urethrocystoscopy, especially where a 30° telescope is used as allowance must be made for the angle of view. When passing

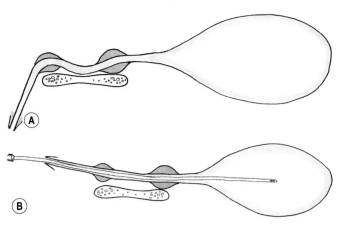

Figure 9-18 Positioning of the male urethra for optimal catheter placement **(A)** normal and **(B)** with the penis extended and dorsal.

such a telescope down the urethra the axis of view is up and away from the light guide post, looking up at the wall of the urethra (if the light guide post is pointing down). Thus the lumen should appear at the bottom of the image on the monitor. If the lumen is kept central the tip of the endoscope will traumatize the ventral wall of the urethra. Urethral rupture will prevent continuation of the procedure, but will usually heal following placement of a Foley catheter for three to five days (Chapter 38).

Hemorrhage from lesions or polyps within the bladder can make visualization very difficult and in some cases replacing the saline irrigant with carbon dioxide from a laparoscopic insufflator will enable a clear view for biopsy or resection of polyps and tumors. Room air may also be considered but carries a higher risk of embolism.

Failure to turn off the flow of irrigant when the cystoscope is in the bladder will lead to over distension and result in small fissures or mucosal tears. Bleeding from these fissures will obscure visualization and a distended bladder makes biopsy very difficult. In rare instances severe over distension may result in rupture of the bladder, especially where there is weakening of the bladder wall due to pathology. Surgical repair will then be necessary (Chapter 37).

Antibiotic cover is not usually required unless there is a pre-existing infection. Analgesia is recommended for two to three days for which NSAIDs or opiates may be used, as indicated.

REFERENCES

1. Lhermette P, Sobel D, editors. BSAVA manual of canine and feline endoscopy and endosurgery. 2008.
2. Hall E, Simpson J, William D, editors. BSAVA manual of canine and feline gastroenterology. 2005.
3. Washabau RJ, Day MJ, Willard MD, et al. Endoscopic, biopsy, and histopathologic guidelines for the evaluation of gastrointestinal inflammation in companion animals. WSAVA International Gastrointestinal Standardization Group. J Vet Intern Med 2010;24:10–26.
4. Willard MD, Mansell J, Fosgate GT, et al. Effect of sample quality on the sensitivity of endoscopic biopsy for detecting gastric

and duodenal lesions in dogs and cats. J Vet Intern Med 2008;22(5): 1084–9.
5. Scott KD, Zoran DL, Mansell J, et al. Utility of endoscopic biopsies of the duodenum and ileum for diagnosis of inflammatory bowel disease and small cell lymphoma in cats. J Vet Intern Med 2011;25:1253–7.
6. Tenwolde AC, Johnson LR, Hunt GB, et al. The role of bronchoscopy in foreign body removal in dogs and cats: 37 cases (2000–2008). J Vet Intern Med 2010;24(5):1063–8.
7. Johnson LR, Drazenovich TL. Flexible bronchoscopy and bronchoalveolar lavage

in 68 cats (2001–2006). J Vet Intern Med 2007;21:219–25.
8. Demko JL, Cohn LA. Chronic nasal discharge in cats: 75 cases (1993–2004). J Am Vet Med Assoc 2007;230:1032–7.
9. Caccamo R, Twedt DC, Buracco P, McKiernan BC. Endoscopic bronchial anatomy in the cat. J Feline Med Surg 2007;9:140–9.
10. Gerber B, Boretti FS, Kley S, et al. Evaluation of clinical signs and causes of lower urinary tract disease in European cats. J Small Anim Pract 2005;46:571–7.
11. Wilson HM, Chun R, Larson VS, et al. Clinical signs, treatments, and outcome in cats with transitional cell carcinoma

of the urinary bladder: 20 cases (1990–2004). J Am Anim Med Assoc 2007;231:101–6.

12. Hotston-Moore A, England G. Rigid endoscopy: urethrocystoscopy and vaginoscopy. In: Lhermette P, Sobel D, editors. BSAVA manual of canine and feline endoscopy and endosurgery. BSAVA Publications; 2008. p. 142–57.

13. Selcer BA. Urinary tract trauma associated with pelvic trauma. J Am Anim Hosp Assoc 1982;18:785–93.

14. McCarthy TC. Cystoscopy for urinary tract assessment in dogs and cats with pelvic fractures. Proceedings of the Veterinary Orthopedic society 21st Annual Conference, 1994. p. 29.

Chapter |10|

Sutures and general surgical implants

S.J. Langley-Hobbs

Knowledge of the properties of the suture materials and implants available is essential to be able to make an informed decision about what to use during surgery. Use of the wrong suture material, use of an inappropriate suture pattern or placement of a loose ligature could cause dehiscence of a surgical incision or hemorrhage in the cat, requiring additional corrective surgery. In some situations where there is inadequate tissue for closure, for example after tumor resection, synthetic materials can be used to fill the defect. Surgical implants have been developed for specific purposes, for example ameroid constrictors for portosystemic shunt closure. In contrast, some readily available inexpensive materials (e.g., cellophane) have also been used with success.

The general properties of suture materials and implants will be covered in this chapter, with specifics of their usage covered in the organ-related chapters.

SUTURE MATERIALS

Suture materials are used to approximate tissues and hold them in apposition while healing occurs. They may be placed to loosely approximate tissue during healing in an area with a good blood supply or low tension or as a tight ligature to seal a blood vessel while a clot is forming. In avascular areas or where there is high tension stress across a wound, the suture needs to retain its strength for a period of time compatible with the healing period of the tissue. In wounds where there is contamination or the risk of infection it may be preferable for the suture to be completely absorbed once its function is complete.

Suture materials are generally categorized as absorbable or non-absorbable, monofilament or multifilament and natural or synthetic. A suture is classified as non-absorbable if its mechanical resistance is constant for 60 days following implantation, even it is eventually absorbed. Although the perfect suture does not exist, ideally a suture should have minimal tissue reactivity, high initial tensile strength, predictable absorption, tie reliably, and be applicable to a wide variety of uses.

Selection of suture materials

Suture material of inadequate strength may result in wound breakdown, while suture material with high memory can lead to knots coming undone unless the surgeon is aware of this and adds additional throws to the knot to counteract this property. Excessively large diameter suture material results in a weaker knot, leading to knot insecurity and also more foreign material at the surgical site.

The smallest diameter suture material that will adequately hold the healing tissue should be used. In cats, size 1.5–3 metric gauge (M) will be suitable for most general use. For either very delicate work or areas where a higher tensile strength is required, sutures outside this size range may be needed. Size conversion for suture materials is shown in Table 10-1.

Multifilament suture material is usually stronger than monofilament and has better knot security due to the higher friction co-efficient. Conversely, multifilament material, particularly if dry, can cause drag which can damage delicate tissue and inadvertently cause the surgeon to tug on the material, which can cause iatrogenic injury and suture pullout. Multifilament suture material also has a greater surface area for bacterial penetration and contains crevices which can harbor bacteria. These characteristics are reduced when the multifilament or braided suture is coated.

Natural materials like silk, cotton, ovine intestinal submucosa, or bovine serosa (catgut) can cause inflammatory reactions within the tissues and their absorption, by phagocytosis, may be variable depending on implant site and patient status. Synthetic materials are usually chemical polymers absorbed by hydrolysis, and thus they often have a more predictable rate of absorption independent of these factors (Table 10-2).

Modifications to several of the generic suture materials include the introduction of rapidly absorbable sutures (the 'Rapide' range) and sutures with improved resistance to bacterial penetration (the 'Plus' range). The 'Plus' range sutures, which include polyglactin 910, polydioxanone and poliglecaprone, are coated with triclosan, which is an inhibitor of bacterial fatty acid synthesis with demonstrable antibacterial activity. The use of triclosan-coated sutures in humans has been associated with a decreased infection rate.[1]

DOI: 10.1016/B978-0-7020-4336-9.00010-X

Table 10-1 Size conversions for suture materials

Actual size (mm)	Metric gauge (M)	United States Pharmacopeia (USP)	Surgical gut (USP)
0.02	0.2	10–0	
0.03	0.3	9–0	
0.04	0.4	8–0	
0.05	0.5	7–0	8–0
0.07	0.7	6–0	7–0
0.1	1	5–0	6–0
0.15	1.5	4–0	5–0
0.2	2	3–0	4–0
0.3	3	2–0	3–0
0.35	3.5	0	2–0
0.4	4	1	0
0.5	5	2	1

Table 10-2 Loss of strength and absorption times of suture materials

Suture material composition	Loss of strength in weeks (percentage loss)	Absorption time in days
Intestinal submucosa (catgut)	2–3 (100%)	14–80 approx
Polyglytone	2–3 (100%)	56
Poliglecaprone	1–2 (50%)	119
Polyglactin 910	2–3 (50%)	56–70
Polyglycolic acid	2–3 (50%)	90
Glycomer 631	2–3 (50%)	90–110
Lactomer	2 (20%)	56–70
Polydioxanone	4–6 (50%)	180

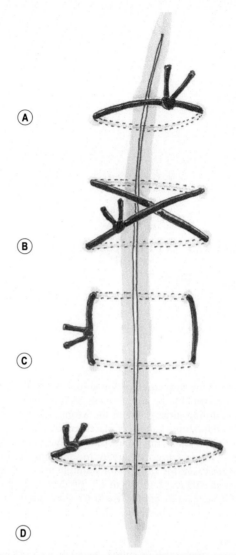

Figure 10-1 Simple sutures: **(A)** simple interrupted; **(B)** cruciate mattress; **(C)** vertical mattress; and **(D)** horizontal mattress.

Suture placement and patterns

Careful attention to proper suturing technique and use of the appropriate suture patterns for wound closure is important in ensuring optimal closure and incisional healing. Careless handling of the suture or the use of damaged instruments can weaken the suture and make it more prone to breakage. Eversion of skin edges or excessively tight skin sutures can encourage self-trauma by the patient, increasing the risk of suture line infection or premature suture removal by the cat. Excess tension on sutures in wound closure can lead to 'cutting out' of sutures or to ischemia of tissue adjacent to the sutures. In areas of tension, the surgeon should consider other techniques such as the use of subcutaneous walking sutures, undermining of the skin, tension-relieving sutures, and then surgical procedures, including relaxing incisions, plasty procedures, or skin flaps (see Chapter 19).

Placing an adequate number of throws is important to minimize the risk of the sutures undoing. Although some manufacturers give guidelines, strict recommendations are not made for individual suture materials, as this is dependent on many factors such as tightness of each throw, length of the cut end(s) or ears and the tissue tension. The knot security of individual suture materials is influenced by the memory, plasticity and pliability of the suture material. Braided material generally has good knot security but this is also influenced by suture coating: some braided material is coated to decrease tissue drag and bacterial penetration but this will tend to decrease knot security. General recommendations for simple interrupted suture placement would be to place four throws, ensuring that the throws are tightened after the third (or second if suturing skin) and subsequent throw. For simple continuous patterns the recommendation is for five to six throws at the start of the suture line with one or two additional throws at the end of the suture pattern, as the suture material becomes damaged during use and the end knots are generally less secure.

Suture patterns commonly used in feline general surgery are shown in Figures 10-1 and 10-2. There are several different suture materials on the market (Table 10-3) with a variety of different properties, indications and contraindications. The materials available in practice will vary according to surgeon preference and procedures commonly performed. The indications and contraindications for the different suture materials are listed in Tables 10-4 and 10-5.

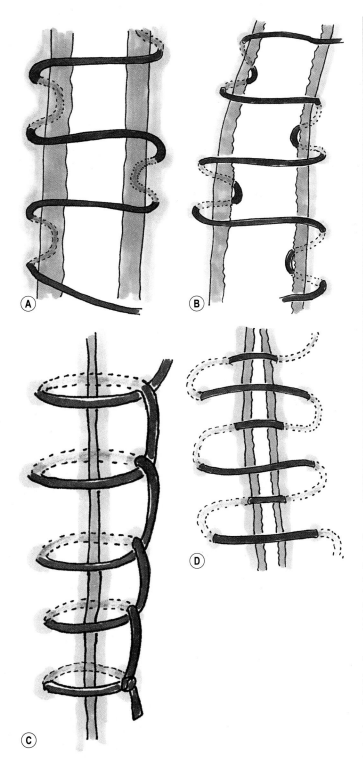

Figure 10-2 Continuous suture patterns: **(A)** Cushing; **(B)** Connell; **(C)** Ford Interlocking; and **(D)** Lembert.

Table 10-3 Suture materials and some commercial manufacturers

Suture material	Manufacturer
Catgut	
Polyglactin 910	Vicryl: Ethicon, Polysorb: USS/DG
Poliglecaprone	Monocryl: Ethicon
Polyglycolic acid	Dexon II: USS/DG, Safil: Braun
Polyglycomers	Maxon: USS/DG, Monosyn: Braun
Polydioxanone	PDS: Ethicon
Glycomer 631	Biosyn: USS/DG
Polyglytone 6211	Caprosyn: USS/DG
Nylon, polyamide	Monosof: Covidien, Ethilon, Nurolon: Ethicon, Dafilon: Braun, Supramid: Braun, Dermalon: USS/DG, Monosof: USS: DG, Surgilon: USS/DG
Caprolactum	Vetafil
Polypropylene	Prolene: Ethicon, Surgiproll: USS/DG, Premilene: Braun
Polyester	Surgidac: USS/DG, Ti.Cron: USS/DG, Mersilene: Ethicon, Ethibond Excel: Ethicon, Miralene: Braun, Dagrofil: Braun, Synthofil: Braun, PremiCron: Braun
Polybutester	Novafil: USS/DG, Vascufil: USS/DG
Silk	Perma-hand: Ethicon, Sofsilk: USS/DG, Silkam: Braun
Stainless steel	Steel: USS/DG, Flexon: USS/DG, Surgical Stainless Steel Suture: Ethicon, Steelex: Braun

ABSORBABLE SUTURE MATERIALS

Catgut

Catgut is made of collagen obtained from bovine intestines. It is naturally degraded by the body's own proteolytic enzymes. It can cause a significant foreign body reaction when implanted in tissues. Absorption is unpredictable, occurring faster in patients with cancer, anemia, and malnutrition or when used in gastric surgery, an infected wound, or highly vascularized tissue.[2] It is also absorbed faster when used in the mouth and in other mucous membranes, e.g., vagina, due to the presence of microorganisms. In one study of 12 cats where suture material was implanted into the oral cavity it completely disappeared between days 3 and 7.[3]

Chromic catgut suture is a variant treated with chromic acid salts. This treatment produces roughly twice the suture-holding time of plain catgut, but greater tissue inflammation occurs. Full tensile strength is extended to 18–21 days. Fast catgut suture is heat-treated to give even more rapid absorption in the body.

Catgut is banned in Europe and Japan because of concern over bovine spongiform encephalopathy (BSE), although the herds from which gut is harvested are certified BSE-free. Catgut has largely been replaced by synthetic absorbable polymers such as polyglactin, polyglytone and poliglecaprone.

Poliglecaprone 25

Poliglecaprone 25 is a monofilament absorbable suture material made of glycolide and epsilon caprolactone copolymer (PGCL). It is pliable, with low tissue drag giving it smooth tissue passage. Knot security is not reliable, hence the ears should not be cut too short and additional throws placed if used for a continuous pattern. It loses its strength relatively quickly, with the tensile strength capability reduced to about

Table 10-4 Some indications and contraindications for use of suture materials in cats

	Indications	Contraindications
Absorbable suture material		
Polyglytone	Soft tissue approximation, subcutaneous, subdermal, intestinal surgery	Areas where there is high tension combined with prolonged healing
Poliglecaprone	Soft tissue approximation, subcutaneous, subdermal, intestinal surgery	Areas where there is high tension combined with prolonged healing
Polyglactin 910	Soft tissue approximation and ligation	Should not be used where extended approximation of tissue is required
Polyglycolic acid	Subcutaneous and dermal sutures, abdominal and thoracic surgery	Elderly anemic and malnourished patients, urinary tract
Glycomer 631	For abdominal closure and soft tissue repair requiring a strong but absorbable material	Should not be used where extended approximation of tissue is required
Polyglyconates	Internal tissues where a long-lasting absorbable suture is preferable (linea alba, hernias). Used for intestinal surgery	Should not be used where extended approximation of tissue is required or for fixation of permanent cardiovascular prostheses or synthetic grafts
Polydioxanone	Internal tissues where a long-lasting absorbable suture is preferable (linea alba, hernias). Used for intestinal surgery	Areas of rapid healing where prolonged suture retention not required
Non-absorbable suture material		
Polyamide	Skin closure	Internally in infected or contaminated areas where non-absorbable material would be ill-advised
Polypropylene	Skin closure and general soft tissue approximation and ligation, tendon and ligament repair	Not necessary in rapidly healing tissue as non-absorbable

Table 10-5 Suture recommendation for various tissue types

Tissue types	Suture recommendation and contraindications
Skin	Monofilament non-absorbable, e.g., polyamide or polypropylene
Subcutaneous	Absorbable, e.g., poliglecaprone, polyglactin 910, polyglytone
Tendon	Strong non-absorbable or slowly absorbable, e.g., polydioxanone, polypropylene, polyamide
Abdominal closure – linea alba	Strong, with good knot security (use extra throws), e.g., polydioxanone, glycomer 631
Muscle	Absorbable, e.g., polyglactin 910, polyglycolic acid, glycomer 631
Parenchymal organs	Absorbable monofilament, e.g., poliglecaprone, glycomer 631
Hollow viscus	Absorbable, e.g., poliglecaprone, polyglactin 910, glycomer 631 Avoid polyglycolic acid in the bladder as it rapidly dissolves in urine
Infected or contaminated wounds	Absorbable g. polyglactin, poliglecaprone. Avoid braided non-absorbable sutures which can fistulate or catgut which rapidly absorbs
Vessels and vascular anastomoses	Ligatures – absorbable suture material Vascular anastomoses – non-absorbable monofilament, e.g., polypropylene and with a needle-to-suture ratio of 1 : 1

60% within a week, 20–30% at two weeks and all strength is lost within three weeks. It undergoes reliable absorbtion by hydrolysis.

It was used in a prospective study for all ligatures and closure of the linea alba in routine ovariohysterectomies in 24 cats.[4] Dehiscence did not occur in any of the cats; however, the author has seen dehiscence of the linea alba after celiotomy closure and would recommend alternative suture material such as polydioxanone or glycomer 631 be used in this situation. Poliglecaprone is commonly used for subcutaneous and subdermal tissue closure. Careful technique ensuring an adequate number of throws, good knot security and sufficient purchase of tissue with each bite should be taken when placing in areas of high tension. It causes a relatively short-lived inflammatory response.

Polyglactin 910

Polylactin 910 is an absorbable, braided suture material made of polyglycolic acid. The suture holds its tensile strength for three to four weeks in tissue, retaining 75% of strength after two weeks, 50% after three weeks and 25% after four weeks and it is completely absorbed by hydrolysis within 70 days. The suture material, being braided, has some tissue drag, particularly if it dries out, but it has good knot security and is good for ligation. The sutures are coated with a copolymer of calcium stearate to allow less drag and better water repellency. The suture material can also be treated to enable more rapid breakdown for its use in rapidly healing tissues such as mucous membranes.

Polyglycolic acid

Polyglycolic acid (PGA) suture is classified as a synthetic, absorbable, braided multifilament. It is coated with N-laurin and L-lysine, which render the thread extremely smooth, soft, and safe for knotting. It is also coated with magnesium stearate and finally sterilized with ethylene oxide gas. It is naturally degraded in the body by hydrolysis and has approximately 60% strength left at 14 days; absorption is completed between 60 and 90 days. It has the advantages of high initial tensile strength, smooth passage through tissue, easy handling, excellent knotting ability, and secure knot tying (better when wet). It is commonly used for subcutaneous sutures, intradermal closure, abdominal and thoracic surgeries. Elderly, anemic and malnourished patients may absorb the suture more quickly. Absorption is faster in urine, and so it is not recommended for urinary tract surgery.[5]

Polydioxanone

Polydioxanone (PDS) or poly-*p*-dioxanone is a slowly absorbable monofilament suture composed of the polyester, poly (p-dioxanone). This is a monofilament with greater strength than monofilament nylon and polypropylene, and with less tissue drag than the multifilament materials. It has good strength retention, with only 20% loss over two weeks and 60% loss after eight weeks. It can sometimes be difficult to handle due to its memory and tendency to coil or 'pig-tail'. Knot security can be relatively poor, and seven throws are advisable at the end of a continuous suture line. Complete absorption occurs by hydrolysis and takes around 200 days.

Polydioxanone was still intact at day 28 in the oral cavity of cats, and it is recommended for procedures in which longer healing time is anticipated[3] such as hernia repair or pexy procedures.

Despite the less than ideal knot security, the strength and predictable rate of absorption make this an ideal suture material for closure of the linea alba and it has become a very popular material for this use.

Polyglyconates

These suture materials are polymers of glyconates (Monosyn: Braun) or combinations such as glycolic acid and trimethylene carbonate (Maxon: USS/DG). The tensile strength and absorption is dependent on the composition. Maxon can be used for linea alba closure; Monosyn has quicker absorption and loses 50% of its tensile strength by two weeks so would be more suitable for subcuticular closure.

Glycomer 631

This monofilament is a copolymer of glycolide, dioxanone, and trimethylene carbonate. It is advertised as the strongest monofilament suture material available, second only to steel. A quarter of the strength is gone by day 14, and only 40% remains at three weeks. Full absorption takes 90 to 110 days. It has fair handling characteristics with low tissue drag and slightly better knot security than polydioxanone, which is a comparable though longer-lasting monofilament. It has slightly less memory compared to polydioxanone. This material is promoted as suitable for abdominal closure and soft tissue repair requiring a strong but absorbable material.

Polyglytone 6211

A synthetic, absorbable polyester material indicated for very short-term wound support. Approximately half of its initial tensile strength is gone at day 5, and only 25% remains at day 10. This suture material is completely absorbed by day 56. Interestingly, the absorption rate for this material is the closest of any synthetic material to catgut, and the handling of the suture material is similar. This suture is suitable for ligature placement, subcuticular closure, intradermal sutures and use in the oral cavity.

NON-ABSORBABLE SUTURE MATERIALS

Stainless steel

An alloy made from natural materials, stainless steel is available as a monofilament or braided multifilament suture material. Steel has the highest strength of any other suture material.[5] It is biologically inert and can easily be sterilized by autoclaving. It incites little tissue reaction other than mechanical irritation from the ends. It has excellent knot security, although the knots can sometimes be difficult to place. Pieces of stainless steel can migrate if loose, and it will break if subject to repeated bending. It can easily cut or tear through sutured tissues if tightened too much. Given its difficult handling properties, it is not commonly used in practice as a suture material, but has a wide range of applications in clips and staples. One area, however, where steel suture is still commonly used is closure of sternotomy wounds, as in dogs it gives increased stability compared to PDS II or prolene.[6]

Silk

Silk has a long history of use as a suture material. It is obtained as a fiber spun from the cocoon of the silk worm, and is available either twisted or as a braided multifilament. Silk has excellent handling characteristics, and is cheap. It has a variety of disadvantages, including tissue reaction, marginal knot security, and poor tensile strength. Many surgeons prefer the feel of silk, and it is still often used to ligate large vessels, although clinical use is limited. It can be moistened in sterile saline before use to improve knot security and reduce tissue drag, although this can slightly decrease its tensile strength. Silk is not recommended in hollow viscera or in infected wounds, as it can potentiate infection by trapping bacteria in its braiding. As with other multifilament materials, use in gall bladder and urinary tract surgery is discouraged, as it can be calculogenic.[7]

Polyamide

Polyamide nylon is a generic designation for a family of synthetic polymers known generically as polyamides. Nylon can be found in both braided and monofilament forms. As a material, nylon is relatively inert, and has no capillary action as a monofilament. Only about 20% of monofilament nylon's initial strength is gone at one year, although in some cases all the tensile strength in a multifilament strand can be gone at six months. Although monofilament nylon has a reputation for relatively poor handling and knot security,[7] it is commonly used in a variety of applications including skin, cornea, fascia, and ligatures, e.g., pedicle ligatures for ovariohysterectomy. Due to its stiffness, it is not recommended within hollow viscera, as the cut ends cause mechanical irritation.[2] A minimum of four throws on nylon is always recommended.

In the same family of materials is polymerized caprolactam, a twisted and coated multifilament material with superior initial tensile strength compared to nylon. It has more tissue reactivity than nylon, however. It has been known to cause sinuses when implanted in tissues, so is best suited for skin. It is generally supplied in bulk rolls, but should not be considered sterile unless processed by ethylene oxide or heat sterilization. Autoclaving can make it more difficult to handle. In general, this family of materials is best suited for skin sutures. Although in general multifilament nylon materials may be easier to handle, the monofilament nylon materials would be preferred for use in the skin because they are less likely to wick outside contaminant bacteria into the deeper tissues of the wound bed.

Polypropylene

Polypropylene is a widely used synthetic monofilament suture material that is composed of polymerized polypropylene. It is non-thrombogenic, and is often used in cardiovascular surgery in human patients. It is available as a mesh material for implantation. Polypropylene is very plastic, meaning that the material will assume a new shape when subject to tension, which contributes greatly to its good knot security if the sutures are tightened appropriately. Some surgeons find this material difficult to handle because of its memory and tendency to break if handled roughly. There is no appreciable loss of tensile strength after implantation. Polypropylene was still intact at day 28 post-implantation in the feline oral cavity[3] and visual inspection showed polypropylene to have the least tissue reaction of all the suture materials tested.

The clinical indications for use of polypropylene are varied and include cardiovascular and microvascular surgery, tracheobronchial surgery (e.g., tracheostomies and closure of bronchial stump after lobectomy), hernias and ruptures (e.g., perineal hernia repair), genitourinary (e.g., perineal urethrostomy), routine skin closure, and as a stay suture material.

Polyester

A synthetic non-absorbable multifilament or monofilament suture material that is usually coated; the suture material has been reported to have some tissue reactivity if the coating is lost. This material has a very high and prolonged tensile strength, although knot security is only fair. Infection in an area where braided polyester suture has been used almost always necessitates removal. Polyester is very strong and has been used most commonly for prosthetic implant placement and large vessel ligation. Given that suture contamination and sinus tract formation with polyester materials can be problematic, other suture materials will provide sufficient strength without this risk.

Polybutester

A special type of polyester material composed of polyglycol terephthalate and polybutylene terephthalate. This makes the material retain many advantages of both polypropylene and polyester. It is delivered as a monofilament, and is commonly used in cardiovascular and ophthalmic procedures. The material is known to have better knot security than polyester alone, with good tensile strength and flexibility.

NEEDLES

Modern sutures feature swaged atraumatic needles where the suture material is provided attached to the eyeless needle. Time does not have to be spent threading the suture on the needle and, more importantly, the suture end of a swaged needle is smaller than the needle body so it passes easily through the tissue. It is essential to use swaged needles for atraumatic surgery in cats, particularly when suturing delicate tissues such as viscera.

There are essentially three types of needle shapes.[8] Straight needles are used in accessible superficial places where the needle can be manipulated directly with fingers, e.g., skin, purse-string suture in the anus. Half-curved needles are straight in their shaft, but have a curved, cutting tip to them. These are not commonly used but are suitable for skin or ophthalmic surgery. Curved needles are manipulated with needle holders. They are formed in an arc of 1/4, 3/8, 1/2, or 5/8 circles. This allows the surgeon access with the needle to smaller

Table 10-6 Needle characteristics

Needle type	Description	Indications
Taper	Needle body is round and tapers smoothly to a sharp point that pierces and spreads tissue without cutting it	Generally used in easily penetrated tissues such as the intestine, subcutaneous tissue or loose fascia; or blood vessels
Cutting	Needle body is triangular and has a sharpened cutting edge on the inside (towards the wound)	Recommended in tough tissue such as skin, fascia, tendons and ligaments
Reverse cutting	Needle body is triangular and has a sharpened cutting edge on the outside (away from wound)	
Taper cut	Has a combination of a reverse cutting point and taper point body	Generally used for suturing tough dense tissue such as a tendon or for vascular grafts
Blunt point	Has a rounded blunt point that can dissect through friable tissue without cutting	For suturing soft parenchyma such as liver or kidney
Side cutting or spatula points	Flat on top and bottom with a cutting edge along the front to one side	For eye surgery

spaces than the straight or half-curved needle, and the arc can be chosen to maximize tissue bite depth and width. 3/8 and 1/2 needles are most commonly used in veterinary medicine, but the 5/8 is slightly easier to manipulate in deep or inaccessible locations.

A needle pierces the tissues by use of a cutting edge or a sharp point (taper) (Table 10-6 and Fig. 10-3) though a blunt-ended round body needle is available for use in friable viscera such as the liver or spleen. Which type of needle to use depends on many factors including the composition of the tissue that it is to be passed through, the thickness of tissue, and its depth in the body. As a general needle the taper point round bodied needle is suitable for most tissues, with the reverse cutting used for tougher tissues such as skin and fascia.

SUTURE REACTIONS IN CATS

Cats appear to be prone to incisional swelling following celiotomy closure[9] independent of the type of suture material used. The associated inflammation and fibrous tissue proliferation usually resolves without treatment over a number of weeks, although complications such as failure of the skin sutures, failure of the skin and subcutaneous sutures, wound dehiscence, and seroma or abscess formation may be associated with severe incisional swelling.[9] Swelling and inflammation along the incision line was observed after elective ovariohysterectomy in 22 of 66 cats in a retrospective study. In a prospective study of 99 feline abdominal incisions closed with surgical gut, polyglactin 910, or polydioxanone, with and without subcutaneous closure, the least inflammation occurred when the linea alba was sutured with polyglactin 910 and the subcutaneous tissues were not sutured. The

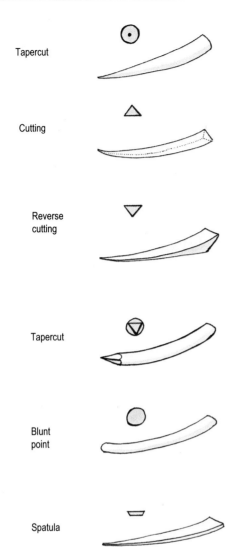

Tapercut

Cutting

Reverse
cutting

Tapercut

Blunt
point

Spatula

Figure 10-3 Needle point types.

inflammatory reaction did not appear to be specifically related to any particular suture material as reactions were seen with all of them.[9] Histologically, reactions in the linea alba of 12 other cats progressed from purulent to fibromononuclear to fibrous within 14 days after closure with gut, polyglactin 910, and polydioxanone. Microscopic evidence of seroma formation was found in nine of 12 animals in which the subcutaneous tissue was not sutured, suggesting that surgical closure of subcutaneous dead space was indicated. Another study found conflicting results, with subcutaneous closure of celiotomy incisions causing increased tissue swelling compared to wounds closed without subcutaneous sutures.[10] The results of this study suggested that placement of subcutaneous sutures in cats may not be the preferred technique in relation to postoperative inflammation. The authors would recommend a subcutaneous layer as it provides additional incisional security and provides an extra barrier to dehiscence, particularly if the cat removes the skin sutures.

TISSUE GLUE

Topical adhesives are made from medical grade cyanoacrylates, a group of rapidly polymerizing adhesives, which polymerize when they come into contact with moisture in the skin. The products may contain dye to allow the user to easily see where the product has been applied. They are provided in single use capsules or bottles or multiple use vials, but the latter have a tendency to block unless used frequently. Cyanoacrylates form a bond across apposed wound edges allowing normal healing to occur below. They should be applied correctly to avoid complications; skin edges need to be accurately apposed and the glue applied over the top to form a bridge. It should not be allowed to enter the incision, where it may cause a foreign body reaction and local inflammation.[11] A spray formulation is also available that forms a thin topical bandage. The adhesive polymerizes on contact with exudates from the wound, forming an occlusive dressing.

Indications

Their use saves time during wound repair, provides a flexible, water resistant protective coating, is less traumatic and eliminates the need for suture removal.[12] They can be used on large wounds concurrently with subcutaneous or subcuticular sutures. They are marketed to replace sutures of size 1 M or smaller or for use on superficial wounds in areas with no tension. They have been used for traumatic lacerations, abrasions, suture/staple line sealing, skin closure after spaying/ neutering and dewclaw removal. N-butyl-cyanoacrylate tissue adhesive was evaluated as a skin closure material in a population control program.[13] The time required for closure of the surgical site with the adhesive was shorter than with nylon, saving approximately one minute per animal. As the adhesive eliminates the need for suture removal and decreases surgery time without additional risk to the cat, it may be indicated for surgical population control programs.[13] Cyanoacrylate has also been used successfully for embolization of an arteriovenous fistula in a cat.[14]

Contraindications

They should not be used for closure of mucous membranes or in areas of tension as they do not provide as strong a closure as a properly sutured incision. Cyanoacrylate was compared with the use of sutures in a study on enteroplication in cats.[13] The inflammation associated with the adhesive persisted for the four weeks of the experiment, and it was concluded that cyanoacrylate tissue adhesive cannot be recommended for this clinical procedure.[13]

IMPLANTS FOR PORTOSYSTEMIC SHUNT CLOSURE

Ameroid constrictor

An ameroid constrictor is a device for gradual occlusion of blood flow. It is composed of a ring of casein, inside a ring of stainless steel (Fig. 10-4). Casein is a hygroscopic substance that swells as it slowly absorbs body fluid. The stainless steel sheath forces the casein to swell inwardly, eventually closing the ring and obliterating the shunt. In cats, ameroid constrictors are most commonly used for gradual constriction of portosystemic shunts, though a higher incidence of multiple acquired shunts has been associated with their use (see Chapter 32). They are gas sterilized and therefore should not be used until 12 to 24 hours after sterilization to allow residual ethylene oxide to be released from the casein.

Before constrictor placement, the 'key', a small column of casein that completes the constrictor ring, is removed from the ameroid constrictor and set aside in a dry cup. The choice of ameroid constrictor size for portosystemic shunt occlusion is based on shunt diameter;

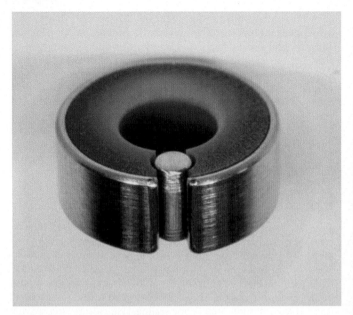

Figure 10-4 An ameroid constrictor.

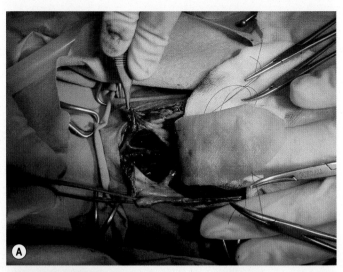

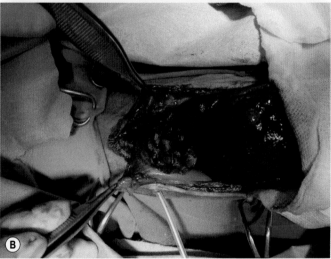

Figure 10-5 Porcine small intestinal submucosa used for reconstruction of a diaphragmatic defect in a kitten. *(From Andreoni AA, Voss K. Reconstruction of a large diaphragmatic defect in a kitten using small intestinal submucosa (SIS). J Fel Med Surg 2009;11:1019–1022, with permission from Elsevier.)*

therefore the surgeon should have a selection of sizes available at each surgery. Ameroid constrictors come in various sizes, with internal diameters ranging from 3.5–9 mm; constrictors with 3.5, 5 and 6.5 mm internal diameters are most frequently used for PSS ligation in cats.[15] To avoid postoperative portal hypertension, a constrictor is selected that does not compress the shunt immediately. After placement around the vessel to be closed, the key is replaced to complete the circle of casein. Ameroid constrictors were thought to gradually close over four to five weeks, but generally thrombus formation in the enclosed vessel will occur earlier, often by ten days to two weeks.[16] Time to occlusion of the vessel is dependent on the size of the vessel and constrictor and the rigidity of the outer ring. Closure is most rapid during the first three to 14 days after implantation; the rate of closure declines thereafter. For further information on the use of ameroid constrictors see Chapter 32.

Cellophane

Gas sterilized strips of cellophane have been used to provide partial occlusion of shunts[17] (see Chapter 32). Cellophane can be obtained from a florist, and is sterilized in ethylene oxide or hydrogen peroxide gas plasma. Strips are cut to size (triple folded 10 mm long by 4 mm wide). After placement around the shunt the strips are secured together with surgical clips or staples. Inflammation caused by the cellophane results in complete occlusion of most shunts in four to six weeks.

SHEETS AND MESHES

Porcine small intestinal submucosa

Small intestinal submucosa (SIS) is a naturally derived biomaterial isolated from the small intestine of pigs. After removal of the mucosal, serosal, and muscular layers of the intestine, a strong, collagenous matrix remains. Following treatment for disinfection, cell removal, and sterilization, SIS is biologically safe, easy to handle, has sufficient tensile strength, is infection resistant, and allows remodeling of replaced tissue. In addition, SIS can be formed into many shapes and

sizes, including large sheets, tubes, cylinders, and cones. This makes it suitable for many surgical applications. SIS comes in multiple sizes (2 cm × 3 cm to 7 cm × 20 cm) and is activated by immersion in sterile water for five to ten minutes. Surgisis Gold is a thicker eight-ply mesh with reinforced suture zones to prevent the suture cutting through the mesh. This thicker mesh has good handling properties and avoids the need for two layers of Surgisis four-ply.[18] SIS has been used successfully in the reconstruction of a large diaphragmatic defect in a kitten (Fig. 10-5)[19] and in feline corneal disease.[20] An advantage of SIS grafts is that are they are absorbed over time, so they should not restrict growth in immature animals.

Surgical meshes

Meshes commonly used for surgical reconstruction include polyglactin, polypropylene and polytetrafluoroethylene (PTFE). Polyglactin is an absorbable mesh and is preferred in contaminated wounds. Polypropylene meshes are non-absorbable and pervious to air and fluid. PTFE is strong, resistant to infection and impervious to air and fluids but it is very expensive. Polypropylene mesh is most commonly used for reconstruction in small animal surgery.

Polypropylene mesh

Polypropylene monofilaments are knitted into an elastic, durable, large pore mesh. This construction permits the mesh to be cut into a desired shape or size without unravelling. Meshes vary in pore size and elasticity. Polypropylene mesh facilitates the reconstruction of large tissue defects and is most commonly used for hernia repair or for reconstruction of the chest or abdominal wall (see Chapter 43).[21] If neoplasms are removed with 1–3 cm margins and a deep margin of at least one fascial plane, then the resulting defect may benefit from closure with mesh.[21] The main complication seen in cats is seroma formation; long-term complications are rarely reported.

SURGICAL STAPLERS

The use of surgical stapling devices in the cat is less widespread than in the dog, due in part to difficulty in placing large stapling units into the chest, but also because resection of organs and tissues using sutures is easier in cats due to their smaller size.

Stapling devices are available for superficial wound closure and intra-abdominal and thoracic resections and anastomoses (Table 10-7). The advantage of surgical staplers is that their use can save time over more conventional or traditional surgical techniques such as suturing. For example, a thoracoabdominal (TA) stapler can be used for pulmonary lobectomy, as it is not necessary to independently isolate or ligate the hilar vessels.[22] The staples are usually composed of stainless steel or titanium and they are therefore minimally reactive.

Selecting the correct size of stapler and staples to create the correct length of staple line is critical. It is important that all the tissue to be ligated lies comfortably within the staple line. It is better to use a stapler that is too long and collect the extra staples on a sponge or swab than to use one that is too short that results in leakage from non-stapled tissue. Experience in the use of the equipment is essential, as is good surgical judgment as to when to use or not to use these techniques.[22]

Skin stapling

Skin stapling devices have become an attractive and affordable alternative to traditional skin closure in small animals. Skin staplers for veterinary use are usually fixed head, disposable and available with varying numbers and sizes of stainless steel staples. Although labeled as for single-patient use, some practices will re-sterilize and reuse them.[23] Staples should be removed with staple extractors. The ideal skin stapler is comfortable to handle, makes a palpable and audible click to signal staple formation is complete, has an open staple view to see how many staples remain in the cartridge, and provides effortless staple alignment. Staples should be consistently formed, secure, and they should not rotate in the skin. Depth of staple penetration should be easy to control and the staples should be easy to remove at the right time. Also, the ideal stapler would be readily re-sterilized for reuse.

Thumb forceps are used to hold skin edges in apposition while the stapler is aligned with the incision, there usually being an arrow to indicate the correct position, then while applying some pressure the staple is fired. It is preferable to start at the proximal end of the incision and work distally so the formed staples are visible, to enable even spacing.

Lung stapling

Lung stapling devices are now routinely used due to the ease and speed of application, safety, and efficacy. Lung stapling devices have been used in cats to perform lobectomies for neoplasia and lung lacerations. In a clinical study in dogs and cats[24] the stapling device was easy to apply accurately and the design generally allowed it to be placed without interference by the lesion. Dissection and ligation of vasculature was not necessary. In many circumstances, the surgeons in the study believed that these factors made the application of staples faster than traditional surgical techniques.[22]

The stapling equipment used most commonly in the cat is the TA30 or TA55/60 (Fig. 10-6). The TA designation stands for thoracoabdominal and the 30 or 55 designation is for length of the staple line in millimeters. The TA apparatus usually places two lines of B-shaped

Table 10-7 Surgical staplers for use in cats

Type of surgical stapler	Abbreviation	Indication or usage	Size for cats
Skin stapler		Wound apposition	4.8 mm × 3.5 mm
Thoracoabdominal – Double staggered rows of staples Triple staggered row for TA 30-V3 Endoscopic version	TA	Partial pulmonary lobectomy Complete lobectomy	30–3.5 mm 55–3.5 mm or 4.8 mm 60–3.5 mm or 4.8 mm
End-to-end anastomosis – places a circular double row of staples that creates a two layer inverting anastomosis and a circular blade within the cartridge simultaneously cuts redundant tissue from each end	EEA	Transrectal colocolostomy	21 mm
Gastrointestinal – Endoscopic version	GIA Linear Proximate Cutter	Few indications due to small size of feline intestine	3.5 mm
Ligating dividing stapler	LDS	Splenectomy Mesenteric vessels Ovariohysterectomy	One size, secures vessels up to 7 mm
Ligating clip appliers Ligaclip (Ethicon) Surgiclip (Covidien)		Splenectomy, limb amputation, vessel sealing	Small Medium

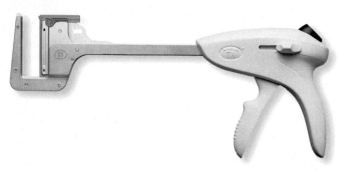

Figure 10-6 A thoracoabdominal stapler; the TA-30 is the size that is most suitable for use in the cat.

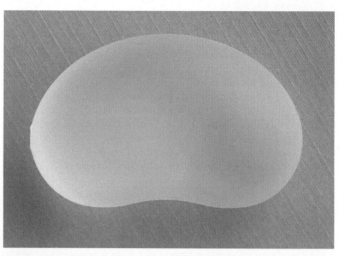

Figure 10-7 Testicular implants for use in cats. (*Courtesy of Neuticles, with permission.*)

staples. The 30 mm staples are available in 3.5 mm heights and the 55 mm staples in 3.5 and 4.8 mm heights. These staples compress to 1.5 mm and 2 mm, respectively. A white vascular cartridge is available for the TA 30, the V3, which fires three lines of 2.5 mm staples, which compress to 1.5 mm. Selection of the height of the 55 mm staples is dependent on the compressed thickness of the tissue. Normal tissues generally have 3.5 mm staples applied, whereas 4.8 mm are generally used on thickened parenchyma. The vascular white cartridge for the TA30 (TA 30-V3) is advised for hilar lung and liver lobectomies. Before cutting the specimen from the staple line, large hemostats are used to clamp the tissue distal to the staples. This avoids spillage of neoplastic or infected cells into the pleural cavity. Any discharged staples that are free on either end of the suture line are removed. The staple line is then inspected. There is usually no indication to routinely oversew staple lines when performing a lobectomy. This may actually increase the chance of air leakage. If point areas of leakage or hemorrhage do occur, these can be independently occluded either with sutures or individual vascular clips.

Thirty-seven dogs and cats were subjected to lobectomy, partial lobectomy, or pneumonectomy, using stapling equipment. The most common indication was neoplasia. No operative, perioperative, or long-term deaths could be attributed to the use of staples; complications were minimal. Staple resection was thus believed to be safe, fast, and efficient for removal of various segments of canine and feline lung.[24]

Abdominal stapling

The use of stapling instruments (TA or GIA/ Proximate Linear Cutter stapler) to perform gastric surgery in small animal patients provides alternate techniques that are often more reliable and are usually performed more quickly than conventional techniques with manual sutures. In addition to reducing anesthetic and operating times, the risk of contamination of the abdominal cavity may be decreased significantly.[25]

The GIA (Covidien) or Proximate Linear Cutter (Ethicon) stapler deploys two staggered rows of staples and sections between them. They are available in a variety of lengths between 50 and 100 mm, with a choice of two different staple sizes. A functional end-to-end intestinal anastomosis can be performed using the GIA stapler (gastrointestinal stapler) placed into the two intestinal ends to be anastomosed and then closing the end of anastomosis with a TA stapler. This technique, though rapid and effective in dogs, is less applicable to most cats due to the size of the arms of the GIA stapler. The linear staplers designed for endoscopic surgery have smaller arms and are more suitable for use in this manner in the cat.

Surgery of the colon and rectum has also been performed in cats using the end-to-end anastomosis (EEA) 21 circular stapler. In an experimental study in cats of caudal rectal resection from a dorsal approach, even this small size of EEA was difficult to insert into the feline anus and its use resulted in anal sphincter impairment postoperatively.[26] The EEA has, however, been used successfully to perform transrectal colocolostomy in a series of cats that had undergone subtotal colectomy for acquired megacolon[27] where the colon is dilated and therefore the size is not such a problem. Regular skin staples have not been successful when used to perform large intestinal anastomosis in cats.

The LDS stapler places two titanium vascular clips and then cuts between them (ligate-divide stapler). It contains 30 staples and thus can be fired 15 times to secure vessels up to 7 mm in diameter. It decreases surgical time in procedures such as splenectomy and can be used to ligate jejunal vessels when performing intestinal resection and anastomosis.

Hemostatic vascular clips, usually of titanium, are available in a variety of different sizes. When applying a clip, the vessel should be isolated and dissected clear of tissue. The diameter of the vessel needs to be between one-third and two-thirds of the length of the clip and the clip should be placed a couple of millimeters from the end of the vessel. Absorbable polymer locking clips are available that do not interfere with MRI signals.

IMPLANTS

Silicone implants are not commonly used or indicated in feline surgery but they are available if owners request their implantation.

There are silicone prostheses for implantation in cats after castration (Neuticles: CTI Neuticles). They are similar in size, shape and weight to the natural testicle. Implants available for use in cats are made of rigid polypropylene. There are two sizes (small and extra small) available for use in cats (Fig. 10-7).

Silicone implants are available for implantation after enucleation in cats. The eyelids can be sutured closed over the prosthetic and its function is to prevent the sunken-in appearance. Alternatively, eyelids can be retained and the gray prosthesis is seen in the socket. An orbital prosthesis would not be recommended in cats with an infected eye socket, and cats with extremely flat faces and very shallow eye sockets such as Persians.

STENTS

A stent is a tube that is used to maintain the patency of different conduits in the body, including the bile ducts, ureters, trachea, and bronchi. There are several different kinds of stents; those used in veterinary medicine are usually made of polyurethane or expandable metal or plastic mesh-like material.

Urinary stent

There are stents specifically designed for placement in the feline ureter (DexStent-PU: Dextronix; Vet Stent-Ureter: Infiniti Medical)[28,29] (Fig. 10-8). They have double-pigtail ends, multiple fenestrations and are

made of polyurethane. The feline ureteral stent is 2.5 Fr tapered to a 0.018 inch wire and is available in three lengths (12, 14 and 16 cm). The multiple fenestrations allow drainage at several sites. The double pigtails are designed to sit in the bladder and renal pelvis.

Urethral stents are self-expanding mesh tubes made of a nickel-titanium alloy (nitinol) (DexStent-UN: Dextronix).[29] The stent mesh is designed for maximum flexibility and minimal shortening. Markers at the proximal and distal ends ensure excellent stent visibility for accurate placement. It can be supplied in two different working lengths: 80 cm or 120 cm. Urethral stents have been used successfully for malignant urethral obstruction and obstructive feline lower urinary tract disease in cats.[30–33]

Respiratory tract

Stents used in the respiratory tract are self-expanding braided systems composed of a highly flexible nickel-titanium alloy (Nitinol) stent with radiopaque markers to assess positioning during fluoroscopy (e.g., DexStent-TN: Dextronix) (Fig. 10-9).[29] Stents are designed to be flexibile yet keep their shape even when the neck is moved. Atraumatic stent endings reduce mucosal trauma/injury and potential inflammation. They have been used for relief of tracheal obstruction[33] and collapsing trachea in the cat.

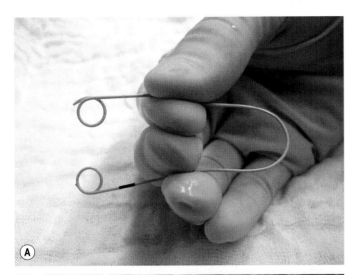

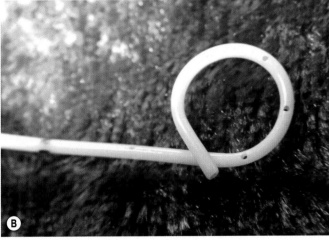

Figure 10-8 A 2.5 Fr double-pigtail, multiple fenestrated, polyurethane stent for use in cats. **(A)** The whole stent showing the double pigtail ends. **(B)** Enlarged view of one of the fenestrated ends. *([A] courtesy of Infiniti Medical, LLC, Menlo Park, CA USA, with permission; [B] courtesy of Dextronix, with permission.)*

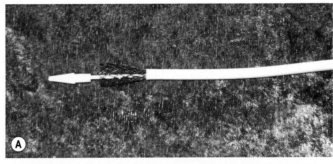

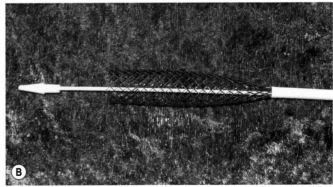

Figure 10-9 The DexStent-TN is a self-expanding braided tracheal stent system composed of a highly flexible Nickel-Titanium Alloy (Nitinol) stent mounted on a coaxial delivery system. **(A)** Stent in delivery system with tip just visible. **(B)** Stent shown after further protrusion from delivery system as it starts to expand. *(Courtesy of Dextronix, with permission.)*

REFERENCES

1. Galal I, El-Hindawy K. Impact of using triclosan-antibacterial sutures on incidence of surgical site infection. Am J Surg 2011;202:133–8.

2. Bellenger CR. Sutures part I. The purpose of sutures and available suture materials. Comp Contin Educ Pract Vet 1982a;4: 507–14.

3. DeNardo GA, Brown NO, Trenka-Benthin S, Marretta SM. Comparison of seven different suture materials in the feline oral cavity. J Am Anim Hosp Assoc 1996;32:164–72.

4. Runk A, Allen SW, Mahaffey EA. Tissue reactivity to poliglecaprone 25 in the feline linea alba. Vet Surg 1999;28: 466–71.

5. Schiller TD. In vitro loss of tensile strength and elasticity of five absorbable suture materials in sterile and infected canine urine. Vet Surg 1993;22:208–12.

6. Stashak TS, Yturraspe DJ. Considerations for selection of suture materials. Vet Surg 1978;7:48–52.

7. Pelsue DH, Monnet E, Gaynor JS, et al. Closure of median sternotomy in dogs: suture versus wire. J Am Anim Hosp Assoc 2002;38:569–76.

8. Bellenger CR. Sutures part II. The use of sutures and alternative methods for closure. Comp Contin Educ Pract Vet 1982b;4:587–600.

9. Freeman LJ, Pettit GD, Robinette JD, et al. Tissue reaction to suture material in the feline linea alba. A retrospective, prospective, and histologic study. Vet Surg 1987;16:440–5.

10. Muir P, Goldsmid SE, Simpson DJ, Bellenger CR. Incisional swelling following celiotomy in cats. Vet Rec 1993;132:189–90.

11. Schmiedt CW. Suture material, tissue staples, ligation devices and closure methods. In: Tobias KM, Johnston SA, editors. Veterinary surgery small animal. Missouri: Elsevier; 2012; p. 187–200.

12. Faria MC, de Almeida FM, Serrão ML, et al. Use of cyanoacrylate in skin closure for ovariohysterectomy in a population control programme. J Feline Med Surg 2005;7:71–5.

13. Nash JM, Bellenger CR. Enteroplication in cats, using suture of N-butyl cyanoacrylate adhesive. Res Vet Sci 1998;65:253–8.

14. Tobias KM, Cambridge A, Gavin P. Cyanoacrylate occlusion and resection of an arteriovenous fistula in a cat. J Am Vet Med Assoc 2001;219:785–8.

15. Kyles AE, Hardie EM, Mehl M, Gregory CR. Evaluation of ameroid ring constrictors for the management of single extrahepatic portosystemic shunts in cats: 23 cases (1996–2001). J Am Vet Med Assoc 2002;220:1341–7.

16. Besancon MF, Kyles AE, Griffey SM, Gregory CR. Evaluation of the characteristics of venous occlusion after placement of an ameroid constrictor in dogs. Vet Surg 2004;33:597–605.

17. Butler LM, Fossum TW, Boothe HW. Surgical management of extrahepatic portosystemic shunts in the dog and cat. Semin Vet Med Surg-Small Anim 1990;5:127–33.

18. Murphy F, Corbally MT. The novel use of small intestinal submucosal matrix for chest wall reconstruction following Ewings's tumour resection. Pediat Surg Int 2007;23:353–6.

19. Andreoni AA, Voss K. Reconstruction of a large diaphragmatic defect in a kitten using small intestinal submucosa (SIS). J Fel Med Surg 2009;11:1019–22.

20. Featherstone HJ, Sansom J, Heinrich CL. The use of porcine small intestinal submucosa in ten cases of feline corneal disease. Vet Ophthalmol 2001;4: 147–53.

21. McAbee KP, Ludwig LL, Bergman PJ, Newman SJ. Feline Cutaneous Hemangiosarcoma: A Retrospective Study of 18 Cases (1998–2003). J Am Anim Hosp Assoc 2005;41:110–16.

22. Walshaw R. Stapling techniques in pulmonary surgery. Vet Clin North Am Small Anim Pract 1994;24(2): 335–66.

23. Smeak DD, Crocker C. Fixed-head skin staplers: features and performance. Compend Contin Ed Pract Vet 1997;19: 1358–68.

24. LaRue SM, Withrow SJ, Wykes PM. Lung resection using surgical staples in dogs and cats. Vet Surg 1987;16:238–40.

25. Clark GN. Gastric surgery with surgical stapling instruments. Vet Clin North Am Small Anim Pract 1994;24:279–303.

26. Fucci V, Newton JC, Hedlund CS, et al. Rectal surgery in the cat: comparison of suture versus staple technique through a dorsal approach. J Am Anim Hosp Assoc 1992;28:519–26.

27. Kudisch M, Pavletic MM. Subtotal colectomy with surgical stapling instruments via a trans-cecal approach for treatment of acquired megacolon in the cat. Vet Surg 1993;22:457–63.

28. http://www.infinitimedical.com/ p_stents_ureter.html.

29. http://www.dextronix.com/ stentscatsanddogs.

30. Choi R, Lee S, Hyun C. Urethral stenting in a cat with refractory obstructive feline lower urinary tract disease. J Vet Med Sci 2009;71:1255–9.

31. Christensen NI, Culvenor J, Langova V. Fluoroscopic stent placement for the relief of malignant urethral obstruction in a cat. Aust Vet J 2010;88(12):478–82.

32. Newman RG, Mehler SJ, Kitchell BE, Beal MW. Use of a balloon-expandable metallic stent to relieve malignant urethral obstruction in a cat. J Am Vet Med Assoc 2009;234:236–9.

33. Culp WT, Weisse C, Cole SG, Solomon JA. Intraluminal tracheal stent placement in three cats. Vet Surg 2007;36:107–13.

Chapter |11|

Surgical drains

L.J. Owen

Surgical drains can be valuable adjuncts to patient management, both in superficial locations and within body cavities; however, their use is not without risks or complications. Used correctly, surgical drains promote wound healing, reduce infection rates, and decrease patient morbidity, but used inappropriately these potential benefits can be reversed. In particular, drains should not be used as an alternative to appropriate wound debridement, lavage and suction, and meticulous wound closure. Surgeons should consider carefully the pros and cons of drain use before placement. A thorough understanding of the types of drain available, their advantages and disadvantages and correct method of placement, will help ensure that they are used in an optimal fashion.

INDICATIONS

Surgical drains perform three main functions:

- Obliteration of dead space
- Removal of pre-existing fluid or air from a wound/body cavity
- Preventing anticipated fluid or air accumulation within a wound/body cavity.

Whilst the first two therapeutic functions are widely accepted, the latter prophylactic use of surgical drains can be a controversial area.

The use of a surgical drain to obliterate dead space is most commonly employed following en-bloc resection of neoplastic masses or chronic, contaminated and infected wounds. The definitive loss of tissue in these situations means that closure of individual wound layers is impractical and placement of a wound drain functions to appose tissue layers and promote healing.

The use of surgical drains to remove pre-existing fluid or air is most commonly from a fluid-filled peripheral swelling, e.g., salivary mucocele or abscess, or from a body cavity. The removal of fluid from a surgical site is desirable due to the negative effects of the fluid on the host's resistance to infection.[1] This occurs via several mechanisms (Box 11-1). Drains are placed routinely during thoracic surgical procedures to evacuate postoperative pneumothorax and to remove either pre-existing or anticipated fluid, which may cause respiratory compromise. In the abdomen, drains are used predominantly for the purposes of removing septic exudate, e.g., in cases of septic peritonitis. Removal

of transudates, modified transudates or blood is rarely of benefit to the patient.

The most common indication for the prophylactic placement of a surgical drain is in combination with reconstructive surgery and the use of cutaneous and myocutaneous flaps. There is evidence within the veterinary literature that seroma formation is a common sequel to these procedures and that drain placement reduces the prevalence of this and subsequently of wound dehiscence and flap failure.[2-4] Whether or not prophylactic drain placement is beneficial following other surgical procedures, however, remains controversial. In human medicine, Cochrane Systematic Reviews investigating the prophylactic use of surgical drains in orthopedic surgery, thyroid surgery, and incisional hernia repairs have failed to show any benefits in drain placement, but have shown some clear disadvantages, e.g., prolongation of hospital stay.[5-7] In veterinary medicine, there is a distinct lack of published data on this subject, eliminating the use of an evidence based approach; thus surgeons are reliant upon anecdotal evidence and their own experience to determine whether a drain should be placed in any individual case.

Experimental studies have documented prolonged tissue healing and reduced blood supply to cutaneous wounds in the cat compared with the dog, which may predispose to seroma formation in cats; however, clinical studies to support this have not been performed.[8-11] In addition, cat owners may be poorly compliant at restricting exercise, allowing behavior such as jumping, which may contribute to problems with wound healing and seroma formation.

ALTERNATIVES TO SURGICAL DRAINS

In some patients or for certain surgical procedures, it may be more appropriate to consider alternatives to the use of a surgical drain, such as incomplete wound closure, omental pedicle flaps or bandaging.

Incomplete wound closure

The most distal portion of a surgical wound can be left open to provide drainage, and is a simple, cheap and usually effective method of preventing fluid accumulation within a surgical site postoperatively.

© 2014 Elsevier Ltd
DOI: 10.1016/B978-0-7020-4336-9.00011-1

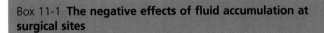

Figure 11-1 Omentum tunneled from a paracostal abdominal exit point for placement into a chronic axillary collar wound. Small arrow, paracostal incision; arrowhead, axillary wound with omentum in place.

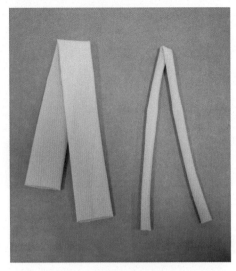

Figure 11-2 Penrose drains: 1 inch and 0.25 inch.

> **Box 11-1 The negative effects of fluid accumulation at surgical sites**
>
> - Reduced ability to opsonize bacteria for phagocytosis
> - Reduced access of phagocytes into the wound
> - Ability of the fluid to act as a substrate to promote bacterial growth
> - Reduced vascular supply to tissues
> - Reduced penetration of systemically administered antibacterial agents into the surgical site

This technique can also be applicable to body cavities, particularly in the treatment of septic peritonitis by open peritoneal drainage. The main disadvantages of this technique are the increased risk of wound infection, reduced wound healing, and requirement for bandaging to collect the fluid.

Omentum

Omentum can be used as an autogenous wound drain (Fig. 11-1). Its beneficial properties include promotion of angiogenesis, improved immune function, and tissue fluid drainage and it has been used successfully to promote healing of a variety of wound types in cats, particularly axillary collar wounds (see Chapter 18) and indolent pocket wounds, which are both challenging to treat by other methods.[12,13] The use of omentum is, however, limited by its availability and the location of the wound: complications such as necrosis of the omental fat and incisional herniation through the omental exit point from the abdominal cavity have been reported.[12] For information on how to create an omental flap see Chapter 19.

Pressure bandage

The use of a bandage to maintain apposition of tissue planes is a suitable alternative to a surgical drain in some locations, e.g., distal limb.[14] However, there are many anatomical locations where application of a bandage is difficult or where it may compromise normal function, e.g., cervical and thoracic regions. In addition, cats are often poorly tolerant of dressings and their presence may reduce feeding and normal behavior postoperatively.

TYPES OF DRAINS

Drains are generally categorized according to function, i.e., whether they act as a passive route for passage of fluids or if they have a more active role in drainage.

Passive drains

Passive drains provide an exit point for fluid from a surgical site postoperatively, but do not actively reduce dead space within a wound and do not provide optimal drainage of air. Several types of passive drain exist, including Penrose drains, tube drains, sump drains, and corrugated drains; however, only the former are commonly in use in companion animal medicine and thus the others will not be considered further here.

Penrose drains

Penrose drains are composed of soft latex and are a flattened tube of variable diameter (0.25–1 inch) (Fig. 11-2). They are readily available, easy to use and cheap, making them a popular choice. This type of drain relies on gravitational forces, capillary action and overflow for wound drainage and therefore is limited to use in locations where these forces can be utilized. Penrose drains placed on the head or dorsum, or exiting from the lateral or dorsal aspects of a surgical site are unlikely to function and will instead contribute to complications of wound healing. The gravitational and capillary action of fluid drainage is related to the surface area of the drain and thus fenestration of these drains is contraindicated. In addition to reducing the efficiency of the drain, fenestration will also predispose to breakage of the drain during removal.

Penrose drains are indicated for use in superficial wounds where there is pre-existing or anticipated fluid production and should have a single ventral exit point. Allowing the drain to have a second exit point proximally is not recommended.[15] This serves only to increase the risk of wound infection and air transmission through the wound, without conferring any advantages to the patient. The main use of the

Box 11-2 **Penrose drain placement**

The drain insertion and surgical site is clipped and aseptically prepared according to standard techniques.

The distal portion of the drain is placed to exit through a stab incision in the most dependent area of the surgical site (Fig. 11-3A). This stab incision must always be separate from the main surgical wound and the size of the drain exit hole should be minimized to reduce the risk of herniation of fat/other organs, although it should not restrict fluid flow. The proximal aspect of the drain is secured to the skin at the dorsal limit of the wound with a single non-absorbable external skin suture (Fig. 11-3B). The ends of this suture are commonly left longer than the standard skin sutures to allow the drain suture to be identified at time of drain removal. The distal portion of the drain is cut to leave approximately 2–3 cm of drain visible from the exit site and the drain is secured at this site with a second single non-absorbable skin suture, to prevent retraction of the drain into the subcutaneous space (Fig. 11-3C). The total length of the drain is recorded at time of insertion so that this can be verified at time of drain removal.

The skin surrounding the drain is protected from fluid scalding with petroleum jelly or similar. A sterile and absorbent bandage is applied over the drain wherever possible to reduce contamination postoperatively.

Penrose drain removal

To remove the drain, the two non-absorbable sutures (proximal and distal) are cut and the drain is gently pulled through its original exit site. The exit site is left to close by secondary intention healing. Consider culture of the drain tubing after removal if there are any concerns about infection.

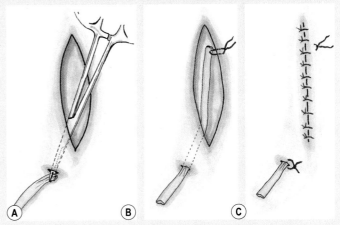

Figure 11-3 Penrose drain placement. **(A)** A stab incision is made away from the main suture line of a surgical wound and a Penrose drain is drawn through this incision into the wound. **(B)** The proximal part of the Penrose drain is secured to the skin by a simple interrupted suture. **(C)** Following closure of the main surgical wound, only a small portion of the distal Penrose drain is visible exiting from a single point in the dependent part of the surgical site and secured by a simple interrupted suture.

double exit technique has traditionally been to prevent subcutaneous emphysema developing in areas of high motion, e.g., the axilla or inguinal region, where air may be sucked into the wound by a single exit point; however, this is not usually considered to be a significant clinical problem.[16]

After placement, where location permits, the drain should be covered by a sterile absorbent contact layer and bandage. This is for collection of the fluid produced, and to reduce the risk of introduction of hospital or environmentally acquired pathogens. The dressing should be changed according to the rate of fluid production from the wound. In locations where bandaging is not possible or would likely result in additional complications, petroleum jelly or similar is applied liberally to the clipped area ventral to the drain to prevent fluid from scalding the skin and to allow easy cleaning of the area. The problems of feline intolerance to dressings and requirements for sedation for dressing changes, thus increasing morbidity and cost, should be taken into consideration when using these drains. The technique of drain placement and removal is described in Box 11-2.

Tube drain

A simple plastic or rubber tube drain can also be used to provide passive drainage. The advantage over a Penrose drain is that the tube does not collapse and thus drainage of fluid may be more rapid and air can more readily be removed from a wound (Fig. 11-4); however, they are likely to cause increased patient discomfort due to their rigidity and they may become occluded during use. Tube drains may also be placed to allow instillation of local anesthetic agents into a surgical site postoperatively, rather than to provide drainage from the wound. The same drain should not be used for both purposes due to the risk of introducing pathogenic organisms.

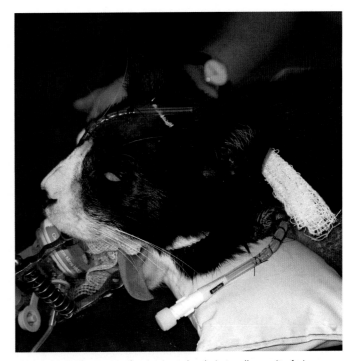

Figure 11-4 Placement of a passive tube drain to allow exit of air following a dorsal rhinotomy in a cat. (© *Adrian Wallace.*)

Active drains

Active drainage is created by application of a vacuum to a wound drain. These drains are generally easier to manage in comparison to passive drains and have reduced risk of ascending infection.

Closed suction drains

This type of drain is commonly used in superficial surgical sites, to obliterate dead space, to remove pre-existing fluid and air, or to prevent formation of fluid within the site postoperatively.

Several commercial suction drains are available, which consist of a rigid, non-collapsible tube drain attached to a collection chamber (compressible or pre-applied vacuum); however, their size and weight need to be considered before their application to cats. The smaller, concertina/grenade type drains are appropriate in most cases and are often very effective (e.g., Mini Red-O-Pack drains or Jackson Pratt drains) (Figs 11-5 and 11-6). As well as being a suitable size, in experimental studies these drains have been shown to operate at a lower pressure and in a more consistent manner compared to rigid drains; thus minimizing the effect of the drain itself on fluid production within the wound.[17] Application of suction to these drains results in a negative pressure of approximately −80 to −120 mmHg within the wound, which is sufficient to obliterate dead space without excessively traumatizing the soft tissues.[1,17,18] As the reservoir becomes filled, the negative pressure generated reduces and the drain becomes less efficient; although the Jackson Pratt and Mini Red-O-Pack drains have been shown to maintain suction at a lower level throughout filling of the reservoir.[17]

Homemade closed suction drains can be particularly useful in cats due to their reduced weight, size, and cost. Two main variations are reported. For both types, the portion of the drain that is to be placed in the wound is made from a 19G butterfly catheter, which has had multiple fenestrations made into the tubing. These fenestrations should not exceed 30% of the tube diameter, to reduce the risk of the tube kinking or breakage of the tubing on removal.[16] The needle from the butterfly catheter can then be placed into a standard blood collection vacutainer (ideally made of plastic rather than glass) to provide suction (Fig. 11-7). Alternatively, the butterfly catheter tubing can be connected to a syringe. The syringe plunger is withdrawn to apply suction and a hypodermic needle is placed across the syringe case to maintain this suction. Both drains are then secured to the trunk with additional sutures or a mesh stockinette. These drains are usually only suitable for use in wounds where minimal fluid production is expected, due to the limited capacity of the collection device.

Continuous suction devices are considered optimal for wound care, but more simple constructions utilizing intermittent suction may have some suitable applications.

Closed suction drains have several advantages over passive drains (Box 11-3). The disadvantages are increased cost (which may be offset

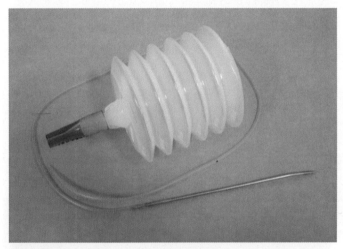

Figure 11-5 Mini Red-O-Pack closed suction drain. *(With permission from Vygon Vet.)*

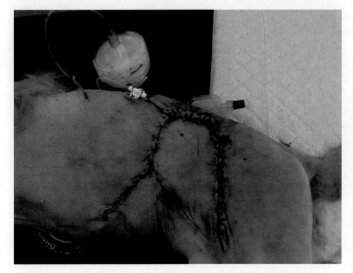

Figure 11-6 Reconstruction of a large soft tissue deficit, following en-bloc resection of a fibrosarcoma from the left flank, using a caudal superficial epigastric skin flap. A mini Red-O-Pack closed suction drain has been placed, in addition to a tube drain for instillation of local anesthetic agents. *(With permission from Vygon Vet.)*

Box 11-3 **Advantages of closed suction drains**
• No bandaging required
• Reduced risk of nosocomial infections
• Work independent of gravity
• Fluid production can readily be quantified
• Fluid can easily be sampled for repeat cytological examination
• Fluid and air are more efficiently removed
• Reduced risk of tube occlusion when continuous suction is used.

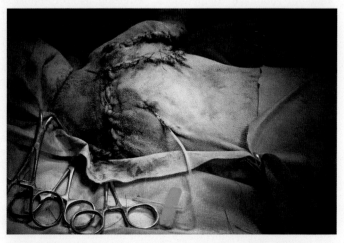

Figure 11-7 Application of a homemade butterfly catheter closed suction drain, following an omocervical axial pattern flap in a cat.

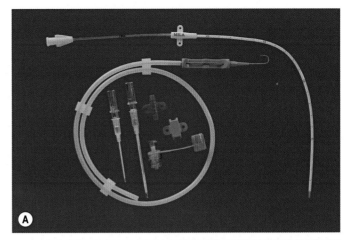

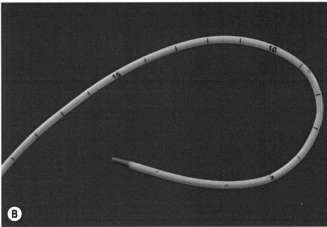

Figure 11-9 **(A)** 14G wire-guided thoracic drain. **(B)** Close up of the tip showing the fenestrations (with permission from MILA International, Inc. www.milaint.com).

The drain insertion and surgical site is clipped and aseptically prepared according to standard techniques.

The drain tubing is placed within the wound so that all fenestrations lie subcutaneously, thus allowing an airtight seal to form. An exit point for this tubing is made away from the main surgical wound via a stab incision or by using the needle attached to the tubing that is provided in some commercial kits. For closed suction drains, the exit point of the drain does not need to be at a dependent point and therefore can be placed so as to make drain management easier and its position more comfortable for the patient. At the exit point, the drain is secured to the skin using a Roman sandal suture (Fig. 11-8).

A sterile adhesive dressing is applied around the exit point of the drain to keep this area as clean as possible. The drain tubing is connected to the collection chamber, which is activated immediately if an airtight seal has been achieved using wound closure alone, or after 6–8 hours once a fibrin seal has formed. The collection chamber is secured to the patient using further sutures or a stockinette dressing or both.

Closed suction drain removal

Removal of the drain is accomplished by cutting all of the securing sutures, followed by withdrawal of the tubing from the wound. The exit site is left to close by second intention healing. Consider culture of the drain tubing after removal if there are any concerns about infection.

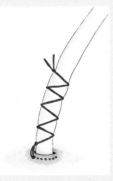

Figure 11-8. A Roman sandal friction suture is used to secure drain tubing to the skin.

by the cost of the dressings and the sedation required for management of a passive drain) and potential occlusion of the drain or reflux of fluid back into the wound.

The technique for insertion of active drains is described in Box 11-4.

THORACIC DRAINS

Three main types of thoracic drain are available for use in small animals: trocar drains, non-trocar drains, and Seldinger-type drains. All three are suitable for use in cats; however, the Seldinger-type is increasing in popularity for use in this species due to the small diameter of the drain, which is associated with a significant reduction in patient discomfort and morbidity.

Trocar and non-trocar drains are available in a range of sizes; 10–16 Fr are most commonly used in cats.[18] Traditionally, the size of drain selected should approximate the diameter of the mainstem

bronchus;[19] however, smaller lumen drains reduce discomfort and thus may be preferable in many situations. Both of these drain types require sedation, or more commonly general anesthesia, for placement in a cat, and can be placed under direct observation during surgery, or as an extra-thoracic technique. Placement of these drains requires considerable force to pass them through the intercostal musculature and a particular concern when dealing with small patients such as cats, with high thoracic wall compliance, is the risk of iatrogenic damage to the heart/lungs/vessels in the thorax during placement.

The Seldinger-type thoracic drains are relatively new in veterinary medicine and are more expensive, but have some significant advantages over the wide-bore drains. The most commonly used drain is 14G in size (Fig. 11-9) and the atraumatic technique with which it is placed means that local anesthesia or mild sedation is often sufficient, avoiding the need for, risks associated with, and cost of general anesthesia. A potential disadvantage often cited is the risk of occlusion of the narrow bore tube with thicker effusions, e.g., pyothorax; however, in a recent veterinary study this was not found to be a significant problem.[20] The small size of these drains results in a significant reduction in postoperative morbidity, particularly in cats due to their relative smaller chest size and therefore the author considers these thoracic drains to be optimal for use in the majority of feline patients.

The technique of placement of thoracic drains is covered in Chapter 41.

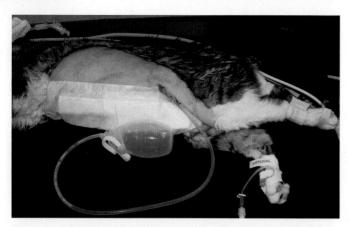

Figure 11-10 Jackson Pratt abdominal drain placed for postoperative management of septic peritonitis in a cat.

ABDOMINAL DRAINS

The Jackson Pratt closed suction drain (Fig. 11-10) is the most common type used for drainage of the abdominal cavity. This is a wide, flat silicone drain, with multiple fenestrations, which reduces the occurrence of drain occlusion during use. The flat portion of the drain merges into tubing, which exits the body wall and attaches to a grenade type collection chamber. Usually, the drain is positioned to lie along the ventral midline of the abdominal cavity, where the majority of fluid will collect due to gravitational forces. Drain use within the abdominal cavity is restricted to situations where ongoing fluid production is expected, e.g., in cases of septic peritonitis where the cause remains unresolved. The advantage of placing a drain is that it allows monitoring of the nature of the fluid produced within the abdomen and repeat cytological analysis to assess for improvement or deterioration of the patient's condition. The main disadvantages are occlusion of the drain by omentum and fibrin, the increased risk of wound dehiscence if the drain is placed too close to an intestinal or other organ incision, and the additional expense of these drains.

More details on indications and placement of this type of drain will be covered in Chapter 26.

POSTOPERATIVE CARE

An Elizabethan collar is mandatory for all patients with a surgical drain in place, to prevent premature removal or damage to the drain. In some cats and depending upon the location of the drain, it may be possible to use a soft collar to allow them to feed more easily and to avoid problems with postoperative anorexia. If a rigid collar is deemed necessary, it may need to be removed under close observation at feeding times.

Drains are likely to add to patient discomfort in the postoperative period and appropriate analgesia should be supplied while they are in place.

Nosocomial infections are a significant risk of drain placement and can lead to multi-resistant wound infections and costly complications. Gloves should ALWAYS be worn when handling the drain or the surgical site. In addition, closed suction drains should only be emptied once they become full, or if suction is lost. More frequent emptying confers no additional advantage, but increases the risk of infection due to increased drain handling. Dressing changes should be performed as aseptically as possible and the drain exit site should be examined at least once daily for the presence of erythema, discharge or swelling.

WHEN TO REMOVE

All surgical drains will act as foreign material within the surgical site and as such will result in soft tissue irritation and inflammation. This inflammatory response will elicit some fluid production independent of the surgical disease and thus fluid production from the drain is rarely expected to reduce to zero after placement. As a general guide, approximately 2–4 mL/kg/24 hours is deemed to be acceptable and likely to be solely due to drain presence; thus when fluid production reduces to this level, the drain can be removed. Alternatively, where this level is not reached, but the quantity of fluid drained remains static over two to three days, the drain should also be removed. In order to use these guidelines, it is important that fluid production is accurately quantified when drains are emptied, and recorded so that the 24 hour rate of fluid production can be calculated.

Because of the difficulty of quantifying fluid production from Penrose drains, these drains are usually removed when fluid production has become serosanguinous/transudate in nature and the amount of fluid is subjectively considered to be decreasing or is unchanged over a number of days. This commonly occurs by day 3 to 5 postoperatively. Delay in removal of the drain beyond this point is generally not recommended, as the advantages of continued drain placement reduce, and the risks of infection and costs of bandaging and hospitalization increase.

COMPLICATIONS

Infection

Removal of fluid from a surgical site is known to be beneficial in reducing infection, because the presence of fluid interferes with opsonization of bacteria, phagocytosis and antibacterial agent penetration. In contrast however, the presence of the drain within the wound may decrease the host's innate resistance to infection and handling of the drain in the postoperative period, often by multiple nursing personnel, carries an inherent risk of introducing nosocomial organisms into the wound. These latter infections may involve organisms with increased pathogenicity compared to original wound contaminants and thus infection with these organisms can greatly increase morbidity or result in patient mortality in the worst case scenario. This means that when drains are used optimally and are active in removing fluid from a wound/resolving dead space, they are likely to be advantageous in fighting infection. If drains are, however, used in a prophylactic setting only, or are poorly managed postoperatively, the overall effect may be more detrimental than beneficial to the individual.

Wound dehiscence

Drains placed to exit through the main wound incision result in increased wound dehiscence and therefore they are always placed to exit at a separate and distant site. Placement of drains within the abdomen adjacent to sites of intestinal anastomosis or incisions into other organs has been shown to increase the risk of wound dehiscence in human beings and the same is likely to be true in animals.

Occlusion

This is a problem of tube drains, which are prone to becoming occluded during use. Occlusion generally occurs by one of three mechanisms: the fluid exiting the drain is too viscous for the size of the drain tubing; fluid production has significantly reduced and thus consolidation of material is allowed to occur within the tubing; or the drain holes within the wound/body cavity have become occluded by fibrous tissue or omentum. Once a drain has become occluded, the clinician must decide upon the next course of action. If fluid production has significantly reduced, removal of the drain would be the most appropriate action. If, however, the function of the drain is still required, the clinician can attempt to aspirate the clot from the tube or a new drain may need to be placed.

Premature drain removal

Cats are fastidious groomers by nature and will show a keen interest or dislike to foreign objects and sutures attached to their body. If the drain is accessible to them, it is likely to be removed by the patient and thus an Elizabethan collar is necessary in all cases to prevent this from occurring. Premature drain removal may result in unwanted fluid build-up within the surgical site or the need for repeat placement of the drain under a second anesthetic or sedation.

Drain retention or breakage

Retraction of the drain back into the wound bed or breakage of the drain during removal can occur. Recording the length of drain initially placed within the wound, using only radio-opaque drains and adequately securing drains at the exit site should limit these complications or allow a problem to be more easily recognized.

Conclusion

In conclusion, when appropriately used, surgical drains may be of significant benefit to the clinician and patient and can optimize wound healing. When used incorrectly, however, at best they are an unnecessary expense and at worst could result in a fatal complication (such as a multi-resistant infection causing septicemia or serious damage to a thoracic drain that could result in pneumothorax, lung collapse, and death).

REFERENCES

1. Hampel NL, Johnson RG. Principles of surgical drains and drainage. J Am Anim Hosp Assoc 1985;21:21–8.

2. Hunt GB, Tisdall PLC, Liptak JM, et al. Skin-fold advancement flaps for closing large proximal limb and trunk defects in dogs and cats. Vet Surg 2001;30:440–8.

3. Lidbetter DA, Williams FA, Krahwinkel DJ, et al. Radical lateral body-wall resection for fibrosarcoma with reconstruction using polypropylene mesh and a caudal superficial epigastric axial pattern flap: A prospective clinical study of the technique and results in 6 cats. Vet Surg 2002;31:57–64.

4. Remedios AM, Bauer MS, Bowen CV. Thoracodorsal and caudal superficial epigastric axial pattern skin flaps in cats. Vet Surg 1989;18:380–5.

5. Gurusamy KS, Samraj K. Wound drains after incisional hernia repair. Cochrane Database Syst Rev 2007;(Issue 1). Art. No.: CD005570.

6. Samraj K, Gurusamy KS. Wound drains following thyroid surgery. Cochrane Database Syst Rev 2007;(Issue 4). Art. No.: CD006099.

7. Parker MJ, Livingstone V, Clifton R, et al. Closed suction surgical wound drainage after orthopaedic surgery. Cochrane Database Syst Rev 2007;(Issue 3). Art. No.: CD001825.

8. Bohling MW, Henderson RA, Swaim SF, et al. Cutaneous wound healing in the cat: a macroscopic description and comparison with cutaneous wound healing in the dog. Vet Surg 2004;33:579–87.

9. Bohling MW, Henderson RA, Swaim SF, et al. Comparison of the role of the subcutaneous tissues in cutaneous wound healing in the dog and cat. Vet Surg 2006;35:3–14.

10. Freeman LJ, Pettit GD, Robinette JD, et al. Tissue reaction to suture material in the feline linea alba. A retrospective, prospective and histologic study. Vet Surg 1987;16:440–5.

11. Runk A, Allen SW, Mahaffey EA. Tissue reactivity to poliglecaprone 25 in the feline linea alba. Vet Surg 1999;28:466–71.

12. Brockman DJ, Pardo AD, Conzemius MG, et al. Omentum-enhanced reconstruction of chronic nonhealing wounds in cats: techniques and clinical use. Vet Surg 1996;25:99–104.

13. Lascelles BDX, Davison L, Dunning M, et al. Use of omental pedicle grafts in the management of non-healing axillary wounds in 10 cats. J Small Anim Pract 1998;39:475–80.

14. Langley-Hobbs SJ, Keller M, Voss K. External coaptation. In: Montavon PM, Langley-Hobbs SJ, Voss K, editors. Feline orthopedic surgery and musculoskeletal disease. Edinburgh: Elsevier; 2009. p. 239–48.

15. Dernell WS. Initial wound management. Vet Clin North Am Small Anim Pract 2006;36:732–4.

16. Ladlow JL. Surgical drains in wound management and reconstructive surgery. In: BSAVA manual of canine and feline wound management and reconstruction. Gloucester UK: BSAVA; 2009. p. 54–68.

17. Halfacree ZJ, Wilson AM, Baines SJ. Evaluation of in vitro performance of suction drains. Am J Vet Res 2009;70:283–9.

18. Lee AH, Swaim SF, Henderson RA. Surgical drainage. Comp Cont Educ Pract Vet 1986;8:94–103.

19. Monnet E. Pleura and pleural space. In: Slatter D, editor. Textbook of small animal surgery. Philadelphia: Saunders; 2003. p. 387–405.

20. Valtolina C, Adamantos S. Evaluation of small-bore wire guided chest drains for management of pleural space disease. J Small Anim Pract 2009;50:290–7.

Chapter 12

Feeding tubes

A. Sparkes

Cats can be notoriously fussy about eating, both while hospitalized and postoperatively, and the importance of maintaining their nutritional status cannot be overemphasized. Adequate nutrition has many benefits including improving the patient's well-being, optimizing healing and preventing re-feeding syndrome (see Chapter 6). This chapter aims to cover the indications and type of feeding tubes that are available for use in cats and the techniques of tube insertion.

GENERAL CONSIDERATIONS

There are many reasons why a surgical patient may become inappetent, anorexic, or have inadequate nutritional intake (Box 12-1).

It is important that a full assessment is made of both the reasons for inadequate nutritional intake and the options available for overcoming these. Due to their unique nutritional requirements, cats should not be allowed to remain significantly inappetent or anorexic for longer than three days,[1] and particular care should be taken of surgical patients where, depending on their condition, nutritional demands may be appreciably higher and inadequate nutritional support may have serious consequences for recovery, morbidity and even mortality.

It is well recognized that providing enteral nutritional support, wherever possible, is far superior to attempting parenteral support,

---

Box 12-1 Reasons for postoperative inappetence in cats

- Medical or surgical conditions directly affecting the alimentary tract
- Presence of uncontrolled pain
- Presence of uncontrolled nausea
- The stress of hospitalization
- Offering unfamiliar or unsuitable foods
- Development or induction of food aversion, e.g., by offering the cat food while it is feeling painful or nauseous
- Side effects of medications being used, e.g., opioids
- Presence of inflammatory cytokines

---

being more physiological, safer, less expensive, and preserving the structure and function of the gastrointestinal tract.[2] There are occasional situations where parenteral or partial parenteral nutrition is the only realistic option available, but for the vast majority of patients some form of enteral nutritional support can be used. However, the technique used may be dictated, at least to some extent, by the patient's condition. The presence of orofacial or esophageal disease may, for example, preclude the use of certain tube feeding techniques such as nasoesophageal or esophagostomy tubes.

Although force-feeding, e.g., syringe feeding, is sometimes advocated for the short-term nutritional support of dogs and cats, this is not a technique that can be recommended, especially for cats. Force-feeding is inevitably a highly stressful procedure, and as such one that is likely to promote further inappetence rather than help resolve the situation. Additionally, it is very difficult to meet nutritional requirements by force-feeding and there is a significant risk of inducing aspiration of food with this technique.

Given the wide availability of other much more suitable forms of nutritional support (tempting of voluntary food intake, pharmacological stimulation of appetite, or tube feeding) there is no rationale for the use of force-feeding with the feline patient. Similarly, orogastric tube feeding is too stressful for the feline patient.

Tube feeding

Tube feeding is an important consideration in inappetent cats. Not every inappetent or anorexic cat will require nutritional support via tube feeding, but many will. Tube feeding should be instituted at an early stage for those cats that do not respond adequately to addressing the underlying causes of the inappetence, together perhaps with the use of appetite stimulants when deemed appropriate; or for those where more conservative measures are considered inappropriate,

In addition, tube feeding may be valuable to avoid inducing food aversion in some cats. Aversion to foods can develop when they are offered to patients when they are experiencing significant pain (especially gastrointestinal pain) or nausea. The cat may subsequently associate those feelings with the food that was offered and therefore refuse the food, even when the pain or discomfort has resolved. Where it is anticipated that pain or nausea may be difficult to fully control, tube feeding may be an important pre-emptive strategy to avoid inducing food aversion.

DOI: 10.1016/B978-0-7020-4336-9.00012-3

Table 12-1 Overview of the three major forms of tube feeding in cats

	Nasoesophageal tubes	Esophageal tubes	Percutaneous endoscopic gastrostomy (PEG) tubes
Advantages	Simple to place Inexpensive Generally well tolerated but usually require an Elizabethan collar No general anesthetic	Simple to place Inexpensive Very well tolerated Wide choice of foods Suitable for long-term use	Very well tolerated Wide choice of foods Suitable for long-term use Can be used in patients with esophageal disease and in some patients with vomiting (does not cause tube displacement)
Size range	3–6 Fr tubes	10–16 Fr tubes	12–20 Fr tubes
Disadvantages	Restricted to specific liquid diets Not suitable with esophageal dysfunction Only short-term use (<7–10 days) Can cause rhinitis Not suitable with esophageal dysfunction or in vomiting patients	Requires anesthesia Not suitable with esophageal dysfunction or in vomiting patients	Technically more demanding Requires anesthesia Have to wait 24 hours to start feeding Peritonitis is potential complication Must wait 14 days before removing

---

Box 12-2 Selection factors for feeding tubes in cats

- The anticipated duration of tube feeding. Nasoesophageal tubes are much less suitable for longer-term support, i.e., longer than one or two weeks
- The type of food available. Choices for nasoesophageal and jejunostomy feeding are much more restricted due to the narrow diameter of the tubes used
- The condition or disease being treated
- The presence or absence of diseases affecting the nose, mouth, pharynx, esophagus, or stomach
- The need for general anesthesia in the placement of any tube other than nasoesophageal tubes
- Owner concerns and abilities, especially if continuation of tube feeding in the home environment is anticipated

---

Box 12-3 Indications and placement for feeding cats via a duodenostomy or jejunostomy tube

Indications

- Where there is persistent vomiting and/or gastric outflow obstruction
- Where there is severe disease of the proximal intestinal tract
- In the face of severe pancreatitis (to reduced neuro-hormonal stimulation of the pancreas)
- Where altered (reduced) levels of consciousness may lead to high risk of aspiration if vomiting was to occur

Placement

- Surgically via the flank into the jejunum
- Transpyloric placement via a nasojejunal tube
- Transpyloric via a gastrojejunal tube, i.e., via a gastrostomy tube

---

The three most common forms of tube feeding in cats are nasoesophageal tube feeding, esophagostomy tube feeding, and gastrostomy tube feeding (Table 12-1). In occasional patients, feeding via a duodenostomy or jejunostomy tube may be indicated. In the past, pharyngostomy tubes have also been advocated for tube feeding of dogs and cats, but these are now not recommended due to complications such as airway obstruction.[2]

FEEDING TUBES

The selection of feeding tube for any individual patient will depend on a variety of factors as listed in Box 12-2.

Duodenostomy and jejunostomy tubes

Orogastric feeding is preferable over feeding that bypasses the stomach, so duodenostomy and jejunostomy tubes are rarely used in cats. There are limited indications for their placement (Box 12-3). Direct surgical placement via the flank is the most common method used,[3] and has been reported to have a low complication rate. A modified jejunopexy technique may reduce the risk of leakage around the site of tube entry into the jejunum.[4] The reader is referred to Heuter (2004)[3] and Daye et al (1999)[4] for further details, but this chapter will focus on the three most commonly used techniques of tube feeding.

Nasoesophageal intubation

Nasoesophageal tubes are very well tolerated by the majority of cats and have the important advantage of being inexpensive, easy to place and requiring no anesthesia (and usually no sedation) for their placement (Box 12-4). The use of nasoesophageal tubes is particularly valuable in providing short-term nutritional support, but esophagostomy or gastrostomy tubes should generally be considered if tube feeding will need to be provided for longer than around seven days. Additionally, other techniques must be used in cases where nasoesophageal tubes are contraindicated, such as esophageal or gastric dysfunction or persistent vomiting, or perhaps where more aggressive nutritional support is required (due to the wider range of feeds that can be used in wider bore tubes).

An additional concern with nasoesophageal tubes is the irritation to the nasal mucosa that can occur or simply the discomfort of having the tube in place. In cats with pre-existing nasal disease and/or with partial nasal obstruction, the use of nasoesophageal tubes can cause further rhinitis as well as physically occluding one nostril, potentially leading to further respiratory problems.

Tube selection

A 3–6 Fr (1.0–2.0 mm diameter) veterinary or human pediatric nasogastric tube is used for most cats, with a 6 Fr generally being

Box 12-4 **Technique of nasoesophageal tube placement**

The length of the tube to be inserted should be pre-measured and marked, by measuring the distance from the tip of the nose to the seventh or eighth intercostal space. This will ensure that the tip of the tube lies in the distal esophagus and not in the stomach itself, which helps to reduce the risk of reflux of gastric juice, vomiting and esophagitis.

Before passing the tube the nasal mucosa should be anesthetized by applying a few drops of a non-irritating local anesthetic, e.g., 0.5% proparacaine/proxymetacaine or 0.5–1% amethocaine. If necessary, the cat may also be sedated lightly to facilitate the procedure.

The tube should be lubricated with a water-soluble gel (a plain gel or 5% lignocaine gel may be used). The head should be held firmly in one hand and the nose tilted up a little, and the tube is then inserted into the anesthetized nose using the other hand in a ventromedial direction, aiming towards the base of the ear on the opposite side of the head (Fig. 12-1A). This should ensure the tube passes along the ventral nasal meatus and into the nasopharynx. If the tube lodges in the dorsal or middle nasal meatus it should be withdrawn and redirected ventrally. Passing the first 1–2 cm is often the most difficult as the skin around the external nare will not be anesthetized.

To help prevent tracheal intubation, as the tube approaches the pharynx the head should be tilted back down and held in a normal position (Fig. 12-1B). The tube is gently advanced until the pre-marked length has been inserted.

Before the tube is secured in place, it is important to confirm it is in the esophagus and has not inadvertently entered the respiratory tree (or, for example, lodged in the oropharynx). To do this the following can be performed:

- Try to aspirate through the tube – if it is in the esophagus, the esophageal wall will collapse around the tube and usually nothing can be aspirated
- Inject a small volume of sterile water or saline through the tube (3–5 mL) – if the tube is in the trachea, this should elicit a cough
- Inject some air through the tube (10–15 mL) and auscultate for borborygmi over the left flank
- If in doubt, radiography can be used to confirm the position

The tube can then be secured in place (Fig. 12-1C). This is usually facilitated by placing small 'butterfly wings' of zinc oxide tape (or similar material) that are then secured to the bridge of the nose and the top of the head with tissue glue or sutures. The tube is taken up over the top of the nose and head to avoid interference with the whiskers, and can then be attached to a collar or neck bandage. Most cats tolerate nasoesophageal tubes well, but an Elizabethan collar is usually required to prevent tube removal by the patient.

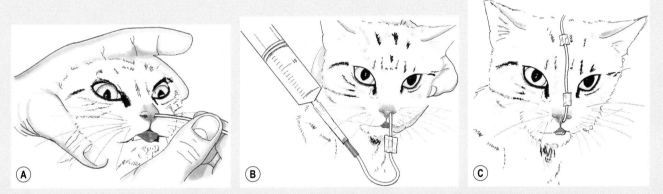

Figure 12-1 (A) Initial placement of a nasoesophageal tube in a cat (sedated with ketamine). **(B)** Checking correct placement of the nasoesophageal tube prior to securing the tube by injecting sterile saline and air. **(C)** Nasoesophageal tube correctly secured in a cat over the bridge of the nose and the head.

suitable for adult cats. Most feeding tubes are made of polyvinyl chloride (PVC), silicone, or polyurethane. Comparative studies evaluating these different materials in cats have not been published; however, based on knowledge of the physical properties of these materials and studies in the human literature several conclusions can be made (Box 12-5).[5–8] For several reasons, polyurethane tubes are regarded as the material of choice by many clinicians.

Esophagostomy intubation

Esophagostomy intubation (O tubes) can be used where nasoesophageal tubes are not tolerated or cannot be used, and it is suitable for either short-term or longer-term nutritional support, e.g., several weeks or even months. Esophagostomy tubes are easily inserted (Box 12.6), inexpensive, and have proved to be remarkably valuable in nutritional support with very few complications reported. Their ease of placement and use, the fact that they are well tolerated and

the wide choice of blenderized feeds that can be used have all meant that O tubes have become the method of choice for tube feeding in many situations where there is a functional esophagus and gastrointestinal tract.

Esophagostomy tubes are generally made of latex, PVC, polyurethane, or silicone. The soft, minimally irritant polyurethane and silicone tubes are likely to be better tolerated, and will not become brittle over time, which can be a problem with latex and PVC tubes. A 12–16 Fr tube (4.0–5.3 mm diameter) is usually suitable.

Alternative placement techniques

As an alternative to the use of Carmalt forceps and cutting down into the esophagus, special metal introducers are available that are put into the esophagus and allow the percutaneous placement of a needle with a peel off sheath directly into the esophageal lumen. The needle is withdrawn and then an esophagostomy tube is inserted through the

Box 12-5 Comparison of polyvinyl chloride (PVC), silicone and polyurethane tubes

- PVC tubes are relatively inflexible and uncomfortable, and the leaching of plasticizers increases their stiffness and discomfort over time
- Silicone and polyurethane tubes are considerably softer and more comfortable, silicone being somewhat better than polyurethane in this respect
- Attempts to aspirate material through a silicone tube may be hampered by a tendency for the walls of the tube to collapse

- Polyurethane tubes are stronger and less prone to kinking
- Polyurethane or silicone tubes can be left in situ for several weeks, whereas it is recommended that PVC tubes are replaced every seven to ten days
- Polyurethane tubes have significantly thinner walls than either silicone or PVC, meaning they have a larger internal diameter allowing the easier administration of liquid diets, higher flow rates, and are less likely to become blocked

Box 12-6 Technique of esophagostomy intubation

Intubation requires a short general anesthetic. The cat should be placed in right lateral recumbency, and the left mid-cervical region clipped and prepared for surgery (from the angle of the mandible to the thoracic inlet). Curved Carmalt forceps are passed into the esophagus, turned outwards to identify the esophagus in the left mid-cervical region (Fig. 12-2A). While pressure is maintained to keep the tip of the forceps tenting the cervical esophagus laterally, a small incision is made through the skin with a scalpel blade directly over the tip of the forceps, ensuring that the jugular vein is avoided. This is carefully deepened until the wall of the esophagus is perforated and the tip of the forceps can be pushed through the skin incision, and the forceps opened.

The length of tube to be inserted is calculated as for nasoesophageal tubes, but measuring the length from the incision site to the seventh or eighth intercostal space, as with nasoesophageal tubes, to ensure the tip of the tube is not too distal in the esophagus.[9] The tip of the tube is then grabbed with the open blades of the

forceps and pulled out through the oral cavity (Fig. 12-2B). The tip of the tube is then repositioned in the forceps and passed back aborally into the esophagus, past the ostomy site, and the pre-measured length of the tube is fed into the esophagus.

The tube is then secured to the cervical skin using a suitable friction suture (Fig. 12-2C). Alternatively, a 'butterfly wing' tape can be applied to the tube at the appropriate site and sutured to the skin to secure the tube in place. A dressing is applied to the ostomy site and then a light neck bandage is placed so that the tube exits dorsally behind the cat's head. The tube should be clamped and/or capped between feeds (Fig. 12-2D).

When the tube is removed (sutures are cut and the tube pulled out), the ostomy site will heal within two weeks, and problems such as esophageal stricture formation have not been reported. The tube can be removed at any time after it has been placed, even the following day.

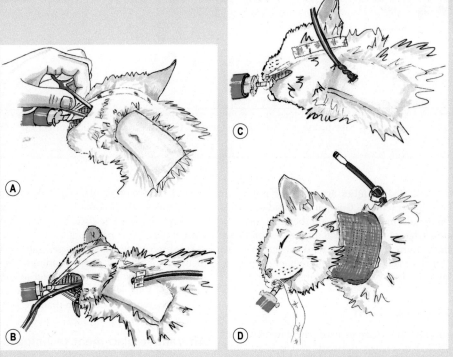

Figure 12-2 (A) Esophagostomy tube placement – Carmalt forceps are placed in the esophagus and rotated so that the tip can be incised down on to. **(B)** The incision through to the esophageal lumen has been made and the tip of the esophagostomy tube has been grasped and pulled through to the mouth. **(C)** The tip of the tube has been placed distally in the esophagus and the tube is secured with a friction suture. **(D)** The esophagostomy tube is secured and protected with a light bandage.

sheath, which is subsequently peeled away (e.g., esophagostomy tube sets, Smiths Medical PM, Inc., Veterinary, Wisconsin, USA). Tubes of up to 14 Fr can be inserted in this way. The procedure time is slightly reduced with this technique, but it has little other advantage in cats (but can be valuable in larger dogs).

Alternatively, a small, e.g., 4 Fr tube, can be inserted through a conventional 14G 'over-the-needle' catheter inserted through the open blades of Carmalt forceps placed in the esophagus.[10] This technique avoids the necessity to purchase any special equipment and is rapid, but has the drawback of only placing a narrow diameter tube, through which only special liquid diets can be used.

Gastrostomy feeding tubes

Large diameter gastrostomy tubes can be placed in the stomach, with most cats tolerating tubes up to 20 Fr (a 12–20 Fr can be used). Gastrostomy tubes are technically more difficult and more time-consuming to place, which is why esophagostomy tubes have become much more popular in many patients unless esophageal disease prevents their use. However, for long-term feeding (over many weeks or months), gastrostomy tubes may have advantages in some cats and be better tolerated by some.

Generally, mushroom tip Pezzar-type catheters are used as gastrostomy tubes, although other designs are also available. Latex, silicone and polyurethane tubes are available, and again silicone and polyurethane are better choices for long-term use, and there is some evidence that polyurethane tubes are better than silicone,[11,12] although for the length of time these are used in most veterinary patients this is not likely to be a major consideration.

Gastrostomy tubes can be placed at surgical laparotomy, but are more commonly placed by percutaneous endoscopic gastrostomy (PEG) intubation (Box 12-7), although this may have a higher rate of complications than open placement.[13] The technique for placement of a gastrostomy tube by open surgery is described in Chapter 28. As with esophagostomy tube placement, anesthesia is required for gastrostomy tube placement whether endoscopically or by open surgery.

If desired, for long-term feeding, the conventional PEG tube can be removed after the first two to four weeks and replaced with a special low-profile gastrostomy tube. These can be placed through the original ostomy site once the original tube has been removed and have the advantage of being easier to maintain and better tolerated on a long-term basis.[14] Purpose-designed low-profile gastrostomy tubes, although more expensive, can also be used for the initial PEG tube placement.[15]

Non-endoscopic placement devices are also available for gastrostomy tubes, but their use has been associated with problems, particularly with incorrect anatomical placement of the tubes,[16] and thus great care should be taken if these are employed.

POST-PLACEMENT CONSIDERATIONS

With any type of tube feeding, if the cat has been significantly inappetent or anorexic over a period of time it is important to slowly increase the food administered over several days, e.g., three to four days, until their full, calculated caloric requirements are being met. Similarly, it is better to start with small (no more than 5–10 mL/kg total volume) frequent meals initially, and then gradually increase the volume of each meal and decrease the frequency (but maintaining four or more meals daily). Volumes of 15–20 mL/kg may be tolerated by cats, but should be given slowly.[1]

Ideally, only liquid medications should be administered via tubes. Crushed tablets are a common cause of tube blockage, especially with smaller diameter tubes.

Every tube should be marked with indelible ink where it exits the body so that tube migration is easy to identify. With nasoesophageal and esophagostomy tubes, care should be taken if the cat vomits to ensure that the tube is still correctly positioned and not kinked.

Owner experience with both gastrostomy and esophagostomy tubes has been reported to be positive, with few complications reported, most owners managing tube feeding well, and with no appreciable differences between the two techniques.[17,18]

COMPLICATIONS OF TUBE FEEDING

Complications of tube feeding are generally mild, such as contact dermatitis around the stoma. However, tube dislodgement or premature removal could result in peritonitis or aspiration pneumonia and therefore potentially be fatal.

Complications of nasoesophageal tubes

The two major disadvantages of nasoesophageal tubes are firstly their narrow diameter, which means that only specifically designed liquid foods can be used (other foods will invariably cause blockage of the tube), and secondly local nasal irritation resulting in rhinitis.

Generally complications of nasoesophageal feeding are rare, and are usually easily overcome. Occasionally, individual cats will not tolerate the tubes and another method of feeding must be chosen, e.g., esophagostomy or gastrostomy. Adequate flushing of the tube with water before and after each feed,[6] followed by temporary plugging of the tube end to prevent the inside drying out, is important to help prevent blockage of the tube. Diarrhea (and less commonly vomiting) occurs in a proportion of cases (see Chapter 5).

Complications of esophagostomy tubes

With the ability to feed blenderized 'standard' foods through an esophagstomy tube, a much wider range of diets is available for use, and gastrointestinal disturbances are less common than with nasoesophageal tubes. The only major complication that has been reported with esophagostomy tubes has been infection at the ostomy site. Careful daily cleaning of the site is thus essential and together with the use of antiseptic creams/gels will help prevent infection.

Although less prone to blockage than the smaller bore nasoesophageal tubes, it is still important to flush the tube with water before and after each feed. The placement of the tube should also be checked if the cat vomits while it is in place.

Complications of PEG tubes

Complications of gastrostomy tubes include infection at the ostomy site, wound breakdown, pneumoperitoneum, peritonitis, and vomiting. As with other techniques, the tube should be flushed with water before and after administration of food, and as with esophagostomy tubes, the larger diameter of gastrostomy tubes means a variety of commercial foods can be blenderized and administered through the tube.

129

Box 12-7 Technique of gastrostomy tube placement endoscopically (PEG)

The cat is placed in right lateral recumbency and the left abdominal wall (over the area of the stomach) clipped and prepared for surgery. A gastroscope is advanced into the stomach, which is then insufflated with air, and the endoscope is directed so that the light can be seen illuminating the skin overlying the stomach (Fig. 12-3A). A 16-gauge 'over-the-needle' intravenous catheter is placed through the skin and into the stomach at this site – the stylet is removed and nylon/polyester suture material is threaded through the catheter into the stomach. The suture material is grasped with biopsy forceps fed through the endoscope's channel (Fig. 12-3B), and the endoscope together with the suture material is then withdrawn via the oropharynx.

The suture material is then secured to the open end of the gastrostomy feeding tube, with another over-the-needle IV catheter usually being threaded over the suture material first to provide a tapering point when it is pulled through the stomach wall (Fig. 12-3C). As an alternative, more expensive but purpose-made gastrostomy tube kits can be purchased that incorporate a tapered end to facilitate the procedure (e.g., MILA PEG kit, Mila International, Kentucky, USA). The suture material is then pulled back through the left flank resulting in the feeding tube being drawn down into the stomach. Gentle traction is applied to pull the tip of the intravenous catheter through the abdominal wall (Fig. 12-3D), and as gentle traction is continually applied a scalpel is used to make a small cut-down incision onto the hub of the catheter to allow passage of the catheter and the feeding tube through the incision.

The mushroom tip or bumper is then drawn up snug to keep the stomach wall in close apposition to the wall of the abdomen (to allow subsequent adhesion of the parietal and visceral peritoneum), and the position of the tube is checked with the endoscope. The tube

is secured to the skin with a suitable friction suture, and a flange is then made by cutting off a 2 cm length of the tube at the distal end. A small horizontal incision is made in the center that allows it to be slid over the catheter and lie at the abdominal wall. This is secured in place with tape or a finger trap suture (Fig. 12-3E) and helps to ensure the gastric wall remains snug against the abdominal wall. It is important that this is neither too tight (so it could cause pressure necrosis) nor too loose (so that gastric contents could leak into the abdomen). It is recommended that with the mushroom tip pulled snug against the stomach wall, there should be approximately a 5mm gap between the external flange and the abdominal wall. Some clinicians, as a precaution, prefer to also put a flange on the gastric side, putting the flange in place before the tube is fed into the stomach. This may be more appropriate in larger dogs, rather than cats, where there may be a greater risk of peritoneal leakage.

The tube is clamped and/or capped, and then secured against the body wall and protected with a light bandage. Ideally, 24 hours should be left before feeding is commenced to allow a fibrin seal to develop, but water can be administered within six to 12 hours. It is recommended that the PEG tube be left in place for a minimum of 14 days before it is removed, to ensure good adhesion between the stomach and the abdominal wall. After this time, the tube can be removed – if there is no inner flange, a rigid stylet can be inserted into the tube and pushed so that the mushroom tip is stretched and thus flattened allowing the tube to be pulled through the ostomy site. Alternatively, the tube can be cut and the mushroom tip (± inner flange) retrieved endoscopically. After removal the ostomy site should heal rapidly and usually seals over within 24 hours.

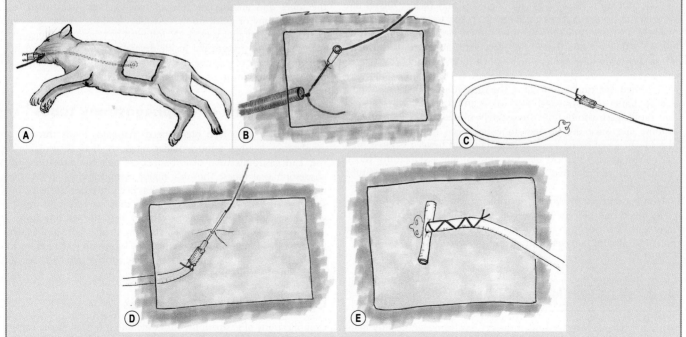

Figure 12-3 (A) Preparation for PEG intubation – the left lateral flank is clipped and surgically prepared. A gastroscope is passed, the stomach is insufflated, and transillumination is used to identify the fundus where the needle can be inserted. **(B)** An over-the-needle catheter is inserted into the stomach lumen and monofilament nylon is passed into the stomach and grasped with the endoscope. **(C)** A silicone mushroom-tipped catheter is used as the PEG tube. An over-the-needle catheter has been threaded over the nylon, and the nylon has been tied to a cut and tapered end of the catheter. **(D)** The nylon has been pulled back through the abdominal wall to pull the catheter into the stomach. The over-the-needle catheter exits through the flank – a small incision is made to facilitate the passage of the hub of the catheter and body of the PEG tube through the flank. **(E)** The PEG tube has been secured with a friction suture. A flange (made from part of the tube) is placed and then secured with tape to ensure the stomach wall remains apposed to the abdominal wall.

REFERENCES

1. Chan D. The inappetent hospitalised cat: clinical approach to maximising nutritional support. J Feline Med Surg 2009;11:925–33.

2. Prittie J, Barton L. Route of nutrient delivery. Clin Tech Small Anim Pract 2004;19:6–8.

3. Heuter K. Placement of jejunal feeding tubes for post-gastric feeding. Clin Tech Small Anim Pract 2004;19:32–42.

4. Daye RM, Huber ML, Henderson RA. Interlocking box jejunostomy: a new technique for enteral feeding. J Am Anim Hosp Assoc 1999;35:129.

5. Minard G, Lysen LK. Enteral access devices. In: Gottschlich MM, Fuhrman MP, Hammond KA, et al, editors. The Science and Practice of Nutrition Support: A Case-Based Core Curriculum. USA: ASPEN; 2001. p. 167–88.

6. Metheny N, Eisenberg P, McSweeney M. Effect of feeding tube properties and three irrigants on clogging rates. Nurs Res 1988;37:165–9.

7. Mensforth A, Nightingale JMD. Insertion and care of enteral feeding tubes. In: Nightingale JMD, editor. Intestinal Failure. London: Greenwich Medical Media Ltd; 2001. p. 281–304.

8. Rees RG, Attrill H, Quinn D, Silk DB. Improved design of nasogastric feeding tubes. Clin Nutr 1986;5:203–7.

9. Balkany TJ, Baker BB, Bloustein PA, Jafek BW. Cervical esophagostomy in dogs: endoscopic, radiographic, and histopathologic evaluation of esophagitis induced by feeding tubes. Ann Otol Rhinol Laryngol 1977;86:588–93.

10. Formaggini L. Normograde, minimally invasive technique for oesophagostomy in cats. J Feline Med Surg 2009;11:481–6.

11. Blacka J, Donoghue J, Sutherland M, et al. Dwell time and functional failure in percutaneous endoscopic gastrostomy tubes: a prospective randomized-controlled comparison between silicon polymer and polyurethane percutaneous endoscopic gastrostomy tubes. Aliment Pharmacol Ther 2004;20:875–82.

12. Sartori S, Trevisani L, Nielsen I, et al. Longevity of silicone and polyurethane catheters in long-term enteral feeding via percutaneous endoscopic gastrostomy. Aliment Pharmacol Ther 2003;17:853–6.

13. Salinardi BJ, Harkin KR, Bulmer BJ, Roush JK. Comparison of complications of percutaneous endoscopic versus surgically placed gastrostomy tubes in 42 dogs and 52 cats. J Am Anim Hosp Assoc 2006;42:51–6.

14. Yoshimoto SK, Marks SL, Struble AL, Riel DL. Owner experiences and complications with home use of a replacement low profile gastrostomy device for long-term enteral feeding in dogs. Can Vet J 2006;47:144–50.

15. Campbell SJ, Marks SL, Yoshimoto SK, et al. Complications and outcomes of one-step low-profile gastrostomy devices for long-term enteral feeding in dogs and cats. J Am Anim Hosp Assoc 2006;42:197–206.

16. Glaus TM, Cornelius LM, Bartges JW, Reusch C. Complications with non-endoscopic percutaneous gastrostomy in 31 cats and 10 dogs: a retrospective study. J Small Anim Pract 1998;39:218–22.

17. Ireland LM, Hohenhaus AE, Broussard JD, Weissman BL. A comparison of owner management and complications in 67 cats with esophagostomy and percutaneous endoscopic gastrostomy feeding tubes. J Am Anim Hosp Assoc 2003;39:241–6.

18. Seaman R, Legendre A. Owner experiences with home use of a gastrostomy tube in their dog or cat. J Am Vet Med Assoc 1998;212:1576–8.

Chapter |13|

Instruments

J. Lapish, S.J. Langley-Hobbs

As the patient size or area of surgery becomes smaller in relation to the surgeon's hand, the tissues must be manipulated, increasingly, through the medium of surgical instrumentation. An extreme example is ophthalmic surgery where the surgeon rarely touches the tissues. Appropriately scaled instruments must be selected to minimize de-vitalization of tissues. Feline soft tissue surgery will therefore require a greater use of instruments than the surgery of larger patients.

GENERAL SURGICAL INSTRUMENTS

General surgical instruments including scalpels, dissecting forceps, scissors, artery forceps, retractors, and needleholders are described in the chapter on Instrumentation in *Feline Orthopedic Surgery and Musculoskeletal Disease* (Chapter 23).[1] An example of the instruments that could be included in a general surgical kit is listed in Box 13-1 and shown in Figure 13-1.

Suction

Suction will contribute to a clear operating field. Many tips are available but the most useful focal tips are the Adson (4 mm diameter) or Frazier (2.6 mm diameter) types, both of which offer fingertip control of suction by an assistant. For suction of larger volumes of fluid from body cavities when performing abdominal or thoracic surgery the Poole is preferred (Fig. 13-2).

Magnification and light

Use of binocular loupes, which magnify while maintaining a normal working distance, will significantly improve visualization of the operative site. A magnification of 2.5× is sufficient for most procedures. The focal distance should be selected to maintain a normal working distance, usually 380 mm or 430 mm. The addition of a loupe light, either fiber optic or the more economic LED type, will automatically provide surgery light where it is needed (Fig. 13-3).

Soft tissue biopsy instruments

Selection of the appropriate soft tissue biopsy devices will be detailed in the relevant organ specific chapters and more generally in Chapter 14. Several types are available. The TruCut type consists of a slim needle which may be inserted relatively atraumatically into an area of parenchymatous tissue, typically within an organ (Fig. 13-4). A spring loaded cutter is fired within the needle, which excises and traps a sample. Where the sample is to be obtained from the surface of a friable tissue, clamshell type biopsy forceps with cutting jaws enclose and remove the sample (Fig. 13-5). Skin biopsies may be obtained using a punch biopsy, available in a variety of sizes. Although available as a reusable instrument it is normally used as a disposable device.

Vessel sealing devices

Accurate hemostasis is of utmost importance to a patient's survival and there are a wide variety of hemostatic tools currently available, all with their inherent advantages and limitations. Considerations should include time taken to achieve hemostasis, reliability in vessel sealing, collateral damage, and expense. Temporary application of pressure with sponges or hemostats may be sufficient for capillary or very small vessels, as clotting should occur. For larger vessels, ligation or the use of diathermy or electrosurgical devices will be required. Diathermy and electrosurgical devices have the advantage of sealing vessels in a shorter period of time than that required to place a ligature, and this might be useful in a situation where time is of the essence. In other situations the surgeon may prefer the security and reliability of a suture, for example for ligation of the femoral artery if performing amputation.

The following were compared for their efficacy and security in achieving vessel ligation: braided suture in a surgeon's knot; a monofilament suture in a granny knot; a metallic clip (Ligaclip, Johnson and Johnson; Fig. 13-6A); a bipolar diathermy system (Ligasure, ValleyLab; Fig. 13-6B); and an ultrasonically activated scalpel (Harmonic Scalpel, Johnson and Johnson).[2] Secure hemostasis was obtained with all the techniques in all vessels below 5 mm in diameter. In vessels over 5 mm, secure hemostasis was obtained with all modalities except the harmonic scalpel. With the harmonic scalpel,

A typical surgical tray might include the following:
Number 3 scalpel handle
Gallipot for warmed flushing solution
Sponges with radio dense marker
Backhouse towel clips 9 cm × 10
Mayo scissors straight 14 cm × 1
Metzenbaum scissor straight 14.5 cm × 1
Metzenbaum scissor curved 14.5 cm × 1
Suture scissors straight
Brown-Adson dissecting forceps 12.5 cm × 2
Straight De Bakey forceps 15 cm × 1
Adson Debakey forceps 12.5 cm × 1
Halstead mosquito artery forceps straight 12.5 cm × 5
Halstead mosquito forceps curved 12.5 cm × 5
Allis tissue forceps 4/5 teeth 15 cm × 2
Mayo-Hegar (T.C.) needleholder 15 cm × 1
Langenbeck or Senn hand held retractor

leaks occurred in vessels greater than 5–6 mm, confirming that the manufacturer's claims for each of the hemostatic methods were accurate. The use of hemostatic tools such as the harmonic scalpel and Ligasure has increased with the use of laparoscopic surgery where it is not easy to place traditional surgical knots.

Vessel sealers

These devices, such as the Ligasure system (EBVS; ValleyLab...) are computer-based, temperature controlled bipolar electrocoagulation systems (otherwise known as electrothermal bipolar vessel sealers). The vessel sealers claim to seal vessels up to 7 mm in diameter by denaturing collagen and elastin within the vessel wall and surrounding connective tissue. Adequate tissue sealing is determined by sensing

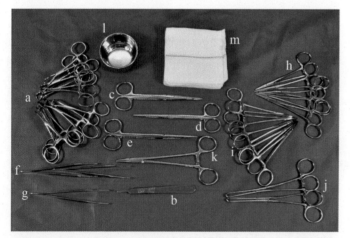

Figure 13-1 Surgical tray. a, Backhouse towel clips 9 cm; b, number 3 scalpel handle; c, Mayo scissors straight 14 cm; d, Metzenbaum scissors straight 14.5 cm; e, Metzenbaum scissors curved 14.5 cm; f, Adson Brown dissecting forceps; g, Adson Debakey dissecting forceps; h, Halstead mosquito artery forceps straight 12.5 cm; i, Halstead mosquito artery forceps curved 12.5 cm; j, Allis tissue forceps 4/5 teeth 15 cm; k, Mayo-Hegar (T.C.) needleholder 15 cm; l, gallipot; m, sponges with radio dense marker.

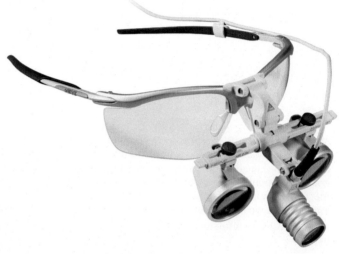

Figure 13-3 Loupes with light.

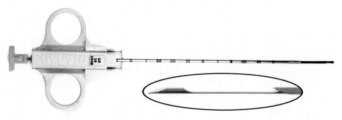

Figure 13-4 TruCut type biopsy needle.

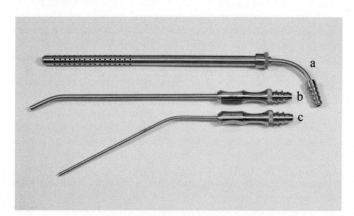

Figure 13-2 Suction tips: a, Poole; b, Adson; c, Frazier.

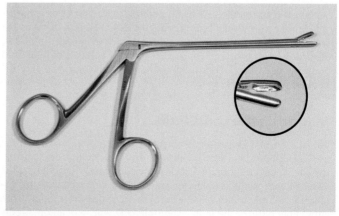

Figure 13-5 Clamshell biopsy forceps.

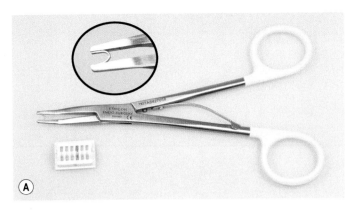

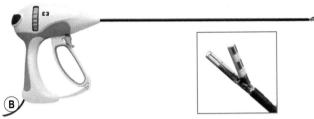

Figure 13-6 (A) Ligaclip vessel sealing clips and applicator. **(B)** Ligasure vessel sealer. *(A, Courtesy of Ethicon Ltd.)*

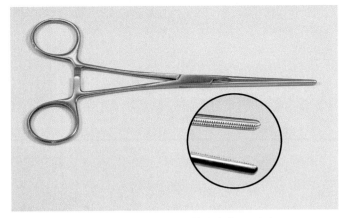

Figure 13-7 Atraumatic 'baby' Doyen with Debakey style jaws.

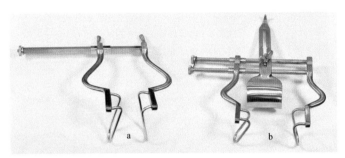

Figure 13-8 Abdominal retractors. **(A)** Gosset; **(B)** 'baby' Balfour.

the resistive index of the tissue. The device notifies the surgeon when the tissue is safe to be cut and the surgeon controls the knife cut of the tissue.

Harmonic scalpel

Using an energy source to excite piezo-electric crystals in the hand piece, the harmonic scalpel employs mechanical energy transmitted and amplified to very high frequency such that at the tip of the blade longitudinal motion frequency reaches 55,500 cycles/second. This rapid movement creates temperatures that denature proteins, creating an area of coagulation and allowing concurrent cutting. This cutting and coagulation occurs without causing a significant rise in temperature at the tissue level, with low smoke formation, no muscular stimulation and without the transmission of energy through the patient. Its safety has been tested extensively in animal experiments and there is now ample evidence to suggest that it produces less thermal damage in vitro than electrosurgery and lasers. Using multifunctional hand pieces and adjusting power levels means that different balances between coagulation and cutting effects are possible. The manufacturers claim efficient and safe hemostasis in vessels < 3 mm using current hand pieces.

ABDOMINAL SURGERY

In addition to the general kit (Box 13-1, Fig. 13-1) the following instruments may be useful for certain abdominal surgical procedures.

Bowel clamps

Doyen bowel clamps (Fig. 13-7) are non-crushing intestinal occluding forceps with longitudinal serrations. They are used to temporarily occlude the lumen of bowel. Standard human bowel clamps are

very large for cats. A pediatric atraumatic version is available and is preferred.

Gosset retractor

The Gosset retractor is a self-retaining retractor suitable for exposure of abdominal viscera (Fig. 13-8A). Two blades are mounted on a bar, the blades are moved apart to open the incision. The blades are a standard P shape with a curved loop to provide retention.

Balfour retractor

The Balfour retractor (Fig. 13-8B) consists of three individually operable, outward-looking curved loops or blades mounted on a bar. By inserting the blades into an incision and spreading them all, the incision is opened to give maximum access to tissues below. Pediatric sizes are suitable for use in the cat's abdomen.

Ring and hook retractor

A novel type of retractor for abdominal wall retraction is of a ring type, which by virtue of an array of slots around the periphery allows the surgeon to use multiple elasticated hooks to retract tissues in a controllable fashion at multiple levels of the approach (Fig. 13-9). These are small and lightweight retractors and therefore suitable for use in cats.

Galiban forceps

It is occasionally necessary to apply sutures under tension. In order to maintain tension it can be useful for an assistant to hold the first throw of the knot using Galiban suture holding forceps. These are designed to atraumatically hold the knot during the tying process. The jaws are angled to allow maximum view of the knot (Fig. 13-10).

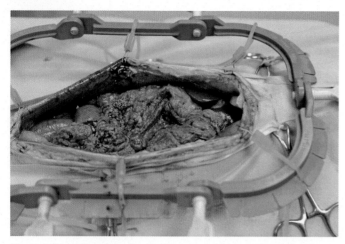

Figure 13-9 Ring and hook retractor. *(Courtesy of Alasdair Hotson-Moore.)*

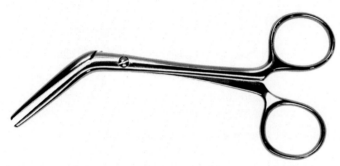

Figure 13-10 Galiban suture forceps.

Liver biopsy

Liver can be sampled using clamshell biopsy forceps (Fig. 13-5) or a skin punch. A 6 mm biopsy instrument is preferred in animals with microvascular disease since the 4 mm instruments are less likely to provide sufficient triads for analysis.[3]

SURGERY OF THE THORAX

In addition to the instruments listed in the general kit the following may be useful for thoracic surgical procedures (Box 13-2 and Fig. 13-11). Thoracic staplers are described in Chapter 10.

Grasping forceps

Although strictly not a surgical instrument, long grasping forceps with a shaft diameter of around 2.5 mm and shaft length 22 cm are useful for removal of foreign bodies in both trachea and esophagus (Fig. 13-12).

Bone cutting

Should access to the chest be made via a sternal osteotomy, instruments for both opening and closing will be required. Liston bone cutters straight 15 cm and wire twister and cutter 16.5cm are suitable for the cat (Fig. 13-11).[1] Alternatively, an oscillating saw could be used.[1]

Box 13-2 **Special thoracic instruments**

Gelpi retractor × 2
Small Finochietto retractor
Beckman retractor
Sterile solution
Poole suction tip + suction
Monopolar or bipolar cautery
Periosteal elevator
Bone cutting forceps (Liston)
Satinsky Forceps

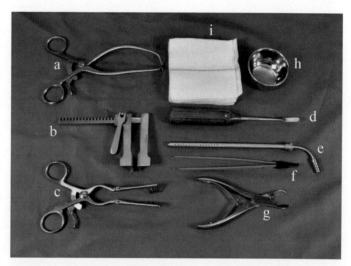

Figure 13-11 Special thoracic instruments: a, Gelpi retractors; b, Finochietto retractor; c, Beckman retractor; d, periosteal elevator; e, Poole suction tip; f, bipolar forceps; g, Liston bone cutting forceps; h, Gallipot for warm Ringer's; i, sponges with radio dense marker.

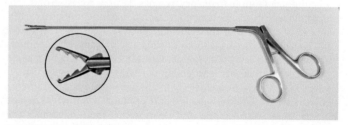

Figure 13-12 Grasping forceps.

Retraction

Retraction of the operative site, whether sternal or intercostal between ribs, can be maintained by multiple Gelpi type retractors (Fig. 13-11), which have the advantage of relatively small atraumatic tips but the disadvantage that the handles and ratchets sit some distance from the patient and they are more likely to dislodge than retractors with multiple prongs. West or Weitlaner are useful self-retaining retractors which have several prongs, making them more secure as intercostal retractors.[1]

Finochietto

The Finochietto is a retractor specifically designed to separate ribs in thoracic surgery. Developed in 1936 by Argentinian surgeon Enrique

Finochietto, it has fenestrated blades and a hand-cranked lever to both separate the parallel arms in a staged fashion and lock them in place at each stop. The small Finochietto with a 9.5 cm spread is suitable for use in cats (Fig. 13-11).

Beckman retractors

These retractors come in a variety of types, e.g., Beckman Weitlaner, Mueller Beckman and Beckman Eaton. They are generally multi-pronged retractors with a varying number of teeth, that are sharp or blunt and with hinged arms (Fig. 13-11). They are useful for retracting ribs for intercostal thoracotomy.

Forceps

Satinsky clamps

These atraumatic elongated C-shaped clamps with fine longitudinal grooves, were designed by the surgeon Victor P. Satinsky. They are in widespread use for temporary vessel closure in cardiovascular surgery. The 15 cm length baby Satinsky clamps are suitable for cats (Fig. 13-13A).

Mixter

These are also known as right-angle forceps. They are small lightweight ratchet-handled hemostats with a sharp angle to the blades near the

tips. They are useful for manipulation of deep intrathoracic structures (Fig. 13-13B).

Debakey forceps

These are a type of atraumatic tissue forceps used for grasping soft tissue, bowel or blood vessels to avoid tissue damage during manipulation of these structures (Fig. 13-14). They have a distinct, coarsely-ribbed grip panel with two rows of microscopic teeth that interfit along slender jaws and they end with blunt tips. These forceps are very useful instruments that should be included in the general surgical kit for all soft tissue surgery (Box 13-1).

Diaphragmatic hernia repair

Repair of diaphagmatic hernias will require rather longer dissecting forceps and needleholders than described in the general section, such as rat-toothed forceps 15 cm and Mayo-Hegar T.C. 16.5 cm or 18 cm.

Box 13-3 **An example of an ophthalmic surgical kit**
Halstead mosquito forceps straight 12.5 cm
Halstead mosquito forceps curved 12.5 cm
Beaver type blade handle plus 65 and 67 blades
Castroviejo needleholder T.C. with catch 15 cm
Stevens tenotomy scissors straight 11 cm
Castroviejo scissors straight 11.5 cm
Colibri forceps 10.5 cm
Graefe fixation forceps 10.5 cm
Roberts tying forceps 10.5 cm
Small Barraquer eyelid speculum 25 mm 'gape' 5 mm blade
Lachrymal cannula straight
Castroviejo needleholders OR
Ryder or Derf needleholders 12 cm (standard action)
Fosters TC miniature (Gillie type action)
Enucleation scissors 14.5 cm

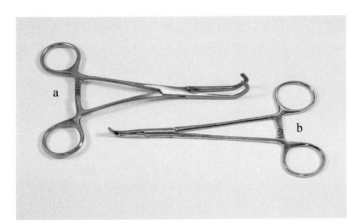

Figure 13-13 (A) Satinsky clamp. **(B)** Mixter clamp.

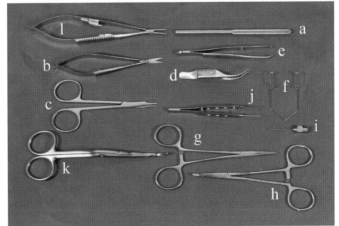

Figure 13-15 Ophthalmic surgical kit: a, Beaver type scalpel blade holder; b, Castroviejo scissors straight 11.5 cm; c, Stevens tenotomy scissors straight 11 cm; d, Colibri forceps 10.5 cm; e, Graefe fixation forceps 10.5 cm; f, Barraquer eyelid speculum; g, Halstead mosquito artery forceps straight 12.5 cm; h, Halstead mosquito artery forceps curved 12.5 cm; i, lachrymal cannula straight; j, Roberts tying forceps 10.5 cm.

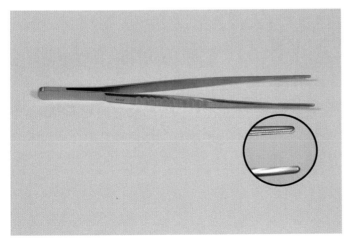

Figure 13-14 Debakey dissection forceps.

SURGERY OF THE HEAD AND NECK

The general kit described (Box 13-1 and Fig. 13-1) is sufficient for most procedures around the head and neck with the addition of small dissecting scissors such as strabismus or iris scissors and two pairs of small self-retaining retractors such as Gelpi retractors.

A ventral bulla osteotomy (VBO) will require a Steinman pin, Jacobs chuck and a small curette.[1] Mandibulectomy or maxillectomy procedures will be aided by an oscillating saw. A freer elevator is useful for retracting nerves or soft tissues in addition to elevating muscle and periosteum.

Ophthalmic surgery is an area where individual surgical training and choice is often exercised to a large degree. The range of ophthalmic instrumentation available is enormous. A kit suitable for most eyelid and periorbital surgery might include the following (Box 13-3 and Fig. 13-15). Some surgeons are not comfortable with the cross action-type Castroviejo needleholders used by some ophthalmologists, so these surgeons might prefer the 12 cm Ryder or Derf needleholder, which has the standard action. For surgeons favoring the Gillie-type action, the miniature Fosters T.C. is the best option. If enucleation is necessary, very curved enucleation scissors 14.5 cm are useful in the cat.

Operating microscope

The use of operating microscopes is becoming increasingly common in veterinary surgery, primarily for ophthalmic procedures but also as a valuable resource in feline soft tissue surgery, particularly when performing vascular surgery, ureteric surgery or where nerves are involved. While extremely expensive if purchased new, operating microscopes are increasing affordable from the pre-owned market.

REFERENCES

1. Lapish JP. Orthopedic instrumentation. In: Montavon PM, Voss K, Langley-Hobbs SJ, editors. Feline orthopedic surgery and musculoskeletal disease. Edinburgh: Elsevier; 2009. p. 249–58.

2. Rajbabu K, Barber NJ, Choi W, Muir GH. To knot or not to knot? Sutureless haemostasis compared to the surgeons knot. Ann R Coll Surg Eng 2007;89:359–62.

3. Tobias KM. Liver Biopsy. In: Manual of small animal soft tissue surgery. Blackwell Publishing; 2010. p. 125–34.

Section | 3 |

J.L. Demetriou, S.J. Langley-Hobbs

Oncological surgery and adjunctive therapy

With the increasing longevity of cats, neoplastic conditions are now identified more frequently in practice. Surgery is often the mainstay of treatment for many feline tumors and the first chapter guides the reader through the principles of surgical oncology, including the necessity for staging, and discussion on guidelines of margins of resection with different tumor types. Multimodal or neoadjuvant treatment can be advantageous for some tumors, and the following two chapters on radiotherapy and chemotherapy aim to give information on which tumors may be responsive to these types of therapy.

Chapter 14

Oncological surgery

J.L. Demetriou

Cancer is known to be an important disease entity in the cat, affecting all age groups. Although a current incidence rate of neoplasia in this species is not available, past data from a US tumor registry report suggests an overall occurrence of 0.5%. Although malignant tumor incidence rates were similar to dogs, the incidence of benign tumors in cats was ten times less than that of dogs.[1] A more recent animal registry from two areas in Italy provided an estimated annual incidence rate of 0.77% for cats. Furthermore, cats had a 4.6-fold higher incidence of malignant than benign tumors, and purebred cats had an almost 2-fold higher incidence of malignant tumors than mixed breeds. Tumor incidence increased with age in the cat populations.[2] With the emergence of oncology as a veterinary specialization and increased public interest in pet cancer it is unsurprising that treatment of feline cancer patients is now commonplace, in both the general practice setting and specialist centres.

This chapter aims to cover the evaluation of the cancer patient, tumor staging, and biopsy techniques. The various methods of surgery that can be utilized in the feline cancer patient will be discussed along with the best practice principles to use when performing surgery.

EVALUATION OF THE CANCER PATIENT

When evaluating the feline cancer patient it is important to focus on the patient as a whole rather than the tumor in isolation to avoid making inappropriate surgical decisions, e.g., mammary tumor excision with unidentified pulmonary metastasis or performing surgery on an anemic cancer patient without recognition of the hematological abnormalities. A suitable diagnostic workup should be planned for each individual patient based primarily on clinical presentation and likely paraneoplastic/concurrent disease processes. This chapter will focus on the biopsy techniques that form an important part of the presurgical diagnosis. However, other aspects of the diagnostic workup are likely to include at least one of the assessments discussed below.

Laboratory assessment

Cancer patients often have other concurrent medical problems in addition to paraneoplastic syndromes. Hematological abnormalities are commonly encountered and identifying the presence of abnormalities such as anemia, disseminated intravascular coagulation or thrombocytopenia will influence treatment planning and basic decisions such as suitability of the patient for anesthesia. Serum biochemical abnormalities will assist in documenting concurrent disease (e.g., renal compromise in elderly cats) or paraneoplastic processes such as hypercalcemia, which has been reported in cats in association with a variety of tumors including carcinomas, lymphoma and multiple myeloma.

Imaging

Diagnostic imaging techniques form a crucial part in the assessment of the cancer patient. It is important to recognize the rapid growth of more sophisticated modalities such as computed tomography (CT), magnetic resonance imaging (MRI), and nuclear imaging (e.g., scintigraphy) and the reader is referred to Chapter 8 for more information. Conventional radiography is still commonly used, partly due to financial reasons, particularly for the assessment of pulmonary metastasis. Ultrasonography is a useful complementary tool and can provide important information regarding tumor location, character and local invasion. CT provides excellent evaluation of bony lesions and is the gold standard for the evaluation of pulmonary metastasis. Three-dimensional reconstruction greatly facilitates surgical planning, and integration of CT scans with radiotherapy allows much more precise and targeted delivery of radiation to the patient (Chapter 15). MRI offers excellent soft tissue contrast and is ideal for evaluation of the brain. Availability and finances are often the two main reasons that limit the routine use of these imaging modalities in general practice.

Minimally invasive techniques

Rhinoscopy for visualizing nasal tumors, cystoscopy for assessing bladder neoplasia and thoracoscopy for examining pulmonary or mediastinal masses are examples of minimally invasive techniques that can combine both presurgical tumor assessment and biopsy procurement in one procedure. Details of these techniques are discussed in Chapters 8 and 24.

DOI: 10.1016/B978-0-7020-4336-9.00014-7

Table 14-1 World Health Organization classification for feline tumors of epidermal origin

Stage	Feature
T = tumor	
T0	No evidence of tumor
Tis	Tumor in situ
T1	Tumor < 2 cm in diameter
T2	Tumor 2–5 cm in diameter or minimally invasive
T3	Tumor > 5 cm in diameter or with invasion of subcutis
T4	Variable diameter; tumor invading fascia, muscle or bone
N = node	
N0	Absence of lymph node metastasis
N1	Presence of lymph node metastasis
M = metastasis	
M0	Absence of distant metastasis
M1	Presence of distant metastasis

(Modified with permission from Owen LN. Classification of Tumors in Domestic Animals. WHO. http://whqlibdoc.who.int/hq/1980/VPH_CMO_80.20_eng.pdf)

Staging

Before treatment can be considered it is important to define the precise extent of the tumor burden of each patient, by means of clinical and histological staging. This provides valuable information not only for treatment planning, but also helps evaluate response to treatment and disease progression. Staging is based on the World Health Organization Program on Comparative Oncology TNM (tumor, node, metastasis) system, with several adaptations for a variety of tumors of domestic animals. An example of such an adaptation is illustrated in Table 14-1 for feline tumors of epidermal origin (carcinomas). Not all tumors lend themselves to staging easily, and in some tumors, with feline mammary tumors being a prime example, it has been shown that the tumor histological grade is significantly linked to prognosis and can be used as an independent prognostic factor.[3,4]

BIOPSY TECHNIQUES

Obtaining a diagnosis is one of the most important steps in the management of the cancer patient. Obtaining a biopsy before the surgical procedure is performed is best clinical practice in the majority of cases as it provides a pre-treatment diagnosis, helps the clinician plan the surgery, and can provide the owner with a more accurate prognosis. There are a number of methods for obtaining samples from the tumor and the choice is based on a number of factors including tumor location, suspected tumor type, safety of the procedure, the patient's clinical status, cost, equipment availability, and surgeon's preference. With the exception of diagnostic cytology, all other techniques listed in Table 14-2 involve tissue sampling and histological interpretation.

Fine needle aspiration

Fine needle aspiration (FNA) is a cost-effective, simple first-line option to obtain a diagnosis from a wide variety of masses, either on the skin

Box 14-1 Requirements for fine needle aspiration

21–23 gauge needles
3–10 mL syringes
Glass microscope slides
Cytological stains
A good microscope with oil immersion

or within body cavities. Enlarged, accessible lymph nodes are easily aspirated and a major advantage of using this method over the histological methods of biopsy is that the sample can be examined 'in-house' after appropriate staining. The equipment that is required is listed in Box 14-1.

The best cytological stains to use in clinical practice are the Romanowsky stains (e.g., Wright stain, Giemsa stain and May–Grünwald–Giemsa stain), as these provide clear detail of both the nuclear and cytoplasmic structures. They are relatively quick to prepare and these stains will also stain bacteria if they are present. The 'rapid' stain kits such as 'Diff-Quik' are very useful and convenient, but one limitation is that they may not consistently stain the granules within mast cells clearly, which could lead to misdiagnosis, particularly in the case of poorly differentiated mast cell tumors in which the granularity can be low. In this instance Toludine blue stain will identify mast cell granules.

Aspiration can be performed using either the needle attached to the syringe or the 'capillary' method, which involves inserting just the needle without the exertion of negative pressure. The act of briskly redirecting the needle hub backwards and forwards within the mass is enough for cells to become detached and move up the core of the needle. This is the author's preferred technique as it is less likely to result in excessive fluid being aspirated that would effectively dilute the cellular component to the sample. Box 14-2 illustrates the steps involved in FNA using both the methods described.

There have been several studies evaluating the accuracy of FNA involving cats. One study found that in ultrasound-guided samples of splenic masses, cytologic diagnoses (by FNA) corresponded with histologic diagnoses in 61% of cases.[5] In another study involving only four cats in which liver aspirates were taken, false results were obtained in all cases when compared with surgical biopsy samples. In these cases hepatic lipidosis was diagnosed by aspiration of samples that were later confirmed as inflammatory or neoplastic.[6] However, in another study of canine and feline patients results suggested that FNA may be a sensitive and specific method of evaluating the regional lymph nodes in dogs and cats with solid tumors, because results correlated well with results of histologic examination of the entire lymph node.[7] In conclusion, these results suggest that the accuracy of FNA may vary considerably and this may be partly dependent on the tissue being sampled. Regional lymph node aspiration appears to be highly specific and sensitive. CT-guided aspiration of bone and lung tissue has also been reported in cats and studies suggest that it may be a safe and accurate procedure.[8,9]

Needle core biopsy

Needle core biopsy provides a quick and easy way of obtaining a tissue sample. It can be used on externally or internally (usually in combination with ultrasound guidance) located masses and can be performed using local anesthetic and sedation, providing a cost effective and less invasive option to clients compared with incisional biopsy. As the initial incision and tract made by the instrument is small, there is little

Table 14-2 Comparison of different biopsy techniques

Biopsy technique	Advantages	Disadvantages	Indications/examples
Cytology	Inexpensive Simple, rapid procedure Minimal equipment Immediate results Minimal restraint	Non-diagnostic specimens Tissue architecture not evaluated	Bone marrow Lymph nodes Cutaneous/subcutaneous masses Body cavity fluids Impression smears
Needle core	Minimally invasive Rapid procedure Well-preserved tissue sample High diagnostic yield Can be done under sedation/local anesthetic Inexpensive Easy procedure	Needle core instruments required Smaller tissue sample compared with incisional technique	Any externally located mass Any internal lesions (kidney, liver, prostate) with the aid of ultrasound guidance or during open surgery
Punch	Larger tissue sample Easy procedure	Sample obtained limited by depth of punch Superficial lesions only Invasive procedure General anesthetic often required	Superficial cutaneous lesions Parenchymatous organ (liver, spleen) biopsy during open surgery
Incisional	Larger tissue mass Useful when needle core or punch methods prove non-diagnostic	Invasive procedure General anesthetic mostly required More expensive Biopsy tract may compromise future surgery	When other biopsy methods have been non-diagnostic Ulcerated and necrotic lesions (e.g., oral masses)
Excisional	Can be both diagnostic and therapeutic May be cost effective Diagnosis always obtained Can evaluate completeness of excision	In most cases may compromise future treatment options and prognosis	Reserve for 'benign' skin lesions and tumor excision where treatment is not dependent on tumor type (mammary masses, single splenic mass, single pulmonary mass)

(Reprinted from Demetriou JL, Foale RD. Small Animal Oncology. London: Saunders Elsevier; 2010, with permission from Elsevier.)

Box 14-2 Fine needle aspiration

The mass is stabilized using two fingers if it is unstable, and basic preparation of the surface is performed. Clipping of the fur will improve the visualization of the mass and a spirit swab is used to clean the surface of the skin.

A 21-23G needle attached to a 5 mL syringe is inserted into the center of the mass and negative suction applied (Fig. 14-1A). The needle is redirected into the mass several times. Negative suction is stopped if fluid appears within the hub of the needle. Negative pressure is released and the needle is withdrawn. The needle is detached from the syringe and the syringe is filled with air. The needle is re-attached and the aspirated material is forced out onto a slide using the air within the syringe. A preparation is made of the sample, which is rapidly dried and then stained.

Another method is using the needle alone without the syringe (Fig. 14-1B). The needle is used to obtain a core of cells from the mass by redirecting the needle several times before attaching it to a syringe filled with air.

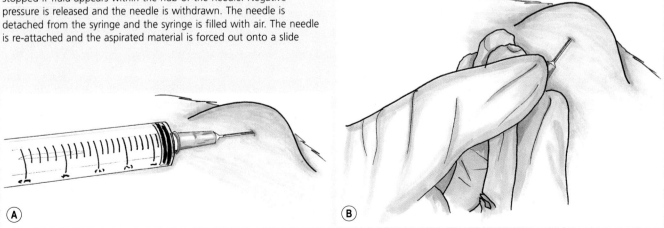

(A) (B)

Figure 14-1 Fine needle aspiration can be performed by **(A)** use of a 5 mL syringe attached to the needle or **(B)** using a needle alone.

Box 14-3 Needle core biopsy technique

An example of a commercially available needle biopsy instrument featuring a 10–20 mm notch size to allow for variable biopsy sample sizes is illustrated in Figure 14-2A. After clipping and aseptic preparation of the biopsy site a number 11 blade is used to make a stab incision (Fig. 14-2B). Sedation in combination with local anesthesia can be used in most patients for this procedure. The needle and sheath is pushed through the skin incision and the subcutaneous tissues and into the mass to be biopsied. The main part of the needle biopsy instrument is held in the left hand and steadied whilst the sheath is withdrawn from the mass using the right hand (Fig. 14-2C). The sheath is then passed over the needle using the right hand, until a 'click' is heard (Fig. 14-2D). Then the needle and sheath are withdrawn together out from the tumor and skin incision. The sheath is once again withdrawn to reveal the biopsy specimen within the notch and the sample is eased off using a fine (25G) needle into a histopathology specimen pot (Fig.14-2E). The steps can be repeated in different areas of the tumor if required.

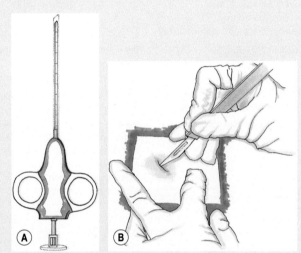

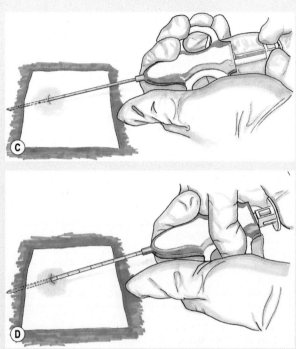

Figure 14-2 (A) A needle core instrument. **(B)** A stab incision is made through the skin with a number 11 needle. **(C)** The needle core instrument is inserted into the tissue to be biopsied and the sheath withdrawn. **(D)** The sheath is reinserted to cut off the biopsy sample. **(E)** After removal of the needle core instrument the sheath is again withdrawn to reveal the biopsy.

risk of disruption of the tumor and subsequent tumor seeding, although removal of the biopsy tract is recommended at the definitive surgery. Although designed as disposable instruments, they can be reused after sterilization with ethylene oxide, and performing the skin incision with a scalpel blade before insertion of the needle will help delay blunting of the tip and extend the life span of the instrument. In core biopsy the typical needle size is 18–14G and comprises an inner notched stylet with an outer cannula (e.g., Tru-cut). Box 14-3 illustrates the steps involved in obtaining a needle core biopsy sample. In one study there was 96% agreement with presurgical Tru-cut results and postsurgical biopsy results when 48 diagnostic tumor samples from dogs and cats were evaluated.[10] The results indicated that needle core biopsy can accurately predict surgical biopsy. Thus, needle core

biopsy performed before surgical excision of masses can facilitate planning and reduce the need for numerous surgical procedures.

Punch biopsy

A punch biopsy is more commonly used for skin or superficial skin masses as the depth of the sample obtained is limited by the length of the punch. The common diameter punch samples obtained range from 2–6 mm, but it would be preferable to aim for the larger size if the location and area of tumor permits. Another indication for the use of punch biopsies is for sampling lesions on the surface of the spleen or liver during exploratory laparotomy. The sample is shorter and wider than a needle core, and hemorrhage from the remaining

Box 14-4 **Punch biopsy technique**

After local anesthesia (in the conscious patient) a 2–6 mm punch biopsy instrument is applied over the area to be sampled and is twisted until the blade has penetrated the epidermis of the skin (Fig. 14-3A). After the blade has penetrated the skin sufficiently it is withdrawn. The skin punch biopsy instrument is only used to penetrate the skin (or other similar biopsy site) and not to remove the biopsy (Fig. 14-3B).

The biopsy is then removed from the rest of the skin. Care must be taken to avoid damaging the sample so fine forceps are used to hold the sample and pull it up to reveal the deep margin and Metzenbaum scissors are used to cut the sample free from the underlying tissues (Fig. 14-3C).

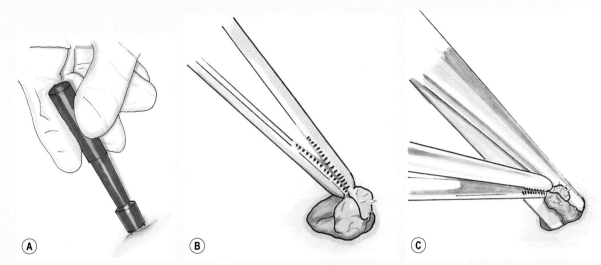

Figure 14-3 **(A)** A Punch biopsy instrument is pressed and rotated in the skin to be biopsied. **(B)** The sample is very carefully held with fine forceps and **(C)** the base cut with Metzenbaum scissors.

deficit can be controlled using a hemostatic agent such as commercially available collagen or gelatin. Box 14-4 illustrates the use of a punch biopsy instrument.

Surgical incisional biopsy

Indications for incisional biopsy are when less invasive biopsy methods yield a non-diagnosis or misdiagnosis, or when the sample to be biopsied is associated with a high proportion of ulceration, necrosis and inflammation that can penetrate deep beyond the surface. An example of such a mass is an oral neoplasm such as a basal cell carcinoma or fibrosarcoma. Often these masses are denervated and a general anesthetic for the incisional biopsy procedure is not necessary.

The procedure is simply carried out with a scalpel blade, under aseptic conditions. If performed in the skin it is preferable to include a portion of normal tissue in addition to the mass that is being sampled. The subsequent deficit can be sutured or left to heal by secondary intention after hemorrhage has been controlled. An important aspect of performing an incisional biopsy is to ensure that future surgery is not compromised by contaminating unaffected tissues or performing the biopsy in a plane that would later make further resection and closure difficult.

Excisional biopsy

In the majority of cancer cases a presurgical biopsy is preferable to an excisional biopsy; however, in some specific situations performing an excisional biopsy is acceptable if the ultimate treatment plan would not be altered without knowledge of the tumor type beforehand. An example of this would be a solitary lung mass. Indeed, performing an

aspirate of this mass could induce unacceptable complications such as hemorrhage or pneumothorax so an excisional biopsy is preferred, either by thoracoscopy or exploratory thoracotomy. Other examples of tumors that lend themselves to excisional biopsy are listed in Table 14-2.

Advanced biopsy techniques

Image guided techniques (ultrasound, CT, MRI, fluoroscopy, endoscopy, laparoscopy and thoracoscopy) are often the procedure of choice for specific tumor types (e.g., gastric mucosal, nasal masses, internal organs). General benefits include improved accuracy and reduced morbidity with minimally invasive techniques. More details of the use of these techniques on certain tumors are described in other individual chapters of this book.

SURGERY FOR CANCER

Despite the increased use and accessibility of chemotherapy and radiotherapy, surgery is still the most prevalent means of treating the majority of feline cancers. Surgery can be used in a number of different areas of cancer management, ranging from diagnosis and effecting a cure, to palliating or preventing cancer.

Surgery to diagnose cancer

Surgery for diagnosis (e.g., incisional or excisional biopsy) is discussed above, but it is important to emphasize that obtaining a preoperative diagnosis is desirable in most cases. Once information regarding tumor type and perhaps grade is obtained and further clinical staging is completed it is worth considering the following questions prior to surgery (Box 14-5).

Whatever the mode of use of surgery, a key element for success is dependent on the surgeon adhering to good basic principles of technique, based on those developed by Halsted in the 1890s (Box 14-6). The biopsy procedure should be performed in such a manner that future surgery is not compromised. For example, an incisional biopsy incision should be planned and orientated in a plane that would make excision of the scar at the definitive surgery simple. Another example is ensuring that the needle core biopsy instrument is inserted in a way that would minimize seeding or contamination of tumor cells through normal tissue planes.

Surgery to treat cancer

There appear to be two major influencing factors that determine the success of surgery as a definitive treatment for cancer: performing appropriate surgery at the first attempt and obtaining 'clean' margins, i.e., removing margins of normal tissue in addition to the main tumor mass. Performing surgery based on a diagnosis ensures that there is a higher probability of complete excision at the first surgery and therefore a higher probability of a potential cure. Furthermore, performing surgery on an undisrupted tumor improves the surgeon's ability to assess the gross margins and reduces the risk of tumor extension into normal tissue planes.

Surgery to palliate cancer

When performing cancer surgery consideration must be given as to whether the procedure is of long-term benefit to the patient or whether the risks of the procedure or postoperative complications outweigh these potential benefits. This debate is even more significant when, from the outset it is known that cure or long-lasting benefits are not possible. In these cases surgery would be performed for short-term palliation of clinical signs (e.g., in cases where metastatic disease is present). Each case must be considered on its own merit with careful consultation and discussion with the owners so that they are fully aware of all risks relating to the surgery and the ultimate prognosis. The final decision in these cases must be left to the owners, who ultimately must give informed consent to the treatment, based on there being some benefit to the patient in terms of improvement of clinical signs and quality of life and/or temporary restoration of function.[11] It is important to note that debulking of a tumor (i.e., partial removal) without any clear, perceived benefits or follow-up treatment is not a recommended palliative procedure as tumor growth following surgery can sometimes be accelerated.

Surgery to prevent or reduce the risk of cancer

Surgery can be used to prevent certain cancers. Although rarely reported in cats, testicular tumor development can be prevented by castration and the risk of uterine tumors is prevented by ovariohysterectomy, although a report of an incomplete ovariohysterectomy with subsequent uterine adenocarcinoma development in a cat has been described.[12] Additionally, ovariohysterectomy/ovariectomy has a prophylactic effect on mammary neoplasia in cats. Cats spayed before 1 year of age have a significantly decreased risk of developing mammary carcinoma, with cats spayed before 6 months of age having only 9% the risk of mammary carcinoma compared with intact cats. Cats spayed between 6 and 12 months had 14% the risk compared with intact cats.[13] However, carcinomas have been reported in cats having ovariohysterectomies before 1 year of age so neutering does not completely eliminate the risk.[14]

SURGICAL PRINCIPLES

Surgical margins

It is clear from the literature that there are a number of feline tumors where survival is correlated with attainment of clean margins. A study investigating prognosis for injection site sarcomas in cats showed that tumors with histologically infiltrative margins recurred ten times more frequently than those with non-infiltrated margins.[15] Another study evaluating colonic malignancies in cats showed that obtaining clean margins from surgery was correlated with improved survival times.[16] However, when reviewing the literature in cats there is a paucity of evidence recommending specific margin measurements for individual tumor types and most data is extrapolated from canine or human studies. One study reviewing injection site sarcomas in cats advocated lateral margins of 5 cm to reduce local recurrence rates.[17] However, this amount would be excessive for tumors such as squamous cell carcinoma of e.g., the pinna or nasal planum, which are often successfully excised using margins of approximately 1 cm. Recommendations regarding deep margins are also generic across species. Often tumors lie over naturally resistant anatomical barriers such as fascia, ligaments and tendons that are resistant to tumor spread and therefore if a fascial plane is included in the deep margin this would normally be considered sufficient as an adequate surgical margin.

There are four basic types of tumor resection depending upon the location of the surgical margin: intracapsular, marginal, wide, and radical (Table 14-3, Fig. 14-4).

Surgical techniques

Good basic surgical principles should be followed in oncologic surgery (Box 14-6). The skin around the tumor should be clipped widely to ensure adequate skin for reconstruction and the skin overlying the tumor prepared gently to avoid excessive handling of the tumor. It is

Table 14-3 Categories of surgical tumor/mass resection

Type of resection	Description	Examples of suitable tumors
Intracapsular	Removal of the mass or tumor from within the capsule	Benign conditions, recurrence unlikely, e.g., abscess, cyst
Marginal	Removal of the tumor through the reactive zone including capsule / pseudocapsule	Benign masses, e.g., lipoma, benign cutaneous mast cell tumors, thyroid adenoma
Wide	Removal of the tumor with the pseudocapsule, including the reactive zone and a margin of normal tissue	Malignant tumors, e.g., mammary gland carcinoma, colonic adenocarcinoma
Radical	Removal of the tumor *en bloc* with the tissue compartment within which it lies	Malignant tumors that have traversed through multiple tissue planes, e.g., mandibulectomy for squamous cell carcinoma, body wall resection for fibrosarcoma

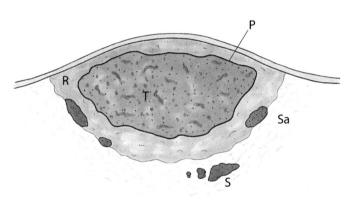

Figure 14-4 Diagram illustrating a feline soft tissue sarcoma and the different types of metastases that can occur. T, tumor; R, reactive zone; P, pseudocapsule; S, skip metastases; Sa, satellite metastases.

particularly important in cancer surgery to avoid trauma and manipulation of the tumor, which could lead to dissemination of tumor cells locally and systemically. The surgeon should consider the principles of cancer surgery to be similar to those of contaminated surgery and precautions should be taken to avoid contact of the tumor, instruments or gloves with surrounding normal tissue. The following principles apply, firstly to reduce manipulation of the tumor and secondly to maintain separation of the tumor from normal surrounding tissue (Box 14-7).

Surgery and regional lymph nodes

The question of whether to routinely perform surgery on regional lymph nodes for the purpose of removing metastatic disease is controversial in both human and veterinary medicine. All accessible regional lymph nodes should be investigated with malignant tumors,

Box 14-7 Principles of oncological surgery

- Use stay sutures on the tumor to avoid unnecessary contact with surgeon's hand or instruments. Stay sutures can also be applied to normal surrounding tissue to provide retraction without contact of potentially contaminated instruments or gloves
- Pack off the tumor with laparotomy sponges or sterile adhesive drapes. The tumor can actually be wrapped in the sponges or drapes so that minimal handling is achieved
- Change gloves and instruments after tumor resection before closing the wound. This is particularly necessary with highly exfoliative tumors such as those derived from epithelial cells
- Avoid excessive hemorrhage by judicious use of electrocautery and ensuring the vascular supply to the tumor is interrupted as quickly as possible during the resection process. Ligating the arterial supply of the tumor is recommended before the vascular supply is interrupted to allow collapse of the venous supply within the tumor. This reduces the risk of embolization of tumor cells. Mass ligation of arteries and veins should be avoided
- Use sharp rather than blunt dissection to minimize surrounding trauma. There has been some evidence suggesting that tissue that has been damaged is more likely to promote tumor growth from implanted tumor cells. Scalpel incisions are preferable to scissor incisions as they result in the least amount of trauma and surrounding necrosis
- Avoid entry into the tumor capsule/pseudocapsule. Grasping the tumor with traumatic forceps can cause bleeding and exfoliation of tumor cells so should be avoided
- Perform 'clean' ('non-tumor') surgeries before excision of the tumor to avoid cross contamination of tumor cells, e.g., perform ovariectomy prior to mammary gland carcinoma excision

which may include fine needle aspirate, needle core aspirate or incisional/excisional biopsy. It has been shown that FNA of lymph nodes shows excellent correlation with histologic findings, with a sensitivity and specificity of 100% and 96%, respectively.[7] Therefore if lymph nodes associated with the tumor are examined for staging purposes only then a fine needle aspirate should suffice in the majority of cases.

The question that is more controversial is whether routine removal of lymph nodes associated with tumor is required in all cases. The exact role of local, draining lymph nodes in preventing further spread of micro-metastasis is not clear, and their routine removal in oncologic surgery may in fact be detrimental by interfering with their immunologic function postoperatively and increasing the surgical morbidity. There is no strong evidence therefore to suggest that excision of regional lymph nodes in oncologic surgery should be performed in every case, particularly if the lymph nodes are not enlarged. However, if the regional lymph nodes are enlarged, accessible and able to be removed without a significant increase in procedural related morbidity, then removal may be beneficial in terms of staging and reduction of total tumor burden, particularly if postoperative adjunctive treatment is considered and the lymph nodes are in close approximation to the tumor. During mastectomy in cats the inguinal lymph nodes are routinely removed 'en bloc' (i.e., in combination with the tumor and draining lymphatics), providing vital information regarding prognosis for that patient. Other examples include excisional biopsy of mesenteric lymph nodes in cases of unconfirmed intestinal neoplasia, tracheobronchial lymph node excision in cases of pulmonary neoplasia, popliteal lymph nodes removal in digital tumor excision.

SURGICAL PATHOLOGY SUBMISSION FORM

External ( )   Internal (X)

Hospital number: _H11/4975_____

Species Feline   Breed ___Domestic Short hair_____

Name _____Molly_____ Age _____5yr_____

Gender: F (x)   M ( )   Entire ( ) Neutered (x) Unknown ( )

Clinician: _____J Demetriou_____.

Address: _____Cat clinic_____.

Phone number: _____ E –mail address: _____.

Owner: _____Smith_____.

Address: _____.

Phone number: _____ E-mail address: _____.

OR STICK LABEL HERE

Specimen submitted : Subcutaneous mass

Date and time taken: ___27th July 2011_____.

Fresh tissue (x)   Fixed tissue ( )   Fixative _____.

Anatomical site of lesion: lateral thorax___.

Completely removed (x)   Incompletely removed ( )

Relevant clinical history (clinical signs, significant haematology and biochemistry, radiology, therapy, duration. Lesion or tissue description: size, shape, colour, appearance and distribution):

Three month history of a slow growing 2 cm mass in the subcutaneous tissues overlying the right thoracic cavity. Appears to be moveable and non painful on palpation. All other clinical parameters are within normal limits. Previous fine needle aspirate suggesting of Mast Cell Tumour. Removed with 1cm lateral margins and 1 fascial layer deep.

Suture tags placed on cranial and ventral tumour margins.

Deep margins inked

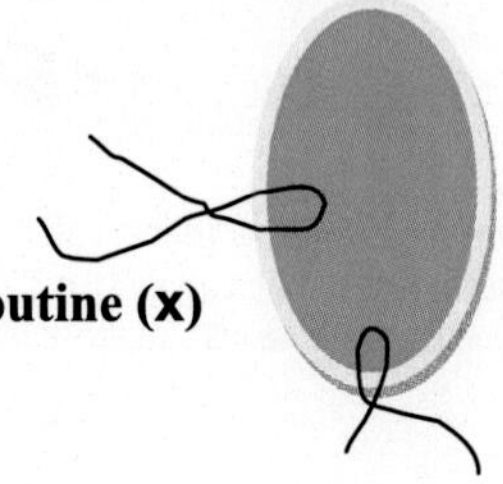

Special concerns (Requests, rule outs, procedures):   **Urgent ( )   Routine (x)**

Please check the tagged lateral and inked deep margins

Submitting Clinician (Print name and signature): __J. Demetriou__ **Date:** ___27th July 2012

Figure 14-5 An example of a fully completed histopathology form, providing the pathologist with as much detail as possible.

Surgery in combination with chemotherapy and/or radiotherapy

Over the past few years in veterinary oncology there has been a drive to treat cancer patients using a multidisciplinary approach. This includes using surgery followed or preceded by either (or both) chemotherapy, radiotherapy or immunotherapy. The advantage of this approach is that less emphasis is placed on achieving a surgical cure in tumors that have an innate sensitivity to chemotherapy and radiotherapy, thereby potentially reducing the extent of surgery and as a result morbidity and complication rates. The aim of postoperative treatment is to target microscopic disease after the bulk of the tumor has been removed. Both chemotherapy and radiotherapy are thought to be effective postoperatively, once the tumor burden has been excised, because the remaining rapidly dividing cells may be more sensitive compared with the slowly dividing cells in the gross tumor mass. In many specialist centers, treatment of certain tumor types with cytoreductive surgery followed by radiotherapy is routine and has resulted in good long-term clinical outcomes with minimal morbidity. For example, soft tissue sarcomas arising on the limb are excised conservatively, with the aim being to remove gross tumor with a tension-free closure, and radiotherapy is commenced once the wound has healed within two to three weeks of surgery. Preoperatively, radiotherapy or chemotherapy can be administered to reduce the tumor to a size that is more amenable to complete surgical excision, and preoperative radiotherapy has been used with success in cases of large injection site sarcomas. With either protocol of radiotherapy there is the potential of impaired wound healing, the effects of which are dose dependent. Further details on adjunctive treatment in multimodal cancer treatment are discussed in Chapters 15 and 16.

Handling of the excised tumor

All excised masses should be submitted for histologic examination. Ideally the entire sample is submitted to allow assessment of margins and to ensure representative sections are examined. If the entire sample cannot be submitted then representative samples are submitted, but the remaining tissue should be stored in-house in case further samples are needed for re-submission at a later date. Representative sections selected from a large sample should include portions from the periphery and the centre of the mass, including portions of normal tissue in the peripheral samples. The most commonly used fixative agent is 10% neutral buffered formalin. Sections should be not be thicker than 1 cm, otherwise the fixative agent will not penetrate adequately. The volume of tissue to fixative should ideally be 1:10. When margins are to be assessed, suture tags or India ink can be used to mark or dye the margins of concern. When using tissue dye the margins are allowed to stand for several minutes so excessive moisture is removed (alternatively, the edges are gently blotted with a swab) and the ink is applied to the cut surface using a swab or cotton buds. The sample is then dried before being fixed in formalin.[18]

It is vital that as much information as possible is provided for the histopathologist and margin assessment and tumor grade requested routinely when appropriate. A detailed history, clinical findings and any other relevant information should be given to allow the pathologist to provide as accurate and detailed information as possible. If possible the tumor and any associated surrounding structures can be drawn on the form, indicating areas of concern and orientation. An example of a histopathology form is provided in Figure 14-5.

REFERENCES

1. MacVean DW, Monlux AW, Anderson PS Jr, et al. Frequency of canine and feline tumors in a defined population. Vet Path 1978;15:700–15.
2. Vascellari M, Baioni E, Ru G, et al. Animal tumour registry of two provinces in northern Italy: incidence of spontaneous tumours in dogs and cats. Biomedcentral Veterinary Research 2009;5:39. http://www.biomedcentral.com/1746-6148/5/39.
3. Giménez F, Hecht S, Craig LE, Legendre AM. Early detection, aggressive therapy. Optimizing the management of feline mammary masses. J Fel Med Surg 2010;12:214–24.
4. Seixas F, Palmeira C, Pires MA, et al. Grade is an independent prognostic factor for feline mammary carcinomas: A clinicopathological and survival analysis. Vet J 2011;187:65–71.
5. Ballegeer EA, Forrest LJ, Dickinson RM, et al. Correlation of ultrasonographic appearance of lesions and cytologic and histologic diagnoses in splenic aspirates from dogs and cats: 32 cases (2002-2005). J Am Vet Med Assoc 2007;230:690–6.
6. Willard MD, Weeks BR, Johnson M. Fine-needle aspirate cytology suggesting hepatic lipidosis in four cats with infiltrative hepatic disease. J Fel Med Surg 1999;1:215–20.
7. Langenbach A, McManus PM, Hendrick MJ. Sensitivity and specificity of methods of assessing the regional lymph nodes for evidence of metastasis in dogs and cats with solid tumors. J Am Vet Med Assoc 2001;218:1424–8.
8. Vignoli M, Ohlerth S, Rossi F, et al. Computed tomography-guided fine-needle aspiration and tissue-core biopsy of bone lesions in small animals. Vet Rad Ultrasound 2004;45:125–30.
9. Zekas LJ, Crawford JT, O'Brien RT. Computed tomography-guided fine-needle aspirate and tissue-core biopsy of intrathoracic lesions in thirty dogs and cats. Vet Radiol Ultrasound 2005;46:200–4.
10. Aitken ML, Patnaik AK. 2000 Comparison of needle-core (Trucut) biopsy and surgical biopsy for the diagnosis of cutaneous and subcutaneous masses: a prospective study of 51 cases (November 1997-August 1998). J Am Anim Hosp Assoc 2000;36:153–7.
11. Moore AS. Managing cats with cancer. An examination of ethical perspectives. J Fel Med Surg 2011;13:661–71.
12. Anderson C, Pratschke K. Uterine adenocarcinoma with abdominal metastasis in an ovariohysterectomised cat. J Fel Med Surg 2011;13:44–7.
13. Overley B, Shofer FS, Goldschmidt MH, et al. Association between ovariohysterectomy and feline mammary carcinoma. J Vet Int Med 2005;19:560–63.
14. Hayes AA, Mooney S. Feline mammary tumors. Vet Clin of N Amer: Sm Anim Pract 1985;15:513–20.
15. Giudice C, Stefanello D, Sala M, et al. Feline injection-site sarcoma: recurrence, tumor grading and surgical margin status evaluated using the three-dimensional histological technique. Vet J 2010;186:84–8.
16. Slawienski MJ, Mauldin GE, Mauldin GN, Patnaik AK. Malignant colonic neoplasia in cats: 46 cases (1990-1996). J Am Vet Med Assoc 1997;211:878–81.
17. Phelps HA, Kuntz CA, Milner RJ, et al. Radical excision with five-centimeter margins for treatment of feline injection-site sarcomas: 91 cases (1998-2002). J Am Vet Med Assoc 2011;239:97–106.
18. Ehrhart EJ, Powers BE. The Pathology of Neoplasisa, In: Withrow SJ, Vail DM, editors. Small Animal Clinical Oncology. Philadelphia: WB Saunders; 2007. p. 54–67.

Chapter |15|

Radiation therapy

J.M. Dobson

The treatment of cancer must always be tailored to suit the individual case, taking into consideration the biology, histology, grade and extent of the tumor, and the general condition and health concerns of the patient. The decision to treat an animal with cancer must be made jointly by the veterinarian and the owner. Owners must be counseled in the nature of the disease, the prognosis, the options for treatment and the expectations of such treatment, and should be given time to consider the options and reach a decision.

For most solid tumors the two main therapeutic considerations are how best to achieve local (and regional) control and what is the risk of metastasis. Local disease treatment options generally include surgery or radiation or both, whereas adjuvant chemotherapy must be considered for systemic or multifocal disease or if the risk of metastasis is high.

Radiotherapy (RT) is widely used in the treatment of human cancer patients and although costly, radiotherapy facilities are becoming increasingly available to treat animals. Most veterinarians in general practice will not have direct access to radiotherapy facilities; however, it is important to have some knowledge of the principles and practice of radiation therapy in order that suitable cases might be identified and referred at an appropriate stage.

THE BASIC PRINCIPLES OF RADIATION PHYSICS AND BIOLOGY

The mode of action of radiation

When absorbed by living tissues, ionizing radiation causes excitation and ionization of component atoms or molecules in the path of the beam. Subsequent chemical reactions result in breaking of molecular bonds and can result in apoptotic cell death if molecules critical for cell viability are disrupted. The 'critical target' is generally regarded as being nuclear DNA, but other molecules in other parts of the cell (e.g., proteins and lipids) may also be damaged and contribute to radiation-induced cellular injury. The damage to DNA prevents normal cell replication but does not lead to immediate cell death; the radiation damage is manifest when the damaged cells attempt to divide. Hence radiation tumor response and toxicity appear delayed.

Radiation biology

The response of living cells and tissues to radiation depends upon the dose of radiation, how this is applied, and the radiosensitivity of the cell population. Radiosensitivity varies according to a number of factors (Box 15-1), one of the most important being the 'growth fraction' of the cell population. Small, rapidly growing tumors tend to respond more favorably to radiation than large, slowly growing tumors. Radiation treatment is unlikely to achieve more than a partial and temporary remission in the latter.

Whilst radiation is a potent means of causing tumor cell death, it is not selective and can be equally damaging to normal tissues; indeed, certain normal tissues may be more sensitive to radiation than many tumors. In order to be of therapeutic benefit, radiation must be employed in such a way as to minimize normal tissue injury whilst achieving maximum tumor cell kill. Various methods may be employed to localize the radiation to the tumor, as outlined later in this chapter.

One way to reduce normal tissue injury is to 'fractionate' the treatment. Following exposure to a single dose of radiation a number of changes occur in the exposed cell population, that are often referred to as the four 'R's' of radiation (Box 15-2).

As normal tissues are able to repair and repopulate better than most tumors and as redistribution (around the cell cycle) and re-oxygenation increase tumor sensitivity, by applying the radiation in multiple small doses (fractions) over a long period of time rather than as one large dose, normal tissue injury is reduced and tumor cell kill increased.

The biological effect of radiation depends on the amount of radiation applied and length of time over which it is applied, hence the term 'biological radiation dose'. The same total dose given in a short time or fewer fractions has greater effect than the same dose given over a longer time in many fractions (applies to both tumor response and toxicity). Fraction size is an important determinant of normal tissue damage. Small fractions minimize normal tissue effects, large fractions increase risk of late tissue effects. Overall treatment time is important in achieving tumor control. Thus by using multiple small fractions of radiation delivered over a long period of time tumor cell kill may be increased whilst normal tissue damage can be limited to some extent.

© 2014 Elsevier Ltd
DOI: 10.1016/B978-0-7020-4336-9.00015-9

Box 15-1 **Factors that cause variation in radiosensitivity**

Dividing cells are generally more sensitive to radiation than non-dividing, differentiated cells

Tissues with a high proportion of dividing cells, e.g., bone marrow and gastrointestinal epithelium, are more radiosensitive than non-proliferating tissues, e.g., fibrous tissue and skeletal muscle

Tumors with a high growth fraction tend to be more sensitive to radiation than those with low growth fractions

Individual cells vary in their radiosensitivity as they pass through the phases of the cell cycle. Cells in the M (mitotic) phase of the cycle being most radiosensitive and those in the S (DNA synthesis) phase being most resistant. The resting (Go) cells are also radioresistant (Fig. 15-1)

Oxygenation is also thought to be significant in determining radiosensitivity. Tumor cells that exist at a low oxygen tension, i.e., hypoxic cells, may be 2.5–3 times less sensitive to radiation than normally oxygenated cells

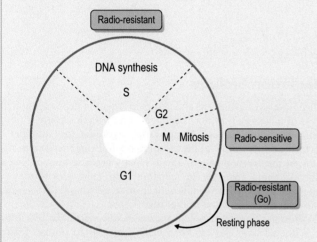

Figure 15-1 The cell cycle and relative radiosensitivity.

Box 15-2 **The 4 'R's' of radiation**

- Repair
- Redistribution
- Repopulation
- Re-oxygenation

At the present time most radical (i.e., definitive, with intent to cure) radiation schedules for human patients employ approximately 30 daily treatments over a period of four to six weeks. In animals, where general anesthesia is required for restraint of the patient during treatment and where radiation facilities are less widely available, larger weekly or biweekly fractions may be used in a more palliative approach. However, many centers do use definitive schedules, e.g., Monday–Wednesday–Friday protocols or daily fractions over several weeks.

In brachytherapy, where implants are placed within the tumor volume, fractionation is not required. Instead the total dose is delivered over a period of time, usually three to four days for implants and up to two to three weeks for systemically administered isotopes, e.g., radioactive iodine (^{131}I) for thyroid tumors in cats.

SOURCES OF RADIATION USED FOR THERAPY

A variety of ionizing radiations may be used for therapeutic purposes including

- X-rays
- gamma-rays
- electrons.

There are essentially two techniques for the application of radiation to tumors:

- **Teletherapy**: radiation is applied in the form of an external beam of X-rays, gamma-rays or electrons that are directed into the tumor
- **Brachytherapy**: radioactive substances, which emit gamma or beta rays, may be applied to the surface of a tumor, implanted within the tumor or administered systemically to the patient.

Each technique has advantages and disadvantages. Whilst external beam therapy is relatively safe for the operator, the equipment is expensive to purchase and maintain and multiple doses of radiation are required over a four to six week course of treatment. Brachytherapy often offers better localization of the radiation and permits the delivery of high doses of radiation to the tumor with minimal normal tissue toxicity. However, the implant and the implanted patient present a radiation hazard for the operator and any staff caring for the patient. Radioactive isotopes can only be used on licensed premises and strict local rules for handling the isotope and patient must be applied. Both techniques require careful planning in consultation with medical physicists to ensure the required dose of radiation is delivered to the tumor.

External beam methods

Various devices exist for generating and delivering radiation to tissues (Box 15-3).

With external beam radiation, the beam can be collimated to the area of the tumor and several treatment ports employed in order to reduce the amount of entry and exit beam radiation affecting the surrounding normal tissues. The prescription and planning of such treatment is facilitated by three-dimensional computerized treatment planning programs (Fig. 15-3). Multi-leaf collimators allow complex planning and shaping of the radiation field to the defined target volume. Intensity modulated radiotherapy (IMRT) allows multiple

Box 15-3 **External radiation generators**

Linear accelerators produce high energy (megavoltage), deeply penetrating radiation that spares the skin and superficial tissues. Photon beam energies range from 4–20 MV. Some linear accelerators produce electron beams, which have a defined range in tissue with a sharp cut-off point at which they deliver their energy, making them more suited to treating soft tissue lesions on chest and abdominal walls and on limbs. Linear accelerators are the mainstay of radiotherapy services in most human hospitals (Fig. 15-2)

Orthovoltage units produce lower energy (kilovoltage), softer radiation that is preferentially absorbed by bone. These are used for treatment of superficial tumors

Cobalt units, housing a radioactive source (Cobalt-60) have been replaced by linear accelerators

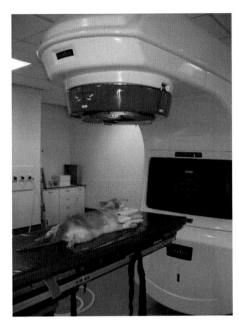

Figure 15-2 Linear accelerator. This unit, installed in the Cancer Therapy Unit at Cambridge Veterinary School, produces a 6 MV photon beam and various electron energies. The cat has been positioned for treatment of an intranasal tumor.

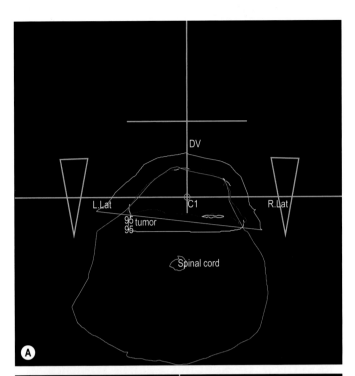

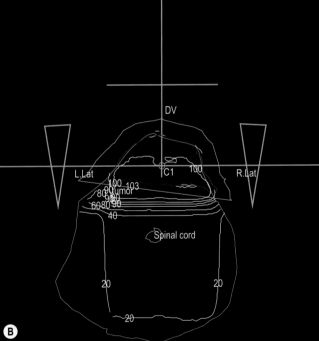

Figure 15-3 Computer generated treatment plan for preoperative radiotherapy of an intrascapular feline injection site sarcoma (FISS). The use of three perpendicular beams (green lines) allows the radiation to be 'focused' into the tumor volume (red line), whilst sparing the surrounding normal tissues to a degree. The white lines are the isodose levels predicted by the computer program. The blue line is the tissue equivalent bolus used to ensure that superficial tumor receives the required dose of radiation. The green triangles are 'wedges' used to reduce the amount of radiation dorsally, where the tumor is narrower. The orange line represents the whole cross-section of the cat.

differently shaped photon beams to be effectively 'painted' onto the tumor, allowing higher doses of radiation to be delivered to the tumor with no increase in the dose delivered to normal tissue. More recent developments in radiotherapy include tomotherapy, which is a form of IMRT that uses a helical delivery system. Stereotactic radiosurgery describes a technique where multiple, highly targeted beams of radiation are delivered in large doses in fewer treatments (usually one to five). Radiosurgery may be delivered by a 'gamma-knife' which uses technology similar to IMRT, or a free standing 'Cyberknife'. Tomotherapy and stereotactic radiosurgery have not been used widely in veterinary medicine to date, although there are some reports of radiosurgery in the treatment of brain tumors.

INDICATIONS FOR AND USE OF RADIATION IN FELINE TUMORS

The main indication for radiation in the treatment of feline tumors is for malignant tumors that, by virtue of their size or site, cannot be controlled by surgery alone. Radiation is most effective and least toxic when used as a local treatment for superficial tumors or those on the extremities of the body. Because of the difficulties in localization and the risk of toxicity, tumors sited in the chest, abdomen or pelvis are not usually treated with radiation in cats (with the exception of thymoma and thymic lymphoma). It is desirable that local and/or distant metastases are not present, although local lymph nodes can be included in the treatment fields. Benign tumors are often not very radiosensitive, and, because radiation is potentially carcinogenic, other means of treatment should always be sought to manage such tumors.

Tumor volume is one of the most important factors in determining tumor response to radiation (as explained above) and generally, for most solid tumors, surgery is the best approach. Radiation may be used as a single means of therapy for tumors that are not amenable to surgical resection due to their site, e.g., in treatment of nasal adenocarcinoma or pituitary macroadenoma. However, radiation is probably most effective when used as an adjunct to surgery for localized, microscopic disease.

Radiation may be combined with surgery in the management of selected tumors that cannot be treated adequately by surgery alone, e.g., soft tissue sarcomas on distal limbs. Radiation can be used prior to, during, or following surgery. Postoperative radiation is the most common method of combining these two modalities. Intentional cytoreductive surgery reduces the tumor burden to microscopic levels leaving small numbers of well oxygenated and rapidly proliferating cells that, in theory, should be sensitive to radiation. Radiation will, however, delay the healing of the surgical wound and must either be commenced immediately following surgery or once the wound has healed. It is important that radiation and surgery should be combined as a carefully planned therapeutic strategy and that the radiation oncologist should be consulted in the management of the case from the outset. The use of radiation as an after-thought to salvage inadequate surgery is fraught with difficulties in planning and application and this practice is strongly discouraged.

Recently preoperative radiation therapy has been shown to be valuable in the management of feline injection site sarcoma (FISS) (Chapter 22).

RESPONSE OF SPECIFIC FELINE TUMORS TO RADIOTHERAPY

Lymphoma

Lymphoma is the most common tumor to affect cats, and whilst many forms of this disease are systemic or multicentric and thus more amenable to treatment with chemotherapy, lymphoma is highly radiosensitive. Thus radiotherapy should be considered as a treatment option for solitary extranodal forms of lymphoma, e.g., nasal and thymic lymphoma. There are very few published studies in the veterinary literature that document the response of extranodal lymphoma to radiotherapy in comparison to chemotherapy or multimodality therapy (radiation and chemotherapy), so it is difficult to advise which option confers greatest survival benefit. A recent study that reported on 97 cats with nasal lymphoma treated with radiotherapy alone (various protocols), chemotherapy alone, or radiotherapy and chemotherapy, failed to show any significant difference in survival between the three treatment groups, with a median survival time regardless of therapy of 536 days. There was a suggestion that higher doses of radiation lead to better local tumor control, hence in theory increasing chance of survival.[1] Similar survival times (median survival 749 days) were reported in 49 cats in the UK with nasal lymphoma treated with chemotherapy alone.[2] The optimal protocol for treatment of feline nasal lymphoma remains a point of debate amongst veterinary oncologists.

Radiotherapy can be used to produce a rapid response in cats with thymic lymphoma and may also be used in combination with surgery in treatment of thymoma (see Chapter 44), although most cats with thymoma do well with surgery alone.

Nasal tumors

Nasal adenocarcinoma

Nasal carcinoma commonly affects the nasal cavity of the cat; usually adenocarcinoma. This is distinct from the sunlight-induced squamous cell carcinoma of the nasal planum, which will also be discussed. In contrast to the numerous reports documenting radiation response of

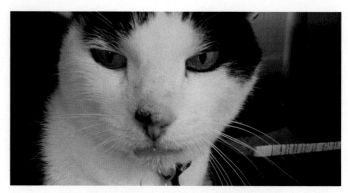

Figure 15-4 Superficial squamous cell carcinoma of the nasal planum.

canine intranasal carcinoma to radiation therapy, there are very few reports on treatment and survival of cats with nasal carcinoma. Eight cats, the majority with nasal adenocarcinoma, were treated with coarsely fractionated radiotherapy (four times weekly fractions to total of 36 Gy) and achieved a median survival time of 382 days, with a one year survival rate of 63%.[3] A similar response was seen in 16 cats treated with a four week Monday–Wednesday–Friday protocol to a minimum of 48 Gy which achieved a one year survival rate of 44%.[4]

Nasal planum squamous cell carcinoma

Squamous cell carcinoma (SCC) of the nasal planum (Fig. 15-4) is a far more common presentation than nasal adenocarcinoma, especially in sunny climates, and this may be managed in a number of different ways depending on the stage or extent of the tumor. Early Tis (carcinoma in situ) or T1 (non-invasive) tumors are amenable to management by surgical excision, cryosurgery, superficial radiation, photodynamic therapy, or topical application of an immunomodulatory agent (Aldara – Imiquimod).[5] Although superficial radiation may be effective in the management of such tumors, a prolonged fractionated course of external beam therapy using either orthovoltage radiation or electrons seems unnecessarily complex and expensive, when other quicker and simpler treatments are equally effective. Strontium-90 plesiotherapy can be used to deliver total radiation doses up to 50 Gy in fewer fractions and has been reported to achieve an 85% complete response rate in 15 cats, 11 of which had stage T2 tumors.[6] Photodynamic therapy (PDT), using a topical application of the photosensitizer 5-amino-levulinic acid (5ALA) followed by 30 minutes' illumination with a high intensity red light also achieved an 85% complete response rate in 55 cats with Tis–T2 tumors.[7] As PDT causes no local tissue injury and is repeatable, this method is the author's preferred first choice for treatment of cats with non-invasive nasal planum SCC (Fig. 15-5). Once tumors become invasive, they are refractory to superficial treatments and surgical resection is the only effective treatment (see Chapter 54).

Oral squamous cell carcinoma

Squamous cell carcinoma is the most common tumor of the feline oral cavity, representing up to 80% of all tumors arising in the mouth of cats. Tumors may arise in the mandibular or maxillary gingiva or at the base of the tongue (Fig. 15-6). Mandibular and maxillary tumors tend to be very invasive and destructive of the underlying bone, and on occasion can stimulate a significant bony reaction (Fig. 15-7). Lingual tumors frequently invade into the tissue of the tongue and cause significant morbidity (Fig. 15-8). Although SCC per se is a reasonably radiosensitive tumor, the extent of the tumor and the associated normal tissue invasion/destruction that is often present at

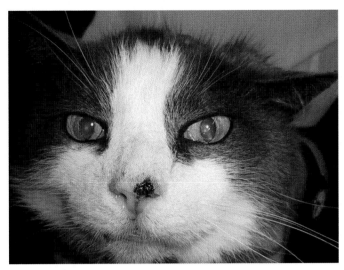

Figure 15-5 Early T1 squamous cell carcinoma of the nasal planum, which is suitable for treatment by topical photodynamic treatment.

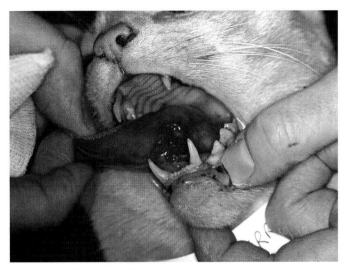

Figure 15-8 Squamous cell carcinoma at base of tongue.

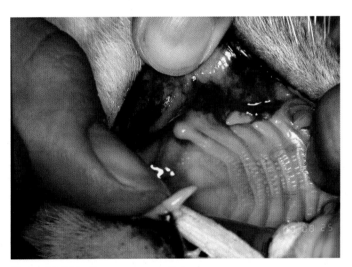

Figure 15-6 Maxillary squamous cell carcinoma.

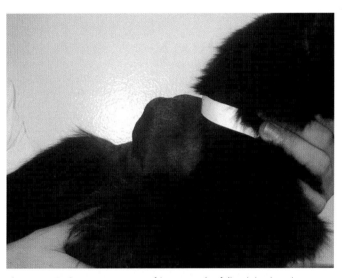

Figure 15-9 Gross appearance of interscapular feline injection site sarcoma.

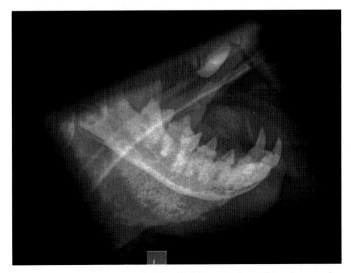

Figure 15-7 Bony reaction associated with squamous cell carcinoma of the mandible.

the time of diagnosis preclude successful treatment of such lesions. There are reports describing the use of orthovoltage or megavoltage radiation in the treatment of feline oral SCC with or without chemotherapy or surgery but response rates are low and survival times short, median 60–86 days.[8,9]

Feline injection site sarcoma

In veterinary medicine the treatment of soft tissue sarcoma by a combination of surgical resection (Chapter 22) followed by local adjuvant radiation has become accepted as an effective method for management of those tumors arising at sites where wide surgical resection is not feasible, e.g., distal limbs. In the cat the 'feline injection site sarcoma (FISS)' or 'vaccine-associated' sarcoma (VAS), which most commonly arises in the dorsal neck/interscapular region, is recognized to be a particularly aggressive, invasive form of soft tissue sarcoma, with a high risk of local recurrence following surgery alone (Figs 15-9 and 15-10). Various combinations of surgery and radiation (and chemotherapy) have been reported in the management of such tumors and there is evidence that the addition of radiation reduces

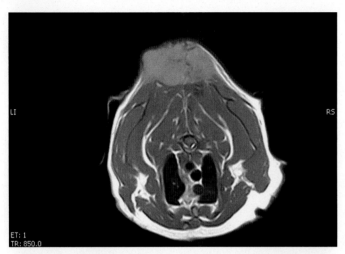

Figure 15-10 Magnetic resonance image of tumor shown in Fig. 15.9. These images were used to generate the treatment plan shown in Fig. 15.3.

local recurrence rate and increases survival time. In a group of 27 cats with macroscopic disease or dirty margins, coarse fractionated radiotherapy achieved a median survival of 24 months and median progression free interval of ten months overall, and those with no macroscopic disease (*n* = 17) had a median survival of 30 months.[10] There is also evidence that preoperative radiation can be particularly beneficial in the treatment of these tumors.[11] The presence of macroscopic tumor facilitates radiation planning and delivery (Fig. 15-3) and this is currently the author's preferred approach.

Pituitary macroadenoma

Tumors of the brain are not common in cats. Meningiomas are one of the commoner tumor types and these are usually amenable to surgical excision (Chapter 58), which is usually curative. There are some reports of radiation treatment of feline pituitary tumors which indicate that radiation is effective in controlling the neurological signs associated with a pituitary mass and can improve the clinical signs associated with hyperadrenocorticism or acromegaly in cats with no neurologic abnormalities.[12,13] In one study of 14 cats with insulin-resistant diabetes mellitus secondary to acromegaly treated with megavoltage radiation three times a week to a total of 37 Gy, 13 cats had improved glycemic control following treatment, which was sustained for up to 60 months.[14]

Radio-iodine for hyperthyroidism

Radiation in the form of brachytherapy using radioactive iodine (^{131}I) has been used extensively for the treatment of feline hyperthyroidism. The majority of cases of feline hyperthyroidism are due to benign adenoma or adenomatous hyperplasia, and only a small 1–2% of cats have malignant thyroid carcinoma. Feline hyperthyroidism may be managed medically (with carbimazole or methimazole) or surgically by removal of the enlarged thyroid gland(s) (Chapter 53). However, neither of these options is ideal. Medical management requires lifelong daily medication and there can be a rapid return to the hyperthyroid state if medication is stopped. The majority of cats with hyperthyroidism have bilateral thyroid involvement; surgical removal of both lobes of the thyroid gland can be very successful therapy but a number of postoperative complications exist including hypoparathyroidism and hypothyroidism (very rare). For these reasons, ^{131}I

therapy is arguably the treatment of choice in most cases, subject to availability and the owner's ability to pay. ^{131}I is preferentially concentrated in the adenomatous areas of the thyroid (Chapter 8); the normal thyroid tissue takes up very little due to normal feedback suppression, making this a highly selective and effective treatment that is not associated with significant side effects. The β (beta) particle emitted by ^{131}I travels an average distance of only 400 μm. This fact guarantees local destruction and spares the surrounding normal tissue. This is particularly relevant to the sparing effect of the parathyroid glands. During the whole duration of treatment the cats have to be hospitalized for radiation protection reasons and handling of cats during treatment has to be restricted to trained personnel. The usual time for elimination of the radionuclide to a level that is considered safe takes about eight to ten days. These levels are dependent on the radiation protection regulations of the country where this treatment is done. A single dose of ^{131}I will return more than 95% of cats with hyperthyroidism to persistent euthyroidism, and no ongoing thyroid medication is required following therapy.

In cats with suspected thyroid carcinoma, thyroidectomy would be the initial treatment of choice because the diagnosis must be confirmed by histopathology and because complete excision can be curative. Treatment with high dose ^{131}I is indicated in cats with non-resectable thyroid carcinoma, evidence of metastasis, or recurrence after thyroidectomy. Higher doses of ^{131}I (10–30 mCi) are required to successfully treat cats with thyroid carcinoma than are required to treat cats with thyroid adenoma.

TUMOR RESPONSE AND NORMAL TISSUE TOXICITY

Whilst the chemical events leading to radiation-induced damage occur almost instantaneously, the biological expression of this injury may take days, weeks or even years to become apparent. Radiation therefore appears to have delayed actions in terms of both tumor response and normal tissue toxicity. Radiation response is therefore assessed at the end of treatment and then at set time periods after this. Response is categorized according to set criteria (Box 15-4).

Normal tissue toxicity

Radiation has a reputation for causing serious toxicity to the patient; however, radiation sickness and severe morbidity only arise when large areas of the body or vital organs are exposed to high doses of radiation. In order to avoid such side effects, radiation is rarely used in this manner in the treatment of animals. Tumors most suitable for irradiation tend to be superficial or those sited on the extremities of the body. The skin, superficial connective tissues, mucous membranes (oral tumors), and bone are therefore the tissues most commonly included in the treatment field and some radiation-induced changes will occur in these tissues.

Radiation toxicity is usually described in terms of 'acute' reactions occurring during and shortly after the radiation treatment and 'late' reactions that are not observed for weeks or even months following treatment. This division is not absolute. Standard guidelines for the reporting of radiation toxicity have been produced by the Veterinary Radiation Therapy Oncology Group and are shown in Tables 15-1 and 15.2.[15]

Acute toxicity

Acute toxicity results from the death of actively dividing cell populations, e.g., epithelium of the skin and mucous membranes. Changes

Table 15-1 Veterinary Radiation Therapy Oncology Group acute radiation morbidity scoring scheme

Organ/tissue	0	1	2	3
Skin/hair	No change over baseline	Erythema, dry desquamation, alopecia/epilation	Patchy moist desquamation without edema	Confluent moist desquamation with edema and/or ulceration, necrosis, hemorrhage
Mucous membrane/oral cavity	No change over baseline	Injection without mucositis	Patchy mucositis with patient seemingly pain free	Confluent fibrinous mucositis necessitating analgesia, ulceration, hemorrhage, necrosis
Eye	No change over baseline	Mild conjunctivitis and/or scleral injection	KCS requiring artificial tears, moderate conjunctivitis or iritis necessitating therapy	Severe keratitis with corneal ulceration and/or loss of vision, glaucoma
Ear	No change over baseline	Mild external otitis with erythema, pruritis secondary to dry desquamation not requiring therapy	Moderate external otitis requiring topical medication	Severe external otitis with discharge and moist desquamation
Lower gastrointestinal tract	No change over baseline	Change in quality of bowel habits not requiring medication, rectal discomfort	Diarrhea requiring parasympatholytic medication, rectal discomfort requiring analgesia	Diarrhea requiring parenteral support, bloody discharge necessitating medical attention, fistula, perforation
Genito/urinary	No change over baseline	Change in frequency of urination, not requiring medication	Change in frequency of urination necessitating medication	Gross hematuria or bladder obstruction
Central nervous system	No change over baseline	Minor neurologic findings not necessitating more than prednisolone therapy	Neurologic findings necessitating more than prednisolone therapy	Serious neurologic impairment such as paralysis, coma, obtunded
Lung	No change over baseline	Alveolar infiltrate, cough requiring no treatment	Dense alveolar infiltrate, cough requiring treatment	Dyspnea

(Reproduced from Bregazzi VS, LaRue SM, Powers BE, et al. Response of feline oral squamous cell carcinoma to palliative radiation therapy. Veterinary Radiology and Ultrasound 2001;42(1):77–9, with permission of John Wiley & Sons.)

Box 15-4 **Response to radiation**

- Complete response (CR): complete disappearance of the tumor
- Partial response (PR): >50% reduction in the tumor mass
- No response/static disease (SD): <50% reduction in tumor mass
- Progressive disease (PD): increase in tumor mass

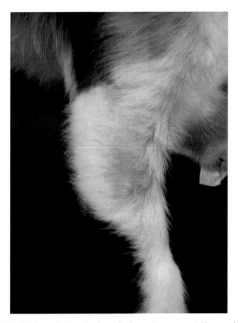

Figure 15-11 Early radiation-induced alopecia, seen at the end of a four week course of postoperative radiotherapy following cytoreductive surgery for a spindle cell tumor, lateral antebrachium.

range from a mild reddening or erythema of the skin/mucosa to vesiculation, desquamation and severe exfoliative dermatitis/ necrosis (the latter is rare). The signs usually resolve spontaneously as the normal cell population regenerates.

Localized hair loss is a common result of irradiation of the skin in animals. This results from damage to the hair follicle epithelium at the time of treatment but the resulting alopecia does not usually occur until the existing hair is shed and not replaced (Figs 15-11 and 15-12). Ultimately some hair usually regrows but this may be patchy and lack pigmentation.

Late toxicity

This is less predictable and more serious than acute toxicity. It tends to occur in slowly proliferating tissues, e.g., connective tissues and bone. Changes are often progressive and irreversible. Examples of late radiation toxicity are listed in Box 15-5.

Table 15.2 Veterinary Radiation Therapy Oncology Group late radiation morbidity scoring scheme

Organ/tissue	0	1	2	3
Skin/hair	None	Alopecia, hyperpigmentation, leukotrichia	Asymptomatic induration (fibrosis)	Severe induration causing physical impairment, necrosis
Central nervous system	None	Mild neurologic signs not necessitating more than prednisolone therapy	Neurologic signs necessitating more than prednisolone therapy	Seizures, paralysis, coma
Eye	None	Asymptomatic cataracts, KCS	Symptomatic cataracts, keratitis, corneal ulceration, minor retinopathy, mild to moderate glaucoma	Panophthalmitis, blindness, severe glaucoma, retinal detachment
Bone	None	Pain on palpation	Radiographic changes	Necrosis
Lung	None	Patchy radiographic infiltrates	Dense radiographic infiltrates	Symptomatic fibrosis, pneumonitis
Heart	None	ECG changes	Pericardial effusion	Pericardial tamponade, congestive heart failure
Joint	None	Stiffness	Decreased range of motion	Complete fixation
Bladder	None	Microscopic hematuria	Pollakiuria, dysuria, hematuria	Contracted bladder

(Reproduced from Bregazzi VS, LaRue SM, Powers BE, et al. Response of feline oral squamous cell carcinoma to palliative radiation therapy. Veterinary Radiology and Ultrasound 2001;42(1):77–9, with permission of John Wiley & Sons.)

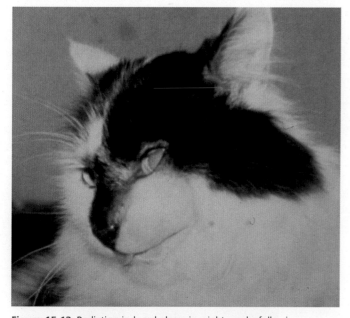

Figure 15-12 Radiation-induced alopecia, eight weeks following radiation of a fibrosarcoma of the left upper lip.

> ### Box 15-5 **Examples of late radiation toxicity in various organs in cats**
>
> **Skin:** In the skin radiation induces fibrosis in the dermal connective tissues resulting in a thickened, rubbery texture and subsequently contraction of the skin and subcutis can occur. As a result of the fibrosis and vascular changes, irradiated skin and soft tissues can be very slow to heal and even the most minor surgical procedure can result in a non-healing, necrotic wound
>
> **Bone:** Osteonecrosis leading to bone pain and pathological fracture is a major concern in fields containing bone, particularly in cases where the bone is already compromised by tumor invasion
>
> **Nervous tissue:** Late reactions in nervous tissues can also be a problem; brain and spinal cord necrosis can have serious consequences, irradiation of the spine should be avoided if at all possible as it can result in paralysis

REFERENCES

1. Haney SM, Beaver L, Turrel J, et al. Survival analysis of 97 cats with nasal lymphoma: a multi-institutional retrospective study (1986–2006). J Vet Int Med 2009;23:287–94.

2. Taylor SS, Goodfellow MR, Browne WJ, et al. Feline extranodal lymphoma: response to chemotherapy and survival in 110 cats. J Small Anim Practice 2009;50(11):584–92.

3. Mellanby RJ, Herrtage ME, Dobson JM. Long-term outcome of eight cats with non-lymphoproliferative nasal tumors treated by megavoltage radiotherapy. J Fel Med & Surg 2002;4: 77–81.

4. Théon AP, Peaston AE, Madewell BR, Dungworth DL. Irradiation of nonlymphoproliferative neoplasms of the nasal cavity and paranasal sinuses in 16 cats. J Aam Vet Med Assoc 1994;204(1):78–83.

5. Gill VL, Bergman PJ, Baer KE, et al. Use of 5% cream (Aldara) in cats with multicentric squamous cell carcinoma in situ: 12 cases (2002–2005). Vet Comp Oncol 2008;6:55–6.

6. Goodfellow M, Hayes A, Murphy S, Brearley M. A retrospective study of (90) Strontium plesiotherapy for feline

squamous cell carcinoma of the nasal planum. J Fel Med & Surg 2006;88: 169–76.

7. Bexfield NH, Stell AJ, Gear RN, Dobson JM.Photodynamic therapy of superficial nasal planum squamous cell carcinomas in cats: 55 cases. J Vet Int Med, 2008;22: 1385–9.

8. Bregazzi VS, LaRue SM, Powers BE, et al. Response of feline oral squamous cell carcinoma to palliative radiation therapy. Vet Radiol Ultrasound 2001;42:77–9.

9. Fidel JL, Sellon RK., Houston RK, et al. A nine-day accelerated radiation protocol for feline squamous cell carcinoma. Vet Radiol Ultrasound 2007;48:482–5.

10. Eckstein C, Guscetti F, Roos M, et al. A retrospective analysis of radiation therapy for the treatment of feline vaccine-associated sarcoma. Vet Comp Oncol 2009;7:54–68.

11. Kobayashi T, Hauck ML, Dodge R, et al. Preoperative radiotherapy for vaccine associated sarcoma in 92 cats. Vet Radiol Ultrasound 2002;43:473–9.

12. Mayer MN, Greco DS, LaRue SM. Outcomes of pituitary tumor irradiation in cats. J Vet Int Med 2006;20:1151–4.

13. Brearley MJ, Polton GA, Littler RM, Niessen SJ. Coarse fractionated radiation therapy for pituitary tumours in cats: a retrospective study of 12 cases. Vet Comp Oncol 2006;4:209–17.

14. Dunning MD, Lowrie CS, Bexfield NH, et al. Exogenous insulin treatment after hypofractionated radiotherapy in cats with diabetes mellitus and acromegaly. J Vet Int Med 2009;23:243–9.

15. LaDue T, Klein MK. Toxicity criteria of the radiation therapy oncology group. Vet Radiol Ultrasound 2001;42: 475–6.

Chapter | 16 |

Chemotherapy

M.J. Brearley

Although not used frequently in cats, chemotherapy can be an important primary or adjunctive therapy in the treatment of feline cancers. However, whilst there are anecdotal comments and single case reports advocating the use of anti-cancer drugs against many cancers in cats, there are only a few tumors for which efficacy has been described with any evidence base. These are the lymphoid malignancies, mammary cancer, vaccine-associated feline sarcoma and, by intralesional administration, squamous cell carcinoma of the mouth and face. It is worth reflecting that even in human oncology there are only a few tumors that are regularly cured by chemotherapy (for example, childhood leukemia and testicular cancer) and indeed the number of patients with other cancers that truly benefit from cytotoxic drugs overall is modest at best. The greatest progress in the treatment of cancer in humans has been by early diagnosis, effective surgical techniques and radiotherapy; it is almost a certainty that this will be true in veterinary oncology also.

Hippocrates is purported to have said, 'First do no harm' and to that end the speculative use of any treatment that can have serious side effects on the chance that it might do some good is not to be encouraged. Just as a radical chest wall resection to treat a cancer that has already metastasized would never be considered, the use of a drug that kills cells, and possibly also the patient, with little to no chance of controlling the disease should not be entertained. The use of a treatment that has potentially devastating side effects has to be based on evidence of efficacy and then with an understanding of all the potential ramifications.

Having given this stark introduction, chemotherapy can help control certain cancers and thereby benefit those individuals with an improved quality of life. This chapter therefore aims to give an insight into some of the drugs that are used, their potential side effects and the management of such problems, and the situations where cytotoxic drugs have been shown to have efficacy in cats. For further information the reader is referred to specialist oncology textbooks.[1-4]

CANCER CHEMOTHERAPY

Cancer chemotherapy is the use of drugs that by some means control the growth of cancer cells either by killing them (cytotoxic) or by preventing their proliferation (cytostatic). To date there are few anti-cancer drugs that are truly specific against cancer cells and therefore their activity against normal cells also gives rise to potential toxicity. Toxicity to normal tissues is not unique to anti-cancer drugs; very few chemicals are totally free of side effects. However, unlike anti-bacterial agents, for example, that utilize the very different biology of bacterial versus eukaryotic cells, anti-cancer drugs are aimed at a cell population that is basically host cells doing something wrong. By a variety of mechanisms the therapeutic gain is the result of either more damage and/or less recovery from damage, in the cancer population compared with the normal host tissues. The therapeutic index, which is the ratio of benefit to toxicity, for most of the current anti-cancer drugs is narrow and indeed the fatal dose is rarely more than double that used therapeutically, thereby highlighting the need to use these medications with care.

How anti-cancer drugs work

Most of the 'conventional' anti-cancer drugs are cytotoxic and work by killing dividing cells (both normal and cancerous) either via damage to DNA synthesis or to a specific mechanism of cell division. The newer so-called targeted therapies, such as the tyrosine kinase inhibitors, act at specific cell surface receptors that promote cell proliferation, hence their cytostatic effect.

Few tumor types are truly insensitive to cytotoxic drugs. However, the cancers arising from cell types whose function is to detoxify or excrete toxic chemicals are relatively resistant; this includes hepatic, renal, and colon cancers. The majority of other cell types are innately sensitive to cytotoxic drugs, but may develop resistance to them either by acquiring mutations as they multiply (because cancer cells are genetically unstable) or by switching on genes in response to repeated exposure to cytotoxic drugs (i.e., an adaptive response). These acquired or activated genes tend to confer resistance to a range of drugs and not just to the chemotherapeutic agent to which they have been exposed. Such multi-drug resistance is the most frequent reason for relapse of a tumor that had apparently achieved complete remission.

Another property of tissues that influences efficacy of cytotoxic drugs is the growth rate (Box 16-1). The rate of clinical tumor growth and the mitotic index given by histology may provide surrogate

© 2014 Elsevier Ltd
DOI: 10.1016/B978-0-7020-4336-9.00016-0

Table 16-1 Weight to surface area conversion chart

Weight (kg)	BSA (m²)	Weight (kg)	BSA (m²)
2.0	0.159	4.2	0.260
2.2	0.169	4.4	0.269
2.4	0.179	4.6	0.277
2.6	0.189	4.8	0.285
2.8	0.199	5.0	0.292
3.0	0.208	5.2	0.300
3.2	0.217	5.4	0.308
3.4	0.226	5.6	0.315
3.6	0.235	5.8	0.323
3.8	0.244	6.0	0.330
4.0	0.252		

BSA, body surface area.

information about the tissue growth rate. In theory, tumors with a high growth fraction and short cell cycle time are the most sensitive to cytotoxic agents. Lymphoblastic lymphoma is an example of a sensitive cell type of this nature, as the cells often exhibit a high mitotic rate, and hence this form of tumor in cats frequently responds to chemotherapy.

A high growth rate is also seen with small or microscopic tumors, which have a high growth fraction and fast cell cycle time. Conversely, large bulky tumors tend to have a low growth fraction, slow cell cycle and increased cell loss. Chemotherapy is therefore more likely to be effective against early microscopic metastases or minimal residual disease following surgery, which is why the adjuvant use of chemotherapy should be actively considered for certain tumor types.

When chemotherapy is indicated

Cytotoxic drugs are used in several scenarios (Box 16-2). In practice, the probability of curing most cancer in dogs or cats with cytotoxic drugs is low because the actual range of tumors that respond to chemotherapy is quite limited, a fact especially true in cats.

Drug dosing issues

There are several principles that should be followed when selecting drugs for chemotherapy (Box 16-3).

The vast majority of anti-cancer agents used in dogs and cats are human drugs; it is only recently that drugs have been developed specifically for veterinary use. Some drug doses have been derived from toxicology data from the pharmaceutical development of human drugs, but this data is more readily available for dogs than cats as the latter are rarely used in the development of human drugs. In addition,

dose escalation as part of phase I and II studies has been performed for some of the cytotoxic drugs used in veterinary oncology. However, most frequently the dose in clinical practice has been derived from clinical experience and the protocols using a single agent or a combination of drugs have often been developed in a rather empirical manner.

As already stated, the therapeutic index of anti-cancer drugs is narrow, which is an important consideration when veterinary surgeons have an ethical obligation to minimize the side effects any treatment may generate. In the main, most drugs are metabolized in a manner proportional to the metabolic rate of the animal. A major function of the basal metabolic rate (BMR) is to maintain the body temperature of the mammal. As heat loss from an object is proportional to its surface area rather than its volume, the BMR is related to the surface area rather than the volume (or weight) of the individual. Larger individuals have a lower surface area to volume ratio, hence a lower BMR and a lower rate of drug elimination. Dosing on a weight basis tends to over-dose larger individuals and under-dose small patients. Using a dose per surface area in theory smoothes this difference, but unfortunately for patients less than 10 kg this may not hold true. There is also species variation, so it is important that the dose for cats should not be simply extrapolated from that for small dogs.

The surface area is derived from the weight by equation in Box 16-4 (see also Table 16.1). The dose interval depends on which drug is being used, the dose given and the recovery time from adverse effects. For most cytotoxic drugs given as a 'high dose' bolus the average time to complete recovery is day 21 following the neutropenic nadir at day 5 to 7, and therefore a dose interval of three weeks is appropriate. However, some drugs (e.g., lomustine and, to a lesser extent, carboplatin)[5,6] have a second weaker nadir around day 20 and may warrant a four week cycle, so it is important to be aware of these individual drug variations when designing a therapeutic plan for individual patients. Drugs may also be given at a lower dose more frequently to give a chronic exposure.

ANTI-CANCER DRUGS

There is a long list of drugs that have anti-cancer effects. Although a dose for many of the drugs suitable for cats can be found in the literature, actual documented evidence of efficacy is either non-existent or at best limited to anecdotal single case reports so this chapter will focus only on the agents which have a reasonably good evidence base for their recommended use. Table 16-2 summarizes the pharmaceutical aspects and dosing issues; Table 16-3 lists the toxicity and indications of the drugs that are used with some frequency in cats.

SIDE EFFECTS AND THEIR MANAGEMENT

Before starting any treatment it is beholden on the attending clinician to be aware of the potential side effects, to discuss these with the owner and to know how to manage them if they occur. However, because the therapeutic index of chemotherapeutic agents is narrow this is particularly important when using anti-cancer drugs.

When discussing the potential side effects with owners it is important to concentrate on those that are common (however minor) and those that are serious or potentially life-threatening (however rare!). The aim of this counseling is not to frighten the owner but to give a balanced view and to ensure they know what is important and when to seek veterinary attention. At the doses used in clinical practice less than 20% of cats will have moderate or severe reactions; however, anorexia and increasing intolerance to intravenous injections can be problematic. Owners are an important part of the caring team and a written list of potential side effects and the action required is preferable to hoping they will remember all that has been discussed.

Fatal and contraindicated

Two drugs are absolutely contraindicated in cats:

* **5-fluorouracil** – will cause a fatal neuropathy
* **Cisplatin** (administered intravenously (IV)) – will cause fatal pulmonary edema.[7]

Some preparations (e.g., oil suspension or in collagen matrix if stable and truly slow release) have been used but there are safety handling issues and these preparations can still not be recommended.

Table 16-2 Summary of anti-cancer drugs: dosing aspects

Drug	Mode of action	Pharmaceutical preparations	Route of admin	Dose	Dose frequency
Vincristine sulphate	Spindle binding	Solution: 1 mg/mL	IV only	0.5–0.7 mg/m²	Not less than q7 days
Cyclophosphamide	Alkylating agent	Powder for reconstitution 50 mg tablet	IV PO	250–300 mg/m² IV; 150 mg/m² PO	High dose: q21 days Low dose: divided weekly equivalent
Chlorambucil	Alkylating agent	2 mg tablet	PO	20 mg/m² or 4–6 mg/m²	High dose: q14–28 days Low dose: eod equivalent
Doxorubicin	Topo-isomerase II inhibitor	Solution: 2 mg/mL Powder for reconstitution	IV only by slow infusion	25 mg/m² or 1 mg/kg	q21 days; cumulative dose limit 180 mg/m²
Cisplatin	Alkylating agent	Powder for reconstitution	Intralesional emulsion	FATAL if IV	Refer to Table 16-3
Carboplatin	Alkylating agent	Solution: 10 mg/mL	Slow IV only	200–240 mg/m²	q21 days
Lomustine (CCNU)	Alkylating agent	40 mg capsules[a]	PO	40–50 mg/m²[a]	q21–28 days

[a]Specialist re-formulation to 10 mg capsules is necessary for clinical use.
IV, intravenous; PO, per os; eod, every other day.

Table 16-3 Summary of anti-cancer drugs – toxicity and indications

Drug	Toxicity	Indications	Comment
Vincristine sulphate	BM, A, V, SI ileus	Lymphoblastic 'large cell' lymphoma	With cyclophosphamide and prednisolone as 'COP' protocol
Cyclophosphamide	BM, A, V, whisker loss	Lymphoblastic 'large cell' lymphoma	With vincristine and prednisolone as 'COP' protocol
Chlorambucil	BM (mild)	Lymphocytic 'small cell' lymphoma	Especially low grade small cell alimentary lymphoma
Doxorubicin	BM, A, V, whisker loss, Cumulative renal damage	High grade sarcoma Mammary carcinoma	Limited efficacy against lymphoma
Cisplatin	FATAL if IV	Carcinoma	Emulsion MUST be stable otherwise potentially fatal! Specialist centres only
Carboplatin	BM, A, V, (renal damage)	Head and neck cancer	Possible radio-sensitizer
Lomustine (CCNU)	BM, A, V	Lymphoma	

A, anorexia; BM, bone marrow suppression; SI, small intestine; V, vomiting.

Issues associated with extravasation

Certain anti-cancer drugs will cause severe irreversible tissue injury after extravasation. The main culprits are doxorubicin and the others in the 'antibiotic' group (epirubicin, mitoxantrone, and actinomycin D) and the vinca alkaloids including vincristine and vinblastine; these drugs are described as having a class 1 extravasation risk. The damage may range from local erythema and phlebitis to progressive necrosis and sloughing of tissue. The latter is particularly true for doxorubicin and similar drugs. The damage is dose dependent, i.e., related to how much drug leaked and how far it spread.

To avoid complications after extravasation of chemotherapeutic agents it is essential to administer these drugs through an intravenous catheter. Accurate 'first stick' and secure placement is essential and the use of a small gauge catheter is recommended in cats. The use of butterfly needles is controversial; although some authorities recommend them for small volume bolus injections, in general the use of intravenous catheters should always be considered the preferable option. Sedation or even anesthesia may also be warranted to adequately restrain some feline patients to reduce the risks of complications for both the animal and the attending clinician and staff. The patency of any catheter should be checked before and during administration of the cytotoxic drug and the area around the catheter site visually monitored for any 'blowing'. Some of the agents are very caustic and will elicit a marked pain reaction if extravasation occurs, but the absence of pain does not mean that extravasation has not occurred, so careful vigilance is essential. At the end of the infusion the catheter should be flushed with normal saline before removal to prevent the creation of a cytotoxic 'catheter tract'.

The result of extravasation may take several days to show. Erythema and swelling are early signs but can progress to necrosis and slough over the following three to four weeks. The vinca alkaloids tend to cause earlier reactions whilst doxorubicin tends to cause later reactions. The sloughing and necrotic lesions that can occur will require extensive debridement and reconstructive surgery to correct and even amputation of the affected limb may be warranted in the case of doxorubicin extravasation, such is the damage this drug can cause.

Immediate response to an extravasation is essential rather than waiting for the full effects to show, so at the first suspicion of an extravasation follow the steps in Box 16-5.

Centrally mediated anorexia and vomiting

Anti-cancer drugs are toxic chemicals that can be recognized by the chemoreceptor trigger zone in the brain. Centrally mediated vomiting with concurrent anorexia is a potential problem common to many of the drugs. However, in the author's experience it is most common with intravenously administered vincristine, cyclophosphamide and doxorubicin. Vomiting and anorexia usually occur within 12 to 24 hours of drug administration but may persist for three to five days. Anorexia tends to be more of a problem than acute vomiting. Tempting with warmed foods such as fish or prawns may help overcome anorexia. Chemical stimulation of the appetite may be necessary, e.g., cyproheptidine (2–4 mg/kg PO q12–24 hours). Mirtazapine (0.5–1.0 mg/kg PO/SQ q72 hours) can be an effective appetite stimulant and it has central anti-emetic properties (for further information on appetite stimulation see Chapter 6). Anti-emetic medications such as metoclopramide or maropitant (Cerenia) should be used in patients who are vomiting or who are considered to possibly be nauseous.

Gastrointestinal toxicity

The epithelial lining of the intestines undergoes constant renewal, with a cell transit time of about three days from the crypt to the villus

Box 16-5 Protocol for extravasation of chemotherapeutic agents

- STOP giving the drug
- Do not remove the catheter but do remove additional tubing such as giving sets, remembering that these are also contaminated with the cytotoxic agent used
- Use syringe suction on the catheter to withdraw as much drug as possible from the site. A temporary tourniquet may help by creating local bleeding into the site to help with this. Again, it must be remembered that any aspirated fluid should be considered as cytotoxic waste and handled appropriately
- If doxorubicin[a] (or similar), apply cold (ice-) pack to limit local spread. If vincristine (or similar) apply hot pack to encourage vasodilatation and absorption
- The use of DMSO and local infiltration with hydrocortisone is controversial, so their use cannot be advocated at the present time
- TELL THE OWNER – it is better to be honest at this stage than when amputation is necessary

[a]A specific 'antidote' to doxorubicin free-radical damage is available (dexrazoxane, Zinecard) that can be used to dramatically reduce the local tissue damage. Dexrazoxane must be given within two to three hours (the sooner the better) intravenously at ten times the dose of doxorubicin administered. It is, however, very expensive with a limited shelf life.

tip. Following a cytotoxic event, villus atrophy occurs and recovery may take a further five to seven days. During the period of villus recovery the increased permeability to outward water transit may cause diarrhea. If the villus atrophy is severe, capillary hemorrhage may result in hemorrhagic diarrhea. During this time the intestinal mucosa will be more permeable to invasion by enteric bacteria. Supportive fluid therapy orally or intravenously may be necessary and the use of microenteral feeding techniques can be beneficial and is to be encouraged. Antibiotics are usually advisable for hemorrhagic diarrhea and intestinal protectants may help with recovery. Cats are, however, relatively resistant to cytotoxic-induced diarrhea and it is a problem less frequently encountered in this species compared to dogs given cytotoxic agents.

Vincristine can cause ileus due to peripheral neurotoxicity. This can lead to abdominal cramps, vomiting and anorexia. This tends to occur five to seven days following a vincristine injection and the effect is cumulative. A delay of a week and dose reduction of the next vincristine injection may be necessary. This problem tends to be more common at the 0.7 mg/m^2 dose than at 0.5 mg/m^2.

Bone marrow suppression

Hemopoetic tissues are continually undergoing cell division to replace the blood cells that have a limited life in the peripheral circulation. These tissues are often dividing more quickly than most cancers and therefore are potentially more susceptible to cytotoxic drugs. However, they also have great powers of recovery from this insult. The effect on the hemopoetic cells is dose dependent and the timing of the result on peripheral cell counts is related to the half-life of the cell type following maturation in the marrow and in the peripheral circulation. In cats it is about 70 days for erythrocytes, 10 days for platelets and four to five days for neutrophils. Recovery of the hemopoetic cell lines from the toxic insult takes three to four days to start. The rapid fall in neutrophils and the delay in recovery results in neutropenia being more common and more serious than thrombocytopenia or anemia. Following a bolus of cytotoxic drug, the nadir for neutrophils is about five to seven days, for platelets around ten to 14 days, but there is generally not an acute problem seen within the erythrocyte series.

The nadir for the neutropenia coincides with the increased permeability of the intestinal mucosa to enteric bacteria. Therefore, what otherwise may have been a transient and insignificant bacteremia can become a full-blown septicemia peaking about seven to ten days following the cytotoxic insult. Typically, the early signs of lethargy, anorexia, vomiting, and a withdrawn character will be obvious in a previously apparently well individual. However, this can progress rapidly over 12 to 24 hours to a state of septic collapse, so these patients need to be monitored carefully. The routine use of prophylactic antibiotics during the at-risk period is controversial as it may lead to antibiotic resistance so their routine use cannot be recommended, although in some susceptible individuals it may be helpful. Left untreated neutropenic sepsis can be fatal, so owners and attending veterinary staff should be aware that early treatment of this acute problem is essential. Supportive fluid therapy, intravenous broad spectrum antibiotics, appropriate nutritional management and hospitalization will usually produce a rapid recovery within 48–72 hours. Antibiotic therapy is usually given for five to seven days and during this time the neutrophil count is likely to have risen well within normal range.

Prior to each round of chemotherapy a complete blood count should always be performed. Neutropenia of less than 1.0×10^9/L is considered serious, but a neutrophil count of less than 2.5×10^9/L should be considered as too low for treatment to be given. Following a septic neutropenic event the next dose of cytotoxic drugs administered should be reduced by 10–25%.

Drug-specific complications

Hair loss

A major concern of most owners before starting their pet on chemotherapy is hair loss, together with vomiting and anorexia (see previously). In the main, significant hair loss does not happen in cats. However, loss of guard hairs and especially of whiskers is common. These usually regrow once the course of treatment has been completed but the whiskers can sometimes regrow kinked and twisted.

Carboplatin

Carboplatin can cause renal damage but this is uncommon in the normal individual. However, patients with reduced renal function are more susceptible and caution should be used in these cases.[7] In humans, dosing is calculated based on glomerular filtration rate, but this is rarely performed in veterinary practice. If there is evidence of reduced renal function (raised serum urea and/or creatinine) then carboplatin should be used with great care, or not at all.

Doxorubicin

Cardiomyopathy associated with doxorubicin, as seen with cumulative dosing in humans and dogs, is rare in cats. This may be due to a true resistance to myocardial toxicity in the species or because most protocols limit the dosing to less than 180 mg/m^2 cumulative dose.

Doxorubicin can, however, cause renal damage as a cumulative dose effect. To that end it should be used to a cumulative dose limit of 180 mg/m^2 and with care in cats with concurrent renal failure. In addition, biochemical renal parameter assessment on a regular basis is a sensible recommendation when doxorubicin is administered to cats. The related drug, epirubicin, may be used in preference to doxorubicin as its efficacy (and dose) is similar in dogs but its cumulative dose limit is higher (+75% in humans). However there are no large series reporting efficacy or toxicity profiles of epirubicin in cats.

Vincristine

Vincristine may cause a peripheral neuropathy; in dogs (and humans); this tends to present as a dragging of the hind paw (foot). In cats intestinal ileus can occur (see above).

Cyclophosphamide

Hemorrhagic cystitis secondary to cyclophosphamide therapy is rare in cats (estimated as 3–4% of all cats receiving cyclophosphamide). If it does occur, discontinuation of cyclophosphamide at an early stage is important as the damage is cumulative and may become irreversible. There is no effective treatment other than symptomatic pain relief and the administration of anti-inflammatory medication.

CHEMOTHERAPY FOR SPECIFIC TUMOR TYPES

As previously stated, there are many single case reports that mention or claim efficacy of a drug against a tumor type; these cannot be taken as a good evidence base for speculative use of anti-cancer agents. Extrapolating from human and dog, there are some tumors that almost certainly will not be treatable in cats with the conventional anti-cancer drugs; for example, adenocarcinomas arising from liver, kidney, gastrointestinal structures and pancreas, and melanomas. Again extrapolating from humans and dog there is another list where efficacy at best is likely to be minimal: these include transitional cell carcinoma (TCC) of the bladder, brain, lung, and oral cavity. An in-depth discussion on the benefit of chemotherapy for every feline tumor type is beyond the scope of this book so the reader is directed to the specific medical oncology literature for an in-depth discussion; or they should seek specialist advice.

Lymphoid malignancies

A variety of chemotherapeutic regimes have been used for treatment of lymphoma in cats.[8-11] The intermediate to high grade lymphoblastic lymphomas seen in cats are in the main responsive to the anti-cancer protocols combining cyclophosphamide, vincristine, and prednisolone; the so-called 'COP' protocol (Table 16-4). There is no evidence of benefit in the addition of doxorubicin to a COP protocol in cats.[11]

Low grade, small T-cell lymphoma of the intestine responds poorly to the COP or single-agent doxorubicin therapy, but by using a metronomic chemotherapeutic approach with chlorambucil and prednisolone, many cats can achieve good, albeit partial remissions that can be durable (more than two years) with minimal risk of side effects.[5]

Feline mammary adenocarcinoma

Mammary cancer in cats is aggressive both locally and also with regards to metastatic spread. By the time that mammary tumors are detected multiple glands are often involved. Radical mastectomy as a full mammary strip unilaterally or as a staged bilateral procedure is recommended (Chapter 21). The use of doxorubicin as adjuvant therapy or as palliative sole therapy has been described but the overall benefit is unfortunately low.[12,13]

Table 16-4 'COP' protocols

	Dose	Comments
Low dose		
Vincristine	0.5 mg/m² IV	Weekly for four to eight weeks, then monthly
Cyclophosphamide	150 mg/m² PO total weekly dose[a]	As 50 mg tablets PO[a] (see below)
Prednisolone	20 mg/m² PO	Daily for seven days then eod
High dose		
Vincristine	0.75 mg/m² IV	Weekly for four weeks, then every three weeks
Cyclophosphamide	250–300 mg/m² IV	Every three weeks
Prednisolone	40 mg/m² reducing to 20 mg/m² PO	Daily for seven days, then reduce dose and frequency

[a]Cyclophosphamide tablets only routinely available as 50 mg and MUST NOT be broken, crushed or divided. To achieve correct oral dosing adjust the interval accordingly to achieve 150 mg/m² total weekly dose. For example:

Cat weighs 3.0 kg, BSA = 0.208 m² × 150 mg/m² = 31 mg required per week = 50 mg every ten days

Cat weighs 5.5 kg, BSA = 0.310 m² × 150 mg/m² = 46 mg required per week = 50 mg every seven days

IV, intravenous; PO, per os; eod, every other day.

Vaccine-associated feline sarcoma

Vaccine-associated feline sarcomas (or feline injection site sarcomas) are very aggressive locally and should be treated at an early stage with aggressive surgery. Beyond this the success of surgery and other modalities is limited. Chemotherapy has been tried for non-resectable lesions with some increase in survival times associated with partial remission.[13] Doxorubicin (or epirubicin) has been described in the neoadjuvant setting to reduce the size of the sarcoma prior to wide excision and then as an adjuvant postsurgery to reduce local recurrence rates[14–16] and this should be considered in such cases.

Intralesional cisplatin emulsion for squamous cell carcinoma

Cisplatin as an emulsion in sesame seed oil has been used intralesionally for some advanced carcinomas of the head in cats (also in dogs and horses). Tumor control has been demonstrated and there may be additional benefit combining this technique with external beam radiation. However, the production of a stable emulsion is essential otherwise rapid release of cisplatin into the extracellular fluid and beyond will have a high risk of fatality. Producing this stable emulsion requires

practice and absolutely must be performed in a safety cabinet for the protection of personnel. It is considered a specialist procedure and its use in general practice cannot be recommended.

Other chemotherapy agents and protocols

The **tyrosine kinase inhibitors** (TKIs) are the first of an exciting new 'targeted' approach. In addition to the human drug imatinib there are two rTKIs, masitinib and toceranib, which have veterinary licenses for use in dogs with mast cell tumors. Clinical trials of these drugs in various cancers in cats are underway, but until these studies are completed and published it remains to be seen whether tyrosine kinase inhibitors will play a significant role in feline oncology.

SAFE HANDLING OF CYTOTOXIC AGENTS

Anti-cancer drugs are toxic and have potentially serious implications for human health. Some of the drugs work by damaging DNA; such damage is mutagenic and therefore potentially teratogenic or even carcinogenic. Other drugs can cause infertility, tissue damage, and cancer. Accordingly, all veterinary staff, owners, and carers must be aware of the need for safe handling of anti-cancer drugs (Box 16-6).

Although there is no known safe limit for exposure, the low doses used in cats mean the potential risk to veterinary staff, carers, and owners is low. However, this is not a reason for complacency.

Protection involves avoidance of contamination—appropriate gloves, over-clothes, eye protection, and mask are the minimum when handling the drugs. The reader should refer to their health and safety advisor for specific guidance. The guidelines produced by ECVIM-CA give an overview of recommended safe handling of cytotoxic drugs[17] but referral to a centre experienced in veterinary oncology and drug handling may be the preferred option.

Box 16-6 Exposure routes for cytotoxic drugs

Exposure to cytotoxic drugs can occur by:
- Inhalation of powder or aerosol
- Ingestion of drug on contaminated food or cigarettes
- Absorption through skin or ocular membranes
- Accidental inoculation (needlestick)

Exposure may be a result of:
- Transfer of drug between containers using an unguarded needle and by stab injury
- Breaking open glass ampoules
- Aerosol from pressurized drug vials when withdrawing needle
- Expulsion of air bubbles from drug-filled syringe
- Accidental spillage or breakage of drug vials
- Exposure to excreta and body fluids (including saliva on hair coat) from treated patient
- Crushing or breakage of tablets or capsules

REFERENCES

1. Ogilvie GK, Moore AS. Feline Oncology. New Jersey, USA: Veterinary Learning Systems; 2001.

2. Withrow SJ, Vail DM. Small Animal Clinical Oncology. 4th ed. St Louis, Missouri: Saunders Elsevier; 2007.

3. Dobson JM, Lascelles BDX. Manual of Canine and Feline Oncology. 3rd ed. Gloucester: BSAVA; 2011.

4. Argyle DJ, Brearley MJ, Turek MM. Decision Making in Small Animal Oncology. Iowa: Wiley-Blackwell; 2008.

5. Kisseberth WC, Vail DM, Yaissle J, et al. Phase 1 clinical evaluation of carboplatin in tumor-bearing cats: a Veterinary Cooperative Oncology Group study. J Vet Int Med 2008;22:83–8.

6. Fan TM, Kitchell BE, Dhaliwal RS, et al. Hematological toxicity and therapeutic efficacy of lomustine in 20 tumor-bearing cats: critical assessment of a practical dosing regimen. J Am Anim Hosp Assoc 2002;38:357–63.

7. Knapp DW, Richardson RC, DeNicola DB, et al. Cisplatin toxicity in cats. J Vet Int Med 1987;1:29–35.

8. Ettinger SN. Principles of treatment for feline lymphoma. Clin Tech Small Anim Pract 2003;18:98–102.

9. Kristal O, Lana SE, Ogilvie GK, et al. Single agent chemotherapy with doxorubicin for feline lymphoma: a retrospective study of 19 cases (1994–1997). J Vet Int Med 2001;15:125–30.

10. Simon D, Eberle N, Laacke-Singer L, Nolte I. Combination chemotherapy in feline lymphoma: treatment outcome, tolerability, and duration in 23 cats. J Vet Int Med 2008;22:394–400.

11. Teske E, van Straten G, van Noort R, Rutteman GR. Chemotherapy with cyclophosphamide, vincristine, and prednisolone (COP) in cats with malignant lymphoma: new results with an old protocol. J Vet Int Med 2002;16:179–86.

12. Novosad CA, Bergman PJ, O'Brien MG, et al. Retrospective evaluation of adjunctive doxorubicin for the treatment of feline mammary gland adenocarcinoma: 67 cases. J Am Anim Hosp Assoc 2006;42:110–20.

13. McNeill CJ, Sørenmo KU, Shofer FS, et al. Evaluation of adjuvant doxorubicin-based chemotherapy for the treatment of feline mammary carcinoma. J Vet Int Med 2009;23:123–9.

14. Barber LG, Sørenmo KU, Cronin KL, Shofer FS. Combined doxorubicin and cyclophosphamide chemotherapy for nonresectable feline fibrosarcoma. J Am Anim Hosp Assoc 2000;36:416–21.

15. Bregazzi VS, LaRue SM, McNiel E, et al. Treatment with a combination of doxorubicin, surgery, and radiation versus surgery and radiation alone for cats with vaccine-associated sarcomas: 25 cases (1995–2000). J Am Vet Med Assoc 2001;218:547–50.

16. Martano M, Morello E, Ughetto M, et al. Surgery alone versus surgery and doxorubicin for the treatment of feline injection-site sarcomas: a report on 69 cases. Vet J 2005;170:84–90.

17. ECVIM-CA Guidelines: Preventing occupational and environmental exposure to cytotoxic drugs in veterinary medicine. http://www.ecvim-ca.org/index.php?option=com_content&view=article&id=72&Itemid=70

Section | 4 |

J.L. Demetriou, S.J. Langley-Hobbs

Skin and adnexa

Cats have abundant loose skin over their body, which aids reconstructive surgery, but there are some anatomic differences and healing properties that are unique to the cat. The clinical relevance of these is described in the first chapter on wound healing. Cats are prone to trauma, from road traffic accidents to cat bite abscesses and axillary injuries from collars. Management of these wounds, including some unusual cryptic and chronic infections that are peculiar to the cat, are described in the subsequent chapter. Some wounds in cats benefit from surgical treatment with flaps or grafts and these are well described with surgical boxes for each procedure.

In the following three chapters, conditions affecting the feline skin and adnexal structures are covered in detail. There are separate chapters on skin tumors, mammary glands, and a final chapter on injection site sarcomas, which can be a particularly problematic condition to manage. This final chapter provides a thorough review of all the literature on this unusual feline problem and comparisons of treatment regimes including surgical resection and adjunctive chemotherapy and radiation.

Chapter 17

Wound healing

M.W. Bohling

There are some fundamental differences in wound healing in cats compared to other species. This chapter will summarize the biology of wound healing, the results of the studies on wound healing in cats, and discuss its clinical relevance.

INTRODUCTION AND OVERVIEW OF WOUND HEALING

Wound healing is the biological process whereby a discontinuity in the tissue is repaired so that function may be restored. With few exceptions the repair takes the form of a scar, rather than regeneration of the exact same as the damaged tissue. Thus the fundamental difference between wound healing (repair) and regeneration is the production of scar tissue, and the study of wound healing is in fact the study of the process of scar formation and remodeling.

Very early in the study of wound healing it was observed that wounds progress through stages: the initial phase of inflammation, followed by the phase of active proliferation (repair), and finally after the defect is closed, the phase of remodeling. Although once thought to be temporally distinct, we now understand that the phases of wound healing occur as a highly overlapping sequence of processes. We can recognize each of the phases in the healing of wounds in all vertebrates, and the phases follow the same chronological order, leading to the assumption that wound healing is more or less homogeneous across species lines, at least among mammals.[1]

Clinical experience reveals that there are significant differences in wound healing between mammalian species. Recently, significant differences between cutaneous healing in the cat and the dog have been described.[2] These differences may cause us to reconsider the validity of long-accepted general small animal wound care recommendations when they are applied to the feline species.

NORMAL CUTANEOUS ANATOMY IN THE CAT

The normal cutaneous anatomy and histology of the cat follows the same general pattern as for other mammalian species. However, interspecies variations in feline cutaneous anatomy and histology may have significant effects on wound healing and other surgical considerations in regard to felines. As with all haired mammals, the epidermis of the cat is much thinner than that of humans, and is slightly thinner than that of the dog. The dermis comprises the majority of the thickness of the skin; it ranges from 0.4–2.0 mm thick in the cat, depending on body location. Like the epidermis, the feline dermis is somewhat thinner than the canine dermis, which ranges from 0.5–5.0 mm thick.[3] The thickness of the subcutis varies greatly with body area and body condition; however, in general the subcutis of the cat is also significantly thinner than the dog. Another feature of feline skin is that the feline skin is very pliable and mobile over most of the body surface, even more so than in the dog, and certainly much more so than for 'tight-skinned' species such as the pig and humans.

Cats also show significant differences from other mammals with respect to their cutaneous vascular supply. In one comparative study, the cutaneous angiosomes of seven mammalian species were evaluated with the purpose of validating the use of animal models for human wound healing research. Comparison of the cutaneous angiosomes of the cat with other mammals revealed that the cat has a relatively low density of tertiary and higher-order vessels, particularly on the trunk.[4] This gross anatomic difference appears to translate to a functional difference based on laser Doppler perfusion studies, in which a significantly lower level of cutaneous perfusion was noted in the trunk skin of normal anesthetized cats than in dogs.[2] The link between tissue perfusion and wound healing has been well established.[5,6]

WOUND HEALING IN CATS

Wound healing can be divided into first intention, i.e., the healing of clean, sutured skin incisions, and second intention healing, i.e., the healing of gaping wounds.

First intention cutaneous healing

First intention cutaneous healing (the healing of clean, sutured skin wounds) has been measured in the cat as part of an overall comparison of cutaneous healing between cats and dogs. Healing of 3 cm

DOI: 10.1016/B978-0-7020-4336-9.00017-2

Table 17-1 Measures of second intention healing in cats compared with dogs

	Cats			Dogs		
	Day 7	Day 14	Day 21	Day 7	Day 14	Day 21
% Contraction	18.2[a]	53.0	75.8	41.2	66.1	70.3
% Epithelialization	0.0	13.0*	34.4[a]	3.2	44.7	89.4
% Total wound healing	18.3[a]	59.0*	83.9[a]	43.1	76.1	97.6

[a]Indicates a significant difference between cats and dogs for the indicated parameter on that day; ($p \leq 0.05$, repeated measures ANOVA)

linear sutured wounds was evaluated via tensiometry at seven days post-wounding. Results demonstrated that the wound breaking strength in healing cat skin is significantly inferior to that of dogs. The mean wound breaking strength for sutured wounds in cats at seven days post-wounding was only one half of the wound breaking strength for dogs.[2] This difference should be taken into consideration when deciding the right time for suture removal. Histologic evaluation of skin biopsies revealed that the observed difference in early first intention healing correlated with significantly lower collagen production in cat wounds compared to those in dogs.[7]

Second intention cutaneous healing

Significant qualitative and quantitative differences between cats and dogs have also been seen in second intention healing. Observable differences begin in the early inflammatory phase of wound healing. On the second day of healing, open wounds in cats have been observed to be relatively less swollen and edematous, and to have a lesser amount of wound fluid produced when compared to similar wounds in dogs.

Interestingly, the grossly observed differences in apparent level of inflammation in open wounds do not correlate well with histopathologic evidence. Based on extensive histologic evaluation of open wound healing in cats and dogs, the picture that has emerged is one of similar levels of inflammatory cell infiltration in the first week of wound healing. However, as healing progresses, the populations of inflammatory cells, (particularly neutrophilic leukocytes and mast cells) in cat wounds appear to remain elevated for a longer period of time (Fig. 17-1 and Table 17-1).[7] This observation supports other experimental and clinical evidence that, in the feline, the inflammatory phase of healing appears to follow a more chronic course compared to other species. The chronicity of inflammation in cat wound healing may in turn be at least partly responsible for delayed onset and slower progression of the proliferative phase of healing.

The production of granulation tissue in the wound is the first gross and histologic evidence of entry into the proliferative or repair phase of wound healing. The cat is notable for a slower rate of production of granulation tissue in open wounds, when compared to other mammals. On average, the first appearance of grossly visible granulation tissue in open wounds in cats and dogs begins at a similar time although is usually about one day later in cats than in dogs. However, once the process of granulation begins, the rate of granulation tissue production is markedly slower in cats. In an experimental model of open wound healing, cats took more than twice as long as dogs to fill the wound cavity with granulation tissue: 19 days for cats vs 7.5 days for dogs (Table 17-2).[2]

The visual character of the granulation tissue also differs between cats and dogs, with the granulation tissue of dogs having a deep red color and that of cats being much paler in comparison. Furthermore, even the original site of granulation tissue is different in the open wounds of cats. Granulation tissue in open wounds of cats appears to

Table 17-2 Inflammatory cell changes in wound healing: cats compared to dogs

		Neutrophils	Macrophages	Mast cells
Day 7	Cats	52	58.6	3.3
	Dogs	14	24.8	0.9
Day 21	Cats	51[a]	35.3	5.1[a]
	Dogs	1.5	21.4	1.3
Overall; Days 0–21	Cats	57.5[a]	47.7[a]	4.0[a]
	Dogs	4.5	19.9	1.1

[a]Indicates a significant difference between cats and dogs for the indicated parameter for the specified time; ($p \leq 0.05$, repeated measures ANOVA)

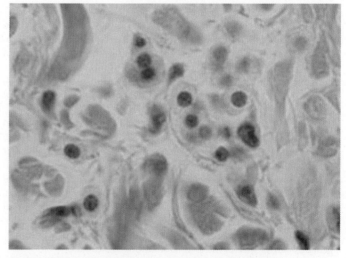

Figure 17-1 Second intention healing in feline skin. Normal uncomplicated healing at 21 days post-wounding. Note the mast cells still present in the wound. (H&E stain, 400× magnification.)

originate at the cut edges of the skin, and then slowly fills in the central part of the wound from the edges. In contrast, granulation tissue develops from the entire surface of the exposed subcutis in the dog (Fig. 17-2).

The aforementioned features of early gross wound appearance and granulation tissue formation in cats are of more than academic interest; in fact they may help explain the slower overall healing rate for open wounds in cats compared to wounds in dogs. The rates of contraction, epithelialization, and total wound healing (overall reduction

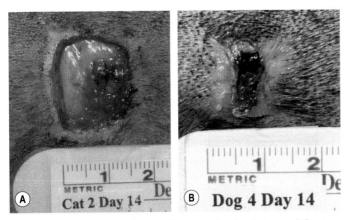

Figure 17-2 Comparison of second intention healing between **(A)** cat and **(B)** dog. The 2 cm × 2 cm open wounds are shown at 14 days post-wounding. Note the relatively smaller amount and paler color of granulation tissue in feline wound and absence of discernable epithelialization at wound margins.

Box 17-1 **The role of the feline subcutis in wound healing**

Removal of the subcutis resulted in no change in the first appearance of granulation tissue, which occurred at about five to six days post-wounding. However, a marked reduction in the rate of production of granulation tissue (time to fill the wound cavity) was noted when the subcutis was excised, and this effect was much greater in cats than in dogs.

Creation of defects in the subcutis resulted in a decrease in cutaneous perfusion that persisted at least until day 14 post-wounding.

The rates of wound contraction and epithelialization were also significantly reduced when the subcutis was removed. As with the rate of granulation tissue production, the negative effect on contraction was significantly more pronounced in cats than in dogs.

in open wound area due to contraction and epithelialization combined) are all significantly slower in cats than in dogs. The currently accepted theory of wound contraction (i.e., the 'pull theory') is that fibroblasts and myofibroblasts within granulation tissue provide the motive power for wound contraction.[8] Therefore, delayed onset and slower rate of accumulation of granulation tissue would be expected to correlate with a slower rate of wound contraction, as seen in the open wounds of cats. Similarly, since granulation tissue provides the substrate for keratinocyte migration during re-epithelialization, a longer time for complete coverage of the wound by granulation tissue should translate into a slower rate of wound epithelialization.

PSEUDOHEALING AND INDOLENT POCKETS

On occasion, routinely managed wounds in cats can have unexpected adverse outcomes. One such outcome is the phenomenon termed 'pseudohealing'. This condition is characterized by a sutured skin incision that initially appears to have healed normally at the time of skin suture removal. However, after suture removal, when the cat places ordinary physiological stress on the closure (e.g., jumping up on a chair), complete dehiscence occurs, usually with little or no bleeding. Examination of these dehisced wounds reveals little if any adhesion of the muscle fascia to the adjacent subcutis.

The skin may heal sufficiently to remain intact when stressed, but if wound re-entry is required (as when a second surgical procedure is required to resect a recurrent neoplasm), it is often found that a chronic pocket has formed in the subcutis. The pocket is lined with mature, smooth collagen and typically contains a thin, serous, modified transudate. This condition has been reported in the veterinary literature in which a granulation tissue-lined pocket forms that fails to contract or fill.[9] The authors termed the condition 'indolent pocket wounds' and hypothesized that this phenomenon occurs when skin has been closed over areas in which the underlying subcutis has been damaged or extensively resected (e.g., major tumor resection).

The role of the subcutis in cutaneous healing

The phenomena of pseudohealing and indolent pocket wounds have led to an interest in, and investigations of, the role of the subcutis in

cutaneous wound healing of cats. In the first of these studies, the role of the subcutis in healing was studied and compared between dogs and cats. Wounds in which the subcutis was completely excised from the wound bed were compared with wounds in which the subcutis was left intact.[10] The comparison of wound healing between treatments and between species has yielded the following observations regarding the role of the subcutis (Box 17-1).

The authors of the study concluded that the subcutis is an important source of precursor cells for granulation tissue and a major contributor to second intention healing. The data did not support a similar direct link between the subcutis and first intention healing, a fact that the authors attributed to a flaw in the study design.[10]

A second study has also examined the role of the subcutis in second intention healing in cats. This work confirmed the findings of the earlier study, i.e., excision of the subcutaneous tissues has a negative impact on wound healing in cats. In the second study, one of three surgical treatments (fascial abrasion, fasciotomy, or fasciectomy) was performed on the open wounds after subcutis removal. The treatments were compared for their ability to ameliorate the negative effects on second intention healing caused by removal of the subcutis. Fasciotomy and fasciectomy increased the rate of granulation tissue formation and were the most successful treatments for restoring wound healing to normal after subcutis removal in cats.[11]

CLINICAL APPLICATION

The clinical applications of our knowledge of feline wound healing are limited, but by no means unimportant. The observation that the seven-day sutured wound strength in cats is only half that in dogs has important implications for feline wound closure and time to suture removal. The mere fact that veterinarians have been closing surgical and natural wounds in cats for a long time does not constitute *a priori* evidence that surgical outcomes would not benefit from special consideration of the feline as a surgical patient. Rather, it may be that incisional dehiscence in cats has been an unrecognized problem that has been incorrectly blamed on characteristics of the individual patient rather than on any inherent weakness or relative indolence in feline cutaneous healing. This may be particularly true in wounds in which a large volume of subcutis has been removed.

Based on our current knowledge of feline cutaneous wound healing, certain recommendations can now be made to improve surgical outcomes and reduce the risk of wound healing complications in cats. For small, uncomplicated wounds, routine apposition of subcutis and skin appears to be sufficient. In cases where complete apposition is not possible, the use of 'tacking' sutures (sutures placed between the

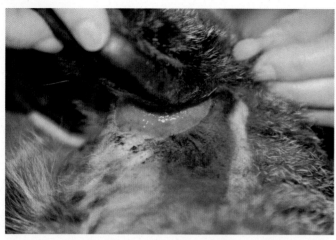

Figure 17-3 An example of an indolent pocket wound in a cat. This chronic axillary wound was observed in a feral cat. Note the deeply under-run wound with somewhat pale chronic granulation tissue lining the pocket, and no adhesion of the walls to each other (hence the formation of an indolent pocket).

subcutis and underlying tissue) would seem a reasonable measure to help ensure adequate skin–subcutis contact and prevent the formation of indolent pocket wounds.

When significant portions of subcutis have been resected, such as one would see with major oncologic resections, extra measures are warranted. The surgical goal should be to ensure a strong and tension-free closure that will provide an extended duration of mechanical support to the coapted wound edges. Specific examples of desirable techniques for these situations may include (but are not limited to) the use of 'walking' sutures, various stenting techniques, multiple layer closures, and slight eversion of the skin (to maximize the surface area of dermal–to–dermal contact). Combinations of factors detrimental to healing can be expected to further increase the overall risk of undesirable outcomes such as pseudohealing or indolent pocket formation. Such conditions exist when substantial resection of subcutis is anticipated and the wound is located in an area of high motion such as the axilla or groin (Fig. 17-3). For these situations, postoperative closed suction drainage and wound immobilization may be beneficial.

When dealing with any chronic wound, the establishment or maintenance of perfusion and an adequate supply of wound healing precursor cells is essential to healing. Often the best success in treating chronic wounds in cats has been achieved with compound flaps that include the subcutis. These flaps supply perfusion from the included capillary subdermal plexus, and wound healing cells in the form of fibroblasts and/or fibroblast precursors. Perhaps even better would be myocutaneous transfer, due to the enhanced blood supply. Though beyond the technical capabilities of most practices, microvascular free tissue transfer provides another option to stimulate healing of chronic wounds in feline patients via improvement in local perfusion.

Finally, it should also be noted that not all of the unique features of feline wound healing are necessarily detrimental to the patient. In particular, wounds and conditions that are characterized by an extensive or excessive inflammatory response may actually heal more rapidly and with fewer complications in feline patients. For example, it has long been generally accepted among veterinary oncologists that feline patients usually recover much more rapidly from the cutaneous effects of radiation therapy than dogs do. The post-radiation therapy inflammatory reaction is usually quite intense when a full course of therapy is administered; therefore it may well be that the overall less exuberant inflammatory response to wounding seen in cats is a likely factor in their more favorable post-radiation treatment outcomes. Another example of favorable healing in cats involves the process of engraftment or 'take' after skin graft placement. The general consensus among veterinary surgeons is that the engraftment process is usually more rapid and complete, with a lower likelihood of complications in feline patients compared to canine patients. The superior engraftment properties of feline skin are probably due to a combination of anatomical and physiologic features of feline skin (Box 17-2).

It was not that long ago when veterinarians began to fully appreciate the feline species and to understand that in regard to the treatment of medical conditions 'cats are not small dogs'. In the same way, optimum surgical care of cats requires knowledge of the unique features of feline cutaneous anatomy and wound healing physiology, and a willingness to allow this knowledge to influence the practice of surgery as applied to our feline patients.

REFERENCES

1. Fretz PB. Traumatic and incisional wounds: how they heal. In: Proc 18th Annual Surgical Forum American College of Veterinary Surgeons. Chicago; 1990. p. 25–7.

2. Bohling MW, Henderson RA, Swaim SF, et al. Cutaneous wound healing in the cat: a macroscopic description and comparison with cutaneous wound healing in the dog. Vet Surg 2004;33: 579–87.

3. Affolter VK, Moore PF. Histologic features of normal canine and feline skin. Clin Dermatol 1994;12:491–7.

4. Taylor GI, Minabe T. The angiosomes of the mammals and other vertebrates. Plast Recon Surg 1992;89:181–215.

5. Jonsson K, Jensen JA, Goodson WH 3rd, et al. Tissue oxygenation, anemia, and perfusion in relation to wound healing in surgical patients. Ann Surg 1991;214: 605–13.

6. Hartmann M, Jönsson K, Zederfeldt B. Effect of tissue perfusion and oxygenation on accumulation of collagen in healing wounds. Eur J Surg 1992;158: 521–6.

7. Bohling MW. Cutaneous wound healing in the cat: a macroscopic and histologic description and comparison with cutaneous wound healing in the dog. PhD dissertation. Auburn University; 2007.

8. Rudolph R, Vande Berg J, Ehrlich HP, et al. Wound contraction and scar contracture. In: Cohen IK, Diegelmann RF, Lindblad WJ, editors. Wound healing: Biochemical and clinical aspects. Philadelphia: WB Saunders; 1992. p. 96–114.

9. Lascelles BD, Davison L, Dunning M, et al. Use of omental pedicle grafts in the management of nonhealing axillary wounds in 10 cats. J Small Anim Pract 1998;39:475–80.

10. Bohling MW, Henderson RA, Swaim SF, et al. Comparison of the role of the subcutaneous tissues in cutaneous wound healing in the dog and cat. Vet Surg 2006;35:1–12.

11. Mitsui A, Mathews KG, Linder KE, et al. Effects of fascial abrasion, fasciotomy, and fascial excision on cutaneous wound healing in cats. Am J Vet Res 2009;70:532–8.

Chapter 18

Wounds and wound management

D.M. Anderson, S.J. Langley-Hobbs

Wound management has been a developing field for thousands of years, with the earliest records dating from ancient Egypt citing remedies of honey, resin, and grease for open wounds. However, it is only in the last 40 years that the role of moist wound healing and the complex interactions of growth factors and vascular supply have become accepted. Wound healing in the cat has unique characteristics (Chapter 17) and this has implications for wound management.[1-3] In general, the principle of more rapid healing in a moist environment is now widely accepted for wound management protocols in all species.

The principles of wound management should revolve around a clear understanding of wound healing in cats. The gross appearance of the different stages of wound healing is important in decision making, as is the recognition of an inflamed wound, a chronic wound, or an infected wound. Direct comparison with wounds seen in other species is unhelpful as cats tend to have paler wounds, when compared with dogs, for example, and the skin and granulation tissue layers are thinner and more fragile. Progression of the wound is slower and responses to wound healing stimulants may be less brisk than seen in the dog (Chapter 17).

Other unique difficulties are found when trying to manage cats with wound dressings. Cats may be distressed by or intolerant of heavy dressings. They may be reluctant to use a litter tray and frequently soil the bandage. Hospitalized cats are often reluctant to eat and this causes problems when trying to maintain nutritional requirements in the face of daily sedation or anesthesia for dressing changes.

HISTORY

Cats are usually very fastidious about grooming and cautious about investigating objects that could cause harm. However, young cats are more likely to injure themselves in road traffic accidents, fall through trees, or be attacked by dogs or other cats. Occasionally, malicious injury is seen when cats present with burns, elastic band induced necrosis of extremities, or ballistic injury. Owners rarely see the accident and the typical history is that the cat returned to the house with the injury, or was found near the house. Close examination of the cat may provide information as to the type of injury and from there the

history can be extrapolated. The etiology of wound types and formation in cats is summarized in Table 18-1.

INITIAL ASSESSMENT AND WOUND MANAGEMENT

A full clinical examination is always necessary; if there is little information as to how the cat has been injured, this is the best way to determine the type of wound and thus ascertain the likely prognosis and appropriate treatment and also to identify further, more serious co-morbidities. It is important not to be distracted by the wound itself but to complete a full physical examination.

A minimum database would involve thoracic auscultation, abdominal palpation, temperature, pulse, respiration, determination of shock, dehydration and a base line packed cell volume/total protein, electrolytes, blood urea nitrogen (BUN) and creatinine. Cats frequently present some time after the original injury, so are often dehydrated on presentation, making interpretation of blood results and assessment of blood loss or electrolyte disorders such as hypokalemia difficult. A minimum hematology and serum biochemistry database is helpful in order to determine the general condition and ancillary disorders that require treatment as well as the wound. Older cats may have previously unrecognized diseases detected at this time, but this should not necessarily preclude treatment of the wounds/injuries. For example, elevated BUN/creatinine results should be interpreted with caution until it is clear whether this is renal or pre-renal in origin. Neurologic examination is carried out if the cat is unable to stand or has deep injuries over or near the spinal column or major peripheral nerves. This is particularly important when it is expected that distal limbs will be bandaged, as determination of neurologic deficits may be important to the prognosis, but difficult to recognize once the cat is bandaged. Furthermore, as subsequent dressing changes may be carried out under anesthesia or sedation, an accurate determination of neurologic status may be difficult at a later date. Thoracic radiographs should also be taken to rule out diaphragmatic rupture, pulmonary contusion, or pleural hemorrhage. On admission, a record is made of the location of the wound and associated injuries together with an accurate description of the condition of the wound. This

DOI: 10.1016/B978-0-7020-4336-9.00018-4

Table 18-1 Wound types and etiologies

Type	Comment
Traumatic	
Shear	Skin loss with underlying tissue loss, often the extremities, which may indicate joint instability or bone loss. Usually heavily contaminated
Avulsion	Skin loss with little underlying tissue loss or damage. Skin may lie back down onto the underlying tissues and initially appear normal despite devascularization
Degloving	Skin loss at the extremities resulting in a circumferential deficit. This is problematic as it cannot contract to heal by second intention and fibrous strictures can result
Laceration	Skin wound with little lateral trauma from the wound. Variable depth, generally little associated tissue damage
Puncture wound	Classic example is cat or dog bite wounds. In the cat, there is potential for deep seated infection and abscessation, or introduction of sepsis into a body cavity causing pyothorax or peritonitis
Ballistic	The damage caused is dependent on the speed and distance of the missile. Soft nosed bullets may 'tumble' on impact and cause widespread damage. Fragments may spread over a wide area underneath the point of impact. Great risk of organ injury
Crush injury	There may be little damage on the skin surface, but underlying organ and muscle damage may be difficult to determine at initial examination. Severe muscle necrosis can have renal consequences
Abrasion	Partial thickness injury with dermal retention, but contamination and denuding of epidermis. Injuries generally heal well, but may cause significant fluid loss if large areas affected. Can be extremely painful. Cats have thin, loosely attached skin and are less likely to suffer these injuries
Skin loss	
Heat/chemical burns	Heat pad burns, malicious injury, extravasation of intravenous medication. The extent of the damage may not be apparent for several days until the skin necrosis is complete
Skin sloughing secondary to necrosis or vasculitis	Unusual acute onset skin loss may be associated with generalized immune mediated vasculitis, drug eruption, venomous bite (e.g., snake/insect bite). The cat may be very depressed due to the systemic effects; skin slough caused by vasculitis may be associated with systemic disorders such as coagulopathy, hypotension, pyrexia, etc. Skin loss depends on type of bite and mechanism of actions. Renal failure can occur secondary to immune complex deposition or secondary to the underlying cause and should be treated aggressively
Chronic wounds	
Fistula/sinus/foreign body tracts	Chronic wounds in cats are not common. Migration of foreign bodies is unusual due to fastidious grooming habits, but may be more common in young cats that are more curious (e.g., sewing needles). Cat bites into the perineal area can cause fistula formation due to penetration of the rectum and heavy contamination of the puncture tract. Bony sequestra or bullet fragments may result in non-healing sinus tracts
Physiologic	
Pressure sore/ulceration	Cats are rarely heavy enough to suffer from pressure sores on recumbency, but skin loss and ulceration can occur secondary to skin thinning and poor repair secondary to hyperadrenocorticism
Frostbite/Sunburn	Usually cats are good at protecting themselves against extreme weather, but where cats have been trapped out of doors, they may suffer skin loss of extremities, especially the pinnae
Iatrogenic	
Surgical wound dehiscence	Cats have thin skin and usually heal well after primary repair, although some data suggests they heal slower than dogs. Wound dehiscence usually occurs secondary to tension, poor suture technique, infection, self-trauma or poor vascularization of the skin edges. Specific areas such as inguinal and axillary wounds may be prone to dehiscence due to movement. These areas may require special reconstruction techniques to be successfully healed. Abdominal wound dehiscence can be treated successfully with prompt intervention[4]
Tourniquet injuries	Malicious tourniquet injuries may be seen when elastic material is tied around extremities causing necrosis. Improper bandage application or management may also result in skin loss due to a tourniquet effect on the limb

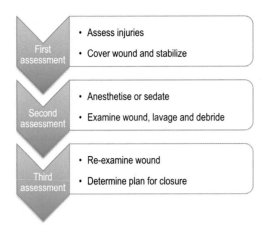

Figure 18-1 A flow diagram illustrating the plan for wound management.

enables objective monitoring of wounds that may continue to progress after treatment has started, due to poor vascular supply. A dated photographic record of the wound should be made in the case of suspected malicious or ballistic wounds. Generally, wounds can be assessed in three stages (Fig. 18-1). These stages may all occur within a few hours, or within days, depending on the nature of the wounds and injuries.

Initial treatment of the wounded cat

All cases showing signs of shock that present with a traumatic injury should be treated appropriately (see Chapter 1). Supplemental oxygen should be provided during handling in the dyspneic patient until the possibility of associated thoracic injury has been ruled out. Hypothermia is a common finding on initial presentation, partly due to shock, but also if the cat has been collapsed outside for a period of time. This will need appropriate management and gradual warming by the use of heat pads, water beds, warming IV fluids, wheat bags, bubble wrap, space blankets, and so on (see Chapter 4).

Analgesics should be initiated immediately on admission, regardless of patient status. This improves patient handling and prevents further 'wind up' of the pain pathways prior to wound management.[5]

First aid treatment of the wound

All wounds are potentially contaminated, either with environmental or endogenous bacteria. However, they are also susceptible to colonization with nosocomial bacteria from the hospital environment or from the owner and staff handling the animal. Cats with open wounds should be handled with gloves and procedures to prevent cross-contamination before and after handling should be in place. On admission, wounds should be immediately covered with a waterproof soft dressing to prevent colonization of the wound with hospital-acquired bacteria prior to definitive treatment. A sterile non-adherent dressing covered with a bandage will suffice, or a waterproof sterile drape may be used for the first one to two hours after admission. The cat is then stabilized prior to a definitive examination of the wound.

Definitive wound assessment

The wound is assessed more thoroughly once the cat is comfortable and can be safely sedated or anesthetized. At this stage, the first aid bandage is removed using gloves, with the surface of the examination table cleaned and covered with a disposable surface (e.g., incontinence

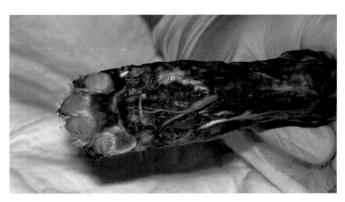

Figure 18-2 This cat presented 24 hours after injury and the digital pads were clearly cyanotic, indicating very poor peripheral perfusion. The foot was cold to touch but the cat was normothermic.

pad). This is important to prevent nosocomial colonization of the wound as well as contamination of the hospital environment with bacteria from the cat. The fur should be carefully clipped away from the edge of the wound, using sterile scissors at the wound edge and fine blade clippers in unaffected areas. It is important to clip a wide area to facilitate keeping the area clean and dry and to be able to see skin changes around the wound as well as adjacent to it. The wound can be protected from loose hair by filling with sterile aqueous jelly that can be easily lavaged away.

The clinical records should list minimum information regarding the wound at this stage (Box 18-1). Photographs of the wound are a useful addition to the clinical records. Some dressings come with paper templates with centimeter grading so an approximate drawing can be made of the wound shape and size. The presence of other injuries whether or not directly associated with the wound (e.g., a jaw fracture which may affect the cat's ability to maintain nutrition during the period of treatment) should also be noted in the patient's record. Sterile instruments are used to investigate the wound, lifting skin flaps and gently probing penetrating injuries. This may prompt further diagnostic procedures such as radiography or ultrasound to determine the involvement of deeper structures. For example, a penetrating injury over the thoracic skin should be carefully assessed to ensure that pleural contamination or injury is not missed.

Assessment of the vascular supply to peripheral injuries can be difficult; although angiography is the definitive way to determine the viability of arterial supply to the distal limb, often animals with this level of injury are not suitable candidates for long procedures under anesthesia, and intravenous contrast agents are contraindicated in cats where the systemic circulation is compromised in any way. Thus assessment of vascular supply often relies on clinical acumen and non-invasive techniques: feeling the toes for warmth, palpating distal pulses, using color flow ultrasound or Doppler detection of blood flow. Visual assessment of the color of non-pigmented pads and needle pinpricks can also be used to assess bleeding (Fig. 18-2). However, the clinician should be aware that extremities will appear cold and pale in cats with shock or hypothermia, and clinical examination should be repeated regularly as resuscitation proceeds. Needle

1. All wounds should be lavaged during and after assessment. The only suitable fluid for lavage, regardless of the degree of contamination, is warm sterile isotonic fluid. The fluid should be sprayed gently into the wound using an 18G needle, ensuring that the pressure does not drive foreign material into the wound, nor cause edema of healthy tissue (Fig. 18-3)

2. Large pieces of foreign material or fascia contaminated with foreign material may be removed or sharply dissected using sterile instruments. Debridement continues at each dressing change until all contaminated or non-viable tissue has been removed (Fig. 18-4A-C)

3. Viable skin flaps may be retained at the first dressing change, but skin that is thin and avascular should be resected, even if this means more open wound is uncovered (Fig. 18-4D)

4. Penetrating injuries should be surgically explored under sterile conditions once the overlying contamination has been removed. Care should be taken with wounds overlying the thorax and abdomen in case the injury enters a body cavity (for example, the anesthetist should be prepared to provide positive pressure ventilation)

5. After lavage a swab is taken for culture and sensitivity in order to direct future decisions regarding antibiotic choice

6. The injury is then re-bandaged pending the next assessment of the wound or definitive closure

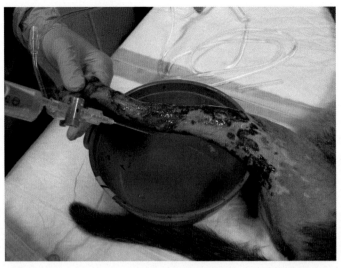

Figure 18-3 Lavage of a wound in a cat with sterile isotonic fluids, using a giving set attached to a three-way tap and a syringe with an 18G needle.

pinpricks should also be interpreted with caution in these circumstances and bleeding due to venous stasis or coagulopathy may be misleading. Needle pinpricks can also introduce infection into healthy tissue.

Each type of wound involves different challenges in terms of assessment, as the risks are inherently different depending on the nature of the injury. In simple lacerations, the tissue is often clearly viable but it is not always easy to determine the degree of damage below the surface and it is very important to assess the possibility of injuries to the underlying tendons and joints in distal limb injuries. However, burns, abrasions, avulsions or crush injuries may involve widespread damage to the skin that is delayed and not obvious on the initial presentation.

Initial wound management

The initial plan of management (Box 18-2) allows time for the full extent of the injury to be assessed prior to establishing a treatment plan, while ensuring that the protocol will not cause more damage.

DAILY WOUND MANAGEMENT

Following first aid and then the initial management, the wound is managed on a daily or as needed basis. Bandages and dressings are often changed daily in the early stages of wound management and then the frequency of changes is reduced according to the contamination and progression of healing. The biggest challenge with open wound management in cats is maintenance of the bandage. Cats tolerate bandages poorly and frequently shake the affected leg or chew at the dressing to try and remove it. Elizabethan, Buster or 'tube' collars may be necessary to maintain the bandage (see Chapter 4), but care should be taken to monitor water and food intake with these collars on. In addition, persistent attempts to remove the bandage may cause

it to slip and then it must be replaced in order to avoid risk of a bandage-related ischemic injury.[6] Hospitalization of cats with wounds ensures close monitoring, but soiling of the bandage due to use of the litter tray or the confined space of the kennel may bring additional challenges.

Sedation or anesthesia for dressing changes is advisable both to reduce the stress and pain for the cat, and also for staff safety. Daily dressing changes can be extremely stressful for both cat and staff if they are done without adequate analgesia. However, this requires careful planning and review of the medications used; regular sedation may result in nausea and inappetence on top of a reluctance to eat in the hospital. Analgesics such as non-steroidal anti-inflammatory drugs (NSAIDs) should not be given on an empty stomach and this makes management of the cat's analgesic protocol more difficult. Nursing staff must weigh the cat daily (taking the dressings into consideration) to monitor any weight loss, and accurate recording of nutritional intake is essential. The aim of the daily management plan should be that the cat is sedated and the dressing changed as early as possible so as to give nursing staff plenty of time during the day to provide the cat with opportunities to eat or be encouraged to do so (see Chapter 6 and 7). Cats that require prolonged wound management may benefit from a feeding tube such as an esophagostomy tube (see Chapter 12). Most of these cases will also benefit from maintenance intravenous fluids for the duration of their treatment, preventing dehydration due to lack of water intake during this period.

A simple mnemonic has been devised by the International Wound Bed Advisory Board,[7] which provides a practical working framework that can be used consistently from one dressing change to the next even if there has been a change in staff. This mnemonic enables consistent wound assessment and treatment plans to be recorded at each dressing change (Box 18-3).

THE BANDAGE

The bandage is constructed of three layers. The primary layer is in contact with the wound and is the layer that most influences the time frame of healing. The secondary and tertiary layers allow protection, absorption, and support of the dressing and prevent any further damage by the animal or the environment. In cats, it is important to

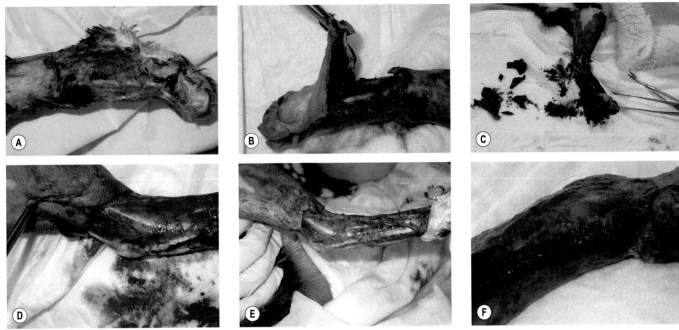

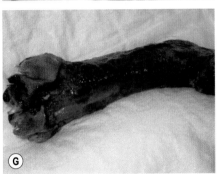

Figure 18-4 The series shows a degloving/avulsion injury at presentation on referral, 24 hours after the injury **(A, B)**. The foot has been incompletely clipped and cleaned and the wound surface is relatively dry. **(C)** During cleaning it became apparent that the plantar skin was avulsed and this skin was sharply debrided using surgical instruments. **(D)** The proximal skin above the hock was also avulsed but as it had a more reliable blood supply, this skin was trimmed but left in situ. **(E)** The wound was dressed with a wet-to-dry dressing and examined under anesthesia the following morning. The proximal skin was found to be healthy and the wound bed showed early signs of granulation. The wound was then dressed with hydrogel under a foam dressing. **(F–G)** Four days later the wound has granulated well and is prepared for full thickness free skin graft.

Box 18-3 **Wound assessment mnemonic used between dressing changes (From the International Wound Bed Advisory Board)**[7]

TIME (tissue; infection, inflammation; moisture; epithelialization) assesses the wound with regard to:

T: The condition of the **t**issue. Necrotic tissue must be debrided, dry tissue must be rehydrated, avascular tissue must be revascularized or debrided

I: Infection or **i**nflammation must be treated. Either treat specifically with antibiotics or non-specifically with saline lavage, antibacterial dressings

M: The level of **m**oisture in the wound. If the tissues are dry, then they may need water delivery in the form of gels or hydrocolloids to maintain tissue humidity. However, exuding wounds will need highly absorbent products to remove exudate, inflammatory fluids from the wound surface, and reduce inflammatory responses as well as maceration of the wound and surrounding skin

E: Ultimately **e**pithelialization results in closure of the wound and healing. Dressings that allow epithelialization to proceed and protect the fragile epithelium from abrasion or desiccation are important in the later stages of wound management

keep these supportive layers as light as possible without compromising security of the bandage. The narrow diameter of cats' limbs, and their thin skin, mean that the bandage must be applied very carefully to prevent ischemic injury.

Primary layer

There are a huge number of primary layer dressings and this makes it confusing for the veterinary surgeon or nurse to know how to apply the principles of wound management to the wound. Nearly all wound dressings have been developed for use in the human market and there is very little objective data on how these dressings perform in cats. Wound dressings can be defined by what they achieve on application to the wound (Table 18-2).[8] There is no perfect wound dressing and many products are able to carry out more than one role. Thus a hydrogel may achieve debridement by enabling autolytic separation of necrotic tissue, but also trap exudate and inflammatory mediators, drawing fluid out of the wound and reducing edema.

Debriding dressings

The single most important step in early wound management is adequate debridement. Not only is this the most effective way to treat infected wounds, but it also prevents infection by removing foreign material and purulent inflammatory exudate, thus preventing the

Table 18-2 Summary of contact layer products for wound dressings

Product type	Examples (not comprehensive)	Action/indications
Polyurethane membranes	Melolin (Smith and Nephew)	A sterile protective surface but does not maintain tissue hydration
Polyurethane foam	Allevyn (Smith and Nephew)	Absorption of fluid from wound surface and controlled evaporation maintaining a humid environment
Hydrogels	Intrasite gel Flexigel (sheet form) (Smith and Nephew)	Rehydration of tissue, absorption of fluid and maintaining a moist environment. May be analgesic if applied cold and may be used combined with other products on the wound surface, e.g., antibacterial drugs, alginates
Hydrocolloid	Granuflex (Convatec)	Water is trapped in the colloid and autolytic debridement is promoted. Debris may be trapped in the colloid gel that is produced on interaction with exudate
Alginates	Kaltostat (Convatec) Tegaderm (3M)	Active stimulation of inflammatory processes in wounds. Must be in a moist environment otherwise may be irritant
Collagens	Biosist (Dechra Veterinary Products)	May improve healing by encouraging fluid flow through the wound and providing a 'scaffold' for granulation tissue
Silver dressings	Acticoat (Smith and Nephew)	Bactericidal and may also stimulate healing
Acemannan	Aloe Vera creams (various)	Stimulation of healing and reduction of inflammatory responses[8]
Honey	Activon (Advancis Medical)	Bactericidal, stimulation of healing, draws fluid through the wound, encourages autolysis

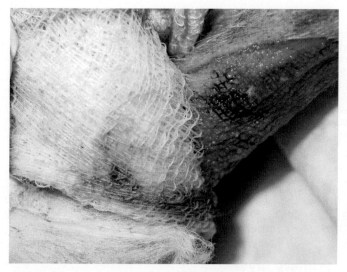

Figure 18-5 A wet-to-dry dressing debrides the wound by pulling exudate and necrotic tissue off the surface at each dressing change. It will also damage healthy granulation tissue.

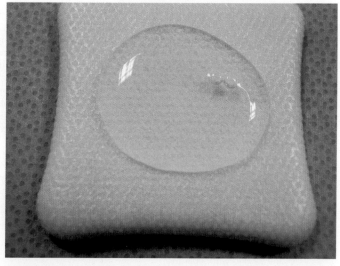

Figure 18-6 A hydrogel in combination with a foam dressing allows gentle debridement, maintenance of a moist but not macerated wound environment and traps exudate and debris in the foam.

perpetuation of inflammatory responses in the wound and encouraging the development of granulation tissue. The most frequently used debriding dressing is the 'wet-to-dry' dressing, where a sterile gauze swab is moistened with sterile isotonic fluid (e.g., Hartmann's solution) and placed onto the wound for 12–24 hours. When the dressing is removed, it pulls away the surface necrotic material, together with trapped exudate and inflammatory mediators (Fig. 18-5). This is a relatively inexpensive and easy treatment for heavily contaminated wounds, but the swabs are painful to remove and few cats will tolerate this dressing change without adequate sedation/analgesia or anesthesia. Wet-to-dry dressings may also damage tissue that is already healthy and in cats may severely damage the thin fragile granulation tissue. Hydrogels can also be used to debride wounds and may be a 'gentler' alternative (Fig. 18-4E). Gels can rehydrate dry necrotic material,

enabling autolytic processes to separate them from the underlying tissue, as well as trap fluid within the gel structure allowing it to be removed from the surface of the wound and flushed away during lavage. Hydrogels are usually applied underneath another dressing (e.g., foam backed with semi-permeable membrane; Fig. 18-6) in order to hold the gel in the wound and prevent desiccation. Cat wounds are rarely very productive and using products that keep the wound moist is important.

Absorbent dressings (Fig. 18-6)

In the management of wounds in human patients, exudation is copious and maintaining fluid balance is a challenge. In cats, however, wounds tend to produce little fluid and although there are occasions

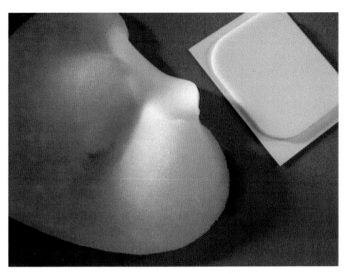

Figure 18-7 A moisture-retaining dressing may play an important role in the cat in maintaining a moist wound environment. This is a hydropolymer dressing showing expansion on contact with fluid. The fluid is retained and maintains a humid environment at the wound surface.

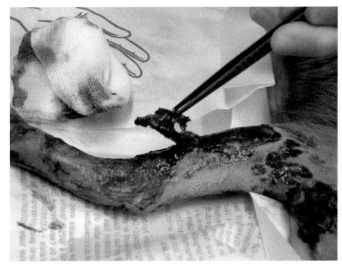

Figure 18-8 Sterile honey was used underneath a foam dressing overnight to facilitate separation of the eschar (necrotic skin) in this cat with a distal shear injury.

where absorption of fluid is necessary, the majority of wounds in cats are more likely to be fairly dry and the challenge is preventing desiccation, rather than maceration. Generally, the foam and absorbent dressings developed for the human market are more than adequate for absorption of the levels of fluid produced in cat wounds. However, using an absorptive dressing with a semi-permeable membrane backing enables the maintenance of a water vapor pressure over the wound environment and this will improve wound surface condition.

Moisture-retaining dressings (Fig. 18-7)

Hydrocolloids, hydrogels, hydroactive are all terms used to describe dressings that have been developed for the human wound market to cope with the challenges associated with chronic distal limb wounds. These products both deliver hydration to wounds and as trap and absorb fluid from the wound, keeping inflammatory mediators off the surface and allowing one-way movement of contaminated exudate out of the wound, without allowing it to dry out. In the cat, moisture-retaining dressings may play a particularly important role in maintaining a moist environment that is most conducive to the development of healthy granulation tissue as well as protecting the epithelialization occurring along the edges of the wound. While it is important to maintain a moist or humid environment, allowing dressings to saturate will result in maceration of the normal surrounding skin as the keratinocytes absorb the excess fluids and slough.

Other categories

There are many miscellaneous wound dressing products that are thought to improve the rate of wound healing, or reduce the incidence of wound infection,[9-11] ranging from nanocrystalline silver, honey, aloe vera, to sterile pathogen-free maggots. It is important to be aware that there is no reported clinical evidence to support the effectiveness of these products in any species, including the cat, and recommendations are based on small series, individual case reports or anecdotal evidence. The products presented here are just a small selection of commercially available dressings that might be useful in the management of wounds in cats.

Honey (Fig. 18-8)

Honey has been used for 5000 years as an effective wound management tool. Medical grade honey is pathogen free and is free from clostridial spores. While honey has an osmotic effect in the wound, drawing fluid through the tissues and reducing bacterial growth, there are also specific antibacterial and anti-inflammatory substances. Debridement of the wound occurs by autolysis and separation of necrotic tissue from viable tissue.[12] In vitro data is available for honey dressing products, but there are no controlled prospective clinical trials in any species. There is no specific data to support honey of any particular origin over another.

Myiasis

Maggots may be used in a controlled way to debride necrotic or non-viable tissue within a wound, using them to digest necrotic material with the secretion of saliva containing a chymotrypsin-like serine protease.[13] They also stimulate fluid production and auto-irrigation of a wound as well as secrete antibacterial substances. Sterile preparations of larvae of the common bluebottle fly (*Lucilia sericata*) are commercially available for use in wounds, with guidelines given as to what quantity is required (www.zoobiotic.co.uk). The larvae are about 2–3 mm long on application, but are 8–10 mm in length two to four days later when they leave the wound seeking a dark dry place to pupate. At this stage, the larvae are removed at the first dressing change and depending on the condition of the wound a second treatment may be used, or the wound may no longer need debridement and other dressings are used (see above). The young larvae are very fragile and must be kept moist for at least 24 hours, but thereafter are more robust. However, maggots may be adversely affected by cytotoxic drugs, and hydrogels appear to reduce larval survival in the wound, so the wound should be thoroughly lavaged prior to each application. The larvae not only secrete enzymes and digest necrotic tissue, but will also ingest and clear multi-drug resistant bacteria from the wound.

Nanocrystalline silver

Silver sulfadiazine cream has long been used for prevention of infection associated with burns and radiation wounds and historically silver vessels were used to make drinking water safe. Modern silver dressings use nanocrystalline silver, which is more labile in the wound and is released more slowly, thus achieving a longer effect.[14] Some studies suggest that there may be improved wound healing in infected chronic wounds and that dressing changes can be reduced.[15] However, while there is established evidence that silver has bactericidal effects, recent data has found silver deposits in distant organs and high serum silver levels that may be toxic, particularly in very small patients such as cats.[16] Bacterial resistance to silver has also been reported, with the acquisition of a *sil* gene.

Vacuum-assisted wound closure (Fig. 18-9)

Controlled negative pressure can be applied to wounds to accelerate the production of granulation tissue and increase exudate removal from the wound surface. Granulation tissue formation is accelerated, but wound contraction and epithelialization may be delayed. This may be a useful approach for very large wounds in locations where it is difficult to maintain dressings, accelerating the formation of granulation tissue and preparing the wound for reconstruction. Vacuum-assisted closure has also been used for complete wound management without reconstruction. In cats, who have loose skin that contracts well, it may be that this technique is more effective than in the distal limb of dogs.[17,18]

WOUND CLOSURE OPTIONS

Surgical closure of wounds results in a more cosmetic final result as well as a more rapid recovery and return to function. However, immediate closure of a wound may be contraindicated and repeat assessment of the wound enables decision making that allows closure of the wound at an appropriate time (Fig. 18-10). There are four options for wound closure (Box 18-4).

BITE WOUNDS

The most common bite wound seen is that from other cats. The injury is different to that seen with wild animal or dog bite wounds, as there is usually very little bruising or crush injury, but a small penetrating wound. Introduction of oral bacteria deep into the underlying tissues usually results in the formation of a painful abscess, the 'cat bite abscess'. Cats present with a history of one to three days of depression,

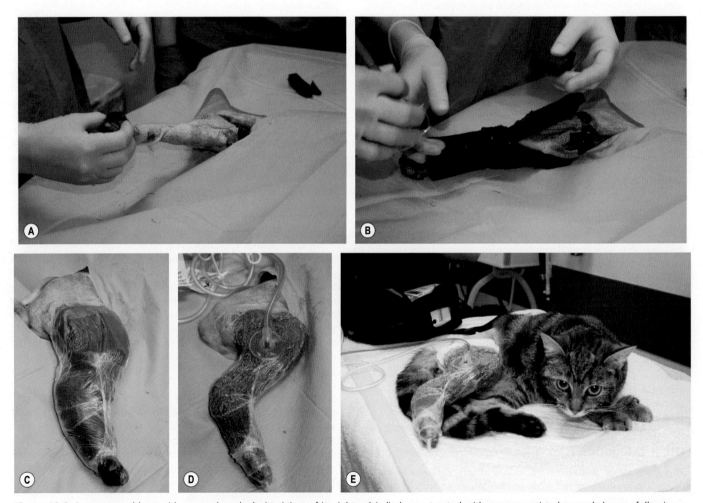

Figure 18-9 A two year old cat with a complete degloving injury of its right pelvic limb was treated with vacuum assisted wound closure, following seven days of standard wound management (combination of surgical debridement and wet-dry dressings). **(A)** Non-adherent paraffin impregnated gauze (Jelonet, Smith & Nephew) is wrapped around the limb, covering the entire wound and preventing injury to exposed blood vessels, nerves and tendons. **(B)** Open-cell polyurethane foam (Smith & Nephew) is cut to fit the shape of the wound and skin staples are used to circumferentially connect the pieces and cover the entire wound area. **(C)** Adhesive, transparent film (Smith & Nephew) is placed over the foam to seal the wound. This is assisted by the application of colostomy tube paste around the proximal wound edge. **(D)** A 2 cm diameter hole is cut in the film and an adhesive suction port (Smith & Nephew) is applied, with the tubing exiting dorsally. **(E)** On recovery from sedation and following application of −80 mmHg pressure, the cat is comfortable with the device, with no attempts at self-trauma. *(Courtesy of Laura Owen.)*

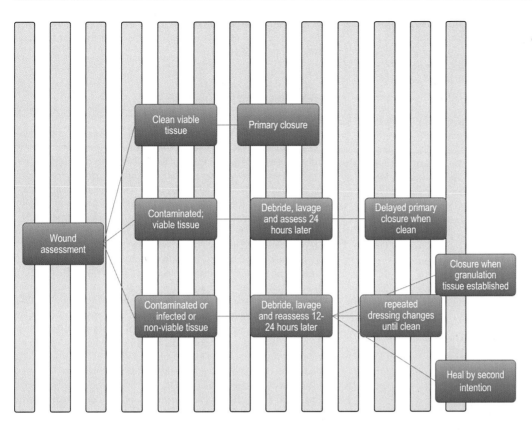

Figure 18-10. Decision making in closure of wounds.

Box 18-4 **Options for wound closure**

1. **Primary closure**: Surgical wounds or simple clean lacerations can be closed primarily (Fig. 18-11). This form of closure is never suitable where there is underlying tissue damage, contamination with foreign material or where there is a possible avulsion injury.

2. **Delayed primary closure**: Many wounds in cats are either heavily contaminated, of unknown etiology, or are presented sometime after the trauma. The wound is managed open for two to four days to allow recovery of the skin, to establish that there is an intact blood supply and to allow drainage of inflammatory fluid, exudate, and removal of foreign material prior to surgical closure of the wound.

3. **Secondary closure**: Heavily contaminated, infected wounds, or wounds with extensive tissue loss such as the shear injuries seen in the distal limb of cats in road traffic accidents, contaminated crush injuries seen with dog bite wounds, or the deficits resulting from ruptured abscesses, benefit from a prolonged period of open wound management prior to attempting closure (Fig. 18-12A,B). The wound is managed open for as long as is necessary for infection to be controlled. When the wound shows evidence that it

is healthy by the development of granulation tissue throughout the wound, it is then considered suitable for surgical closure. In the cat this is often difficult to determine (see Chapter 17), as granulation tissue may be sparse and slow to form, developing from the edges, but being slow to establish in the center.

4. **Healing by second intention**: Some wounds, particularly partial thickness wounds, or small wounds, may heal quickly with simple, careful wound management, and it rapidly becomes apparent that surgical intervention is not going to be necessary. However, in the cat some wounds heal very poorly and will always require surgical closure (e.g., axillary and inguinal wounds and wounds with little subcutaneous tissue). Open wound management is not a cheap option and the pros and cons should be carefully established with the owner at the outset, so as not to compromise care of the wound (for example, by trying to reduce the frequency of dressing changes which is often counterproductive). Distal limb shear and avulsion injuries require enormous commitment and time, but can be successfully treated provided the owner understands what is involved from the start.[19]

---

anorexia, and pyrexia and there is often a painful swelling associated with the injury. The commonest bacteria isolated from these injuries are *Pasteurella multocida* and obligate anaerobes. Ninety-five per cent of these abscesses will resolve with a short (seven to ten days) course of amoxicillin.[20] Large abscesses should be lanced or aspirated and lavaged with warm sterile isotonic saline to relieve the pain associated with the pressure and inflammation. Anti-inflammatory medication improves recovery, achieving resolution of pyrexia, pain, and inflammation associated with the abscess. Abscesses over vital structures such as joints should be explored carefully in case there is joint sepsis,

which would require specific treatment.[21] Cats should be evaluated for feline immunodeficiency virus and feline leukemia virus status with serologic testing six months after the bite.

Dog and wild animal bite wounds are more commonly associated with tissue loss and crush injury. Contaminating bacteria will include obligate anaerobes, but less commonly the *Pasteurella* species found after cat bites. Generally, a broad-spectrum antibiotic with activity against anaerobes would be appropriate; however, culture of an infected wound on admission can be useful. One report of a dog bite found a canine-specific *Mycoplasma* species, which allowed successful treatment of the infection with ciprofloxacin, which was not the first choice of antibiotic on presentation.[22] The crush injury associated with dog bite wounds may cause continued tissue necrosis for some days after the injury. Bruising and hematoma formation may be widespread, providing a medium for the development of cellulitis and widespread sepsis (see Chapter 3), and avulsion injuries to cutaneous vessels may result in cutaneous ischemia and further tissue loss or infection. Crush injuries can also cause damage to lymphatic vessels and long-term complications include lymphedema.

Cats with suspected bite wounds should be carefully assessed for body cavity or spinal injury with thoracic and abdominal radiographs.[23,24] Ultrasound examination of the body wall may be useful to determine injuries to abdominal organs and body wall defects, and CT imaging may be used to accurately detect and characterize injuries to the skull (Fig. 18-13). Injuries to the limbs should be evaluated for peripheral nerve injury as well as more obvious orthopedic injury, which may be difficult to determine once the injuries are bandaged. Vascular injury may be assessed with Doppler examination of major vessels, angiography, or bleeding from a toenail.

Initial treatment should include analgesics, intravenous broad-spectrum antibiotics and exploration and lavage of crush injuries.

Body wall defects should be repaired, but skin wounds may be better treated with delayed primary or secondary closure, to allow resolution of infection prior to closure.

BURN WOUNDS

Burns have been reported in cats trapped in burning buildings, when resting on warm car engines, or in malicious circumstances. However, it is more common that they are injured when placed on heating pads during anesthetic procedures or from prolonged exposure to operating lights or heat lamps. Iatrogenic injuries usually only result in skin damage; however, other etiologies may have associated life-threatening complications such as smoke inhalation or orthopedic injuries.

Cat skin is unlikely to blister in response to heat pad burns and the injury is often overlooked for a few days after the incident. The skin becomes white or hard to the touch and the hair epilates easily. Eventually, as the eschar forms it separates from the underlying subcutaneous tissue and discharge may be noticed at the edges. In the absence of noting the injury acutely, the extent of damage should be assessed at seven days; at this stage further skin loss is unlikely and the eschar may be surgically removed. Partial thickness eschars (scabs) may already show signs of epithelialization underneath and will heal quickly provided the cat is prevented from self-excoriation. Eschars can also be removed using hydrogels, honey, or other hydrating/debriding dressing materials (see Fig. 18-8). Full-thickness injuries are covered with silver sulfadiazine ointment or managed with moisture controlling wound dressings and systemic antibiotics. All cases should be given adequate analgesia and cats with large injuries will need to be hospitalized for intravenous fluid therapy.

BALLISTIC INJURIES

Ballistic injuries are generally rare in cats, but most likely to be related to malicious intent. The injury sustained depends on the type of projectile and the velocity (kinetic energy). The commonest ballistic injury seen in cats in the UK is from air powered rifles. The projectile is an hourglass shape and made of a soft metal. They should be low velocity, but adaptations to the pellet and/or the barrel of the air rifle may make them a higher velocity and thus much more harmful. Low velocity injuries (considered to be <1000 ft/second) result in smaller

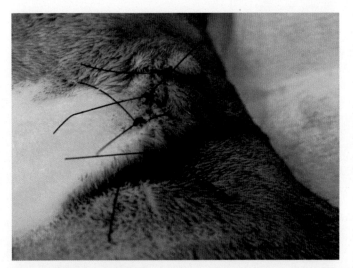

Figure 18-11 Wounds suitable for primary closure should be clean and not contaminated or infected. Most traumatic wounds would not be suitable for primary closure.

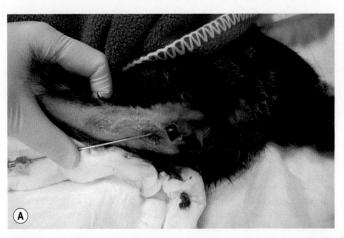
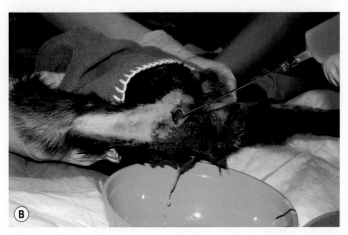

Figure 18-12 (A) A perineal cat bite resulted in a recto-cutaneous fistula. (B) Daily flushing allowed the wound to heal uneventfully by second intention, although secondary closure could also have been used once the rectal surface had closed.

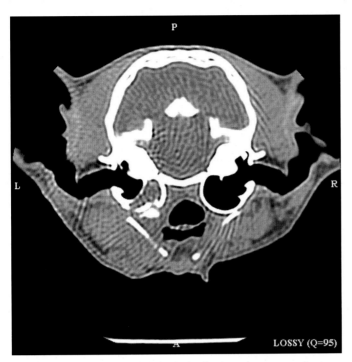

Figure 18-13 This cat presented with dysphagia and Horner syndrome after sustaining bite injuries to the ventral neck. The CT scan shows a comminuted fracture of the left tympanic bulla.

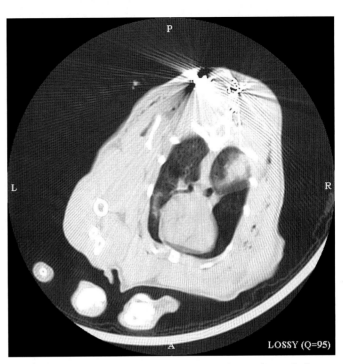

Figure 18-14 A CT image of a cat presented with a medium velocity ballistic injury. The bullet fragments create radiodense artefacts showing the scatter of the fragments of the missile and the extent of tissue involvement, including pulmonary contusion adjacent to the site of impact.

injuries, with less fragmentation of projectile material on impact and less shock wave injury through the tissue. High velocity injuries are likely to pass right through cats. However, if the projectile has a tumbling trajectory it may not pass through the exit wound. All ballistic injuries should be regarded as contaminated, with a vacuum effect on entry that sucks tissue, skin, and fur into the wound. The track of the projectile/fragments may be unpredictable and all entry wounds should be carefully explored and lavaged. Radiographs or CT help to identify fragments, as they are likely to be radiodense and will identify potential risks such as abdominal or thoracic organ injury (Fig. 18-14).

Due to the contaminated nature of these injuries, they are ideally treated with delayed primary or secondary closure, with removal of a wide area of fur around the injury and cleaning and lavage/bandaging at initial presentation. Photographic recording of injuries, together with patient and date identification in the image may be important for prosecution of the perpetrator and projectile fragments should be saved (in a plastic container, not a metal one) and handed to the police (not to the owner).

NON-HEALING WOUNDS

Non-healing wounds can be very problematic to treat in cats. A list of possible causes of non-healing wounds is provided in Table 18-3. This is not a completely comprehensive list, but indicates suggestions for further diagnostic workup that may be helpful when carrying out investigations.

History and signalment

The signalment, history of presentation, management, and response to treatment are essential to understand a non-healing wound. This is a time-consuming process and the owner needs to reveal all aspects of how the cat lives at home, what happens with the dressing, how frequently it has been changed, how active the cat is, the general health of the cat, other injuries, and signs of stress (e.g., FLUTD). This builds up a picture of issues (that may not be central to the wound management per se) that could be improved upon in order to achieve the expected rate of wound healing.

Further investigations

Hematology, biochemistry, and serology may identify other underlying diseases that are contributing to the etiology of delayed wound healing. Diagnostic imaging may help to identify foreign body involvement or sequestra (Fig. 18-15).

Biopsy

During surgical wound debridement all tissue that is removed or a biopsy should be submitted for histopathological analysis and culture (Fig. 18-16). On occasion, an underlying tumor may be present or the wound bed may transform to a neoplastic phenotype. Furthermore, there may be organisms, foreign body reaction, or other pathological signs that may indicate a cause for non-healing. A complete clinical history is helpful for the pathologists in order to enable them to suggest appropriate immunostaining or other tests.

Culture and sensitivity testing

Wound infection is a common cause of non-healing wounds so culture and sensitivity testing should be considered. Wounds with healthy granulation tissue, no odor and little exudate are unlikely to be infected. Infected wounds often produce an inflammatory exudate

Table 18-3 Causes of non-healing in chronic wounds

Source	Investigation
Infection: Bacterial L forms, mycobacteria, fungal granuloma, multi-resistant bacteria	Tissue culture; PCR Take biopsies from the chronic part of the wound, deep in the granulation tissue or in the thickened skin around the wound
Neoplasia: squamous cell carcinoma or sarcoma	Tissue biopsy
Self-trauma	History taking, hospitalization, observation
Poor wound management	Review clinical history. Look for multiple veterinary surgeon involvement, infrequent bandage changes, poor home care instructions/compliance
Medical disease: cachexia, malnutrition, protein losing disease, endocrinopathy	History and medical investigations, hematology, biochemistry, abdominal ultrasound, radiography, fecal/urine analysis Monitor weight loss during treatment, calculate caloric intake
Viral disease: feline leukemia virus, feline immunodeficiency virus, feline cowpox	Serologic and tissue testing
Foreign body or sequestra	Ultrasound, CT, MRI, radiography In some cases, sino-endoscopy may be helpful
Therapy for other diseases: immunosuppressants, long-acting corticosteroid treatments, cytotoxic drugs, radiotherapy	Review treatments and ensure you are aware of treatments that the cat may have received from other veterinary surgeons

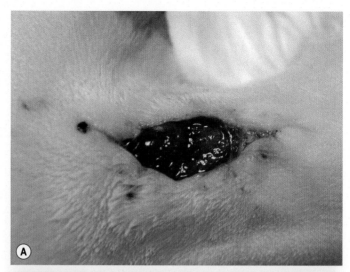

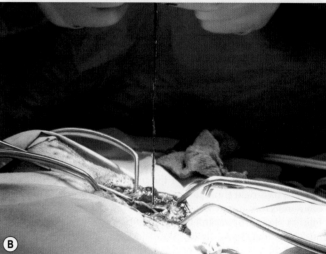

Figure 18-15 (A) This cat had a chronic wound on the ventral neck that had been sutured four times. Clinical examination found a dense structure in the tissues beneath the wound and ultrasound examination confirmed a dense linear foreign body. **(B)** A sewing needle and thread were removed and the wound healed uneventfully.

that causes an inflammatory response in the intact skin surrounding the wound, which can be seen as erythema, pain, and swelling at the wound edges. Enlarged regional lymph nodes are also suspicious for infection (although not definitive) and this should be confirmed with lymph node aspirates for cytology. A swab taken from the surface of a granulating wound bed may produce a positive culture that has no clinical significance and indeed may not even warrant antibiotic therapy. It is best to sample after sterile lavage to avoid culturing surface contaminants. A swab rolled across the surface of the wound may, however, produce a useful sample for cytological analysis, identifying filamentous organisms, for example.[25]

Culture of a tissue sample may be more accurate of the underlying infection and therefore more useful than culture of a superficial swab sample of a chronic wound. A positive culture with an unusual resistance pattern or a culture from an inflamed exudative wound is more likely to be a significant finding. Nosocomial infections (hospital acquired) are more likely to have an unusual pattern of resistance, but these infections should be prevented with good hospital protocols for managing patients with open wounds. Some infections such as MRSA (methicillin-resistant *Staphylococcus aureus*) are most often acquired from the owner, particularly if they work in the healthcare industry.

Extended culture requests

Occasionally it is necessary to request extended culture on tissue biopsies, particularly if the presence of organisms has been identified on histopathology or cytology (Fig. 18-17). Some organisms are very fastidious and difficult to culture and polymerase chain reaction techniques (PCR) have been used to successfully identify mycobacteria and leishmaniasis in tissue biopsies that had sterile culture results.[26] While PCR results do not provide any information on sensitivity, knowledge that a specific organism is involved can guide therapeutic decisions, particularly the duration of therapy required.[27]

Treatment

Treatment of non-healing wounds is determined by a final diagnosis of the limitation on the normal healing processes. Wound healing in cats, for the most part, is very efficient and the commonest cause of delayed healing is poor wound management. Increasing the frequency

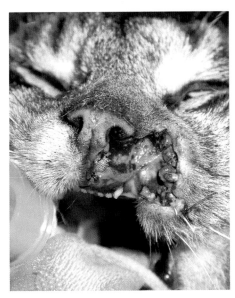

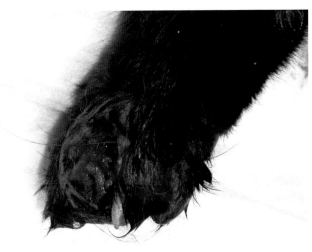

Figure 18-17 This interdigital wound failed to heal for some months despite repeated attempts at closure and dressings. Tissue culture identified a *Nocardia* infection in the soft tissues of the foot.

Figure 18-16 This non-healing wound on the lip of a tabby cat was biopsied and found to be a squamous cell carcinoma.

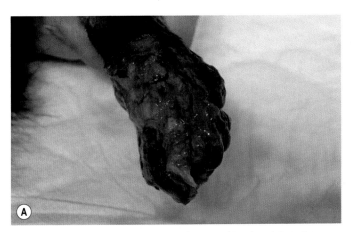

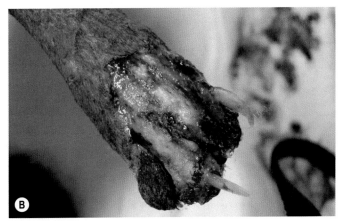

Figure 18-18 (A) A cat was referred after a multi-resistant *Pseudomonas* was cultured from the wound. Daily lavage, with wet-to-dry dressings followed by hydrogel dressings and no other antibiotic or antiseptic treatment resolved the infection satisfactorily. **(B)** The wound after five days of management.

of dressing changes, monitoring nutrition and cat welfare, and ensuring appropriate dressings are used are the most effective ways of managing chronic wounds. However, in some cases there will be a specific diagnosis and this would need to be addressed.

Wound infection is also a common cause of delayed healing and often administration of antibiotics is ineffective as a single solution to what is essentially a multi-faceted problem. Wound debridement and lavage followed by daily dressing changes is the single most effective way to manage wound infection (Fig. 18-18). Unless there is evidence of systemic infection (depression, limb edema, pyrexia), treatment with oral or topical antibiotics/antiseptics is unlikely to be as effective. Sampling wounds for culture is important, particularly in non-healing chronic wounds, and may be used as an objective measure of the 'health' of the wound. Surface swabs or fluid samples are unreliable and may not represent the clinically significant infection, and tissue biopsies are preferred to bacterial culture. Treatment of infected wounds should be carried out based on specific culture and sensitivity

results and the laboratory should be notified to use a suitable panel of antibiotics in the in vitro tests, i.e., antibiotics that are suitable for oral administration in cats.

AXILLARY WOUNDS

S.J. Langley-Hobbs

Axillary wounds in cats are usually caused by entrapment of a forelimb in a neck collar or wire loop.[28,29] The usual presentation is of an active cat that has been missing for a period of time, often several weeks or even months.[29] The cat may return home with the front leg still trapped in the collar; alternatively, the collar is missing but the cat has a typical, unilateral, indolent, axillary wound.[29] Axillary wounds generally do not heal spontaneously and they pose a particular problem for complication-free healing despite aggressive and extensive medical and surgical treatment. Primary closure often results in wound breakdown even if flaps are used and irrespective of surgeon experience.[28,30]

Surgical anatomy

The cat has loose and thin skin around the axilla, an essential prerequisite for climbing and jumping. The well-developed elbow skin fold consists of two opposing layers of skin, triangular in shape, consisting of a laterally facing outer layer and a medially facing inner layer, separated by loose connective tissue. Each fold has four attachments: the outer layer has a lateral attachment to the brachium and a dorsal attachment to the trunk; the inner layer has medial attachments to the brachium and a ventral attachment to the trunk. The blood supply is thought to derive from the lateral thoracic artery as well as from the subdermal plexus. Due to this abundance of loose skin between the forelimb and trunk, when the cat's front leg is fully flexed, the elbow lies within a pocket formed by the two layers of skin fold: there is no skin closely adhering to the caudal and medial brachium.[29]

Etiology

Axillary wounds classically form a non-healing wound. At presentation the wounds are usually granulated and exudative. They commonly extend from the cranial axilla towards the point of the elbow and dorsally up to a point mid-way up the thorax, level with the shoulder joint. In each case loss of the elbow skin fold[28,29] and puckering of skin adjacent to the medial brachium are noticeable.[29] The surrounding skin is very thin and is under tension because of the mobility around the axilla.

The delayed healing can be associated with under-running or pocketing.[31] The formation of a pocket wound, in which epithelialization fails due to separation of the skin edges from the underlying wound bed, has been suggested as a reason for the chronic nature of axillary lesions.[31] Wound contraction is often impeded because of the tension and shearing forces of movement as one side of the wound moves against the other as the cat walks.[32] Another possible cause of chronicity and wound breakdown might be excessive skin-to-wound, or skin-to-suture line contact within the axilla. In a study evaluating a free latissimus dorsi muscle flap in cats, the donor site consistently broke down only where the suture line entered the caudal aspect of the axilla.[33] This may have been partly due to excessive skin-to-suture line contact. Poor vascularity and excessive dead space may also contribute to the chronicity of these wounds.[28]

Preoperative investigations and preparation for surgery

Chronic axillary wounds should be assessed as non-healing wounds with appropriate preoperative investigations, including virus serology, biopsy, and culture (see above). For heavily contaminated wounds, primary wound care should be instigated first to reduce contamination and hence the chance of postoperative infection (Box 18.2).

Surgical treatment

Historically, primary repair of axillary flaps in cats has a high failure rate[28,30] and various techniques have been described for repair of these wounds. Success has been achieved in five cats with a simple technique where the wound was closed primarily and the elbow flap was reconstructed.[29] These cats had wounds of between three weeks' and four months' duration and had not had previous surgery. For chronic wounds with previous unsuccessful attempts at repair, the combination of omentalization and skin flaps has been successful. There is a single case report on the use of the omocervical axial pattern flap (see Chapter 19) in combination with an omental pedicle graft, this offers a useful alternative where the use of a thoracodorsal axial pattern flap is not possible due to the extent of the lesion.[34]

After anesthesia the wound should be packed with a water soluble jelly before a wide area is clipped and prepared for surgery. Hair should be clipped from the forelimb distally to the carpus, proximally to the midline, cranially to the neck and caudally to the abdomen, including the ventral abdomen if omentalization is planned. The cat is usually positioned in lateral recumbency with the affected axilla uppermost; if omentalization is planned the cat can be tilted slightly off lateral to improve access to the abdomen.

Reconstruction of elbow skin fold[29]

Hunt originally described the surgical unfolding and advancement of the elbow fold to reconstruct cranioventral skin deficits and axillary wounds in cats.[35,36] Restoring the elbow skin fold before closing the wound may improve the chances of a successful reconstruction at the first surgical intervention (Box 18-5).[29]

Omental pedicle flap and primary closure

For chronic wounds with previous unsuccessful attempts at repair, the combination of omentalization and primary closure[28,30] or a thoracodorsal axial pattern flap[37] have been successful (Box 18-6).

Postoperative care, complications and prognosis

Analgesia should be provided pre- and postoperatively with opioids and NSAIDs. The wounds are usually dirty or infected so cats are usually given antibiotics pre- and postoperatively (e.g., clavulanate amoxicillin for ten days) which can be changed dependent on culture results. It should not be necessary to place a drain after placement of an omental pedicle as the omentum acts as a natural drain.[37] If the omentum is not used then a closed suction drain or a Penrose drain placed in the dependent part of the right axilla can be used for 24–72 hours. Bandaging should not be necessary. A Velpeau-type bandage[38] can be placed on the right thoracic limb for two weeks, but as cats do not tolerate bandages well this may result in a fraught and anxious cat that could self-traumatize its surgical repair in its efforts to remove its bandage.

Complications include seroma, partial or complete necrosis of skin flaps, wound breakdown at the donor or recipient site (Fig. 18-21A). Possible complications after omental transposition include a visible subcutaneous swelling over the omentum as it passes from the laparotomy to the axilla (Fig. 18.21B), seroma formation, herniation of abdominal contents through the omental exit hole, and flap necrosis.

Axillary wounds in cats represent a significant challenge to the surgeon to achieve uncomplicated healing. Collars should not be used in cats unless they are of the quick release type; collars with an elasticated portion in them will still cause injury.

Box 18-5 **Reconstruction of the elbow skin fold**

The surgery aims to restore the normal structure of the elbow skin fold allowing the elbow to move freely in this pocket of skin. The skin edges and all the granulation tissue are excised en bloc by sharp dissection. A sufficient margin of skin is removed to include all tissue that appears scarred, unduly thin or poorly vascularized. Skin adhered to the caudal and medial brachium is undermined and separated from the deeper tissues by blunt dissection. The skin of the lateral thorax caudal to the brachium is undermined deep to the cutaneous musculature in a similar manner. Blunt dissection to detach the adhered skin is continued until the elbow skin fold is reconstructable (Fig 18-19).

A 6 mm Penrose drain is positioned in the dead space beneath the skin of the lateral thorax, exiting through a stab incision placed ventrally. The buried proximal end of the drain is anchored dorsally with an external skin suture. The distal end of the drain is trimmed to allow 2 cm to protrude ventrally and sutured with another skin suture. The wound is closed primarily using two layers of sutures. No attempt is made to close dead space. A subdermal simple interrupted or continuous suture pattern of 2M polyglactin or polydioxanone and simple interrupted skin sutures of 2M polyamide are used for closure. After closure the forelimb should be fully flexed and extended to ensure that the elbow is able to move freely within the recreated skin fold and beneath the lateral thoracic skin. The Penrose drains are removed after three days.

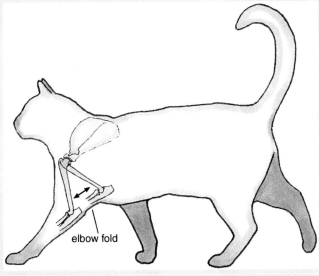

elbow fold

Figure 18-19 Diagram illustrating the elbow skin fold in a cat. The antebrachium moves freely in this fold of skin and re-establishing this normal anatomical feature in the cat can be part of a successful means of repairing axillary wounds.

Box 18-6 **Omental pedicle flap combined with primary closure or a thoracodorsal axial pattern flap**

The cat is positioned with the affected axilla uppermost, and slightly tilted 'off' lateral recumbency to provide access to the ventral midline and the area over the scapula and up to the dorsal midline (Fig 18-20A). Surgical debridement is performed first (Fig 18-20B). This consists of resection of the entire wound bed, including all grossly abnormal tissue and a margin of skin from the edge of the wound. Instrumentation is changed before the omentalization procedure.

Omentalization

A cranial midline celiotomy is performed and a vascularized omental pedicle created (see Chapter 19).

A paracostal incision is then made on the same side as the axillary wound, by incising full thickness through the skin and body wall just behind the costal arch, about two-thirds of the way up the body wall. The omental pedicle is passed out of the abdomen through this incision. During handling of the omentum, great care is taken to prevent excessive handling or twisting of the pedicle. Desiccation is prevented by wrapping the omentum in saline-soaked swabs.

Passage of the omentum is facilitated by wrapping the pedicle in a longitudinally split, saline lubricated, 1 inch Penrose drain (Fig 18-20C). A subcutaneous tunnel is created between the axillary wound and the paracostal incision using Roberts artery forceps, which can be used to grasp the Penrose drain and gently pull it through (Fig 18-20D). Another Penrose drain can also be used to gather the two ends of the subcutaneous tunnel together to make the distance that the omental pedicle had to be pulled subcutaneously as short as possible. The free end of the omental pedicle is used to fill the axillary deficit.

Omentopexy is performed by means of synthetic absorbable sutures placed:

1. Between the free edge of omentum and the body wall at the site of the abdominal exit incision. These sutures are placed to prevent the omentum from returning to the abdominal cavity and in a manner that does not interfere with its vascular supply.
2. The omentum is spread out to cover the wound site and sutured to the surrounding subcutaneous tissue with fine synthetic absorbable suture material (Fig. 18-20E).
   The remainder of the laparotomy incision is closed routinely.

Primary closure

The local skin is undermined and mobilized and the wounds closed over the omentum using subdermal sutures (2M Polyglactin 910 or polyglycolic acid) and skin sutures of 2 or 1.5M monofilament nylon.

A thoracodorsal flap, which extends to the dorsal midline, is created using previously described landmarks (see Fig. 19-8). The thoracodorsal artery is visualized during the dissection (Fig. 18-20F). The axial pattern flap is rotated into the axillary region and sutured in place with simple interrupted polyglactin 910 sutures (2M) in the subcutaneous fascia, and simple interrupted monofilament polyamide sutures (2M) in the skin. The donor site is closed routinely with interrupted polyglactin 910 sutures (2M) in the subcutaneous fascia and simple interrupted monofilament polyamide sutures (2M) or staples in the skin (Fig. 18-20G).

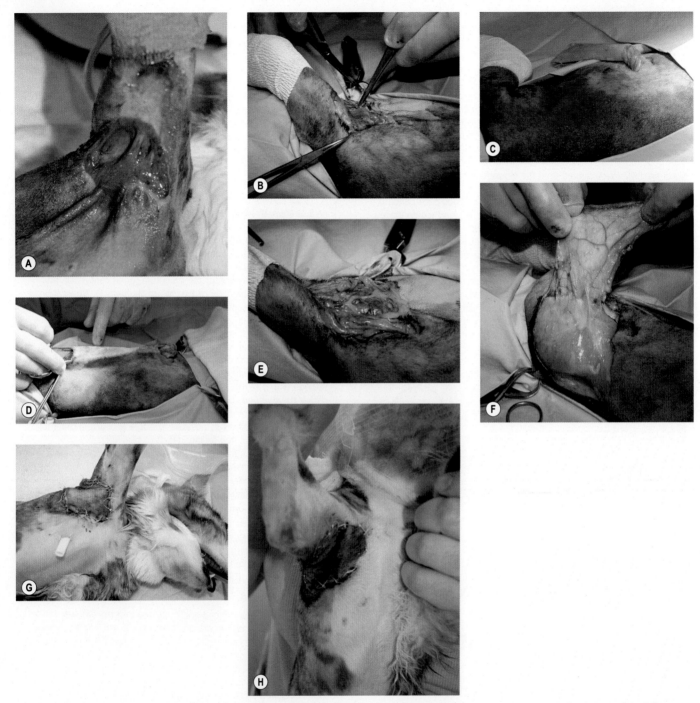

Figure 18-20 Axillary wound management in a two-year-old female tortoiseshell cat. **(A)** The axillary wound has been prepared for surgery. **(B)** The skin is sharply incised around the periphery of the chronic wound and the wound and skin edges are debrided. **(C)** The omentum is exteriorized through a small paracostal laparotomy and placed inside a large Penrose drain. **(D)** It is passed subcutaneously to the axillary wound. **(E)** The omentum is sutured over the debrided axillary wound. **(F)** The thoracodorsal artery is clearly seen in the thoracodorsal axial pattern flap. **(G)** The thoracodorsal axial pattern flap is sutured in place and the donor site closed. A Penrose drain is shown protruding caudally. The drain should not be necessary with omentalization. **(H)** Three weeks after surgery at the time of suture removal there is good evidence of healing. *(Courtesy of Jon Hall.)*

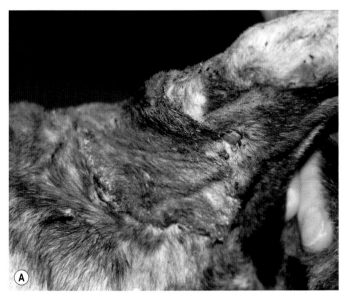
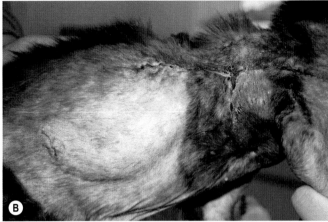

Figure 18-21 (A) A small area of wound breakdown after omentalization and thoracodorsal flap performed in a cat with a chronic axillary wound three weeks previously. This resolved without specific treatment. **(B)** There is a visible swelling where the omentum has been passed under the skin from the paracostal laparotomy to the axilla.

REFERENCES

1. Bohling MW, Henderson RA, Swaim SF, et al. Cutaneous wound healing in the cat; a macroscopic description and comparison with cutaneous wound healing in the dog. Vet Surg 2004;33: 579–87.

2. Bohling MW, Henderson RA. Differences in cutaneous wound healing between dogs and cats. Vet Clin North Am Small Anim Pract 2006;36:687–92.

3. Bohling MW, Henderson RA, Swaim SF, et al. Comparison of the role of the subcutaneous tissues in cutaneous wound healing in the dog and cat. Vet Surg 2006;35:3–14.

4. Gower SB, Weisse CW, Brown DC. Major abdominal evisceration injuries in dogs and cats: 12 cases. J Am Vet Med Assoc 2009;234(12):1566–72.

5. Kaestner S. Analgesia. In: Montavon PM, Voss K, Langley-Hobbs SJ, editors. Feline Orthopedic Surgery and Musculoskeletal disease. Edinburgh: Elsevier; 2009. p. 199–205.

6. Anderson DM, White, RAS. Ischaemic bandage injuries; a case series and review of the literature. Vet Surg 2000;29: 488–98.

7. Schultz GS, Sibbald RG, Falanga V, et al. Wound bed preparation: systematic approach to wound management. Wound Rep Reg 2003;11:1–28.

8. Roberts DB, Travis EL. Acemannan-containing wound dressing gel reduces radiation induced skin reaction in C3H

mice. Int J Radiat Oncol Biol Phys 1995;32(4):1047–52.

9. Majno G. The Healing Hand. Man and Wound in the Ancient World. Cambridge, Massachusetts: Harvard University Press; 1975. p. 69–140.

10. Krahwinkel DJ, Boothe HW. Topical and Systemic Medications for Wounds. Vet Clin Small Anim 2006;36:739–57.

11. Thomas S. Formulary of Wound Management Products. 10th ed. Passfield, Hampshire: Euromed Communications Ltd; 2009. p. 1–195.

12. Mathews KA, Binnington A. Wound Management: using honey. Compend Contin Educ Pract Vet 2002;24:53–60.

13. Hendrix C.M. Facultative myiasis in dogs and cats. Compend Contin Educ Pract Vet 1991;13(1):86–94.

14. Fong J, Wood F. Nanocrystalline silver dressings in wound management: a review. Int J Nanomedicine 2006;1(4): 441–9.

15. Lo SF, Hayter M, Chang CJ, et al. A systematic review of silver-releasing dressings in the management of infected chronic wounds. J Clin Nurse 2008;17:1973–85.

16. Wang XQ, Kempf M, Mott J, et al. Silver absorption on burns after the application of Acticoat: data from pediatric patients and a porcine burn model. J Burn Care Res 2009;30:341–8.

17. Guille AE, Tseng LW, Orsher RJ. Use of vacuum assisted closure for management

of a large skin wound in a cat. J Am Vet Med Assoc 2007;230:1669–73.

18. Owen L, Hotston-Moore A, Holt P. Vacuum-assisted wound closure following urine induced skin and thigh muscle necrosis in a cat. Vet Comp Orthop Traumatol 2009;22:417–21.

19. Corr S. Intensive, extensive, expensive. Management of distal limb shearing injuries in cats. J Feline Med Surg 2009;11(9):747–57.

20. Roy J, Messier S, Labrecque O, Cox WR. Clinical and in vitro efficacy of amoxicillin against bacteria associated with feline skin wounds and abscesses. Can Vet J 2007;48(6):607–11.

21. Voss K, Langley-Hobbs SJ. Diseases of Joints. In: Montavon PM, Voss K, Langley-Hobbs SJ, editors. Feline Orthopedic Surgery and Musculoskeletal disease. Edinburgh: Elsevier; 2009. p. 63–74.

22. Walker RD, Walshaw R, Riggs CM, Mosser T. Recovery of two mycoplasma species from abscesses in a cat following bite wounds from a dog. J Vet Diagn Invest 1995;7(1):154–6.

23. Chai O, Johnston DE, Shamir MH. Bite wounds involving the spine: characteristics, therapy and outcome in seven cases. Vet J 2008;175:259–65.

24. Risselada M, de Rooster H, Taeymans O, van Bree H. Penetrating injuries in dogs and cats: a study of 16 cases. Vet Comp Orthop Traumatol 2008;21:434–9.

25. Barfield D, Rich S, Pegrum S, Malik R. What is your diagnosis? Nocardia infection. J Small Anim Pract 2007;48(6): 353–4.

26. Santoro D, Prisco M, Ciaramella P. Cutaneous sterile granulomas/ pyogranulomas, leishmaniasis and mycobacterial infections. J Small Anim Pract 2008;49(11):552–61.

27. Studdert VP, Hughes KL. Treatment of opportunistic mycobacterial infections with enrofloxacin in cats. J Am Vet Med Assoc 1992;20(19): 1388–90.

28. Lascelles BD, Davison L, Dunning M, et al. Use of omental pedicle grafts in the management of non-healing axillary wounds in 10 cats. J Small Anim Pract 1998;39:475–80.

29. Brinkley CH. Successful closure of feline axillary wounds by reconstruction of the elbow skin fold. J Small Anim Pract 2007;48:111–15.

30. Brockman DJ, Pardo AD, Conzemius MG, et al. Omentum-enhanced reconstruction of chronic nonhealing wounds in cats: techniques and clinical use. Vet Surg 1996;25:99–104.

31. Pavletic M.M. Common complications in wound healing. In: Pavletic MM, editor. Atlas of small animal wound management and reconstructive surgery. 3rd ed. Iowa: Wiley-Blackwell; 1994. p. 127–57.

32. Swaim SF, Hinkle SH, Bradley DM. Wound contraction: basic and clinical factors. Compend Contin Educ 2001;23:20–33.

33. Nicoll SA, Fowler JD, Remedios AM, et al. Development of a free latissimus dorsi muscle flap in cats. Vet Surg 1996;25: 40–8.

34. Gray MJ. Chronic axillary wound repair in a cat with omentalisation and omocervical skin flap. J Small Anim Pract 2005;46:499–503.

35. Hunt GB. Skin fold advancement flaps for closing large sternal and inguinal wounds in cats and dogs. Vet Surg 1995;24: 172–5.

36. Hunt GB, Tisdall PL, Liptak JM, et al. Skin-fold advancement flaps for closing large proximal limb and trunk defects in dogs and cats. Vet Surg 2001;30:440–8.

37. Lascelles BDX, White RAS. Combined omental pedicle grafts and thoracodorsal axial pattern flaps for the reconstruction of chronic, nonhealing axillary wounds in cats. Vet Surg 2001;30:380–5.

38. Langley-Hobbs SJ, Voss K, Montavon PM. External coaptation. In: Montavon PM, Voss K, Langley-Hobbs SJ, editors. Feline Orthopedic Surgery and Musculoskeletal disease. Edinburgh: Elsevier; 2009. p. 239–48.

Chapter 19

Flaps and grafts

P. Nelissen, D. White

Ongoing advances in oncological and trauma surgery ensure that the indications for advanced reconstructive surgery in the cat continue to increase. Large skin wounds present the feline clinician with reconstructive challenges and a range of further options can be considered where local skin tension or lack of adjacent skin preclude primary closure. These include promoting second intention healing and the use of local skin flaps, distant skin flaps, axial pattern flaps, and free skin grafts. Although second intention healing may be suitable for many smaller wounds, its use in larger skin deficits is associated with prolonged healing times, a fragile long-term result, and potentially undesirable wound contraction that may impair function. Feline skin, however, lends itself particularly well to the use of random and axial pattern flaps and both can be used early in wound reconstruction even with suboptimal wound beds. Free skin grafts have more fastidious needs; they require an optimal recipient bed and meticulous postoperative management to achieve a favourable outcome.

The indications for muscle flaps are far fewer than the indications for skin flaps but after large oncological resection there may be the requirement for both a muscle flap and a skin flap. For completeness, another flap that is used for reconstructive surgery, amongst other indications, is the omental pedicle and a description of this will be included.

SURGICAL ANATOMY

Skin is composed of two layers, an outer epidermis consisting of stratified squamous epithelium and an inner dermis of dense connective tissue. The skin is loosely attached to the hypodermis composed of loose connective tissue, which in turn connects to underlying muscles.[1] When considering using skin for flaps or grafts it is essential to have an understanding of the blood supply.

Cutaneous vascular supply (Fig. 19-1)

Direct cutaneous arteries travel through intermuscular fascial planes and then run parallel with the overlying skin before connecting to the cutaneous circulation. Direct cutaneous arteries supply angiosomes composed of cutaneous musculature, subcutaneous tissue and skin.

The cutaneous vascular system divides further into three interconnecting levels:[1]

- the deep, subdermal plexus
- the middle, cutaneous plexus
- the superficial, subpapillary plexus.

The subdermal plexus is the major route of arterial supply to the skin.

SKIN FLAPS

A skin flap is a piece of skin that retains at least one source of vascular support from the donor site during its transfer. The terms 'skin flap' and 'pedicle graft' are synonymous. They are termed 'subdermal plexus' or 'random' where the integrity of the vascular supply is maintained through an intact attachment of the deep or subdermal plexus. Where a layer of cutaneous muscle is present, the subdermal plexus lies both superficial and deep to this and it should be incorporated when creating a flap. Flaps that derive their primary vascular support from direct cutaneous arteries alone are termed 'axial', or 'island' where no cutaneous attachment is maintained. Flaps are most commonly moved immediately from donor to recipient site. They provide tissue to achieve coverage of open wounds while redistributing tension away from wound margins. Ideal flap donor sites have ample skin available without excessive tension and motion so as to allow the secondary defect created by the transfer of the flap to be closed readily. Careful planning and meticulous, atraumatic surgical technique to ensure that excessive tension, kinking and circulatory compromise do not develop are necessary for survival of the flap.

Random pattern or subdermal plexus flaps

Random flaps are dependent for their vascular support on the terminal branches of the cutaneous circulation and may be developed anywhere in the skin. Although the vascular integrity of random flaps is somewhat less consistent than axial pattern flaps, they remain a very reliable method of reconstruction. It may be beneficial to align the base of random flaps when possible in the direction of any known direct cutaneous vessels to take advantage of this additional vascular support. Although it is sensible to avoid narrow or excessively long

DOI: 10.1016/B978-0-7020-4336-9.00019-6

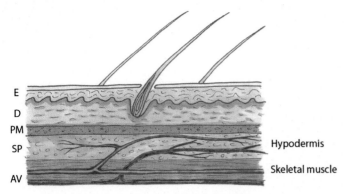

Figure 19-1 Cutaneous vascular supply. Cross section of the skin and the vascular supply. Direct cutaneous artery and vein supplying an angiosome. AV, direct cutaneous artery and vein; D, dermis; E, epidermis; PM, panniculus muscle; SP, subdermal plexus.

Box 19-1 Classification of random flaps

Relationship with the recipient site

Local: Are used to reconstruct wounds in the immediate adjacent vicinity. Local flaps are developed immediately adjacent to the recipient bed and represent one of the simplest and most efficient methods of closing skin defects not amenable to primary closure. They are likely to maintain a similar pattern of local hair growth and color

Distant: Are used to reconstruct wounds at a remote site (e.g., flank donor to limb recipient site) and are less likely to provide a similar pattern of hair growth or color

Attachment at the donor site

Single pedicle: Maintain one cutaneous donor site attachment
Double or bipedicle grafts: Maintain two cutaneous attachments

Method of local flap transfer

Advancement flaps are moved in a forward direction away from their base attachment
Rotation and transposition flaps pivot into position around their base attachment

---

flaps, there is no viability limit to the length of random flaps and predicted base width/flap length ratios are not relevant to flaps in the cat.[2] Random flaps may be classified in a number of ways (Box 19-1).

Advancement flaps

Single pedicle advancement flaps (Fig. 19-2) are probably the most commonly used local flap employed in veterinary medicine because of their simplicity and the lack of a significant secondary defect requiring closure. Advancement (or sliding) flaps are rectangular in shape and are created parallel to lines of tension with an attachment at the base opposite the edge covering the wound. Paired advancement flaps resulting in an H-pattern of closure can also be employed although they are more complex. They may have better viability than one large flap, otherwise there is little significant advantage (Fig. 19-3). The single relaxing or release incision is a bipedicle advancement flap by design (Fig. 19-4).

Advancement flaps provide wound coverage by stretching the flap skin along its long axis over the defect, and as a result there is an opposing elastic retraction in the surrounding skin.

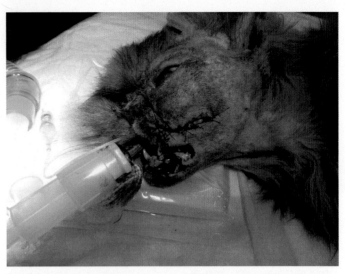

Figure 19-2 Single pedicle advancement flap. Elevation of a single pedicle flap to reconstruct the cutaneous surface of the upper lip after resection of a large skin tumor.

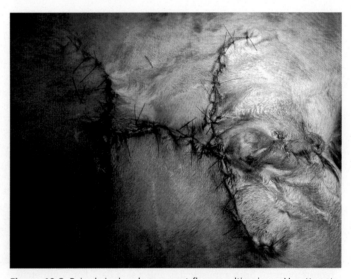

Figure 19-3 Paired single advancement flaps resulting in an H-pattern to close a large rectangular defect on the thorax of a cat.

Rotating/transposition flaps

Rotation flaps are created by releasing the skin along an arc-shaped incision before moving it along the same axis. They are of limited use in feline reconstruction since relatively large areas of skin need to be raised to achieve wound coverage. The transposition flap is a rectangular pedicle graft, which instead of being moved along its long axis is rotated up to 90 degrees of the wound axis (Fig. 19-5). This is the most common type of rotating flap and is by far the most useful technique to close a variety of small sized problematic wounds. A modification of this flap is the front or hind limb fold flap.

Distant flaps

Direct distant flaps are raised at a location remote from the skin defect and ultimately transferred to the recipient bed by approximating the wound with the donor site. This technique is used almost exclusively for reconstruction of wounds involving the middle or lower extremities and provides durable full thickness skin coverage without

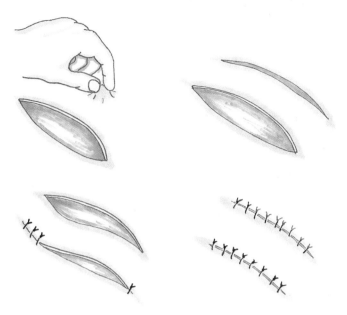

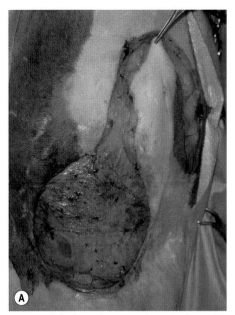

Figure 19-4 Bipedicle advancement flap. The releasing incision creates a flap with vascular supply on both ends of the flap. The resulting defect is left to heal by second intention.

the need for skin grafts.[3] Flaps are normally raised on the flank and the affected limb brought alongside to allow the flap to be sutured to the recipient bed. Flaps may be single pedicle (hinge; Fig. 19-6) or bipedicle (pouch; Fig. 19-7) grafts. The limb must then be secured against the flank over a ten to 14 day period while the flap attaches to the wound. The pedicle(s) are divided, often in two stages, to complete the transfer.[4] Cats are generally well suited to this technique and tolerate the period of limb immobilization better than dogs because of their size, flexible limbs, and the availability of ample loose elastic skin. Distant flaps are multi-staged procedures and consequently are time consuming and expensive. The transplanted skin assumes the same hair growth as its donor site despite its new location. Some patients will not tolerate their limb being immobilized against their flank and this is particularly evident if the limb is positioned in an elevated position. Occasionally, moist dermatitis caused by skin-to-skin contact and moisture accumulation is encountered; transient muscle atrophy of the limb may be noticed in some cases.

Axial pattern flaps (Fig. 19-8)

An axial pattern flap is a pedicle graft based primarily or solely on the vascular supply of a direct cutaneous artery and vein.[5] The vessels, of which terminal branches supply blood to the subdermal plexus, extend the length of the flap. Therefore axial pattern flaps have better perfusion compared to subdermal plexus flaps. Large axial pattern flaps can be safely elevated and transferred in a single-stage procedure for closure of major cutaneous defects. These flaps have excellent survival rates and they can be used to reconstruct wounds associated with less optimal conditions such as contamination, uneven surfaces, exposed bone, tendon, and cartilage. Axial or island pattern flaps are classified according to the vascular territory supplied by the direct cutaneous artery (angiosome). These vessels and territories including the thoracodorsal artery, lateral thoracic artery, omocervical artery, caudal superficial epigastric artery have been researched and mapped for clinical use as axial pattern flaps in the cat. Although the location and relative size of each angiosome are similar for both dogs and cats, the extreme elasticity of feline skin and the relative increase in body size to limb length often facilitates more distal coverage of limb

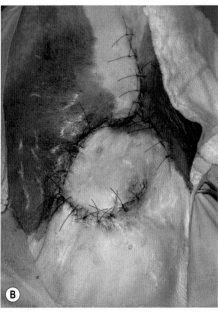

Figure 19-5 (A) 90 degrees rotating flap. Two parallel skin incisions are made at an equal distance from the nipples. The length of the flap depends on the length of the defect that needs to be covered. **(B)** A 90 degree transposition flap. These flaps are used to reconstruct large rectangular defects involving adjacent sites.

wounds in cats.[6] Axial pattern flaps sometimes require extensive dissection of the donor site for flap elevation; because of their relatively large size, axial pattern donor sites may require undermining and walking sutures to appose the defect created by the raised flap. The cosmetic appearance of the recipient bed differs from the donor site with regard to hair direction, color, length, glandular tissues, and amount of subcutaneous tissues.

FREE SKIN GRAFTS

Free grafts are areas of skin that are completely detached from the donor site and hence lose their original vascular supply before being

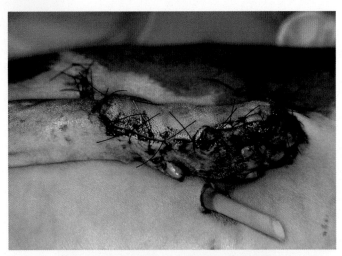

Figure 19-6 Single pedicle direct distant flap (hinge). These flaps are used to cover defects on the lower forelimb and hindlimb. The flap can be dorsally or ventrally employed depending on the location of the skin defect.

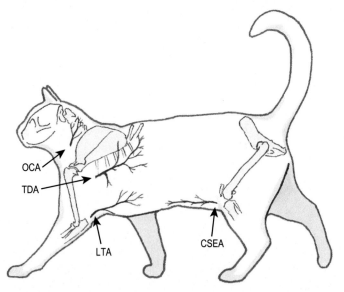

Figure 19-8 Axial pattern flaps. Identification of commonly used axial pattern flaps based on the location of the direct cutaneous artery. CSEA, caudal superficial epigastric artery; LTA, lateral thoracic artery; OCA, omocervical artery; TDA, thoracodorsal artery.

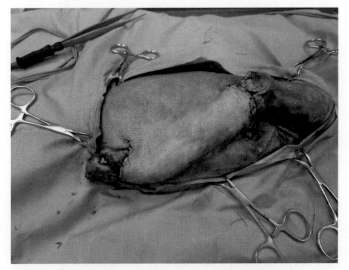

Figure 19-7 Bipedicle direct distant flap (pouch). Two incisions equal to the width of the skin deficit are made. The flap is undermined below the panniculus muscle. The limb is then secured beneath the flap and sutured.

transferred to resurface a recipient site. In feline surgery the use of free skin grafts is confined almost exclusively to reconstruction of large skin defects of the extremities where few alternate options are available.[7] Secondary healing of limb wounds can lead to unsightly scar tissue development and may also lead to impaired limb function if formed in the vicinity of joints. The use of random flaps is often restricted by the limited availability of adjacent skin. Direct flaps offer an alternative solution although the temperament of some cats may not always be conducive to this option.

Free grafts lack vascular support in the period after transfer and must survive for at least the following 48 hours by absorbing protein-containing fluid from the recipient bed by capillary action, a process known as plasmatic imbibition. During this period the graft becomes attached to the underlying tissue by the development of an interposed fibrin seal that acts as a biological 'glue' and provides a scaffold across which capillaries from the recipient bed begin to anastomose with

those of the exposed graft plexus to re-establish circulation (inosculation). New capillaries later grow into the graft and the vascular channels remodel (revascularization). Free skin grafts therefore require a vascularized recipient bed and preparation of the recipient bed is a major determinant of successful skin grafting. Fresh active pink granulation tissue is the ideal recipient bed and provides excellent vascular support and the growth factors necessary for these processes to occur. Granulation tissue is not, however, essential for graft survival and any well-vascularized tissue is theoretically capable of accepting and supporting a skin graft. Grafts can therefore be applied over surgically clean and fresh surgical wounds since periosteum, peritenon, and muscle normally have sufficient vascular supply to support skin grafts (Fig. 19-9).

The accumulation of any material such as blood, serum, pus, or foreign material between the graft and the recipient bed will interfere with the early nutrition processes and may ultimately prevent revascularization. It is essential, therefore, that all tissue debris, contamination and superficial infection should be controlled before the graft is applied since the early fibrin seal that fixes the graft to the recipient bed can be easily destroyed by the fibrinolytic activity of proliferating bacteria in the wound. Immobilization of the graft is similarly important, since this attachment can also be mechanically damaged by excessive motion in the graft site during the first week. Methods to immobilize the surgical site include: Robert Jones bandages, splints, or external skeletal fixation. Bandaging and splinting methods vary with the type and location of the graft. Any areas of early epithelialization should be removed from the surface of the granulation tissue because this can prove remarkably resistant to the establishment of the fibrin seal. Grafts are applied with sufficient tension to ensure good contact with the recipient surface; excessive tension may limit capillary circulation while inadequate surface-to-surface contact may prevent interdigitation and delay revascularization.

Meshed or pie-crusted sheets have perforations through the entire thickness of the skin. Perforated grafts have greater flexibility and conform better to an uneven surface than unmeshed skin while permitting the ongoing drainage of any sub-graft exudate. Unmeshed sheets have less flexibility and hence need to be pre-cut more

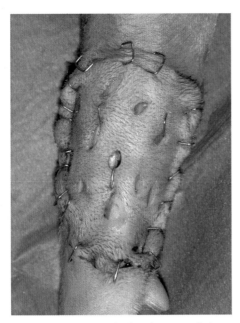

Figure 19-9 Free skin graft. A meshed graft was applied over a fresh surgical wound to cover a larger defect after a tumor had been resected. *(Courtesy of Georgio Romanelli.)*

accurately to the outline of the defect. Additionally, they provide no route for drainage, necessitating temporary placement of active suction drains under larger grafts.

Healthy grafts may appear swollen and dark during the first 48–72 hours due to the process of imbibition of hemoglobin degradation products but become pinker and less edematous as a rudimentary circulation becomes established. Non-viable grafts will, however, progress to become white or black and necrotic over a period of three to five days. Occasionally, grafts lose their epidermal layer during the first week, giving rise to the appearance of an apparently complete graft failure. This can be disconcerting but usually an outline of the dermal graft will appear within the next week and the graft will progress satisfactorily to complete coverage of the defect.

In feline surgery, full thickness grafts are preferred for virtually all reconstructive procedures because they are more robust, durable and withstand considerable handling during graft elevation and positioning. Full thickness grafts contain all dermal structures and therefore can provide a better cosmetic appearance. Although they have more demanding nutritional requirements than split-thickness grafts, well-prepared full-thickness grafts can achieve survival rates comparable to thinner grafts. Split-thickness grafts contain the epidermis and only a variable amount of dermal structures. They have a number of disadvantages and are rarely used since they are rather fragile, require more care during collection and transfer and grafted sites tend to have poor durability, sparse hair growth and a greater tendency to contracture due to the absence of dermal structures.

Likewise, almost all grafts are applied as a sheet providing complete wound coverage since this provides the most functional and cosmetically acceptable result. Partial coverage techniques (e.g., stamp, pinch, strip, and mesh) are used only very infrequently and provide a poorer long-term result with significant contribution from epithelialization.

Ideal donor sites for skin grafts have an abundance of easily mobilized durable skin of suitable thickness with hair of a similar color, length and thickness to that it replaces at the recipient site. In practice, the flank usually satisfies most of these criteria and offers the best opportunity to remove sufficient skin for the reconstruction while permitting simple closure of the donor site.

PREOPERATIVE CONSIDERATIONS

The etiology and type of wounds are important preoperative considerations that influence the appropriate timing of closure. Surgically created or clean wounds can be immediately managed with local flaps, axial pattern flaps, or skin grafts. Traumatic wounds are often contaminated and usually require several days of open wound management before surgical reconstruction can be attempted.

Adequate planning must be undertaken prior to surgical dissection and reconstruction of large skin defects. It is essential to know which technique or method is most appropriate given the size, dimension, and location of the wound. A second important factor to take into account is the proper preparation of the recipient bed.

Preoperative measurements should be taken to ensure adequate length, width and total size of the flap so it can reach and cover the entire wound. Using sterile paper, cloth, gauze, or foam rubber, a template is made of the recipient bed, pressing the material in the wound and outlining the defect. The template is cut to the desired shape and positioned on the selected donor site to represent the proposed dimensions of the defect and additional skin required for the flap to reach the recipient bed. The graft outline is drawn on the skin with a felt-tipped marker pen to provide reference lines for the proposed incision. As one becomes more familiar with certain reconstruction techniques, the measurements can be drawn directly on the skin without resorting to templates.

Atraumatic technique and Halsted principles of surgery are essential to the execution of successful reconstructive surgery. Because of the limited blood supply, great care should be taken during the dissection and transfer of flaps and grafts.

SURGICAL TECHNIQUES

Single pedicle advancement flap
(Fig. 19-10, Box 19.2)

Advancement, or sliding, single pedicle flaps are rectangular in shape and are created parallel with lines of tension, with an attachment at the base opposite the edge covering the wound. They commonly are used to close square or rectangular wounds when tissue for closure is only available on one side of the defect.

Direct distant single pedicle (hinge) flap
(Figs 19-11–19.13, Box 19.3)

Distant flaps are used to reconstruct wounds at a remote site (e.g., flank donor to limb recipient site) and with the single pedicle one cutaneous donor site attachment is maintained. The patient's ability to tolerate immobilization of the affected limb against the flank should be assessed preoperatively. This flap is used in preference to the bipedicle flap when the wound is confined to either the medial or lateral aspect of the limb.

Direct distant bipedicle (pouch) flap
(Figs 19-14 and 19-15, Box 19.4)

Distant direct bipedicle (pouch) flaps are used to cover distal limb wounds which are not amenable to cover by axial pattern flaps or random flaps. The patient's ability to tolerate immobilization of the affected limb against the flank should be assessed preoperatively. The direct distant bipedicle flap is used in preference to the single pedicle

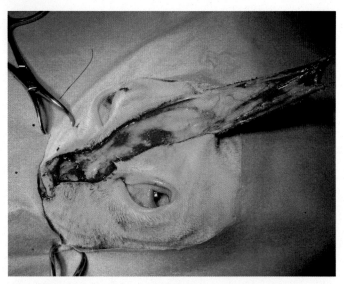

Figure 19-10 Single pedicle advancement flap. A single pedicle advancement flap is created to close a defect on the dorsal nasal bridge. There is plenty of skin that can be retrieved from the dorsal surface of the head.

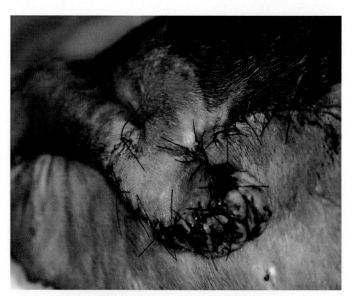

Figure 19-11 Single pedicle direct distant flap. A single pedicle direct distant flap is created to close a defect on the dorsal lateral aspect of the foot of a cat after a road traffic accident.

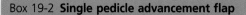

Box 19-2 Single pedicle advancement flap

Flap width equals the width of the defect and flap length is dictated by the amount of skin required to stretch and advance into the defect.

The skin is grasped to assess the direction of regional skin tension. Where possible, the long axis of the flap is oriented parallel with the lines of greatest tension. Two parallel incisions are made from the opposing wound edges equal to the width of the defect. The flap is carefully undermined and the incisions are extended in a staged fashion until the flap is sufficiently mobile to stretch over the defect. The leading corners of the flap are anchored to the distal edge of the wound defect. The surrounding skin is drawn back towards the flap base and anchored at the base. The flap is sutured into position to complete the transfer. A simple continuous suture pattern using 2M absorbable suture material such as polyglecaprone or polyglyconate is used for the subcutaneous layer and simple interrupted sutures of monofilament Nylon 2M for dermal closure. Skin folds created at the base of the flap will rapidly disappear without surgical interference.

---

flap when the wound is involving the entire circumference of the extremity. Bipedicle flaps are often impossible to use for proximal limb defects because the joints cannot usually be flexed enough to rotate the limb beneath the flap.

Thoracodorsal (TD) flap
(Figs 19-16 and 19.17, Box 19-5)

This flap is based on the cutaneous branch of the thoracodorsal artery and vein.[8,9] The TD vessels emerge from the intermuscular fascia at the caudal edge of the shoulder at the level of the acromion. The moderately sized artery arborizes in a caudodorsal direction. The cranial limit of the angiosome is defined by a line extending along the scapular spine. The caudal edge is parallel to the cranial edge and originates at a point equidistant from the scapular spine to the caudal shoulder depression. The ventral limit is marked by a line from the acromion to the axilla. The dorsal border is defined by the dorsal midline. Thoracodorsal flaps are robust and can be used to reconstruct

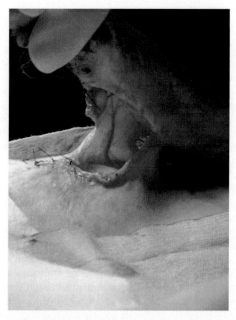

Figure 19-12 The pedicle is divided ten to 14 days after the initial transfer in stages. One-half to one-third is cut initially to avoid ischemia.

defects involving the shoulder, forelimb, elbow, axilla and thorax.[9] In some cats it is even possible to use this flap for reconstructions that extend to the level of the carpus.[8]

Lateral thoracic (LT) flap
(Figs 19-18–19.20, Box 19.6)

The lateral thoracic artery is the second branch of the axillary artery, is caudally directed, and initially runs deep to the axillary lymph node.[10] The artery becomes superficial caudal to the triceps muscle and continues in the subcutaneous tissue to the level of the last rib. This point can be palpated on careful examination and is defined as the centre of the flap in the dorsoventral direction. The ventral border of the flap is defined as the ventral midline. The dorsal border is defined

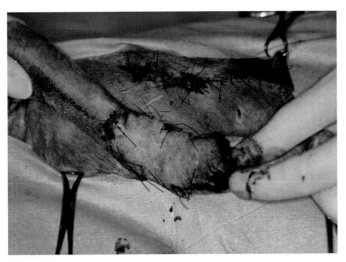

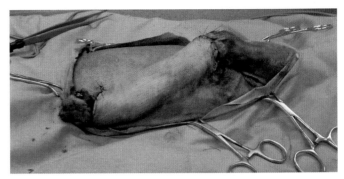

Figure 19-14 Bipedicle advancement direct distant flap. This flap was created after this cat had sustained a car accident and had one hindlimb amputated; one front leg had a comminuted fracture and the other front leg had a 360° circumferential degloving injury.

Figure 19-13 The end result after the remaining part of the pedicle is divided and the skin is sutured in place. This provides a robust full-thickness skin coverage.

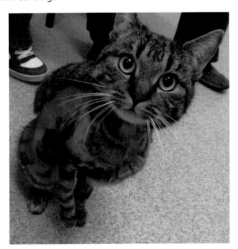

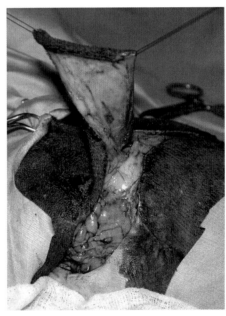

Figure 19-15 The same patient after the direct distant flap had completely healed. A good functional and cosmetic end result was achieved.

Figure 19-16 Thoracodorsal axial pattern flap. The borders of the flap are incised. Dissection begins at the dorsal edge and proceeds ventrally. Care should be taken at the vascular pedicle.

Box 19-3 **Direct distant single pedicle (hinge) flap**

The affected limb is positioned temporarily against the surface of the flank. For the forelimb this means drawing the limb caudally and for the hind limb drawing the limb cranially. The flap width is determined by the length of the limb deficit. The flap length is determined from the flap base to the most distal edge of the defect (circumferential size of deficit). The flap is incised and elevated below the cutaneous trunci muscle. The flap is sutured to the edges of the defect with subcutaneous and cutaneous sutures. The donor bed is partially closed, especially the subcutaneous tissues. Padding is placed between the limb and the trunk to prevent moist dermatitis. Retaining sutures can be placed to help support and prevent movement of the extremity. Large loop simple interrupted sutures with 3.5M Nylon are placed dorsal to the limb that needs supporting and wide Nylon tape can be looped around the limb and tied to the suture.

The leg is bandaged in place; bandages are changed and the graft assessed every 48 hours. The base of the flap is divided in two stages over the next ten to 14 days. Half of the flap is detached after five to six days and the remaining attachment divided by ten days. The free edges of the flap are sutured to the opposing wound border.

Box 19-4 **Distant direct bipedicle (pouch) flap**

Bipedicle flaps are created by two parallel incisions at the level of the desired donor site. The skin of the flap is undermined below the cutaneous trunci muscle but remains attached at each base. The limb is positioned under the flap by passing it under the elevated tunnel of skin. The flap is sutured to the proximal and distal borders of the defect.

A few additional mattress sutures can be placed to provide additional contact between skin of donor site and granulation tissue of recipient bed. The leg is immobilized as described above.

Both flap bases are divided in stages beginning five to six days after surgery. One-half of the lower pedicle and one-half of the upper pedicle at the opposite site are incised and sutured to the opposing wound border, followed by the remaining second halves two to three days later.

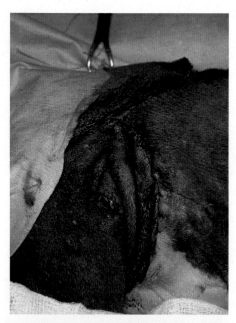

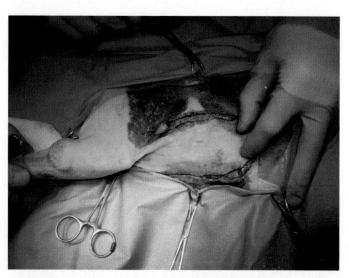

Figure 19-18 Lateral thoracic flap. The borders of the flap are incised. *(Courtesy of Laurent Findji.)*

Figure 19-17 The thoracodorsal axial pattern flap was used in this cat to cover a chronic axillary wound.

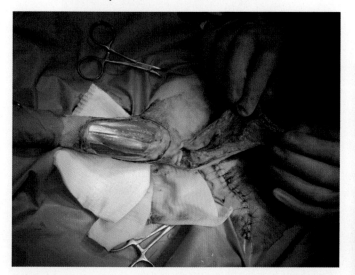

Figure 19-19 Lateral thoracic flap. A large tumor on the lateral aspect of the antebrachium was resected and a bridging incision was made to allow the axial pattern flap to be fit in place. *(Courtesy of Laurent Findji.)*

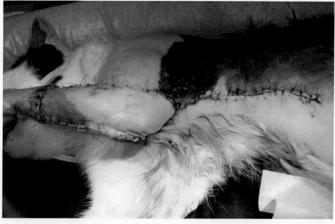

Figure 19-20 Lateral thoracic flap. The axial pattern flap was sutured in place and the donor site was closed. *(Courtesy of Laurent Findji.)*

Box 19-5 Thoracodorsal axial pattern flap

The patient is in lateral recumbency with the forelimb in relaxed extension (normal standing position). The cranial limit is defined by a line extending along the scapular spine. The caudal edge is parallel to the cranial edge and originates at a point equidistant from the scapular spine to the caudal shoulder depression. The dorsal border is defined by the dorsal midline. The borders of the flap are marked with a felt-tipped marker. The skin is incised and the flap is elevated below the level of the cutaneous trunci muscle beginning at the dorsal end of the flap. Great care must be taken to avoid damaging the thoracodorsal artery and vein. The vascular pedicle does not need to be completely isolated from the surrounding fat. This flap can then be pivoted into a variety of positions. A bridging incision can be made to traverse the skin interposed between donor and recipient site. The flap is sutured in place with subcutaneous and skin sutures.

Box 19-6 Lateral thoracic axial pattern flap

The lateral thoracic artery and vein enter the skin cranial and ventral to the thoracodorsal artery. The borders of the flap are outlined as shown in Figures 19-18 and 19-19. The ventral border of the flap is defined as the ventral midline. The dorsal border is defined as a line parallel to the ventral border at a distance equal to the distance from the centre of the flap, which is an area just caudal to the triceps muscle. The caudal border coincides with the last rib. Elevation of the lateral thoracic axial pattern flap under the cutaneous muscle and mammary tissue allows closure of defects within its arc of rotation. A small bridging incision can be made to facilitate flap placement onto the recipient bed. The flap is sutured in place with subcutaneous and skin sutures.

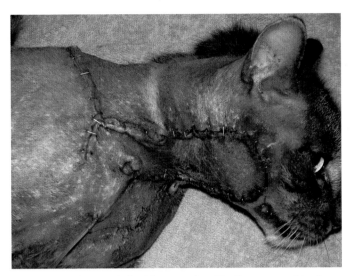

Figure 19-21 Omocervical axial pattern flap. The flap was used to close a large defect in the cervical region of this patient after resection of a large skin tumor.

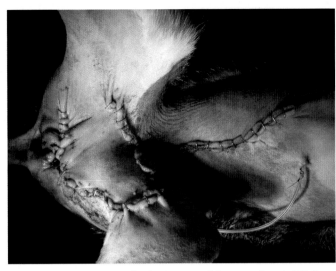

Figure 19-22 Caudal superficial epigastric axial pattern flap. A CSE flap was created for this cat to cover a large chronic non-healing wound on the medial thigh after a cat bite.

Box 19-7 Omocervical axial pattern flap

The cranial shoulder depression is identified and this point denotes the emergence of the superficial branch of the omocervical artery. The caudal border is incised over the scapular spine. The cranial shoulder depression is palpated and the cranial incision is made parallel to the caudal incision equal to the distance from the cranial shoulder to the caudal incision line. The dorsal midline incision extends between the cranial and caudal incision. The flap is undermined below the level of the superficial cutaneous muscle. The flap is sutured into the recipient bed with subcutaneous and skin sutures. The donor site is closed in a routine fashion.

Box 19-8 Caudal superficial epigastric axial pattern flap

Two skin incisions are made, midline and a lateral parallel incision at an equal distance from the nipples. The cranial extent of the flap depends on the length required to incorporate the second mammary gland and the length required to cover the intended deficit. The flap is undermined below the supramammarius muscle and above the aponeurosis of the external abdominal oblique muscle. The flap can be rotated into a variety of positions, taking care to preserve the vascular bundle from excessive kinking or twisting. A bridging incision may be necessary. Wider flaps may be possible as long as there is adequate skin left to close the donor bed.

---

as a line parallel to the ventral border at a distance equal to the distance from the centre of the flap. The caudal border coincides with the last rib and the cranial border lies adjacent to the caudal border of the triceps muscle. The proximity of the LT flap to the thoracic limb facilitates reconstruction in this region. The area of the LT skin flap is one-third larger than the TD flap and this can be used to cover skin defects extending distally to the carpus.[10]

Omocervical (OC) flap (Fig. 19-21 and Box 19.7)

The superficial cervical branch of the omocervical artery originates at the prescapular lymph node and radiates craniodorsally. This flap is robust and is very useful for head and neck reconstruction. The ventral limit of this flap is defined by a line from the prescapular lymph node to the acromion. The dorsal edge is formed by the dorsal midline. The cranial edge is defined by a line equidistant to a point between the cranial shoulder depression and the scapular spine. The caudal border is a line parallel to the scapular spine. This flap is versatile and can be used to cover defects of the face, head, axilla, and ear.[11]

Caudal superficial epigastric (CSE) flap
(Fig. 19-22, Box 19.8)

This flap includes the tissue of the second, third and fourth mammary glands and is based on the caudal superficial epigastric artery, a branch

of the external pudendal artery. This vessel emerges from the inguinal ring and travels cranially along the mammary chain. The caudal border is defined by the inguinal ring. The cranial border extends to the second mammary gland. The medial limit is delineated by the ventral midline and the lateral edge extents from a point twice the distance from the nipple to the midline. This flap is a highly versatile option for closure of major skin defects of the abdomen, flank, inguinal area, perineum, thigh, and hind limbs.[8] Flap length and width will vary according to the patient's body conformation, elasticity of the skin and the size required to cover or to reach the defect. The CSE flap can extend to, or even below, the level of the feline tarsus. Bilateral CSE flaps have been used to repair large defects of the hindlimb[12] and perineal area[13] in the cat.

Sheet skin grafts
(Figs 19-23 and 19-24, Box 19.9)

The use of free skin grafts is confined almost exclusively to reconstruction of large skin defects of the extremities. The use of random flaps for these distal limb wounds is often restricted by the limited availability of adjacent skin. Direct flaps offer an alternative solution although the temperament of some cats may not always be conducive to this option. The use of axial pattern flaps for distal limb wounds is limited by the length of the vascular pedicle and the size of the flap, which is often not long enough to cover distal wounds.

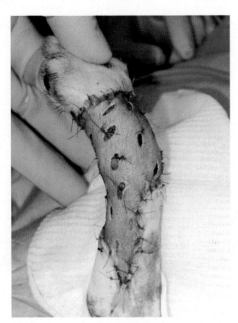

Figure 19-23 Free skin grafts. A free skin graft was applied for a 360° defect of the distal extremity of this patient. *(Courtesy of Laurent Findji.)*

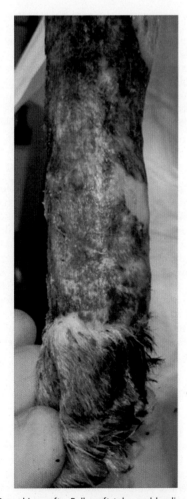

Figure 19-24 Free skin grafts. Full graft take and healing of the skin graft with a complete functional and good cosmetic end result. *(Courtesy of Laurent Findji.)*

Box 19-9 Free skin grafts

A template is made from the wound defect and then positioned over the donor site to match the hair growth at the recipient site. Ideally, the longest aspect of the template should be orientated along the tension lines of the donor site. An area of skin to include the area of the template is incised; in possible, elliptical areas are removed since this provides for simplest reconstruction of the donor wound. In general, skin incisions are made slightly larger than the template outline to ensure wound coverage. The underlying hypodermis and loose adipose tissue is carefully removed with scissors from the graft until the dermal layer is apparent. This can be most easily performed by laying the skin over a roll of sterile Vetrap (Smith and Nephew) to keep the skin flap under slight tension while performing this dissection. Damage to the dermal layer itself should be avoided. Depending on the type of graft, one or more stab incisions can be made in the graft. Grafts should be kept moist by rinsing them with sterile saline. The graft is laid over the wound and anchored with sutures to one side of the wound. The opposite side of the graft is now anchored with slight stretching of the graft to result in slight tension that ensures good contact with the wound surface and eliminates dead space. Redundant areas of graft are excised. The graft is carefully bandaged with a low adherent to non-adherent contact layer such as a silicone dressing. These dressings are usually comprised of an absorbent layer of cotton and acrylic fibre heat bonded with a thin perforated polyester film. An example of such a dressing is Mepitel (Molnlycke Health Care).

MUSCLE FLAPS

Pedicled muscle flaps have been used for a wide range of purposes in small animal surgery including coverage after large oncological resections (see Chapter 43), perineal hernia repair (see Chapter 25), diaphragmatic hernia,[14] bone coverage, and for combating infections. Free muscle flaps are not commonly performed in small animals due to the need and expense of being able to perform microvascular transfer,[15] and compared to humans small animals have considerable amounts of loose skin and a number of direct cutaneous arteries for local flaps, axial pattern flaps and free skin grafts. Several individual muscles in cats and dogs are expendable without compromising function and these muscles can be pivoted into an adjacent defect.[16] Muscles are capable of contributing additional circulation to ischemic areas. Individual muscles have different vascular supplies and muscles are classified according to their vascular anatomy. There are five major vascular patterns. Preservation of muscle function and bulk will depend upon preservation of the blood supply and the innervation. A muscle flap involves elevating part or all of a muscle while preserving its vascular supply and transposing it into a recipient bed. The most useful muscles are superficial and should be accessible through a standard surgical approach (Box 19.10). The dissection of the muscles should be easy and with minimal trauma to surrounding structures. Examples of muscle flaps include: internal obturator transposition for ventrolateral augmentation of perineal hernia, cranial sartorius flap to fill dead space, close over pressure sore, repair of abdominal hernias or prepubic tendon avulsion, semitendinosus flap to augment complicated perineal hernias, latissimus dorsi muscle flap to reconstruct defects left after trauma or tumor resection of the thoracic wall and cranial and caudal portions of the sternocephalic, sternothyroid, and sternohyoid muscles to repair wounds in the cervical region or to patch defects in the trachea or esophagus.

An ideal muscle flap should have the following properties:
Easily accessible
Expendable function
Consistent vascular supply
Single pedicle vascular supply
Sufficiently far away from recipient bed
Reasonable size and bulk
Available bilaterally

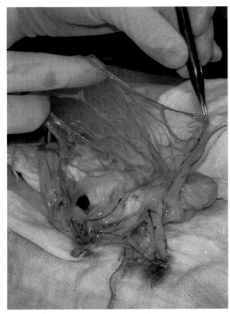

Figure 19-25 Omental pedicle flaps. The greater omentum is a double leaf of peritoneal mesothelial tissues. The omentum is composed of connective tissue and fat and has a rich vascular and lymphatic network.

OMENTAL PEDICLE FLAP

The greater omentum is a thin double peritoneal mesothelial sheet composed of connective tissue and streaks of fat that surround fine arteries and a rich lymphatic network. This double sheet folds onto itself in the caudal abdomen forming a ventral and dorsal leaf (Fig. 19-25). The omentum attaches ventrally to the greater curvature of the stomach and dorsally to the greater curvature of the stomach and the pancreas and spleen. The blood supply derives from peripheral vessels of the right and left gastroepiploic arteries. The lesser omentum connects the lesser curvature of the stomach and a part of the duodenum with the liver. The greater omentum is used for pedicle flaps.

Omentum has been extensively used in surgical applications and can be useful for closure of problematic defects by improving circulation to ischemic or compromised tissues.[17] This tissue effectively obliterates dead space, acts as a natural drain, and the rich vascular and lymphatic networks provide the cells and humoral factors required to control infection, promote adhesion, and stimulate angiogenesis. The omentum is used widely in humans in situations where rapid neovascularization is needed, to enhance immune function and provide local tissue support and lymphatic drainage, and to achieve hemostasis.[17]

Omentum provides a permanent drain and improved ability to resist infection.[18]

Creation of an omental pedicle flap was first described in veterinary medicine by Ross & Pardo.[19] The omentum can be transferred to all sites within the abdominal cavity and outer abdominal wall (Box 19-11); however, lengthening procedures are required for transferring the omentum to more distant sites such as the axillary or inguinal areas. The dorsal or ventral surfaces of the omentum can be unfolded and divided to increase its length. Major limitations of using the omentum are its relatively fragility and lack of bulk tissue for closure of large defects. Indications for omental flaps include axillary wounds (see Chapter 18), non-healing wounds, drainage of pancreatic or prostatic cysts, placement over intestinal incisions, and after thoracic wall resection (see Chapter 43).

POSTOPERATIVE CARE

Passive or active suction drains can be placed for two to four days after surgery to prevent or manage seroma formation.[20] Soft padded bandages can protect the drains from contamination, decrease dead space, help prevent fluid accumulation, and prevent mutilation by the patient. Buster (Elizabethan) collars are mandatory to prevent interference with or mutilation of the surgical site (see Chapter 3).[20]

The role of microbial agents in wound management is based on the disease process, contamination, microorganisms involved, and surgical procedures. Acute infections are usually due to one microorganism, but chronic wounds are often polymicrobial. Therefore the choice whether to use antibiotics pre- and/or postoperatively is dictated by the patient, disease, and surgical procedure.[20]

Postoperative analgesia is very important in patients undergoing reconstructive surgery. Skin tension, swelling, inflammation, and infection can all contribute to increased pain. A multimodal approach to pain management is therefore recommended. Pre-, intra- and postoperative pain control using opioids, non-steroidal inflammatory drugs and local anesthetic protocols should be tailored to each individual cat.

The postoperative care of skin grafts is extremely important. The survival of a skin graft largely depends on optimization of adherence and nutrition of the graft. Few bandages require more exact application than a bandage used to secure and immobilize an area after application of a free graft. Most free grafts are performed on extremities and suitable dressings and bandages are critical during the period of graft take.[20] The different components of the bandage promote good contact between graft and recipient bed, minimize graft movement, remove exudates from the wound bed, and prevent soiling, contamination and patient interference.

The dressing may be changed as early as 48 hours; however, it is safer to wait for three days to assure the period of revascularization is not disturbed. Care must be taken not to pull or lift the graft from the recipient bed during the dressing change. If the dressing is adhered to the graft, the dressing can be softened with warm sterile saline.

The frequency of bandage changes varies with patient and graft techniques used. Generally, bandage changes can be performed every three to four days after the initial change.

Viable grafts assume lavender to pink color depending on the state of vascularization. Dead skin assumes a white or black color. Early signs of graft necrosis are not always catastrophic, because hair follicles and cutaneous adnexa can survive in the dermal layers and may serve as a source for wound epithelialization.

Experimental treatments to rescue a failing flap or graft using hyperbaric oxygen have shown some encouraging results, including improved color and decreased exudate production by the skin flap in

Box 19-11 **Omental pedicle flaps**[19]

A midline laparotomy is performed (see Chapter 23); alternatively, a paracostal incision can be made. The omentum is lifted upward and cranially to expose the dorsal surface. The omentum can be used by creating a vascular pedicle involving either the right or left gastroepiploic artery or by releasing the omentum from the pancreas and then lengthening it with an inverted L-shaped incision.

Vascularized pedicle: The vascularized omental pedicle or flap is created by ligation of the segmental gastric arteries as they leave the gastroepiploic artery and enter the greater curvature of the stomach (Fig. 19-26A). Either the right or left gastroepiploic artery has to be ligated or additional attachments to the pancreas and spleen have to be incised. A pedicle of the ventral omental sheet is created based on the right or left gastroepiploic artery, respectively.

Release from pancreas: An alternative technique involves traction of the omental leaf cranially and release of the dorsal leaf from the pancreas by sharp dissection (Fig. 19-26B,C). Vessels originating from the splenic artery are ligated and the omentum is unfolded caudally.

Further lengthening can be performed by creating an inverted L incision beginning on the left side of the omentum caudal to the gastrosplenic ligament and crossing to half the width of the omental sheet (Fig. 19-26D,E). The encountered omental vessels have to be double ligated. The incision is continued caudally parallel to the omental vessels along two-thirds of the length of the omentum.

Omentalization outside the body: An incision is made in the abdominal wall relevant to the region where the omentum is required and a subcutaneous tunnel can be created (Fig. 19-27). The omentum is packed into a large Penrose drain to facilitate its passage to the desired area without damaging this friable tissue. The omentum is sutured, using simple interrupted 3M absorbable suture material such as poliglecaprone, into the recipient wound bed. The laparotomy wound is closed and the exit wound for the omentum should be partially closed but left large enough so as not to cause vascular compromise.

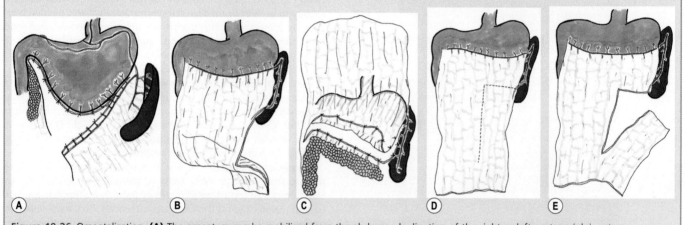

Figure 19-26 Omentalization. **(A)** The omentum can be mobilized from the abdomen by ligation of the right or left gastroepiploic artery, depending on which side of the body the omentum is to be used. **(B)** Alternatively, the omentum can be unfolded by retracting the dorsal omental leaf cranially by exteriorizing the spleen. **(C)** The omentum is separated from its attachments on the pancreas and spleen by ligating the vessels as they are encountered. **(D, E)** An inverted L-shaped incision can be performed to further lengthen the omentum. One-half to two-thirds of the omental width can be cut. The omentum should be handled with care to prevent occlusion of the remaining vessels to maintain its viability.

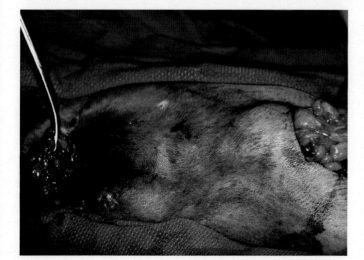

Figure 19-27 An incision is made at the region where the omentum is required and a Penrose drain can be useful to help guide the omentum through a subcutaneous tunnel. The omentum is then sutured in place in the recipient bed.

the early postoperative period but clinical data in small animals is lacking.[21]

COMPLICATIONS

The most common postoperative complications following local flaps and axial pattern flaps are edema, seroma formation, and poor wound drainage.[20] The problems arise due to extensive soft tissue dissection at the donor and recipient sites. Hematoma and seroma formation can predispose to wound infection, may cause discomfort, and prevent healing of tissues on to wound beds. Prevention of intraoperative hemorrhage is more prudent than postoperative management of a hematoma.

Creation of dead space through trauma or surgical dissection can lead to accumulation of fluid within the subcutaneous space. Prevention of seroma formation is achieved by gentle tissue handling and elimination of dead space by using active suction drains, subcutaneous sutures and bandages.

Exudation of fluid into the interstitial space of the subcutaneous tissue is associated with early wound healing processes. Traumatic wounds generally exhibit more edema than surgical wounds. Depending on the dissection and the nature of the procedure, surgical wounds can also appear edematous in the first three to four days postoperatively.

Wound dehiscence may be the result of several factors including wound closure under excessive tension, sutures placed too close to the incision site, improper suture material, closure of compromised skin, compromised cutaneous circulation, underlying infection, necrosis, foreign material, neoplasia, lack of postoperative protection and support, premature suture removal, delayed healing due to steroid use, or delay in healing due to metabolic disorders.

Infection is uncommon if aseptic techniques are adhered to. Pasteurella is a common isolate from soft tissue infections in cats and these are mostly related to cat bites. Two to three days after surgery clinical signs of infection become apparent. The affected area is warm, erythematous, edematous, and painful. The incision may be gaping with serosanguinous, mucoid or purulent discharge.

Omentalization

Possible complications after omental transposition include seroma formation, herniation of abdominal contents through the omental exit hole, and flap necrosis.

REFERENCES

1. Bohling MW, Henderson RA, Swaim SF, et al. Comparison of the role of the subcutaneous tissues in cutaneous wound healing in the dog and cat. Vet Surg 2006;35:3–14.

2. Pavletic MM. Vascular supply to the skin of the dog, a review. Vet Surg 1980;9:77.

3. Lemarié RJ, Hosgood G, Read RA, et al. Distant abdominal and thoracic pedicle skin flaps for treatment of distal limb skin defects. J Small Anim Pract 1995;36: 255–61.

4. Yturraspe DJ, Creed JE, Schwach RP. Thoracic pedicle skin flap for repair of lower limb wounds in dogs and cats. J Am Anim Hosp Assoc 1976;12:581.

5. Pavletic MM. Axial pattern flaps in small animal practice. Vet Clin North Am 1990;20:105.

6. Waldron DR. Feline axillary pattern skin flaps. NAVC Conference, 2008.

7. Siegfried R, Schmökel H, Rytz U, et al. Treatment of large distal extremity skin wounds with autogenous full thickness mesh skin grafts in five cats. Schweizer Arch.Tierheilkunde 2004;146:277–83.

8. Remedios AM, Bauer MS, Bowen CV. Thoracodorsal and caudal superficial epigastric axial pattern skin flaps in cats. Vet Surg 1989;18:380–5.

9. Lascelles BDX, White RAS. Combined Omental Pedicle Grafts and Thoracodorsal Axial Pattern Flaps for the Reconstruction of Chronic, Nonhealing Axillary Wounds in Cats. Vet Surg 2001;30:380–5.

10. Benzioni H, Shahar R, Yudelevich S, et al. Lateral thoracic artery axial pattern flap in cats. Vet Surg 2009;38:112–16.

11. Gray MJ. Chronic axillary wound repair in a cat with omentalisation and omocervical skin flap. J Small Anim Pract 2005;46:499–503.

12. Woods S, de C Marques AI, Yool DA. Simultaneous bilateral caudal superficial epigastric flaps in a cat. Vet Rec 2009;164: 434–5.

13. Clarke BS, Findji L. Bilateral caudal superficial epigastric skin flap and perineal urethrostomy for wound reconstruction secondary to traumatic urethral rupture in a cat. Vet Comp Orthop Traumatol 2011;24:142–5.

14. Furneaux RW, Hudson MD. Autogenous muscle flap repair of a diaphragmatic hernia. Feline Pract 1985;6:20–4.

15. Nicoll SA, Fowler JD, Remedios AM, et al. Development of a free latissimus dorsi muscle flap in cats. Vet Surg 1996;25: 40–8.

16. Gregory CR, Gourley IM, Snyder JR, Ilkiw J. Experimental definition of the gracilis musculocutaneous flap for distant transfer in cats. Am J Vet Res 1992;53:153–6.

17. Brockman DJ, Pardo AD, Conzemius MG, et al. Omentum-enhanced reconstruction of chronic nonhealing wounds in cats: techniques and clinical use. Vet Surg 1996;25:99–104.

18. Lascelles BDX, Davison L, Dunning M. Use of omental pedicle grafts in the management of non-healing axillary wounds in 10 cats. JSAP 1998;39:475–80.

19. Ross WE, Pardo AD. Evaluation of an omental pedicle extension technique in the dog. Vet Surg 1993;22(1):37–43.

20. Amsellem P. Complications of reconstructive surgery in companion animals. Vet Clin North Am Small Anim Pract 2011;41:995–1006.

21. Kerwin SC, Hosgood G, Strain GM, et al. The effect of hyperbaric oxygen treatment on a compromised axial pattern flap in the cat. Vet Surg 1993;22:31–6.

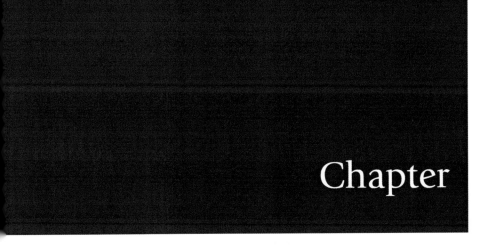

Chapter |20|

Skin tumors

J.M. Dobson, J.L. Demetriou

The skin is the largest and most easily observed organ in the body and therefore it is not surprising that the skin is a common site for tumor diagnosis in the cat. According to one large study, skin tumors comprised 9.6% of feline necropsy or biopsy specimens.[1] Due to its complex structure, a large variety of tumors may arise in the skin and it is also a possible site for the development of secondary, metastatic tumors. This chapter will consider tumors arising from or within the epidermis, dermis and related structures and soft tissue tumors, which may arise within dermal connective tissue; the reported incidence of these tumors in the cat is summarized in Table 20-1.[2]

PATHOGENESIS

Etiology

Several external agents and biologic factors are recognized to be important in the development of certain tumors of the skin but for the majority the etiology is unknown. Long-term exposure to ultraviolet light (especially UVB) is implicated in the development of squamous and basal cell tumors in unprotected, non-pigmented and lightly haired skin. Papilloma viruses may, in some cats, give rise to viral plaques and these can progress to form 'Bowenoid' in situ carcinoma which can in turn progress to invasive squamous cell carcinoma (SCC).

Pathology

The skin is a complex organ essentially comprising two layers:

- The epidermis, a stratified squamous epithelium
- The dermis, of vascular dense connective tissue.

In addition, there are associated sebaceous and sweat glands and hair follicles, collectively termed the 'adnexae', plus melanocytes, histiocytes, and dermal mast cells. Any of these tissues and cells may give rise to benign or malignant tumors. Squamous cell carcinoma is the most frequent malignant tumor of the skin in the cat. Benign skin tumors, e.g., lipoma and adenoma, are less common in the cat as compared with the dog, with the exception of basal cell tumors.

GENERAL CLINICAL APPROACH

Clinical examination

A presumptive diagnosis of a solitary skin tumor may be made on the clinical examination, including visual inspection and palpation. Skin tumors that present as multifocal lesions may be harder to distinguish from other dermatological conditions. In both cases skin tumors must be differentiated from other skin lesions (Box 20-1).

A useful clinical approach to a lesion affecting the skin is to determine the location of the lesion, i.e., whether it is epidermal, dermal or subcutaneous, as this will give some indication of its origin and thus its possible histogenesis. The distinction between solitary and multiple lesions is also of clinical value. However, a definitive diagnosis can only be made upon histopathological examination of representative tissue.

Blood analysis

Routine hematological and biochemical analysis of blood is not generally very helpful in the diagnosis of skin tumors, although some skin tumors may be associated with hematological or paraneoplastic complications and these investigations would be indicated in the general evaluation of such tumors.

Imaging techniques

Radiography of the primary tumor is not usually necessary unless the lesion is invasive and sited close to bone (e.g., SCC of the digit). Radiography of the thorax and ultrasound evaluation of abdominal organs (liver, spleen, and kidneys) is important in the clinical staging of malignant tumors. Both techniques may be used to assess the internal iliac and sub-lumbar lymph nodes for staging malignant skin tumors sited on the hind limbs and perianal region.

Biopsy and fine needle aspiration

Cutaneous masses are easily accessible for fine needle aspiration and this is a quick, minimally invasive and useful technique for assessing

© 2014 Elsevier Ltd
DOI: 10.1016/B978-0-7020-4336-9.00020-2

Table 20-1 The reported incidence of skin tumors in the cat

Skin tumors and tumor-like lesions (n = 3260)		Mesenchymal skin tumors (n = 1550)	
Epithelial tumors	43% (60% benign, 40% malignant)	Fibrosarcoma	36%
Melanocytic tumors	1% (58% benign, 42% malignant)	Giant cell tumor of soft tissue	2%
Mesenchymal tumors	47% (20% benign, 80% malignant)	Myxomatous tumors	2%
Tumor-like lesions	9%	Neural tumors	3%
Epithelial skin tumors (n = 1400)		Lipoma	12%
Basal cell tumor	34%	Liposarcoma	<1%
Basal cell carcinoma	3%	Hemangioma	4%
Basosquamous carcinoma	<1%	Hemangiosarcoma	6%
Squamous cell carcinoma	23%	Lymphangioma	<1%
Sebaceous adenoma	4%	Mast cell tumor	27%
Sebaceous carcinoma	2%	Lymphosarcoma	6%
Meibomian gland adenoma	<1%	Plasmacytoma	<1%
Apocrine gland adenoma	7%	Others	<1%
Apocrine ductal adenoma	5%	**Non-neoplastic skin lesions (n = 280)**	
Apocrine gland carcinoma	6%	Epidermal cyst	42%
Ceruminous gland adenoma	6%	Follicular cyst	10%
Ceruminous gland carcinoma	7%	Apocrine cyst	13%
Anal sac gland carcinoma	<1%	Ceruminous cyst / hyperplasia	20%
Trichoepithelioma	2%	Sebaceous hyperplasia	11%
Pilomatrixoma	<1%	Meibomian hyperplasia	<1%
		Adnexal nevus	1%
		Skin tag	3%

Reprinted from Goldschmidt MH and Shofer FS, Skin Tumours of the Dog and Cat. 2008. Copyright ©John Wiley and Sons, with permission.

Box 20-1 Differential diagnoses for skin lesions

Tumor, benign or malignant
Hyperplastic lesions
Granulomatous lesions
Inflammatory lesions
Immune-mediated lesions
Developmental lesions

---

any mass within the skin. In some cases (e.g., mast cell tumors, cutaneous lymphoma) cytology may provide a diagnosis, although histological examination of the tumor may still be required to assess the grade of the lesion. Fine needle aspiration of local lymph nodes is also useful to assess metastatic spread.

Skin punch, needle, or incisional biopsies are required for a definitive histological diagnosis. Collection of a representative sample of tissue is important. Areas of ulceration and necrosis should be avoided and it is important to collect a deep enough sample of the tumor. Careful planning of the biopsy procedure should be made so that seeding of tumor cells through normal tissue planes is avoided.

Definitive surgery should include the biopsy tracts, as they are regarded as contaminated. Excisional biopsy (i.e., local resection of the whole mass) is not generally recommended, except as a diagnostic procedure in a case with multiple skin lesions. More details on biopsy techniques can be found in Chapter 14.

Staging

Clinical staging of primary tumors of the skin is by clinical examination and imaging of body cavities where indicated by the nature of the primary tumor. The primary tumor is assessed on the basis of its size, infiltration of the subcutis, and involvement of other structures such as fascia, muscle, and bone (Box 20-2). For more information on tumor staging see Chapter 14.

EPITHELIAL TUMORS

Papilloma/cutaneous papillomatosis

Cutaneous papillomatosis is a viral disease that is rare in dogs and very rare in cats, but papilloma viruses may be implicated in the etiology of some carcinomas of the feline skin.

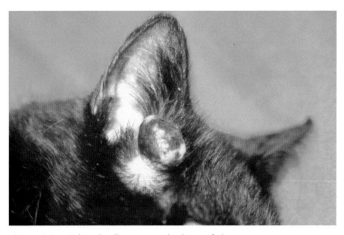

Figure 20-1 A basal cell tumor at the base of the ear. *(Courtesy of David Grant.)*

indicated that quantitative analysis of the nuclei of basal cell carcinoma neoplastic cells (by nuclear morphometry) is able to predict recurrent tumor growth and helps to differentiate histological subtypes in cats, which may be of practical value.[5]

Tumors of the adnexae

Benign adnexal tumors are relatively common in the dog but appear to be less common in the cat and they include:

- Tumors of hair follicles (trichoelipthelioma and pilomatricoma)
- Glandular tumors (sebaceous, apocrine, meibomian, ceruminous).

In one survey of feline follicular tumors in Italy trichoblastoma was reported as the most common form, representing 26% of cases. Follicular tumors and tumor-like lesions together represented 8% of all skin tumors in the cat.[6] All these tumors are slow growing, non-invasive and benign in their behavior. Malignant tumors arising from the adnexal structures of the skin are extremely rare in the cat.

Treatment and prognosis

Treatment is surgical (if required) and the prognosis is good. Sebaceous epithelioma may recur following incomplete surgical excision.

Squamous cell carcinoma

Squamous cell carcinoma is the most common malignant skin tumor in the cat, accounting for 15–50% of all skin neoplasms. It usually affects older animals and there is no known breed predisposition, although white-coated cats have a higher incidence. SCC is a locally invasive tumor that infiltrates the underlying dermal and subcutaneous tissue. Metastasis tends to be via the lymphatic route but the incidence of metastasis is low.

Feline cutaneous SCC most frequently occurs on the head, affecting particularly the pinnae, nasal planum, and eyelids (Figs 20-2 to 20-4). The etiology in the majority of cases is related to long-term exposure of unprotected skin (non-pigmented, hairless regions) to ultraviolet light, with lesions initially of solar dermatitis progressing to actinic keratitis (actinic carcinoma in situ) to carcinoma in situ to invasive SCC, often over quite a long course of time. Ultraviolet-related p53 lesions have been identified in feline SCC. Clinically these lesions are crusty, scabby, ulcerated to plaque-like. Diagnosis is made by tissue biopsy and histology. Staging beyond local disease is not usually necessary.

Basal cell tumor/carcinoma

This tumor is relatively common in the cat and usually affects middle-aged to older animals. It is reported to account for 14– 26% of feline skin tumors[1,2] or for 34% of feline epithelial tumors.[3]

Tumors are usually solitary, discrete, firm, well-circumscribed masses, sited in the dermis and subcutis of the head and neck (Fig. 20-1). The overlying skin may be ulcerated. Most tumors are small, 0.5–2.0 cm in diameter, although on occasion they may reach up to 10 cm in size. Some feline basal cell tumors contain abundant melanin pigment and may therefore be confused on gross inspection with melanoma. Various subtypes have been described based on the histological appearance, e.g., solid, cystic, adenoid, and medusoid. Diagnosis can be made on cytological examination; however, the occurrence of cells with characteristic basal cell-like appearance has been shown to be an inconsistent finding in cats.[4]

Treatment and prognosis

These are usually slow-growing, non-invasive tumors that follow a benign course and rarely metastasize. Occasionally, more invasive tumors may be seen that are similar to the human 'rodent ulcer'. Local/wide local surgical excision is the treatment of choice and in most cases is curative so the prognosis is good. Local recurrence can occur following incomplete surgical excision. Results from one study

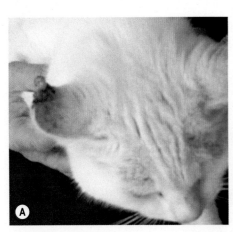
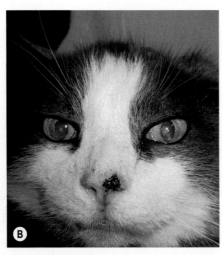
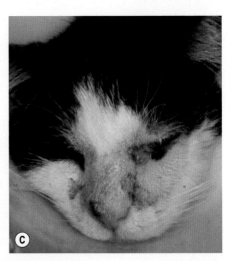

Figure 20-2 Squamous cell carcinoma **(A)** on the pinna of a white cat, **(B)** on the nasal planum, and **(C)** on the eyelid.

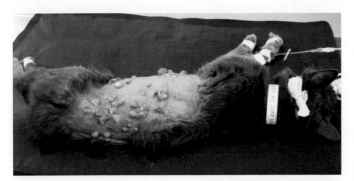

Figure 20-3 Diffuse form of squamous cell carcinoma affecting the trunk.

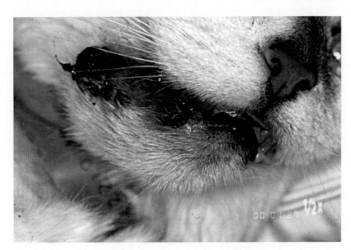

Figure 20-4 A lip melanoma.

Treatment and prognosis

These sunlight-induced lesions are generally slowly progressive, locally invasive and very rarely metastasize. Wide local surgical excision is the treatment of choice, and in cases where this can be achieved, the prognosis is favorable. Early diagnosis and prompt and effective treatment are recommended for these lesions as, if left, over time they can become more invasive and less responsive to treatment. Surgery is the only effective means of management of more extensive lesions (see

Chapters 50 and 54). For early lesions, local control may be also achieved by a number of other methods including cryosurgery and strontium radiotherapy. Superficial lesions may also be treated successfully with photodynamic therapy (PDT) that offers the advantage of excellent cosmetic results. One of the authors (JMD) has experience of using a topical method of applying the photochemical, 5-aminolevulinic acid (ALA) and excitation using a high intensity red light. An 85% complete response rate was seen in 55 cats with superficial Tis–T1 tumors, treated with topical PDT, and at a median follow up of 1146 days 45% of cats were alive and disease free.[7] There are also reports in the literature of use of an immunomodulatory agent imiquimod (Aldara) as a topical cream in cats with superficial or multicentric SCC.[8] Electrochemotherapy, involving the administration of a chemotherapeutic agent alongside the delivery of appropriate waveforms that induce and increase uptake of the drug by cancer cells, has also been described as a successful treatment in cats, with some cats responding for up to three years.[9] However, a larger scale trial is required before this therapy can be recommended.

One study evaluating the prognosis of feline cutaneous SCC looked at the role of epidermal growth factor receptors (EGFR). Results indicated that 74% of tumors were positive for EGFR and this did not correlate with tumor differentiation or mitotic activity. However, patients with EGFR-positive tumors had a significantly worse outcome with decreased disease free intervals (DFIs) and survival times. It was postulated that using EGFR inhibitors in addition to conventional treatments may therefore improve outcomes for some cats with SCC.[10]

Multicentric SCC

A muticentric SCC in situ has been described in cats. Biologically, this is a premalignant lesion that is histologically similar to Bowen disease in humans (and hence sometimes referred to as Bowenoid carcinoma). This tends to affect middle-aged to older mixed breed cats with lesions developing in haired, pigmented regions of the skin including the trunk, limbs, feet, head, and neck. As with the human Bowen's disease papilloma virus may be implicated in the etiology, and the lesion can progress to invasive SCC.

Other forms of SCC

Multiple digital carcinomas have been reported in cats. The digital lesions appear to be secondary, metastatic tumors from a primary pulmonary carcinoma, a so-called 'lung-digit' syndrome.[11] Other rare carcinomas that have been reported in cats include Merkel Cell

Carcinoma, a cutaneous neuroendocrine tumor[12] and an intraepidermal adenocarcinoma in the perianal skin.[13]

MELANOMA

Melanocytic tumors are relatively uncommon tumors of the skin in the cat, representing 1–2% of all feline skin tumors.[2,3] Older cats are affected, with a mean age of 8 years; there is no sex or breed predisposition. Grossly, tumors may appear as flat, plaque-like to domed masses, up to 2 cm in diameter, sited within the dermis. They are usually dark brown to black and quite well defined. Malignant tumors, which comprise 35–45% of cutaneous melanocytic tumors in cats, may attain a larger size, contain less pigment and frequently ulcerate. Cutaneous melanoma must be distinguished from the more common pigmented basal cell tumor.

Treatment and prognosis

Wide surgical excision is the treatment of choice for benign dermal melanoma and the prognosis following complete surgical excision is good. Tumors may recur locally if excision is incomplete, so regular follow-up examinations are recommended. Surgical excision is also indicated for local control of malignant tumors but the prognosis in such cases is guarded to poor because of the high incidence of metastasis. These tumors are not considered to be chemosensitive. The efficacy of radiation therapy and immunotherapy is unknown for this tumor in cats.

MAST CELL TUMORS

Mast cell tumors are less common in the cat than in the dog and are also less of a diagnostic problem. Two forms of mast cell tumor are recognized in the cat: cutaneous and visceral.

Cutaneous mast cell tumors

Cutaneous mast cell tumors account for up to 21% of all feline cutaneous tumors. The majority of feline cutaneous mast cell tumors are solitary cutaneous/dermal nodules (Fig. 20-5). The most common sites of occurrence are on the head and trunk. These tumors are usually histologically well differentiated and have a benign clinical course. On occasion a cat may be affected by multiple skin nodules (Fig. 20-6) or a solitary lesion may be invasive (Fig. 20-7). However, the majority of cutaneous mast cell tumors in the cat are benign and histological grading of feline cutaneous mast cell tumors has not been shown to be clinically useful.

Treatment and prognosis

Surgical resection is the treatment of choice for feline cutaneous mast cell tumors and the prognosis is usually good.[14] Prognosis for the cutaneous form of this disease is significantly better than the visceral/

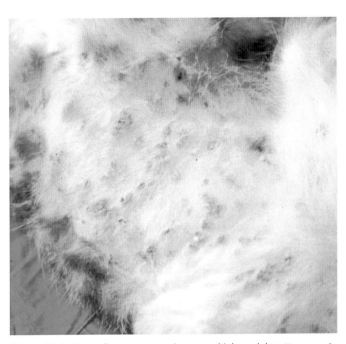

Figure 20-6 Mast cell tumor presenting as multiple nodules. *(Courtesy of David Grant.)*

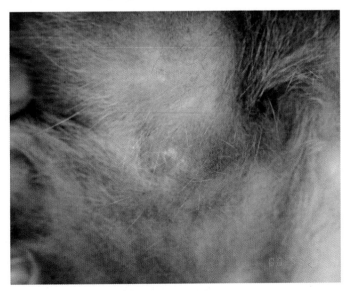

Figure 20-5 A typical solitary mast cell tumor.

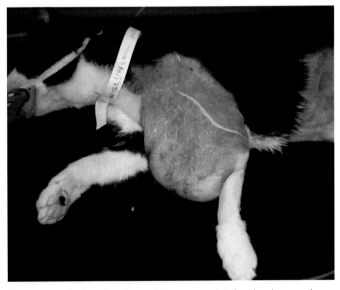

Figure 20-7 An invasive mast cell tumor associated with edema and seroma.

systemic form. Furthermore, cats with single cutaneous tumors have better outcomes compared with cats with multiple tumors.[15] This study also showed that there was a recurrence of mast cell neoplasia in approximately one-third of cats that had complete excision of their tumors, which was about the same proportion of recurrence in cats that had incomplete excisions. This supports previous studies showing that incomplete excision is not associated with a higher rate of tumor recurrence. A study on periocular cutaneous mast cell tumors in cats treated with surgery reported excellent local tumor control despite incomplete margins in nearly half the cases. All cases were classified as low-grade and metastatic disease involving peripheral lymph nodes or abdominal viscera was not detected in any cat.[16]

In cats with multiple or unresectable tumors corticosteroids may be of palliative value. The use of lomustine (CCNU) at a dose of 50 mg/m² has been reported in cats with mast cell tumors. Twenty-six of 38 cases in one study were cutaneous, an overall response rate of 50% was achieved with median response duration of 168 days.[15]

Invasive or incompletely excised tumors may be treated with adjunctive radiotherapy. Strontium 90 has been used in cutaneous mast cell tumors, providing local tumor control in 53/54 cases (median follow up of 783 days). Adverse effects were infrequent and mild.[17]

A variant of feline mast cell tumor has been reported predominantly affecting Siamese cats.[18] This tumor, which may be multicentric, is characterized histologically by sheets of histiocyte-like mast cells with scattered lymphoid aggregates and eosinophils. These tumors may regress spontaneously without therapy.

Visceral and systemic mast cell tumors

Lymphoreticular mast cell tumors are occasionally seen in cats, although this is the rarer form of mast cell disease seen in this species. In this condition, also called systemic mastocytosis, the tumor primarily involves the spleen (see Chapter 34). Presenting signs are usually vomiting and anorexia with common clinical findings of mastocytosis, marked splenomegaly and bone marrow infiltration, the latter often leading to anemia and other cytopenias. Occasionally, mediastinal involvement can lead to a pleural effusion and lymph nodes elsewhere may also be involved. A diffuse cutaneous infiltration has sometimes been reported with this form of the disease, and this has been the cause of some confusion regarding the clinical behavior of cutaneous mast cell tumors (most of which are benign). The diagnosis may be confirmed by fine needle aspirates from the enlarged spleen.

Treatment and prognosis

Splenectomy is the treatment of choice (see Chapter 34). In one study mast cell neoplasia was the most common reason for splenectomy in cats (53%) and the only prognostic risk factor for survival was the existence of preoperative weight loss.[19] Long-term survival has been reported in cats receiving no other therapy.[20] It has been postulated that the systemic response to splenectomy alone may be mediated by the immune system, hence the use of postoperative corticosteroids in these animals is controversial.

Intestinal mast cell tumor

Intestinal mast cell tumor in the cat is distinct from systemic mastocytosis (which does not involve the bowel). This form of feline mast cell tumor is malignant, with widespread metastases and carries a poor prognosis. Recently a variant of intestinal mast cell tumor, feline intestinal sclerosing mast cell tumor, was reported in 50 cats.[21] Histologically, the tumors were described as having a significant stromal component. Neoplastic cells had poorly discernible

intracytoplasmic granules. Lymph node and hepatic metastasis was evident in 66% of cases and the majority of patients who were followed up either died or were euthanized within two months of diagnosis.

SOFT TISSUE SARCOMAS (NON-INJECTION SITE)

Soft tissue tumors arise from mesenchymal connective tissues and are classified accordingly. Benign soft tissue tumors such as fibroma, lipoma, etc. are rare in the cat but their malignant counterparts, sarcomas, account for 7–10% of all feline tumors and fibrosarcoma is the most common diagnosis (Figs 20-8 and 20-9). Cutaneous hemangiosarcomas appear to be uncommon in the cat, accounting for approximately 2% of all cutaneous neoplasms,[1] with the majority located on the head. In a further study evaluating hemangiosarcomas in 53 cats the majority of tumors were either cutaneous or subcutaneous rather than visceral.

Treatment and prognosis

While there is established evidence to differentiate clinical and histopathological features between 'injection site' and spontaneous soft tissue sarcomas in cats, it is unknown whether outcomes following

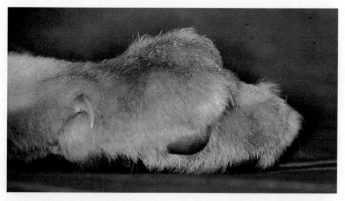

Figure 20-8 A fibrosarcoma ('non-injection site' sarcoma) on the foot.

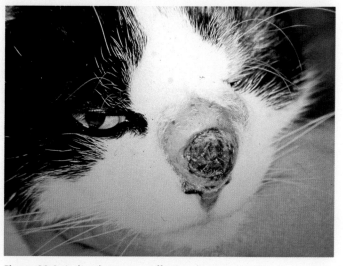

Figure 20-9 A chondrosarcoma affecting the nose.

treatment (either radiation or surgery) differ between the two categories as studies often combine the groups or else focus solely on injection site sarcomas. One study involving a questionnaire to veterinary surgeons who had submitted a fibrosarcoma from a cat for histopathology attempted to compare results from cats with vaccine site (VS) tumors and non-vaccine site (NVS) tumors.[22] It was found that VS tumors developed in younger cats and were larger than NVS tumors. Interestingly, although the VS tumors were biologically more aggressive and recurred with higher frequency, the NVS tumors had a reduced survival. It would appear from studies that non-injection site sarcomas occur less frequently in cats compared with dogs; however, diagnosis and treatment with early surgical excision, using wide or radical surgery to obtain tumor-free margins is the treatment of choice. One study that looked at a group of cats with soft tissue sarcoma (including both injection site and non-injection site variants) treated with preoperative or postoperative curative intent radiation therapy in combination with surgery reported relatively long-term survival (310 days following preoperative and 705 days following postoperative radiotherapy).[23] Anemia was found to be common in these cats and was associated with decreased survival.

Surgical excision was the primary treatment in most cases and both clean margins and increased survival were more likely in the cutaneous tumors compared with the subcutaneous tumors.[24] Injection site sarcomas are discussed in detail in Chapter 22.

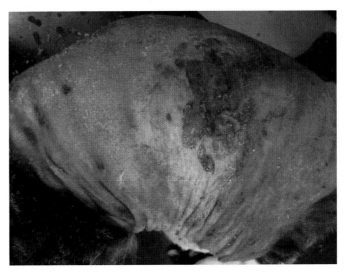

Figure 20-10 Cutaneous lymphoma affecting the dorsum and flank.

MULTIFOCAL/DIFFUSE CUTANEOUS NEOPLASIA

As a result of the increasing use of skin biopsies in the investigation of skin disease, disseminated neoplastic infiltration of the skin is assuming increasing importance in the differential diagnosis of ulcerative, nodular, or crusting skin lesions. Although mast cell tumor and metastases from both carcinomas and sarcomas can present as multiple, nodular skin lesions, lymphoproliferative diseases are those most commonly associated with multifocal or diffuse skin lesions.

Cutaneous lymphoproliferative disease

The cutaneous form of lymphoma is rare in the cat. In one study of 110 cats with extranodal lymphoma, only five cases of cutaneous lymphoma were recorded, and most of these were solitary skin lesions.[25] In the cat, cutaneous lymphoproliferative diseases may manifest in many different ways. Lesions may be benign or malignant and may be epitheliotrophic or confined to the dermis; rarely is there association with leukemia (c.f., Sezary syndrome). Most occur in older cats that are generally feline leukemia virus seronegative.

Feline cutaneous lymphocytosis is an uncommon disease characterized by slowly progressing single or multiple alopecic, erythematous, scaling/crusting lesions that are often intensely pruritic. This is described as a benign condition that rarely progresses to systemic involvement,[26] but may be difficult to distinguish from small cell cutaneous lymphoma. Feline cutaneous lymphomas are malignant proliferations of T-lymphocytes, non-epitheliotrophic variants appear more common than epitheliotrophic and are characterized by diffuse or nodular growths which are not usually associated with scaling or pruritis (Fig. 20-10).[27]

Treatment and prognosis

Feline cutaneous lymphoma lesions eventually progress to involve regional lymph nodes or viscera and are poorly responsive to chemotherapy, although use of lomustine has been reported in one case.[28]

Epitheliotrophic lymphoma

True epitheliotrophic lymphoma appears very rare in cats and its behavior is not well characterized in this species. A review article including five cases of feline cutaneous epitheliotropic T-cell lymphoma reported a predilection for older cats but no predilection for breed, sex, or location of lesions. Diagnosis is challenging and relies upon good histopathological examination. Survival times appear to be more variable in the cat compared with the dog.[29]

Feline cutaneous histiocytosis

Various forms of dendritic cell, 'histiocytic' proliferations have been documented in humans and dogs, but such conditions are not well characterized in cats. Affolter & Moore described a series of 30 cats with both epitheliotrophic and non-epitheliotrophic histiocytic infiltrates of the superficial and deep dermis with variable extension into the subcutis.[30] Animals presented with solitary or multiple non-pruritic papules, nodules and plaques with a predilection for feet, legs, and face. There was no age or breed association but females were more often affected than males. Although in most cases the condition was progressive, lesions could be limited to the skin for prolonged periods. Terminal dissemination to internal organs was documented in seven cases.

Treatment and prognosis

Treatment with chemotherapy, immunosuppressive or immunomodulatory drugs was not successful in the aforementioned study.[30] The authors called the condition feline progressive histiocytosis and suggested it is best considered an initially indolent cutaneous neoplasm which is mostly slowly progressive but may spread beyond the skin in terminal stages. This is in contrast to malignant histiocytosis or disseminated histiocytic sarcoma, which has been described as a multifocal systemic condition often associated with anemia due to erythrophagia, with similarities to the hemophagocytic form of histiocytic sarcoma recognized in the dog.[31]

CUTANEOUS PARANEOPLASTIC CONDITIONS

Tumors may cause metabolic disturbances through production of hormones or hormone-like substances that act on organs distant to the site of the tumor; the resulting conditions are termed paraneoplastic syndromes. Whilst rare, several cutaneous paraneoplastic syndromes have been documented in the cat: feline paraneoplastic alopecia and feline thymoma associated exfoliative dermatitis. Feline paraneoplastic alopecia has mainly been described in association with pancreatic carcinoma, especially tumors that have metastasized to the liver and other distant sites,[32,33] although there is one report of a similar syndrome associated with hepatocellular carcinoma in a cat.[34] This syndrome manifests as a non-pruritic, progressive alopecia involving the limbs, ventrum, and perineum. The alopecic skin has a shiny appearance and the hair in non-alopecic areas is easily epilated. In one case resolution of the alopecia occurred within ten weeks of resection of the pancreatic mass.[33] An exfoliative dermatitis with pruritis and erythroderma has been reported in cats in association with thymoma. This dermatopathy has also been shown to resolve following resection of the thymoma.[35-37] Symmetrical ischemic cutaneous necrosis of the skin of the hind feet of a 7-year-old domestic short haired cat with alimentary–hepatic lymphoma was considered a paraneoplastic syndrome as has been seen in people with lymphoma or other internal malignancies.[38]

SURGICAL MANAGEMENT

Surgical management of a skin tumor in a cat should only be considered following a cytological or histopathological diagnosis and once staging has been completed, where appropriate. It is only once this information has been obtained that correct decision making regarding surgical technique and indeed whether surgery is the most appropriate treatment can be made. If the tumor is deemed to be 'unresectable' then consideration should be given to other forms of management. For example, a large sarcoma on the limb may respond well to a combination of a marginal resection surgery followed by radiotherapy. Unfortunately, conclusive information on the use of adjunctive treatments in the cat is not as readily available as in the dog and for further information the reader is directed towards chapters on individual tumor types and the chemotherapy (see Chapter 16) and radiotherapy chapters (see Chapter 15). The other area of controversy is that of skin 'margins' (see Chapter 14). Clear and defined recommendations for margins of excision (lateral and deep) are not available for every tumor type in this species. Furthermore, veterinary histopathologists would not usually examine more than four to eight sections of margins and therefore the accuracy of margin assessment of the entire tumor is not high. This assessment is further complicated by fixation techniques, type of tissue planes examined (as not all normal tissues are equal barriers to tumor invasion), and how the sample is presented to the pathologist. However, it is known that the rate of recurrence of tumors is reduced (but not eliminated) with reported histologically clear margins. Benign tumors are usually well defined and demarcated and the probability of complete removal with several millimeters of margins is good. Equally, it is important to remember that even benign tumors can recur with 'dirty' margins. With malignant tumors, the margins of excision are less well defined (see Chapter 14). However, it is recommended that excisions are performed with a minimum of 1 cm (for epithelial skin tumors and benign mast cell tumors) to a minimum of 3–5 cm (for non-injection site and injection site sarcomas). For most malignant tumors that overlie a fascial plane then removal of this fascia would usually be considered adequate for the deep margin although for injection site sarcoma two fascial planes would be best practice (see Chapter 22).

General principles of oncological surgery should be applied when performing the surgery (see Chapter 14), with consideration of skin tension lines in the cat when specifically excising skin tumors.

GENERAL COMPLICATIONS AND PROGNOSIS

Complications of skin tumor excision depend on the location and extent of the surgery but may include infection, seromas, wound dehiscence, draining tracts, and tumor recurrence. Each complication should be fully investigated and treated early as it may lead to the development of a non-healing wound which could potentially be more challenging to manage compared with any of the above early complications. For more information on wound healing and management of the non-healing wound see Chapters 17 and 18.

Prognosis is dependent on the tumor type and is discussed in the relevant sections above.

REFERENCES

1. Miller MA, Nelson SL, Turk JR, et al. Cutaneous neoplasia in 340 cats. Vet Path 1991;28:389–95.
2. Bostock DE. Neoplasms of the skin and subcutaneous tissues in dogs and cats. Brit Vet J 1986;142:1–18.
3. Goldschmidt MH, Shofer FS. Skin tumors of the dog and cat. Pergamon Press; 1992. p. 2–3.
4. Stockhaus C, Teske E, Rudolph R, Werner HG. Assessment of cytological criteria for diagnosing basal cell tumors in the dog and cat. J Small Anim Pract 2001;42:582–6.
5. Simeonov R, Simeonova G. Nucleomorphometric analysis of feline basal cell carcinomas. Research in Veterinary Science 2008;84:440–3.
6. Abramo F, Pratesi F, Cantile C, et al. Survey of canine and feline follicular tumors and tumor-like lesions in central Italy. J Small Anim Pract 1999;40:479–81.
7. Bexfield NH, Stell AJ, Gear RN, Dobson JM. Photodynamic therapy of superficial nasal planum squamous cell carcinomas in cats: 55 cases. J Vet Int Med 2008;22:1385–9.
8. Gill VL, Bergman PJ, Baer KE, et al. Use of imiquimod 5% cream (Aldara) in cats with multicentric squamous cell carcinoma in situ: 12 cases (2002–2005). Vet & Comp Onc 2008;6:55–64.
9. Spugnini EP, Vincenzi B, Citro G, et al. Electrochemotherapy for the treatment of squamous cell carcinoma in cats: A preliminary report. Vet J 2009;179:117–20.
10. Sabattini S, Marconato L, Zoff A, et al. Epidermal growth factor receptor expression is predictive of poor prognosis in feline cutaneous squamous cell carcinoma. J Feline Med Surg 2010;12:760–8.
11. Scott-Moncrieff JC, Elliot GS, Radoveky A, Blevins WE. Pulmonary squamous cell carcinoma with multiple digital metastasis in a cat. J Small Anim Pract 1989;30:696–9.

12. Ozaki K, Narama I. Merkel cell carcinoma in a cat. J Vet Med Sci 2009;71:1093–6.

13. Hargis AM, Baldessari AE, Walder EJ. Intraepidermal adenocarcinoma in the perianal skin of two cats, a condition resembling human extramammary Paget's disease. Vet Dermatol 2008;19(1):31–7.

14. Molander-McCrary H, Henry CJ, Potter K, et al. Cutaneous mast cell tumors in cats: 32 cases (1991–1994). J Am Anim Hosp Assoc 1998;34:281–4.

15. Litster AL, Sorenmo KU. Characterisation of the signalment, clinical and survival characteristics of 41 cats with mast cell neoplasia. J Feline Med Surg 2006;8: 177–83.

16. Montgomery KW, van der Woerdt A, Aquino SM, et al. Periocular cutaneous mast cell tumors in cats: evaluation of surgical excision (33 cases). Vet Ophthalmol 2010;13:26–30.

17. Turrel JM, Farrelly J, Page RL, McEntee MC. Evaluation of strontium 90 irradiation in treatment of cutaneous mast cell tumors in cats: 35 cases (1992–2002). J Am Vet Med Assoc 2006;228:898–901.

18. Wilcock BP, Yager JA, Zink MC. The morphology and behavior of feline cutaneous mastocytomas. Vet Pathol 1986;23(3):320–4.

19. Gordon SS, McClaran JK, Bergman PJ, Liu SM. Outcome following splenectomy in cats. J Feline Med Surg 2010;12:256–61.

20. Liska WD, MacEwen EG, Zaki FA, Garvey M. Feline systemic mastocytosis: A review and results of splenectomy in seven cases. J Am Anim Hosp Assoc 1979;15:589–97.

21. Halsey CH, Powers BE, Kamstock DA. Feline intestinal sclerosing mast cell

tumour: 50 cases (1997–2008). Vet Comp Onc 2010;8:72–9.

22. Hendrick MJ, Shofer FS, Goldschmidt MH, et al. Comparison of fibrosarcomas that developed at vaccination sites and at nonvaccination sites in cats: 239 cases (1991–2). J Am Vet Med Assoc 1994;205:1425–9.

23. Mayer MN, Treuil PL, LaRue SM. Radiotherapy and surgery for feline soft tissue sarcoma. Vet Rad & Ultra 2009;50:669–72.

24. Johannes CM, Henry CJ, Turnquist SE, et al. Hemangiosarcoma in cats: 53 cases (1992–2002). J Am Vet Med Assoc 2007;231:1851–6.

25. Taylor SS, Goodfellow MR, Browne WJ, et al. Feline extranodal lymphoma: response to chemotherapy and survival in 110 cats. J Small Anim Pract 2009;50: 584–92.

26. Gilbert S, Affolter VK, Gross TL, et al. (2004) Clinical, morphological and immunohistochemical characterization of cutaneous lymphocytosis in 23 cats. Vet Derm 2004;15:3–12.

27. Day MJ. Immunophenotypic characterization of cutaneous lymphoid neoplasia in the dog and cat. J of Comp Path 1995;112:79–96.

28. Komori S, Nakamura S, Takahashi K, Tagawa M. Use of lomustine to treat cutaneous non-epitheliotropic lymphoma in a cat. J Am Vet Med Assoc 2005;226: 237–9.

29. Fontaine J, Heimann M, Day MJ. Cutaneous epitheliotropic T-cell lymphoma in the cat: a review of the literature and five new cases. Vet Derm 2011;22:454–61.

30. Affolter VF, Moore PF. Feline progressive histiocytosis. Vet Pathol 2006;43:646–55.

31. Friedrichs KR, Young KM. (2008) Histiocytic sarcoma of macrophage origin in a cat: case report with a literature review of feline histiocytic malignancies and comparison with canine haemophagocytic histiocytic sarcoma. Vet Clin Pathol 2008;37:121–8.

32. Brooks DG, Campbell KL, Dennis JS, et al. Pancreatic paraneoplastic alopecia in three cats. J Am Anim Hosp Assoc 1994;30:557–63.

33. Tasker S, Griffon DJ, Nuttall TJ, Hill PB. Resolution of paraneoplastic alopecia following surgical removal of a pancreatic carcinoma in a cat. J Small Anim Pract 1999;40:16–9.

34. Marconato L, Albanese F, Viacava P, et al. Paraneoplastic alopecia associated with hepatocellular carcinoma in a cat. Vet Dermatol 2007;18:267–71.

35. Forster-Van Hijfte MA, Curtis CF, White RN. Resolution of exfoliative dermatitis and Malassezia pachydermatitis overgrowth in a cat after surgical thymoma resection. J Small Anim Pract 1997;38:451–4.

36. Godfrey DR. Dermatosis and associated systemic signs in a cat with thymoma and recently treated with an imidacloprin preparation. J Small Anim Pract 1999;40: 333–7.

37. Singh A, Boston SE, Poma R. Thymoma-associated exfoliative dermatitis with post-thymectomy myasthenia gravis in a cat. Can Vet J 2010;51:757–60.

38. Ashley PF, Bowman LA. Symmetrical cutaneous necrosis of the hind feet and multicentric follicular lymphoma in a cat. J Am Vet Med Assoc 1999;214:211–14.

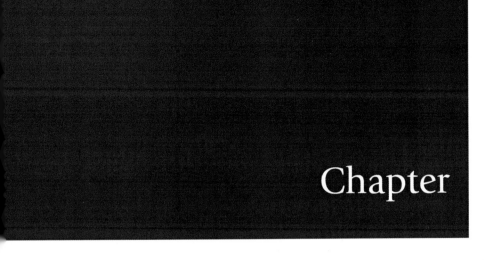

Chapter |21|

Mammary glands

P. Buracco

The high prevalence of neutered female cats ensures that mammary gland problems in cats are not common. However, in the un-neutered queen the incidence and severity of mammary gland disease is relatively high. When mammary neoplasia occurs it is more often malignant. Benign conditions such as fibroepithelial hyperplasia can occur in young cats and the mammary glands can reach a spectacular size. Other benign lesions are rare. For malignant tumors (i.e., adenocarcinoma) an early diagnosis and clinical staging are essential for planning the best treatment in order to improve prognosis. At present the mainstay of treatment of adenocarcinoma is aggressive surgery; the benefit of neoadjuvant and adjuvant therapeutic measures is still unknown.

SURGICAL ANATOMY

Cats normally have eight mammary glands, four on each side: two thoracic (T1, T2) and two abdominal (A1, A2; A2 also referred to as the inguinal or the second abdominal mammary gland). When comparing feline and canine mammary glands, the first three pairs would be thoracic and the caudal pair abdominal or inguinal; numbered first to fourth (cranial to caudal).[1-4] The terminology T1-2 and A1-2 will be used in this chapter. The nipples have five to seven lactiferous pores with one to three openings on the top and the remaining ones on the side.[5] Queens may have additional rudimentary mammary glands.[3] One or two rudimentary mammary glands may be found in male cats.[5]

Knowledge of the blood and lymphatic supply of the feline mammary glands is important, particularly in relation to mammary gland malignancy, staging, treatment, and prognosis.

Blood supply

The epigastric arteries supply the mammary glands. There are two arteries (cranial and caudal) that anastomose in the umbilical area, with some branches crossing the midline. The venous drainage mirrors the arterial pattern, but veins cross the midline more frequently than arteries. This makes extension of malignancy from one side to the other possible.[1,6] Malignant cells from A1 and A2 may also be spread hematogenously directly via the internal thoracic and/or intercostal veins[1,7] that flow into the vertebral veins.[8] A summary of the blood supply is detailed in Table 21-1.

Lymphatic drainage

The axillary glands drain to the axillary lymph nodes and the inguinal glands to the inguinal lymph nodes (Table 21-2). The exact lymphatic drainage pattern is still debatable and there is controversy as to whether it is possible to have lymphatic spread of feline mammary malignancy from one mammary gland to other mammary glands. A summary of the conclusions relating to lymphatic drainage and potential means of metastasis is shown in Box 21-1.[1,3,4,9-11]

DIAGNOSIS AND GENERAL CONSIDERATIONS

Signalment, history and physical examination

Clinical features of mammary gland disease include a change in shape, size, appearance, or consistency of one or more mammary glands. The signalment of the cat and a full history should be taken from the owner. The cat's age, neuter status, signs of estrus, mating history, whether it has had any hormonal therapy, and previous history of surgery in the area are of particular relevance.

A full physical examination should be performed including a thorough palpation of all mammary glands and regional lymph nodes. The vulva should be inspected for evidence of enlargement or discharge and abdominal palpation performed to manually evaluate the uterus and the entire abdomen.

Further investigations

Fine needle aspiration of any mammary mass and especially of any enlarged regional/sentinel lymph node(s) may give useful information regarding the type of tumor and therefore be an aid to planning further investigations and treatment.

© 2014 Elsevier Ltd
DOI: 10.1016/B978-0-7020-4336-9.00021-4

Table 21-1 The arterial blood supply of feline mammary glands[1]

Region	Arteries
T1–T2	Axial: perforating branches of the internal thoracic arteries; cutaneous branches of the intercostal arteries from T7 caudally Abaxial: Lateral thoracic arteries
A1	Cranial superficial epigastric artery Cutaneous branches of the caudal intercostal arteries Some cutaneous branches of phrenicoabdominal and deep circumflex iliac arteries
A2	Caudal superficial epigastric artery (from external pudendal artery) Some cutaneous branches of phrenicoabdominal and deep circumflex iliac arteries

Box 21-1 Lymphatic drainage of feline mammary glands[1,3,4,9–11]

- The axillary and inguinal lymph nodes are the primary lymphatic nodes
- Axillary lymphatics drain T1, T2 and possibly A1
- Inguinal lymphatics drain A2 but may also drain A1
- Neither an interglandular nor a right/left connection has been definitively demonstrated
- Local spread (to one side to the other) is more likely to occur through venous rather than lymphatic vessels
- Whether direct (primary) spread to sternal and medial iliac lymph nodes occurs is debatable. If the axillary and/or inguinal lymph nodes are not involved, the probability that the sternal and medial iliac (secondary lymph) nodes are involved is likely to be low and, therefore, they should only be investigated as a potential secondary lymphatic center. The purported order of drainage is axillary–sternal and inguinal–medial iliac

Based on the initial cytological results, further investigations might include thoracic radiographs (both right and left lateral and dorsoventral views) to check for pulmonary metastasis; abdominal ultrasound to check for pregnancy, ovarian remnants, uterine disease or lymphatic, splenic or hepatic metastasis. Computed tomography is useful for detecting pulmonary metastatic disease and for staging the tumor more effectively (Table 21-3).[12]

Blood tests might include FIV/FeLV status, general hematological and biochemical evaluation in the older cat prior to anesthesia, and if ovarian remnant syndrome is suspected then a progesterone assay can be useful.

SURGICAL DISEASES

Feline mammary glands can be affected by benign non-neoplastic lesions (non-inflammatory and inflammatory) and tumors (benign and malignant). The diseases affecting cats are listed in Table 21-4.[13,14] An accurate diagnosis is critical for staging, treatment, and prognosis.

Benign non-neoplastic lesions

Benign non-neoplastic non-inflammatory lesions in cats include cysts, ductal ectasia or hyperplasia, focal fibrosis or fibroepithelial hyperplasia (lobular hyperplasia).

Fibroepithelial hyperplasia

The most common benign non-neoplastic lesion in the cat is fibroepithelial hyperplasia (also known as fibroadenomatous or lobular hyperplasia) with or without ductal ectasia. There is a rapid and abnormal stromal and epithelial duct proliferation of one or more mammary glands.[15] It usually affects young intact female cats at puberty, sometimes occurring after a silent estrus.[16] Pseudopregnant and pregnant queens of any age can be affected due to the effects of ovarian progesterone. The condition has also been described in both male and female cats after treatment with synthetic progestagens.[17–20] The exaggeratedly enlarged mammary glands (Fig. 21-1) are non-lactating, with a firm and elastic consistency. They may be edematous

Table 21-2 Axillary and inguinal lymphatic centers[1]

Lymph nodes	Number of lymph nodes	Frequency in cats	Location
Axillary lymph center			
Axillaris proprius (proper axillary LN)	1	100%	Junction of v. thoracica lateralis with v. axillaris
Axillaris accessorius (accessory axillary LN)	2 (1–3)	97%	Caudal to the proper axillary LN adjacent to a. and v. thoracica lateralis
Axillaris primae costae (axillary first rib LN)	Variable	5%	Adjacent to v. axillaris
Inguinal lymph center			
Inguinalis superficialis (superficial inguinal LN)	1 (2–3)	100%	Near the junction of v. epigastrica caudalis superficialis with v. pudenda externa
Epigastricis cranialis (cranial epigastric LN)	2 (1–3)	7%	On the m. rectus abdominis adjacent to v. epigastrica cranialis superficialis
Epigastricis caudalis (caudal epigastric LN)	2 (1–3)	98%	Adjacent to v. epigastrica caudalis superficialis

a., artery; LN, lymph node; m., muscle; v., vein.

Table 21-3 Clinical staging of feline mammary tumors

T: primary tumor		N: regional lymph nodes (RLN)		M: distant metastasis	
T1	<2 cm of diameter	N0	RLN not involved (cytology, histology)	M0	No evidence
T2	2–3 cm of diameter	N1	RLN involved	M1	Present
T3	>3 cm of diameter				
Stages					
I	T1 N0 M0				
II	T2 N0 M0				
III	T1 or T2 N1 M0 T3 N0 or N1 M0				
IV	Any T Any N1 M0				

(Modified from Owen LN. Classification of tumors in domestic animals. Geneva: World Health Organization; 1980. http://whqlibdoc.who.int/hq/1980/VPH_CMO_80.20_eng.pdf)

RLN, regional lymph node.

Table 21-4 Classification of feline neoplastic and non-neoplastic mammary lesions

Lesion	Common	Less common / Rare
Mammary tumors: malignant	Non-infiltrating (in situ) carcinoma Tubulopapillary carcinoma Solid carcinoma Cribriform carcinoma	Squamous cell carcinoma Mucinous carcinoma[73] Sarcoma and carcinosarcoma[74] Carcinoma or sarcoma in a benign tumor Inflammatory carcinoma[75] Lipid-rich carcinoma[76] Lymphangiosarcoma[77] Histiocytic sarcoma[58]
Mammary tumors: benign	Simple adenoma Complex adenoma Fibroadenoma	Benign mixed tumor Duct papilloma
Inflammatory lesions	Mastitis	Abscessation
Benign lesions	Duct ectasia Lobular hyperplasia (fibroadenomatous hyperplasia or fibroepithelial hyperplasia)	Cyst Focal fibrosis (fibrosclerosis) Ductal hyperplasia

(Modified from Hampe JF, Misdorp W. Tumours and dysplasias of the mammary gland. Bull World Health Organ 1974;50:111–33; and Misdorp W, Else RW, Hellmen E, Lipscomb TP. Histological classification of mammary tumors of the dog and the cat. In Schulman FY, editor. World Health Organization International Histological Classification of Tumors of the Domestic Animals, second series, vol. 7. Washington DC: Armed Forces Institute of Pathology; 1999. p. 11–56.)

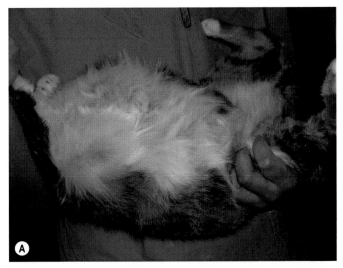

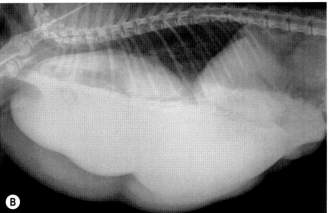

Figure 21-1 Fibroepithelial hyperplasia in a 13-month old female cat. **(A)** Gross and **(B)** radiographic appearance.

Box 21-2 Fibroepithelial hyperplasia

Patient signalment – usually young female cats
History – previous administration of synthetic progesterone or mating
Abdominal palpation and ultrasound:
  – Exclude pregnancy
  – Exclude ovarian remnant syndrome (see Chapter 40)

in Box 21-2. The treatment of fibroepithelial hyperplasia is summarized in Box 21-3.

Mammary tumors

Feline mammary tumors are the third most common tumors after lymphoproliferative and skin tumors in cats. They account for about 17% of neoplasia in the queen and 1–5% of all tumors in male cats.[16,27–29]

Benign tumors

Benign tumors (Table 21-4) account for about 10–15% of all mammary lesions seen in cats. They occur in queens ranging in age from 1 to 9.5 years.[6,16] Once the benign nature of the lesion has been

(with swelling extending to the pelvic limbs and potentially causing lameness), hot, painful and ulcerated, with areas of localized and superficial necrosis. Systemic signs may also be present.[15,16,21] Acute mastitis should be considered as a differential diagnosis; both conditions can occur concurrently.[22] A summary of the condition is listed

ascertained, marginal surgical excision is the treatment of choice (simple mammectomy). Surgical resection is recommended as these lesions could undergo malignant transformation.[15] Histology should be performed on the excised specimen, including evaluation of excision margins.

Malignant tumors

Malignancy is recognized histologically in 85–93% of all mammary lesions and more than 80% are adenocarcinomas but other tumors are occasionally seen (Table 21-4).[16,30,31] A viral cause has been advocated but not proven for adenocarcinomas.[32,33] Predisposition has been advocated for domestic shorthaired and Siamese cats;[27] in the latter breed even younger cats may be affected.[31] Mammary tumor incidence increases after six years of age;[34,35] the reported mean age of

affected queens is 10–12 years;[16] males may be a little older.[28] No definitive predilection for any specific gland has been demonstrated. Adenocarcinoma may involve one (Fig. 21-3) or more glands, with at least half of the cats having more than one gland affected.[16] The rate of growth is usually rapid and cats are usually presented at an advanced

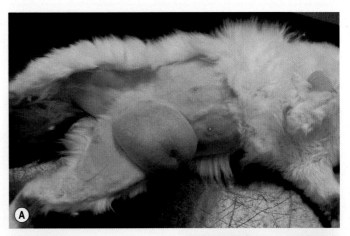

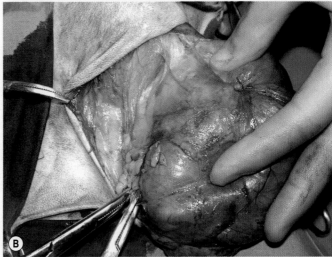

Figure 21-2 **(A)** The gross appearance of fibroepithelial hyperplasia affecting a single mammary gland in a one-year-old cat. **(B)** Introperative view of a marginal excision. *(Courtesy of Nick Bacon.)*

Box 21-3 **Treatment of fibroepithelial hyperplasia**

- Treat ulceration and/or pain as appropriate
- Drain abscesses and administer antibiotics in cases with concurrent mastitis[22]
- In pregnant or pseudopregnant queens the disease may regress spontaneously after the end of pregnancy or luteolysis[15,23,24]
- Discontinue exogenous synthetic progestin administration. If disease does not regress, partial (Fig. 21-2) or total mastectomy has been recommended.[15] If mammary glands are very enlarged, surgery may be problematic and should be avoided if possible[15]
- Ovariectomy/ovariohysterectomy (OVH) by median celiotomy or through the flank (when mammary glands are so enlarged as to impede the midline approach).[16] OVH is effective in most cases, but regression may take up to 6 months.[15] In cats treated with long-acting injectable progestins, regression may only be partial or not at all, even after spaying[20]
- Antiprogestins such as aglepristone[15,21,25,26] can be tried. Complete remission is achieved in a variable time but with a mean of about four weeks.[26] Before its use, pregnancy should be ruled out as these drugs will have an abortive effect.[15] The protocol proposed by Gorlinger et al (2002)[21] (aglepristone, 20 mg/kg once a week until remission) should be effective for cases induced by both long-acting progestins and endogenous progesterone. One important advantage of using antiprogestins is preservation of fertility, if this is a concern[15]

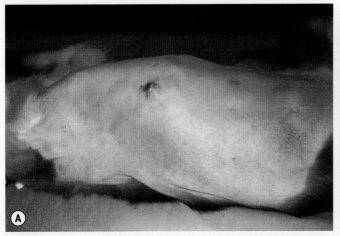

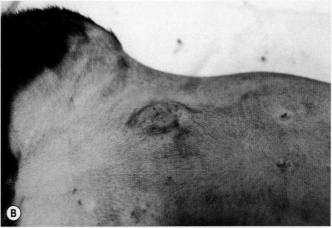

Figure 21-3 Feline mammary adenocarcinoma affecting single mammary glands. Gross appearance in two different elderly female cats. Fine needle aspiration should be performed in order to confirm the diagnosis. *((B) Courtesy of Lisa Mestrinho.)*

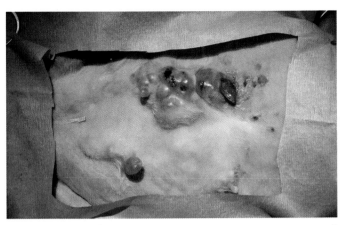

Figure 21-4 Ulcerated cystic mammary adenocarcinoma affecting several glands in a 12-year-old female entire cat.

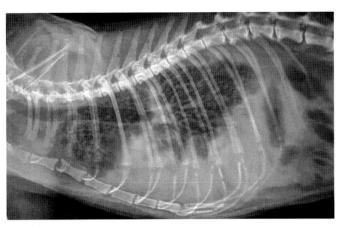

Figure 21-6 Lateral thoracic radiograph showing disseminated miliary metastasis and pleural effusion secondary to a mammary adenocarcinoma.

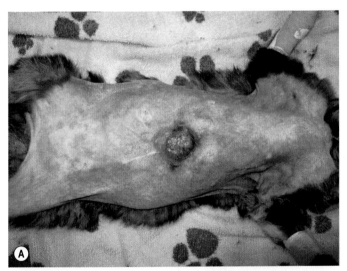

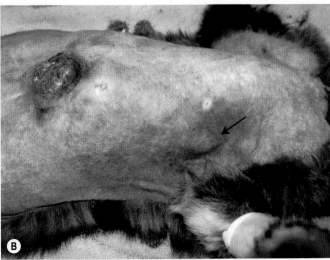

Figure 21-5 (A) A single ulcerated adenocarcinoma that had metastatized to both the axillary lymph nodes; **(B)** clinical appearance of the left axillary lymph node (arrow). *(Courtesy of Julius Liptak.)*

stage with lesions adherent to the skin and/or deep muscular fascia. Ulceration develops in over 25% of cases, and even in small lesions nipples may be swollen and exude fluid (Fig. 21-4).[2,15,16] Pelvic limb thromboembolism has been reported.[15] Metastasis occurs in 50–90% of cats, most commonly to regional lymph nodes (Fig. 21-5), lungs, pleura (Fig. 21-6), liver and less commonly to the adrenal glands, kidneys, diaphragm, and other organs.[2,6,15,16,31,35,36] If the tumor is left untreated, the reported mean survival of cats is about one year.[15,36]

Two studies have shown a significant decrease in the risk of developing a mammary tumor if ovariohysterectomy is performed before the cat is 6 months of age[34,37] and a slightly reduced risk, but still significant, if ovariohysterectomy is done when the cat is between 6 months and 1 year of age (86% risk reduction).[37] There is at least a threefold increased risk of mammary tumor development (and fibroepithelial hyperplasia) in intact queens when progestagens or estrogen/progesterone combinations have been administered;[32,38] this has been also documented in male cats[29,39] and in zoo felids.[40,41] The hormonal influence implies a receptor activity in feline mammary tumors, usually low for estrogen and moderate for progesterone receptors.[18,42–46] In undifferentiated tumors the receptors are absent or only present in low numbers. Feline mammary adenocarcinoma has been proposed as a model for human mammary disease.[43,47]

PREOPERATIVE CONSIDERATIONS AND PLANNING

Mammary carcinoma should be staged according to the TNM clinical staging system as described in Chapter 13 (see Table 21-3).[12] If feasible, aggressive surgery is the treatment of choice, but unfortunately it is rarely curative as mammary adenocarcinoma is often presented at too advanced stage. Surgery may be combined with other therapeutic options, especially in more advanced cases. A unilateral or preferably a bilateral mastectomy should always be planned in cats. Bilateral mastectomy may be performed in one single stage or four to eight weeks apart (two-staged total mastectomy, performing a unilateral mastectomy each time).

Antibiotics are given intravenously at induction of anesthesia (20 mg/kg of cephazolin).

The inguinal lymph node should be removed together with A2 mammary gland and both submitted for histopathological analysis. Through a supplemental and cranial incision (or cranial extension of the mastectomy incision) the axillary node(s) are removed if enlarged and submitted for histological analysis. If not enlarged, their prophylactic removal is controversial as it is unclear whether it results in any clinical benefit.[16,48,49]

No real benefit has been demonstrated to performing concurrent ovariohysterectomy from an oncologic point of view.[15,16,31]

Histologic evaluation of margins is important for prognosis so the entire excised specimen should be prepared for this purpose. Some full thickness sutures should be applied to avoid any tissue layer sliding; other sutures should be applied to orientate the pathologist (cranial vs. caudal); finally, the sample should be inked on its excision surface (particularly in areas where the surgeon believes the excision may have been more marginal).

SURGICAL MANAGEMENT AND TECHNIQUES

The surgical options for mammary masses in cats include excision of the lesion (simple lumpectomy or mammectomy), unilateral

mastectomy or bilateral mastectomy. For small benign lesions a simple elliptical excision of the lesion can be performed but it is preferable to excise the entire mammary gland involved (mammectomy) (see Fig. 21-2). Even with a benign lesion, it is recommended that a small amount of unaffected mammary tissue is removed with the tumor.

Particular care must be paid to meticulous hemostasis of the cranial and caudal epigastric vessels in addition to the other minor vessels. As a general rule, veins should be ligated before arteries to limit neoplastic spread. Excessive use of electrocautery may delay healing and complicate both identification and histologic evaluation of the excision margins. Dead space should be eliminated by 'walking' sutures[50] of 3/0 absorbable monofilament material applied in a continuous pattern to close the subcutaneous tissues, with the sutures engaging the deep fascia. Meticulous hemostasis and obliteration of any dead space during closure should help prevent seroma formation. A drain is not usually applied.

Unilateral mastectomy

Simple lumpectomy and mammectomy should be reserved only for a single confirmed benign nodule. A unilateral mastectomy (Box 21-4), as part of a two-staged (four to eight week) bilateral

---

Box 21-4 Unilateral mastectomy

The cat is placed in dorsal recumbency with a wide area of the abdominal hair clipped and aseptically prepared. If the plan is to also remove the axillary lymph node(s) then the clip must extend cranially enough to incorporate this.

Surgery starts with a skin incision encircling all four mammary glands to be removed (Fig. 21-7), taking a minimum of a 2 cm margin all around the tumor(s) (Fig. 21-8A). Muscular fascia deep to the tumor may be excised if the neoplasm appears to be fixed to it, again aiming to remove a minimum of 2 cm of macroscopically sound tissue from around the neoplasm. The tissue is undermined in a cranial to caudal direction using Metzenbaum scissors (mammary stripping); if fascia is to be included with the excision it is sharply incised with a scalpel. Excision of the tumor together with the underlying fascia is recommended in an attempt to respect the oncological principle of removal of 2cm of normal tissue from the periphery.

Excision of the axillary lymph node is performed by extending the skin incision cranially when a palpable lymphatic tract is present. If the tract is not palpable then a single lymph node, without tract, is removed through a supplementary, more cranial incision. The inguinal lymph node is removed together with the most caudal mammary gland.

During surgery, the exposed tissue is protected from drying with saline soaked sponges. The cranial epigastric vessels are ligated first, followed by the caudal epigastric vessels. Careful hemostasis of all the minor vessels encountered is warranted. Excessive use of electrocautery should be avoided, as it may delay healing and complicate both identification and histologic evaluation of the excision margins. The caudal epigastric vessels are encountered in the inguinal region, and are usually surrounded by fat; careful and delicate dissection with fine Metzenbaum scissors is necessary to identify them. Once identified, they are ligated (or double ligated if desired) with 3/0 monofilament absorbable material, forceps are applied distal to the ligature(s) and the vessels transected between the forceps and ligature(s). Inadvertent transection of these vessels before they are visualized is problematic as they can retract into the inguinal canal. Hemorrhage may be significant so, if the latter occurs, it may be necessary to perform a caudal celiotomy (see Chapter 23) to locate, grasp and ligate these vessels.

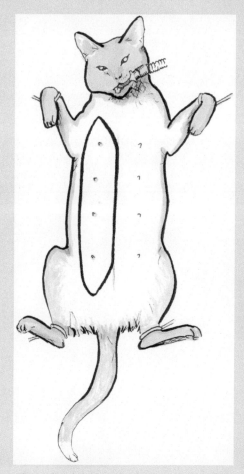

Figure 21-7 The outline for the surgical incision for a unilateral mastectomy is shown on the diagram.

Box 21-4 **Continued**

Once mammary excision is completed, the surgical instruments and gloves are changed, and the area thoroughly lavaged with warm saline.

To close the wound a 'walking suture' may be performed with a 3/0 monofilament absorbable suture material in order both to eliminate dead space and appose skin margins. This is done taking alternate bites of the subcutaneous tissue close to the skin margins and then fascia up to the middle of the wound; this is performed on both sides of the wound so the skin margins are brought together. These sutures can be placed in a continuous pattern or, if desired, the continuous suture on each side may be divided into two or three partial continuous sutures. Skin closure should be absolutely tension free and can be performed with intradermal (rarely applied by the author in these cases), simple interrupted, metal staples, horizontal (Fig. 21-8B) or vertical (preferable to horizontal as they interfere less with vascularization) mattress sutures.

Before submitting the excised specimen for histological evaluation the cranial and caudal borders of the sample should be tagged with sutures.

The lymph node(s) removed should be clearly identified, and the parts where the excision may have been marginal ideally inked.

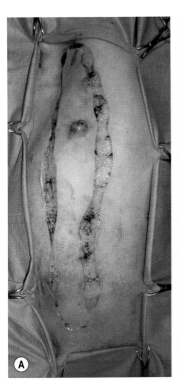 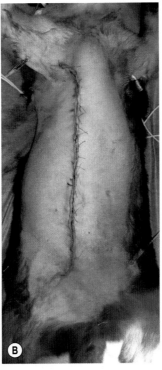

Figure 21-8 Unilateral mastectomy for a cat with a single adenocarcinoma. **(A)** Intraoperative view of the incision encircling all the mammary glands on one side. **(B)** After the final skin closure with horizontal mattress sutures. The cat was scheduled to be returned for a contralateral unilateral mammary strip four weeks later.

mastectomy, should be performed for single or multiple malignant tumors that need to be removed with a minimum of 2 cm margins. A unilateral mastectomy is still acceptable only for very small (stage 1) and single malignant tumors, identified early. The bilateral mastectomy may be performed as a two-staged procedure (two unilateral mastectomy's done four to eight weeks apart) in obese cats or those with large lesions where there is concern regarding the ability to achieve tension free closure of the skin.

Bilateral mastectomy

Bilateral mastectomy (Box 21-5) should be performed for single (over 2 cm diameter) or multiple malignant tumors that need to be removed with a minimum of 2 cm margins. If a one-stage bilateral mastectomy

has been planned, it is not always easy to remove the tumor(s) with a minimum of 2 cm margins as both reconstruction and tension may be relevant concerns. For these reasons, it may be preferable to perform bilateral mastectomy as two-staged unilateral mastectomies, four to eight weeks apart (see Box 21-4).

Achieving adequate margins and tension free closure

When performing a single stage total mastectomy reconstruction problems and tension during closure may arise as all the skin between the two mammary chains is removed.

For malignant tumors at least 2 cm of macroscopically healthy tissue around the tumor should be excised independent of size and adherence. It is often appropriate to include at least one fascial plane deep to the tumor. It is the author's opinion that this may be easier and therefore increase the probability of getting 'clean' margins, when a two-stage radical bilateral mastectomy is planned. If the tumor is fixed to the underlying fascia, an en-bloc resection should be performed, if necessary entering the abdominal cavity (full thickness wall excision; Fig. 21-12A). If the abdominal cavity is not breached and if excessive tension is present at closure, a tract of fascia may be left unsutured. If the abdominal cavity is breached and part of the entire wall is excised, reconstruction may be performed exploiting the abdominal wall's elasticity (Fig. 21-12B) but if tension is excessive, the defect may be closed either with a muscular flap or a polypropylene mesh (Fig. 21-13). If mesh (or a muscle flap) is used omentalization of the area can be performed (Fig. 21-13B). A tract of the greater omentum is exteriorized through a 1–1.5 cm hole in the abdominal wall (left unsutured) and spread over the external mesh surface. The fascial or fascial/mesh borders are closed with a 3/0 slowly absorbable monofilament material applied in an interrupted pattern.

Staged skin suture removal should be planned during the ten to 20 postoperative days.

POSTOPERATIVE MANAGEMENT

Postoperative antibiotics are usually not necessary unless preoperative infection is present. Analgesia should be administered until postoperative pain has resolved (see Chapter 2) and the cat continued on intravenous fluids, particularly after bilateral mastectomy. The cat should be monitored for adequate renal function and for complications such as disseminated intravascular coagulation (see Chapter 4).

In order to prevent self-trauma, the use of an Elizabethan collar is imperative. Postoperative bandaging is optional; the bandage should

Box 21-5 Bilateral mastectomy

The cat is placed in dorsal recumbency with a wide area of the abdominal skin clipped of hair and aseptically prepared. If the plan is to also remove the axillary lymph node(s) then the clip must extend cranially enough to incorporate this.

Preoperatively, tension may be tentatively tested by pinching the skin in folds and evaluating its elasticity and potential for tension-free closure.

In the one-stage bilateral mastectomy, surgery starts with a skin incision encircling all eight mammary glands, taking a minimum of a 1–2 cm margin all around the tumor(s). Preservation of one triangle of skin between the two mammary lines, especially cranially but also caudally, may aid wound closure (Fig. 21-9). In an attempt to plan both the surgical removal and reconstruction, it can help to draw the area to be removed with a sterile surgical marker (Fig. 21-10). To achieve adequate margins for malignant mammary gland tumors then deep excision may require excision of the body wall and the surgeon must be prepared as to how to close this, e.g., using a muscle flap or mesh.

The remainder of the surgery is performed in a similar manner as for unilateral mastectomy, but more careful consideration should be given to acheiving tension-free closure (Fig. 21-11).

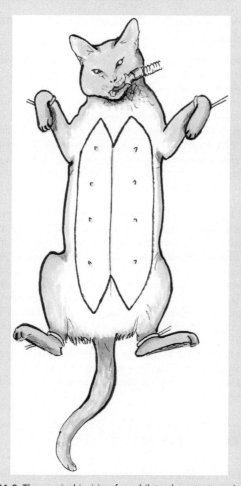

Figure 21-9 The surgical incision for a bilateral mastectomy is shown. A small triangle of skin can be spared, both cranially and caudally, to facilitate wound closure.

be changed every 24–48 hours, to check the wound, and the bandage maintained for a total of 3–5 days.

Ancillary therapy

Chemotherapy

The efficacy of chemotherapy is still debatable but there is some evidence that the use of doxorubicin ± cyclophosphamide may prolong survival in originally non-metastatic cats[51] while there is limited benefit when metastasis is already established.[52–54] A retrospective study[52] has shown that adjuvant doxorubicin prolonged survival in comparison with surgery alone. However, in a more recent study these results were not validated.[55] Multidrug resistance-associated P-glycoprotein has been found in feline mammary tumors so a significant response to chemotherapy would not be expected.[56] Doxorubicin is nephrotoxic and this may limit its regular use in elderly cats. In a further study, the combination of chemotherapy, surgery, and meloxicam, as a COX-2 inhibitor, did not improve survival.[57] In a case report, a cat with pleural effusion from a metastatic mammary histiocitic sarcoma experienced a 13-month survival after both chemotherapy (doxorubicin) and thoracic omentalization.[58]

Radiation therapy

At present there is no study demonstrating an increase in survival using radiation. This is not surprising, as the reason for death of cats with mammary tumors is usually distant metastasis rather than local recurrence.

Other treatments

The few studies dealing with the use of biologic response modifiers (levamisole, bacterial vaccines, L-MTP) following surgery have failed to demonstrate a real improvement in prognosis.[16,59] It is likely that future and alternate treatment options will be directed towards gene therapy and novel immunologic strategies.[60,61]

COMPLICATIONS

Most of the problems after mammary gland surgery are related to tension at wound closure.

Tension

This is mainly a concern when a bilateral mastectomy has been performed, especially in obese cats. Tension can be a problem at both the cranial and (less frequently) the caudal aspect of the excision area. To minimize tension during surgery a triangle of skin[50] (see Fig. 21-9) may be spared. Tension may cause transitory postoperative discomfort, ventilatory impedance and pain. Tension may also result in limb edema, partial or complete skin suture dehiscence, ulceration (especially at the incisional intersection), necrosis, seroma formation, and inflammation.

Seroma

If a seroma develops, NSAIDs and antibiotic administration are recommended as infection may potentially occur. If the seroma is small, it should be left untreated as it may resolve spontaneously in a variable period of time. Aseptic aspiration of the fluid by syringe may result in infection and the seroma may reform as the dead space still

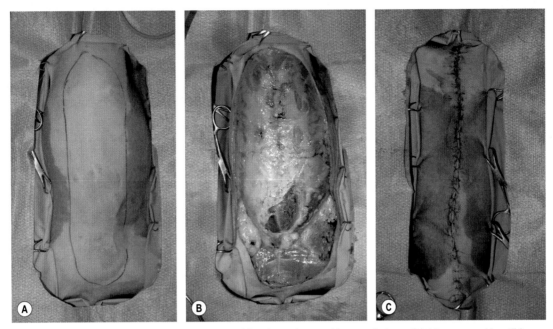

Figure 21-10 Bilateral mastectomy. **(A)** The area to be removed has been drawn with a surgical pen (in this case no skin will be spared) cranially, caudally and between the two mammary lines. **(B)** Intraoperative view after all eight mammary glands have been excised; reconstruction is similar to that described after a unilateral mastectomy. The 'walking suture' is performed from each side of the incision. **(C)** After the final skin closure. *(Courtesy of Julius Liptak.)*

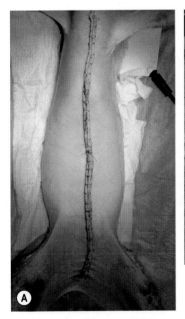

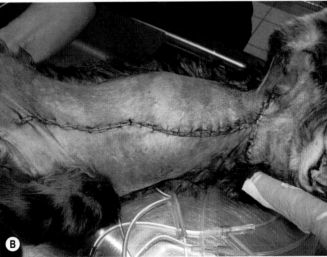

Figure 21-11 (A, B) Two cats following bilateral mastectomy surgery. (B) the cranial incision has been extended on each side for excision of the metastatic axillary lymph nodes (the same cat in Fig 21-5). *(Courtesy of Julius Liptak.)*

remains. If a large seroma is present, treatment options include suture removal, drainage and second intention healing, passive or active drain application, and a padded abdominal bandaging.[62]

Other complications

Dehiscence may result from tension and/or seroma. Wound revision and resuturing are rarely necessary and second intention healing (protected with a tie-over bandage) is monitored until complete healing has occurred. Herniation may occur in cases with unsutured abdominal fascia, deep suture failure or through holes made for omentalization of mesh. This requires corrective surgery. Hemorrhage may occur due to failure of a vessel ligature. The use of a postoperative bandage may partially control it; alternatively, surgical revision is warranted.

PROGNOSIS

The prognosis is excellent in cats with benign lesions while it is guarded in cats with mammary gland adenocarcinoma because animals are usually presented at an advanced stage and this tumor has a high metastatic rate and stromal invasiveness.[16] The prognostic factors to consider are listed below.

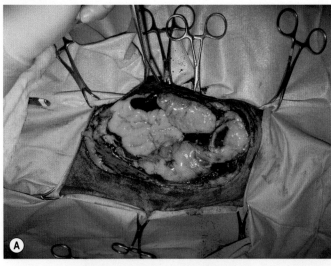
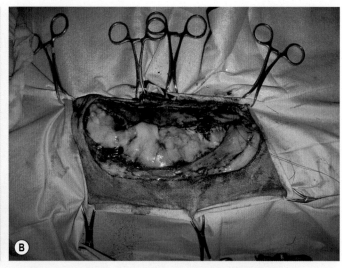

Figure 21-12 **(A)** An example of a full thickness excision of the abdominal wall. **(B)** Closure is achieved by exploiting the elasticity of the cat's abdominal wall. Sutures should engage the fascia rather than the muscular tissue.

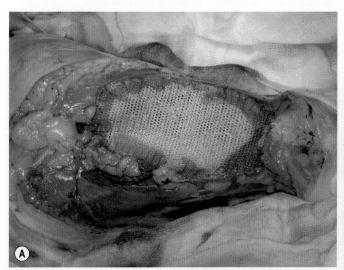
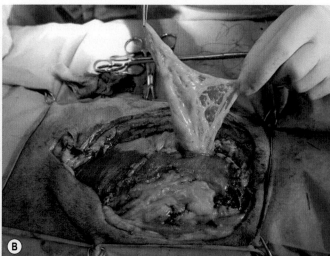

Figure 21-13 Full thickness excision of mammary tumors involving the body wall. **(A)** Polypropylene mesh has been used to cover the defect in this cat; it is sutured to fascia with interrupted sutures. **(B)** The full thickness defect has been filled with a transposed muscular flap and then omentalized. *([A] Courtesy of Giorgio Romanelli.)*

Tumor size

Reported mean survival time for T1 (tumor <2 cm) and T2 (tumor of 2–3 cm) staged cats was 54 and 24 (15–24) months, respectively; for T3 (tumor >3 cm) staged cats survival ranged between 4 and 12 months.[15,16,35,49–51,63,64] These results emphasize the need for an early diagnosis and treatment.

Histologic grade

The classical distinction to well, moderately, and poorly differentiated adenocarcinoma may help in predicting survival at one year, ranging from 100% in well-differentiated tumors to 0% for poorly differentiated lesions; variable results are expected for the intermediate forms.[15,35,48,49,52,64,65] Specific histologic phenotypes may carry different prognoses: that is, poor in cases of invasive micropapillary carcinoma[66] (Fig. 21-14) and more favorable in cases of complex (biphasic

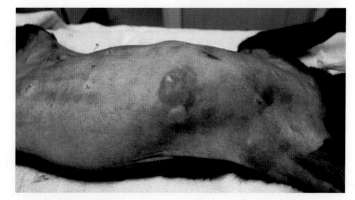

Figure 21-14 A papillary mammary adenocarcinoma in a queen; this cat also had an adenocarcinoma affecting a different mammary gland (the same cat in Fig. 21-3B). *(Courtesy of Lisa Mestrinho.)*

Table 21-5 Molecular studies relating to feline mammary carcinoma as a comparative model of study[a]

Target	Function	Result	References
HER2/neu (c-erbB-2)	Proto-oncogene implicated in cell growth and differentiation	Overexpressed in feline, associated with shorter survival time, similar to women. More recently this conclusion was not validated	78–82
Cyclin A	Cycle regulating gene	Present in about 50% of carcinomas but not in benign lesions	83
VEGF	Vascular endothelial growth factor implicated in tumor angiogenesis, tumor growth and metastasis	Higher immunohistochemical staining correlated with poorer prognosis, both in women and queens	84,85
E-cadherin	Cell adhesion	Reduced or absent in mammary malignancy	86
p53	Cycle regulating gene, tumor suppression	Mutated in many human and animal tumors. Altered in some feline mammary carcinoma, less so in benign lesions	83,87–89
RON	Macrophage-stimulating protein receptor, family of receptor tyrosine kinases. Exacerbation of invasive properties of carcinoma cells	Similar to humans, high level also in feline mammary carcinoma (20% of cases)	90,91
COX2	Conversion of arachidonic acid into prostaglandins	COX-2 overexpression seen in many human and animal tumors, including feline mammary carcinoma (87% of cases). Usually associated with more aggressive tumors	92,93
TopBP1	Topoisomerases are implicated in DNA control, replication, etc.	Increased expression in more malignant lesions	94
PTEN (phosphatase and tensin)	Tumor suppressor genes	Feline mammary carcinoma: loss of PTEN expression associated with lymphatic invasion	95
STAT3-p-tyr705	Cytoplasmic transcription factors play a role in cell-cycle; induced by cytokines and growth factors	Potential role in malignancy as reported in humans and for other sporadic tumors. Correlation between nuclear positivity and histologic grade, tubular formation and mitotic activity	96

[a]Often these studies identify prognostic factors useful to predict survival.

epithelial and myoepithelial) carcinoma.[67] A high ki-67 has been associated with reduced survival.[65,68]

Extent of surgery

Based on one study, aggressive surgery alone may decrease the recurrence rate[48] but it does not necessarily improve the overall survival time.[49] A further study[51] indicated that survival length was associated with extent of surgery (917 days after radical bilateral mastectomy, 428 after regional mastectomy and 348 after unilateral mastectomy); however, in this retrospective study doxorubicin chemotherapy was also given. More recently, another study[10] suggested that surgical resection should be limited to neoplastic gland(s) and sentinel lymph node(s) (see Box 21-1). The draining lymphatic vessels and the exact location of the sentinel lymph nodes relative to the neoplastic gland should be demonstrated preoperatively by radiographic indirect lymphangiography and/or CT-indirect lymphangiography.[11] It is argued that the lymphatic pattern may be locally modified by the tumoral growth, at least in dogs.[69] However, a recent study[70] evaluating VEGFR-3 (vascular endothelial growth factor)-mediated lymphangiogenesis in feline mammary cancer concluded that metastasis to the regional lymph node occurs through pre-existing and not new lymphatic vessels. Given the lack of evidence in favor of one technique over another, the author would still recommend bilateral mastectomy.

Clinical stage

The influence of metastases and their location on outcome may be intuitive. One study[71] has shown that median survival of stage I, II, III and IV mammary carcinoma was 29, 12.5, 9 and 1 months, respectively. Based on another retrospective case series, survival of cats developing metastases after treatment depended on the location of metastases: 331 days for animals with pulmonary metastasis and over 1500 days for those developing nodal metastasis.[51] The latter finding was unexpected and it was attributed to the use of chemotherapy, potentially able to influence the overall metastatic pattern. This also occurs in women.[72]

Molecular markers

Many molecular markers (Table 21-5) in mammary gland tumors can be used to try and determine prognosis.[78–96]

REFERENCES

1. Silver IA. The anatomy of the mammary gland of the dog and cat. J Small Anim Pract 1966;7:689–96.

2. Moore AS, Ogilvie GK. Mammary tumors. Feline oncology. 1st ed. Trenton: Veterinary Learning System; 2001. p. 355–67.

3. Raharison F, Sautet J. Lymph drainage of the mammary glands in female cats. J Morphol 2006;267(3):292–9.

4. Raharison F, Sautet J. The topography of the lymph vessels of mammary glands in female cats. Anat Histol Embryol 2007;36:442–52.

5. Bruni AC, Zimmerl U. Anatomia degli animali domestici. 1st ed. Milan: Dr. Francesco Vallardi; 1974. Vol I. p. 182.

6. Hayden DW, Nielsen SW. Feline mammary tumors. J Small Anim Pract 1971;12:687–98.

7. Ogilvie GK. Feline mammary neoplasia. Compend Contin Educ Pract Vet 1983;5:384–91.

8. Merighi A. Anatomia applicata e topografia regionale veterinaria. 1st ed. Padova: Piccin Nuova Libraria; 2005. p. 118.

9. Mailot JP, Lagneau F, Parodi AL, André F. Particularités des tumeurs mammaires de la chatte. Point Vétérinaire 1980;11:107–8.

10. Papadopoulou PL, Patsikas MN, Charitanti A, et al. The lymph drainage pattern of the mammary glands in the cat: a lymphographic and computerized tomography lymphographic study. Anat Histol Embryol 2009;38(4):292–9.

11. Patsikas MN, Papadopoulou PL, Charitanti A, et al. Computed tomography and radiographic indirect lymphography for visualization of mammary lymphatic vessels and the sentinel lymph node in normal cats. Vet Radiol Ultrasound 2010;51(3):299–304.

12. Owen LN. Classification of tumours in domestic animals. Geneva: World Health Organization; 1980.

13. Hampe JF, Misdorp W. Tumours and dysplasias of the mammary gland. Bull World Health Organ 1974;50:111–33.

14. Misdorp W, Else RW, Hellmen E, Lipscomb TP. Histological classification of mammary tumors of the dog and the cat. In: Schulman FY, editor. World Health Organization International Histological Classification of Tumors of the domestic animals, second series, vol. 7. Washington DC: Armed Forces Instistute of Pathology; 1999. p. 11–56.

15. Giménez F, Hecht S, Craig LE, Legendre AM. Early detection, aggressive therapy: optimizing the management of feline mammary masses. J Feline Med Surg 2010;12(3):214–24.

16. Lana SE, Rutteman, GR, Withrow, SJ. Tumors of the mammary gland. In: Withrow SJ, Vail DM, editors. Withrow & MacEwen's small animal clinical oncology. 4th ed. Saunders Elsevier; 2007. p. 619–35.

17. Hinton M, Gashell CJ. Non-neoplastic mammary hypertrophy in the cat associated with either pregnancy or with oral progestogen therapy. Vet Rec 1977;100:277–80.

18. Hayden DW, Johnston SD, Kiang DT, et al. Feline mammary hypertrophy/fibroadenoma complex: clinical and hormonal aspects. Am J Vet Res 1981;42:1699–703.

19. Hayden DW, Barnes DM, Johnson KH. Morphologic changes in the mammary gland of megestrol acetate-treated and untreated cats: a retrospective study. Vet Pathol 1989;26:104–13.

20. Loretti AP, Ilha MR, Ordás J, Martín de las Mulas J. Clinical, pathological and immunohistochemical study of feline mammary fibro epithelial hyperplasia following a single injection of depot medroxyprogesterone acetate. J Feline Med Surg 2005;7:43–52.

21. Görlinger S, Kooistra HS, van den Broek A, Okkens AC. Treatment of fibroadenomatous hyperplasia in cats with aglepristone. J Vet Intern Med 2002;16:710–13.

22. Burstyn U. Management of mastitis and abscessation of mammary glands secondary to fibroadenomatous hyperplasia in a primiparturient cat. J Am Vet Med Assoc 2010;236(3):326–9.

23. Center SA, Randolph JF. Lactation and spontaneous remission of feline mammary hyperplasia following pregnancy. J Am Anim Hosp Assoc 1985;21:56–8.

24. Mandel M. Spontaneous remission of feline benign mammary hypertrophy. Vet Med Small Anim Clin 1975;70:846–7.

25. Wehrend A, Hospes R, Gruber AD. Treatment of feline mammary fibroadenomatous hyperplasia with a progesterone antagonist. Vet Rec 2001;148:346–7.

26. Jurka P, Max A. Treatment of fibroadenomatosis in 14 cats with aglepristone – changes in blood parameters and follow-up. Vet Rec 2009;165(22):657–60.

27. Kessler M, Vonbomhard D. Mammary tumors in cats: epidemiologic and histologic features in 2,386 cases (1990–5). Kleintierpraxis 1997;42:459.

28. Skorupski KA, Overley B, Shofer FS, et al. Clinical characteristics of mammary carcinoma in male cats. J Vet Intern Med 2005;19:52–5.

29. Jacobs TM, Hoppe BR, Poehlmann CE, et al. Mammary adenocarcinomas in three male cats exposed to medroxyprogesterone acetate (1990–2006). J Feline Med Surg 2010;12(2):169–74.

30. Bostock DE. Canine and feline mammary neoplasms, Br Vet J 1986;142:506–15.

31. Hayes HM Jr, Milne KL, Mandell CP. Epidemiological features of feline mammary carcinomas. Vet Rec 1981;108:476–9.

32. Misdorp W, Romijn A, Hart AA. Feline mammary tumors: a case control study of hormonal factors. Anticancer Res 1991;11:1793–7.

33. Hsu WL, Lin HY, Chiou SS, et al. Mouse mammary tumor virus-like nucleotide sequences in canine and feline mammary tumors. J Clin Microbiol 2010;48(12):4354–62.

34. Dorn CR, Taylor DO, Schneider R, et al. Survey of animal neoplasms in Alameda and Contra Costa Counties, California. II. Cancer morbidity in dogs and cats from Alameda County. J Natl Cancer Inst 1968;40:307–18.

35. Weijer K, Hart AA. Prognostic factors in feline mammary carcinoma. J Natl Cancer Inst 1983;70:709–16.

36. Hahn KA, Adams WH. Feline mammary neoplasia: biological behavior, diagnosis, and treatment alternatives. Feline Pract 1997;25:5–11.

37. Overley B, Shofer FS, Goldschmidt MH, et al. Association between ovarihysterectomy and feline mammary carcinoma. J Vet Intern Med 2005;19:560–3.

38. Keskin A, Yilmazbas G, Yilmaz R, et al. Pathological abnormalities after long-term administration of medroxyprogesterone acetate in a queen. J Feline Med Surg 2009;11(6):518–21.

39. Spugnini EP, Mezzanotte F, Freri L, et al. Cyproterone acetate-induced mammary carcinoma in two male cats. J Feline Med Surg 2010;12(6):515–16.

40. McAloose D, Munson L, Naydan DK. Histologic features of mammary carcinomas in zoo felids treated with melengestrol acetate (MGA) contraceptives. Vet Pathol 2007;44(3):320–6.

41. Munson L, Moresco A. Comparative pathology of mammary gland cancers in domestic and wild animals. Breast Dis 2007;28:7–21.

42. Hamilton JM, Else RW, Forshaw P. Oestrogen receptors in feline mammary carcinomas. Vet Rec 1976;99:477–9.

43. Martin PM, Cotard M, Mialot JP, et al. Animal models for hormone-dependent human breast cancer. Relationship between steroid receptor profiles in canine and feline mammary tumors and survival rate. Cancer Chemother Pharmacol 1984;12(1):13–17.

44. Rutteman GR, Blankenstein MA, Minke J, Misdorp W. Steroid receptors in mammary tumours of the cat. Acta Endocrinol 1991;125:32–7.

45. Millanta F, Calandrella M, Vannozzi I, Poli A. Steroid hormone receptors in normal, dysplastic and neoplastic feline mammary tissues and their prognostic significance. Vet Rec 2006;158:821–4.

46. Millanta F, Calandrella M, Bari G, et al. Comparison of steroid receptor expression in normal, dysplastic, and neoplastic canine and feline mammary tissues. Res Vet Sci 2005;79(3):225–32.

47. Burrai GP, Mohammed SI, Miller MA, et al. Spontaneous feline mammary intraepithelial lesions as a model for

human estrogen receptor- and progesterone receptor-negative breast lesions. BMC Cancer 2010;10:156.

48. MacEwen EG, Hayes AA, Harvey HJ, et al. Prognostic factors for feline mammary tumors. J Am Vet Med Assoc 1984;185: 201–4.

49. Hayes AA, Mooney S. Feline mammary tumors. Vet Clin North Am Small Anim Pract 1985;15:513–20.

50. Pavletic MM. Atlas of small animal wound management and reconstructive surgery. 3rd ed. Philadelphia: Wiley-Blackwell; 2010.

51. Novosad CA, Bergman PJ, O'Brien MG, et al. Retrospective evaluation of adjunctive doxorubicin for the treatment of feline mammary gland adenocarcinoma: 67 cases. J Am Anim Hosp Assoc 2006;42(2):110–20.

52. Jeglum KA, deGuzman E, Young KM. Chemotherapy of advanced mammary adenocarcinoma in 14 cats. J Am Vet Med Assoc 1985;187:157–60.

53. Mauldin GN, Matus RE, Patnaik AK, et al. Efficacy and toxicity of doxorubicin and cyclophosphamide used in the treatment of selected malignant tumors in 23 cats. J Vet Intern Med 1988;23:60–5.

54. Stolwijk JA, Minke JM, Rutteman GR, et al Feline mammary carcinomas as a model for human breast cancer. II. Comparison of in vivo and in vitro adriamycin sensitivity. Anticancer Res 1989;9:1045–8.

55. McNeill CJ, Sorenmo KU, Shofer FS, et al Evaluation of adjuvant doxorubicin-based chemotherapy for the treatment of feline mammary carcinoma. J Vet Intern Med 2009;23(1):123–9.

56. Van der Heyden S, Chiers K, Vercauteren G, et al. Expression of multidrug resistance-associated P-glycoprotein in feline tumours. J Comp Pathol 2011;144(2–3):164–9.

57. Borrego JF, Cartagena JC, Engel J. Treatment of feline mammary tumours using chemotherapy, surgery and a COX-2 inhibitor drug (meloxicam): a retrospective study of 23 cases (2002–2007)*. Vet Comp Oncol 2009;7(4):213–21.

58. Talavera J, Agut A, Fernández Del Palacio J, et al. Thoracic omentalization for long-term management of neoplastic pleural effusion in a cat. J Am Vet Med Assoc 2009;234(10):1299–302.

59. Fox LE, MacEwen EG, Kurzman ID, et al. Liposome-encapsulated muramyl tripeptide phosphatidylethanolamine for the treatment of feline mammary adenocarcinoma: a multicenter randomized double-blind study. Cancer Biother 1995;10:125–30. Erratum in Cancer Biother 1995;10(3):249.

60. Vannucci L, Chiuppesi F, di Martino F, et al. Feline immunodeficiency virus vector as a tool for preventative strategies against human breast cancer. Vet Immunol Immunopathol 2010;134(1–2): 132–7.

61. Penzo C, Ross M, Muirhead R, et al. Effect of recombinant feline interferon-omega alone and in combination with chemotherapeutic agents on putative tumour-initiating cells and daughter cells derived from canine and feline mammary tumours. Vet Comp Oncol 2009;7(4):222–9.

62. Waldrom DR, Zimmermam-Hope N. Superficial skin wounds. In: Slatter B, editor. Textbook of small animal surgery. vol. 1. 3rd ed. Philadelphia: Saunders Elsevier Science; 2003. p. 259–73.

63. Viste JR, Myers SL, Singh B, Simko E. Feline mammary adenocarcinoma: tumor size as a prognostic indicator. Can Vet J 2002;43:33–7.

64. Seixas F, Palmeira C, Pires MA, et al. Grade is an independent prognostic factor for feline mammary carcinomas: A clinicopathological and survival analysis. Vet J 2011;187:65–71.

65. Castagnaro M, Casalone C, Bozzetta E, et al. Tumour grading and the one-year post-surgical prognosis in feline mammary carcinomas. J Comp Pathol 1998;119:263–75.

66. Seixas F, Palmeira C, Pires MA, Lopes C. Mammary invasive micropapillary carcinoma in cats: clinicopathologic features and nuclear DNA content. Vet Pathol 2007;44:842–8.

67. Seixas F, Pires MA, Lopes CA. Complex carcinomas of the mammary gland in cats: pathological and immunohistochemical features. Vet J 2008;176:210–15.

68. Castagnaro M, De Maria R, Bozzetta E, et al. Ki-67 index as indicator of the post-surgical prognosis in feline mammary carcinomas. Res Vet Sci 1998;65:223–6.

69. Patsikas MN, Karayannopoulou M, Kaldrymidoy E, et al. The lymph drainage of the neoplastic mammary glands in the bitch: a lymphographic study. Anat Histol Embryol 2006;35:228–34.

70. Sarli G, Sassi F, Brunetti B, et al. Lymphatic vessels assessment in feline mammary tumours. BMC Cancer 2007;7:7.

71. Ito T, Kadosawa T, Mochizuki M, et al. Prognosis of malignant mammary tumor in 53 cats. J Vet Med Sci 1996;58: 723–6.

72. DeVita VT Jr. Cancer of the breast. In: Devita VT Jr, Hellman S, Rosenberg SA, editors. Cancer principles and practice of oncology. 5th ed. Philadelphia: Lippincott Williams & Wilkins; 1997. p. 1692–706.

73. Sarli G, Brunetti B, Benazzi C. Mammary mucinous carcinoma in the cat. Vet Pathol 2006;43(5):667–73.

74. Matsuda K, Kobayashi S, Yamashita M, et al. Tubulopapillary carcinoma with spindle cell metaplasia of the mammary gland in a cat. J Vet Med Sci 2008;70(5): 479–81.

75. Pérez-Alenza MD, Jiménez A, Nieto AI, Peña L. First description of feline inflammatory mammary carcinoma: clinicopathological and immunohistochemical characteristics of three cases. Breast Cancer Res 2004;6:R300–7.

76. Kamstock DA, Fredrickson R, Ehrhart EJ. Lipid-rich carcinoma of the mammary gland in a cat. Vet Pathol 2005;42(3): 360–2.

77. Sugiyama A, Takeuchi T, Morita T, et al. Lymphangiosarcoma in a cat. J Comp Pathol 2007;137:174–8.

78. Sahin AA. Biologic and clinical significance of HER-2/neu (cerbB-2) in breast cancer. Adv Anat Pathol 2000;7: 158–66.

79. Winston J, Craft DM, Scase TJ, Bergman PJ. Immunohistochemical detection of HER-2/neu expression in spontaneous feline mammary tumours. Vet Comp Oncol 2005;3(1):8–15.

80. De Maria R, Olivero M, Iussich S, et al. Spontaneous feline mammary carcinoma is a model of HER2 overexpressing poor prognosis human breast cancer. Cancer Res 2005;65:907–12.

81. Millanta F, Calandrella M, Citi S, et al. Overexpression of HER-2 in feline invasive mammary carcinomas: an immunohistochemical survey and evaluation of its prognostic potential. Vet Pathol 2005;42:30–4.

82. Rasotto R, Caliari D, Castagnaro M, et al. An immunohistochemical study of HER-2 expression in feline mammary tumours. J Comp Pathol 2011;144(2–3):170–9.

83. Murakami Y, Tateyama S, Rungsipipat A, et al. Immunohistochemical analysis of cyclin A, cyclin D1 and p53 in mammary tumors, squamous cell carcinomas and basal cell tumors in dogs and cats. J Vet Med Sci 2000;62:743–50.

84. Gasparini G. Prognostic value of vascular endothelial growth factor in breast cancer. Oncologist 2000;5(suppl 1):37–44.

85. Millanta F, Lazzeri G, Vannozzi I, et al. Correlation of vascular endothelial growth factor expression to overall survival in feline invasive mammary carcinomas. Vet Pathol 2002;39:690–6.

86. Pereira PD, Gartner F. Expression of E-cadherin in normal, hyperplastic and neoplastic feline mammary tissue. Vet Rec 2003;153:297–302.

87. Mayr B, Blauensteiner J, Edlinger A, et al. Presence of p53 mutations in feline neoplasms. Res Vet Sci 2000;68:63–70.

88. Nasir L, Krasner H, Argyle DJ, Williams A. Immunocytochemical analysis of the tumour suppressor protein (p53) in feline neoplasia. Cancer Lett 2000; 155:1–7.

89. Nakano M, Wu H, Taura Y, Inoue M. Immunohistochemical detection of

Mdm2 and p53 in feline mammary gland tumors. J Vet Med Sci 2006;68: 421–5.

90. Maggiora P, Marchio S, Stella MC, et al. Overexpression of the RON gene in human breast carcinoma. Oncogene 1998;16:2927–33.

91. De Maria R, Maggiora P, Biolatti B, et al. Feline STK gene expression in mammary carcinomas. Oncogene 2002;21:1785–90.

92. Millanta F, Citi S, Della Santa D, et al. COX-2 expression in canine and feline invasive mammary carcinomas: correlation with clinicopathological features and prognostic molecular markers. Breast Cancer Res Treat 2006;98(1):115–20.

93. Sayasith K, Sirois J, Doré M. Molecular characterization of feline COX-2 and expression in feline mammary carcinomas. Vet Pathol 2009;46: 423–9.

94. Morris JS, Nixon C, Bruck A, et al. Immunohistochemical expression of TopBP1 in feline mammary neoplasia in relation to histological grade, Ki67, ERalpha and p53. Vet J 2008;175: 218–26.

95. Ressel L, Millanta F, Caleri E, et al. Reduced PTEN protein expression and its prognostic implications in canine and feline mammary tumors. Vet Pathol 2009;46(5):860–8.

96. Petterino C, Ratto A, Podestà G, et al. Immunohistochemical evaluation of STAT3-p-tyr705 expression in feline mammary gland tumours and correlation with histologic grade. Res Vet Sci 2007;82(2):218–24.

Chapter |22|

Injection site sarcomas

B. Séguin

Sarcomas developing at the injection sites of vaccines have been recognized in cats since the early 1990s.[1,2] They can be highly invasive tumors with a tendency for local recurrence. Early aggressive multimodality treatment after advanced imaging gives the best chance for a cure.

EPIDEMIOLOGY

There is strong epidemiologic evidence that links the administration of inactivated feline vaccines and subsequent development of sarcomas at the site of injection. Other causes have been implicated, including sites of antibiotic and lufenuron administration.[3–5] A fibrosarcoma, with features of a vaccine-associated tumor, developed at the site of a deep non-absorbable suture in a cat.[6] It is now believed that vaccines are not the only agents capable of causing the development of sarcomas at the injection site, but instead virtually anything that produces local inflammation has the potential in susceptible cats.[5] A leading hypothesis for the etiopathogenesis is that the inflammatory reaction leads to uncontrolled proliferation of fibroblasts and myofibroblasts that undergo malignant transformation in a subset of cats.[7] Transition zones from inflammatory granuloma to sarcoma have been identified on histopathology as well as microscopic foci of sarcoma located in areas of granulomatous inflammation, which again strongly supports the idea that inflammation precedes the sarcoma development.[8,9] As the incidence is relatively low and vaccines are the compounds that are given to most cats in the population with any frequency to make any correlation, vaccines have received the most attention as potential causative agents and hence most of the research has focused on vaccines.[10]

Strong epidemiologic evidence has demonstrated an association between the administration of inactivated feline leukemia virus (FeLV) and rabies vaccines and subsequent development of soft tissue sarcomas.[2,11–13] Associations have also been reported between feline panleukopenia and feline rhinotracheitis vaccines.[7,11,14,15] The true incidence of sarcoma development after vaccination is unknown. Some studies report an incidence of sarcomas per vaccines administered,[13] whereas others report a prevalence of sarcoma per cat.[12] The incidence is estimated to be between 1/1000 and 1/10 000 vaccines administered.[7,8] One epidemiologic study determined the incidence of post-vaccination injection site sarcoma to be 0.63 sarcoma/10 000 cats vaccinated and 0.32 sarcoma/10 000 doses of all vaccines administered.[16] Therefore, the incidence is now believed to be 1 case/10 000 to 30 000 cats vaccinated.[16]

It appears that the reaction to vaccines is additive and that the likelihood of sarcoma development increases with the number of vaccines given simultaneously at the vaccine site.[13] In a retrospective study, it was determined that the risk a cat would develop a sarcoma after administration of a single vaccine in the cervical–interscapular region (a site not recommended any more by the Vaccine-Associated Feline Sarcoma Task Force and American Association of Feline Practitioners[8,17]) was 50% higher than the risk a cat not receiving any vaccines at this site would have. The risk for a cat given two vaccines at the same site was approximately 127% higher, and the risk for a cat given three to four vaccines was 175% higher.[8,13] Time to tumor development in cats following vaccination has been reported to be between four weeks and ten years.[7,16] It has been postulated that most tumors will develop within three years after vaccination.[16] Tumor types that have been reported at the sites of vaccination are fibrosarcoma (most common), malignant fibrous histiocytoma, extraskeletal osteosarcoma, rhabdomyosarcoma, myofibrosarcoma, undifferentiated sarcoma, liposarcoma, and chondrosarcoma.[5,18,19]

CLINICAL SIGNS AND TUMOR STAGING

Feline injection site sarcomas are usually highly aggressive, poorly circumscribed, not encapsulated, and more invasive locally than non-injection site sarcomas, making them more challenging to treat;[20,21] they are also more likely to recur after surgical excision than non-injection site sarcomas.[11] When compared to non-injection site sarcomas, injection site sarcomas have a higher inflammatory response, as characterized histologically by a predominately lymphocytic infiltration, along with increased necrosis and mitotic rates and the presence of multi-nucleated giant cells.[20,22,23] Injection site sarcomas have a propensity for higher histologic grade than non-injection site sarcomas.[23] Although in one study, more injection site sarcomas were of lower grade,[24] in two other studies, high grade sarcomas (grade III) were the most common, accounting for 46% and 59%, respectivelty.[21,25]

© 2014 Elsevier Ltd
DOI: 10.1016/B978-0-7020-4336-9.00022-6

A biopsy-confirmed injection site sarcoma needs to be staged. Cats with suspected injection site sarcoma based on history and location of the tumor can have the staging process started (see Chapter 14) before or after the biopsy procedure is performed but always before definitive treatment is initiated. Complete blood count, serum biochemistry panel, urinalysis, along with FeLV and feline immunodeficiency virus (FIV) tests will determine the overall health status. Although no association is apparent between viral status (FeLV, FIV) and tumor development, the course of the disease may be altered because of compromise of the immune system.[7]

IMAGING

The chest should be evaluated for evidence of metastasis, which occurs in 5–24% of cases.[3,19,24,26–28] Chest radiographs can be performed using three views or alternatively computed tomography (CT) can be performed to evaluate the chest and lungs. CT is more sensitive than radiographs in detecting pulmonary metastatic lesions.[29] Regional lymph nodes should be evaluated through palpation, radiographs, or ultrasonography, and cytology where applicable. Metastasis occurs primarily to the lungs but other sites such as regional lymph nodes, mediastinum, pericardium, liver, skin, and pelvis have also been reported.[7,19,30–32]

Advanced imaging techniques such as CT or magnetic resonance imaging (MRI) are extremely helpful, and considered by many to be mandatory in planning a surgical resection and potentially deciding to perform radiation therapy in the neoadjuvant setting (Fig. 22-1). In a study to evaluate the usefulness of CT imaging of vaccine-associated sarcomas, the CT image revealed the tumor to be, on average, twice as large as determined by physical examination and caliper measurement, and recommendations regarding the treatment were often altered based on the CT results.[7,33] In another study, the

use of CT resulted in the reclassification of 17/26 subcutaneous neoplasms in dogs to a more advanced clinical stage as compared to physical examination.[34] Even patients that have had a previous surgical excision can benefit from advanced imaging as it can provide information regarding the extent of the previous surgical field and therefore the area that needs to be re-excised or included in the radiation treatment field.[7]

TREATMENT OPTIONS

Surgery is one of the most important components of the treatment regime for these tumors. However, attempts at simple excision (i.e., debulking or marginal excision) are rarely curative and ultimately lead to local recurrence with a more difficult second surgery.[5,7] Therefore wide to radical excision is the recommended surgical approach. Multimodal treatment consists of a combination of surgery, radiation and/or chemotherapy, and a multimodal treatment to include irradiation is considered the standard of care to treat injection site sarcomas.[5] However, results of studies evaluating radical surgical excision alone question the necessity and the benefit of radiation therapy with this type of surgery.

Decision making

As with any tumor, vaccine-associated sarcomas should be treated early when small. Unfortunately, these tumors can be very fast growing and the cat is often presented when the tumor is relatively large (Fig. 22-2). Given that these tumors grow in the subcutaneous areas (where natural barriers to tumor growth are absent), there are no definitive criteria that define a resectable versus a non-resectable tumor. The locally invasive nature of these tumors necessitates wide to radical excision to achieve the longest disease-free intervals (see surgical treatment and prognosis sections). These tumors do not invade bone, but the locally invasive injection site sarcomas can extend to the soft tissue–bone interface, necessitating removal of bone as a deep surgical margin with radical excision (see Fig. 22-1).[21] In one study, 57% of

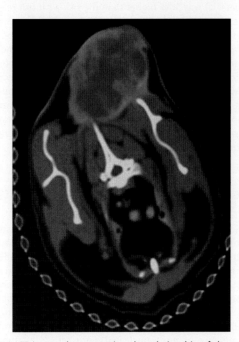

Figure 22-1 CT image demonstrating the relationship of the tumor with local anatomical structures. The tumor is seen extending to the soft tissue–bone interface with the scapula and spinous process of the vertebra. For a curative-intent surgery, this will necessitate removal of those structures (osteotomy of the spinous process and partial scapulectomy) to achieve an adequately deep surgical margin.

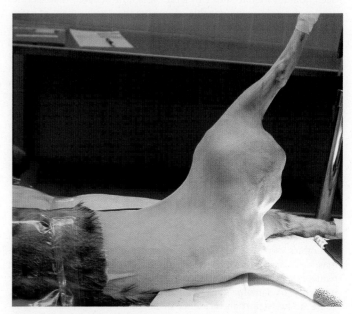

Figure 22-2 A cat with a large tumor on the caudal aspect of the pelvic limb. Because of the proximal extension of the tumor, a mid to caudal hemipelvectomy was performed (see Fig. 22-5).

cats that had an injection site sarcoma removal required an ostectomy of some sort.[21]

Aggressive surgeries are generally well tolerated by cats.[21,24] With the advancement of reconstructive surgical techniques and the availability of polypropylene mesh, in conjunction with advancements made in critical care, extensive body wall resections are possible. When performing a thoracic wall resection as many as eight ribs can be successfully removed (Charles Kuntz, personal communication).

Cats can survive massive resections, even following tumor removal resulting in a wound of over 15 cm in diameter.[21] Therefore relatively large tumors can still be amenable to wide or radical surgical excision and the size of the tumor is rarely a limiting factor in the decision to perform surgery.

SURGICAL EXCISION

For the purpose of feline injection site sarcomas, wide excision is the removal of the tumor with 2–3 cm of normal tissue beyond the edges of the tumor and one fascial plane (one muscle) deep to the tumor, whereas radical excision is the removal of the tumor with 5 cm of normal tissue beyond the edges of the tumor and two fascial planes (two muscles) deep to the tumor, including bones that are part of these margins.[21] The rationale to remove muscles, which are covered by fascia, deep to the tumor is that fascia is a collagen-rich, vascular-poor tissue that has been shown to be a natural barrier against cancer and it is more difficult for tumors to grow across these collagen-rich, vascular-poor tissues.[35] Sometimes it is possible to remove the fascial layer only without having to remove the muscle. This is possible when the fascia peels easily away from the muscle it covers. But in most instances, the fascia is too intimate to be peeled from the muscle and it is best to remove the entire muscle thickness.

Because of the variation in anatomic location and tumor size, the technical details of the surgical excision will vary from cat to cat (Box 22-1). Adherence to sound principles of surgical oncology is important throughout the surgical procedure (see Chapter 14).

Osteotomies

If the tumor comes close to a bone such as a dorsal spinous process or scapula (see Fig. 22-1), these bony structures are excised en bloc with the tumor. Therefore osteotomies are performed as part of the tumor excision as opposed to removing the tumor by peeling off the soft tissues from the bone and then performing the osteotomies. Even though a tumor might not be in contact with a bony structure, osteotomies may still be required to achieve appropriate and adequate deep margins. This is particularly applicable for tumors that cross the dorsal midline in areas where there are no single fascial/muscle planes. Therefore for these tumors, it is best to remove the dorsal spinous processes of the vertebrae in the surgical field of resection. Osteotomies of the dorsal spinous processes can be performed with Liston bone cutting forceps, power burr, power oscillating saw, or gigli wire saw; the latter option is not usually recommended. The best excision of any malignant tumor is one where entry into the tumor or its capsule is avoided. If the tumor, or its capsule, is visualized or entered during the dissection there is the risk of contamination of the surgeon's gloves and/or instruments with tumor cells resulting in potential seeding of these cells to other areas of the surgical wound bed.

Scapulectomy

Tumors growing in the interscapular area can require scapulectomy. Typically, a partial scapulectomy is performed (Box 22-2). If a

---

Box 22-1 **Vaccine-associated tumor excision**

A wide area should be clipped and aseptically prepared for surgery. After the cat has been draped, if the tumor is ulcerated, it is covered with a sterile surgical gauze or laparotomy sponge and care is taken not to touch the ulcerated area. A sterile marker pen is used to delineate the palpable borders of the tumor or landmarks to which tumor extension was seen on advanced imaging. Another line (line of excision) is made 3 cm (for wide excision) to 5 cm (for radical excision) from the first line (Fig. 22-3) The line of excision can be made in an elliptical shape to help with closure if closure can be performed without a skin reconstruction technique (see Chapter 19). The ellipse should be in the appropriate orientation based on skin tension and availability. An incision is made in the skin along the line of excision with a scalpel blade. Subcutaneous tissue and muscles are incised. Sharp dissection is used preferentially over blunt dissection. The incision will include one (for wide excision) or two muscles (for radical excision) deep to the tumor as the deep margin. Depending on the anatomic location, there may not be one or two layers of muscle that are deep to and continuous under the entire surface of the tumor. In those cases, as the incision in the muscles is performed circumferentially around the tumor, other muscle planes are incised as well to provide as complete a deep margin made up of one or two muscle layers across the entire surface area under the tumor. Once the muscles are excised, they are elevated from the underlying tissues to remove the tumor out of the body. It may not be possible to first incise the muscles completely circumferentially before working under the deep margin. Often, a plane of the deep margin is determined in one area of the surgical field (e.g., cranially or dorsally to the tumor) and the dissection under the tumor is made concurrently with the circumferential incision in the muscles around the tumor. To achieve wide or radical excision it may also be necessary to perform osteotomies. Hemostasis during the surgery can be achieved with a combination of cautery, hemostatic clips, and suture ligation.

Box 22-2 **Partial scapulectomy**

For a partial scapulectomy, most often the osteotomy is performed at or dorsal to the neck of the scapula. Muscles that still have an attachment on the scapula after incising around the tumor are transected. These include the trapezius and deltoid muscles at the dorsolateral aspect of the scapula. Dorsomedially, the rhomboideus and serratus ventralis muscles are transected. The teres major muscle, which is caudodorsal, is also transected. If an osteotomy is made more ventrally on the scapula, the long head of the triceps, omotransversarius, and teres minor muscles may need to be transected as well. At the site of the proposed osteotomy on the scapula, the muscle attachments are elevated with a periosteal elevator and the osteotomy is performed with an oscillating saw. After the tumor is removed en bloc with the partial scapulectomy, remaining muscles at the site of the scapulectomy are used to cover the dorsal osteotomized border of the scapula. This will provide as much support as possible to the scapula and help minimize the dorsal motion of the scapula that will happen with weight-bearing on the limb.

---

complete scapulectomy is deemed necessary, it is best to perform a full forelimb amputation. The reason for this is not that cats cannot do well with a complete scapulectomy, but rather because better margins are achieved with a full amputation of the limb. Partial scapulectomy involves the excision of the dorsal aspect of the bone. As a general rule, the less bone removed, the better the limb function.

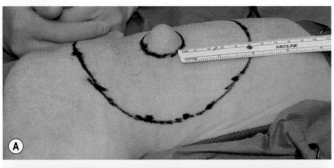

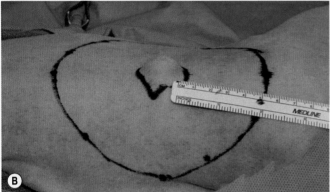

Figure 22-3 A sterile marker pen was used to delineate the edges of the tumor. Then another line was made circumferentially around the tumor 5 cm from the first line in preparation for a radical excision. **(A)** Ventrolateral view; **(B)** dorsolateral view.

However, bone should not be preserved for the sake of function as this may compromise the completeness of excision of the tumor. Tumor excision with adequate margins is the priority.

Hemipelvectomy

Excision of tumors located on the caudal aspect of the trunk, over the pelvis, may require hemipelvectomy (Box 22-3). A total hemipelvectomy is the removal of the limb and entire hemipelvis (os coxae) including the ilium, acetabular bone, and pubis and ischium to midline (Fig. 22-4A). A middle-to-caudal partial hemipelvectomy is removal of the hemipelvis including the acetabulum with amputation of the hind limb and a portion of the ischium to the midline (Fig. 22-4B). A middle-to-cranial partial hemipelvectomy includes removal of the hemipelvis from immediately caudal to the acetabulum to the sacroiliac joint combined with pelvic limb amputation (Fig. 22-4C). Caudal partial hemipelvectomy is defined as removal of the ischium with preservation of the acetabulum and limb (Fig. 22-4D). For tumors that are located more cranially, removal of the wing of the ilium alone may be sufficient, with a single osteotomy performed cranial to the sacroiliac joint.

Body wall excision

Some tumors will require a full-thickness body wall excision (Fig. 22-6A). Depending on the anatomic location this will either involve abdominal or thoracic wall or a combination of the two (for more information on surgery of these areas see Chapters 25 and 43). Thoracic wall excision requires the removal of ribs. As previously mentioned, as many as eight ribs have been removed successfully in a cat (Charles Kuntz, personal communication). When the caudal ribs are removed it may be possible to advance the diaphragm cranially and

Box 22-3 **Hemipelvectomy**

In order to perform the proposed ostectomy, muscles are transected as part of the excision of the tumor down to the level of the pelvic bones. Muscle attachments are elevated from the bones and the different bones are osteotomized with an oscillating saw (Fig. 22-5). Remaining muscle attachments are transected to free the tumor en bloc with the segment of pelvis. The reader is referred to more complete descriptions of the surgical techniques involved with hemipelvectomy and amputation.[36,37]

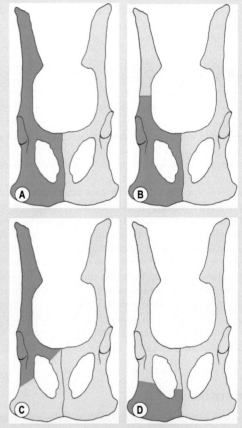

Figure 22-4 Categories of hemipelvectomy. **(A)** Total hemipelvectomy; **(B)** mid-to-caudal partial hemipelvectomy; **(C)** mid-to-cranial hemipelvectomy; **(D)** caudal partial hemipelvectomy. *(Redrawn from Kramer, A., Walsh, P., and Seguin, B. 2008. Hemipelvectomy in dogs and cats: technique overview, variations and description. Vet Surg 37:413-419, with permission from John Wiley and Sons.)*

attach it to the most caudal rib left intact. Cranial advancement of the diaphragm may require partial or complete removal of the caudal lung lobe. Otherwise it will be compressed and can lead to ventilation/perfusion mismatch and the potential for pneumonia.

Large body wall defects, both thoracic and abdominal, can be reconstructed with autogenous tissues (Fig. 22-6B), synthetic materials such as polypropylene mesh, or a combination of both (Fig. 22-7). This author favors the use of autogenous muscle flaps to reconstruct body wall defect in cats. In dogs it has been demonstrated that reconstruction with synthetic material alone leads to a higher complication rate.[38] However, because of the aggressive nature of the surgical excision with injection site sarcomas, the potential muscle flaps available locally might be sacrificed as part of the excision, which will leave few options to reconstruct body wall.

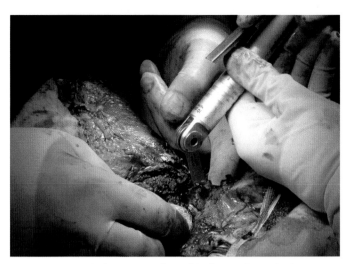

Figure 22-5 Hemipelvectomy performed in the cat shown in Figure 22-2. The oscillating saw is used to perform the osteotomy of the pubis.

Amputation

Tumors located on a limb are treated with limb amputation. It is best to perform a complete amputation, meaning removal of the scapula for the thoracic limb and disarticulation of the coxofemoral joint for the pelvic limb.[37] For tumors that are close enough to the greater trochanter, an en-bloc acetabulectomy with the pelvic limb amputation is indicated to allow better soft tissue margins. The acetabulectomy is a form of partial hemipelvectomy that requires three osteotomies: one in the body of the ilium cranial to the acetabulum, one in the ischium just caudal to the acetabulum, and one in the pubis ventral to the acetabulum. The osteotomies in the ilium and pubis need to end up in the obturator foramen. In some instances, even though the tumor is mainly located on a limb, in order to achieve a wide or radical excision it may be necessary to perform a body wall excision en bloc with the amputation (Fig. 22-8).

Closure

After removing the tumor, the surgeons and the assistants need to change gloves and use new instruments. If the drapes are soiled, new drapes are used to cover the soiled ones. Hemoclips are placed in the surgical bed created from having removed the tumor to delineate the surgical bed later on with radiographs (Fig. 22-6B). This will help planning of radiation therapy if necessary.[39] The surgical bed is lavaged copiously throughout the closure. Closure is performed with monofilament absorbable materials for the muscle layers and subcutaneous tissues. Tumor cells adhere the most to multifilament suture materials.[40] It is best to eliminate the dead space as much as possible to reduce the risk or size of a postoperative seroma. However, given the extensive nature of the excision and the volume of tissues that can be removed with the excision of these tumors, it can be difficult to impossible to eliminate all the dead space. In spite of this, the use of drains is generally discouraged and if one is used, it should be done judiciously. It is best to use closed suctions drains and the skin exit site of the drain should be planned carefully. The drain tract can become seeded with tumor cells and if postoperative radiation therapy is to be performed, the drain tract must be included in the radiation field.

Skin is closed routinely using non-absorbable suture material or staples (Fig. 22-6C). When excessive tension exists on the suture line, a tension-relieving tie-in bandage can be placed over the incision in the area of excess tension (Fig. 22-9). Skin flaps may be required to close large defects although this is uncommon given the relatively

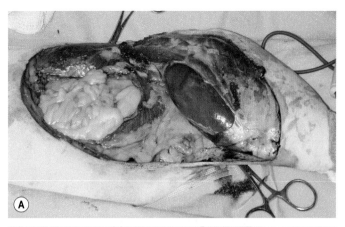

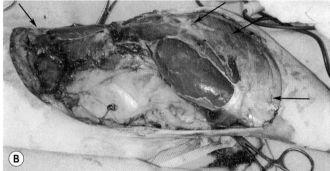

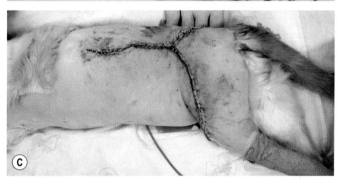

Figure 22-6 (A) A radical excision has been performed to include the lateral body wall of the abdomen and fascia lata with part of the tensor fascia lata muscle. **(B)** The abdominal wall has been closed by simply apposing the cut edge of the abdominal wall muscles to the muscles surrounding the spine. Hemoclips have been placed to delineate the surgical field (black arrows). **(C)** The final appearance of the surgical wound after closure of the skin. The skin was closed by apposing the cut edges. This is often possible in cats in spite of radical excision, due to the copious surface area of skin present.

loose and elastic skin in most cats. If a skin flap is necessary (see Chapter 19), new gloves and new instruments are to be used. The instruments that are used for the closure, although different than those used for the excision, should not be used for the creation of the flap. If there are any tumor cells in the surgical bed and the instruments come in contact with these cells, the instruments may seed the donor site of the skin flap with tumor cells and allow the formation of a new tumor at a different site.

Before placing the tumor sample that has been removed in formalin, the surgical margins (edges of the tissues that were incised to allow removal of the tumor) are covered with ink (Fig. 22-10).[41] This allows a more accurate assessment of the surgical margins by the pathologist.

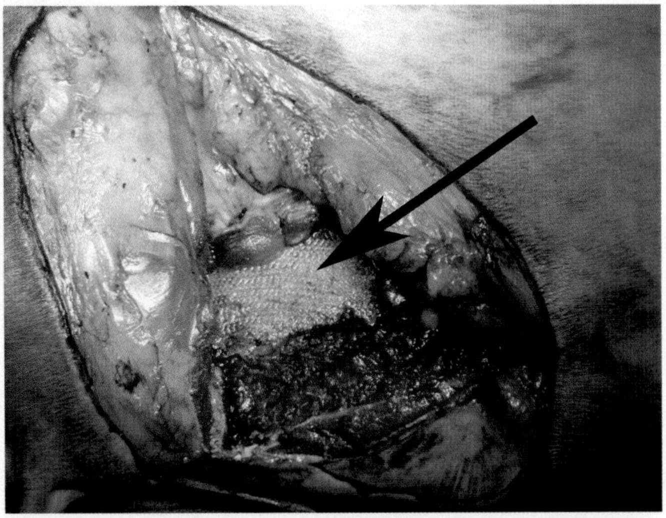

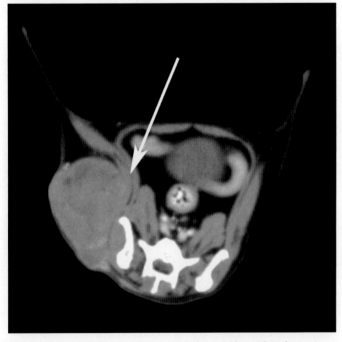

Figure 22-7 A combination of autogenous and synthetic mesh (arrow) was used to close the body wall defect. *(Courtesy of Dr Milan Milovancev.)*

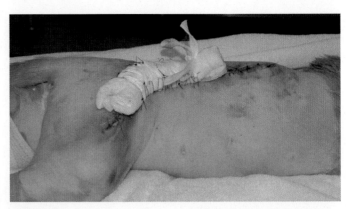

Figure 22-9 A tension-relieving tie-in bandage is applied over the incision in the area of most tension. This helps prevent dehiscence in the postoperative period. Loops of non-absorbable sutures are placed on either side parallel to the surgical incision. A laparotomy sponge is rolled and placed over the incision, between the two rows of suture loops. A string of umbilical tape is used to connect the two rows of suture loops in a shoe-lace fashion and the umbilical tape is tightened to take most of the tension away from the incision line itself. The bandage is usually left in place for seven to 14 days.

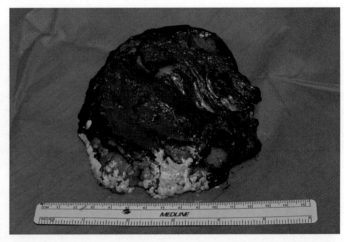

Figure 22-10 Tumor specimen turned upside down. The surgical margins have been inked with different colors to help the pathologist evaluate them for the presence of tumor cells.

Figure 22-8 CT image showing a tumor that was located at the proximal aspect of the hind limb but on CT it can be seen that the tumor extends over the abdominal wall (arrow). To achieve a radical excision, the body wall will need to be removed en bloc with the limb amputation to achieve a radical excision. The wing of the ilium will also need to be excised en bloc.

Buster collars (see Chapter 3) should not be used as an alternative to pain relief but can be used in conjunction with analgesia.

Skin suture or staple removal is performed two to three weeks after the surgery, when the surgical incision has healed appropriately. If radiation therapy was delivered before surgery, it is best to leave the sutures or staples longer (three to four weeks) as radiation delays wound healing.

POSTOPERATIVE CARE

Proper analgesia must be provided in the postoperative period.[42] Pain relief is imperative following surgery, particularly following wide and radical excisions. Cats are maintained on intravenous fluids until they can drink and eat well. Blood transfusions or component therapy (i.e., packed red blood cells or plasma) may be needed during or after the surgery if blood loss is significant (see Chapter 5). Bandaging is not usually necessary; devices to prevent wound interference such as

Radiation

Once the wound has healed well, radiation therapy (see Chapter 15) can be started (if not performed in the neoadjuvant setting), which is typically two weeks after surgery. Any complications with wound healing can delay the start of radiation therapy. The debate as to which is the better approach between preoperative and postoperative irradiation remains open. No clinical study has evaluated this issue for feline injection site sarcomas. There are advantages and disadvantages for each (Table 22-1).[43]

Table 22-1 Advantages and disadvantages of postoperative and preoperative radiation therapy[43]

	Preoperative xrt	Postoperative xrt
Delay in performing or delivering therapy	**A:** no delay in staring xrt from wound healing problems **D:** delay performing Sx if acute side effects of xrt persist	**A:** no delay in performing Sx because of acute side effects from xrt **D:** delay start of xrt from wound healing complications (e.g., seroma). Allows more time for tumor cell repopulation
Wound healing	**D:** impaired from xrt	**A:** not impaired from previous xrt
Size of radiation treatment field	**A:** smaller because no Sx has been performed	**D:** larger because must include all tissues handled at Sx, including entire incision line and draining sites if present. The larger the field, the greater the morbidity
Circulating cancer cells released because of manipulation of tumor at surgery	**A:** cancer cells entering circulation less likely to be viable because killed from xrt	**D:** cancer cells released are more likely to be viable. May increase risk of developing metastasis
Blood supply to tumor, especially to cells at periphery	**A:** blood supply to cancer cells at periphery of tumor is at its best. Therefore cells are most radiosensitive from the oxygenation standpoint	**D:** surgery disrupts blood supply to tumor cells, especially the ones at the periphery of the tumor since these are the cells that are mostly targeted by xrt. Hypoxic cells are more radioresistant
Size of tumor	**A:** tumor *may* regress in size from xrt and make it more amenable to surgical resection. However, making an inoperable tumor operable with xrt should *not* be the main goal of xrt	**D:** the tumor is as large as can be and may be difficult to resect

A, advantage; D, disadvantage; xrt, radiation therapy; Sx, surgery.

Preoperative radiation refers to radiation delivered before surgery. The surgery involves removing the tumor in toto at some predetermined time rather than waiting to see if radiation was effective or not in controlling the tumor locally. Typically, surgery is performed three to four weeks after the end of the radiation treatments.[43] Radiation therapy alone is not considered an appropriate treatment for these tumors. Irradiation alone should only be considered in the palliative setting.[7,44]

Postoperative radiation therapy refers to the planned delivery of radiation following surgery. Typically, the radiation is started ten to 14 days after the surgery although it can be started as early as 24 hours postoperatively.[43] For more information on radiation see Chapter 15.

Chemotherapy

Chemotherapy alone should not be considered definitive therapy,[45] but similar to radiation therapy, chemotherapy alone can be considered palliative therapy. In the adjuvant or neoadjuvant setting, chemotherapy may play an important role in the multimodal approach to treatment. The use of various chemotherapeutic protocols has resulted in some partial and less frequently complete responses.[7] Chemotherapy in the preoperative setting may reduce tumor size thereby facilitating surgical resection; or chemotherapy can also be used as a radiation sensitizer. Agents that have been used clinically include doxorubicin, cyclophosphamide, carboplatin, mitoxantrone, vincristine, and ifosfamide.[7,27,46–49] Typically, when used in the adjuvant setting, chemotherapy is started two weeks after surgery. For more information on chemotherapy see Chapter 16.

Follow up

Patients that have been treated for an injection site sarcoma should be rechecked with a physical examination performed monthly for three months, then at least every three months for the first year, and then every three to six months thereafter. Additional diagnostic procedures should be performed as indicated by the clinical signs and findings on the physical exam.

COMPLICATIONS

Complications are varied and are, to some degree, dependent on the type of surgery that was performed. Complications include dehiscence, surgical site infection, seroma formation, development of chronic draining tracts following the use of mesh for reconstruction, laryngeal paralysis (after resection of a tumor in the cervical area and transection of the recurrent laryngeal nerve), pneumothorax following thoracic wall resection, pneumonia, constipation following hemipelvectomy or high tail amputation, hypovolemic shock, acute renal failure, and death.[21,50]

In one study where wide or radical excision was performed, the non-fatal complication rate was 15.7% and 4.6% of cats died in the perioperative period.[50] In another study where radical excision was performed, major complications occurred in 11% of cats.[21] In both studies, wound complications were the most common finding. Four per cent had dehiscence of their surgical incision in the study where wide or radical excisions were performed and 8% had dehiscence in the study where radical excisions were performed. In the study where only radical excisions were performed, all dehiscences had interscapular tumors. Size of tumor was not prognostic for developing a dehiscence.[21]

PROGNOSIS

Rates of local tumor recurrence for injection site sarcomas with surgery alone range from 14– 69%[21,25,48,51] and from 26–52% with adjuvant therapies, including pre- or postoperative radiation and chemotherapy.[3,24,26–28,47–49,52]

Complete surgical margins correlate with increased survival times (ST) and disease-free interval (DFI).[26–28,52] Radical excisions can lead to complete surgical margins in 95% to 97% of cases.[21,24] In spite of clean surgical margins, local recurrence is still possible.[21,25]

In one study, the rate of local recurrence for tumors resected with incomplete margins was 69% whereas the rate was 19% for tumors resected with complete margins.[25] In another study where tumors were resected with a radical excision, 97% of tumors had clean surgical margins and the rate of local recurrence was 14%, demonstrating that a number of tumors will recur in spite of clean margins.[21]

With surgery alone, median ST has been reported as >16 months,[52] 576 days,[19] 804 days,[24] and 901 days.[21] Cats with wide excision at first attempt have longer TFIs than marginal excision (419 days versus 66 days)[19] and cats with complete excision have a longer tumor-free interval (>16 months versus four months) and survival time (>16 months versus nine months) than those with incomplete excision.[52] Tumors located on a limb that are amenable to being treated by amputation have a better prognosis. Median time to first recurrence for appendicular tumors was significantly greater than that for tumors located on the trunk (325 days versus 66 days).[19] From the Kaplan Meier product limit method, it was estimated that approximately 45% of the cats with tumors located on the limbs treated by amputation can be considered cured whereas less than 10% of cats with tumors on the trunk treated by wide or marginal excision can be considered cured.[19] Time to local tumor recurrence can range from a couple of weeks to years.

Both local tumor recurrence and metastasis are negative prognostic factors for survival time.[3,21,24,53] In one study of cats treated by radical excision of the tumor, median survival time of cats with and without recurrence was 499 and 1,461 days, respectively, and median survival time of cats with and without metastasis was 388 and 1,528 days, respectively.[21]

The prognostic value of tumor grade is not very well determined for injection site sarcomas in cats. Grading criteria can differ from one study to another, making comparisons difficult.[21,24,25] In one study, grade was prognostic for metastasis,[24] while other studies were not able to correlate grade to recurrence or survival.[21,25]

The type of surgery that has been reported with the best outcome for local control and survival is the radical excision where 5 cm margins laterally all around the tumor and two fascial planes or bone for the deep margin are achieved. The rate of local recurrence was 14% and overall survival was 901 days; the survival time was 1528 days when no metastasis developed.[21]

Radiotherapy combined with surgery in the non-radical excision setting appears to increase the tumor control rate.[7] Studies evaluating pre- or postoperative radiation in addition to surgical excision reported median time to local recurrence to range between 5.7 months and 37 months.[3,26,49,54] Local recurrence rates are between 41% and 52%.[3,26,27,49] Survival times range from 600 to 1300 days.[3,26,47,49,54]

Conflicting results exist regarding the prognosis associated with completeness of surgical margins when radiation therapy is performed. In two studies, cats that had tumors removed with complete margins had a prolonged DFI. In one, the DFI for cats with incomplete surgical margins was 112 days versus 700 days for cats with complete surgical margins.[26] In the other the DFI was 986 days versus 292 days for complete and incomplete margins, respectively.[27] In the latter study, however, some cats received chemotherapy. Conversely, in another study, the status of the surgical margins was not a prognostic factor for local recurrence or survival time.[3]

The role and benefit of chemotherapy in the treatment of injection site sarcomas in cats remains ill-defined and controversial. In one study evaluating the use of combination doxorubicin and cyclophosphamide in cats with tumors considered non-resectable, half had a 50% or greater decrease in gross tumor burden.[45] Seventeen per cent had resolution of all clinically detectable tumor. Unfortunately, the responses were not durable, with a median response duration of 125 days. Median survival for responders was 242 days versus 83 days for non-responders.[45] Another study where doxorubicin (to include liposome-encapsulated doxorubicin) was given to cats with measurable disease, similar results were obtained. Fifteen percent of cats achieved a complete response and 24% achieved a partial response for an overall response rate of 39%. Thirty-nine per cent of cats had stable disease and 21% had progressive disease.[28] The median time to progression was 84 days for cats that had a response.

Two studies evaluated the use of doxorubicin following surgery. One study concluded that the administration of doxorubicin after surgery did not affect median DFI or overall survival compared to surgery alone.[48] Another study concluded that administering doxorubicin (to include liposome-encapsulated doxorubicin) after surgery prolongs median DFI compared to historical control of surgery alone (388 days versus 93 days, respectively). In this particular study, cats with complete surgical margins had a longer DFI (median not reached) compared to cats with an incomplete excision (median 281 days).

Another study comparing surgery and radiation therapy with or without doxorubicin found no significant difference between the group receiving adjuvant chemotherapy and the group that did not.[47] Another study had similar results where cats treated with surgery and irradiation, with or without chemotherapy (doxorubicin and cyclophosphamide) did not have a significant difference in rate of local recurrence, rate of metastasis, and survival time.[3] A different conclusion was reached in another study. When doxorubicin was given to cats undergoing surgical excision and radiation therapy, the median DFI was significantly longer than when doxorubicin was not administered (15.4 months versus 5.7 months). However, survival time was not significantly different between groups.[49] Another study did not find an improvement in DFI and the administration of chemotherapy with preoperative radiation therapy and surgery except potentially for carboplatin alone.[27]

PREVENTION

One of the only ways to help prevent the genesis of injection site sarcomas is to not give unnecessary injections, particularly vaccines. Every injection intended to be administered should be carefully justified based on risk versus benefit. Vaccination protocols should be tailored to the individual risk of each cat.[8,17,55,56] A determination must be made for every individual cat if the relative risk of disease excludes the cat from being vaccinated.[55] The one exception might be vaccination against rabies where some public health authorities make vaccination against rabies mandatory regardless of risk (e.g., a cat that remains completely indoors), for public health reasons. Most other recommendations are to help treat the tumor with a better chance for success.

Where to vaccinate

Different vaccines should be injected in different anatomic locations to potentially reduce the level of inflammation and to be able to keep track of which vaccines might be a greater risk. Good record keeping is essential to be able to make these determinations later in time. The choice of distal limbs was also chosen to help achieve a cure with the excision by amputating the limb. The Vaccine-Associated Feline Sarcoma Task Force (a task force formed in November 1996 by the

American Veterinary Medical Association, American Animal Hospital Association, American Association of Feline Practitioners, and Veterinary Cancer Society) has recommended the following (Box 22-4).[17.]

Client education

Client education is imperative. First the clients should be warned of the risk of vaccine/injection-associated sarcomas and the occurrence of local vaccine/injection reactions. The owner should be taught how to examine the injection site and seek veterinary assistance if any of the three following scenarios occur (Box 22-5).[7,8,57]

The client should not hesitate to seek veterinary assistance if there is any doubt. After confirmation of one of those three scenarios by the veterinarian, a biopsy should be performed to find out if it is a granuloma/reactive mass or a sarcoma. A Trucut needle biopsy, punch biopsy, or wedge biopsy are preferred. It is mandatory to follow sound principles of performing a biopsy (see Chapter 14). Cytologic evaluation of fine needle aspirates is considered unreliable for the diagnosis of vaccine-associated sarcomas and is not recommended.[8,57]

Vaccination reactions or granulomas

If the mass is a vaccine reaction (granuloma), the course of action to be undertaken is controversial. Based on one study it appears safe to leave the granuloma.[16] In this study, the incidence of postvaccinal reaction was 11.8 reactions/10 000 vaccine doses. Approximately 98% of the postvaccinal reactions resolved without medical intervention; 96% of these did so within three months of vaccination, and 100% did so within four months of vaccination. The size of the reactions was reported to range from less than 1 cm and up to 6 cm in diameter.[16] In addition, the impact of excision of a vaccine reaction on subsequent tumor development at the site has not been elucidated. Fibrosarcomas have allegedly occurred in areas that had been previously excised and determined on histopathology to be injection site reactions, raising the question of the utility of excising vaccine reactions or the type of excision that would be required (i.e., marginal vs wide).[1,2,7] Based on these results, it is cautiously recommended to not remove reactive granulomas unless they persist for more than four months.[16] It has been postulated that removing an injection site granuloma may interfere with the body's development of immunity.[16] These recommendations regarding the management of granulomas may be shown to be erroneous as we learn more about this clinical entity and may need to be revised as new information becomes available. If the mass is a sarcoma, proper treatment planning becomes essential, which re-emphasizes the importance of performing a biopsy first before making any kind of treatment decisions.

REFERENCES

1. Hendrick MJ, Goldschmidt MH. Do injection site reactions induce fibrosarcomas in cats? J Am Vet Med Assoc 1991;199(8):968.
2. Hendrick MJ, Goldschmidt MH, Shofer FS, et al. Postvaccinal sarcomas in the cat: epidemiology and electron probe microanalytical identification of aluminum. Cancer Res 1992;52(19):5391–4.
3. Cohen M, Wright JC, Brawner WR, et al. Use of surgery and electron beam irradiation, with or without chemotherapy, for treatment of vaccine-associated sarcomas in cats: 78 cases (1996–2000). J Am Vet Med Assoc 2001;219(11):1582–9.
4. Gagnon A. Drug injection-associated fibrosarcoma in a cat. Feline Pract 2000;28:18–21.
5. Liptak JM, Forrest LJ. Soft tissue sarcomas. In: Withrow SJ, Vail DM, editors. Withrow and MacEwwen's small animal clinical oncology. 4th ed. St Louis: Saunders Elsevier; 2007. p. 425–53.

6. Buracco P, Martano M, Morello E, Ratto A. Vaccine-associated-like fibrosarcoma at the site of a deep nonabsorbable suture in a cat. Vet J 2002;163(1):105–7.
7. McEntee MC, Page RL. Feline vaccine-associated sarcomas. J Vet Intern Med 2001;15(3):176–82.
8. Morrison WB, Starr RM. Vaccine-associated feline sarcomas. J Am Vet Med Assoc 2001;218(5):697–702.
9. Hendrick MJ, Kass PH, McGill LD, Tizard IR. Postvaccinal sarcomas in cats. J Natl Cancer Inst 1994;86(5):341–3.
10. MacEwen EG, Powers BE, Macy D, Withrow SJ. Soft tissue sarcomas. In: Withrow SJ, MacEwen EG, editors. Small animal clinical veterinary oncology. Philadelphia: W.B. Saunders Co.; 2001. p. 283–304.
11. Hendrick MJ, Shofer FS, Goldschmidt MH, et al. Comparison of fibrosarcomas that developed at vaccination sites and at nonvaccination sites in cats: 239 cases (1991–2). J Am Vet Med Assoc 1994;205(10):1425–9.

12. Coyne MJ, Reeves NC, Rosen DK. Estimated prevalence of injection-site sarcomas in cats during 1992. J Am Vet Med Assoc 1997;210(2):249–51.
13. Kass PH, Barnes WG Jr, Spangler WL, et al. Epidemiologic evidence for a causal relation between vaccination and fibrosarcoma tumorigenesis in cats. J Am Vet Med Assoc 1993;203(3):396–405.
14. Burton G, Mason KV. Do postvaccinal sarcomas occur in Australian cats? Aust Vet J 1997;75:102–6.
15. Lester S, Clemett T, Burt A. Vaccine site-associated sarcomas in cats: clinical experience and a laboratory review (1982–1993). J Am Anim Hosp Assoc 1996;32(2):91–5.
16. Gobar GM, Kass PH. World Wide Web-based survey of vaccination practices, postvaccinal reactions, and vaccine site-associated sarcomas in cats. J Am Vet Med Assoc 2002;220(10):1477–82.
17. Richards JR. Feline sarcoma task force meets. J Am Vet Med Assoc 1997;210(3):310–11.

18. Hendrick MJ, Brooks JJ. Postvaccinal sarcomas in the cat: histology and immunohistochemistry. Vet Pathol 1994;31(1):126–9.

19. Hershey AE, Sorenmo KU, Hendrick MJ, et al. Prognosis for presumed feline vaccine-associated sarcoma after excision: 61 cases (1986–1996). J Am Vet Med Assoc 2000;216(1):58–61.

20. Doddy FD, Glickman LT, Glickman NW, Janovitz EB. Feline fibrosarcomas at vaccination sites and non-vaccination sites. J Comp Pathol 1996;114(2): 165–74.

21. Phelps HA, Kuntz CA, Milner RJ, et al. Radical excision with five-centimeter margins for treatment of feline injection-site sarcomas: 91 cases (1998–2002). J Am Vet Med Assoc 2011;239(1): 97–106.

22. Couto SS, Griffey SM, Duarte PC, Madewell BR. Feline vaccine-associated fibrosarcoma: morphologic distinctions. Vet Pathol 2002;39(1):33–41.

23. Aberdein D, Munday JS, Dyer CB, et al. Comparison of the histology and immunohistochemistry of vaccination-site and non-vaccination-site sarcomas from cats in New Zealand. N Z Vet J 2007;55(5):203–7.

24. Romanelli G, Marconato L, Olivero D, et al. Analysis of prognostic factors associated with injection-site sarcomas in cats: 57 cases (2001–7). J Am Vet Med Assoc 2008;232(8):1193–9.

25. Giudice C, Stefanello D, Sala M, et al. Feline injection-site sarcoma: recurrence, tumour grading and surgical margin status evaluated using the three-dimensional histological technique. Vet J 2010;186(1):84–8.

26. Cronin K, Page RL, Spodnick G, et al. Radiation therapy and surgery for fibrosarcoma in 33 cats. Vet Radiol Ultrasound 1998;39(1):51–6.

27. Kobayashi T, Hauck ML, Dodge R, et al. Preoperative radiotherapy for vaccine associated sarcoma in 92 cats. Vet Radiol Ultrasound 2002;43(5):473–9.

28. Poirier VJ, Thamm DH, Kurzman ID, et al. Liposome-encapsulated doxorubicin (Doxil) and doxorubicin in the treatment of vaccine-associated sarcoma in cats. J Vet Intern Med 2002;16(6):726–31.

29. Nemanic S, London CA, Wisner ER. Comparison of thoracic radiographs and single breath-hold helical CT for detection of pulmonary nodules in dogs with metastatic neoplasia. J Vet Intern Med 2006;20(3):508–15.

30. Esplin DG, Campbell R. Widespread metastasis of a fibrosarcoma associated with vaccination site in a cat. Feline Pract 1995;23:13–16.

31. Esplin DG, Jaffe MH, McGill LD. Metastasizing liposarcoma associated with a vaccination site in a cat. Feline Pract 1996;24:20–3.

32. Rudmann DG, Van Alstine WG, Doddy F, et al. Pulmonary and mediastinal metastases of a vaccination-site sarcoma in a cat. Vet Pathol 1996;33(4):466–9.

33. McEntee MC, Samii VF, editors. The utility of contrast enhanced computed tomography in feline vaccine-associated sarcomas: 35 cases. Vet Radiol and Ultrasound 2000;41(6):575.

34. Hahn KA, Lantz GC, Salisbury SK, et al. Comparison of survey radiography with ultrasonography and x-ray computed tomography for clinical staging of subcutaneous neoplasms in dogs. J Am Vet Med Assoc 1990;196(11): 1795–8.

35. Gilson SD, Stone EA. Principles of Oncologic Surgery. Compend Contin Educ Vet. [review]. 1990;12(6): 827–38.

36. Kramer A, Walsh PJ, Seguin B. Hemipelvectomy in dogs and cats: technique overview, variations, and description. Vet Surg 2008;37(5): 413–9.

37. Langley-Hobbs SJ, Voss K, Montavon PM. In: Montavon PM, Voss K, Langley-Hobbs SJ, editors. Orthopedic surgery and musculoskeletal disease. Edinburgh: Saunders Elsevier; 2009. p. 527–33.

38. Liptak JM, Dernell WS, Rizzo SA, et al. Reconstruction of chest wall defects after rib tumor resection: a comparison of autogenous, prosthetic, and composite techniques in 44 dogs. Vet Surg 2008;37(5):479–87.

39. McEntee MC, Samii VF, Walsh P, Hornof WJ. Postoperative assessment of surgical clip position in 16 dogs with cancer: a pilot study. J Am Anim Hosp Assoc 2004;40(4):300–8.

40. Reinbach D, McGregor JR, O'Dwyer PJ. Effect of suture material on tumour cell adherence at sites of colonic injury. Br J Surg 1993;80(6):774–6.

41. Kamstock DA, Ehrhart EJ, Getzy DM, et al. Recommended guidelines for submission, trimming, margin evaluation, and reporting of tumor biopsy specimens in veterinary surgical pathology. Vet Pathol 2011;48(1):19–31.

42. Kaestner S. Perioperative analgesia. In: Montavon PM, Voss K, Langley-Hobbs SJ, editors. Feline orthopedic surgery and musculoskeletal disease. Edinburgh: Saunders Elsevier; 2009. p. 199–205.

43. McLeod DA, Thrall DE. The combination of surgery and radiation in the treatment of cancer. A review. Vet Surg 1989;18(1): 1–6.

44. Ogilvie GK. Recent advances in the treatment of vaccine-associated sarcomas. Vet Clin North Am Small Anim Pract 2001;31(3):525–33, vi–vii.

45. Barber LG, Sorenmo KU, Cronin KL, Shofer FS. Combined doxorubicin and cyclophosphamide chemotherapy for nonresectable feline fibrosarcoma. J Am Anim Hosp Assoc 2000;36(5): 416–21.

46. Rassnick KM, Rodriguez CO, Khanna C, et al. Results of a phase II clinical trial on the use of ifosfamide for treatment of cats with vaccine-associated sarcomas. Am J Vet Res 2006;67(3):517–23.

47. Bregazzi VS, LaRue SM, McNiel E, et al. Treatment with a combination of doxorubicin, surgery, and radiation versus surgery and radiation alone for cats with vaccine-associated sarcomas: 25 cases (1995–2000). J Am Vet Med Assoc 2001;218(4):547–50.

48. Martano M, Morello E, Ughetto M, et al. Surgery alone versus surgery and doxorubicin for the treatment of feline injection-site sarcomas: a report on 69 cases. Vet J 2005;170(1):84–90.

49. Hahn KA, Endicott MM, King GK, Harris-King FD. Evaluation of radiotherapy alone or in combination with doxorubicin chemotherapy for the treatment of cats with incompletely excised soft tissue sarcomas: 71 cases (1989–1999). J Am Vet Med Assoc 2007;231(5):742–5.

50. Davis KM, Hardie EM, Martin FR, et al. Correlation between perioperative factors and successful outcome in fibrosarcoma resection in cats. Vet Rec 2007;161(6): 199–200.

51. Banerji N, Kanjilal S. Somatic alterations of the p53 tumor suppressor gene in vaccine-associated feline sarcoma. Am J Vet Res 2006;67(10):1766–72.

52. Davidson EB, Gregory CR, Kass PH. Surgical excision of soft tissue fibrosarcomas in cats. Vet Surg 1997;26(4):265–9.

53. Sorensen KC, Kitchell BE, Schaeffer DJ, Mardis PE. Expression of matrix metalloproteinases in feline vaccine site-associated sarcomas. Am J Vet Res 2004;65(3):373–9.

54. Eckstein C, Guscetti F, Roos M, et al. A retrospective analysis of radiation therapy for the treatment of feline vaccine-associated sarcoma. Vet Comp Oncol 2009;7(1):54–68.

55. Kirpensteijn J. Feline injection site-associated sarcoma: Is it a reason to critically evaluate our vaccination policies? Vet Microbiol 2006;117(1): 59–65.

56. CVMP advice on injection-site fibrosarcomas in cats. Vet Rec 2003;152(13):381–2.

57. Vaccine-Associated Feline Sarcoma Task Force guidelines. Diagnosis and treatment of suspected sarcomas. J Am Vet Med Assoc 1999;214(12):1745.

Section | 5 |

J.F. Ladlow, S.J. Langley-Hobbs

The abdomen

This part of the book is divided into four sections: abdominal surgery and the abdominal wall, the gastrointestinal tract, the hepatosplenic and endocrine system, and the urogenital system.

In the first chapter the reader is guided through performing an exploratory celiotomy. It is important to be able perform a thorough and methodical inspection of the abdomen and take biopsies when appropriate, particularly if the disease process affecting the cat is of an unknown etiology. Some abdominal procedures in the cat are now being performed endoscopically and the equipment required for laparoscopy and how to perform the more routine procedures in this minimally invasive manner is described in the next chapter. The final two chapters in this section cover conditions of the abdominal wall, such as hernias and traumatic ruptures and diseases of the peritoneal cavity.

In the second section of this part of the book, surgical management of diseases affecting the entire gastrointestinal tract is covered. Cats are fastidious eaters and are therefore unlikely to ingest large objects that can cause intestinal obstructions. However, due to their grooming habits and barbed tongue they are more likely to ingest linear foreign bodies such as pieces of string. As this is a relatively common condition and is particularly associated with cats it is described in detail in this section. The commonest surgical condition affecting the large intestine in cats is megacolon and the etiopathogenesis and treatment of this condition is thoroughly described.

In the third section, conditions affecting the liver and spleen, including hepatic shunts, are described. Cats are prone to liver disease and in many cases surgery would not be a first line treatment option but surgical biopsy may be necessary to obtain a specific diagnosis and therefore direct appropriate management. Portosystemic shunts are conditions that can be managed both surgically and medically. The surgical management of portosystemic shunts in cats is covered in detail. In subsequent chapters surgical management of conditions of the pancreas, spleen and adrenal glands is described. Historically adrenal gland surgery in the cat is not a commonly performed technique but with the increasing diagnosis of hyperaldosteronism (Conn syndrome) adrenalectomy may be become more frequent.

In the final section of this part of the book conditions of the genitourinary tract are covered. Cats are frequently affected by urinary conditions, and obstruction of the urinary tract can be life threatening. New developments in the surgical management of this system include placement of stents in both the ureters and the urethra. The final two chapters on the male and female genital tracts include commonplace procedures such as castration and ovariohysterectomy, which are techniques that are often not covered in detail in some surgical texts, along with more complex diseases such as pyometra and uterine torsion.

Chapter **|23|**

Celiotomy

C. Shales

Surgical exploration of the abdomen can provide invaluable information to help achieve a diagnosis of a large number of disease processes. Progress in the fields of imaging, minimally invasive biopsy techniques, and endoscopy and laparoscopy (Chapter 24) has significantly reduced the indications for open exploration of the abdomen. Despite these techniques, the ability of the surgeon to perform both a visual and manual examination of all abdominal organs and obtain biopsies from multiple sites during open exploratory surgery can be invaluable.[1-3]

Celiotomy refers to an incision into the abdomen; laparatomy, a term often used interchangeably with celiotomy, can also refer to surgery performed through a flank incision, which is rarely performed in cats except for ovariohysterectomy. Exploratory celiotomy cannot be considered a benign procedure and therefore, whenever possible, the clinician should ensure that all other diagnostic possibilities have been considered prior to surgery. While the limitations of preoperative diagnostic procedures should be appreciated (ultrasonography failed to identify the causative pathology in 25% of cases in one study[4]), preoperative investigations can reduce the incidence of unnecessary surgery and should minimize the risk of 'peak-and-shriek' intervention where the pathology proves to be beyond the experience level of the surgeon. At the very least, the principal surgeon involved in an exploratory procedure should be familiar with and have the necessary equipment available to assess and biopsy any abnormal tissue.

In addition to facilitating a global assessment of the abdomen and biopsy of tissue, in some cases the exploratory celiotomy also offers the opportunity to treat the pathology.[2,3] It is inevitable, therefore, that the experience and competence level of the surgeon in recognition of abnormality, application of biopsy techniques and in the surgical treatment of disease will have an impact on whether the procedure can be judged as a success.

SURGICAL ANATOMY

A more detailed account of the abdominal anatomy of the cat is provided in the chapters on the relevant organs (see Chapters 27 to 40). In this section, for the benefit of the surgeon who is more accustomed to operating on the dog, anatomical differences between the feline and canine abdominal cavity and viscera that are relevant to exploratory celiotomy surgery will be briefly highlighted.

Midline

The *linea alba* is generally relatively wider and more readily visible in the cat than the dog, especially caudal to the umbilicus. Care is required when gaining access to the abdominal cavity as the fascia is significantly thinner and more delicate than in the dog.

Liver

The liver consists of seven major lobes, which in the cat are separated by particularly deep fissures, rendering them more mobile relative to each other than in the dog.[5] The feline gallbladder is situated between the right medial and quadrate lobes as in the dog and can be double as a normal variation.[6] The cystic duct of the cat is usually longer and more undulating in its course than in the dog, and the common bile duct shares a common opening at the major duodenal papilla with the dominant pancreatic duct (see below).[5]

Pancreas

The pancreas is similar in appearance to its canine counterpart and occupies the same anatomical location and blood vessel arrangement as in the dog. Drainage of secretions from the feline exocrine pancreas differs in two respects from the situation in the dog, the first being that most cats (approximately 80%) only have one duct, with the result that all of, or the significant majority of, the secretions enter the duodenum at the proximal (major) duodenal papilla (the canine pancreas drains predominantly via the minor duodenal papilla). The second difference is that the pancreatic duct can join with the common bile duct in cats and therefore share the same opening into the duodenal lumen.[5] These differences combine to make both the common bile duct and pancreatic duct prone to secondary obstruction in the presence of disease involving the region of the major duodenal papilla.

DOI: 10.1016/B978-0-7020-4336-9.00023-8

Urogenital system

The left renal artery can divide before it enters the kidney (resulting in two or more renal arteries) in approximately 10% of cats.[7] The right renal artery usually remains undivided outside the capsule. The vessels running over the surface of the renal capsule (both arteries and veins) are significantly more prominent in the cat than in the dog.

Venous drainage occurs into the caudal vena cava via the renal veins. There are commonly several renal veins visible at the feline hilus, particularly on the right-hand side.[8]

Feline ureters are comparable to those of the dog although their significantly smaller diameter renders surgery very challenging except in the presence of significant dilatation.

The bladder neck/preprostatic urethra is significantly longer in the cat than the dog. As in other species, the feline urethra can be divided into different sections of which only the preprostatic and prostatic parts are intra-abdominal. Unlike in the dog, the feline urethra is not completely enclosed within the prostate gland.

HOW TO PERFORM AN EXPLORATORY CELIOTOMY

Preparation for surgery

Despite diagnostic information that might indicate disease in only one organ, the surgeon should be prepared for the necessity to extend the incision from the xiphisternum to the pubis as indicated during the procedure. Hair removal should therefore be performed to include a 10–15 cm margin from the incision that may be required. Preparation for the 'worst case scenario' in terms of skin preparation is always preferable to compromise of exposure or remedial preparation.

Before the procedure begins, as with all surgery, it is important that the surgeon is aware of exactly what equipment is on the instrument trolley and what is available on request if required. Swab numbers should be checked and noted to ensure that no errors occur at the end of the procedure.

The exploratory celiotomy

In order to perform a complete exploration of the abdomen the skin incision is made from the xiphisternum to the pubis. Reduced length incisions either cranial or caudal to the umbilicus can be used to access the cranial or caudal viscera, respectively, but will not provide access suitable for complete exploration of the entire cavity. In cats, the linea alba is wider than in the dog (up to 4 mm wide) and usually obvious after incision of the subcutaneous tissue and thus the temptation to undermine the fat or skin edges lateral to midline should be avoided in order to minimize the potential for dead space following closure.

In the presence of significant volumes of abdominal free fluid a Poole suction tip can be placed through a stab incision in the linea alba caudal to the umbilicus to remove fluid in a controlled fashion. It is important to minimize fluid leakage over the animal due to the increased potential for heat loss during the procedure. The *linea alba* incision can then be extended to match the skin incision.

Retraction of the abdominal wall can be performed by mini Balfour, Gosset, Gelpi, or other self-retaining retractors (Chapter 13), ensuring that no viscera become trapped between the retractor and the body wall. Moist swabs or laparotomy swabs are used to protect the abdominal wall from trauma that can be caused during retraction. Lightweight self-retaining retractors with elasticated hooks are versatile and can be very useful in small animals due to their reduced weight

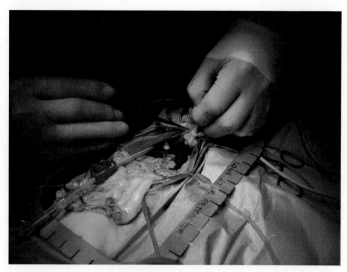

Figure 23-1 A versatile lightweight retractor in position during excision of the falciform fat using bipolar diathermy forceps. There is a transdiaphragmatic thoracic drain in place.

(Fig. 23-1). Excision of the falciform fat can be very helpful in gaining unimpaired access to the cranial abdomen in some cats (Fig. 23-1) and can be performed with judicious use of electrocautery or bunch-ligation at its cranioproximal extent.

The order in which viscera are examined is not itself important, but each surgeon should adopt a logical systematic exploration technique that is performed each time that an exploratory celiotomy is undertaken. Adherence to a rehearsed exploration technique will minimize the risk of pathology being missed, and serve to familiarize the surgeon with natural variations of normal anatomy.

Abdominal exploration includes evaluation of the abdominal surface of the diaphragm, the distal extent of the esophagus, the entire stomach, duodenum, jejunum, ileum, colon, cecum, pancreas (both limbs), liver, gall bladder, kidneys (the duodenal and colonic maneuvers are useful; Figs 23-2 and 23-3), ureters (observe peristalsis if relevant), bladder and proximal urethra, and any genital organs that are present or likely to be relevant. Table 23-1 gives details of a suitable approach to abdominal exploration although other techniques have been described.[9]

The jejunum can be temporarily arranged on a moist swab if necessary to make room within the abdominal cavity or to facilitate surgery involving the intestine itself (Fig. 23-4). Retraction of the bladder is best performed using a stay suture in the cranial pole if repeat or prolonged handling is necessary (Fig. 23-5). The spleen can also be exteriorized in most cats although care is required to ensure that the short gastric blood vessels are preserved at its head (Fig. 23-6).

It is important that all of the intra-abdominal organ systems are explored even if the diagnosis is immediately obvious once access to the abdominal cavity has been obtained. This additional information can become extremely useful in the postoperative treatment period and as an aid for the clinician in interpretation of biopsy results. In some cases the disease process will need to be addressed before the remainder of the exploration is performed to improve access or avoid life-threatening complications.

The surgeon is required to decide whether immediate treatment of pathology identified during an exploratory surgery is appropriate. Any tissue excised during treatment should be considered for submission for histopathology and additional biopsies from other tissue taken as appropriate (e.g., regional lymph nodes, splenic nodules, etc.). In the event that the primary source of pathology cannot be identified,

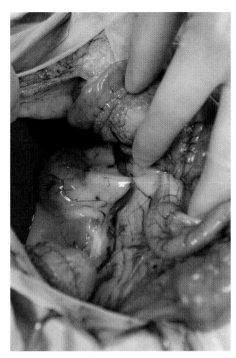

Figure 23-2 The duodenal maneuver. The right kidney and associated vasculature are visible. Retention of the remainder of the abdominal viscera was achieved using the mesoduodenum as a 'dam'. The duodenum is grasped gently, ensuring that the right limb of the pancreas is not damaged. The pancreatic appearance was not associated with clinical signs and was considered acceptable.

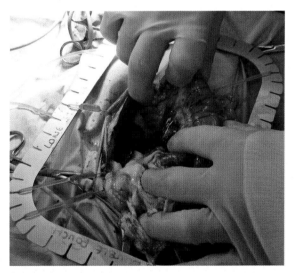

Figure 23-3 The colonic maneuver. The mesocolon acts as a 'dam' providing the surgeon with an excellent view and access to the left kidney and sublumbar gutter.

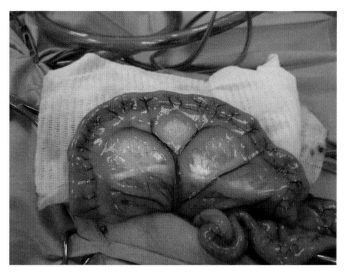

Figure 23-4 A loop of jejunum is shown arranged on a moist swab. The arboreal nature of the blood supply can be readily seen.

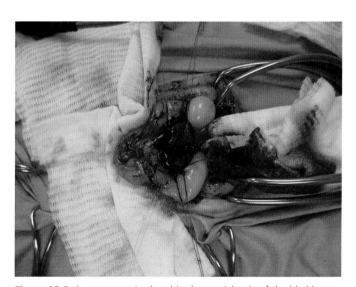

Figure 23-5 A stay suture is placed in the cranial pole of the bladder to stabilize the viscera during a ventral cystotomy procedure. Four stay sutures have also been placed at the edges of the cystotomy incision to minimize tissue handling. Note the abnormally thick bladder wall; multiple calcium oxalate uroliths were recovered.

multiple organ biopsies should be obtained based on the preoperative clinical signs and laboratory results.

In the majority of cases it is unacceptable to complete an exploratory celiotomy without either achieving treatment of the pathology or obtaining biopsies of tissue thought likely to be involved. Failure to advance the diagnostic process or achieve treatment at surgery suggests that the decision to perform exploratory celiotomy was inappropriate.

Abdominal lavage prior to closure with warmed saline or lactated Ringer's solution can be a useful way of reducing the level of contaminants such as bacteria or inflammatory mediators. However, it should be remembered that the entire volume of lavage solution must be recovered due to the potential detrimental effect on neutrophil efficacy caused by residual fluid. Local lavage of biopsy sites packed-off from the remainder of the abdominal cavity may be preferable, particularly in the absence of suction equipment. Lavage solution should always be warmed due to the potential for hypothermia associated with abdominal surgery, especially in relatively small species.

Closure of celiotomy

Prior to closure the surgeon may want to use the opportunity to place an open gastrostomy feeding tube (see Chapter 27) if there is any doubt about the cat's ability or willingness to eat postoperatively.

Table 23-1 Example of a protocol to achieve systematic exploration of the abdomen

Area of exploration	Technique
Gastric cardia, distal esophagus, left diaphragm, cranial pole of the left kidney and left adrenal gland	The left medial and lateral liver lobes are retracted towards midline to reveal the diaphragm and distal esophagus. Both surfaces of the left side of the liver can be assessed. The colonic maneuver (described below) can be used to increase exposure of the left kidney and adrenal gland if necessary
Right liver lobes, right diaphragm	The quadrate, right medial and right lateral liver lobes are retracted towards midline. The surgeon can then palpate and assess those liver lobes, and make a visual inspection of the surface of the right diaphragm
Gall bladder and extrahepatic biliary system. Portal vein	The stomach is then retracted caudally slightly, facilitating inspection of the gall bladder, cystic duct and common bile duct. Great care is taken over performing or interpreting manual gall bladder emptying due to the potential for reflux into the hepatic ducts
Gastric assessment	The entire stomach is then palpated, including the fundus, body, pyloris and assessment continued to include the proximal duodenum. The proximal duodenum is tethered by the duodenohepatic ligament
Pancreas	The right limb of the pancreas is elevated by grasping the descending duodenum. Care is required in order not to handle the pancreas excessively. The left pancreatic lobe can be inspected by reflecting the greater omentum ventrally and cranially or opening the omentum itself
Small intestines	The duodenum is followed to the duodenocolic ligament that tethers it to the dorsal abdomen. A loop of jejunum is grasped and followed in one direction. The surgeon will then either encounter the distal duodenum and duodenocolic ligament again or the ileocecocolic junction. The surgeon then proceeds by following the jejunum in the other direction from the start point. The ileum is identified by its antimesenteric vessel
Large intestines	The cecum can be palpated and inspected along with the ascending, transverse and descending colon. The proximal ascending colon is relatively immobile as it is secured dorsally in the abdomen by the duodenocolic ligament
Proximal urinary tract	Duodenal maneuver: the descending duodenum is grasped, taking care to avoid handling of the pancreas, and the mesoduodenum is used as a barrier to gently retract the jejunum etc. towards midline. The right kidney, adrenal gland and proximal ureter can be examined, palpated if appropriate and observed. A similar maneuver making use of the descending colon and mesocolon (colonic maneuver) will allow inspection of the left kidney
Distal urinary tract	The bladder is palpated and reflected ventrocaudally to inspect its dorsal surface and ureteric insertion points. The neck of the bladder can be gently palpated
Genital system	The ovaries or stumps should have been visualized during the duodenal or colonic maneuvers. The uterus or uterine stump(s) can be identified/palpated dorsal to the bladder and ventral to the colon, assisted by caudoventral retraction of the bladder if necessary

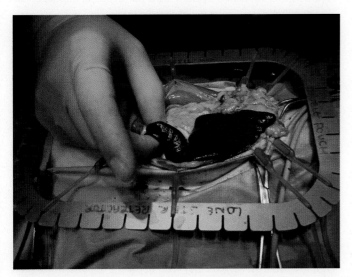

Figure 23-6 The spleen can usually be exteriorized with care. Notice that the spleen is an irregular shape as part of normal variation.

Closure can be achieved using either a simple interrupted or a simple continuous appositional suture pattern. For exploratory celiotomy where the patients may have underlying debilitating disease, two or three metric absorbable materials such as polyglyconate or polydioxanone offer suitable absorption profiles to provide sufficient support for the six weeks likely to be necessary for the avascular *linea alba* fascia to heal. There are prospective experimental studies that have demonstrated poliglecaprone and polyglactin 910 to be safe for *linea alba* closure following ovariohysterectomy in cats.[10,11] However, these were elective procedures on young healthy cats. Most incisional hernias are a result of surgical error rather than incorrect choice of suture material. The rectus sheath represents the tension holding layer that must be engaged when closing a midline incision. The sutures should include 3–5 mm of rectus sheath either side of the incision and bites should be approximately 3–5 mm apart along the incision. There is no requirement to close the peritoneum.

It is generally accepted that closure of the linea alba in cats should include the external sheath of the rectus abdominis muscle as in other species. However, there is a lack of consensus in the literature regarding suture placement within the subcutaneous tissues. As one would expect, the absence of subcutaneous closure is likely to increase the risk of seroma formation[10] but the inclusion of a subcutaneous layer has been proposed to increase the risk of incisional postoperative swelling.[12] Subsequent work and clinical experience have supported the relatively high incidence of incisional swelling following abdominal surgery in cats,[13] but in reality the degree of swelling that occurs is not usually clinically significant. In the opinion of the author, the abdominal closure should adhere to Halsted's principles and therefore include a subcutaneous layer except in very lean cats. One and a half or two metric monofilament poliglecaprone, polyglycomer 631, polydioxanone and polyglytone 6211 are common selections for the subcutaneous tissue and multifilament polyglactin 910 also offers suitable characteristics. The third layer of closure usually consists of intradermal continuous absorbable suture or more conventional monofilament non-absorbable skin sutures, depending on surgeon preference and the nature of the individual case.

BIOPSY PROCEDURES

Full thickness biopsy of the intestine

In the presence of the correct equipment and a skilled endoscopist, endoscopic intestinal biopsies are often preferred for mucosal disease of the proximal or distal intestinal tract due to the increased morbidity associated with an open procedure.[14-16] Full thickness biopsy of abnormal intestinal tissue with reduced capacity for suture holding in animals that may be compromised in terms of healing ability carries a significant risk of complications that require careful consideration prior to the procedure.[15]

However, in contrast to partial thickness intestinal biopsies obtained by endoscopy, surgical biopsy of the small intestine (Box 23-1) usually yields samples of adequate quality regardless of the surgeon and can offer greater sensitivity when diagnosing lymphoma and inflammatory bowel disease.[17-21]

Standard protocol for surgical biopsy as part of an investigation for small intestinal disease commonly involves samples from the duodenum, jejunum, and ileum with the stomach, liver, and pancreas sampled as indicated. Full thickness large intestinal biopsy is rarely performed due to the poor healing and high bacterial load in this area. Biopsies of the regional lymph nodes and spleen can be obtained as the pathology dictates.

Biopsy of the liver

A biopsy of the liver should be performed routinely during any procedure involving confirmed or suspected hepatobiliary disease. There are a number of techniques available for sampling hepatic tissue, depending on the location and nature of the intended site. While agreement between cytology and histopathology samples has been reported to be approximately 80% of cases,[24] hepatic tissue needle aspirates are usually avoided in open surgery due to the risk of insufficient information being available.

Nodules or masses within the liver can be biopsied using a Tru-Cut biopsy needle, Keyes skin biopsy punch[25,26] or sampled as an excisional biopsy if the location and size is considered suitable (i.e., using partial or complete lobectomy techniques). Histologic data gained using Tru-Cut type biopsy needles has the potential to be significantly less reliable than that available from wedge biopsy techniques[25,26] with the result that multiple core biopsies or an alternative technique should be considered. Bleeding from penetration-type biopsy sites, particularly punch biopsy sites, can be more severe than with other techniques,[26] but can usually be controlled effectively by application of pressure for two to five minutes or alternatively

---

Box 23-1 **Full thickness intestinal biopsy technique**

The section of intestine intended for biopsy is gently 'milked' free from intraluminal ingesta and liquid. Doyen bowel forceps or an assistant's fingers are placed approximately 3–5 cm orad and distad to the biopsy site and the area is packed-off from the remainder of the surgical field using damp swabs.

A number 11 scalpel blade is then used to create a full thickness stab incision (approximately 5–10 mm long) in the anti-mesenteric aspect parallel to the long axis of the intestine. A second incision is then made parallel to the first, resulting in a full thickness biopsy of approximately 2–3 mm width. The blade can then be used to incise away from the lumen to section one end of the biopsy, at which point the tissue tends to evert into a curve based on the one end that remains attached (Fig. 23-7). Adson or DeBakey forceps can then be used to stabilize the free end of the biopsy to facilitate section of the remaining attachment. An elliptical incision achieves the same end result[22] but can require additional handling of the tissue. The surgeon should check to ensure that the sample comprises mucosa before arranging for it to be fixed in 10% formal saline solution.

Alternate techniques include use of a Keyes skin biopsy punch[23] (but these need to be very sharp); or use of a stay suture to elevate a small section of tissue and a scalpel blade to excise a wedge. Whichever technique is used, the key is to minimize or avoid handling the biopsy and to ensure that a full thickness sample is obtained.

Several closure techniques are acceptable including appositional simple interrupted/continuous or inverting interrupted/continuous (e.g. Lembert or Connell) patterns. The suture-holding layer in the intestine is the submucosa and ensuring its inclusion usually requires full thickness bites with the needle.

If necessary, gastric biopsy can be performed using the same technique and closed in one or two layers.

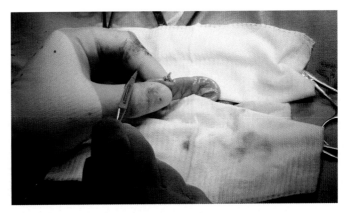

Figure 23-7 A full thickness intestinal biopsy is being taken from the feline jejunum. Notice how the sample has curled and everted due to the mucosal layer. *(Photograph courtesy of Robert N. White.)*

---

placing a plug of hemostatic material (e.g., gelatin sponge) over the bleeding area.

It is useful to note that samples from the periphery of the liver (Box 23-2) are generally considered representative for the generalized changes seen with most hepatobiliary disease processes.[27]

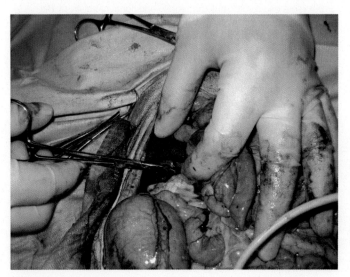

Figure 23-8 Liver biopsy. Most biopsies can be obtained from the periphery of a lobe at a suitable location to apply curved hemostatic forceps.

Biopsy of the pancreas

Handling of the pancreas must be particularly gentle in all species to minimize the risk of iatrogenic pancreatitis. Pancreatic biopsies do not usually form part of the standard protocol for exploratory surgery but should not be avoided if there is significant evidence to suggest pathology.

A biopsy can be obtained by careful isolation of the tip of one limb (usually the right which is easier to access) or a suitable lobe, using a combination of sharp and blunt dissection (see Box 33-2) to separate it from the mesoduodenum, major vessels and adjacent pancreatic lobes. Monofilament suture (e.g., polydioxanone, polyglyconate or polypropylene) of suitable size (e.g. 1.5 metric (4/0)) can be used to ligate the base of the proposed biopsy tissue as a simple encircling ligature or as two sutures used to isolate a 'V-shaped' section.[28] Titanium clips placed in a similar orientation to sutures can also be used to achieve hemostasis.[29]

As for all biopsies, handling of the sample with forceps should be minimized to avoid crush artifact. The surgeon must take additional care to ensure that there is minimal damage to pancreatic tissue remaining within the animal and that the ligation avoids the cranial or caudal pancreaticoduodenal vessels that can be intimately associated with the right limb.

Biopsy of the lymph nodes

Regional lymph nodes should be visually and manually assessed and biopsies obtained if there is a suspicion of abnormality. Palpation can be a useful technique to determine whether the node(s) feel firmer or larger than would be considered normal. Nodes can be sampled by needle aspirate, core biopsy needle, or by excision, depending on the location and the individual case. The surgeon should bear in mind that many nodes are situated in close approximation to regional blood vessels and care is required to avoid hemorrhage.

Biopsy of the kidneys

Advances in imaging and availability of blood tests have significantly improved the non-invasive investigation of renal disease. Furthermore, the results of renal biopsy do not usually alter the treatment protocol, with the result that it is not a common procedure during exploratory surgery.

Renal biopsy can be performed using a Tru-Cut style core biopsy needle oriented along the long axis of the organ, with care taken to confine the sample to the outer cortical tissue (see Chapter 36). The needle should not cross into the medullary region due to the risk of severe hemorrhage. Digital pressure over the resultant small hole in the capsule is usually sufficient to achieve hemostasis.

POSTOPERATIVE CARE

The degree of analgesia and supportive nursing care required following exploratory laparotomy inevitably depends on the degree of intervention necessary during the procedure itself and the recovery of the animal from both the surgery and the disease process. The reader is referred to Chapters 3 and 4 for detailed information on postoperative monitoring and nursing. Surgeons should pay particular attention to the more subtle signs of pain that cats display when compared with dogs, and use opioids in conjunction with non-steroidal analgesics when appropriate. The importance of early enteral feeding has already been discussed but has additional significance when considering cats at risk from hepatic lipidosis.

Recovery and duration of hospital stay following intestinal surgery are improved by achieving effective postoperative enteral nutrition[30] and there is evidence to suggest that enteral nutrition is essential for enterocyte function.[31] Voluntary oral feeding is always preferable but the general anesthetic and celiotomy used to perform the exploratory procedure may represent an ideal opportunity to place a feeding tube in appropriate cases (see Chapters 12 and 27).

Hypokalemia can result from anorexia and can in turn contribute to poor intestinal motility, nausea, and poor appetite. Supplementation of fluids in appropriate cases is usually worthwhile.

COMPLICATIONS AND PROGNOSIS

The surgeon must monitor carefully for signs of complications that could result from the celiotomy procedure. The incidence of herniation of abdominal wall contents is very low in small animals compared to humans and is usually associated with technical error or inappropriate suture selection (Fig. 23-9). Postoperative complications are two to three times more likely to be caused by the underlying disease process rather than the exploratory procedure itself.[2,3] Conditions reported to be associated with the highest complication rates

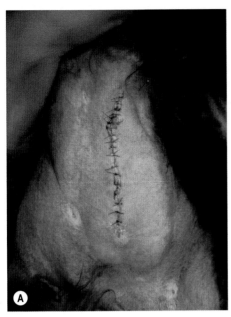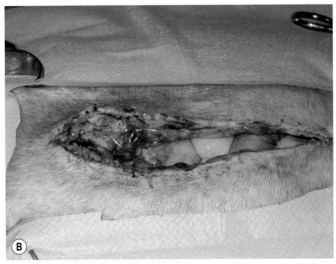

Figure 23-9 (A) Abdominal wound dehiscence in a cat. **(B)** The simple continuous poliglecaprone closure failed at the knot but the skin closure prevented catastrophic evisceration.

include gastrointestinal foreign body, hepatic lipidosis, ureteral abnormalities, intussusception, pancreatitis, hepatic neoplasia, and lymphoreticular neoplasia.[2] Complication rates attributed to the exploratory celiotomy procedure alone are approximately 7–9%.[2,3]

Full thickness intestinal biopsy or enterectomy can risk development of septic peritonitis, of which the signs and pathophysiologic changes can be both subtle and varied in both dogs and cats following open surgery. Clinical signs displayed by cats suffering from septic peritonitis can differ from dogs in that abdominal pain can be absent (see Chapter 26). A minority of cats experiencing septic shock secondary to peritonitis have been reported to be bradycardic rather than tachycardic.[32]

REFERENCES

1. Harvey CJ, Lopez JW, Hendrick MJ. An uncommon intestinal manifestation of feline infectious peritonitis: 26 cases (1986–1993). J Am Vet Med Assoc 1996;209:1117–20.

2. Boothe HW, Slater MR, Hobson HP, et al. Exploratory celiotomy in 200 nontraumatized dogs and cats. Veterinary Surgery 1992;21:452–7.

3. Lester S, Welsh E, Pratschke K. Complications of exploratory coeliotomy in 70 cats. J Small Anim Pract 2004;45:351–6.

4. Pastore GE, Lamb CR, Lipscomb V. Comparison of the results of abdominal ultrasonography and exploratory laparotomy in the dog and cat. J Am Anim Hosp Assoc 2007;43:264–9.

5. Grandage J. Functional Anatomy of the Digestive System. In: Slatter D, editor. Textbook of Small Animal Surgery. 3rd ed. Philadelphia: WB Saunders; 2003. p. 499–521.

6. Carlisle CH. Radiographic anatomy of the cat gall bladder. Vet Radiol Ultrasoun 1977;18:170–2.

7. Rieck AF, Reis RH. Variations in the pattern of renal vessels and their relation to the type of posterior vena cava in the cat *Felis domestica*. Am J Anat 1953;93:457–74.

8. Cáceres AV, Zwingenberger AL, Aronson LR, Mai W. Characterization of normal feline renal vascular anatomy with dual-phase CT angiography. Vet Radiol Ultrasoun 2008;49:350–6.

9. House A, Brockman D. Emergency management of the acute abdomen in dogs and cats 2. Surgical treatment. In Practice 2004;26:530–7.

10. Freeman LJ, Pettit GD, Robinette JD, et al. Tissue reaction to suture material in the feline linea alba. A retrospective, prospective, and histologic study. Vet Sur 1987;16:440–5.

11. Runk A, Allen SW, Mahaffey EA. Tissue reactivity to poliglecaprone 25 in the feline linea alba. Vet Surg 1999;28:466–71.

12. Muir P, Goldsmid SE, Simpson DJ, Bellenger CR. Incisional swelling following coeliotomy in cats. Vet Rec.1993;32:189–90.

13. Papazoglou LG, Tsioli V, Papaioannou N, et al. Comparison or absorbable and nonabsorbable sutures for intradermal skin closure in cats. Can Vet J 2010;51:770–2.

14. Elwood C. Best practice for small intestinal biopsy. Editorial. J Small Anim Prac 2005;46:315–16.

15. Shales CJ, Warren J, Anderson DM, et al. Complications following full thickness small intestinal biopsy in 66 dogs: a retrospective study. J Small Anim Prac 2005;46:317–21.

16. Day MJ, Bilzer T, Mansell J, et al. Histopathological standards for the diagnosis of gastrointestinal inflammation in endoscopic biopsy samples from the dog and cat: A report from the World Small Animal Veterinary Association Gastrointestinal Standardization Group. J Comp Pathol 2008;138:(Supplement 1):S1–S43.

17. Baez JL, Hendrick MJ, Walker LM, Washabau RJ. Radiographic, ultrasonographic, and endoscopic findings in cats with inflammatory bowel disease of the stomach and small intestine: 33 cases (1990–1997). J Am Vet Med Assoc 1999;215:349–54.

18. Willard MD, Jergens AE, Duncan RB, et al. Interobserver variation among histopathologic evaluations of intestinal tissues from dogs and cats. J Am Vet Med Assoc 2002;220:1177–82.

19. Kleinschmidt S, Meneses F, Nolte I, Hewicker-Trautwein M. Retrospective study on the diagnostic value of full thickness biopsies from the stomach and intestines of dogs with chronic gastrointestinal disease symptoms. Vet Pathol 2006;43:1000–3.

20. Evans SE, Bonczynski JJ, Broussard JD, et al. Comparison of endoscopic and full thickness biopsy specimens for diagnosis of inflammatory bowel disease and alimentary tract lymphoma in cats. J Am Vet Med Assoc 2006;229:1447–50.

21. Willard MD, Mansell J, Fosgate GT, et al. Effect of sample quality on the sensitivity of endoscopic biopsy for detecting gastric and duodenal lesions in dogs and cats. J Vet Int Med 2008;22:1084–9.

22. Cimino Brown D. Small intestines. In: Slatter D, editor. Textbook of Small Animal Surgery. 3rd ed. Philadelphia: WB Saunders; 2003. p. 644–64.

23. Keats MM, Weeren R, Greenlee P, et al. Investigation of Keyes skin biopsy instrument for intestinal biopsy versus a standard biopsy technique. J Am Anim Hosp Assoc 2004;40:405–10.

24. Roth L. Comparison of liver cytology and biopsy diagnoses in dogs and cats: 56 cases. Vet Clin Path 2001;30: 35–8.

25. Cole TL, Center SA, Flood SN, et al. Diagnostic comparison of needle and wedge biopsy specimens of the liver in dogs and cats. J Am Vet Med Assoc 2002;220:1483–90.

26. Vasanjee SC, Bubenik LJ, Hosgood G, Bauer R. Evaluation of haemorrhage, sample size and collateral damage for five hepatic biopsy methods in dogs. Vet Surg 2006;35:86–93.

27. Martin RA, Lanz OI, Tobias KM. Liver and biliary system. In: Slatter D, editor. Textbook of Small Animal Surgery. 3rd ed. Philadelphia: WB Saunders; 2003. p. 708–26.

28. Allen SW, Cornelius LM, Mahaffey EA. A comparison of two methods of partial pancreatectomy in the dog. Vet Surg 1989;18:274–8.

29. Barnes RF, Greenfield CL, Schaeffer DJ, et al. Comparison of biopsy samples obtained using standard endoscopic instruments and the harmonic scalpel during laparoscopic and laparoscopic-assisted surgery in normal dogs. Vet Surg 2006;35:243–51.

30. Lewis SJ, Egger M, Sylvester PA, Thomas S. Early enteral feeding versus 'nil by mouth' after gastrointestinal surgery: systematic review and meta-analysis of controlled trials. Brit Med J 2001;323:773–6.

31. Souba WW. Glutamine: A key substrate for the splanchnic bed. Annu Rev Nutr 1991;11:285–308.

32. Costello MF, Drobatz KJ, Aronson LR, King LG. Underlying cause, pathophysiologic abnormalities, and response to treatment in cats with septic peritonitis: 51 cases (1990–2001) J Am Vet Med Assoc 2004;225: 897–902.

Chapter 24

Endoscopic surgery in cats: Laparoscopy

S.A. van Nimwegen, J. Kirpensteijn

Laparoscopy is becoming increasingly popular in veterinary medicine for performing investigative and surgical procedures in small animals. Cats have a flexible abdominal wall that allows sufficient distension for laparoscopic procedures at relatively low intra-abdominal pressures. The advantages, disadvantages, and indications for laparoscopy in cats will be discussed in this chapter.

LAPARASCOPIC SURGERY IN CATS

Rigid endoscopy enables visualization of the abdominal cavity in a minimally invasive approach.[1,2] Laparoscopy and celioscopy are terms used for the abdominal cavity and thoracoscopy for the chest. Laparoscopic surgery is performed with special instruments through small-diameter access-points (portals) in the abdominal wall (Fig. 24-1). Apart from the advantage of minimally invasive access causing less incisional trauma, the use of an optical laparoscope enables a close-up view of abdominal tissues, improving visibility compared to open

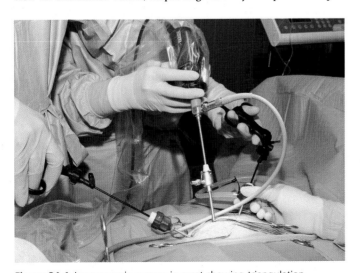

Figure 24-1 Laparoscopic surgery in a cat showing triangulation. An assistant holds the camera.

surgery. Thus, laparoscopy can improve access to abdominal tissues without requiring extensive manipulation (e.g., exteriorization of tissues) resulting in reduced pain and trauma of tissues compared to open surgery. In human evidence-based medicine, laparoscopy has become the preferred approach for a growing number of surgical procedures, including cholecystectomy,[3] ovariectomy,[4] and appendectomy.[5,6] Likewise, laparoscopy is increasingly used in veterinary medicine and surgery,[7–9] including in smaller animals such as reptiles, ferrets, and rodents.[10,11] Several advantages of laparoscopic surgery compared to open surgery that have been described for humans, have also been reported in dogs, including reduced peri- and postoperative pain,[12–14] less postoperative adhesion formation,[15–17] a shorter convalescence period and faster return to normal activity level,[18–21] and reduced surgery-induced physical stress and inflammatory response.[13,14,16,22–25]

In cats, descriptions of laparoscopic procedures are sparse and include exploratory laparoscopy for observation of abdominal organs,[1] biopsy of abdominal organs,[26–28] ovariectomy,[29–31] ovariohysterectomy,[32] and abdominal cryptorchidectomy.[33,34] Few case reports of other procedures exist.[35,36] The smaller size of cats and their different conformation of skin and abdominal wall, compared with dogs, require a different approach to minimally invasive surgery in this species. However, adapting to these differences enables minimally invasive surgical approaches similar to those in other species to be performed, with comparable advantages.

The main disadvantages of laparoscopic surgery are the associated costs of investment in equipment, specific anesthetic requirements, and the need for an assistant, especially in more advanced procedures. Furthermore, the acquisition of minimally invasive surgery skills is known to be associated with a distinct learning curve, requiring considerable training. Practice on low-cost box-trainers or cadavers can be very useful,[37,38] particularly in cats with their relatively small abdominal cavity. However, the anatomy of the abdominal wall in cats also has advantages that will be discussed later.

Basic surgical principles

The owner should always be informed that in cases where laparoscopic access is limited, or if unforeseen difficulties or complications occur, the procedure may have to be converted to an open approach.

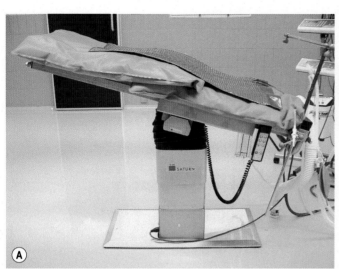
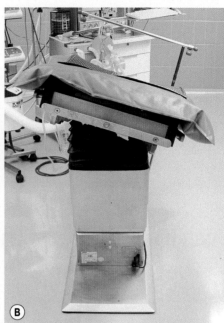

Ⓐ Ⓑ

Figure 24-2 Motorized surgery table showing Trendelenburg position and lateral tilt. On top are two moldable vacuum cushions and a heating pad.

Anticipation of conversion during aseptic preparation of a patient is warranted. Laparoscopy should always be performed under sterile conditions. The type of surgery (including endoscopic) can never be an excuse for breaks in sterility or decreased vigilance.

The operating room is set up according to the surgical procedure to be performed. Ideally, the surgeon, the operating field, and the monitor displaying the image of the laparoscope are positioned in a straight line. This so-called coaxial set-up maximizes spatial awareness and hand–eye co-ordination. Deviation from this line increases perceptual distortion and makes operating more difficult. Changes in position of the surgeon or operating field during the operation should be accompanied by changing the position of the monitor/endoscopy tower. The use of a second (or third) monitor may improve surgical circumstances in specific procedures. An assistant should preferably hold the laparoscope while the surgeon uses both hands to control instrument manipulation, as would be the case in open surgery. The assistant should also be positioned in a more or less straight line with the monitor. The instrument cannulas should ideally be in a 30°–60° angle with the axis of the laparoscope port and surgical field, also referred to as 'triangulation' (Figs 24-1 and 24-8). If the angle is too small, instruments may obscure the operative site inside the abdomen and the accompanying short distance between the portals may reduce manipulation freedom of the instruments outside the abdomen. With a larger angle, depth perception is impaired and fine movements are more difficult.[39,40]

Pneumoperitoneum, patient positioning, and anesthetic considerations

In order to create a comprehensive space for visualization, manipulation, and surgery, the abdominal cavity is insufflated with gas. Carbon dioxide is the preferred gas for the creation of pneumoperitoneum because it is inexpensive, highly soluble, chemically stable, rapidly eliminated, physically inert, suppresses combustion, and at physiological levels it is non-toxic. To further enhance access to certain tissues, the patient, lying in supine position, can be tilted into a head-down

(Trendelenburg) or head-up (reverse Trendelenburg) position and towards a right or left lateral position, using gravity to move abdominal organs away from the area of interest. A motorized table that allows tilting is very useful for endoscopic surgery. In order to freely tilt the patient during surgery, the patient needs to be securely adhered to the table. Apart from tying the patient's legs to the table, a moldable vacuum cushion greatly improves positioning (Fig. 24-2). Because of the obvious advantage of the small size of cats, positioning is relatively easy and repositioning during surgical procedures is possible if necessary. The need to move the animal should not impede the need to keep the procedure aseptic.

In the presence of CO_2 pneumoperitoneum, transperitoneal absorption will cause an increase in partial arterial CO_2 pressure ($PaCO_2$), which may require mechanical ventilation to increase ventilation minute volume to facilitate expulsion of CO_2. The most important event during laparoscopy that may negatively affect cardiovascular and respiratory function is the increase in intra-abdominal pressure (IAP) caused by pneumoperitoneum. Abdominal insufflation causes pressure on the diaphragm and abdominal blood vessels, resulting in a pressure-dependent increase in intrathoracic pressure, pulmonary vascular resistance, and systemic vascular resistance; and a pressure-dependent decrease in venous return, portal-venous blood flow, and abdominal visceral blood flow. These events result in an increase in peak-inspiratory airway pressure, heart rate, mean arterial blood pressure, and pulmonary arterial blood pressure; and a decrease in pulmonary compliance, tidal volume, minute ventilation, cardiac output, hepatic arterial, and renal arterial blood flow.[41]

In dogs and humans, an IAP up to 12 mmHg causes minimal cardiovascular and respiratory changes and is considered safe for laparoscopy.[42,43] Higher pressures (>14 mmHg) may cause significant changes and should be avoided if possible.[41,43–48] In humans, an IAP of <12 mmHg, caused less postoperative pain and discomfort than an IAP of >12 mmHg.[49] Furthermore, an increase in IAP is not linearly related to an increase in abdominal space.[50] Therefore, the lowest IAP providing adequate surgical space should be used, avoiding any unnecessary hemodynamic alterations. In dogs, an IAP of 8–10 mmHg was sufficient for laparoscopic ovariectomy (lapOVE).[51,52] Of the few available descriptions of laparoscopic procedures in cats, most authors used an IAP of 8–12 mmHg,[26,30,33–35] or up to 15 mmHg,[28] which is merely a result of extrapolation of the technique that is used in dogs. In cats, however, effects of increased IAP have never been investigated. Furthermore, cats have a much more flexible body wall and skin that allows the creation of sufficient laparoscopic surgical space at much lower IAPs compared to dogs. We have found that a reduction in IAP to around 4–6 mmHg is sufficient in cats.[29] A higher IAP is not needed for most procedures and may cause significant detrimental effects in this species and put them at an increased risk for complications.

A Trendelenburg position may also cause cardiovascular changes. Depending on the amount (angle) of tilting, an increase in intrathoracic pressure compromises pulmonary function and baroreceptor reflexes cause generalized vasodilation and reduced heart rate and cardiac output. The reverse Trendelenburg position triggers baroreceptor reflexes resulting in vasoconstriction, increased heart rate and arterial blood pressure. Cardiac output is decreased, probably because of a decreased venous return.[41] However, a 10–15° head-up or -down tilt is usually sufficient, and it does not cause major physiological changes, and the cardiovascular and respiratory effects of increased IAP generally dominate the situation.[53,54]

Because of the expected alterations in hemodynamic and respiratory function, cats should be carefully monitored during the application of pneumoperitoneum. Increased $PaCO_2$ and intrathoracic pressure require increased ventilatory support, anticipating higher ventilation pressures and reduced lung volume, and aiming for normocapnia. Mechanical intermittent positive pressure ventilation (IPPV) should be considered. Positive end expiratory pressure ventilation (PEEP) should not be used because it further increases intrathoracic pressure, depressing cardiopulmonary function.[55,56]

One should be aware that in unstable cardiovascular or pulmonary patients, the effects of increased IAP and tilting of the body can be more severe and even dangerous. Furthermore, general anesthesia aggravates the effects of increased IAP and tilting and one could consider a combination of sedation and local anesthesia for laparoscopic procedures in critical patients.[57] The use of local anesthetic infiltration of portal sites using lidocaine, bupivicaine or chirocaine has been shown to significantly improve postoperative analgesia in humans.[58] However, a significant advantage of bupivacaine infiltration of portal sites was not found in a recent controlled clinical trial in dogs.[59]

Abdominal access

Introduction of the first trocar into the abdomen can be performed using an open or closed technique. A closed technique implies *blind* insertion of the first trocar, either after establishment of pneumoperitoneum by pre-inserting a needle through which CO_2 is introduced into the abdomen, or by direct insertion of the primary trocar while pulling up the abdominal wall. An open technique refers to performing a small skin incision and subcutaneous dissection, identifying and incising the abdominal fascia, and inserting a sharp or blunt trocar under visualization, through which the abdomen is inflated. The most commonly used closed technique is the use of a Veress needle. After a small skin incision, the needle is inserted through the abdominal wall. Once the sharp Veress needle has penetrated the abdominal wall and peritoneum, the blunt spring-loaded obturator protrudes past the sharp edge of the needle, protecting abdominal tissues from injury by the tip of the needle. The hollow obturator can then be connected to a mechanical insufflator to initiate CO_2 inflow into the abdominal cavity. The point of insertion is usually caudal to the umbilicus to avoid the falciform ligament but alternatively, insertion close to the rib cage edge away from the midline to the right has been described in dogs. In cats, the edge of the rib cage can be lifted up with fine

towel clamps to allow some counter pressure while inserting the needle. Depending on the location, aiming the needle somewhat craniolaterally or caudolaterally while manually lifting the abdominal wall may reduce the risk of injury to the spleen, bladder, or liver. In cats, it is essential to always palpate the abdomen and evacuate the urinary bladder prior to needle insertion.

A Trendelenburg position may reduce the chance for splenic trauma, because the spleen tends to slide craniolaterally away from the insertion point.[28,60] Proper placement of the Veress needle into the abdominal cavity can be checked by the 'hanging drop' test. Using this test, a drop of sterile saline solution is applied to the hub of the needle and should be sucked into the abdomen by the negative IAP. The test is not fail-safe due to occlusion of the tip of the needle from contact with an organ or omentum. Possible occlusion can be judged by first flushing the Veress needle with 1–2 mL of sterile saline or lifting up the abdominal wall to move the tip away from any organ and then repeating the hanging drop test.[28,60] The use of a low IAP, which is preferred in cats, may limit the possibilities for primary trocar insertion because the abdominal wall is under relatively low tension and will move inwards with pressure exerted on it when trying to puncture it with a trocar, increasing the chance for iatrogenic damage. Some authors overcome this difficulty by using a higher IAP for initial port placement, after which IAP is set to a lower value.[9,52] However, trocar insertion can be facilitated using stay sutures to stabilize the abdominal wall during insertion or by using threaded cannulas that can be screwed through a small stab incision in skin and fascia.

Abdominal wall-lifting techniques have been described for direct primary trocar insertion in cats.[29] We prefer to perform direct trocar insertion using a semi-open technique: first a small skin incision is made (about the diameter of the trocar to be inserted) and the subcutaneous tissue bluntly dissected to reveal the linea alba. The linea alba is carefully lifted with forceps, and stay sutures placed at both corners (cranial and caudal) of the incision. To ensure enough strength, the stay sutures pass through both skin and linea alba. A 2–3 mm incision is made through the abdominal wall at the linea alba. This incision is kept smaller than the cannula diameter to provide a good tight fit of the cannula. Incising the abdominal wall facilitates entry of air, which together with lifting the abdominal wall, should prevent abdominal organs from being lifted with the abdominal wall which could occur due to negative pressure-adherence with the closed approach. The abdominal wall is lifted up while the trocar is inserted (Fig. 24-3). Using a blunt trocar or threaded cannula is the safest entry technique.

To check proper placement, initiate insufflation at a low flow (1 L/minute): in cases with improper placement, pressure will rapidly rise above 10–20 mmHg (because there is no available space to fill) and it will not fall back to <10 mmHg immediately when insufflation stops. If an open or direct trocar technique was used, proper placement should be checked with the laparoscope. Intact muscle fascia or peritoneum will be visible at the end of the cannula in cases of improper placement, or abdominal organs when the procedure has been performed correctly. If a Veress needle was incorrectly placed, it should be re-inserted.

The placement of a second or more trocars is then safely performed under laparoscopic guidance (Fig. 24-3). Transillumination from within the abdomen helps to avoid puncturing blood vessels in the abdominal wall during trocar insertion. This is very easy and useful in cats because of their thin abdominal wall. If the low IAP complicates proper entry of a sharp trocar, stay sutures may be used to stabilize the abdominal wall during trocar insertion (Fig. 24-3). In order to reduce the number of cannulas needed for a specific procedure, transabdominal suspension sutures may be used to keep tissues lifted up for surgical access without using extra laparoscopic forceps.[61] This creates a fixed position of the tissues and decreases freedom of

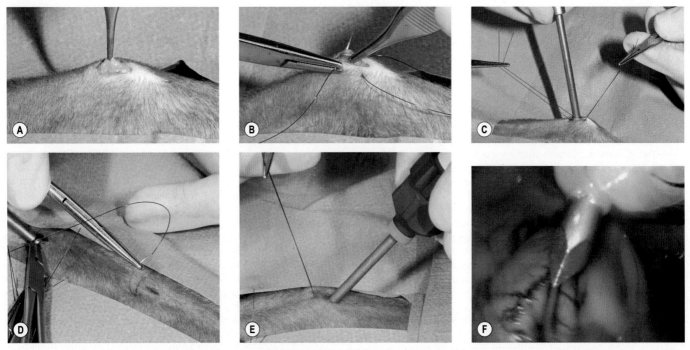

Figure 24-3 Abdominal entry. **(A)** The linea alba is grabbed and lifted up while **(B)** stay sutures are placed in the cranial and caudal border of the skin incision, penetrating skin, subcutaneous tissue, and linea alba/external rectus fascia. **(C)** The stay sutures are used to pull up the abdominal wall while inserting the trocar. After trocar placement, the stay sutures can be used to fixate the cannula. **(D,E)** Stay sutures can also be used for insertion of secondary trocars, which are placed under laparoscopic guidance **(F)**.

manipulation. The flexible abdominal wall of cats facilitates 'lifting up' procedures, but care needs to be taken not to apply too much tension, which could result in the stay suture being pulled out of the tissue.

An alternative to pneumoperitoneum has been evaluated in five cats using a custom-made abdominal wall-lifting device to pull the abdominal midline upwards to create a surgical space for laparoscopy without using gas insufflation. However, this technique seemed to be associated with poorer visualization of the abdominal cavity compared to pneumoperitoneum, necessitating conversion to laparotomy in one cat. In particular, lateral intra-abdominal space was reduced because of the upward 'tenting' effect of abdominal wall lifting compared to the dome-shape of pneumoperitoneum.[62]

After entering the abdomen for the first time, condensation of water vapor on the cold surface of the endoscope may blur the image. Warming up the laparoscope (with warm saline for instance) before-hand will prevent 'fogging-up' of the scope. A blurred image can also occur from blood or fat adhered to, or dripping down the laparoscope. The tip of the laparoscope may be cleared by *gently* touching the serosal surface of an intestinal loop, the spleen, or the body wall. Commercially available anti-condensation solutions may also be of benefit. Holding the scope tip too close to the cannula tip is a frequent reason for the scope to blur and should be avoided. This is difficult in cats because of their small size and also because the cannula often moves with the scope during insertion and retraction. Holding the cannula during these manipulations or the use of threaded cannulas will prevent this.

At the end of the procedure, the abdomen is properly deflated before cannula removal. For portal incisions of 5 mm we recommend closing the abdominal fascia with one or two sutures to prevent herniation of omentum or other viscera. For smaller portals, closure of only subcutaneous tissue and skin may be sufficient.

EQUIPMENT

Insufflation

For use in cats, an automatic CO_2 insufflation device should be at least capable of switching between low (1 L/minute) and moderate (6 L/minute) gas flow rates and automatically regulate insufflation rate to maintain a constant, manually adjustable pressure level, allowing low pressure settings (4–8 mmHg).

Optical and video set-up

The rigid optical laparoscope preferably is composed of a Hopkins rod lens system, which has a relatively wide field of view and bright image. A laparoscope with 0° or 30° viewing angle is adequate for most laparoscopic procedures. The 30° viewing angle allows observation of abdominal organs from different angles by rotating the telescope. The diameter of the scope determines the maximum width of the field of view and the amount of light passing through. For cats we recommend a 2.7–5 mm diameter endoscope for laparoscopic and thoracoscopic procedures (Fig. 24-4). In our opinion, the advantage of a further decrease in size does not compensate for the smaller and less bright field of view. We commonly use a 3.9 mm diameter laparoscope (Hopkins II, Storz) with 4.5 mm diameter cannula because of its superb image quality compared to smaller diameter scopes. Furthermore, smaller scopes are usually used with a protective sheath, increasing the total diameter without enhancing the image. The endoscope is connected to a camera system with monitor. Camera resolutions range from single CCD-chip (450 horizontal lines, poor color reproduction) to three CCD-chips (750 horizontal lines and good color quality) to full HD (1080 horizontal lines and 16:9 widescreen

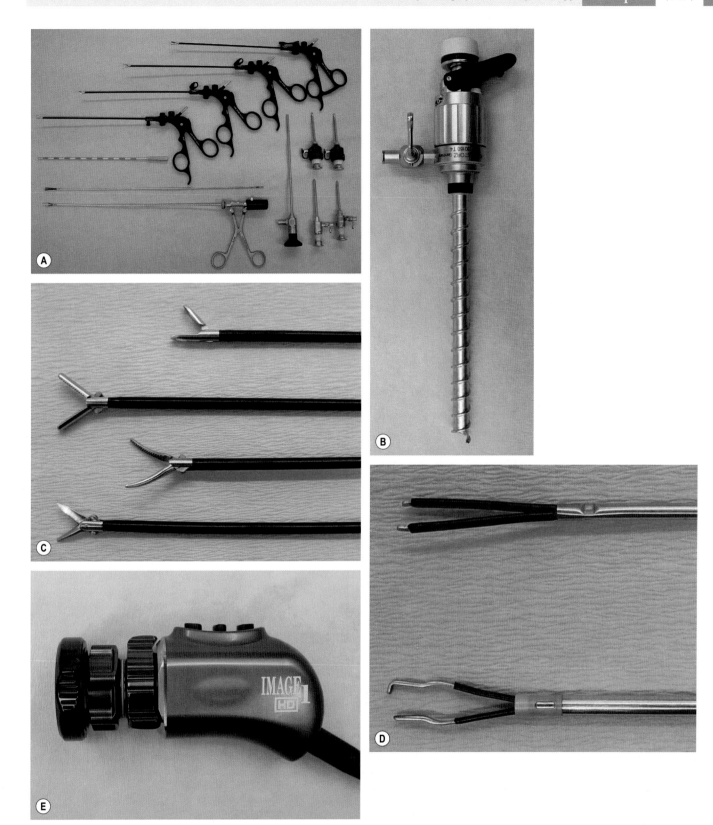

Figure 24-4 Endoscopic surgery instruments. **(A)** Basic pediatric instrument set with 3 mm diameter instruments, a 3.9 mm diameter laparoscope (Hopkins II, Storz), 3.8 mm and 4.5 mm outer diameter trocars. **(B)** Ternamian EndoTip threaded cannula (Storz). **(C)** Biopsy cup forceps, straight grasping forceps, curved Kelly forceps, and scissors; **(D)** two types of bipolar forceps; **(E)** HD camera (Storz).

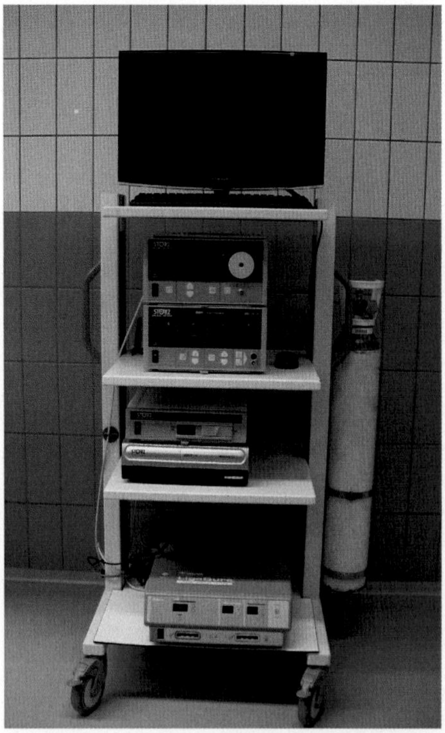

Figure 24-5 Endoscopic surgery equipment on cart. From top to bottom: Widescreen monitor, xenon light source, insufflator, camera power source, image and video capture device, and Ligasure power source. The CO$_2$ gas reservoir is on the right-hand side.

image; Fig. 24-5). The most popular light sources use xenon lamps, being much brighter and whiter than halogen.[7,9,63] It can be helpful to be able to capture images and video clips of your laparoscopic procedures. Although dedicated devices are on the market, digital recording devices can be bought relatively inexpensively nowadays and several laptop computers enable digital video capturing as a standard feature.

Standard instruments

A basic set of instruments for laparoscopic surgery contains grasping forceps (Kelly, Babcock, etc), a biopsy forceps, a palpation probe, scissors, and bipolar forceps or other vessel-sealing device (Fig. 24-4). For cats we recommend the use of 3 mm pediatric instruments.[64] A suction/irrigation device can be helpful to maintain visualization of tissue structures in case of hemorrhage, which can dramatically obscure the surgical field. Because the smallest vessel-sealing devices are 5 mm in diameter, port size needs to be sacrificed for ease and speed of surgery in certain cats.

Trocars/cannulas

A trocar is the combination of a cannula (or sleeve) and obturator. Cannulas function as instrument portals in the abdominal wall. Placement through the abdominal wall can be facilitated by the use of a sharp obturator. Puncturing the abdominal wall with a sharp trocar has the advantage of creating a tight fit between cannula and body wall. A disadvantage is the risk of damaging an organ iatrogenically during blind entry (i.e., placement of primary trocar). A safer entry may be facilitated by using a blunt threaded cannula without an obturator, which has the benefit of also resulting in a tight fit.[65] A blunt trocar can be used with an open entry technique. A cannula for

laparoscopy contains an automatic valve to prevent leakage of CO$_2$ gas when no instrument is inserted and a rubber washer to prevent gas leakage between instrument and cannula. A cannula with a Luer lock valve can be used for insufflation of the abdomen and instillation of fluids.

Cats have a thin and flexible skin and abdominal wall. Smaller and lighter cannulas reduce surgical trauma (incision length) and reduce problems such as cannulas slipping in and out of the abdomen and the weight of the cannula pushing onto the abdominal wall, reducing surgical space. Because of the small size of cats, smaller-sized instruments greatly improve surgical performance. Figure 24-4A displays a basic pediatric instrument set that may be used for endoscopic surgery in cats, containing 3 mm diameter laparoscopic equipment with 3.8 mm outer diameter cannulas. Specially designed reusable cannulas containing silicone leaflet valves and plastic casing further reduce weight. Because of the abdominal wall anatomy of cats, slipping of cannulas in and out of the abdominal wall incisions can pose a problem.[28,29] To avoid this, it is important to make the initial portal incisions smaller than the cannula size, which can be challenging when using an open entry technique. The use of threaded cannulas (Ternamian EndoTip, Storz, Fig. 24-4B) or Hasson trocars that can be sutured to skin can improve cannula stability in the abdominal wall. Threaded cannulas also have the advantage of not needing a sharp obturator to facilitate placement through the abdominal wall. Instead, the cannula is 'screwed' in place through a small incision, which can be visualized by inserting a 0° laparoscope.[65] Threaded cannulas are also available in pediatric sizes (3.9 mm inner diameter; see also Chapter 42). Another option is the use of a purse-string suture around the incision to tighten the cannula in the abdominal wall. When stay sutures are used for primary trocar entry, they can be wound around the cannula and secured with mosquito forceps to add stability (Fig. 24-3). Surgeons that perform arthroscopy can use some of the available 2.7 mm equipment on cats. The size and length of the equipment is of course also an important consideration.

Hemostasis

The biggest challenge in laparoscopic surgery is conducting hemostasis during tissue dissection. Intracorporeal suturing and knot tying can be performed using laparoscopic needle holders, but this may be considered an advanced laparoscopic skill. Placing ligatures can also be done through extracorporeal knot tying in which each throw of a surgeon's knot is made outside the body and pushed down into the abdominal cavity using a knot pusher. Another way is to push down an extracorporeally tied slip-knot or to use commercially available pre-tied loops (Endoloop, Ethicon).[9,66] Pre-tied loops are made for human surgery and may be too big in suture size and length for the small feline patient. Alternatively, most procedures can be performed using electrosurgery or other devices designed for hemostasis, greatly improving the ease of surgery and decreasing surgery duration.[67]

The most economical, relatively safe and good quality hemostatic technique is the use of bipolar electrocoagulation. Regular bipolar devices are available as reusable autoclavable equipment and these can be connected to a standard bipolar electrocoagulation unit. Another advantage is that bipolar forceps come in a 3 mm diameter size. Bipolar devices enable faster and better hemostasis of blood vessels compared to monopolar devices.[68] A major disadvantage of monopolar electrocoagulation is the chance of alternate site burns due to capacitive coupling, conduction through metal instruments, and coagulation at a location of highest electrical resistance (thinnest point) away from the intended location of instrument contact in pedicle-like structures.[69,70] Other means of energetic tissue dissection and hemostasis are ultrasonic energy (Harmonic scalpel, Ethicon), impedance-controlled pulsed bipolar energy vessel sealer/divider forceps combined with sharp dissection (Ligasure, Tyco/ValleyLabs; PlasmaKinetic, Gyrus Medical), and surgical laser[29] (see Fig. 24-9).

There are also several more economical vessel sealer/divider devices combining regular bipolar forceps with sharp dissection (BiCOAG, Gyrus Medical; HotBlade, Patton Surgical). Vessel sealer/divider instruments are very useful for laparoscopic tissue dissection because coagulation and dissection is performed with the same instrument (see Fig. 24-9). These devices do measure at least 5 mm in diameter and thus require larger cannulas. Additionally, most devices have a relatively large beak, making application in a small space difficult. Most laparoscopic staplers and clip appliers are 10 mm in diameter (some 5 mm versions exist) and are expensive. Impedance-controlled vessel sealer/dividers are relatively expensive and, although they are disposable they can be gas sterilized a number of times (up to ten times or more when cared for diligently). The blood vessels encountered in the cat during the procedures described in this chapter are usually easily manageable using standard pediatric bipolar forceps. More advanced surgeries are only performed with vessel-sealing devices in our hands. The advantage of the laser is obvious: its small fiber size (0.6–1.0 mm diameter) makes it very useful for feline endoscopic surgery. Air leakage can happen if an adequate washer size is not available. The use of laser and electrosurgery may occasionally cause a significant amount of smoke or fog obscuring the laparoscopic image, which can be cleared by releasing some of the gas from the abdomen while fresh CO_2 from the insufflator enters the abdominal cavity.

INDICATIONS

Indications for laparoscopy may be diagnostic or therapeutic. Laparoscopic evaluation and biopsy of abdominal abnormalities has the advantage over ultrasound-guided percutaneous biopsies in that better quality tissue samples can be obtained, the lesions are clearly visible and magnified through the endoscope allowing observation and biopsy of smaller (metastatic) lesions. Furthermore, because of excellent control of hemorrhage from biopsy sites, larger biopsies can be obtained. The advantage of laparoscopy over laparotomy is obvious, except that laparoscopy cannot always replace a complete exploratory laparotomy. On the other hand, a laparoscopic exploration of the abdomen may prevent an unnecessary laparotomy, such as with tumor staging.[71] The list of surgical indications is growing as knowledge and experience are expanding. Because of its minimally invasive nature there are few contraindications for laparoscopy. Absolute contraindications include diaphragmatic herniation with severe respiratory complications, septic peritonitis, severe cardiac or pulmonary dysfunction, and conditions in which open surgery is clearly indicated.[72] Relative contraindications include ascites, extreme obesity, poor patient condition, and lack of skills. Ascitic fluid can be removed before or during laparoscopy; however, obesity will also complicate conventional open surgery, and poor patient condition may benefit from a less invasive surgical approach. Furthermore, one can always convert to open surgery when necessary. Adhesions from prior surgery may also pose an increased risk of complications.

LAPAROSCOPIC PROCEDURES

Tissue biopsy

Laparoscopy is used for biopsy (Box 24-1) of a variety of tissues in cats including the pancreas (Box 24-2), liver (Box 24-3), and kidney (Box 24-4). Pancreatic biopsy is a safe means to obtain a definite diagnosis of pancreatic disease in cats and a laparoscopic approach

---

Box 24-1 **Laparascopic biopsy**

Dorsal recumbency

For most feline exploratory and biopsy procedures we prefer to position the animal in dorsal recumbency. Depending on the organ of interest, the cat can be tilted in any direction that improves access. Some examples of the laparoscopic view in a cat in dorsal recumbency and Trendelenburg position are displayed in Fig. 24-6. The initial (camera) port in a dorsal recumbent cat is usually placed in the midline to minimize trauma to muscle layers and caudal to the umbilicus to avoid penetrating falciform fat. Distention of the stomach by fluid or gas may limit access to the cranial abdomen, necessitating the use of an orogastric tube to empty the stomach. Depending on the ease of access to the tissue of interest, two or three portals are used: one for the laparoscope, one for the biopsy forceps, and one for an additional instrument, such as a palpation probe, laparoscopic forceps, or hemostatic device. Positioning of secondary ports is directed by intra-abdominal findings, using a triangulated access to the tissues of interest. The portals are placed caudal to the last rib to avoid opening the thoracic cavity. Most solid organs can be biopsied using a biopsy cup forceps, either by grasping the edge of an organ or tissue mass or by entering perpendicular to the tissue surface. After the instrument is closed, a delay of 10–30 seconds allows clotting to start and reduces bleeding after specimen removal. The tissue sample is then gently removed by pulling the forceps back. Care should be taken not to pull in an asymmetrical direction to prevent accidental laceration of remaining tissue, especially in cats with, for instance, a fatty liver. A quick but careful twisting motion may improve sample removal. Proper hemostasis should be observed before ending the laparoscopic procedure. Hemostasis may be improved by inserting a piece of collagen sponge or gel foam into the defect. In case of excessive bleeding, other options include the use of electrosurgery or vessel sealer, clips, or a suture loop device. The use of pre-tied loops is advocated by some authors for improved hemostasis with biopsies of the pancreas or liver, especially when hemostasis may be impaired, such as in cats with liver disease. An edge of the organ is grasped with forceps and pulled through the pre-tied loop, which is tightened, crushing through the parenchyma and ligating blood vessels and ducts. Our experience is that pre-tied loops are too big and custom-made loops of smaller material work better and are cheaper. The tissue sample is cut with scissors just distal to the ligature.[8,28,71,73]

Left lateral recumbency

A left lateral position has been described for laparoscopic abdominal organ biopsies in cats.[28] Lateral recumbency can be used to review the organs located in the retroperitoneal and lumbar troughs. In a left lateral recumbent cat, the initial port is usually made halfway between the caudal border of the ribs and the wing of the ilium and midway between the spine and ventral midline.[8,71]

Sternal recumbency

There is limited experience with the use of sternal recumbency in cats, but adrenal visualization may be improved this way. When a cat is placed in sternal recumbency, both the hips (ventral pelvic area) and the chest need to be supported, while minimalizing the pressure on the abdomen. The position of the camera port in sternal recumbency is 3 cm caudal to the rib cage, midbelly.

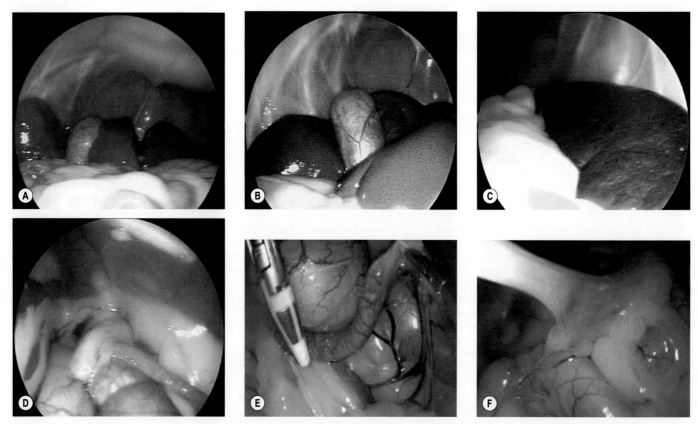

Figure 24-6 Images of feline laparoscopy. **(A-C)** cranial and caudal abdomen with liver, gall bladder, spleen and intestines. **(D)** Caudal abdomen showing uterus, colon, urinary bladder. **(E)** Caudal vena cava and left ureter (pointed out by forceps). **(F)** Adhesion of omentum to abdominal wall in previously operated cat.

Box 24-2 **Pancreatic biopsy**

A two-portal technique may be used for inspection and biopsy of the right pancreatic lobe with the cat in left lateral or dorsal recumbency.[28,72,73] However, for access to the corpus or left lobe of the pancreas, dorsal recumbency and a three-portal technique are advised (Fig. 24-7).[8,26] Biopsies are preferably obtained from the margin of the pancreas and care should be taken to avoid the pancreatic ducts and major vessels, especially in the corpus and proximal right lobe area.[8,28,73] The distal end of the right lobe in a cat ends closer to the larger abdominal veins compared to dogs. A vessel sealer or suture loop device may be used for larger specimens. Grasping the descending duodenum and pulling it medially allows access to the right lobe. Access to the left lobe and corpus may be enhanced by a reverse Trendelenburg position.[8] The dorsal aspect of the left lobe of the pancreas can be exposed by maneuvering the spleen and associated omentum in a cranial direction and to the right.[26] The ventral aspect of the body and left lobe may be exposed by grasping and elevating the great curvature of the stomach with Babcock forceps and opening the omental bursa by creating a window in an avascular part of the ventral leaf of the greater omentum, caudal to the gastroepiploic vessels. The cranial part of the greater omentum is retracted over the stomach to enter the lesser omental sac. If necessary, the stomach can be retracted cranially to expose the body and left lobe of the pancreas.[8]

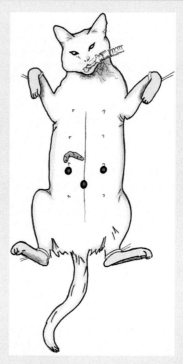

Figure 24-7 Trocar placement for laparoscopic biopsy of the pancreas.

Box 24-3 Liver biopsy

A right lateral approach with the cat in left lateral recumbency is the approach preferred by several authors, because it gives good access to the majority of the liver.[28,72,74] However, unless a liver biopsy is the only intended procedure, we recommend dorsal recumbency and tilting of the patient in any direction to access different parts of the liver combined with a routine exploration of the abdomen.[8,71,73] The falciform ligament can partially block the cranial field of view in dogs, but is less of a problem in cats (Fig. 24-6). If necessary, the falciform ligament can be removed with the use of a vessel-sealing device. The gall bladder can be percutaneously aspirated under laparoscopic guidance using a 22G spinal needle or can be removed laparoscopically if necessary.

Box 24-4 Renal biopsy

Laparoscopic kidney biopsies are usually obtained using core-type biopsy needles, such as Tru-Cut needles. Biopsy cup forceps are not used for kidney biopsies, except for focal superficial lesions. If only one kidney has to be biopsied, a right lateral approach can be used because the right kidney is less mobile and thus more suitable for biopsy. For observation and/or biopsy of both kidneys a ventral midline approach is preferred.

The cat is placed in dorsal recumbency in reversed Trendelenburg position with 30–60° lateral tilt. A second trocar is placed to insert an instrument (palpation probe or forceps) to exert pressure at the biopsy site after tissue collection to aid hemostasis. Gel foam or electrosurgery can be applied if hemostasis is insufficient. A 2 mm skin incision is made to allow insertion of the biopsy needle perpendicular to the skin surface at the desired location (usually close to the kidney). The needle is inserted at a shallow angle into the renal capsule, directing it away from the hilus, to avoid entering the medulla with associated blood vessels.[8,72] Remember that these instruments are forward tracking, so the stylet is pushed into the tissue for the complete length of the stylet, possibly injuring tissue that is not visible. The chance that this happens of course increases with decreasing size of the animal.

Box 24-5 Laparoscopic-assisted intestinal biopsy

A three-portal midline approach with the cat in dorsal recumbency is preferred to explore the entire intestinal tract by 'running' along the bowel using two grasping forceps. If combined with laparoscopic abdominal exploration and biopsies of other organs, these procedures should be performed first because pneumoperitoneum will be lost. In case of a focal lesion, the intestine is grasped nearby and brought near the instrument cannula opening, which is subsequently enlarged under laparoscopic vision using a number 11 scalpel blade. The cannula, forceps, and grasped loop of intestine are exteriorized through the enlarged incision (approximately 2 cm) in the abdominal wall and a standard full thickness intestinal biopsy can be performed.[28,73] In case of several intestinal biopsies, the peri-umbilical midline portal incision is enlarged to 2–4 cm. A loop of intestine is grasped and the entire intestinal tract up to the stomach and down to the colon is inspected before taking full thickness biopsies. If indicated, intestinal resection with end-to-end enterostomy can also be performed outside the abdominal wall. It may be helpful to place a small Balfour wound retractor or a specially designed laparoscopic wound retractor (designed for hand-assisted laparoscopic surgery). Because of the flexibility of the feline abdominal wall, biopsies can also be taken from stomach, right lobe of the pancreas, and mesenteric lymph nodes if indicated,[71,73] without the need of a larger incision. The biopsy sites are wrapped in omentum prior to routine closure of the wounds in three layers. The benefit of an exploratory laparoscopy before the procedure is that the total incision length can be kept to a minimum. Also, the flexible abdominal wall makes laparoscopic-assisted exploration of benefit in these cases.

for animals <7 kg,[52] and does not decrease total incision length compared to a two-portal approach, but considerably decreases freedom of manipulation and access to the ovary and is therefore not commonly used in cats. An advantage in cats compared to dogs is the small amount of fat deposited in the ovarian ligament. In obese dogs, a large amount of fat may be deposited in the ovarian ligament, completely covering the blood vessels and ovary, which significantly increases surgery duration,[51] whereas in cats fat is not typically present in the ovarian ligament, even in obese animals (Fig. 24-9).[29]

Laparoscopic ovariohysterectomy

Elective ovariohysterectomy (OVH) is not commonly performed in most European countries, because it is more invasive and has no significant advantage over ovariectomy.[78] OVH can be performed as a fully laparoscopic or laparoscopic-assisted procedure (Box 24-7). Because the uterus and ovaries have to be exteriorized for removal anyway, the laparoscopic-assisted approach is not markedly different from the fully laparoscopic approach in respect of invasiveness. And in the case of laparoscopic ligation, exteriorization of the uterine body and cervix will reduce surgery duration. In order to facilitate exteriorization of the uterine body and cervix, care has to be taken that the caudal portal is made at a point midway between umbilicus and pubic bone or even more caudally. However, a too caudal position may interfere with the ventral bladder ligament. We tend to place this port after determination of the correct location of the cervix and under endoscopic guidance.

Laparoscopic cryptorchidectomy

Feline (or canine) endoscopic diagnosis and treatment of abdominally retained testicles (Box 24-8) is relatively straightforward and

will minimize surgical morbidity.[27,28] In healthy cats, laparoscopic pancreatic biopsy using biopsy forceps did not negatively affect pancreatic health or clinical status in a controlled trial.[26] The most important advantages of a laparoscopic renal biopsy approach are direct visualization of the kidney and control of hemorrhage, as severe post-biopsy renal hemorrhage has been reported to occur in 17% of the cats, with 3% hemorrhage-related mortality in a retrospective study.[75] The significant advantage of surgical full thickness intestinal biopsies compared to endoscopically obtained mucosal biopsies of the stomach and duodenum (Box 24-5) has been clearly demonstrated in cats with intestinal malignant lymphoma.[76]

Laparoscopic ovariectomy

In contrast to dogs, cats are most commonly gonadectomised independent of their gestation status.

Laparascopic ovariectomy (lapOVE) can be performed using a two- or three-portal approach (Box 24-6). In a one-portal approach described for dogs[52] and cats,[77] a relatively large diameter (12 mm) portal is required to accommodate a laparoscope with working channel. This large diameter device is not considered to be practical

Box 24-6 **Laparoscopic ovariectomy**

The abdominal skin is clipped and prepared for surgery from the xiphoid process to the pubic bone. For the two-portal technique, the width of the skin preparation must exceed the level of the mammary glands, while for the three-portal technique the width may be within the level of the mammary glands. Cats are placed in dorsal recumbency in a 10–15° Trendelenburg position. The operating room set-up for removal of the left ovary is displayed in Figure 24-8. The surgeon and assistant are on the right-hand side of the cat, the monitor/endoscopy tower on the left-hand side. A primary (camera) portal is made just below the umbilicus (see section on abdominal access). After establishment of pneumoperitoneum and insertion of the laparoscope, the abdominal cavity is inspected for abnormalities and entry-related complications. A second portal is made under visual guidance halfway between the umbilicus and pubic bone, taking care not to traumatize the ventral bladder ligament. In the three-portal approach, a third portal is made halfway between umbilicus and xiphoid process. The third trocar is commonly angled in a lateral direction during insertion or placed slightly paramedian to avoid entering the falciform ligament. The cat is tilted 20–45° to the right side. The ovary is located using either the uterus or round ligament that originates from the inguinal canal. The uterus or round ligament is grasped using a 3 mm diameter self-retaining grasping forceps through the cranial portal and a 3 mm diameter curved Kelly grasping/dissecting forceps through the caudal portal. The uterus or its round ligament is followed cranially until the ovary is visualized. The ovary is then grasped and lifted upward using the self-retaining grasping forceps through the cranial portal (Fig. 24-9). In the two-portal approach, manipulation is performed by use of a pair of single grasping forceps, passed through the caudal portal. The ovary is then lifted upward and attached to the ventrolateral abdominal wall by use of a transabdominal suspension suture. The suspension suture is applied from outside the abdomen, puncturing skin and abdominal wall and ovarian ligament just proximal to the ovary, pulling the ovary to the abdominal wall.[61] Care is taken not to puncture the ovary while applying the stay suture. Ovariectomy is performed using bipolar electrosurgery forceps and endoscopic scissors or another hemostatic/dissecting device through the caudal portal. We prefer the use of standard pediatric bipolar forceps in combination with endoscopic scissors or a vessel sealer/divider forceps (such as Ligasure) to coagulate and cut in a caudal-to-cranial direction the proper ligament or uterus just caudal to the proper ligament, the ovarian pedicle with associated blood vessels, and the suspensory ligament (Fig. 24-9). Please note that the uterine vessels attaching to the ovarian vessels are relatively bigger in cats compared with dogs, which may be caused by differences in gestation status. The ovary is then placed in the left caudal quadrant (or held attached to the transabdominal suspension suture in the two-portal approach) to be removed after excision of the right ovary. The surgeon and assistant move to the left-hand side of the cat, and the monitor/endoscopy tower is placed at the right-hand side of the cat. This last step is not necessary if a second monitor is available at the right-hand side of the cat (Fig. 24-8). The cat is tilted to the left side and the procedure is repeated for the right ovary. Both ovaries can be removed under visual guidance through the caudal portal by pulling them into the portal with the grasping forceps and removing the cannula. If the portal incision is too small, the incision is somewhat enlarged so that the ovaries can be removed. However, the ovaries are usually small enough to be exteriorized through the original portal, sometimes by applying gentle force (Fig. 24-10). The procedure ends with a routine exploration of the abdomen (while manually closing the caudal portal if necessary). The abdomen is deflated and the incisions are closed routinely (see section on abdominal access) with 4-0 absorbable suture material.

One advantage of the two-portal approach is that the procedure may be performed without an assistant. However, the fixed position of the ovary and the absence of a second pair of forceps greatly reduces freedom of manipulation. Furthermore, care has to be taken not to injure the abdominal wall during electrosurgical use because of the close proximity of the ovarian ligament due to the transabdominal suspension suture. Whether the advantage of a decreased incision length with the two-portal technique outweighs the reduction in surgical freedom compared to the 3-portal technique has not been investigated in cats.

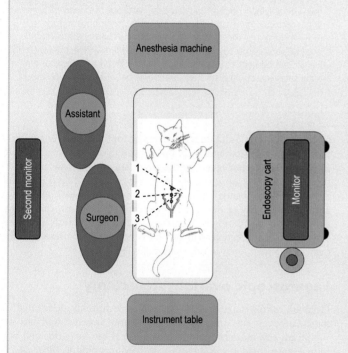

Figure 24-8 Operating room set-up for laparoscopic ovariectomy of the left ovary through three portals, showing triangulation of instruments and a coaxial configuration of surgeon, operating field, and monitor. 1, laparoscope; 2, self-retaining grasping forceps to grab ovary; 3, electrosurgery forceps/scissors for tissue coagulation and dissection.

greatly reduces invasiveness and surgical trauma compared to open laparotomy. Furthermore, the use of a small laparotomy incision for cryptorchidectomy is strongly discouraged because of the need to properly identify all associated tissue structures before excision of any tissue to prevent complications.[34,80,81] After a thorough patient work-up, cryptorchidectomy can be performed using a laparoscopic or laparoscopic-assisted approach.[8,33,34]

OTHER PROCEDURES

If performed by an experienced endoscopic surgeon, multiple other procedures can be performed in felids. As mentioned before, the feline abdomen is quite expandable, allowing a great space to work in.

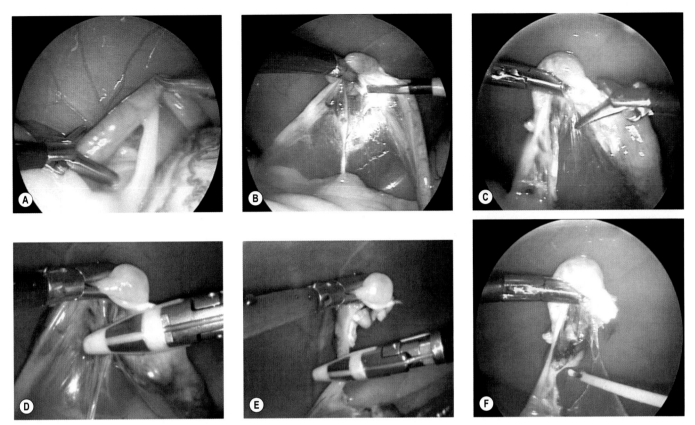

Figure 24-9 Laparoscopic ovariectomy. **(A)** The uterus is grasped and followed cranial. **(B)** The ovary is fixated using self-retaining grasping forceps. **(C-F)** Examples of dissection of the ovarian pedicle are shown using bipolar forceps and scissors, vessel sealer/divider, and surgical laser.

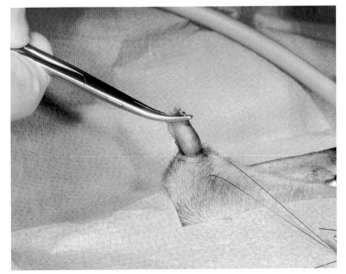

Figure 24-10 Removal of ovary or uterus through caudal portal.

Procedures can vary from organ resections (liver lobe, pancreas), video-assisted procedures (cystotomy, cystectomy, cystopexy, gastrotomy, gastropexy, gastric tube placement), tumor excisions, to organ excisions (adrenalectomy, nephrectomy and splenectomy). All such procedures have been performed at the authors' institution but require additional instruments and expertise. The benefit to the patient needs to be weighed against the increase in procedural time.

COMPLICATIONS

Data on complication rates of feline laparoscopic surgery is limited.[82] Anesthetic complications may be associated with respiratory or circulatory derangement due to pneumoperitoneum or Trendelenburg position, especially in respiratory or circulatory compromised animals (see above). In human laparoscopic surgery, the overall complication rates in large study groups generally range from <1–5%. However, rates are strongly related to the difficulty of the procedure performed (ranging from <1–>15%). There are no differences found in major complication rates between laparoscopic and open surgical approaches. Mortality is generally less than 0.1%.[83–85] One of the most important factors is experience of the surgeon, the complication rate being almost four times higher during the first 100 procedures compared with the subsequent complication rate.[84] Up to 50% of complications occur during abdominal entry, either by the Veress needle or primary trocar, resulting in injury to blood vessels, spleen, intestinal tract, urinary tract, or other abdominal organs. In dogs, reported incidence of mild splenic hemorrhage from trauma during abdominal entry from either Veress needle or trocar insertion (both closed and open technique) ranges from 5–19%.[12,52,67,86] We do not expect the numbers to be different in the cat.

Other injuries may occur during surgical dissection, manipulation, or the use of energetic devices, especially monopolar electrosurgery.

Box 24-7 Laparascopic ovariohysterectomy

Laparoscopic-assisted ovariohysterectomy

The same three-portal configuration can be used as for lapOVE (see Box 24-6). An important difference with lapOVE is that excision of the ovaries and mesometrium is performed in a cranial-to-caudal direction. The cat is in dorsal recumbency, 10–15° Trendelenburg position, and 20–45° right lateral tilt. After establishing pneumoperitoneum and inserting the three midline cannulas as for lapOVE, the left ovary is localized and grasped using a self-retaining grasping forceps through the caudal portal. Tissue dissection is performed using a vessel sealer/divider or by exchanging a bipolar forceps with scissors through the cranial portal. Thus, the suspensory ligament, ovarian pedicle, and broad ligament are transected in a cranial-to-caudal direction up to the level of the cervix. The same procedure is performed for the right ovary and uterine horn.

In the laparoscopic-assisted approach, the caudal portal is now slightly enlarged (5–10 mm, depending on the size of the uterus) and

the right ovary and uterine horn are exteriorized. Following the bifurcation, the left uterine horn and ovary are also exteriorized. The uterus and associated blood vessels can now be routinely ligated and transected at the level of the cervix. The uterine stump is returned into the abdomen and a routine laparoscopic exploration of the abdomen is performed before routine closure of the portals (see section on abdominal access).

Full laparascopic ovariohysterectomy

In the fully laparoscopic approach, ligation of the uterine body/cervix and associated vessels may be performed inside the abdomen using extracorporeally tied ligatures or laparoscopic suture loops followed by laparoscopic scissors excision. If the size of the uterine body/cervix permits, excision may be facilitated using the same laparoscopic bipolar or vessel sealer/divider device as was used for the ovarian pedicle.[79] The excised uterus and ovaries are exteriorized through a slightly enlarged portal.

Box 24-8 Laparascopic cryptorchidectomy

The cat is prepared for laparoscopy and placed in dorsal recumbency and 10–15° Trendelenburg position. A wide surgical preparation of the abdomen and inguinal region should be performed. The primary cannula for laparoscopy is placed just caudal to the umbilicus and the abdomen is inspected. Usually, the abdominal testicles are readily seen after entry of the laparoscope. However, if a retained testicle is not apparent, both internal inguinal ring areas should be inspected. If the vas deferens and testicular vessels are entering the inguinal ring, the testicle is located outside of the abdomen in the inguinal canal or inguinal fat. In that case, gentle external pressure is applied on the inguinal canal to see if the testicle can be pushed through the internal inguinal ring. If not, a surgical approach to the inguinal canal is considered.[81] If the gubernaculum is seen entering the inguinal ring, it is followed into the abdomen to locate the testis, which could be obscured by other organs. Both inguinal areas are inspected, even in unilateral cryptorchidism, to rule out other abnormalities.

Full laparascopic cryptorchidectomy

In a full laparoscopic approach for bilateral cryptorchidism, a three-portal technique is used (Fig. 24-11). The second and third cannulas are placed under visual guidance and transillumination in a paramedian position midway between umbilicus and pubic bone. The testicle is grasped with laparoscopic forceps through the nearest portal, while a bipolar forceps (alternately exchanged with scissors) or vessel sealer/divider device is used through the other instrument portal to seal and transect the vas deferens, testicular vessels, and associated ligaments close to the testicle. It is sometimes useful to switch the camera and instrument portals around to enhance surgical access to the testicle. In a case of bilateral cryptorchidism, the procedure is repeated on the other side. Both testicles can be exteriorized through one portal, which may have to be slightly enlarged. After routine exploration of the abdomen, CO_2 is expelled and the portals are routinely closed (see section on abdominal access). An approach through three caudal midline portals may also be used.

Laparascopic-assisted cryptorchidectomy

This can be performed via a two-portal approach. The second portal is placed in a paramedian location at the side of the retained testicle in unilateral cryptorchidism. With bilateral cryptorchid testicles, the second

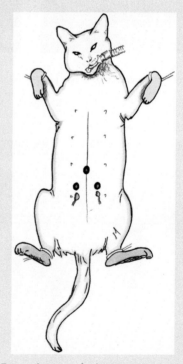

Figure 24-11 Trocar placement for laparoscopic cryptorchidectomy.

portal is made in the midline, midway between umbilicus and pubic bone. The testicle is grabbed and pulled towards the portal opening to be exteriorized, enlarging the portal if necessary. With the testicle outside the abdomen, the testicular vessels and vas deferens duct are identified, separately ligated, and transected to remove the testicle. In a bilateral cryptorchid cat, this procedure can be performed for both testicles through the same midline portal, the abdominal wall being flexible enough to exteriorize the testicles from both locations.

The most common intestinal injuries are thermal or associated with abdominal entry[87] and less than 50% are diagnosed during surgery.[88] There is no consensus concerning differences in safety between open or closed entry techniques for laparoscopy in human literature.[89] However, differences in anatomy in smaller animals may imply different risks of complications between techniques. No matter which entry technique is used, the abdomen should always be thoroughly inspected for entry-related injury at initial entry with the endoscope. The abdomen is then again thoroughly inspected for unforeseen injury before ending the procedure.

REFERENCES

1. Wildt DE, Kinney GM, Seager SW. Laparoscopy for direct observation of internal organs of the domestic cat and dog. Am J Vet Res 1977;38:1429–32.

2. Rothuizen J. Laparoscopy in small animal medicine. Vet Q 1985;7:225–8.

3. Keus F, de Jong JA, Gooszen HG, van Laarhoven CJ. Laparoscopic versus open cholecystectomy for patients with symptomatic cholecystolithiasis. Cochrane Database Syst Rev 2006:CD006231.

4. Medeiros LR, Rosa DD, Bozzetti MC, et al. Laparoscopy versus laparotomy for benign ovarian tumour. Cochrane Database Syst Rev 2009:CD004751.

5. Li X, Zhang J, Sang L, et al. Laparoscopic versus conventional appendectomy – a meta-analysis of randomized controlled trials. BMC Gastroenterol 2010;10:129.

6. Sauerland S, Lefering R, Neugebauer EA.. Laparoscopic versus open surgery for suspected appendicitis. Cochrane Database Syst Rev 2004:CD001546.

7. McCarthy TC. Veterinary endoscopy for the small animal practitioner. St. Louis, Mo: Elsevier Saunders; 2004.

8. Freeman LJ. Veterinary endosurgery. St. Louis: Mosby; 1999.

9. Lhermette P, Sobel DS, British Small Animal Veterinary Association. BSAVA manual of canine and feline endoscopy and endosurgery. Gloucester: British Small Animal Veterinary Association; 2008.

10. Divers SJ. Exotic mammal diagnostic endoscopy and endosurgery. Vet Clin North Am Exot Anim Pract 2010;13: 255–72.

11. Divers SJ. Reptile diagnostic endoscopy and endosurgery. Vet Clin North Am Exot Anim Pract 2010;13:217–42.

12. Davidson EB, Moll HD, Payton ME. Comparison of laparoscopic ovariohysterectomy and ovariohysterectomy in dogs. Vet Surg 2004;33:62–9.

13. Devitt CM, Cox RE, Hailey JJ. Duration, complications, stress, and pain of open ovariohysterectomy versus a simple method of laparoscopic-assisted ovariohysterectomy in dogs. J Am Vet Med Assoc 2005;227:921–7.

14. Hancock RB, Lanz OI, Waldron DR, et al. Comparison of postoperative pain after ovariohysterectomy by harmonic scalpel-assisted laparoscopy compared with median celiotomy and ligation in dogs. Vet Surg 2005;34:273–82.

15. Schippers E, Tittel A, Ottinger A, Schumpelick V. Laparoscopy versus laparotomy: comparison of adhesion-formation after bowel resection in a canine model. Dig Surg 1998;15: 145–7.

16. Szabo G, Mikó I, Nagy P, et al. Adhesion formation with open versus laparoscopic cholecystectomy: an immunologic and histologic study. Surg Endosc 2007;21: 253–7.

17. Gamal EM, Metzger P, Szabó G, et al. The influence of intraoperative complications on adhesion formation during laparoscopic and conventional cholecystectomy in an animal model. Surg Endosc 2001;15:873–7.

18. Culp WT, Mayhew PD, Brown DC. The effect of laparoscopic versus open ovariectomy on postsurgical activity in small dogs. Vet Surg 2009;38:811–17.

19. Mayhew PD, Brown DC. Prospective evaluation of two intracorporeally sutured prophylactic laparoscopic gastropexy techniques compared with laparoscopic-assisted gastropexy in dogs. Vet Surg 2009;38:738–46.

20. Böhm B, Milsom JW, Fazio VW. Postoperative intestinal motility following conventional and laparoscopic intestinal surgery. Arch Surg 1995;130:415–19.

21. Nickel R, Stürtzbecher N, Kilian H, et al. Postoperative Rekonvaleszenz nach laparoskopischer und konventioneller Ovariektomie: eine vergleichende Studie. Kleintierpraxis 2007;52:413–24.

22. Naitoh T, Garcia-Ruiz A, Vladisavljevic A, et al. Gastrointestinal transit and stress response after laparoscopic vs conventional distal pancreatectomy in the canine model. Surg Endosc 2002;16: 1627–30.

23. Matsumoto ED, Margulis V, Tunc L, et al. Cytokine response to surgical stress: comparison of pure laparoscopic, hand-assisted laparoscopic, and open nephrectomy. J Endourol 2005;19:1140–5.

24. Marcovich R, Williams AL, Seifman BD, Wolf JS Jr. A canine model to assess the biochemical stress response to laparoscopic and open surgery. J Endourol 2001;15:1005–8.

25. Yoder B, Wolf JS, Jr. Canine model of surgical stress response comparing standard laparoscopic, microlaparoscopic, and hand-assisted laparoscopic nephrectomy. Urology 2005;65:600–3.

26. Cosford KL, Shmon CL, Myers SL, et al. Prospective evaluation of laparoscopic pancreatic biopsies in 11 healthy cats. J Vet Intern Med 2010;24:104–13.

27. Webb CB, Trott C. Laparoscopic diagnosis of pancreatic disease in dogs and cats. J Vet Intern Med 2008;22:1263–6.

28. Webb CB. Feline laparoscopy for gastrointestinal disease. Top Companion Anim Med 2008;23:193–9.

29. van Nimwegen SA, Kirpensteijn J. Laparoscopic ovariectomy in cats: comparison of laser and bipolar electrocoagulation. J Feline Med Surg 2007;9:397–403.

30. Alves AE, Ribeiro AP, Filippo PA, et al. Evaluation of creatine kinase (CK) and aspartate aminotransferase (AST) activities after laparoscopic or conventional ovariectomy in queens. Schweiz Arch Tierheilkd 2009;151:223–7.

31. Alves AE, Ribeiro APC, Di Filippo PA, et al. Leucogram and serum acute phase protein concentrations in queens submitted to conventional or videolaparoscopic ovariectomy. Arq Bras Med Vet Zootec 2010;62:86–91.

32. Schiochet F, Beck CAC, Silva APFF, et al. Laparoscopic ovariohysterectomy in healthy felines: comparative study of three hemostatic methods. Arq Bras Med Vet Zootec 2009;61:369–77.

33. Vannozzi I, Benetti C, Rota A. Laparoscopic cryptorchidectomy in a cat. J Feline Med Surg 2002;4(4):201–3.

34. Miller NA, Van Lue SJ, Rawlings CA. Use of laparoscopic-assisted cryptorchidectomy in dogs and cats. J Am Vet Med Assoc 2004;224:875–8.

35. Mouat EE, Mayhew PD, Weh JL, Chapman PS. Bilateral laparoscopic subtotal perinephric pseudocyst resection in a cat. J Feline Med Surg 2009;11: 1015–8.

36. Schiochet F, Beck CAC, Stedile R, et al. Ovariectomia laparoscópica em uma gata com ovários remanescentes. Act Sci Vet 2007;35:245–8.

37. Munz Y, Kumar BD, Moorthy K, et al. Laparoscopic virtual reality and box trainers: is one superior to the other? Surg Endosc 2004;18:485–94.

38. Al-Abed Y, Cooper DG. A novel home laparoscopic simulator. J Surg Educ 2009;66(1):1–2.

39. Jones DB, Wu JS, Soper NJ. Laparoscopic surgery: principles and procedures.

St, Louis: Quality Medical Publishing; 1997.

40. Mayhew PD. Advanced laparoscopic procedures (hepatobiliary, endocrine) in dogs and cats. Vet Clin North Am Small Anim Pract 2009;39:925–39.

41. Bailey JE, Pablo LS. Anesthetic and physiologic considerations for veterinary endosurgery. In: Freeman LJ, editor. Veterinary Endosurgery. St. Louis: Mosby; 1999. p. 24–43.

42. Gutt CN, Oniu T, Mehrabi A, et al. Circulatory and respiratory complications of carbon dioxide insufflation. Dig Surg 2004;21:95–105.

43. Ishizaki Y, Bandai Y, Shimomura K, et al. Safe intraabdominal pressure of carbon dioxide pneumoperitoneum during laparoscopic surgery. Surgery 1993;114: 549–54.

44. Windberger UB, Auer R, Keplinger F, et al. The role of intra-abdominal pressure on splanchnic and pulmonary hemodynamic and metabolic changes during carbon dioxide pneumoperitoneum. Gastrointest Endosc 1999;49:84–91.

45. Dexter SP, Vucevic M, Gibson J, McMahon MJ. Hemodynamic consequences of high- and low-pressure capnoperitoneum during laparoscopic cholecystectomy. Surg Endosc 1999;13:376–81.

46. Williams MD, Murr PC. Laparoscopic insufflation of the abdomen depresses cardiopulmonary function. Surg Endosc 1993;7:12–16.

47. Marathe US, Lilly RE, Silvestry SC, et al. Alterations in hemodynamics and left ventricular contractility during carbon dioxide pneumoperitoneum. Surg Endosc 1996;10:974–8.

48. Duke T, Steinacher SL, Remedios AM. Cardiopulmonary effects of using carbon dioxide for laparoscopic surgery in dogs. Vet Surg 1996;25:77–82.

49. Gurusamy KS, Samraj K, Davidson BR. Low pressure versus standard pressure pneumoperitoneum in laparoscopic cholecystectomy. Cochrane Database Syst Rev 2009:CD006930.

50. Rayman R, Girotti M, Armstrong K, et al. Assessing the safety of pediatric laparoscopic surgery. Surg Laparosc Endosc 1995;5:437–43.

51. Van Nimwegen SA, Kirpensteijn J. Comparison of Nd:YAG surgical laser and Remorgida bipolar electrosurgery forceps for canine laparoscopic ovariectomy. Vet Surg 2007;36:533–40.

52. Dupré G, Fiorbianco V, Skalicky M, et al. Laparoscopic ovariectomy in dogs: comparison between single portal and two-portal access. Vet Surg 2009;38: 818–24.

53. Rauh R, Hemmerling TM, Rist M, Jacobi KE. Influence of pneumoperitoneum and patient positioning on respiratory system compliance. J Clin Anesth 2001;13: 361–5.

54. Rist M, Hemmerling TM, Rauh R, et al. Influence of pneumoperitoneum and patient positioning on preload and splanchnic blood volume in laparoscopic surgery of the lower abdomen. J Clin Anesth 2001;13:244–9.

55. Kraut EJ, Anderson JT, Safwat A, et al. Impairment of cardiac performance by laparoscopy in patients receiving positive end-expiratory pressure. Arch Surg 1999;134:76–80.

56. Luz CM, Polarz H, Böhrer H, et al. Hemodynamic and respiratory effects of pneumoperitoneum and PEEP during laparoscopic pelvic lymphadenectomy in dogs. Surg Endosc 1994;8:25–7.

57. Hewitt SA, Brisson BA, Sinclair MD, Sears WC. Comparison of cardiopulmonary responses during sedation with epidural and local anesthesia for laparoscopic-assisted jejunostomy feeding tube placement with cardiopulmonary responses during general anesthesia for laparoscopic-assisted or open surgical jejunostomy feeding tube placement in healthy dogs. Am J Vet Res 2007;68: 358–69.

58. Coughlin SM, Karanicolas PJ, Emmerton-Coughlin HM, et al. Better late than never? Impact of local analgesia timing on postoperative pain in laparoscopic surgery: a systematic review and metaanalysis. Surg Endosc 2010;24: 3167–76.

59. Fitzpatrick CL, Weir HL, Monnet E. Effects of infiltration of the incision site with bupivacaine on postoperative pain and incisional healing in dogs undergoing ovariohysterectomy. J Am Vet Med Assoc 2010;237:395–401.

60. Kolata RJ, Freeman LJ. Access, port placement, and basic endosurgical skills. In: Freeman LJ, editor. Veterinary endosurgery. St. Louis: Mosby; 1999. p. 44–60.

61. Rosin D, Kuriansky J, Rosenthal RJ, et al. Laparoscopic transabdominal suspension sutures. Surg Endosc 2001;15:761–3.

62. Fransson BA, Ragle CA. Lift laparoscopy in dogs and cats: 12 cases (2008-2009). J Am Vet Med Assoc 2011;239:1574–9.

63. Van Lue SJ, Van Lue AP. Equipment and instrumentation in veterinary endoscopy. Vet Clin North Am Small Anim Pract 2009;39:817–37.

64. Divers SJ. Endoscopy equipment and instrumentation for use in exotic animal medicine. Vet Clin North Am Exot Anim Pract 2010;13:171–85.

65. Ternamian AM. Laparoscopy without trocars. Surg Endosc 1997;11:815–18.

66. Stoloff DR. Laparoscopic suturing and knot tying techniques. In: Freeman LJ, editor. Veterinary endosurgery. St. Louis: Mosby; 1999. p. 73–91.

67. Mayhew PD, Brown DC. Comparison of three techniques for ovarian pedicle hemostasis during laparoscopic-assisted

ovariohysterectomy. Vet Surg 2007;36: 541–7.

68. Van Goethem BE, Rosenveldt KW, Kirpensteijn J. Monopolar versus bipolar electrocoagulation in canine laparoscopic ovariectomy: a nonrandomized, prospective, clinical trial. Vet Surg 2003;32:464–70.

69. Hunter JG. Laser use in laparoscopic surgery. Surg Clin North Am 1992;72: 655–64.

70. Thompson SE, Potter L. Electrosurgery, lasers, and ultrasonic energy. In: Freeman LJ, editor. Veterinary endosurgery. St. Louis: Mosby; 1999. p. 61–72.

71. Freeman LJ. Gastrointestinal laparoscopy in small animals. Vet Clin North Am Small Anim Pract 2009;39:903–24.

72. Monnet E, Twedt DC. Laparoscopy. Vet Clin North Am Small Anim Pract 2003;33:1147–63.

73. Mayhew P. Surgical views: techniques for laparoscopic and laparoscopic assisted biopsy of abdominal organs. Compend Contin Educ Vet 2009;31:170–6.

74. Rothuizen J, Twedt DC. Liver biopsy techniques. Vet Clin North Am Small Anim Pract 2009;39:469–80.

75. Vaden SL, Levine JF, Lees GE, et al. Renal biopsy: a retrospective study of methods and complications in 283 dogs and 65 cats. J Vet Intern Med 2005;19:794–801.

76. Evans SE, Bonczynski JJ, Broussard JD, et al. Comparison of endoscopic and full-thickness biopsy specimens for diagnosis of inflammatory bowel disease and alimentary tract lymphoma in cats. J Am Vet Med Assoc 2006;229:1447–50.

77. Kim YK, Lee SY, Park SJ, et al. Feasibility of single-portal access laparoscopic ovariectomy in 17 cats. Vet Rec 2011;169:179.

78. van Goethem B, Schaefers-Okkens A, Kirpensteijn J. Making a rational choice between ovariectomy and ovariohysterectomy in the dog: a discussion of the benefits of either technique. Vet Surg 2006;35:136–43.

79. Austin B, Lanz OI, Hamilton SM, et al. Laparoscopic ovariohysterectomy in nine dogs. J Am Anim Hosp Assoc 2003;39: 391–6.

80. Millis DL, Hauptman JG, Johnson CA. Cryptorchidism and monorchism in cats: 25 cases (1980–1989). J Am Vet Med Assoc 1992;200:1128–30.

81. Birchard SJ, Nappier M. Cryptorchidism. Compend Contin Educ Vet 2008;30: 325–36; quiz 36–7.

82. McClaran JK, Buote NJ. Complications and need for conversion to laparotomy in small animals. Vet Clin North Am Small Anim Pract 2009;39:941–51.

83. Keus F, Gooszen HG, van Laarhoven CJ. Open, small-incision, or laparoscopic cholecystectomy for patients with symptomatic cholecystolithiasis. An overview of Cochrane Hepato-Biliary

Group reviews. Cochrane Database Syst Rev 2010:CD008318.

84. Fahlenkamp D, Rassweiler J, Fornara P, et al. Complications of laparoscopic procedures in urology: experience with 2,407 procedures at 4 German centers. J Urol 1999;162:765–70; discussion 70-1.

85. Makai G, Isaacson K. Complications of gynecologic laparoscopy. Clin Obstet Gynecol 2009;52:401–11.

86. Fiorbianco V, Skalicky M, Dörner J, et al. Right intercostal insertion of Veress needle for laparoscopy in dogs: a comparative study of two entry points. American college of veterinary surgeons 19th Annual Scientific Meeting; Helsinki; 2010.

87. Breda A, Finelli A, Janetschek G, et al. Complications of laparoscopic surgery for renal masses: prevention, management, and comparison with the open experience. Eur Urol 2009;55:836–50.

88. Lam A, Khong SY, Bignardi T. Principles and strategies for dealing with complications in laparoscopy. Curr Opin Obstet Gynecol 2010;22:315–19.

89. Ahmad G, Duffy JM, Phillips K, Watson A. Laparoscopic entry techniques. Cochrane Database Syst Rev 2008:CD006583.

Chapter 25

Abdominal wall hernias and ruptures

K.M. Pratschke

Cats are prone to abdominal wall hernias and ruptures either as congenital abnormalities or more often as a result of trauma. Concurrent and frequently more severe life-threatening injuries may mask the rupture and it may only become apparent when the owner notices a swelling, or secondary signs due to strangulation of herniated organs occur. This chapter aims to cover the anatomy, diagnosis, and treatment of the reported abdominal wall hernias and ruptures in cats.

SURGICAL ANATOMY

Abdominal wall[1,2]

The muscles of the abdominal wall fall into two groups, the ventrolateral and the sublumbar. The sublumbar group are more properly considered part of the girdle division of hind limb musculature. The muscles within the ventrolateral group comprise the flank and abdominal wall muscles which are of more immediate relevance for abdominal hernias.

The intrinsic musculature of the flank and abdominal wall comprises three broad, fleshy sheets that lie one on top of the other, with contrasting orientation of muscle fibers. Ventrally each is continued by means of an aponeurotic tendon that has a main insertion along the linea alba. A fourth muscle, the rectus abdominis, lies along the ventral abdominal wall to either side of the linea alba, where it is ensheathed by these aponeurotic tendons.

The *external abdominal oblique* (EAO) muscle has its origin over the lateral surfaces of the ribs and the lumbar fascia from where the bulk of the fibers run caudoventrally, radiating outwards slightly. The aponeurosis of the EAO divides into two crura, with the larger medial crus terminating on the linea alba after passing around the rectus abdominis. The smaller lateral crus attaches to fascia over the iliopsoas, and the pubic brim lateral to the insertion of the rectus abdominis.

The *internal abdominal oblique* (IAO) muscle arises predominantly from the tuber coxa, with smaller points of origin from the lateral crus of the EAO, thoracolumbar fascia and the transverse processes of the lumbar vertebrae. The fibers of the IAO run largely caudoventrally, and the central fascicles insert via an aponeurotic tendon to the linea alba after passing round the rectus abdominis. Towards the midline insertion there is usually some interchange of fibers between the aponeurosis of the IAO and EAO. The IAO has a free caudal margin, which is important with regard to the formation of the inguinal canal. In the dog, the cremaster muscle is formed from a caudal slip of muscle from the IAO, but in the cat the levator scroti muscle replaces the cremaster, which is absent. The levator scroti muscle is formed from fibers of the caudoventral border of the external anal sphincter and the pars caudalis of the external anal sphincter.[3]

The *transversus abdominis* (TAB) arises from the inner surfaces of the last ribs and the transverse processes of the lumbar vertebrae. The fibers run transversely internal to the rectus abdominis to their aponeurotic insertion at the midline.

The *rectus abdominis* (RA) is a broad band of muscle on either side of the linea alba that has a segmental appearance caused by irregular transverse septae. It takes its origin from the ventral surfaces of the rib cartilages and inserts at the pelvic brim via the strong prepubic tendon in dogs. It has been speculated that in cats the strong attachments of the crura of the superficial inguinal ring on the iliopubic eminence, plus the EAO muscle aponeurosis to the medial thigh may serve the same function as the prepubic tendon does in the dog.[4,5] Despite the anatomic difference, it is standard practice to refer to a prepubic tendon in cats (Fig. 25-1).

The *rectus sheath* is the term used for the anatomic arrangement of the aponeuroses from the IAO, EAO and TAB around the RA. The EAO aponeurosis always lies external to the RA, but the IAO aponeurosis may lie either internal or external, depending on the portion of the abdominal wall studied. In the cranial third of the abdomen, fibers pass both internal and external to the RA, but from the umbilicus caudally all fibers pass external. All fascial structures lying external to the RA are termed the *external sheath or external leaf*, while those lying internal to the RA are termed the *internal sheath or leaf*. The internal rectus sheath is lined by a thin layer of transversalis fascia and peritoneum.

The *linea alba* is the ventral midline fibrous zone where the right and left abdominal walls meet. In cats the linea alba is a broad white band, typically up to 3–4 mm wide, whereas in the dog the linea alba is a shallow trough rarely more than 2 mm wide.

The *inguinal canal* is located adjacent to the groin, between the fleshy part of the IAO on one side and the lateral crus of the EAO

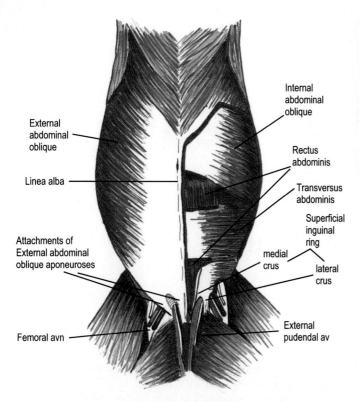

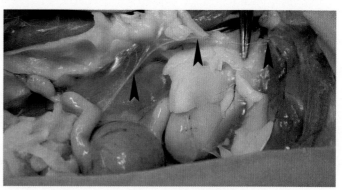

Figure 25-2 The arrowheads in this figure show the line of the peritoneal sheet that covers the entrance to the inguinal canal in a female cat cadaver. There is no extension or pouch of peritoneum extending into the inguinal ring, and no visible vaginal process. *(Courtesy of Joshua Milgram.)*

Figure 25-1 Cats do not have a structure that fits the precise description and appearance of the prepubic tendon in dogs. However, the strong attachments of the medial and lateral crura of the superficial inguinal ring on the iliopubic eminence, plus the external abdominal oblique (EAO) muscle aponeurosis to the medial thigh may serve the same function as the prepubic tendon does in the dog. The EAO is pictured excised on the right side of this diagram to show the relationship of the underlying rectus abdominis (RA) to the crura of the superficial inguinal ring and EAO aponeurosis. The location of the femoral artery and vein, and external pudendal artery and vein, are important to note from the point of view of surgery in this area.

on the other. Other than where the external pudendal vessels, the genitofemoral nerve, and the spermatic cord (male) or vaginal process (female) pass through the canal, it contains only fatty tissue. In male dogs the peritoneum evaginates through the inguinal canal, to form the vaginal tunic around the spermatic cord and testis while in the bitch it envelops the round ligament of the uterus and is called the vaginal process. Recent dissection of eleven embalmed adult female cats, however, failed to identify any evidence of either a vaginal ring or process.[6] Similar anatomic information is not currently available in the literature for male cats; however, anatomic dissection of three male cadavers identified a consistent vaginal tunic, with no evidence of a vaginal process (personal communication, Joshua Milgram; also Fig. 25-2).

The deep inguinal ring is a slit-like entrance to the abdomen along the free caudal edge of the IAO, while the superficial inguinal ring is contained between the two crura of the EAO aponeurosis.

Pelvic diaphragm[1–3]

The perineum describes the part of the body wall that covers the pelvic outlet, and surrounds the anal and urogenital canals. The sacrotuberous ligaments in the dog form the lateral borders; cats, however, do

not have a sacrotuberous ligament.[3] The principal structure contained within the perineum is the pelvic diaphragm. This is a muscular structure consisting of the coccygeal and levator ani muscles, together with their internal and external fascial coverings. These muscles are anchored to the caudal vertebrae and pelvis. The ischiorectal fossa is a wedge-shaped depression formed between the external anal sphincter, levator ani and coccygeal muscles medially, the internal obturator muscle ventrally, and the superficial gluteal muscle laterally. The pudendal nerve and internal pudendal artery and vein pass into the fossa on the ventrolateral surface of the coccygeus before passing across the dorsal surface of the internal obturator muscle.

CLASSIFICATION OF HERNIAS AND RUPTURES

The term hernia is used where the defect is congenital, due to a failure of embryonic signaling and fusion, and a distinct hernia ring and sac will exist. The term rupture is used where the defect is acquired, typically traumatically. Ruptures do not have a distinct hernia ring and sac. Therefore, although the terms 'hernia' and 'rupture' are not synonymous, for certain conditions they are used interchangeably, e.g., diaphragmatic hernia/diaphragmatic rupture, or perineal hernia/perineal rupture. In this chapter the term hernia will be used, although the reader should understand that this also includes ruptures (Table 25-1).

Anatomical location

Describing the anatomical locations is probably the most common way of classifying hernias, e.g., umbilical, inguinal, or perineal. *External abdominal hernias* are defects in the external abdominal wall that allow protrusion of abdominal contents; *internal abdominal hernias* are those that occur through a ring of tissue contained within the abdomen, e.g., hiatal hernia.

Congenital or acquired

A congenital defect is present from birth and is usually due to failure of embryonic signaling and fusion, such as with certain umbilical hernias. Although the defect or hernia ring is present from birth, herniation may not necessarily manifest until later in life. An acquired hernia occurs sometime after birth, and is usually traumatic or iatrogenic in origin, although some may be degenerative.

Table 25-1 Definition of common terms used in relation to hernias

Term	Comments
Hernia	Protrusion of an organ, in whole or in part through a defect in the wall of the anatomical cavity within which it normally lies. The terms 'hernia' and 'rupture' are not synonymous, although for certain conditions they are used interchangeably e.g., diaphragmatic hernia/ diaphragmatic rupture or perineal hernia/perineal rupture
True hernia	Consists of a *hernia ring/defect* and a *hernia sac*, which contains the hernia contents
False hernia	Does not necessarily imply the presence of either a hernia ring or sac
Hernia defect or ring	This may be a normal opening such as the inguinal ring; an iatrogenic opening such as with incisional hernia; or an abnormal defect as in prepubic tendon avulsion
Hernia sac	This is a thin serosal lining surrounding and covering the contents of the hernia. In the case of abdominal hernias this lining will be peritoneum. There may be additional layers of muscle, fascia and skin outside the hernia sac depending on the location and type of hernia
Incisional hernia	This occurs when surgical closure of any body cavity fails or disrupts

Contents

A hernia is *reducible* when its contents lack adhesions, are freely moveable and can be readily manipulated back into the anatomic cavity from whence they came. If hernia contents cannot be replaced readily then it is considered *non-reducible*. *Incarceration* occurs when adhesions form between the hernia contents and surrounding structures, such as between intestinal loops and the body wall in inguinal hernias. *Strangulation* occurs when vascular supply to structures within the hernia is compromised. This can be from direct compression on viscera/vessels; torsion of a long vascular pedicle; or contraction of the hernia ring around the contents.

DIAGNOSIS AND GENERAL CONSIDERATIONS

The diagnostic approach to an abdominal hernia starts with a thorough history and clinical examination, but thereafter is largely dictated by the specific type of hernia present.

Physical examination

Initial observation should cover the animal's demeanor, mentation and gait, hydration, and nutritional state. A thorough systematic examination of all core elements should always be performed. Gentle abdominal palpation may assist in identifying organomegaly, displacement of organs, or localizing pain, although in painful or obese patients palpation may be unrewarding. If there is pain in response to palpating the hernia this can suggest ischemic damage or excessive pressure accumulation, while color changes over the skin surface may reflect deeper vascular compromise or inflammation secondary to fat or other tissue necrosis. Gastrointestinal signs such as anorexia or vomiting may develop with entrapment of intestinal loops, or urinary tract obstruction with post-renal azotemia where the bladder is involved. Rectal examination is essential if there is any suspicion of perineal hernia.

Further comments specific to each type of abdominal hernia follow later in this chapter.

Laboratory tests

Laboratory tests will not specifically diagnose the presence of a hernia, but they may form an important part of assessment and planning or provide a baseline against which to assess postoperative progress. The extent of testing required preoperatively will obviously depend both on the patient and the presenting complaint. A young animal in good health undergoing an elective surgery will require less testing than one due to undergo a more complex procedure, or an emergency procedure.[7]

Diagnostic imaging

For patients with uncomplicated, small, reducible hernias, routine abdominal imaging is unlikely to be of significant benefit unless there is a specific indication, e.g., checking for peritoneopericardial hernia with a supraumbilical defect. If the history and/or physical examination are suspicious for entrapment or strangulation of organs within hernia sacs, then ultrasound examination is most likely to be helpful. Plain and contrast radiography may be useful in specific cases, such as where bladder involvement is suspected (Fig. 25-3). Where traumatic body wall ruptures are encountered, further imaging is always warranted to investigate not only the abdominal injury but also concurrent pathologies such as possible pulmonary contusions, pneumothorax or orthopedic injuries. Advanced imaging modalities such as CT or MRI can provide excellent levels of detail, and a CT scan is strongly recommended for investigation of traumatic abdominal wall hernias in humans.[8] These modalities are unlikely to be necessary for routine investigation of abdominal hernias in veterinary patients unless the hernia is traumatic and concurrent neurological injury is suspected.

UMBILICAL HERNIAS

These are usually congenital, and are often identified as inconsequential findings during routine pre-vaccination examination. The abdominal wall develops from migration of the cephalic, caudal and lateral folds, with the umbilical aperture remaining as a normal defect after migration and fusion of the folds.[8] Umbilical vessels, the vitelline duct, and the stalk of the allantois pass through this umbilical ring in the fetus, but the opening should close at birth, leaving the umbilical cicatrix. If the aperture fails to contract, is excessively large or improperly formed, then a hernia may result. Umbilical hernias are usually congenital and are thought to be inherited. The Cornish Rex breed is listed as over-represented for umbilical hernias although this is largely based on a high incidence that was reported within one family.[9] Umbilical hernias should not be confused with congenital cranial abdominal hernias or supraumbilical hernias, which can be associated with peritoneopericardial hernia. Two reports have documented the incidence of congenital hernias per 1000 cats as between 1.43–1.66 (umbilical) and 0.25–0.2 (inguinal);[10,11] however, these

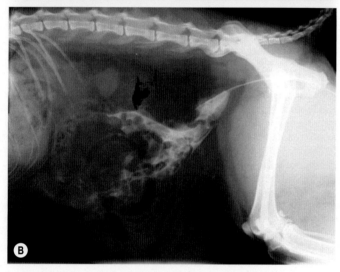

Figure 25-3 Plain and contrast radiography can be useful for identifying specific injuries. **(A)** In this case the plain films show loss of the ventral abdominal wall line with loops of small intestine outside the normal confines of the body wall. **(B)** The ruptured bladder/urethra is not, however, evident without administration of contrast.

reports reflect the hospital population in the US and Canada in the early 1970s and may not be generally applicable. Acquired umbilical hernias may result from excessive traction during assisted parturition, or from clamping and severing the umbilical vessels too close to the body wall.

Omphaloceles are large midline umbilical and skin defects that result in evisceration of abdominal organs. Most affected neonates either die or are euthanized at birth. Attempted repair has been reported in a litter of five-day-old kittens; however, treatment was unsuccessful as the abdominal wall was too thin and fragile to hold sutures.[12] Gastroschisis (this is a congenital defect characterized by a defect in the abdominal wall through which the abdominal contents freely protrude) may appear similar to an omphalocele, but the condition is paramedian rather than midline. It has been reported only rarely in cats, and typically results in early neonatal death.[13]

Physical findings

Umbilical hernias are usually identified soon after birth, unless the defect is very small. A very small hernia ring that contains only

falciform fat is unlikely to cause major problems in the short term, allowing repair to be postponed until the patient is older (Fig. 25-4). If, however, the defect is large enough to allow herniation of intestinal loops or this is already happening then the hernia should be addressed regardless of age. In dogs there is a known association between umbilical hernia and cryptorchidism; similar information is not available for cats but the presence of other concurrent congenital anomalies should be carefully evaluated as these may affect prognosis as well as an owner's willingness to treat.

Treatment and surgical techniques

It is recommended not to correct umbilical hernias in puppies less than 6 months of age as there is potential for delayed closure up to this time; no similar recommendations are available for kittens.[14] The surgical technique is described in Box 25-1.

Aftercare and prognosis

Following repair of an uncomplicated umbilical hernia, the prognosis is excellent, with recurrence being uncommon and aftercare being as for any routine elective abdominal surgery. Where there is an incarcerated or strangulated hernia, then the aftercare and monitoring required may be intensive and the prognosis accordingly will be more guarded.

INGUINAL AND FEMORAL HERNIAS

Inguinal hernias may be either indirect or direct. Indirect inguinal or scrotal hernias occur when hernia contents pass through the hernia ring to lie within the cavity of the vaginal tunic. In male dogs these hernias are particularly associated with incarceration, strangulation, and organ dysfunction because of compression. This condition has not yet been reported in a cat. Anatomic dissections in female cats have confirmed that there is no vaginal process present; the literature is vague on the subject in male cats but anecdotal information suggests that a vaginal tunic exists similar to that seen in the dog. The apparent rarity of scrotal hernia in the cat may merely reflect the differing anatomic arrangement of external genitalia between the two species. Direct hernias exist where the hernia contents pass through the hernia ring but then lie adjacent to the cavity of the vaginal tunic and are not compressed by it. These hernias tend to be large and are less prone to incarceration and strangulation. Inguinal hernias are rare in cats and whether they are inherited is unknown.

In dogs the contents of inguinal hernias can include omentum, fat, ovaries, uterus, small intestine, colon, bladder, and spleen.[15] There are only 16 cases of feline inguinal hernia reported in the literature, and other than one case report with bladder herniation the contents of the inguinal hernias were not reported specifically.[11,16,17] In the case report in question, both inguinal canals were apparently larger than normal, at 20 mm for the left and 25 mm for the right. This was based on measurements obtained by the authors from ten cats undergoing surgery for reasons unrelated to inguinal hernia, which suggested an average 5 mm diameter.

Congenital inguinal hernias in dogs are more common in males than females, possibly due to delayed inguinal ring narrowing associated with testicular descent,[18,19] while acquired inguinal hernias are far more common in females, associated with estrogen levels. It is commonly thought that in cats there is no sex or breed predilection,[12] but reported numbers are too low for meaningful conclusions to be drawn. Contributing factors for inguinal hernia may include

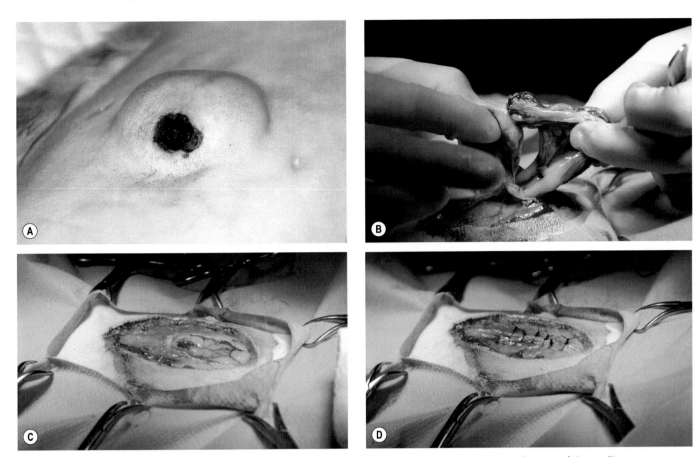

Figure 25-4 (A) A large umbilical hernia in an adult cat that developed an area of ulceration on the most ventral aspect of the swelling.
(B) Adhesions were present between the ulcerated area and the falciform fat. **(C)** The hernia was resected and **(D)** closed with simple interrupted sutures of polydioxanone.

Box 25-1 **Umbilical hernia repair**

The patient is positioned in dorsal recumbency with the legs gently extended caudally.

Many umbilical hernias will be corrected at the time of other elective surgery, often ovariohysterectomy. If this is the case then the ventral midline abdominal incision is continued cranially to encompass the hernia.

The hernia sac is bluntly dissected free of surrounding skin and either removed following ligation across the neck of the hernia sac or inverted within the abdomen prior to abdominal wall closure. Umbilical hernias are repaired with tension-relieving suture patterns such as the horizontal mattress, using heavy gauge synthetic monofilament sutures such as polydioxanone, nylon or polypropylene.

Large umbilical hernias containing abdominal viscera require a more extensive surgical approach, with the skin incision usually following an elliptical shape around the base of the hernia to remove redundant skin, taking care not to resect so much skin that wound closure is

difficult. If adhesions are present they are carefully broken down, and any tissues that show devitalization are debrided.

If the hernia is incarcerated it may be necessary to carefully enlarge the hernia ring along the linea alba to facilitate treatment.

In rare cases umbilical hernias may be associated with large defects in the abdominal wall, such that primary closure is not possible. Although tension-relieving techniques for local myofascial tissues are described,[14] the author's preference is to use prosthetic mesh for such cases. If the hernia is supraumbilical, and associated with a diaphragmatic defect, then the diaphragmatic defect should be closed first, followed by closure of the midline defect as described previously. Any associated sternal defects should preferably be reconstructed with orthopedic wire of a suitable diameter to ensure rigid stability, although the use of heavy gauge monofilament suture material has also been described.[14]

---

weakening of the abdominal wall structures from nutritional or metabolic problems, and obesity.[14]

Femoral hernias occur through a defect in the femoral canal. They are considered uncommon in humans[20] and there are only anecdotal citings in both dogs and cats.[13,14] The femoral canal is in the caudal abdominal wall just lateral to the inguinal ligament, and consists

of a muscular lacuna (containing the femoral nerve within the substance of the iliopsoas muscle) and a vascular lacuna (containing the femoral artery and vein and saphenous nerve). Femoral hernia may be confused with inguinal hernia; however, the two may also occur together. One study of 258 people identified an almost 50% incidence of concurrent femoral and inguinal hernia.[20] It has been suggested that femoral hernias in small animals are usually acquired, secondary to trauma (associated with prepubic tendon rupture) or surgery (pectineus myectomy in dogs), although there is no evidence to support this.[14]

Physical findings

The most common presentation and history is that of a painless, soft swelling in the inguinal ring, although if contents are strangulated then the patient can present with vomiting, depression, abdominal pain, and evidence of sepsis. In one study of inguinal hernia in 35 dogs, vomiting of two to six days' duration was predictive for intestinal necrosis.[19] If the gravid uterus or the urinary bladder is involved in the hernia then the swelling may be large, fluctuant and painful on palpation, or may be associated with hematuria or vaginal bleeding. Reduction of hernia contents (unless incarcerated) and palpation of the femoral and inguinal rings is facilitated by laying the patient in dorsal recumbency then elevating the hindquarters. Even if a hernia appears, unilateral careful palpation of the contralateral side is advisable to avoid missing a small or occult hernia. When palpating suspected hernias over the medial thigh, inguinal hernias are typically identified craniomedial to the pelvic brim, whereas a femoral hernia should be located ventrolateral to the pelvic brim. If the suspected hernia cannot be reduced then palpation alone is unlikely to be sufficient to differentiate femoral from inguinal hernia.

Treatment and surgical techniques

Inguinal hernias should be repaired as soon as they are diagnosed, as delayed treatment increases the risk of complications. Surgical repair mandates good knowledge of anatomy, to ensure appropriate suture placement and high hernia sac ligation. Straightforward inguinal hernias can be managed by a direct approach, but large or complicated hernias such as those with incarceration or following abdominal trauma should be managed through a combination of an abdominal approach and a direct approach over the hernia (Box 25-2).

The abdominal approach for repair has the advantage of familiarity for most surgeons, and where there is a complicated hernia it can provide better exposure and access (Box 25-2).

Aftercare and prognosis

Seroma or hematoma formation is the most common complication of inguinal hernia repair, typically from inadequate hemostasis or excessive tissue handling during surgery, complicated by the high motion nature of the site. Exercise restriction and wound hygiene are important after surgery, and gentle massage with warm compresses may help to reduce fluid retention. Entrapment of neurovascular structures passing through the canal will cause obvious pain postoperatively, and in people a chronic pain syndrome is well recognized as a complication of inguinal and femoral hernia repair.[20]

As with all hernias, strangulation and incarceration can have a significant adverse effect on prognosis. A complication rate of 17% was described in one report of 35 dogs, with a 3% mortality rate.[19] Peritonitis, sepsis, incisional infection, and recurrence of hernia were responsible for most of the complications. There is little information available regarding success rates, complications, or prognosis for cats with inguinal or femoral hernias. Anecdotally, pelvic limb swelling due to edema is common after surgery for femoral hernia and should be self-limiting within five to seven days unless there is iatrogenic obstruction to lymphatic and venous drainage, in which case revision surgery is needed. Nerve entrapment or compression is possible within the hernia repair, and will cause postoperative pain and/or femoral nerve deficits.[14]

Box 25-2 Repair of inguinal and femoral hernias

Depending on the intended procedure, the patient may be positioned in either dorsal or lateral recumbency, although most surgeons prefer to work with the patient in dorsal recumbency without caudal traction applied to the hind limbs. Complicated hernias or those with incarceration or strangulation should be approached both intra- and extra-abdominally.

An incision is made over the lateral aspect of the swelling, roughly parallel to the flank fold. The hernia sac is carefully separated from attachments to skin and subcutis using blunt dissection, and if possible the contents are reduced through the inguinal canal by direct gentle pressure and manipulation. If the contents are non-reducible then the hernia sac is opened and dissection continued to the entrance of the inguinal canal to be enlarged. This should be done in a craniomedial direction, taking care to avoid traumatizing tissues that will be required for closure.

Once the hernia contents have been reduced, the hernia sac is ligated as close to the internal inguinal ring as possible, and the sac is resected. Sutures of synthetic monofilament material such as polydioxanone, nylon or polypropylene are placed through the parietal peritoneum, the aponeurosis of the transversalis, the IAO muscle and the RA to close the hernia.

Inguinal hernia

The majority of inguinal hernias can be closed using the patient's own tissues without the necessity for prosthetic mesh. The use of the cranial sartorius muscle with synthetic mesh has been reported for reconstruction of large chronic caudal abdominal defects in two cats[21] and may be considered as an alternative.

If the inguinal ligament is intact, the hernia may be closed by placing sutures of synthetic monofilament material between the inguinal ligament and the pectineus fascia.

If the inguinal ring is enlarged or damaged, synthetic monofilament sutures can be placed between the inguinal ligament, external rectus fascia and the IAO muscle to close it to approximately 5 mm diameter.[17]

Femoral hernia

The approach to a femoral hernia is similar to that for inguinal hernia repair. Good knowledge of regional anatomy is essential to avoid iatrogenic trauma and allow appropriate suture placement.

TRAUMATIC ABDOMINAL HERNIAS

The most common causes of traumatic abdominal wall hernias (TAWH) are vehicular trauma, and animal bite injuries, most often involving the caudoventral abdominal wall and paracostal area.

In one report of traumatic abdominal hernias only 18% of feline hernias were due to dog-bite wounds;[22] however, a subsequent report identified a 40% incidence.[23] This difference may merely have been a reflection of the different patient populations seen by the two centers in question. TAWH are thought to have a relatively low incidence overall, with one report of 600 vehicular accidents documenting only two TAWH, and another of 123 cats with high rise syndrome injuries again identifying only two.[24,25]

It has been postulated that pressure from blunt force trauma must be distributed over a relatively large surface area in order to prevent penetration of the relatively elastic skin, yet cause disruption of deeper less elastic tissues such as muscle and fascia (Fig. 25-5). TAWH may also result from shearing forces across bony prominences such as the

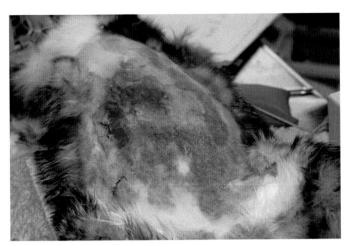

Figure 25-5 Where blunt force trauma is distributed over a relatively large area of the abdominal wall, it is possible to see rupture of deeper muscle and fascial structures with the overlying skin and subcutis remaining intact. This can mean that on external examination all that is present is severe extensive bruising without immediate evidence of penetrating wounds or disruption of the abdominal wall.

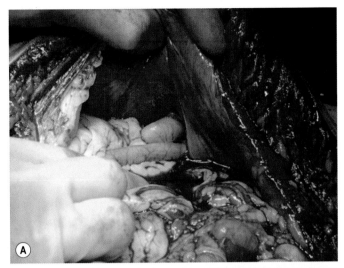

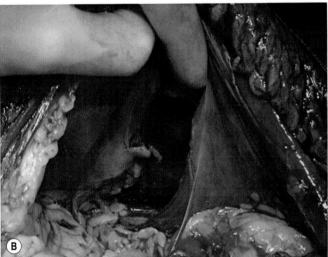

Figure 25-6 These pictures were taken intraoperatively from the patient shown in Figure 25-3. The muscular layers of the abdominal wall show a longitudinal tear through which intestinal loops and omentum have herniated to lie beneath the panniculus muscle and skin.

pelvis or the caudal rib cage, which tear muscle/tendon away from bone.[26,27] Where TAWH is caused by an animal bite wound the hernia is likely to be complicated by contamination, infection, devitalization, and hemorrhage. Animal bite wounds often involve trauma to internal organs, including perforation of the gastrointestinal tract, and these cases will require emergency surgical intervention as soon as stabilized.

When there is blunt abdominal trauma in the presence of a closed glottis, hernias result from rupture of the wall from within-out, because intra-abdominal pressure rises rapidly while abdominal muscles are still contracted (Fig. 25-6). If pressure is applied while the glottis is open, then the rise in intra-abdominal pressure is limited and avulsion-type injuries are more likely, such as prepubic tendon avulsion or traumatic inguinal hernia.[14] Paracostal hernias occur when the origin of the EAO and transversus abdominis muscle separate from their rib or costal cartilage attachments. Paracostal hernia has been associated with diaphragmatic rupture in people[28] and it has been suggested that it is more common in cats than in dogs. TAWH associated with pelvic fracture gaps have occasionally been reported in dogs but not in cats.[29,30] In most cases with prepubic tendon rupture there is either partial or complete avulsion of the tendinous attachments from the iliopubic eminence, although occasional cases are caused by rupture of the musculotendinous junction.

Unlike congenital hernias, traumatic hernias do not typically have a peritoneal lining although chronic cases may demonstrate 'peritonealization'. It has been suggested that TAWH may be more prone to adhesion formation and incarceration due to this absence of a serosal lined hernia sac, although this does not seem to be borne out by clinical experience.[14]

Physical findings

The most obvious manifestation of TAWH is visible swelling or abdominal asymmetry. Depending on the location of the hernia, viscera may move subcutaneously under the influence of gravity post-herniation, in which case the location of the swelling may not be the same as the location of the hernia. Movements that increase abdominal pressure through contraction, such as coughing or vomiting, may cause the size of the swelling to increase transiently, while progressive

steady enlargement is more likely to reflect secondary obstruction. Prepubic tendon ruptures are often associated with pelvic fractures, and sometimes concurrent inguinal and/or femoral hernia.

In many cases the clinical signs of TAWH are non-specific and for this reason they can be overlooked initially.[4,31] In some cases, despite diagnostic evaluation, the diagnosis of prepubic hernia may not be made until surgery is performed for exploration and management of other associated abdominal injuries.[4] The presence and exact site of an abdominal wall rupture can be very difficult to identify on initial clinical examination due to the combination of local tissue swelling and pain, so where there is a reasonable index of suspicion physical examination should be combined with appropriate diagnostic imaging, bearing in mind that ultrasound is likely to be more rewarding than plain radiography. Partial thickness body wall ruptures are a particular challenge to diagnose.

As a general rule, acute traumatic hernias will be painful, and are usually reducible, at least to some extent. Clipping the hair coat will facilitate recognition of bruising and other wounds, which may help with localization. Chronic hernias in comparison are often not painful, and may no longer be reducible.

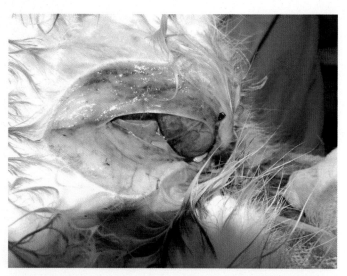

Figure 25-7 This cat was the victim of an animal bite injury from a fox, resulting in extensive skin lacerations as well as a full thickness abdominal wall rupture with the bladder lying in an exposed subcutaneous position. In this case the result was partial obstruction of the bladder neck in addition to the traumatic injuries received.

Treatment and surgical techniques

Acute trauma cases require rapid evaluation for life-threatening problems and stabilization of cardiopulmonary function. A penetrating or impaling abdominal wound, evidence of intra-abdominal trauma, or a patient that does not respond to stabilization are all indications for emergency surgery (Fig. 25-7). In these cases, priority is given to dealing with organ damage, displacement, or dysfunction unless the hernia is directly contributing to the emergent problem. If the patient is stable and the hernia is not associated with any breaks or devitalization in overlying skin, then conservative management for several days may be warranted to allow conditions such as myocardial or pulmonary contusions to resolve. With prepubic hernias the defect that results is usually very large, and therefore the incidence of incarceration and strangulation is quite low, meaning that repair can usually be safely delayed for several days if required.[14] There is no firm agreement regarding the optimal timing of surgery for non-emergency TAWH. Some surgeons favor waiting three to five days to allow revascularization and reduction in inflammation,[14] while others prefer to operate as soon as the patient is stable to avoid further problems.[13]

A large area should be clipped and prepared for aseptic surgery, particularly with acute hernias where the exact location and number of defects in the abdominal wall may be difficult to pinpoint and full abdominal exploration is required. Such cases should be approached by a standard midline celiotomy that facilitates repair of multiple TAWH, e.g., animal bite injuries, and allows management of concurrent intra-abdominal injuries. With chronic hernias it may be appropriate to make an approach directly over the site of the hernia provided there is no other damage present.

Muscle, fat, fascia, and dermal tissues that are clearly devitalized are carefully debrided around the hernia, and all foreign material identified and removed. Hernias that result from sharp injuries without significant tissue loss can usually be closed primarily following copious sterile lavage. Where the hernia results from blunt trauma there may be extensive bruising, but usually little tissue loss, and again primary closure should be feasible. Where the injury is caused by a high velocity injury or animal bite injury, there is typically more extensive tissue trauma, with bruising, contamination, and often marked tissue loss. Wherever possible, the defect is closed using the

Box 25-3 **Prepubic hernia repair**

It is important to position the patient correctly to facilitate a tension-free repair; this can be achieved either through standard dorsal recumbency without caudal traction applied to the hind limbs, or in a modified dorsal recumbency where the hind limbs are actively flexed and pulled cranially.[14] The disadvantage to this latter approach is that it does not mimic natural body position in a conscious patient, so what appears to be a relatively tension-free repair in modified recumbency may come under significant pressure once the patient is awake. The initial approach is by ventral midline celiotomy so that assessment of damaged, devitalized or malpositioned organs can take place first, and only then should the herniorrhaphy be performed (Fig. 25-8). In cats it is important to check the crura of the superficial inguinal ring and the aponeurosis of the EAO muscle in addition to the lateral margins of the prepubic tendon. If there are concurrent inguinal or femoral hernias present then the prepubic tendon rupture should be addressed first in order to restore normal topography. The femoral artery and vein and the genitofemoral nerve should be identified within the femoral triangle and protected during hernia repair.

A tension-relieving suture pattern such as the horizontal or cruciate mattress suture should be used, with a synthetic monofilament non-absorbable suture such as polypropylene or nylon. Absorbable monofilament sutures such as polydioxanone can be used but it has been suggested that despite providing reliable wound support for up to six weeks after surgery polydioxanone may not retain sufficient tensile strength to support healing of a prepubic rupture.[32] Absorbable sutures such as poliglecaprone 25 or polyglactin 910 should not be used as they lose most of their tensile strength within two to three weeks, while muscle fascia takes approximately three weeks to regain even 20% of its original strength and up to a year to regain 80% of pre-injury strength.[32] Nylon will retain 81% of its tensile strength at one year and 72% at two years, while polypropylene is not significantly degraded within the body and will therefore maintain almost all of its tensile strength at two years.

Holes are predrilled through the cranial brim of the pubis to allow passage of secure sutures without excessive soft tissue dissection. This is recommended even where it appears that there may be sufficient tissue attached to the brim of the pelvis to allow direct tissue apposition as the holding power of injured tendon is questionable. In the cat, sutures are placed through the fascia of the EAO and then through the holes in the pubis, unlike in the dog where sutures are placed through the avulsed prepubic tendon first. All sutures are preplaced to facilitate placement and subsequent closure. Once all sutures are tied, the linea alba can be closed as normal.

patient's own tissues as vascularized autogenous tissue is far more likely to survive without medium- or long-term complications in an infected or contaminated environment than with a prosthetic mesh.

Many variations in surgical technique for prepubic hernia repair have been described; the most common method is the only one that will be discussed in detail here (Box 25-3).[4]

Other techniques for repair of prepubic tendon rupture include the *obturator foramen suture placement method*, whereby sutures are passed through the obturator foramina rather than predrilling holes, and the use of a *cranial sartorius muscle flap*.[14] The risk with the obturator foramen technique is that if any soft tissues are caught under the suture loops, then fixation will loosen as the sutures progressively cut through these tissues down to bone. The cranial sartorius muscle flap was first described in dogs,[33] and then subsequently in cats for prepubic tendon ruptures.[21] To use it in this way the muscle flap must be

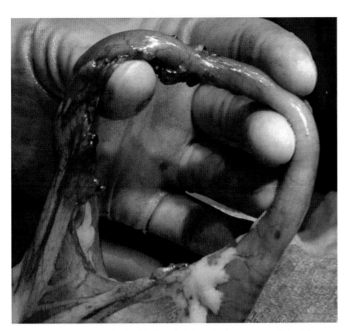

Figure 25-8 Severe intestinal ischemic injury is demonstrated in this case following a penetrating abdominal wound, which resulted in avulsion of the mesenteric blood supply from a 6 cm length of jejunum amongst other injuries. Intervention for this injury should be prioritized, as it is potentially and imminently life threatening.

rotated through 180°, and then secured with sutures. This technique may be useful if there is a large defect or very little tendon left for reconstruction, but there is the risk of devitalization following rotation. In both the reported cats, there was abdominal bulging at the flap site long term although not at the adjacent prosthetic mesh which was used in each case. This may reflect a difference in muscle fiber types between the sartorius (type II) and the postural abdominal muscles (type I), or denervation atrophy, both of which could lead to weaker support. This weakness was not associated with recurrence of herniation in either case.

The use of synthetic mesh is indicated where there is excessive tension along the suture line when using autogenous tissues alone. Either a mesh cuff, or a double layer mesh onlay can be used to augment any of the aforementioned techniques.

Porcine small intestinal submucosa (SIS) has been described for repair of perineal hernias and its use has been suggested to augment prepubic tendon repair.[4] However, the expected pressure that might be brought to bear on a prepubic tendon repair is quite different to that within a perineal hernia, and there is currently no evidence to show whether porcine SIS can actually provide adequate support in this location.

It is usually unnecessary to place wound drains in prepubic hernia repairs, and the potential for additional complications should be carefully weighed against their likely benefit before using them.

The failure rate for prepubic tendon repair is approximately 15%, and in the majority of cases morbidity and mortality are related to concurrent abdominal or musculoskeletal injuries. Complications directly relating to the prepubic tendon repair include urethral entrapment within sutures and wound infection.

Treatment: conservative management

Conservative management has been documented in two cats for prepubic tendon rupture[31] due to concurrent open wound management.

There are obvious risks involved in choosing not to manage this type of injury surgically, however, and it is very difficult to recommend a non-surgical approach as standard.

PERINEAL HERNIA

Perineal hernia is relatively uncommon in cats, and in contrast to dogs the available information suggests that the condition is more common in neutered than intact animals.[34–37] Bilateral herniation is more common than unilateral, and in many cases there are pre-existing medical problems that could increase the risk of perineal hernia, or a history of trauma.[35–37] Conditions associated with perineal hernia include feline urologic syndrome requiring perineal urethrostomy, megacolon, perineal masses, chronic fibrosing colitis,[34,35] and cutaneous asthesia.[36]

Contents of perineal hernias most often include rectal sacculation or dilation, fluid, connective tissue, and retroperitoneal fat that may contain small nodules and cystic structures. Rectal sacculation implies expansion into a unilateral hernia, and dilation a bilateral expansion. Flexure or deviation implies rectal herniation into the hernia and is uncommon. Many perineal hernias are covered with a mesothelial membrane, but it is not known whether this represents a true peritoneal outpouching, or peritonealization as seen with chronic traumatic hernias.[38]

Physical findings

A visible perineal swelling may be present together with a history of straining and constipation, but in many of the reported cats there were no clinical signs prior to development of a perineal bulge.[34] Where bladder retroflexion exists, then signs of dysuria and urinary tract obstruction will be present, and the case should be treated as an emergency. If perineal hernia develops subsequent to trauma, then triage and stabilization may be necessary as discussed in the section covering TAWH. Other clinical signs will vary depending on the presence of predisposing or concurrent conditions.

Given how many cats have additional medical problems, a thorough history and a comprehensive physical examination including rectal examination are mandatory. Routine hematology and serum biochemistry plus abdominal imaging are advisable in every case and in some cases additional lab tests such as fecal parasitology and bacteriology should be carried out.

Treatment and surgical techniques

Medical and dietary measures should be viewed as an adjunct to surgical management, and not the preferred treatment option. Without surgery, conservative measures will only temporarily control the clinical signs, while allowing the condition to progress.

There are several techniques described for perineal hernia repair, of which those described in cats include the anatomical reduction technique, the internal obturator muscle flap (IOMF) and the semitendinosis muscle flap (SMF).[34–38] The IOMF is now widely considered the standard technique for perineal hernia repair in dogs.[38]

Some surgeons recommend administering enemas up to 12 hours prior to surgery; however, the author does not favor this approach as any residual fecal material will form liquid slurry that increases the risk of surgical site contamination. Digital evacuation of fecal material within the terminal rectum followed by placement of a rectal plug or tampon, and/or a purse-string suture will maintain a satisfactorily clean surgical field.

Whether it is necessary to neuter patients that are intact at the time of repair is not at all clear in cats. In dogs, it is well accepted that failure to neuter male animals results in a significantly higher risk of recurrence,[38] but no such information exists for cats.

If the anatomic reduction technique is used, surgeons should bear in mind that the cat has no sacrotuberous ligament to incorporate in the repair and the perineal muscles of cats are considerably less substantial than those of dogs. Sutures are placed between the external anal sphincter (EAS) medially, the levator ani (LA) and coccygeus (CO) muscles dorsally, and the internal obturator muscle (IOM) ventrally.[38] In dogs, the use of this technique is associated with a higher failure rate than the IOMF, but the small numbers and lack of detailed description in reported feline cases mean comparable information is not available.

The technique for the IOMF is essentially identical to that described for the dog and is described in Box 25-4.[38]

The *semitendinosis muscle flap* (SMF) was initially described in 1991[39] and specifically for ventral perineal hernias in dogs in 2007.[40] There is only one report to date of the use of this technique in a cat.[37] In this case the semitendinosus (ST) was dissected and transected at its midbelly, and then rotated to the ventral perineum. The authors used the right ST to repair a left sided hernia, with the original medial border of the ST sutured to the ventral border of the EAS, and the original lateral border sutured to the ventral aspects of the IOM, LA

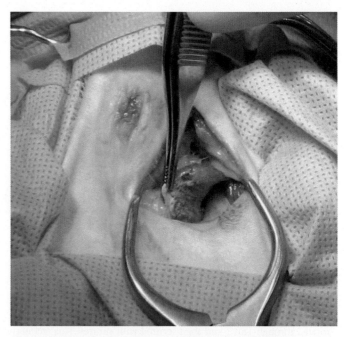

Figure 25-9 The internal obturator muscle should be elevated subperiosteally in order to ensure maximum hold for sutures. Relative to dogs, the internal obturator muscle in cats often seems to be a more robust structure with a large muscle belly.

Box 25-4 Perineal hernia repair using an internal obturator muscle flap

The cat is placed in sternal recumbancy with the tail pulled cranially and the hind limbs suspended over the edge of the table. Care should be taken to ensure that good padding is placed between the hind limbs and the table to reduce the risk of neuropraxia or muscle damage postoperatively. Either a purse-string suture or anal plug is used to prevent fecal contamination during surgery, and both anal sacs should be emptied and flushed as part of aseptic preparation.

A skin incision is made from the tail base to just medial to the ischial tuberosity, and the hernia sac opened carefully by blunt dissection. Great care must be taken to identify the internal pudendal artery and vein, the pudendal nerve and its branch, the caudal rectal nerve. These typically lie in the ventral part of the hernia sac but may be displaced by adhesions in chronic cases. The motor supply to the external anal sphincter (EAS) must be preserved in order to avoid postoperative fecal incontinence. The EAS, the rectum, the levator ani (LA) and coccygeus (CO) muscles are identified. A sharp incision is made in the periosteum along the dorsocaudal border of the ischial tuberosity to allow subperiosteal elevation of the IOM (Fig. 25-9). A common technical error is failure to elevate the entire muscle, leaving the medial and lateral borders firmly attached to the ischium, thereby limiting the degree of mobilization possible. The IOM may be elevated as far as the caudal margin of the obturator foramen, taking care not to damage the ischiourethralis muscle. If required, the tendon of insertion can be transected where it passes lateral to the ischium to allow greater movement, but in the author's experience this is rarely necessary and carries an increased risk of damage to the pudendal and sciatic nerves. Once the IOM has been satisfactorily elevated, sutures are preplaced between it and the LA/CO; the IOM and the EAS; and the EAS and the LA/CO. A synthetic monofilament suture such as polydioxanone, nylon or polypropylene should be used, and all sutures are preplaced then closed sequentially from dorsal to ventral (Fig. 25-10). The hernia repair is palpated for any areas of weakness or defects, which can be closed with additional sutures as needed. Despite the fact that elevation of the IOM leaves a visible space over the ischial tuberosity, placement of drains is not required and will increase the risk of postoperative complications and infection. Following apposition of subcutaneous tissues the skin incision can be closed with either skin sutures or a buried intradermal suture. Where there are bilateral hernias it is routine practice to repair both simultaneously, although some surgeons prefer to stage the procedures a few weeks apart.

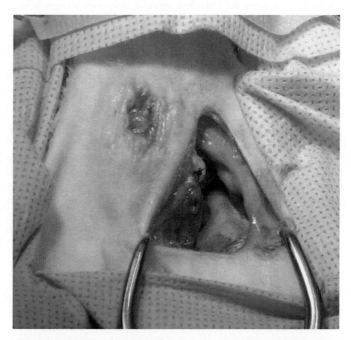

Figure 25-10 Once elevated the internal obturator muscle is secured in position by means of sutures placed between it and the levator ani, coccygeus, and external anal sphincter. As a general rule fewer sutures are required to achieve a secure herniorrhaphy than are required when using the same technique in dogs.

and CO muscles. The distal end of the muscle flap was secured to the dorsal part of the LA and CO muscles. A concurrent left sided perineal hernia was not repaired; however, despite this, at follow up one year later there were no recorded problems with defecation.

Needless to say, regardless of technique selected, it is vital to remember to remove the purse-string suture and the rectal plug/tampon after surgery! It is good practice to make a note on the anesthetic record, or write a reminder on adhesive tape stuck to the patient's head, to ensure that this is not forgotten.

Bladder retroflexion with perineal hernia is unusual in cats,[35] but where present a ventral midline celiotomy approach should be made first to allow repositioning of the bladder without torsion. Cystopexy has been recommended to prevent recurrence of displacement. The use of additional techniques recommended in dogs with large or recurrent perineal hernia, such as colopexy and vas deferensopexy has not been reported in cats.[38] The author has, however, encountered two young cats with bilateral perineal hernias and recurrent severe rectal prolapse, which were treated with a combination of bilateral IOMF transposition and colopexy (Fig. 25-11). The use of porcine SIS, fascia lata grafts and synthetic mesh to augment hernia repair has yet to be reported in cats.[38,41,42]

Aftercare and prognosis

Broad-spectrum antibiotic prophylaxis is recommended for the immediate perioperative period, and antibiotic cover is typically continued for five to seven days after surgery. The use of stool softeners and/or laxatives such as psyllium or lactulose is based on individual surgeon preference, as is the type of diet recommended postoperatively. The surgical site should be kept clean to reduce the risk of contamination and infection, and an Elizabethan collar or similar used to prevent licking and self-trauma, which is a significant problem following perineal surgery.

The prognosis is generally good following repair of perineal hernia in cats, with a 73% success rate for bilateral perineal hernia repair in

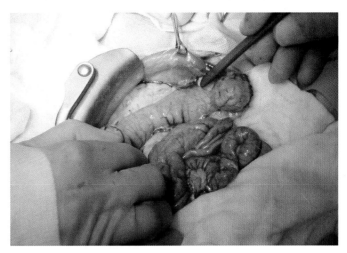

Figure 25-11 Colopexy has been described as part of the treatment for large or severe perineal hernias in dogs, and for management of recurrent rectal prolapse in cats. The cat in this picture had a history of severe recurrent rectal prolapse and also had large bilateral perineal hernia. The colopexy was specifically included for management of rectal prolapse, but may also contribute in such a case to prevent recurrence of perineal herniation.

one study,[34] and successful outcomes recorded in case reports by other authors.[35-37]

In dogs, factors that influence recurrence include surgeon competence, failure to neuter, follow-up time (recurrence rates are greater after the first year) and the number of times hernia repair has been attempted.[38] Whether some or all of these factors are also relevant to feline perineal hernia is unknown as the numbers documented are too small for meaningful analysis. Intuitively, it seems likely that factors such as the length of follow up, surgeon competence and number of attempted repairs may be important.

REFERENCES

1. Dyce KM, Sack WO, Wensing CJG. The locomotor apparatus. In: Textbook of Veterinary Anatomy. 1st ed. Philadelphia: W.B. Saunders Company; 1987. p. 51–5.

2. Crouch JE, Lackey MB. In: Text-Atlas of Cat Anatomy. Philadelphia: Lea and Febiger; 1969. p. 177.

3. Martin WD, Fletcher TF, Bradley WE.. Perineal musculature in the cat. Anatom Rec 1974;180:3–14.

4. Beittenmiller MR, Mann FA, Constantinescu GM, Luther JK. Clinical anatomy and surgical repair of prepubic hernia in dogs and cats. J Am Animal Hosp Assoc 2009;45:284–90.

5. Beittenmiller MR, Mann FA, Constantinescu IA. Clinical anatomy of the prepubic tendon in the dog and a comparison with the cat. J Exp Med Surg Res 2007;14:79–83.

6. Watson A. Vaginal ring and round ligament of the uterus in the female cat. Anat Hist Embryol 2009;38:319–20.

7. Alef M, von Praun F, Oechtering G. Is routine pre-anaesthetic haematological and biochemical screening justified in dogs? Vet Anaesth Analg 2008;35:132–40.

8. Henrotay J, Honoré C, Meurisse M. Traumatic abdominal wall hernia: case report and review of the literature. Acta Chir Belg 2010;110:471–4.

9. Klein MD, Hertzler JH. Congenital defects of the abdominal wall. Surg Gynecol Obstet 1981;152:805–8.

10. Robinson R. Genetic aspects of umbilical hernia incidence in dogs and cats. Vet Rec 2007;100:9.

11. Priester WA, Glass AG, Waggoner NS. Congenital defects in domesticated animals: general considerations. Am J Vet Res 1970;31:1871–9.

12. Howard DR. Omphalocele in a litter of kittens. Vet Med Small Animal Clin 1973;68:879.

13. Crowe DT, Archibald J. Abdominal wall and cavity. In: Crowe DT, Catcott EJ,

editors. Canine and Feline Surgery, Vol 1. Santa Barbara: American Veterinary Publishers; 1984. p. 23.

14. Smeak DD. Abdominal hernias. In: Slatter DG, editor. Textbook of Small Animal Surgery. 3rd ed. Phildelphia: WB Saunders; 2003. p. 449–71.

15. Bellenger CR. Inguinal and scrotal herniation in 61 dogs. Austr Vet Pract 1996;26:58.

16. Hayes HM. Congenital umbilical and inguinal hernias in cattle, horses, swine, dogs and cats: Risk by breed and sex among hospital patients. Am J Vet Res 1974;35:839.

17. Zulauf D, Voss K, Reichler IM. Herniation of the urinary bladder through a congenitally enlarged inguinal canal in a cat. Schweizer Archiv fur Tierheilkunde 2007;149:559–62.

18. Fox MW. Inherited inguinal hernia and midline defects in the dog. J Am Vet Med Assoc 1963;143:602–4.

19. Waters DJ, Roy RG, Stone EA. A retrospective study of inguinal hernia in 35 dogs. Vet Surg 1993;22:44–9.

20. Chan G, Chan CK. Longterm results of a prospective study of 225 femoral hernia repairs: indications for tissue and mesh repairs. J Am Coll Surg 2008;207:360–6.

21. Sylvestre A, Weinstein MJ, Popovitch C, et al. The Sartorius muscle flap in the cat: an anatomic study and two case reports. J Am Animal Hosp Assoc 1997;33:91–6.

22. Waldron DR, Hedlunh CS, Pechman R. Abdominal hernias in dogs and cats: a review of 24 cases. J Am Animal Hosp Assoc 1986;22:817–22.

23. Shaw SP, Rozanski EA, Rush JE. Traumatic body wall herniation in 36 dogs and Cats. J Am Animal Hosp Assoc 2003;39: 35–46.

24. Kolata RJ, Johnson DE. Motor vehicle accidents in urban dogs: A study of 600 cases. J Am Vet Med Assoc 1975; 167:938.

25. Whitney WO, Mehlhaff CJ. High rise syndrome in cats. J Am Vet Med Assoc 1987;191:1399–403.

26. Damschen DD, Landercasper J, Thomas CH, et al. Acute traumatic abdominal hernia: case reports. J Trauma 1994;36: 273–6.

27. Perez VM, McDonand DA, Ghani A, et al. Handlebar hernia: a rare traumatic abdominal wall hernia. J Trauma 1998;44:568.

28. Dubois PM, Freeman MD. Traumatic abdominal wall hernia. J Trauma 1981;21: 72–4.

29. Dorn AM, Olmstead ML. Herniation of the urinary bladder through the pubic symphisis in a dog. J Am Vet Med Assoc 1976;168:688.

30. Mann FA, Herron MR. What is your diagnosis? J Am Vet Med Assoc 1989;187:955.

31. Friend EJ, White RAS. Rupture of the cranial pubic tendon in the cat. J Small Animal Pract 2002;48:522–5.

32. Boothe HW. Suture materials, tissue adhesives, staplers and ligating clips. In: Slatter DG, editor. Textbook of Small Animal Surgery. 3rd ed. Philadelphia: WB Saunders; 2003;235–43.

33. Weinstein MJ, Pavletic MM, Boudrieau RJ, Engler SJ. Cranial sartorius muscle flap in the dog. Vet Surg 1989;18:286–91.

34. Welches CD, Scavelli TD, Aronsohn MG, et al. Perineal hernia in the cat: a retrospective study of 40 cases. J Am Animal Hosp Assoc 1992;28:431–8.

35. Risselada M, Kramer M, Van de Welde B, et al. Retroflexion of the urinary bladder associated with a perineal hernia in a female cat. J Small Animal Pract 2003;44:508–10.

36. Benitah N, Matousek JL, Barnes RF, et al. Diaphragmatic and perineal hernias associated with cutaneous asthenia in a cat. J Am Vet Med Assoc 2004;5:706–9.

37. Vnuk D, Babic T, Stejskal M, et al. Application of a semitendinosus muscle flap in the treatment of perineal hernia in a cat. Vet Record 2005;156:182–4.

38. Bellenger CR, Canfield RB. Perineal hernia. In: Slatter DG, editor. Textbook of Small Animal Surgery. 3rd ed. Philadelphia: WB Saunders; 2003. p. 487–98.

39. Chambers JN, Rawlings CA. Application of a semitendinosus muscle flap in two dogs. J Am Vet Med Assoc 1981;199: 84–6.

40. Bottcher P, Thiel C, Kramer M, et al. Transposition of the semitendinosus muscle for ventral perineal hernia repair in dogs. Retrospective analysis of six cases (2003–2005). Tierartzle Praxis Kleintiere 2007;2:93–102.

41. Stoll MR, Cook JL, Carson WL, et al. The use of porcine small intestinal submucosa as a biomaterial for perineal herniorrhaphy in the dog. Vet Surg 2002;31:379–90.

42. Bongartz A, Carofiglio F, Balligand M, et al. Use of autogenous fascia lata graft for perineal herniorrhaphy in dogs. Vet Surg 2005;34:405–13.

Chapter | 26 |

Peritoneum

D. Holt, K.A. Agnello

Peritonitis in cats is a serious problem that can often prove fatal. Mild or non-specific clinical signs can delay definitive diagnosis and treatment. Therefore awareness of the possibility of peritonitis, careful examination, and appropriate diagnostic tests are necessary for a timely diagnosis. Even with prompt and aggressive treatment the prognosis for survival is still guarded.

SURGICAL ANATOMY

The peritoneum is a closed cavity that contains all of the abdominal organs except for the kidneys and the adrenal glands. The parietal peritoneum covers the abdominal wall and diaphragm. The visceral peritoneum covers the abdominal organs (Fig. 26-1). The peritoneum consists of a single layer of mesothelial cells covering a basement membrane.[1] The peritoneal mesothelial cells have the same embryological origin as vascular endothelial cells[2] and produce surfactant that acts as a lubricant.[3] The basement membrane is a fibroelastic tissue containing glycosylated proteins, mast cells, macrophages, and lymphocytes and it covers a well-defined network of elastic fibers. The basement membrane is absent in parts of the diaphragm, omentum, and mesentery.[1] The absence of the basement membrane in the diaphragm allows large gaps between the mesothelial cells ('stomata') to communicate directly with underlying lymphatic channels, facilitating absorption of fluid and particulate matter.

PHYSIOLOGY

The majority of the peritoneum behaves as a semi-permeable membrane allowing bidirectional diffusion of water and solutes. A small amount of serous fluid, formed by the action of Starling forces across the peritoneal capillaries, is normally present in the space between the parietal and visceral peritoneal surfaces. The fluid has a low protein concentration (<3 g/dL protein) and resembles an ultrafiltrate of plasma. In humans, normal peritoneal fluid has antibacterial activity against Gram positive and Gram negative bacteria.[4] A normal peritoneal cavity contains approximately 300 cells/mm³, which are largely lymphocytes and macrophages.

Fluid injected into a normal peritoneal cavity is dispersed throughout the entire peritoneal space over a period of between 15 minutes and two hours.[5] Contraction of the diaphragm promotes a cranial flow of peritoneal fluid.[6] Relaxation of the diaphragm generates a subatmospheric pressure that draws fluid and small particles into the large openings between the peritoneal mesothelial cells covering the diaphragm ('stomata') that communicate with the underlying lymphatic system. Contraction of the diaphragm closes the stomata and forces fluid into the lymphatic system.[1] This lymphatic system transports fluid and other absorbed material into the internal thoracic (or 'parasternal') mediastinal lymphatic system and mediastinal and parasternal lymph nodes, then to the thoracic duct system, and eventually to the systemic venous circulation.[7] Fluid is normally also absorbed through other sites in the peritoneum, including the omentum.[1,8]

PATHOPHYSIOLOGY

A physical, chemical, or microbiological injury to the peritoneum activates local defense mechanisms. These defense mechanisms fall into three broad categories (Table 26-1).[9–18]

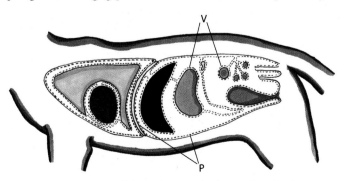

Figure 26-1 Illustration of the peritoneum in the cat. P, parietal peritoneum; V, visceral peritoneum.

© 2014 Elsevier Ltd
DOI: 10.1016/B978-0-7020-4336-9.00026-3

Table 26-1 Local defense mechanisms of the peritoneum

Defense mechanism	Pathogenesis
Removal of bacteria and particulate matter from the peritoneal cavity	Bacteria and small particles are rapidly absorbed by the diaphragm through the stomata
Immune cells and systems designed to kill bacteria	Peritoneal mast cells release histamine, resulting in vasodilation and the exudation from peritoneal capillaries of fluid that contains complement proteins and opsonins capable of coating bacteria Activation of complement system by endotoxin, other components of bacterial cell walls, damaged cells, and antigen–antibody complexes Bacteria are rapidly ingested by peritoneal phagocytes at the same time as they are cleared by the diaphragmatic lymphatic system Acute inflammatory response with neutrophils serves to eliminate bacteria that have not been cleared by macrophage phagocytosis or the diaphragmatic lymphatic system[9] Activation of peritoneal mesothelial cells, resident macrophages, mast cells, lymphocytes, and complement initiates the production of protein mediators called cytokines Cytokines regulate the complex interactions between the inflammatory cells and result in chemoattraction and phagocyte recruitment to the peritoneal cavity[1,11,16]
Sequestration of infection locally.	Fluid exuded into the peritoneal cavity is rich in fibrinogen. Injured cells release tissue thromboplastin, promoting the conversion of prothrombin to thrombin, stimulating fibrin formation from fibrinogen The normal fibrinolytic system is down regulated in peritonitis, leading to the accumulation of fibrin, which walls off bacteria[17]

The inflammatory response within the peritoneal cavity and the associated increased peritoneal vascular permeability result in the effusion of a large volume of protein-rich fluid into the peritoneal space. This results in a substantial loss of intravascular volume. In addition, systemic activation of the inflammatory and coagulation cascades causes further loss of fluid and protein and often disregulation of vascular tone and decreased tissue perfusion.[19]

Systemically, macrophages and other cells in the immune system respond to endotoxin and other bacteria-derived molecules ('pathogen-associated molecular patterns' or PAMPS) and endogenous mediators released from dead or dying cells[20] through Toll-like receptors to initiate a complex systemic inflammatory response (SIRS). The SIRS response is referred to as 'sepsis' when initiated by bacteria. Binding of endotoxin from Gram negative bacteria to the lipopolysaccharide (LPS)-binding protein on macrophages stimulates the release of multiple cytokines.[21] The mechanisms by which Gram positive bacteria induce systemic inflammation are less well characterized but several substances they contain, including peptidoglycan, teichoic acid, and their polysaccharide-hyaluronic acid capsules have pro-inflammatory effects, including the production of cytokines (tumor necrosis factor [TNF], interleukin-1 [IL1]) and nitric oxide.[22,23]

The macrophage is the main cell initiating the systemic response to bacteria and proteins from damaged cells.[19] IL1 and TNFα are rapidly released after macrophage stimulation and promote activation of many of the inflammatory and coagulation cascades. A detailed discussion of cytokines involved in sepsis is beyond the scope of this chapter and the reader is referred elsewhere for a more detailed review.[19]

The net result of sepsis in peritonitis is a decrease in intravascular volume, decreased cardiac output as a result of decreased preload, abnormal vascular tone, and vascular thrombosis, leading to maldistribution of blood flow, poor tissue perfusion, and organ damage. For more information on shock and SIRS the reader is referred to Chapter 3.

Gastrointestinal tract leakage

The gastrointestinal tract is the most frequent source of peritoneal contamination in cats.[24] Usually, only two or three bacterial species are grown in culture, although numerous species of bacteria are found in the gastrointestinal tract. Polymicrobial infections present a significant problem because of bacterial synergism. This appears to be most important in mixed infections with Gram negative and anaerobic bacteria. Anaerobic bacteria alone (such as *Bacillus fragilis*) seem to cause minimal pathology in experimental models. However, when combined with Gram negative enteric bacteria, the resulting infection is considerably more severe.[25] Ingesta, exfoliated cells, blood, gastric mucin, and bile salts are adjuvant substances that worsen peritonitis. Blood is an excellent growth medium for bacteria and hemoglobin interferes with chemotaxis and phagocytosis. Bile salts destroy peritoneal mesothelial cells and inhibit neutrophil function.

Urinary tract leakage

Uroperitoneum occurs when the bladder or peritoneal urethra is damaged by external or iatrogenic trauma. Severe trauma to the kidneys or ureters often damages the peritoneum, allowing urine to leak into the abdominal cavity from the retroperitoneal space. Urine is hyperosmotic and pulls fluid from the vascular space into the peritoneal cavity, resulting in dehydration. Failure to excrete urine also causes acidosis and progressively worsening hyperkalemia. Severe hyperkalemia is truly life threatening. For the effects and treatment of hyperkalemia see Chapters 1 and 3.

DIAGNOSIS AND GENERAL CONSIDERATIONS

The historical and physical examination findings of cats with peritonitis are usually associated with the SIRS syndrome. The historical findings most commonly reported by owners tend to be non-specific. However, a history of trauma or penetrating abdominal wounds may increase the clinician's suspicion of peritonitis. Gastrointestinal signs may be associated with primary gastrointestinal problems (i.e., foreign body) or may solely be due to peritonitis. An icteric animal may suggest primary biliary disease or associated pancreatitis. In both primary (not associated with feline infectious peritonitis [FIP]) and secondary bacterial peritonitis in the cat, common historical findings include lethargy, vomiting, anorexia, and diarrhea.[26] Weight loss is another clinical sign reported that appears to be more frequently associated with secondary peritonitis than with primary.[26]

Physical examination findings

On physical examination, pertinent findings in cats with peritonitis tend to be associated with dehydration and shock, and can include depressed mentation, inadequate hydration, pale mucus membranes, tachypnea, tachycardia, weakness, hyperthermia, and poor nutritional condition.[26–28] Cats with peritonitis and sepsis are often bradycardic and/or hypothermic.[26–28] Abdominal distension, which has been reported to be a common finding in cats with peritoneal effusion, can be identified by owners or on palpation during physical examination.[29]

In humans, abdominal pain is an early clinical sign of primary peritonitis,[30,31] but it appears not to be a good indicator of peritonitis in cats.[24,27] The overall incidence of abdominal pain elicited in cats with peritonitis ranged from 38–62%.[24,27]

Diagnostic procedures

Radiography

Survey abdominal radiographs are often taken to evaluate cats with clinical signs of gastrointestinal, urinary, or non-specific abdominal disease. The presence of free abdominal gas with no history of recent abdominal surgery or penetrating trauma warrants immediate stabilization and surgical exploration (Fig. 26-2).[32] It can be difficult to definitively diagnose small volumes of free peritoneal gas; close attention should be given to the diaphragmatic crura, as they are often highlighted by gas in the lung cranially and in the peritoneal cavity caudally. Loss of serosal detail and ileus also suggest intraperitoneal disease. Plain abdominal radiography may also diagnose diseases underlying peritonitis, including gastrointestinal foreign bodies, pyometra, cholelithiasis, and abdominal neoplasia.

Ultrasonography

Abdominal ultrasonography (Fig. 26-3) is very useful for obtaining samples of free peritoneal fluid. Blind, four quadrant tapping and diagnostic peritoneal lavage have been described for the same purpose. Although these three techniques have not been rigorously compared, ultrasound-guided aspiration has a subjectively higher diagnostic yield than a four quadrant tap and allows fluid to be directly analyzed without the dilutional effect of diagnostic peritoneal lavage. The hair over the abdomen is clipped and prepared with aseptic technique. A fluid accumulation is located with ultrasound and aspirated using a syringe and needle. The fluid's pH, glucose, lactate, and cytology are evaluated (Table 26-2).[33] Ultrasonography can also evaluate the

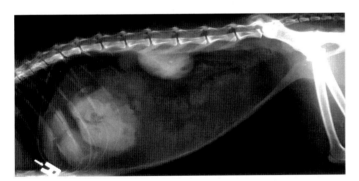

Figure 26-2 Pneumoperitoneum in a cat secondary to intestinal perforation. *(Courtesy of Dr Adrienne Bentley.)*

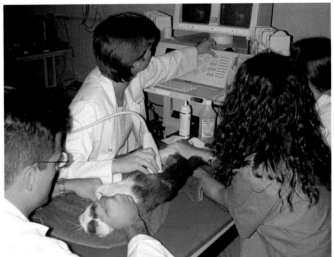

Figure 26-3 A cat with suspected peritonitis undergoing abdominal ultrasound.

Table 26-2 Cytological analysis of peritoneal fluid[48,62,63]

	Levels	Does the cat have peritonitis?
Nucleated cell count	>13,000 cells/µL	100% sensitivity and specificity*
Glucose concentration	<20 mg/dL or more lower than peripheral blood glucose	86% sensitive, 100% specific*
Peripheral venous blood lactate	1.3–10.6 mmol/L (median = 6.2 mmol/L)	Affected cats
	1.2–1.6 mmol/L (median = 1.4 mmol/L)	Unaffected cats
Bile crystals	Presence of intra- and extracellular bile crystals	Bile peritonitis
Bilirubin	Two to three times higher than peripheral blood levels	Bile peritonitis
Creatinine	Increased levels compared to serum. Mean abdominal fluid creatinine-to-serum creatinine ratio = 2:1 (range, 1.1:1 to 4.1:1)	Uroperitoneum
Potassium	Increased levels compared to serum. Mean abdominal fluid K⁺ to serum K⁺ ratio was 1.9:1 (range, 1.2:1 to 2.4:1)	Uroperitoneum

*, for diagnosing peritonitis.

abdominal organs for masses and abscesses and evaluate the urinary and biliary systems.

Cytological analysis

Cytological analysis has traditionally been used to evaluate peritoneal fluid (Table 26-2). Septic peritoneal effusions generally contain degenerate neutrophils and macrophages. The presence of intracellular bacteria is diagnostic for septic peritonitis.[34] A comparison of peritoneal fluid and peripheral blood lactate and glucose concentrations is also useful for confirming the diagnosis of septic peritonitis. Bile peritonitis is diagnosed based on cytological and biochemical analysis of peritoneal fluid. The diagnosis of uroperitoneum is based on a history of either blunt abdominal trauma, recent catheterization, or recent expression of the bladder. In the majority of cats with uroperitoneum, the peritoneal fluid creatinine and potassium levels are higher than those in the serum (see Chapter 3).[35]

SURGICAL DISEASES OF THE PERITONEUM

Peritonitis (inflammation or infection of the peritoneum) is the most common disease affecting the peritoneum in the cat. It occurs subsequent to systemic infection or leakage of gastrointestinal tract contents. Peritonitis can be subdivided into primary, secondary, or tertiary peritonitis, reflecting the cause or source of the infection. Neoplasia of the peritoneum is rare, but both primary mesothelioma[36–38] and secondary metastases to the peritoneum have been reported in the cat.

Primary peritonitis

Primary or spontaneous peritonitis is defined as an infection of the peritoneal cavity where no cause for the intraperitoneal bacterial contamination has been identified.[30,31,39] In primary peritonitis, bacterial contamination of the peritoneal cavity occurs via blood-borne or lymphatic spread or by bacterial translocation from the intestinal tract.[30] The true origin of bacterial contamination is difficult or impossible to determine in many instances. Primary peritonitis is more commonly reported in human than veterinary patients and is usually associated with diseases that cause ascites, such as cirrhosis.[30,31,40,41] In veterinary medicine, FIP is the most common cause of primary peritonitis.[39,42] FIP is caused by infection with a feline coronavirus and presents in two forms, the granulomatous (dry) form or the effusive (wet) form, which is the form that results in abdominal effusion and peritonitis.[43] In a retrospective study on cats with peritonitis, four out of 65 cats had primary peritonitis resulting from the effusive FIP.[44] There are numerous reports of primary peritonitis in cats due to other pathogens besides FIP; however, the true source of the infection in most cases is unclear.[45–49]

Secondary peritonitis

Secondary peritonitis is the most common form of peritonitis seen in veterinary medicine.[31] Bacterial contamination results from penetrating abdominal trauma, bite wounds, contamination from surgery or diagnostic aspiration procedures. Leakage of bacteria from abdominal organs into the peritoneal cavity is another frequent source of contamination in secondary peritonitis.[31] While all of the abdominal organs can be potential septic sources of contamination, leakage of contents from the gastrointestinal tract is the most common cause of peritonitis.[27,50–53] In cats, gastrointestinal leakage causing septic peritonitis is most often the result of neoplasia.[27] In one study, neoplasia was the underlying cause of gastrointestinal leakage and subsequent

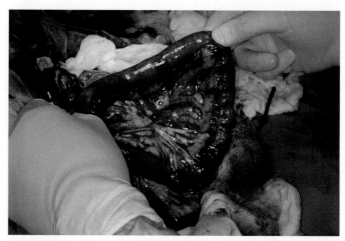

Figure 26-4 Peritonitis secondary to intestinal perforations from a linear foreign body. *(Courtesy of Dr Karen Tobias.)*

septic peritonitis in 54% of cats.[27] Adenocarcinoma and lymphosarcoma were the most common neoplasms identified.[27] Other reported causes of gastrointestinal leakage include perforation of the bowel due to a foreign body (Fig. 26-4), leakage from a previous surgical site, and perforation of the colon due to megacolon and enteritis.[27]

Leakage from an enterotomy, gastrotomy, or a resection and anastomosis site is another potential cause of secondary peritonitis.[54,55] Dehiscence occurred in 14% of cases in one study of dogs and cats, although none of the 25 cats had surgical dehiscence and leakage.[55] It is difficult to interpret the significance of these findings due to the limited numbers of cases in this study specifically evaluating cats. In a second study, no anastomosis or biopsy site leaked in 70 cats with alimentary lymphosarcoma.[56] In dogs, factors suggesting an increase in the risk of postoperative dehiscence include presence of a foreign body or a traumatic injury, preoperative peritonitis, and hypoalbuminemia.[54,55] Perforation of a gastrointestinal ulcer, perhaps associated with carprofen ingestion, has been reported in one cat with peritonitis.[57]

Secondary peritonitis in cats may occur following bite wounds, gunshot wounds or vehicular trauma.[27] Bacteria enter the peritoneal cavity directly from the environment or from trauma resulting in rupture of a viscus. Penetrating wounds warrant emergency surgical exploration to evaluate for possible bowel damage, wound debridement, and lavage.

Septic peritonitis from urinary tract infection is rare and urine is not considered an adjuvant substance in peritonitis.[58] In a retrospective study of 51 cases of septic peritonitis in cats, only four cases of peritonitis appeared to have resulted from a urinary tract infection.[27] Feline pyometras occasionally rupture and cause secondary peritonitis. In a retrospective study of cats with pyometra, seven out of 183 cats (3.8%) had a uterine rupture, and four of the seven cats died as a result of the septic peritonitis.[59]

Secondary septic peritonitis can also occur because of biliary leakage resulting from trauma anywhere along the biliary tract, necrotizing cholecystitis, cholelithiasis, or iatrogenic injury from aspiration or surgical manipulation.[24,60–63] In dogs, it appears that animals with septic bile peritonitis had a decreased survival rate and increased mortality as compared to those with aseptic peritonitis.[60,63]

Other potential sources of secondary peritonitis include abscessation of the pancreas, liver, or spleen[64] or iatrogenic contamination of the abdominal cavity after abdominal surgery. In 51 cats with secondary peritonitis, three developed septic peritonitis due to septic pancreatitis or a pancreatic abscess, and one due to liver lobe necrosis.[27]

Tertiary peritonitis

Tertiary or recurrent peritonitis is diagnosed when there is persistent infection of the peritoneal cavity after an effort has been made to treat either primary or secondary peritonitis.[65] Tertiary peritonitis can occur even after optimal, standard-of-care treatment and often cases present with systemic sepsis without an obvious focus of infection.[66,67] In humans, the mortality rate is greater than 60%.[68] The lack of peritoneal inflammation due to immune paralysis and derangement in the endocrine stress response has been tentatively linked with the occurrence of tertiary peritonitis in people.[67] The organisms that are generally found in cases of tertiary peritonitis in humans tend to be from the gastrointestinal tract or lesser pathogens such as *Candida* spp. or *Staphylococcus epidermidis*.[30,68] Tertiary peritonitis has currently not been truly described in cats or dogs.

Mesothelioma

Primary tumors of the peritoneal serosal surfaces are uncommon in cats. They occur within the thoracic or abdominal cavities and are regularly associated with pleural or peritoneal effusions; involvement of the pleura in the cat (see Chapter 44) has been reported more commonly than involvement of the peritoneum. Mesothelial neoplasms can be benign or malignant, and are classified as predominantly epitheloid, mixed (biphasic), or fibrous (spindle cell, fibrosarcomatous).[36,37] Affected cats range in age from 1–17 years and may present with ascites, weakness, and collapse.[36] Diagnosis is aided by imaging, fine needle aspiration, and peritoneal fluid analysis.

Surgical findings include infiltration of the omentum, which can form an irregular mass that extends onto the stomach, pancreas, spleen, and proximal intestinal tract.[36,38] The visceral and parietal peritoneal surfaces can be affected and appear thickened with off-white friable material and occasionally firm fibrous plaques.[36] Immunohistochemistry may be necessary for confirmation of the suspected diagnosis.[36,37]

PREPARATION FOR SURGERY

Cats with peritonitis usually require emergency management and stabilization prior to surgery.

Intravenous fluids

Stabilization of the cat with bacterial peritonitis requires intravenous access, generally with two peripheral catheters or one central catheter. The type of fluid and the rate of resuscitation depend on an assessment of the cat's perfusion, initial laboratory data, and the presence of concurrent respiratory and cardiac diseases. In general, colloids are often used with crystalloids, as endothelial dysfunction and increased vascular permeability are common. Synthetic colloids (Hetastarch, Dextran 70) are administered as a bolus (5 mL/kg) with 20–30 mL/kg of crystalloid. When available, fresh frozen plasma provides albumin and clotting factors. Ongoing resuscitation is determined by the response to therapy, measured by clinical and laboratory parameters, including heart rate, direct or indirect blood pressure, acid/base status, and blood lactate levels. In some cases blood pressure and tissue perfusion do not improve despite apparently adequate intravascular volume expansion. This may occur because of sepsis-associated disruption of vascular tone. In these instances, careful use of a vasopressor (dopamine: 5 µg/kg/minute; norepinephrine: 0.1 µg/kg/minute) can be effective in restoring vascular tone and tissue perfusion.

Antibiosis

Antibiotics are administered perioperatively in all cases of suspected bacterial peritonitis. Samples for bacterial culture and sensitivity testing are taken during surgery. Until these results are obtained, the choice of antibiotics is based on knowledge of the normal bacterial flora of the organ suspected to be the source of the contamination, and antimicrobial pharmacokinetics. Intestinal bacteria are commonly coliforms, enterococci, and anaerobes. Appropriate antibiotics for these bacteria include a combination of ampicillin and either an aminoglycoside or fluoroquinolone. Metronidazole is often added to target anaerobes. Penicillin and cephalosporin antibiotics are 'time dependent' as they rely on maintaining serum concentrations above the minimum inhibitory concentration (MIC) by frequent dosing, generally every six hours. Aminoglycosides and fluoroquinolones depend on obtaining the highest possible drug concentration ('concentration dependent') by using a single daily dose for their bactericidal effect.

Uroperitoneum

In cats with uroperitoneum, rehydration should begin immediately, using warm intravenous fluids. The rate of fluid administration is based on the severity of dehydration. Severely dehydrated animals with no underlying heart disease can be given 40–60 mL/kg over the first hour; subsequent rates of 5–15 mL/kg/hour are used depending on hydration status. Although some clinicians use 0.9% NaCl to avoid administering potassium, it is clear that more balanced electrolyte solutions (lactated Ringer's, Normosol R) allow for a more rapid correction of acid–base status without affecting normalization of serum potassium levels.[69,70] In cases of marked hyperkalemia, calcium gluconate (a functional antagonist of potassium) should be administered slowly, intravenously (0.5 mL/kg). Although it does not lower serum potassium, calcium changes the threshold potential and returns membrane excitability to normal for approximately 20 to 30 minutes. Regular insulin (1 unit/kg) and/or glucose (1–2 g/unit of insulin) can also be administered. Animals are often also severely acidotic. Sodium bicarbonate can be administered (3–9 mEq/kg) to correct acidosis; however, this can paradoxically lower ionized calcium and so worsen the effects of hyperkalemia. Correction of the hyperkalemia and acidosis depends on re-establishing urine flow to allow effective potassium and acid excretion from the body. In animals with uroperitoneum this involves placement of a catheter to drain urine from the peritoneal cavity and ideally placement of a catheter into the bladder via the urethra. In cases where the urethra is completely transected a cystostomy tube is placed surgically or by using interventional radiology techniques.

SURGICAL MANAGEMENT AND TECHNIQUES FOR PERITONITIS

The goals of surgery for septic peritonitis are to remove the source of infection, decrease the infectious pathogen load, remove foreign material and other adjuvants, and prevent recurrence or persistence of infection in the peritoneal cavity. Surgery may also include the placement of feeding tubes (i.e., gastrostomy or enterostomy tubes) for postoperative nutritional support (see Chapters 12 and 28).

Celiotomy

A standard ventral midline celiotomy from just caudal to the xiphoid to just cranial to the pubis is recommended to allow for maximum

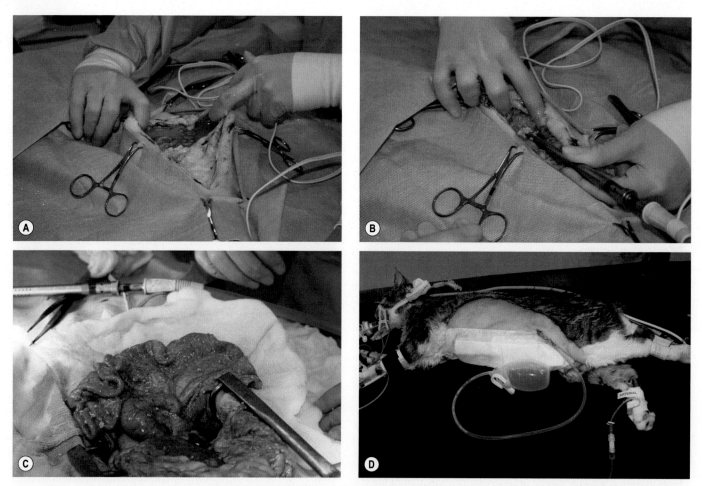

Figure 26-5 An 8-year-old domestic short-haired cat presented with a chronic history of peritonitis. **(A)** After celiotomy the abdominal wall is maintained in an elevated position by finger retraction to prevent spillage of peritoneal fluid prior to suction. **(B)** The fluid is suctioned out using a Poole suction tip. Fibrinous material was present in the fluid. **(C)** The mesentery and peritoneal surface has a granular appearance with fibrin deposits throughout the abdomen. **(D)** Multiple biopsies were taken, and following celiotomy closure a closed-suction drain (Jackson–Pratt) was placed. A *Nocardia* type organism was cultured, thought to be a secondary pathogen; the primary cause was not identified. *(Courtesy of the University of Cambridge.)*

exposure to perform complete exploration of the peritoneal cavity (Fig. 26-5) (see Chapter 23). Complete exploration is crucial for determination of the underlying primary cause, correction and elimination of continued contamination, and adequate lavage of the peritoneal cavity. The hepatobiliary, gastrointestinal, and urogenital systems are carefully evaluated to identify the underlying cause of peritonitis. Resection and anastomosis of a gastrointestinal lesion, a cholecystectomy, or ovariohysterectomy to remove a pyometra, may be necessary to treat the primary cause. Debridement of abnormal tissue and removing foreign material and adjuvants such as hemoglobin are also performed during surgery. This will decrease the concentrations of intra-abdominal pathogens, adjuvants, and fibrin, minimizing the risk of persistent infections and clinical deterioration.

Omentalization and serosal patching

Peritonitis is associated with an increased risk of surgical dehiscence and leakage after closure of a viscus.[55,71] Degradation of collagen and the extracellular matrix by the proteolyic enzymes in peritonitis is thought to predispose enterotomies and intestinal anastomoses to dehiscence.[72] The omentum plays an important role in the body's defense against injury and infection in the peritoneal cavity. The

omentum provides a rich blood supply, has absorptive capabilities, and stimulates angiogenesis.[1] The omentum will also form adhesions to help seal off or isolate sources of contamination. Omentalization can be used when the source of the infection cannot be entirely removed, such as prostatic or pancreatic abscesses. The abscess cavity is located by palpation, intraoperative ultrasound, or aspiration. It is opened, drained, and the abscess cavity is gently debrided with a moistened gauze sponge. After thorough local lavage with a warm, balanced electrolyte solution, the omentum is packed loosely into the cavity and the abdominal incision is closed. The immunologic and angiogenic properties of the omentum promote local infection control and healing. The technique has been associated with some success in (six of 12; 50% survival) dogs with pancreatic abscesses.[73] Results of a large clinical study of omentalization for abdominal abscesses in cats are lacking.

Omental wrapping involves placing the omentum around the suture line of an enterotomy or anastomosis and has been described for animals with an increased risk of postoperative bowel leakage.[55,74] Serosal patching involves suturing loops of jejunum over the closure site of the viscus. It can be used over suture lines that are at a high risk of dehiscence.[71] The technique for making an omental graft is described in Chapter 19.

Peritoneal lavage

The current standard of practice holds that the contaminated perito-neal cavity is thoroughly lavaged after surgery. Whilst the concept of treating the peritoneal cavity in a similar manner to any other con-taminated wound seems reasonable, peritoneal lavage has both ben-eficial and detrimental effects.[75] Peritoneal lavage does not necessarily decrease peritoneal bacterial contamination. Once bacteria have colo-nized and adhered to the peritoneum, they are difficult to remove by lavage.[76,77] Lavage fluid remaining in the peritoneal cavity dilutes com-plement and other opsonins and suspends bacteria away from neu-trophils and macrophages, making phagocytosis more difficult. Lavage, then, should ideally be used to remove blood, purulent mate-rial, bile, mucus, and gross intestinal content from the peritoneal cavity but all fluid should be aspirated before the abdominal cavity is closed. The best fluid to use for peritoneal lavage has not been deter-mined. The addition of antiseptics to lavage fluid is not recommended in clinical cases because of toxicity (povidone iodine) or a lack of perceived clinical efficacy in spite of benefits in some experimental models (chlorhexidine). The addition of antibiotics to lavage fluid has no benefit over parenteral antibiotics administered intravenously at the appropriate doses.

PERITONEAL DRAINAGE

Once the source of the peritonitis has been addressed, access for enteral nutrition should be provided if necessary (see Chapter 11). The surgeon must then decide whether the abdomen should be closed primarily or if some type of local or more general peritoneal drainage is required. Local drainage has largely been recommended for pancre-atic abscess or prostatic abscesses in dogs. Localized drainage is used to limit accumulation of a large volume of ongoing infected exudate as this might limit the efficacy of local peritoneal defense mechanisms, prevent localization of the contamination, and speed the systemic absorption of bacteria and endotoxin.[75] However, the technique of placing one or more drains into an intra-abdominal abscess has largely been replaced in clinical practice by omentalization (see above).

In generalized peritonitis the surgeon must choose to close the abdomen primarily, close the abdomen after placing drains, or leave the abdomen open. There are no objective criteria and few subjective criteria to guide this decision, and no large scale, randomized clinical trials of these treatment methods in cats with peritonitis.

Primary closure without drainage

A decision to close the peritoneal cavity without drainage is based on control of the source of contamination and adequate decontamina-tion of the peritoneal cavity. The clinician then relies on the body's peritoneal drainage and immune defense systems to resolve residual infection and peritoneal contamination. Fifty-four per cent of dogs with septic peritonitis treated by primary closure survived in one study.[78] This form of management is most appropriate when the source of contamination can be controlled definitively and peritonitis is not severe.

Closed-suction drainage

The use of closed-suction drains in generalized peritonitis has been reported in cats and dogs. Some type of suction or vacuum system is necessary for drains to be potentially effective because the peritoneal

space within the abdomen is at a sub-atmospheric pressure. Even with experimental insufflation of air, the intraperitoneal pressure never exceeds atmospheric pressure.[79] Unless either the intraperitoneal pres-sure becomes higher than atmospheric or air can enter the peritoneal cavity postoperatively through a vent, drainage from the peritoneal cavity will not occur without the use of a vacuum system. The use of drains within the peritoneal cavity is somewhat controversial because of the discrepancy between reasonable clinical results from their use and experimental studies clearly showing that the omentum and viscera rapidly encase drains inserted into the peritoneal cavity.[80] It is therefore not clear if drainage occurs from the peritoneal cavity proper or, more likely, from the area around the encased drain. In an experi-mental study in dogs, sump-Penrose drains were found encapsulated and isolated from the peritoneal cavity at necropsy performed after 48 hours.[5] Despite this isolation, the drains continued to remove radio-opaque contrast material from the peritoneal cavity. In a clinical study of closed-suction silicone drains for septic peritonitis, drains continued to accumulate fluid for up to eight days, seeming to indicate adequate function. However, it is not clear if closed-suction drains are encased to the same extent as sump-Penrose drains and are draining a localized area, or if they retain functional drainage of the peritoneal cavity despite being encased.[81] This study reported 70% survival in a cohort of 30 dogs and ten cats with septic peritonitis managed with closed-suction drains. Drains were in place for a mean of 3.6 days with a range of two to eight days. The volume of fluid produced was vari-able but decreased with time. The drains remained patent until removal, as evidenced by ongoing fluid collection. However, it is unclear what percentage of the total peritoneal fluid volume they drained. No significant complications were reported with clinical use of the closed-suction drains.

Closed-suction drains are relatively inexpensive, easy to place, and seem to be free of significant complications (see Fig. 26-5 and Chapter 11). It should be noted, however, that experimentally, latex drains can significantly impair bowel wound healing. It is not clear if silastic closed-suction drains impair bowel healing in a similar manner. Advantages of closed-suction drainage over open peritoneal drainage include the ability to quantify the volume of effusion and decreased cost and labor.

Commercially available closed-suction drains consist of a fenes-trated silicone drain connected to an external reservoir by a non-fenestrated tube (Jackson–Pratt drain, Cardinal Health Australia, Sydney, Australia). The drain is typically positioned near the dia-phragm and liver in the most dependent portion of the peritoneal cavity, although a more caudal position may be appropriate, depend-ing on the source of the contamination. The non-fenestrated portion of the drain is exited through a small paramedian incision in the body wall and is secured with a purse-string and finger trap of non-absorbable suture. Compression of the bulb reservoir creates negative pressure within the peritoneal cavity. A bandage is typically applied to cover the exit site of the drain and to provide a means of attaching the bulb reservoir to the patient (see Chapter 4). The contents of the reservoir are easily emptied, typically every 6 hours or when the res-ervoir is half full.

Open peritoneal drainage

Historically, open peritoneal drainage (Box 26-1) has been reserved for the most severe cases of generalized septic peritonitis, which are anecdotally associated with a large volume of effusion postoperatively. Assessment of the severity of peritonitis is largely subjective and based on individual experience.

Clinical studies report a mean duration of open peritoneal drainage of four to five days, with a range of less than one day to up to two weeks.[82,83] Hypoproteinemia and nosocomial infection are reported

Box 26-1 Open peritoneal drainage

Open peritoneal drainage is established through a long abdominal incision, extending from the xiphoid process to the pubis and including the most dependent portion of the abdomen. The falciform fat should be excised according to standard exploratory laparotomy technique (see Chapter 23), but omentectomy is not necessary or desirable. The linea alba is closed with non-absorbable suture in a simple continuous pattern with a gap of 1–3 cm between the edges (Fig. 26-6), depending on the patient's size. The subcutaneous tissues and skin are not closed. A sterile bandage consisting of a non-adherent contact layer, such as petrolatum impregnated gauze, laparotomy sponges, and surgery towels underneath routine bandage material is applied and changed at least daily. If the bandage becomes wet from peritoneal effusion or urine, or if the bandage becomes displaced, the bandage should be replaced as soon as possible. The bandage should be changed in the operating room with the patient sedated or anesthetized. During each bandage change, adhesions at the incision are digitally disrupted and the incision is checked for organ evisceration. The decision to close the peritoneal cavity is based on reassessment of the same factors used in selecting open peritoneal drainage or cytological analysis of the effusion. Closure is performed as a complete laparotomy.

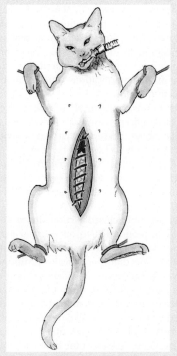

Figure 26-6 Illustration of closure for open peritoneal drainage in a cat. A simple continuous suture is placed leaving a gap of 1–3 cm between the fascia lata. The skin and subcutaneous tissue is left unsutured. The open abdomen is protected by a sterile bandage.

complications of open peritoneal drainage, although their clinical significance is not well established.

POSTOPERATIVE CARE

The postoperative care of the cat with peritonitis is a critical part of the management of the case and will influence its chances of recovery. Particular attention should be paid to the cat's fluid status, electrolyte balance, analgesia, and nutritional balance. The cat should be monitored frequently for complications associated with the procedures performed. The reader is referred to Chapter 3 on postoperative monitoring and management of complications, and Chapter 4 on postoperative nursing for more information.

Perioperative nutrition

Once the primary source of peritonitis has been controlled, the surgeon must consider options for postoperative nutrition (see Chapter 6). In cases of uncomplicated bladder rupture and uroperitoneum the clinician might reasonably expect a cat to eat within one to two days of a successful surgery. However, in cases of generalized bacterial peritonitis, voluntary food intake is unlikely. At the same time, generalized peritonitis is associated with a significant hypermetabolic state, intraperitoneal protein loss, and protein/energy malnutrition. An esophagosotomy, gastrostomy, or jejunostomy tube allows early enteral feeding (see Chapter 12). Enteral feeding maintains mucosal enterocyte health and minimizes bacterial translocation from the gut. In cases where enteral feeding is not tolerated, total parenteral nutrition is considered; ideally, a multiple lumen catheter is placed immediately before or after surgery.

PROGNOSIS FOR PERITONITIS

In a study examining 26 cats that were treated surgically for septic peritonitis, 46% of the cats survived to discharge; the remainder of the cats either died or were euthanized due to deterioration of their clinical status.[24] Similarly, the survival rate in a study of nine cats was 44% and no differences were detected between cats that had primary or secondary peritonitis.[29] In another study, a 30% mortality rate was reported in 23 cats having surgical treatment of septic peritonitis.[27] Lastly, when specifically examining primary septic peritonitis in 13 cats where treatment included surgery, the overall mortality rate was 31%.[28]

REFERENCES

1. Hall JC, Heel KA, Papadimitriou JM, Platell C. The pathobiology of peritonitis. Gastroenterology 1998;114: 185–96.

2. Le Gros Clark WE. The tissues of the body: an introduction to the study of anatomy. Oxford, England: Oxford University; 1958. p. 62–3.

3. Beavis J, Harwood JL, Coles GA, Williams JD. Synthesis of phospholipids by human peritoneal mesothelial cells. Perit Dial Int 1994;14:348–55.

4. Bercovici B, Michel J, Miller J, Sacks TG. Antimicrobial activity of human peritoneal fluid. Surg Gynecol Obstet 1975;141:885–7.

5. Hosgood G, Salisbury SK, Cantwell HD, DeNicola DB. Intraperitoneal circulation and drainage in the dog. Vet Surg 1989;18:261–8.

6. Last M, Kurtz L, Stein TA, Wise L. Effect of PEEP on the rate of thoracic duct lymph flow and clearance of bacteria from the peritoneal cavity. Am J Surg 1983;145:126–30.

7. Abu-Hijleh MF, Habbal OA, Moqattash ST. The role of the diaphragm in lymphatic absorption from the peritoneal cavity. J Anat 1995;186:453–67.

8. Flessner MF, Parker RJ, Sieber SM. Peritoneal lymphatic uptake of fibrinogen and erythrocytes in the rat. Am J Physiol 1983;244:H89–96.

9. Dunn DL, Barke RA, Knight NB, et al. Role of resident macrophages, peripheral neutrophils, and translymphatic absorption in bacterial clearance from the peritoneal cavity. Infect Immun 1985;49:257–64.

10. Dunn DL, Barke RA, Lee JT Jr, et al. Mechanisms of the adjuvant effect of hemoglobin in experimental peritonitis. VII. Hemoglobin does not inhibit clearance of Escherichia coli from the peritoneal cavity. Surgery 1983;94:487–93.

11. Heemken R, Gandawidjaja L, Hau T. Peritonitis: pathophysiology and local defense mechanisms. Hepatogastroenterology 1997;44:927–36.

12. Hau T, Ahrenholz DH, Simmons RL. Secondary bacterial peritonitis: The biologic basis of treatment. Curr Probl Surg 1979;16:1–65.

13. Rohrer RJ. Basic immunology for surgeons. In: O'Leary PJ, editor. The Physiologic basis of surgery. 3rd ed. Philadelphia: Lippincott Williams and Wilkins; 2002. p. 169–77.

14. Heel KA, Hall JC. Peritoneal defences and peritoneum-associated lymphoid tissue. Br J Surg 1996;83:1031–6.

15. Fry DE. Surgical infection. In: O'Leary JP, editor. The Physiologic basis of surgery. Philadelphia: Lippincott, Williams & Wilkins; 2002. p. 213–34.

16. Culp WTN, Holt DE. Septic peritonitis. Comp Contin Ed Pract Vet 2010;32: E1–15.

17. Vipond MN, Whawell SA, Thompson JN, Dudley HA. Effect of experimental peritonitis and ischemia on peritoneal fibrinolytic activity. Eur J Surg 1994;160:471–7.

18. Van Goor H, de Graaf JS, Kooi K, et al. Effect of recombinant tissue plasminogen activator on intra-abdominal abscess formation in rats with generalized peritonitis. J Am Coll Surg 1994;179:407–11.

19. Silverstein D, Otto CM. Sepsis. In: Greene CE, editor. Infectious diseases of the dog and cat 4e. Philadelphia: Saunders Elsevier; 2012. p. 359–69

20. Lotze MT, Zeh HJ, Rubartelli A, et al. The grateful dead: damage-associated molecular pattern molecules and reduction/oxidation regulate immunity. Immunol Rev 2007;220:60–81.

21. Evans TJ. The role of macrophages in septic shock. Immunology 1996;195:655–9.

22. Cohen J. The immunopathogenesis of sepsis. Nature 2002;420:885–91.

23. Srisskandan S, Cohen J. Gram positive sepsis. Infect Dis Clin North Am 1999;13:397–412.

24. Parsons K J, Owen LJ, Lee K, et al. A retrospective study of surgically treated cases of septic peritonitis in the cat (2000-2007). J Small Anim Pract 2009;50:518–24.

25. Onderdonk AB, Bartlett JG, Louie T, et al. Microbial synergy in experimental intra-abdominal abscess. Infect Immun 1976;13:22–6.

26. Culp WT, Zeldis TE, Reese MS, Drobatz KJ. Primary bacterial peritonitis in dogs and cats: 24 cases (1990-2006). J Am Vet Med Assoc 2009;234:906–13.

27. Costello MF, Drobatz KJ, Aronson LR, King LG. Underlying cause, pathophysiologic abnormalities, and response to treatment in cats with septic peritonitis: 51 cases (1990-2001). J Am Vet Med Assoc 2004;225:897–902.

28. Ruthrauff CM, Smith J, Glerum L. Primary bacterial septic peritonitis in cats: 13 cases. J Am Anim Hosp Assoc 2009;45:268–76.

29. Wright KN, Gompf RE, DeNovo RC Jr. Peritoneal effusion in cats: 65 cases (1981-1997). J Am Vet Med Assoc 1999;214:375–81.

30. Johnson CC, Baldessarre J, Levison ME. Peritonitis: update on pathophysiology, clinical manifestations, and management. Clin Infect Dis 1997;24:1035–47.

31. Laroche M, Harding G. Primary and secondary peritonitis: an update. Eur J Clin Microbiol Infect Dis 1998;17:542–50.

32. Smelstoys JA, Davis GJ, Learn AE, et al. Outcome of and prognostic indicators for dogs and cats with pneumoperitoneum and no history of penetrating trauma: 54 cases (1988-2002). J Am Vet Med Assoc 2004;225:251–5.

33. Bonczynski JJ, Ludwig LL, Barton LJ, et al. Comparison of peritoneal fluid and peripheral blood pH, bicarbonate, glucose, and lactate concentration as a diagnostic tool for septic peritonitis in dogs and cats. Vet Surg 2003;32:161–6.

34. Alleman AR. Abdominal, thoracic, and pericardial effusions. Vet Clin North Am Small Anim Pract 2003;33:89–118.

35. Aumann M, Worth LT, Drobatz KJ. Uroperitoneum in cats: 26 cases (1986-1995). J Am Anim Hosp Assoc 1998;34:315–24.

36. Heerkens TM, Smith JD, Fox L, Hostetter JM. Peritoneal fibrosarcomatous mesothelioma in a cat. J Vet Diagn Invest 2011;23:593–7.

37. Bacci B, Morandi F, De Meo M, Marcato PS. Ten cases of feline mesothelioma: an immunohistochemical and ultrastructural study. J Comp Pathol 2006;134:347–54.

38. Kobayashi Y, Usuda H, Ochiai K, Itakura C. Malignant mesothelioma with metastases and mast cell leukaemia in a cat. J Comp Pathol 1994;111:453–8.

39. Kirby BM. Peritoneum and peritoneal cavity. In: Slatter D, editor. Textbook of small animal surgery. Philadelphia: WB Saunders; 2003. p. 414–45.

40. Evans LT, Kim WR, Poterucha JJ, Kamath PS. Spontaneous bacterial peritonitis in asymptomatic outpatients with cirrhotic ascites. Hepatology 2003;37:897–901.

41. Boixeda D, De Luis DA, Aller R, De Argila CM. Spontaneous bacterial peritonitis. Clinical and microbiological study of 233 episodes. J Clin Gastroenterol 1996;23:275–9.

42. Seim HB. Management of peritonitis. In: Bonagura JD, Kirk RW, editors. Current veterinary therapy xii: small animal practice. Philadelphia: WB Saunders; 1995. p. 933–7.

43. Gaskell R, Dawson S. FIP-related disease. In: Ettinger SJ, Feldman EC, editors. Textbook of veterinary internal medicine. Philadelphia: WB Saunders; 2000. p. 137–9.

44. Wright KN, Gompf RE, DeNovo RC Jr. Peritoneal effusion in cats: 65 cases (1981-1997). J Am Vet Med Assoc 1999;214:375–81.

45. Culp WT, Zeldis TE, Reese MS, Drobatz KJ. Primary bacterial peritonitis in dogs and cats: 24 cases (1990-2006). J Am Vet Med Assoc 2009;234:906–13.

46. Costello MF, Drobatz KJ, Aronson LR, King LG. Underlying cause, pathophysiologic abnormalities, and response to treatment in cats with septic peritonitis: 51 cases (1990-2001). J Am Vet Med Assoc 2004;225:897–902.

47. Ruthraff CM, Smith J, Glerum L. Primary bacterial septic peritonitis in cats: 13 cases. J Am Anim Hosp Assoc 2009;45:268–76.

48. Ingham B, Brentnall DW. Acute peritonitis in a kitten associated with Salmonella typhimurium infection. J Small Anim Pract 1972;13:71–4.

49. Dickie CW, Sniff ES. Chlamydia infection associated with peritonitis in a cat. J Am Vet Med Assoc 1980;176:1256–9.

50. Woolfson JM, Dulisch ML. Open abdominal drainage in the treatment of generalized peritonitis in 25 dogs and cats. Vet Surg 1986;15:27–32.

51. Greenfield CL, Walshaw R. Open peritoneal drainage for treatment of contaminated peritoneal cavity and septic peritonitis in dogs and cats: 24 cases (1980-1986). J Am Vet Med Assoc 1987;191:100–5.

52. Mueller MG, Ludwig LL, Barton LJ. Use of closed-suction drains to treat generalized peritonitis in dogs and cats: 40 cases (1997-1999). J Am Vet Med Assoc 2001;219:789–94.

53. Staatz AJ, Monnet E, Seim HB 3rd. Open peritoneal drainage versus primary closure for the treatment of septic peritonitis I dogs and cats: 42 cases (1993-1999). Vet Surg 2002;31:174–80.

54. Allen DA, Smeak DD, Schertel ER. Prevalence of small intestinal dehiscence and associated clinical factors: a retrospective study of 121 dogs. J Am Anim Hosp Assoc 1992;28:70–6.

55. Ralphs SC, Jessen CR, Lipowitz AJ. Risk factors for leakage following intestinal anastomosis in dogs and cats: 115 cases (1991-2000). J Am Vet Med Assoc 2003;223:73–7.

56. Smith AL, Wilson AP, Hardie RJ, et al. Perioperative complications after full-thickness gastrointestinal surgery in cats with alimentary lymphoma. Vet Surg 2011;40:849–52.

57. Runk A, Kyles AE, Downs MO. Duodenal perforation in a cat following the administration of non-steroidal anti-inflammatory medication. J Am Anim Hosp Assoc 1999;35:52–5.

58. Hardie EM. Peritonitis from urogentital conditions. Prob Vet Med 1989;1:36–49.

59. Kenney KJ, Matthiesen DT, Brown NO, Bradley RL. Pyometra in cats:183 cases (1979-84). J Am Vet Med Assoc 1987;191: 1130–2.

60. Ludwig LL, McLoughlin MA, Graves TK, Crisp MS. Surgical treatment of bile peritonitis in 24 dogs and 2 cats: a retrospective study (1987-1994). Vet Surg 1997;26:90–8.

61. Kirpensteijn J, Fingland RB, Ulrich T, et al. Cholelithiasis in dogs: 29 cases (1980-90). J Am Vet Med Assoc 1993;202: 1137–42.

62. Moores AL, Gregory SP. Duplex gall bladder associated with choledocholithiasis, cholecystitis, gall bladder rupture and septic peritonitis in a cat. J Small Anim Pract 2007;48: 404–9.

63. Mehler SJ, Mayhew PD, Drobatz KJ, Holt DE. Variables associated with outcome in dogs undergoing extrahepatic biliary surgery: 60 cases (1988-2002). Vet Surg 2004;33:644–9.

64. Sergeeff JS, Armstrong PJ, Bunch SE. Hepatic abscesses in cats: 14 cases (1985-2002). J Vet Intern Med 2004;18: 295–300.

65. Malangoni MA. Evaluation and management of tertiary peritonitis. Am Surg 2000;66:157–61.

66. Broche F, Tellado JM. Defense mechanisms of the peritoneal cavity. Curr Opin Crit Care 2001;7:105–16.

67. Buijk SE, Bruining HA. Future directions in the management of tertiary peritonitis. Intensive Care Med 2002;28:1024–9.

68. Nathens AB, Rotstein OD, Marshall JC. Tertiary peritonitis: clinical features of a complex nosocomial infection. World J Surg 1998;22:158–63.

69. Cunha MG, Freitas GC, Carregaro AB, et al. Renal and cardiorespiratory effects of treatment with lactated Ringer's solution or physiologic saline (0.9% NaCl) solution in cats with experimentally induced urethral obstruction. Am J Vet Res 2010;71: 840–6.

70 Drobatz KJ, Cole SG. The influence of crystalloid type on acid-base and electrolyte status of cats with urethral obstruction. J Vet Emerg Crit Care 2008;18:355–61.

71. Crowe DT. The serosal patch: Clinical use in 12 animals. Vet Surg 1984;13: 29–38.

72. Tani T, Tsutamoto Y, Eguchi Y, et al. Protease inhibitor reduces loss of tensile strength in rat anastomosis with peritonitis. J Surg Res 2000;88: 135–41.

73. Johnson MD, Mann FA. Treatment for pancreatic abscesses via omentalization with abdominal closure versus open peritoneal drainage in dogs: 15 cases (1994-2004). J Am Vet Med Assoc 2006;228:397–402.

74. McLachlin AD, Denton DW. Omental protection of intestinal anastomoses. Am J Surg 1973;125:134–40.

75. Platell C, Papadimitriou JM, Hall JC. The influence of lavage on peritonitis. J Am Coll Surg 2000;191:672–80.

76. Haagen IA, Heezius HC, Verkooyen RP, et al. Adherence of peritonitis-causing staphylococci to human peritoneal mesothelial cell monolayers. J Infect Dis 1990;161:266–73.

77. Edmiston CE Jr, Goheen MP, Kornhall S, et al. Fecal peritonitis: microbial adherence to serosal mesothelium and resistance to peritoneal lavage. World J Surg 1990;14:176–83.

78. Lanz OI, Ellison GW, Bellah JR, et al. Surgical treatment of septic peritonitis without abdominal drainage in 28 dogs. J Am Anim Hosp Assoc 2001;37:87–92.

79. Gold E. The physics of the abdominal cavity and the problem of peritoneal drainage. Am J Surg 1956;91:415–17.

80. Yates JL. An experimental study of the local effects of peritoneal drainage. Surg Gynecol Obstet 1905;1:473–92.

81. Mueller MG, Ludwig LL, Barton LJ. Use of closed-suction drains to treat generalized peritonitis in dogs and cats: 40 cases (1997-1999). J Am Vet Med Assoc 2001;219:789–94.

82. Woolfson JM, Dulisch ML. Open abdominal drainage in the treatment of generalized peritonitis in 25 dogs and cats. Vet Surg 1986;15:27–32.

83. Greenfield CL, Walshaw R. Open peritoneal drainage for treatment of contaminated peritoneal cavity and septic peritonitis in dogs and cats: 24 cases (1980-1986). J Am Vet Med Assoc 1987;191:100–5.

Chapter | 27 |

Esophagus

J.M. Williams

The most frequently diagnosed esophageal surgical conditions are foreign body obstructions and stricture formation, though vascular ring anomalies and intramural masses are also found. Diagnosis is based on good history taking combined with contrast radiography and or esophagoscopy (endoscopy). Though esophageal conditions are rare in the cat, their early recognition and intervention gives the best opportunity for a successful outcome. The esophageal anatomy together with the diagnosis and surgical management of these conditions is discussed in this chapter.

SURGICAL ANATOMY

The esophagus is a hollow distensible muscular tube, some 18–19 cm in length in the cat,[1] which dilates and propels food from the pharynx to the stomach. The wall of the esophagus has four components, but differs from other intestinal structures in having a loose outer adventitial layer but no serosa.[2–4] In common with other viscera it has muscularis layers, a submucosa and a mucosa. The mucosa is plentiful and thrown into longitudinal folds cranially (Fig. 27-1). In the distal third the mucosa is folded transversely to create the herringbone pattern that is seen on contrast radiography and esophagoscopy. The mucosa is covered by stratified squamous epithelium that is continuous with the oropharynx. Distally the intra-abdominal esophagus is lined with columnar epithelium. Tubuloacinar glands, that maintain luminal lubrication, are confined to the cervical portion of the feline esophagus.[3] The folds of the mucosa may have a role to play in closure of the distal esophagus, as a true cardiac sphincter has not been identified in the cat.[2] Based on pressure manometry the functional lower esophageal sphincter is at the level of the diaphragm in the cat and is approximately 1.4 cm long.[5]

The thick submucosa has a rich vasculature and elastic tissue, though the presence of neural tissue in this layer is debated.[2] The submucosa is the suture-holding layer of the esophagus.[6] The rich plexus of intramural vessels in the submucosa can support the thoracic esophagus even if the segmental blood supply is compromised.[7] The majority of the muscle in the esophageal wall is striated but in the distal few centimeters, in the cat, the muscle is smooth.

Centrally, there are two spiral layers of muscle that cross over at right angles and change from superficial to deep by means of dorsal and ventral decussation of the fibers; this is less well defined cranially and caudally. Cranially, the esophageal muscle is a continuation of the cricopharyngeal muscle and the cricoesophageal tendon. The cranial esophageal sphincter is formed by the cricopharyngeal muscle and associated elastic tissues. The esophagus does not have a distinct outer serosal layer but is covered by adventitia, a layer of connective tissue, which adheres to adjacent structures but also allows a degree of mobility.

Though the presence of a neural network in the submucosa is a matter of debate, there is a well-defined myenteric plexus of Auerbach between the muscle layers. The vagal nerve supplies the special visceral efferent fibers to the esophagus via its various branches. The cervical esophagus receives its blood supply predominantly from the cranial

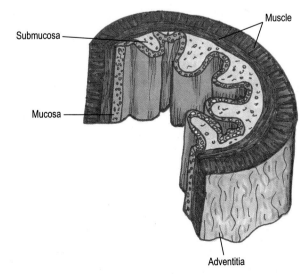

Figure 27-1 Anatomy of the esophageal wall showing the outer adventitia, two muscle layers (outer longitudinal and inner circular), the submucosa and mucosa.

DOI: 10.1016/B978-0-7020-4336-9.00027-5

and caudal thyroid arteries together with smaller branches from the carotid arteries. The bronchesophageal artery supplies the majority of the intrathoracic portion, while the terminal portion is vascularized by the esophageal branch of the left gastric artery. Venous drainage is via the jugular veins in the cervical portion and the thoracic portion drains into the azygous vein.

DIAGNOSIS AND GENERAL CONSIDERATIONS

Esophageal disorders in cats are rare, comprising only 1% of referred feline cases in a recent study.[8] As the majority of the esophagus is intrathoracic, diagnosing esophageal disorders requires good history taking and the use of ancillary diagnostic aids, in particular esophagoscopy and radiography. Masses or dilatation of the cervical esophagus are potentially palpable and cats with esophagitis may resent palpation of the cervical area.[9]

It is essential to carry out a full and thorough examination of the patient as concurrent conditions may also be present, e.g., laryngeal paralysis, peritoneo-pericardial diaphragmatic hernia, gastroesophageal reflux, esophageal hiatal hernia and inflammatory bowel disease. A summary of disorders causing esophageal dysmotility in the cat is listed in Box 27-1.[10]

Clinical signs of esophageal disease include the following, either singly or in combination: vomiting/regurgitation, dysphagia, anorexia, coughing, noisy breathing, nasal discharge, dyspnea, weight loss and poor growth. It should be noted that differentiating between true vomiting and regurgitation can be difficult in the cat, though the observant owner may note the lack of retching that is classically associated with vomiting in cats. It should also be noted that cats may vomit 'casts' of material that mimic esophageal contents.

Diagnostic aids

The decision whether to use endoscopy and/or radiography will depend on the clinician's experience and the equipment available, though both modalities are now commonplace.[8,9] The use of CT or MRI has been advocated in diagnosing esophageal tumors.[11]

Radiography

When initially assessing the esophagus radiographically, it is important that sedation and anesthesia are avoided as they may lead to relaxation of the esophagus and a false positive diagnosis of a gas-filled dilated esophagus.[8] Plain or survey radiographs should always be taken before carrying out contrast studies. For most cases barium sulphate is used as a positive contrast medium, but if an esophageal perforation is suspected water-soluble iodine based contrast medium should be used. The herringbone pattern seen with positive contrast

is normal in the distal third of the feline esophagus. If there is concern over the motility of the esophagus (see Box 27-1) (e.g., in the pouch cranial to a vascular ring anomaly) consideration should be given to using fluoroscopy, if available.

Esophagoscopy (endoscopy)

Both rigid and flexible endoscopes are suitable for examination of the cat's esophagus (Fig. 27-2). Endoscopy is particularly valuable in confirming the presence of strictures, foreign bodies and masses. If barium contrast studies have been carried out, endoscopy should not be performed until 24 hours later as the barium may obscure any abnormality. For further information on endoscopy, see Chapter 9.

SURGICAL DISEASES OF THE ESOPHAGUS

Though esophageal disease is not common, in a recent study nearly 60% of cases required surgical intervention.[8] The majority of those cases had esophageal strictures, foreign bodies or intramural neoplasia. Disorders associated with the esophageal hiatus are rare; conditions such as gastroesophageal intussusception and hiatal hernias are covered in Chapters 28 (Stomach) and 45 (Diaphragm), respectively.

Intramural strictures

An intramural esophageal stricture is the end stage of the submucosa and muscular layers healing by fibrosis as a consequence of severe deep esophagitis. The possible causes of intramural esophageal stricture in the cat are listed in Box 27-2. Clinical signs are seen within five to 14 days of the injury or onset, with dysphagia, regurgitation and weight loss being the most common signs. Confirmation is by positive contrast radiography (Fig. 27-3) and/or esophagoscopy; in some cases radiographic evidence of aspiration pneumonia may be seen (Fig. 27-4).

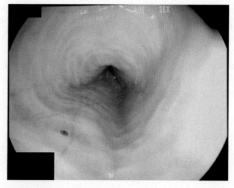

Figure 27-2 Herringbone pattern due to transverse mucosal folds seen on esophagoscopy. *(Courtesy of Ian Hopkins.)*

Box 27-1 **Causes of esophageal dysmotility**[10]

Idiopathic megaesophagus
Foreign bodies
Vascular ring anomalies
Esophageal stricture
Myasthenia gravis
Dysautonomia
Mediastinal/esophageal mass

Box 27-2 **Causes of intramural esophageal strictures**[4,10,12]

Gastroesophageal reflux
Drug-induced esophageal disorder, e.g., doxycycline, clindamycin[8,13–15]
General anesthesia[12,16,17]

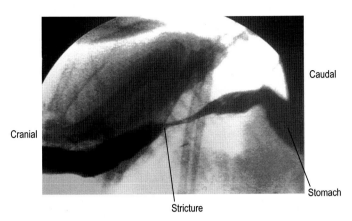

Figure 27-3 Fluoroscopy showing an esophageal stricture.

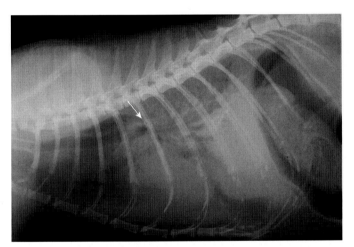

Figure 27-4 Thoracic radiograph of the cat in Figure 27-3 showing evidence of aspiration pneumonia with consolidated dorsal lung lobes. The gas-filled stomach is due to aerophagia. The site of esophageal stricture is indicated by an arrow. *(Courtesy of Ian Hopkins.)*

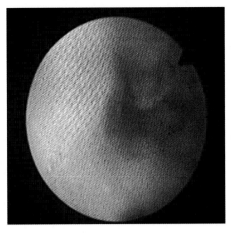

Figure 27-5 Chronic esophageal stricture. *(Courtesy of Ian Hopkins.)*

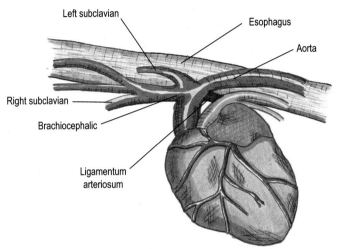

Figure 27-6 Normal anatomical arrangement of the aortic arch and vessels in the cat.

Endoscopically, a ridge, ring, or web of fibrous tissue (Fig. 27-5), is seen, which dramatically narrows the lumen (average diameter is 3–4 mm); this cannot be distended with insufflation and the endoscope will not pass through. Over 75% are in the caudal thoracic esophagus;[12] multiple strictures may be present.

A number of techniques have been proposed for managing esophageal strictures; these include dilatation with an endoscope, serial bougienage, balloon dilatation, stents, and surgical resection and anastomosis. The median number of dilatation procedures per patient is two to three, with ranges varying from one to 20 attempts to dilate the stricture.[8,12,18–21]

Complications and prognosis

Balloon dilatation of a single stricture is successful in up to 80% of patients; there is no correlation between the number of attempts and long-term success.[18] A recent report showed that the outcome of serial bougienage was good in 75% of cats.[22] Retrospective studies have shown no difference in complication rates between bougienage and balloon dilatation, with perforation rates reported to be from 0–3.9%.[4,22]

Resection and anastomosis of strictures has not been well described in the cat, though Shamir and others[32] report success in one cat. With the relatively high success rate of serial dilatation/bougienage, surgical resection can currently only be recommended when other techniques have failed.

Vascular ring anomalies

Vascular ring anomalies have been rarely described in the literature.[24,25] Affected cats are usually presented as kittens for regurgitation of solid food that began at the time of weaning. Most cats are presented before 6 months of age. Regurgitation of undigested food usually occurs immediately after eating, but is sometimes delayed as ingesta is retained in a large esophageal pouch that may develop cranial to the obstruction. Liquids and semi-solid food are preferentially retained. On physical examination, most cats are underweight. Esophageal dilatation cranial to the base of the heart in young kittens is normally the result of an extramural constriction secondary to a vascular ring anomaly (Fig. 27-6). A persistent right aortic arch is by far the most common anomaly, accounting for 81% of cases, but others have been reported, such as anomalous subclavian artery, double aortic arches and left aortic arch with right ligamentum arteriosum.[25] Early diagnosis and surgical intervention is required if the prognosis is to be favorable. Aggressive supportive therapy including, if required, rehydration, nutritional support and antibiotic management for any respiratory complications must be initiated prior to surgical intervention.

Prognosis

The degree of megaesophagus and hypomotility preoperatively are important prognostic indicators. Those kittens demonstrating comparatively minor dilatation and demonstrable motility on fluoroscopy

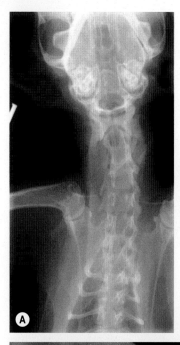

Figure 27-7 Cervical esophageal foreign body. **(A,B)** A 2-year-old female entire stray domestic short-haired cat presented with dysphagia. A hard percutaneous foreign body was palpable in the ventrolateral mid to cranial cervical region. The cat was anesthetized and orthogonal radiographs showed a bony foreign body in the mid cervical area. **(C)** The cervical area was clipped of hair and aseptically prepared for surgery. The bony foreign body **(D)** was removed by passing long handled forceps into the proximal esophagus, the percutaneous portion of the bone was then cut and then the reminder of the foreign body was carefully withdrawn using the forceps. The esophagus should be checked endoscopically 5 days post bone removal. The skin wound was left to granulate. *(Courtesy of Jon Hall.)*

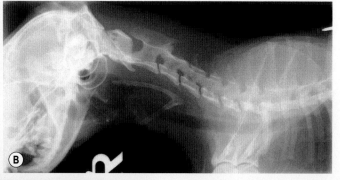

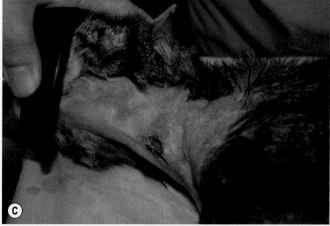

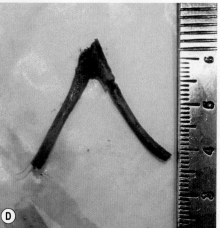

are likely to have a significantly improved prognosis compared to those with major redundant sacculation. A proportion of cases will require permanent feeding from a height; the prognosis is therefore guarded in some cases and owners should be made aware of this prior to surgery. Resection or plication of redundant esophageal tissue has not proved successful and the technique is not recommended. Recurrence of clinical signs may be due to postsurgical scarring around the esophagus. In such cases bougienage may be attempted or repeat surgery may be necessary to remove the scar tissue. The prognosis for such cases is generally guarded.

Esophageal foreign bodies

Foreign body obstruction of the esophagus is common in the dog but rare in the cat, due to their more fastidious eating habits. A variety of foreign bodies have been described in the esophagus of the cat, which are commonly acquired during hunting or play behavior. String, bone, trichobezoars (hairballs), needles, and fishhooks have all been seen.[26,27] Bones that cause obstruction tend to be 'V-shaped' avian bones (wishbones; Fig. 27-7),[28] though others may be seen (Fig. 27-8). Obstructions reportedly occur in one of three portions of the esophagus, namely the thoracic inlet, the heart base (or proximal to the cardia) and the diaphragmatic hiatus. The presenting signs are those

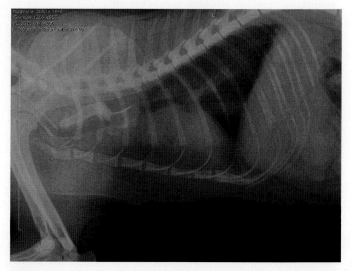

Figure 27-8 Cat with a bone esophageal foreign body as a result of being fed a bone and raw food (BARF) diet. *(Courtesy of Ian Hopkins.)*

commonly seen with esophageal disease, i.e., dysphagia, hypersaliva-tion, gagging, and retching. The severity of signs and the rate of onset will depend on whether the obstruction is partial or complete. Respi-ratory signs due to aspiration pneumonia or mediastinitis, secondary to esophageal perforation, may be encountered in severe cases.

Esophageal foreign bodies may present acutely due to total occlu-sion. Such cases not only regurgitate and gag, but also may show hypersalivation, signs of discomfort on swallowing, or collapse. Rapid deterioration may occur due to electrolyte imbalances, inhalation pneumonia, or perforation of the esophagus.[27] Prompt diagnosis and management is required. Prior to any definitive management it is essential to correct any dehydration and electrolyte changes with appropriate fluid therapy. Where cats ingest foreign bodies that cause incomplete obstruction, liquid or semi-solid food will pass in to the stomach and it can be some time before a diagnosis is made, with veterinary attention only being sought when there are signs of chronic wasting.[28]

Prognosis

The prognosis following removal is generally excellent. However, the presence of perforation or the breakdown of esophageal incisions, with the risk of developing mediastinitis and pleuritis, carries a poor prognosis and requires aggressive management. With long-standing foreign bodies or where there is gross compromise of the esophageal wall there are the risks of permanent proximal dilatation or esopha-geal strictures forming.

Neoplasia

Esophageal neoplasia is rare in the cat, and is reported as accounting for less than 0.5% of primary neoplasms.[29] Squamous cell carcinoma (SCC) is the most commonly reported neoplasm predominantly seen in older cats and usually but not exclusively seen in the distal third of the esophagus.[9,11,30] Neuroendocrine esophageal carcinomas have also been described in the cat.[31] Cats usually present with a history of progressive anorexia, dysphagia and regurgitation, weight loss, and depression. Plain radiographs may demonstrate a soft-tissue mass in the distal esophagus, with contrast studies showing marked mucosal filling defects. Confirmation of the diagnosis requires endoscopic evaluation and biopsy, though confirmation of the diagnosis may be difficult.[11] The prognosis is generally poor as the lesions are often extensive at the time of diagnosis.

The esophagus may be compressed by extraluminal masses, particu-larly mediastinal lymphoma or thymoma.

Prognosis

There is very little data available on feline esophageal neoplasia, but from the limited number of cases reported the prognosis is grave.[11,30] Resection may be feasible in some cats, dependent on the location and size of the intramural mass. In one case balloon dilatation was not successful but the cat survived four months with a gastrostomy tube.[11] The esophagectomy technique described by Ranen and others[32] can be used, but there is little data on survival post resection in the cat.[29]

PREOPERATIVE CONSIDERATIONS FOR ESOPHAGEAL SURGERY

Cats should be prepared for surgery by correction of any dehydration and electrolyte imbalances. Surgery that involves incising the esopha-gus is considered clean contaminated and intravenous perioperative antibiotics are recommended. Antibiotics should also be considered if the patient has aspiration pneumonia. If megaesophagus is present

then there is a risk of sequestered food being regurgitated after anesthesia induction. Personnel should be ready for this possibility with suction apparatus close to hand and with the aim of trying for rapid endotracheal tube placement so as to minimize the risk of aspi-ration pneumonia as a result of the anesthetic. The patient should also be checked at the end of surgery or anesthesia and the pharynx aspi-rated if required.

For lesions in the caudal cervical esophagus the possibility of needing to perform a thoracotomy should be prepared for (see Chapter 25).

Esophageal healing and closure

The esophagus can be closed in one or two appositional layers but it is essential that the submucosa is included as it is the layer of strength.[23,28,33] It has been suggested that a two-layer (simple inter-rupted) appositional technique results in the greatest immediate wound strength and best tissue apposition and healing,[33] although clinically a single layer has proved to be satisfactory in the cat.[23,29] A double layer of two continuous suture patterns, using a monofilament suture with little friction between itself and the tissue has the advan-tage of distributing the tension equally along the entire length of the incision and resists dehiscence as well as simple interrupted sutures.[34] The choice of suture materials is one of personal choice; the studies by Oakes[33] and Shamir[23] used polydioxanone. In one recent clinical report in the cat, poliglecaprone 25 was used for single layer closure[28] while Sale & Williams[35] used a two-layer closure with poliglecaprone 25 in mucosa/submucosa and glycomer 630 in the outer layer. If there is evidence of severe contusion or necrosis at the surgical site, the esophageal wound can be reinforced by using the caudal or cranial portions of the sternohyoideus muscle.[36]

SURGICAL MANAGEMENT AND TECHNIQUES FOR ESOPHAGEAL SURGERY

Surgical management for esophageal disease can be carried out in three ways. Esophageal strictures and foreign bodies are best approached endoscopically initially. If this is unsuccessful, considera-tion is given to esophagotomy that may or may not be combined with a thoracotomy, depending on the location of the lesion. Extraluminal obstructions, such as vascular ring anomalies, require surgical inter-vention that does not enter the esophageal lumen, but will require a thoracotomy (see Chapter 41).

Esophageal strictures: bougienage and balloon dilatation

Surgery is generally not recommended for the management of esopha-geal strictures, rather dilatation of the narrowing by ballooning or bougienage is usually attempted. Balloon dilatation (Box 27-3) is generally preferred to serial bougienage as the former applies an even radial force and there are theoretically less shear forces applied to the stricture (Fig. 27-14).[27]

Bougies are long narrow rounded instruments that are available in a number of sizes (Fig. 27-12). Some are designed to pass over a guide wire and are most easily used with rigid endoscopes or fluoroscopy. The aim is to start with the smallest size and progressively increase the diameter of the bougie used in steps of 2 French gauge. In human surgery, there is a 'rule of three' where it is recommended to dilate only by three sizes at each procedure. Such a rule should always be tempered by clinical judgment and it is advisable to stop once hemor-rhage is seen at the stricture site.

Box 27-3 Balloon dilatation of an esophageal stricture

The cat is anesthetized for mechanical dilatation of the stricture under endoscopic visualization. Balloon catheters with a balloon size (when inflated) of 10 or 20 mm in diameter and 6–8 cm in length are used (Fig. 27-9). The catheter diameter when deflated is 2.8 mm and it can either be passed via the operating channel of a flexible endoscope or guided alongside the endoscope. The deflated balloon is inserted into the lumen of the stricture, with a small part of the balloon visible proximally (Fig. 27-10A,B), it is then inflated to 40–50 psi for 60–90

seconds with the pressure monitored (Fig. 27-11). The balloon is deflated and withdrawn allowing the stricture to be reassessed (Fig. 27-10C) and the procedure repeated if necessary. Some hemorrhage is inevitable, but if it seems excessive then assess for any evidence of esophageal tearing. The procedure is repeated at three to five day intervals for a minimum of three treatments. Serious complications (hemorrhage, perforation) are rare.

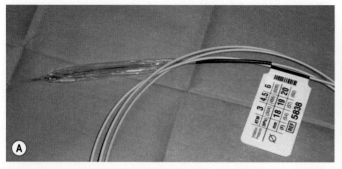 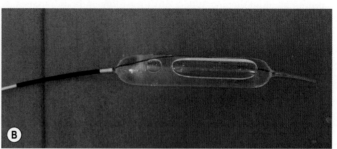

Figure 27-9 Balloon catheters. **(A)** Deflated balloon catheter. The attached pressure scale corresponds to the balloon diameter. **(B)** Inflated balloon catheter.

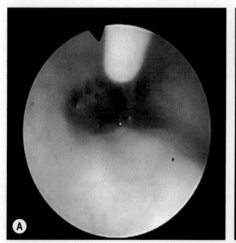 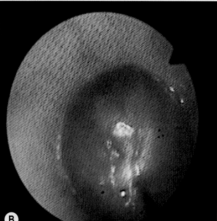 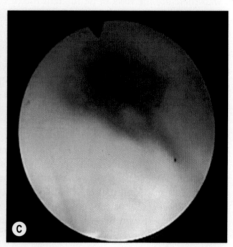

Figure 27-10 Endoscopic images of **(A)** an esophageal stricture in a cat and **(B)** balloon placement. **(C)** After dilation. *(Courtesy of Ian Hopkins.)*

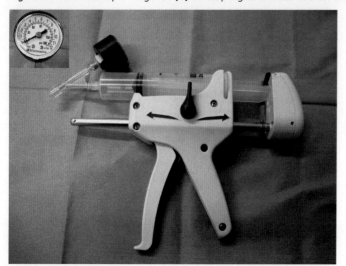

Figure 27-11 Inflation handle with syringe and pressure gauge.

Recently, the use of intraluminal esophageal stents has been described with limited success.[18,37] The use of a suitable biodegradable stent after two or three attempts at balloon dilatation may be a viable option in the future, though further work is needed in this area before it can be recommended as a routine treatment.[18]

Vascular ring anomalies

For the majority of vascular ring anomalies a left-sided fourth intercostal thoracotomy is employed, which provides the best access for the left-sided ligamentum arteriosum found with a persistent right-sided aortic arch (Box 27-4). For further information on thoracotomy see Chapter 41.

Esophageal foreign bodies

In most cases, esophagoscopic retrieval with forceps is the safest and most effective means of recovering esophageal foreign bodies.[28,38] Open, rigid esophagoscopes (Fig. 27-15) in combination with long

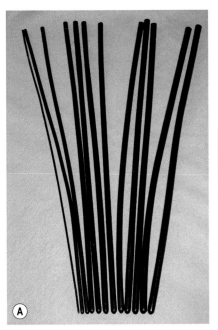

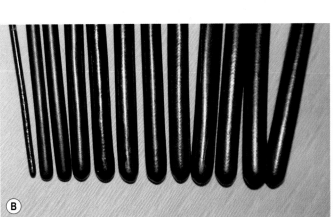

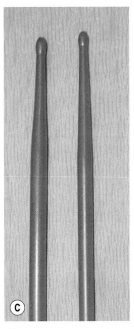

Figure 27-12 Bougies are thin cylinders that are inserted into the esophagus to widen a stricture. **(A,B)** Rubber blunt-ended bougies in a range of sizes from 20 to 60 French Gauge. **(A)** full length, **(B)** close up of tips, **(C)** silicone bougies that are tapered.

Box 27-4 **Thoracotomy for left-sided ligamentum arteriosum found with a persistent right-sided aortic arch**

The cat is positioned in right lateral recumbency for a left-sided fourth intercostal thoracotomy (see Chapter 41, Box 41-3). The lungs are gently displaced from the surgical field and held away by moist surgical swabs. The pericardium is incised longitudinally between the vagosympathetic trunk and the phrenic nerve. In order to facilitate localizing the esophagus and the stricture, an esophageal tube is inserted per os. The ligamentum arteriosum is identified (Fig. 27-13) and dissected free of the esophageal wall, then two encircling ligatures of 3M silk are tied distally and proximally on the ligamentum, which is then divided. It is essential at this stage to break down the periesophageal fibrous tissue proximal and distal to the stricture; failure to do this will result in inadequate dilatation of the narrowed portion of the esophagus. Dilatation can be aided by bougienage or balloon dilatation from within the esophageal lumen, if required.

The defect in the pericardium is left unsutured and all swabs removed from the thoracic cavity. Three to four sutures of polypropylene (3 or 3.5M) are pre-placed and passed bluntly around adjacent ribs either in a simple interrupted or cruciate mattress pattern. Care is taken to avoid the intercostal vessels. Muscles are reattached and sutured with a synthetic absorbable suture and skin closure is routine. The thorax should be drained of air using a wide bore cannula and three-way tap; in kittens, tube thoracostomy is not required.

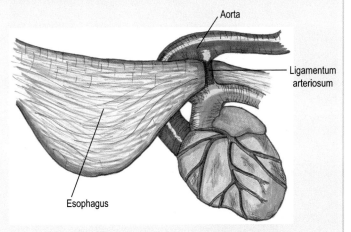

Figure 27-13 Persistent right aortic arch. Ligamentum arteriosum runs from the pulmonary artery to the anomalous right-sided aorta.

---

forceps (Chevalier-Jackson pattern; Fig. 27-16) have the advantage of allowing dilatation of the esophagus sufficiently to recover the foreign body. It is also possible to use a flexible endoscope in combination with a basket retrieval system for small foreign bodies, but this has the disadvantage of not being able to dilate the esophagus around the foreign body. It is essential that care be taken not to lacerate or perforate the mucosa on withdrawal of the foreign body. With some distal foreign bodies it is easier to retropulse the foreign body into the stomach as bony foreign bodies can be left in the stomach to be digested, while non-digestible foreign bodies should be retrieved via a gastrotomy or endoscopy. It has been suggested that hairballs can be managed by oral laxatives once in the stomach.[26] Following removal of a foreign body the esophagus should be inspected for evidence of ulceration or perforation. If there is any doubt regarding viability a gastrostomy tube should be placed. Esophagotomy is required if forceps delivery is not possible.

Esophagotomy for intramural masses[39]

Resection may be feasible in some cats, dependent on the location and size of the intramural mass. Small esophageal masses can be excised with a margin of unaffected muscle and the remaining esophagus closed with a single or double layer of interrupted simple continuous sutures (Boxes 27-5 and 27-6).[39] The diameter of the esophagus

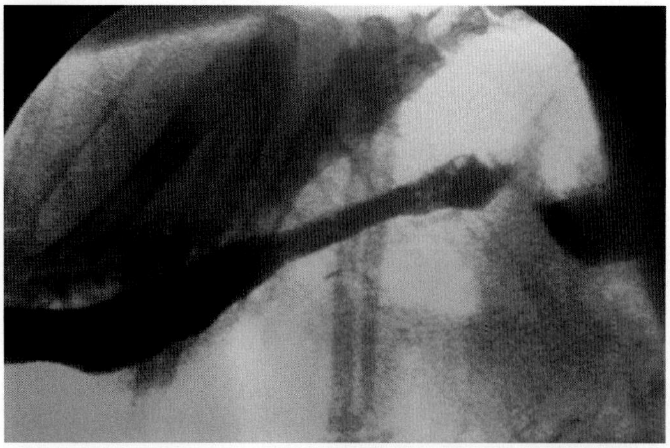

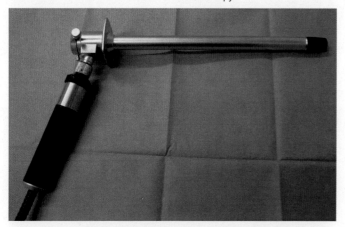

Figure 27-14 Fluoroscopy after a barium swallow showing successful dilation of the esophageal stricture seen in Figure 27-4. The barium is black rather than white because it is a fluoroscopy.

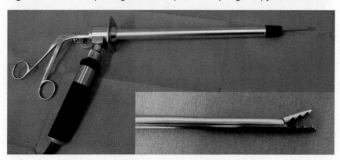

Figure 27-15 An open rigid endoscope for esophagoscopy in the cat.

Figure 27-16 Chevalier–Jackson forceps passed down the endoscopy instrument channel and **(inset)** close up view of the tips. These are useful for foreign body retrieval.

can be maintained by making an additional transverse incision or by closing the longitudinal incisions in a transverse fashion (Fig. 27-18).

POSTOPERATIVE CARE AFTER ESOPHAGEAL SURGERY

Postoperative or procedure pain relief is achieved in the first 24 hours with systemic opioids (see Chapter 2). All cats can be fed small volumes of a soft tinned proprietary diet 12 hours postoperatively. Following surgery for management of a vascular ring anomaly the cat should initially be fed from a height until it is certain that no further regurgitation occurs. Some cats will have a persistent dysfunctional esophagus due to the dilatation and will require long-term postural feeding.

During the course of stricture dilatation ongoing medical therapy for esophagitis is essential. Concurrent use of corticosteroids systemically is not likely to be beneficial though their use intralesionally may have some merit.[4] It is further recommended that following the last dilatation procedure or esophagotomy, medical management for esophagitis should be continued for at least three weeks. This should include oral mucosal protectants and antacids (either an H2 blocker or a proton pump inhibitor). The use of ranitidine as the antacid has the added advantage of accelerating gastric emptying and so further reducing the risk of gastroesophageal reflux.[4]

There is some debate as to whether a gastrostomy tube should be placed routinely following esophagotomy or bougienage.[41] It has been advocated to divert food and to allow healing of the esophagus,[23] but movement of the esophagus is unavoidable postoperatively.[35] Augusto[28] placed a gastrostomy tube, but the cat was fed orally after two days and recovered well. None of the dogs in one series of transthoracic esophagostomies had a tube placed and all healed uneventfully.[35] There is some anecdotal evidence that the esophagus is less prone to postsurgical stricture formation if early function is maintained.

COMPLICATIONS AND PROGNOSIS AFTER ESOPHAGEAL SURGERY

Complications after esophageal surgery in general are rare, but can include incisional breakdown, stricture formation, and megaesophagus. The prognosis is dependent on the severity of the disease preoperatively and specifically the degree of megaesophagus and the presence and size of esophageal necrosis or perforation as well as the location of the lesion. If mediastinitis and pleuritis develops this carries a poorer prognosis and requires aggressive management, which includes placement of thoracic drains and lavage of the pleural cavity.

Box 27-5 **Cervical esophagotomy**

The cat is positioned in dorsal recumbency with the head extended. A ventral midline approach is used to access the cervical esophagus.[28]

Foreign bodies

The site of foreign body lodgment is identified visually and by palpation and the area is carefully examined for contusions or perforation. An incision should be made longitudinally over the foreign body; stay sutures of 2 or 1.5M polypropylene can be used to facilitate retraction and handling of the esophageal wound. Once the foreign body has been removed, the esophagus is reassessed for evidence of perforation

and any defects sutured, though experimental evidence suggests that even defects up to 12 mm may heal spontaneously.[40] The esophagus can be closed in one or two appositional layers (Fig. 27-17) using either simple interrupted or continuous suture patterns, but it is essential that the submucosa is included as it is the layer of strength.[23,28,33] The author uses a two-layer closure with poliglecaprone 25 in mucosa/submucosa and glycomer 630 in the outer layer. If there is evidence of severe contusion or necrosis at the surgical site, the esophageal wound can be reinforced by using the caudal or cranial portions of the sternohyoideus muscle.[36]

Box 27-5 **Continued**

Intramural masses

A longitudinal incision is made in the esophageal wall opposite where the bulk of the mass is present. A full thickness incision is then made around the base of the mass with a margin of approximately 1 cm of unaffected esophagus. After mass removal, there are two incisions in the esophageal wall, which are closed longitudinally, but if necessary a short transverse closure is carried out to maintain esophageal diameter (Fig. 27-18). After closure of the closest incision, the esophagus is rotated using the stay sutures, to allow closure of the other side. Closure is either by a single or double layer of simple interrupted sutures, or interrupted simple continuous sutures as described previously.[32]

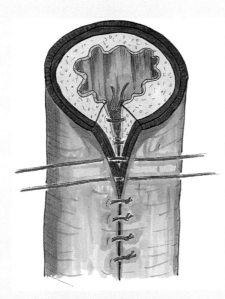

Figure 27-17 Closure of the esophageal wall can be achieved in one or two layers. In this diagram the inner layer is closed with simple interrupted sutures, ensuring the sutures engage the submucosa. The outer layer is closed with a separate layer of simple interrupted sutures.

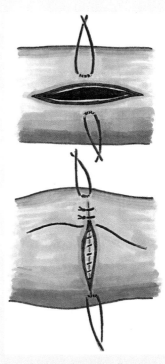

Figure 27-18 Longitudinal esophageal wall incisions can be closed transversely to maintain esophageal diameter.

Box 27-6 **Transthoracic esophagotomy**

Cats are positioned in right lateral recumbency and a standard left intercostal thoracotomy performed at the level of the intercostal space overlying the foreign body or mass (see Chapter 41).[39] The esophagus is identified, the vagus retracted where necessary, and stay sutures (2 or 1.5M polypropylene) placed either side of the affected site to provide traction and stability during handling. Saline soaked swabs are packed around the affected esophageal site to limit contamination of the pleura.

Foreign bodies

A longitudinal incision is made overlying the foreign body. A suction cannula is inserted into the incision to remove esophageal fluid content. The foreign body is grasped with Kocher forceps and removed from the lumen by gentle manipulation and traction. Post removal the distal esophageal wall is checked for perforation and necrotic tissue and debrided as necessary. The esophagotomy site and any perforations are closed using a double or single layer appositional technique. If a perforation is present the site and pleura should be lavaged with warm physiologic saline. An intercostal thoracostomy tube (8 or 10 Fr gauge) is placed through the dorsocaudal thoracic wall prior to thoracic closure. The thoracotomy is closed routinely (see Chapter 41) using monofilament 3 or 3.5M polydioxanone sutures. These are pre-placed and passed bluntly through adjacent intercostal spaces in a cruciate mattress pattern. The subcutaneous tissues and skin are closed routinely. Air and fluid are drained from the pleural cavity via the thoracostomy tube immediately after closure. Where there is no local contamination due to perforation the thoracostomy tube can be removed immediately. If an effusion is present it should be left in situ and aspirated as required until the effusion resolves.

Intramural masses

After thoracotomy, esophageal masses are readily identified by palpation and the affected part of the esophagus packed off from the thorax with moistened swabs. Polypropylene stay sutures can be used proximal and distal to the mass to facilitate manipulation. A longitudinal incision is made in the esophageal wall opposite where the bulk of the mass is present. A full thickness incision is then made around the base of the mass with a margin of approximately 1 cm of unaffected esophagus. After mass removal, there are two incisions in the esophageal wall, which are closed longitudinally but if necessary a short transverse closure is carried out to maintain esophageal diameter (Fig. 27-18). After closure of the closest incision, the esophagus is rotated using the stay sutures, to allow closure of the other side. Closure is either by a single or double layer of simple interrupted sutures, or interrupted simple continuous sutures as described above.[32]

REFERENCES

1. Reynolds RP, El-Sharkawy TY, Diamant NE. Lower esophageal sphincter function in the cat: role of central innervation assessed by transient vagal blockade. Am. J Physiol 1984;246:G666–74.

2. Grandage J. Functional anatomy of the digestive system. In: Slatter D, editor. Textbook of small animal surgery. 3rd ed. Philadelphia: Saunders; 2002. p. 504.

3. Ellenport CR. Carnivore digestive system. In: Getty R, editor. Sisson and Grossman's The anatomy of the domestic animals. 5th ed. Philadelphia: W. B. Saunders Co.; 1975. p. 1547.

4. Glazer A, Walters P. Oesophagitis and Oesophageal Strictures. Compend Continuing Educ 2008;30:281–92.

5. Hasim MA, Waterman AE. Determination of the length and position of the lower oesophageal sphincter (LOS) by correlation of external measurements with combined radiographic and manometric estimations in the cat. Br Vet J 1992;148: 435–44.

6. Dallman MJ. Functional suture-holding layer of the oesophagus in the dog. J Am Vet Med Assoc 1988;192:638–40.

7. Macmanus JE, Dameron JT, Paine JR. The extent to which one may interfere with the blood supply of the esophagus and obtain healing on anastomosis. Surgery 1950;28:11–23.

8. Frowde PE, Battersby IA, Whitley NT, Elwood CM. Oesophageal disease in 33 cats. J Feline Med Surg 2011;13:564–9.

9. Ruaux CG, Steiner JM, Williams DA. The gastrointestinal tract. In: Chandler EA, et al, editors. Feline medicine and therapeutics. 3rd ed. Oxford: Wiley-Blackwell; 2007. p. 397.

10. Moses L, Harpster NK, Beck KA, Hartzband L. Esophageal motility dysfunction in cats: a study of 44 cases. J Am Anim Hosp Assoc 2000;36:309–12.

11. Berube D, Scott-Moncrieff JC, Rohleder J, Vemireddi V. Primary esophageal squamous cell carcinoma in a cat. J Am Anim Hosp Assoc 2009;45:291–5.

12. Adamama-Moraitou KK, Rallis TS, Prassinos NN, Galatos AD. Benign esophageal stricture in the dog and cat: a retrospective study of 20 cases. Can J Vet Res 2002;66:55–9.

13. McGrotty YL, Knottenbelt CM. Oesophageal stricture in a cat due to oral administration of tetracyclines. J Small Anim Prac 2002;43:221–3.

14. German AJ, Cannon MJ, Dye C, Booth MJ, et al. Oesophageal strictures in cats associated with doxycycline therapy. J Feline Med Surg 2005;7:33–41.

15. Beatty JA, Swift N, Foster DJ, Barrs VR. Suspected clindamycin associated oesophageal injury in cats: five cases. J Feline Med Surg 2006;8:412–19.

16. Pearson H, Darke PG, Gibbs C, et al. Reflux oesophagitis and stricture formation after anaesthesia: a review of seven cases in dogs and cats. J Small Anim Prac 1978;19:507–19.

17. Galatos AD, Rallis T, Raptopoulos S. Post anaesthetic oesophageal stricture formation in three cats. J Small Anim Prac 1994;35:638–42.

18. Glanemann B, Hildebrandt N, Schneider MA. Recurrent single oesophageal stricture treated by a self-expanding stent in a cat. J Feline Med Surg 2008;10:505–9.

19. Harai BH, Johnson SE, Sherding RG. Endoscopically guided balloon dilation of benign esophageal strictures in 6 cats and 7 dogs. J Vet Int Med 1995;9:332–5.

20. Melendez L, Twedt DC, Weyrauch EA, et al. Conservative therapy using balloon dilation for intramural, inflammatory esophageal strictures in dogs and cats: a retrospective study of 23 cases (1987-1997). Eur J Comp Gastroenterol 1998;3:31–6.

21. Leib MS, Dinnel H, Ward DL, et al. Endoscopic balloon dilation of benign esophageal strictures in dogs and cats. J Vet Int Med 2001;3:139–43.

22. Bissett SA, Davis J, Subler K, Degernes LA. Risk factors and outcome of bougienage for treatment of benign oesophageal strictures in dogs and cats: 28 cases (1995–2004). J Am Vet Med Assoc 2009;235:844–50.

23. Shamir MH, Merav H, Shahar R, et al. Approaches to oesophageal sutures. Compend Continuing Educ 1999;21: 414–20.

24. Urich SJ. Report of a persistent right aortic arch and its surgical correction in a cat. J Small Anim Prac 1962;4:337–8.

25. White RN, Burton CA, Hale JS. Vascular ring anomaly with coarctation of the aorta in a cat. J Small Anim Prac 2003;44: 330–4.

26. Squires RA. Oesophageal obstruction by a hairball in a cat. J Small Anim Prac 1989;30:311–14.

27. Barrs VR, Beatty JA, Tisdall PL, et al. Intestinal obstruction by trichobezoars in five cats. J Feline Med Surg 1999;1: 199–207.

28. Augusto M, Kraijer M, Pratschke KM. Chronic oesophageal foreign body in a cat. J Feline Med Surg 2005;7:237–40.

29. Ridgway R, Suter P. Clinical and radiographic signs in primary and metastatic esophageal neoplasms of the dog. J Am Vet Med Assoc 1979;174: 700–4.

30. Gualtieri M, Monzeglio MG, Di Giancamillo M. Oesophageal squamous cell carcinoma in two cats. J Small Anim Prac 1999;40:70–83.

31. Patnaik AK, Erlandson RA, Lieberman PH. Oesophageal neuroendocrine carcinoma in a cat. Vet Pathol 1990;27:128–30.

32. Ranen E, Shamir MH, Shahar R, Johnston DE. Partial oesophagectomy with single layer closure for treatment of oesophageal sarcomas in 6 dogs. Vet Surg 2004;33: 428–34.

33. Oakes MG, Hosgood G, Snider TG 3rd, et al. Oesophagotomy closure in the dog. A comparison of a double layer appositional and two single layer appositional techniques. Vet Surg 1993;22:451–6.

34. Poole GV Jr, Meredith JW, Kon ND, et al. Suture technique and wound bursting strength. Am Surg 1984;50:569–72.

35. Sale CSH, Williams JM. Results of transthoracic oesophagotomy retrieval of oesophageal foreign body obstructions in dogs: 14 cases (2000–2004). J Am Anim Hosp Assoc 2006;42:450–6.

36. Purinton PT, Chambers JN, Moore JL. Identification and categorization of the vascular patterns to muscles of the thoracic limb, thorax, and neck of dogs. Am J Vet Res 1992;53:1435–45.

37. McLean GK, LeVeen RF. Shear stress in the performance of oesophageal dilation: comparison of balloon dilation and bougienage. Radiology 1989;172:983–6.

38. Houlton JEF, Herrtage ME, Taylor PM, et al. Thoracic oesophageal foreign bodies in the dog: a review of ninety cases. J Small Anim Prac 1985;26:521–36.

39. Orton EC. Surgical diseases of the thoracic wall. In: Slatter D, editor. Textbook of small animal surgery. 3rd ed. Philadelphia: Saunders, 2002. p. 373.

40. Killen DA, Pridgen W. Tolerance of the dog to esophageal perforation. J Surg Res 1961;1:315–17.

41. Williams JM, White RAS. Tube gastrostomy in dogs. J Small Anim Prac 1993;34:59–64.

Chapter |28|

Stomach

Z. Halfacree

This chapter discusses the surgical diseases of the stomach in the cat. Simple gastric surgery, in particular gastrotomy for foreign body removal or full-thickness gastrointestinal biopsy, is sometimes indicated in the cat. More involved gastric surgery, such as gastric resections and pyloroplasty are encountered less frequently. This chapter includes an overview of the preoperative and perioperative considerations for cats undergoing gastric surgery and a summary of the indications for gastric surgery. The surgical techniques for commonly indicated procedures, including gastrotomy and tube gastrostomy, are discussed in detail and the techniques used for pyloric surgery are summarized.

SURGICAL ANATOMY AND PHYSIOLOGY

The stomach is positioned in the cranial abdomen at the level of the costal arch, sitting within the concavity of the visceral surface of the liver (Fig. 28-1). The position of the stomach varies depending upon filling and the size of the surrounding viscera. A cat's stomach can accept 300–350 mL of liquid.[1] Ingesta enters the stomach at the cardia, passing through the lower esophageal sphincter. In the cat this sphincter is comprised of an oblique gastric sling muscle, which lies on the left lateral aspect of the sphincter, and a circular muscle that fully encircles the distal esophagus.[2] Ingesta exits the stomach via the pylorus; although the exact mechanisms are not clear, it is evident that the pylorus plays an essential role in coordinating gastric motility and gastric emptying.[3]

The vascular supply of the stomach is derived from the celiac artery, which branches into the hepatic artery, left gastric artery, and splenic artery. The right and left gastric arteries are situated along the lesser curvature and the right and left gastroepiploic arteries situated along the greater curvature of the stomach. A few branches from the splenic artery (short gastric arteries) supply the fundus. The hepatic artery gives rise to the gastroduodenal artery before continuing as the right gastroepiploic artery. In turn, the gastroduodenal artery supplies the cranial pancreaticoduodenal artery, which is responsible for the vascular supply to the proximal duodenum.[4]

The parasympathetic innervation is supplied by the vagus nerve and its dorsal and ventral vagal trunks that supply branches to the stomach as they pass through the esophageal hiatus. The sympathetic innervation arises from the splanchnic nerves, with the post-ganglionic fibres from the celiacomesenteric ganglion traveling along the branches of the celiac artery. The feline enteric nervous system is composed of two ganglionated plexuses.[5] The gastric lymphatic system drains to the gastric, hepatic, or splenic lymph nodes.[1] The gastric lymph nodes are located on the lesser curvature of the stomach within the lesser omentum and are inconsistently present.[6]

The mesenteric structures supporting the stomach are known as the greater and lesser omentum. The greater omentum is composed of parietal and visceral layers and each layer is composed of two peritoneal sheets. A meshwork of blood vessels and lymphatics running within strands of adipose tissue lies between the fine sheets, creating a net-like appearance. The visceral layer of the greater omentum originates at the dorsal abdominal wall in common with the transverse mesocolon and extends caudally, covering the ventrolateral aspect of the small intestines. At the level of the pelvic inlet the omentum is reflected upon itself to form the parietal layer of the greater omentum

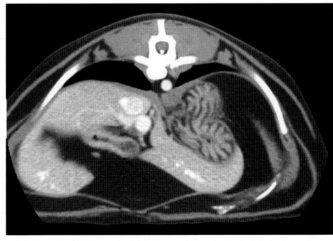

Figure 28-1 A computed tomography scan in transverse section of an adult domestic short-haired cat demonstrating the position of the stomach within the concavity of the visceral surface of the liver.

DOI: 10.1016/B978-0-7020-4336-9.00028-7

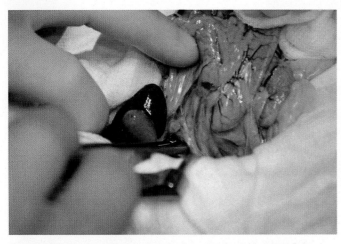

Figure 28-2 Topographic anatomy in the normal cat: the tips of the forceps are inserted into the epiploic foramen in the craniodorsal abdomen.

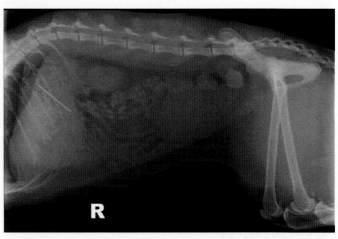

Figure 28-3 A needle foreign body in the stomach of a cat. The cat had ingested a needle and thread and the radiopaque needle is clearly visible.

that lays adjacent to the ventrolateral abdominal wall and continues cranially to insert on the greater curvature of the stomach.

The stomach sits between the two sheets of the greater omentum and these then converge at the lesser curvature of the stomach to form the lesser omentum. The potential space between the visceral and parietal layers of the omentum is called the omental bursa. Access to this space is gained via the epiploic foramen (Fig. 28-2) in the craniodorsal abdomen, or surgically by gently creating a small opening through the greater omentum, into the omental bursa. The left limb of the pancreas is present between the sheets of the visceral layer of the greater omentum adjacent to the dorsal aspect of the stomach and the spleen is situated between the sheets of the parietal layer of the greater omentum. The portion of greater omentum extending between the greater curvature of the stomach and the spleen is referred to as the gastrosplenic ligament.

DIAGNOSIS AND GENERAL CONSIDERATIONS

Hematology, serum biochemistry, serum electrolytes, and urinalysis are routinely performed in cats with gastric disease. Gastric ulceration may lead to anemia and serum electrolytes may be deranged in any patient suffering from vomiting. Vomition and loss of chloride, potassium, and acid-rich gastric secretions can lead to hypochloremic hypokalemic metabolic alkalosis; however, acid–base imbalances can be complex and hypovolemia may lead to metabolic acidosis.[7]

Diagnostic imaging

Plain abdominal radiography can be valuable in diagnosis of intraluminal foreign bodies (Fig. 28-3) and gastric distension. In order to identify gastric mucosal or mural lesions using radiography, contrast studies may be necessary. However, ultrasonography is frequently rewarding for evaluating these lesions (Fig. 28-4) and often eliminates the need for contrast studies of the stomach in these patients. Approximately 30% of normal cats have submucosal fat which appears as a radiolucent line within the gastric wall on radiography;[8] it is important to note that this is a normal finding.

Studies of gastric motility and gastric emptying often rely upon fluoroscopic contrast studies.[9] Nuclear scintigraphy is the gold standard for monitoring of gastric transit times and gastric emptying.[10]

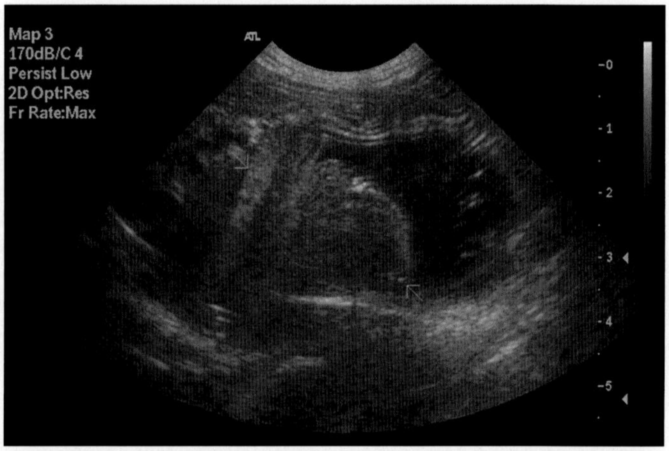

Figure 28-4 An ultrasound image demonstrating a mass involving the cardia of the stomach in a 1-year-old domestic short-haired cat. (Courtesy Alison Moores; © Anderson Moores Veterinary Specialists.)

Inflated thoracic radiography, including both lateral projections, is indicated in patients in which neoplasia is suspected to screen for metastatic pulmonary disease. In patients suffering from regurgitation thoracic radiography is advised to identify evidence of aspiration pneumonia.

Gastroscopy

Gastroscopy can be extremely useful in the management of gastric disease. It provides an unrivalled perspective of the gastric lumen and mucosal surface and may reveal lesions eluding other imaging modalities, which could also be missed on external evaluation of the stomach at laparotomy. Endoscopy allows biopsy samples to be obtained for histopathology, thereby providing prognostic information and aiding surgical planning if appropriate (Fig. 28-5). Unfortunately, the mucosal surface of neoplastic lesions may be necrotic or inflamed and histopathology can be misleading.[11] Gastroscopy is also a useful technique to allow retrieval of foreign bodies without the need for surgery. However, the withdrawal of very large or sharp objects through the cardia and esophagus should be avoided.

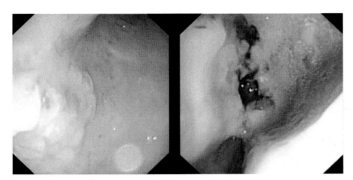

Figure 28-5 Two images captured during gastroscopy performed in an 11-year-old domestic short-haired cat with a history of weight loss and vomiting. Cytologic and histopathologic specimens obtained at gastroscopy confirmed a diagnosis of large cell lymphoma.

SURGICAL DISEASES

Full thickness gastric biopsy and gastric foreign body removal are the most common reasons for performing gastric surgery in the cat. Other less common indications include surgery for management of gastric outflow disease, neoplasia, and gastroduodendal perforation and addressing gastric dilatation associated with diaphragmatic rupture.

Gastric foreign bodies

Gastric foreign bodies are occasionally seen in the cat, but due to the relative dietary discretion of this species they are far less common than in the dog. The most common gastric foreign bodies include trichobezoars (fur balls) and linear foreign bodies, such as a needle and thread (see Fig. 28-3). Foreign bodies may be responsible for vomiting secondary to gastric outflow obstruction, initiation of gastritis or intestinal plication. They may be seen as incidental findings on abdominal radiographs in the absence of clinical signs.

Where facilities and expertise permit, endoscopic retrieval of gastric foreign bodies is preferable to surgery unless the nature of the foreign body suggests that damage to the cardia or esophagus may occur during retrieval.

Linear foreign bodies

The most common site of anchorage of linear foreign bodies in the cat is under the tongue (Fig. 28-6); however, anchorage at the gastric pylorus is also seen.[12] Plication of the duodenum and jejunum occurs as intestinal peristalsis attempts to move the anchored foreign body aborally, resulting in a functional and/or structural intestinal obstruction; however, unlike the dog, secondary intussusception has not been observed.[12,13] The radiographic appearance of linear foreign bodies does not conform to the classical picture of dilated loops of small intestine normally associated with intestinal obstruction and could lead to the diagnosis being overlooked. Thorough patient evaluation together with inspection of the abdominal radiographs for bunching of the small intestine, potentially in an abnormal position, and irregular accumulations of small intestinal gas should alert the clinician to the diagnosis.

Removal of the linear foreign body requires release of the anchorage point, which is commonly at the base of the tongue or the gastric pylorus. Surgical management should be performed promptly following release at the base of the tongue, since loss of intestinal plication may expose areas of intestinal perforation and allow leakage of intestinal contents. When the anchorage site is at the pylorus a

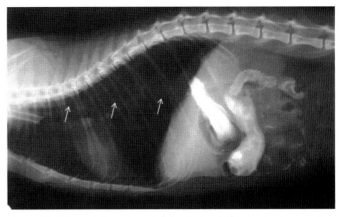

Figure 28-6 Lateral thoracic and abdominal radiograph of a 1-year-old female neutered domestic short-haired cat with a cotton thread linear foreign body lodged under the cat's tongue. A barium study had previously been performed. The small intestines appear bunched in the cranial abdomen with an irregular contrast pattern. Barium has been absorbed by the cotton thread, highlighting the path of the cotton through the thoracic esophagus from the oral cavity to the abdomen (arrows).

combination of gastrotomy and one or more enterotomy incisions may be required. Initially, a gastrotomy is performed in the distal aspect of the gastric body allowing access to the most proximal portion of the foreign body. Gentle traction can be applied to attempt retrieval via the gastrotomy site; however, caution must be exercised to prevent further damage to the mesenteric border of the small intestine. If any resistance is experienced the foreign body must be removed in pieces; the large portion present within the gastric lumen is sectioned from the portion extending into the small intestine allowing the plication effect to be released. The remaining portion of the linear foreign body is removed through additional enterotomy incisions as required and gastrotomy and enterotomy sites are closed routinely. Careful inspection of the mesenteric border of the small intestine is essential to determine if perforation or necrosis of the intestinal wall has occurred. Multiple sites of intestinal resection and anastomosis can be necessary; however, the incidence of intestinal perforation and requirement for intestinal resection anastomosis is far lower in the cat compared to the dog.[12,13] It has been theorized that the thinner, less bulky, nature of linear foreign bodies in cats is responsible for a lesser degree of intestinal plication, resulting in a lower morbidity and mortality in this species in comparison to the dog.[13] Based upon review of the literature, it is suggested that the probability of septic peritonitis and death secondary to a linear foreign body is approximately half that in a cat in comparison to a dog.[12,13]

A technique has been described via which linear foreign bodies may be removed through a single enterotomy in the cat.[14] The linear foreign body is secured to a red rubber catheter that is inserted into the intestinal lumen and milked towards the anus, together with the intestinal foreign body. Due to the difference in the nature of the foreign bodies they ingest, this technique is unlikely to be applicable to the dog, but it should always be considered in the cat. The authors describe that this technique would be applicable when the anchorage site was within the stomach; however, the catheter would be introduced via the gastrotomy and advanced aborally towards the anus.

Conservative management of linear foreign bodies in the cat has been described with successful outcome.[15] This involved identifying the anchorage site of the foreign body under the tongue and releasing it, therefore allowing the foreign body to pass. This could be considered if surgical intervention is not possible due to financial constraints; however, due to the risk of gastrointestinal perforation the author would advocate surgical management via exploratory laparotomy.

Pyloric stenosis

Gastric dysfunction is seen in young, pure bred cats, in particular Siamese cats.[16] They are generally less than 6 months old at presentation. The presenting clinical signs include vomiting, which may be projectile, and weight loss; regurgitation may also be present. Investigations reveal gastric distension and a functional delay in gastric outflow associated with pyloric stenosis (Fig. 28-7). Normal gastric emptying should start within 15 minutes of barium ingestion and the stomach is generally empty in four hours.[9] Concurrent megaesophagus is often present (Fig. 28-7) and while primary megaesophagus is suspected, it can be unclear if this is due to secondary esophagitis. Postmortem examination of one cat has documented gastric heterotopia, with secretory gastric mucosa within the distended esophagus, presumably contributing to esophagitis.[17] Some cats have been successfully managed medically with postural feeding and gastroprotection; however, when delayed gastric emptying or pyloric stenosis are documented, pyloroplasty is warranted. As this appears to be largely a functional obstruction, pyloromyotomy or Y to U pyloroplasty are likely to be sufficient; a Billroth procedure is not warranted. Tube gastrostomy (see Box 28-3) is recommended due to the potential for altered gastric motility following pyloroplasty in a patient where gastric motility may already be abnormal.

The outcome is likely to be influenced by presence of megaesophagus, but the prognosis for resolution of megaesophagus is unclear until resolution of vomiting has been achieved, together with an appropriate period of medical management for esophagitis.

Gastroduodenal ulceration and perforation

Gastroduodenal ulceration is occasionally seen in the cat.[18-21] Predisposing factors include stress associated with surgery, administration of steroid or non-steroidal anti-inflammatory medication, and as a paraneoplastic syndrome (e.g., systemic effects of mast cell neoplasia or pancreatic gastrinoma).[18-21] Several cases reported in the literature have failed to identify an underlying cause. Gastric ulceration and perforation may also occur secondary to primary gastric disease, including neoplasia and inflammatory bowel disease. Clinical signs include inappetence, vomiting, hematemesis, and melena; progression to gastric perforation may result in depression and collapse due to sepsis. Anemia is a common clinical finding in cats with gastrointestinal blood loss; however, it is important to note that hematemesis or melena were present in less than a third of cats with gastrointestinal ulceration in one review.[18]

Cats that have suffered from gastric perforation may present with depression and abdominal distension due to pneumoperitoneum. Radiographic evidence of marked spontaneous pneumoperitoneum in the cat should raise the suspicion of gastric perforation (Fig. 28-8). Ultrasonographic findings of gastric perforation can be quite nonspecific, with bright regional mesenteric fat and peritoneal effusion noted most frequently.[22] Abdominal radiography is advocated to facilitate detection of pneumoperitoneum.

Tension pneumoperitoneum causing respiratory embarrassment has been described in a cat with concurrent upper respiratory tract obstruction.[23] Therapeutic abdominocentesis may be required in this situation to achieve stabilization; however, this is uncommon.

Indications for surgery in cats with gastroduodenal ulceration are listed in Box 28-1. Surgery is invariably required as cats tend to present when disease is advanced and gastric perforation has occurred.

Septic peritonitis is a life-threatening condition with a guarded prognosis; its presence necessitates careful patient stabilization and prompt surgical intervention (see Chapter 26). In one study looking at septic peritonitis in cats, with a range of underlying causes, only 12 of 26 cats survived to discharge.[24] Thorough exploratory laparotomy, gastric resection at the site of perforation (see Box 28-4), copious lavage, and empirical antibiosis (while pending culture results) are

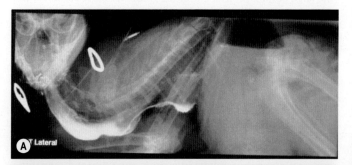

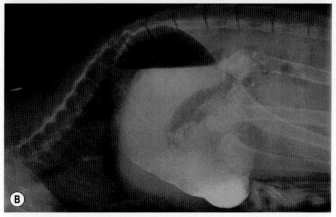

Figure 28-7 Fluoroscopic barium swallowing study in a 6-month-old male neutered Siamese kitten. **(A)** The esophagus is moderately dilated along its length. **(B)** The stomach is distended with food particles, fluid and gas. There is no evidence of barium passing into the small intestines after 15 minutes, suggestive of pyloric stenosis.

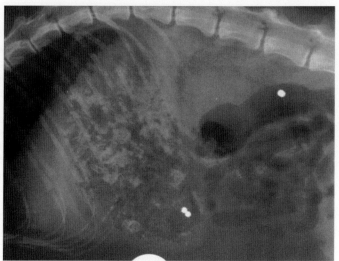

Figure 28-8 A lateral abdominal radiograph of a 5-year-old male entire domestic short-haired cat that presented following discovery of small focal penetrating wounds. The cat had been shot with an air rifle and one of the airgun pellets had perforated the gastric wall.

essential. The site of gastric perforation can be challenging to identify and thorough inspection must be performed.

Perforation of a gastric ulcer involving the pylorus can present a surgical challenge. The morbidity associated with a Billroth I (pylorectomy and gastroduodenostomy) or Billroth II (pyloroduodenectomy and gastrojejunostomy) is ideally avoided in patients with potentially benign disease. When possible, local debridement and primary closure should be performed in the first instance, avoiding more radical gastric resection which is potentially unnecessary. It is essential that the repair is augmented with omentum or a serosal patch. Tissue must always be obtained for histopathology to rule out gastric neoplasia.

Gastric perforation may be caused by trauma; due to the protected site of the stomach within the costal arch the most common traumatic lesion is a ballistic projectile, such as an airgun pellet (Fig. 28-8).

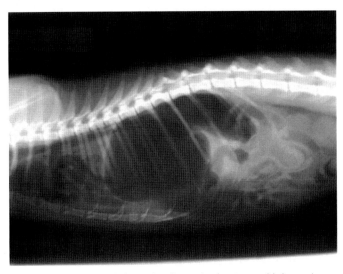

Figure 28-9 A lateral abdominal radiograph of a 4-year-old domestic short-haired cat that presented with acute collapse and dyspnea. The cat has a traumatic diaphragmatic rupture and herniation of the stomach into the pleural cavity with subsequent development of tension gastrothorax. *(Courtesy Victoria Lipscomb.)*

Disorders associated with the esophageal hiatus

Gastric disease associated with the esophageal hiatus occurs infrequently in the cat, with only a few case reports available in the literature.[25–28] Gastroesophageal intussusception is the term used to describe invagination of the stomach into the lumen of the distal esophagus. Predisposing factors are reported to be megaesophagus, an incompetent lower esophageal sphincter, and chronic vomiting. Presenting signs include regurgitation, vomiting, dyspnea and collapse. The prognosis is considered guarded, but successful outcome has been reported in the dog following prompt diagnosis and intervention.[29] Surgical management involves an exploratory laparotomy, reduction of the intussusception, gastropexy, and placement of a stomach tube. Non-surgical management with endoscopic reduction of the intussusception intraluminally and percutaneous endoscopic gastrostomy tube placement has been reported in one puppy.[30] In contrast to the dog, in which gastroesophageal intussusception is predominantly a life-threatening condition requiring rapid intervention, intermittent gastroesophageal intussusception with mild chronic clinical signs represents two of the four individual case reports in the cat.[26,28]

Congenital sliding hiatal hernia has been reported in a small number of cats.[31–33] Surgical management, by herniorrhaphy, esophagopexy and incisional gastropexy is reported,[31,32] although there was no long term follow up. Successful management by dietary change, with resolution of regurgitation, has also been reported.[33] Surgical management of sliding esophageal hiatal hernia has been reported in a lynx, cougar, and a lion.[34] For more information on management of hiatal hernia, see Chapter 45.

Gastric disorders associated with diaphragmatic rupture

Traumatic diaphragmatic rupture is frequently encountered in the cat (see Chapter 45) and is associated with herniation of abdominal contents, often including the stomach, into the pleural cavity. Rarely, herniation of the stomach into the pleural cavity can result in the life-threatening complication of 'tension gastrothorax' (Fig. 28-9). Respiratory compromise occurs due to occupation of the pleural space by the stomach which, depending upon position, can become markedly distended by trapped air.[35,36] Emergency decompression of the distended stomach is required via passage of a nasogastric tube or percutaneous gastrocentesis. Following stabilization, surgery to reduce the herniated viscera and repair the diaphragmatic rupture must also be performed.

Abdominal viscera, including the stomach, may become incarcerated following diaphragmatic rupture and non-viable tissue must be resected (Fig. 28-10).

Gastric dilatation and volvulus occurs rarely in cats and diaphragmatic rupture, with the stomach remaining within the peritoneal cavity, appears to be a predisposing factor.[37,38] Successful outcome has been reported following appropriate stabilization and gastric derotation at surgery, following the same management approach as for the dog. Gastropexy is advocated; however, the literature indicates this is not consistently performed when the predisposing factor of diaphragmatic rupture has been identified. Sliding hiatal hernia has been reported as a complication following diaphragmatic rupture and diaphragmatic herniorrhaphy in the cat;[33] successful surgical management is reported with hiatal herniorrhaphy and tube or incisional gastropexy.

Gastric neoplasia

Gastric neoplasia is uncommon in the cat and is generally seen in older animals. Lymphoma is the most commonly reported gastric tumor in the cat and it is not amenable to surgical resection due to the diffuse nature of disease. In comparison to lymphoma at other sites, a histopathologic diagnosis is often required to achieve a diagnosis in visceral lymphoma.[39] Even then, it can be difficult to differentiate low grade lymphoma from lymphoplasmacytic enteritis on the basis of cytology and histopathology and therefore other tests such as clonality may be required.[40] Most cats are feline leukemia virus negative. Feline gastric adenocarcinoma is rare and the stomach is the least commonly affected gastrointestinal site in the cat.

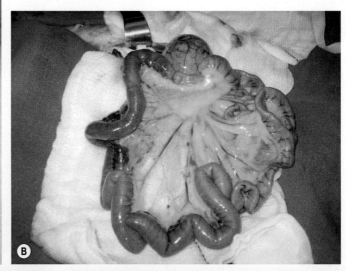

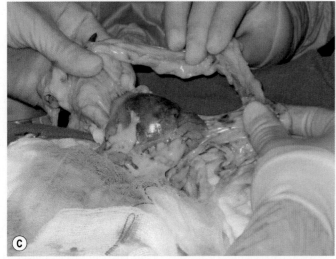

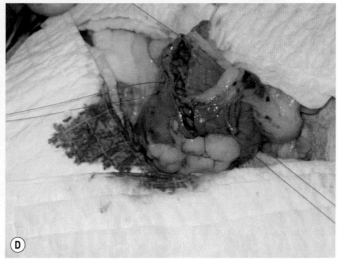

Figure 28-10 A chronic traumatic diaphragmatic rupture in an 8-year-old domestic short-haired cat with herniation of the stomach, small intestines and omentum into the pleural cavity. **(A)** The diaphragmatic defect in the tendinous portion of the diaphragm following reduction of the herniated abdominal contents. **(B, C)** A section of jejunum and a region of the gastric wall had become strangulated. **(D)** The portion of devitalized gastric wall was resected and closed in two layers. *(Courtesy Matthieu Cariou.)*

PREOPERATIVE CONSIDERATIONS

Thorough preoperative investigations are essential to attempt to achieve a diagnosis prior to surgery, therefore allowing a surgical plan to be formulated. Adequate preparation can then be made to prepare the cat for surgery, decide on therapeutics and anesthetic needs, and also to consider the postoperative conditions that will be required.

Surgical considerations

Despite preoperative investigations, additional findings may be made at surgery and it is important to perform a full systematic abdominal exploration. Evaluation of a gastric mucosal lesion and its extent can be facilitated by inspection through a gastrotomy made opposite the lesion, thereby aiding intraoperative decision making.

Perioperative antibiotic use

Gastric surgery in which the gastric lumen is entered is classified as clean contaminated surgery, provided appropriate care is taken to ensure minimal intraoperative contamination. Perioperative prophylactic antibiosis is therefore appropriate but postoperative antibiotic administration is not justified.[41] Minimal intraoperative contamination is achieved by use of stay sutures to manipulate the gastrotomy, use of laparotomy swabs to isolate the gastrotomy site from the rest of the abdomen, designation of both clean and contaminated areas for surgical instruments, and use of copious peritoneal lavage. Septic peritonitis, due to pre-existing gastric perforation or necrosis, necessitates the use of therapeutic antibiosis postoperatively. This will initially be empirical but should be adjusted based upon culture and sensitivity results from bacteriology samples obtained at surgery.

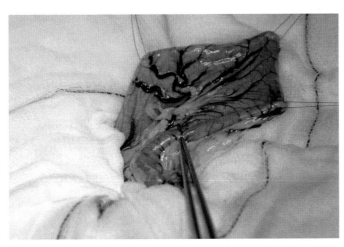

Figure 28-11 Stay sutures have been placed in the ventral surface of the stomach to aid in atraumatic manipulation and to reduce the risk of spillage of gastric contents following gastrotomy.

Anesthesia considerations

Gastric fluid retention may result in regurgitation with the risk of aspiration at the time of induction. It is important to achieve a smooth induction and intubate the patient promptly; stomach tubes and suction apparatus should be made available.

Multimodal analgesia should be provided where possible in patients undergoing a laparotomy. Non-steroidal anti-inflammatory medication is contraindicated in patients that may be suffering from gastrointestinal ulceration and in patients that are hypovolemic. Premedication with systemic gastroprotectant medication (cimetidine or ranitidine) may be indicated in cats with a high risk of gastrooesophageal reflux or regurgitation; elevation of the pH of gastric fluid ameliorates the potential effects upon the esophagus or lungs should regurgitation and/or aspiration occur. For further information on anesthesia see Chapter 2.

SURGICAL MANAGEMENT AND TECHNIQUES

The surgical approach to the stomach is via a routine ventral midline celiotomy (see Chapter 23), extending cranially to the level of the xiphoid. Removal of falciform fat is recommended to improve visualization. Increased mobilization of the stomach may be achieved by transection of the hepatogastric ligament and the avascular peritoneal reflection. Manipulation of the stomach is facilitated by placement of stay sutures in the ventral aspect of the stomach to reduce tissue trauma and reduce the risk of gastric contents spillage. The stay sutures should be passed full thickness through the gastric wall to engage the submucosa, with a bite 1 cm in length to avoid suture pull through (Fig. 28-11).

Gastrotomy

Gastrotomy (Box 28-2) is commonly indicated for foreign body retrieval, inspection of lesions within the gastric lumen and to obtain full thickness biopsies. The principles of gastrotomy that should be applied prior to performing a gastric resection state that a simple gastrotomy is performed at a site that allows initial luminal inspection without interfering with the subsequent surgical plan.

Box 28-2 **Gastrotomy**

Isolate the stomach using moistened laparotomy swabs to pack off other abdominal contents. Place stay sutures in the ventral stomach wall using monofilament suture material, full thickness bites and sutures placed 1 cm apart. Make a stab incision at a non-vascular part of the ventral gastric wall into the gastric lumen, using the stay sutures to 'tent' the gastric wall (Fig. 28-12). The stomach wall naturally separates into two distinct layers, with the outer layer including the serosa and muscularis and the inner layer including the submucosa and mucosal layer. Extend the incision using Metzenbaum scissors, making a full thickness cut through the gastric wall. Use suction apparatus to aspirate gastric contents and prevent spillage.

If indicated, a full thickness gastric biopsy can be obtained at this stage by excising a portion from the edge of the gastrotomy wound using Metzenbaum scissors. The serosa muscularis and the submucosa mucosal layers will naturally separate. It is recommended to tack the two together with a suture to avoid loss of one half of the biopsy sample. Place additional stay sutures at either wound edge to minimize tissue trauma and facilitate manipulation of the gastrotomy. Remove gastric foreign bodies using swab holding forceps or Allis tissue forceps.

Any instruments that were used within the gastric lumen should be discarded and if gloves have become contaminated with gastric contents they should be changed. The gastric wall should be closed in two layers. The author uses a simple continuous appositional suture in both the mucosa/submucosa layer and the outer muscularis/serosa layer. Absorbable monofilament suture (e.g., polydioxanone, poliglecaprone 25) in 1.5 or 2M is appropriate. Chromic catgut is not recommended. Whenever a gastric foreign body is removed ensure that the stomach and the entire gastrointestinal tract are carefully checked for additional foreign bodies.

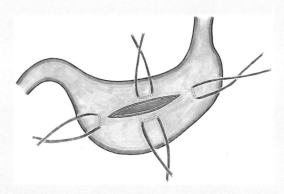

Figure 28-12 Stay sutures are placed prior to performing a gastrostomy. The stay sutures are used for atraumatic manipulation of the stomach.

Gastrostomy

Gastrostomy tube placement in the cat has several indications (Box 28-3). The tube can be inserted per endoscopically (see Chapter 12) or by open surgery (Box 28-4). The latter technique is indicated if the cat is having a celiotomy, if there are not facilities for endoscopic tube placement, or the tubes are not of the type that are ideally placed endoscopically. The major advantage of surgically placed gastrostomy tubes in comparison to percutaneous endoscopic gastrostomy tubes is the reduced risk of peritoneal leakage.[42]

The patient can be fed orally with the tube in place and, if ongoing enteral nutrition is required, the cat can be discharged with the tube in place, following appropriate client education.[43]

The gastrostomy tube should not be removed earlier than ten days postoperatively to ensure satisfactory healing resulting in an adhesion between the gastric and body walls, and therefore avoiding intraperitoneal contamination. While early adhesion formation is promoted in surgically placed gastrostomy tubes by suturing the gastric wall to the abdominal wall, the author still does not recommend early removal. Experimental studies in healthy dogs have reported that the risk of peritoneal contamination is low after three days postoperatively due to adequate adhesion formation;[44] however, it is unclear how adhesion formation may be affected by debilitation of the patient. The tube is removed by traction and the stoma is left to heal by second intention. The insertion of a trocar into the lumen of the tube to efface the mushroom tip can be useful to facilitate removal. Sedation or general anesthesia is advisable in the cat. Foley catheters are unsuitable for use as gastrostomy tubes, as degradation of the balloon by exposure to gastric acid may cause premature failure and leakage of gastric contents to occur.

Gastric resection

Gastric resection (Box 28-5) is rarely indicated in the cat. It may be indicated for excision of a perforated gastric ulcer (Fig. 28-15), excision of a focal neoplastic lesion, or a devitalized region of gastric wall (see Fig. 28-10).

Pyloric surgery

Pyloric surgery is infrequently indicated in the cat. Pyloroplasty (Fig. 28-17) is indicated for management of congenital pyloric stenosis (Fig. 28-18), which is associated with delayed gastric emptying. Surgical procedures involving the pylorus may be indicated for management of a discrete gastric tumor or for resection of a perforated area of ulceration (Table 28-1).

POSTOPERATIVE CARE

Multimodal postoperative analgesia is provided where appropriate, combining a pure (methadone) or partial (buprenorphine) opioid agonist together with a non-steroidal anti-inflammatory drug if

---

Box 28-3 Indications for tube gastrostomy

Nutrition

Indications
  Prolonged inappetence or inability to eat
  To bypass the oral cavity, pharynx or esophagus
Contraindications
  Primary gastric disease
  Vomiting patient
  Used with caution in patients with esophageal dysfunction or altered mentation due to risk of aspiration

Gastric decompression

Surgery involving the pylorus commonly affects pyloric function and gastric motility postoperatively which may cause gastric retention and inappetence. Placement of a tube gastrostomy allows gastric decompression to be achieved and enteral nutrition to be provided where necessary.

Gastropexy

Gastropexy is seldom indicated in the cat. However, it is recommended in cases of gastric dilatation and volvulus, esophageal hiatal hernia and gastrooesophageal intussusception, that are reported rarely. Tube gastropexy is ideal in these patients both to prevent recurrence of dilation and volvulus and provide nutrition.

Box 28-4 Tube gastrostomy technique (Fig. 28-13)

Choose an appropriate position for the tube gastrostomy between the body of the stomach and the left body wall, approximately one third of the distance from ventral to dorsal along the body wall and just behind the last rib (Fig. 28-14A).

Make a stab incision through the body wall with a number 10 or 15 blade. Pass the external end of the mushroom tipped tube through the body wall using Kelly artery forceps (note the tube is not tunneled at all) (Fig. 28-14A,B). Now block the end of the tube to prevent contamination of the surgical field. Place a purse-string suture in the gastric body at the site where the tube will enter, prior to creating the stab incision (Fig. 28-14C).

Insert the mushroom tube via the stab incision. The mushroom tip must be folded within the jaws of a pair of artery forceps to achieve this. Once the tube is inserted (Fig. 28-14D), withdraw it until the mushroom abuts the gastric wall and tie the purse-string suture tight. The stomach is then secured to the body wall using four horizontal mattress sutures between the stomach wall and the body wall, placed around the tube in sequence to create a box of sutures (Fig. 28-14E,F).

Omentalize the stoma site by wrapping some omentum around the tube and sutures.

Secure the tube externally using a finger trap suture. Additional fixation of the tube is essential prior to recovery from anesthesia to prevent inadvertent removal. This can be achieved using a stockinette dressing or bandaging material.

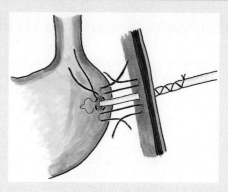

Figure 28-13 Diagram summarizing placement of a gastrostomy tube. Only two sutures are shown between the stomach and body wall; usually four would be placed.

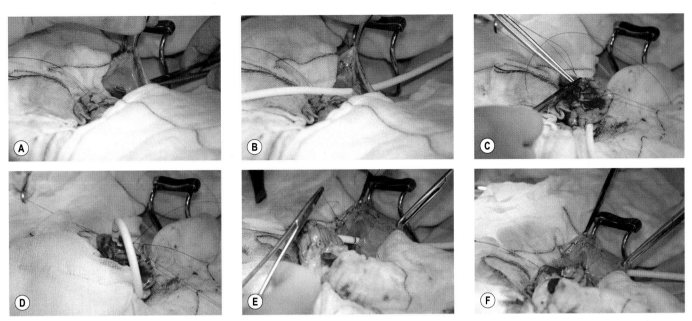

Figure 28-14 Surgical placement of a tube gastrostomy in a cat. See Box 27-4 for details of the technique with a description of parts **(A)** to **(F)**.

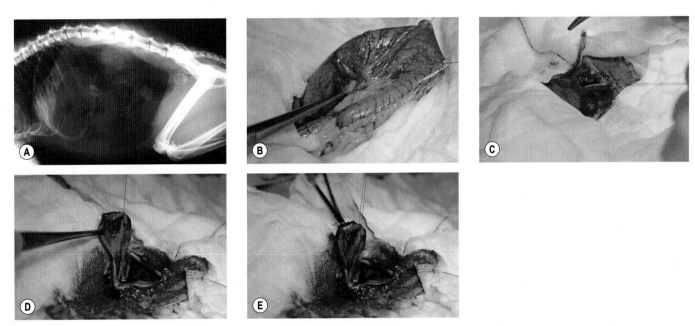

Figure 28-15 Gastric ulceration and perforation in a 5-year-old female neutered Persian cat. **(A)** Lateral abdominal radiography revealing a pneumoperitoneum. **(B)** DeBakey forceps indicate the site of gastric perforation on the lesser curvature of the stomach. Local inflammation of the serosal surface is the only apparent abnormality on initial inspection. **(C)** A full thickness incision is made through the gastric wall adjacent to the lesion to allow inspection of the mucosal surface and evaluate the extent of the lesion. **(D, E)** A focal area of mucosal erosion is identified on the luminal surface. A focal area of gastric wall with a margin of normal tissue surrounding the ulcer is resected. This will be closed in two layers, as for a standard gastrotomy incision.

appropriate. Cats that are hypotensive or have evidence of gastrointestinal ulceration should not receive non-steroidal anti-inflammatory drugs.

Early enteral nutrition is recommended as soon as the cat has fully recovered from general anesthesia. Intravenous fluid therapy should be continued until normal oral intake of fluid and food is resumed.

COMPLICATIONS AND PROGNOSIS

Complications associated with gastric surgery include routine surgical complications such as bleeding, wound infection, and wound

Box 28-5 Gastric resection (Fig. 28-16)

Perioperative assessment of the gastric mass or lesion, at the time of exploratory laparotomy, is often necessary to establish if resection is feasible. Evaluation of the extent of a focal mass lesion, and feasibility for resection, is often aided by inspection of the mucosal surface of the lesion via a gastrostomy on the opposite side. In some cases (e.g., benign adenomatous polyps), submucosal resection may be appropriate and can be useful for resection of lesions within the pylorus, thereby avoiding more radical surgery. If surgical excision is not straightforward, incisional biopsy of the gastric lesion and regional lymph nodes should be performed to achieve complete surgical staging.

Lesions involving the greater curvature may be amenable to resection using surgical stapling equipment (gastrointestinal anastomosis stapler; see Chapter 10). Alternatively, the area that requires resection should be removed using scissors or a scalpel blade. The use of Doyenne bowel clamps, careful use of stay sutures, and a surgical assistant aid the procedure and reduce the risk of gastrointestinal spillage. The stomach should be closed in two layers as for gastrotomy; an additional layer of inverting sutures (e.g., interrupted or continuous Cushing or Lembert sutures) may be used to over-sew the site and reinforce the closure.

dehiscence. Dehiscence of gastrotomy wounds and subsequent septic peritonitis is uncommon; in one study describing the underlying cause of septic peritonitis in cats, none of the cats had developed septic peritonitis due to gastrotomy dehiscence, while five of 26 cats had developed septic peritonitis due to enterotomy dehiscence.[25]

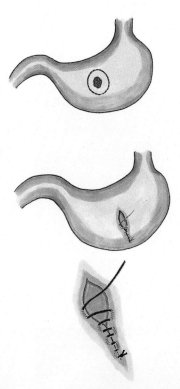

Figure 28-16 A small lesion can be removed by partial gastrectomy. Closure is achieved by placement of a continuous appositional suture in the two distinct layers of the gastric wall, reinforced by an inverting suture if required.

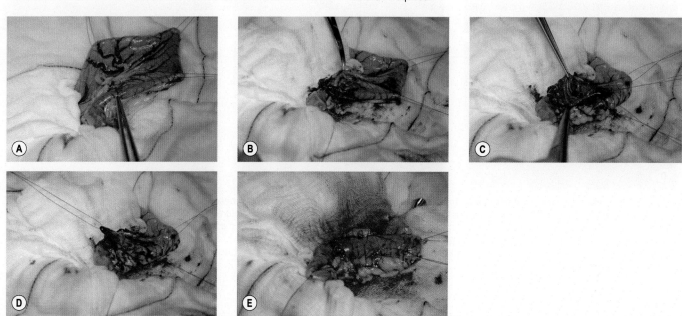

Figure 28-17 A 6-month-old male neutered Siamese kitten undergoing a Y-to-U pyloroplasty. **(A)** The pyloric region of the stomach appears relatively unremarkable on external examination. **(B)** A full thickness Y-shaped incision is made over the pylorus with the centre of the Y situated at the pylorus. **(C)** The luminal surface of the pylorus is inspected. **(D)** The top portion of the Y created a U-shaped flap, which is advanced aborally to widen the pylorus. **(E)** The Y-to-U pyloroplasty is complete. *(Courtesy Dr Stephen Baines.)*

Table 28-1 Summary of the options for pyloric surgery in the cat

Surgical technique	Technique	Indications	Disadvantages	Comments
Fredet–Ramstedt pyloromyotomy	Longitudinal incision over the pylorus through the serosa and muscularis layers only, leaving submucosa and mucosa intact	This technique is of limited use	Does not allow inspection of mucosal surface Does not allow full thickness biopsy Improvement in outflow may be short-lived due to narrowing during healing	
Heineke Mikulicz Pyloroplasty (HMP)	Full thickness longitudinal incision over the pylorus which is then closed transversely to create widening	Pyloric stenosis	These are preferable first-line procedures due to simplicity and reduced disruption of pyloric function. Subjectively, the Y-U pyloroplasty creates a greater degree of widening than the HMP and allows greater access to achieve mucosal resection. These techniques may afford limited benefit in patients with severe disease, in particular if muscular hypertrophy is advanced and pylorectomy may therefore be indicated	
Y-U advancement pyloroplasty (see Fig. 28-18)	A full-thickness Y-shaped incision is made over the pylorus with the leg of the Y oriented towards the duodenum. The created flap is used as an advancement flap creating a U-shaped wound			
Pylorectomy and gastroduodenostomy (Billroth I)	End-to-end anastomosis of the distal stomach to the duodenum. Luminal disparity must be corrected and can be achieved by spatulation of the duodenal end or partial closure of the gastrotomy	Severe pyloric stenosis Gastric resection due to neoplasia or severe gastroduodenal ulceration	For neoplastic lesions margins of 1–2 cm should ideally be achieved, but close proximity to the common bile duct and pancreas may preclude this	Take great care to avoid damage to the common bile duct in its course through the lesser omentum
Partial gastrectomy and gastrojejunostomy (Billroth II)	The distal stomach and proximal duodenum are closed and a side-to-side anastomosis of the jejunum to the diaphragmatic surface of the stomach is created. Surgical stapling equipment can be used Biliary diversion and potentially ligation of the pancreatic duct are also necessary	Gastric resection due to neoplasia or severe gastroduodenal ulceration	Complex surgical procedure resulting in significant long-term postoperative morbidity This technique should be avoided unless all other options have been ruled out Careful client communication regarding morbidity and the need for long-term medical management is essential	

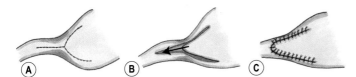

Figure 28-18 Y-to-U pyloroplasty for pyloric stenosis. **(A)** A Y-shaped incision full thickness incision is made just proximal to the pylorus. **(B)** The first suture, indicated by the arrow, converts the Y to U. **(C)** Additional sutures are placed to close the gastrotomy.

Surgery involving the esophageal hiatus or the gastric pylorus may interfere with regulation of gastric motility in the postoperative period and therefore patients should be monitored for gastric distension. Occasionally, gastric decompression may be required and is facilitated by prior placement of a tube gastrostomy. Careful monitoring of serum electrolytes is essential if gastric decompression is performed. The feeding of a low fat diet will reduce gastric retention and may ameliorate gastric motility dysfunction.[45]

Complications of gastrostomy tube placement include peristomal inflammation or infection, premature tube removal, septic peritonitis, and fistula formation after tube removal.[42] Stoma site metastasis has been reported associated with gastrostomy tube placement in the human and dog.[46] Fungal colonization precipitating tube failure has been reported with long-term use.[47]

REFERENCES

1. Barone R. Système lymphatique du chat. In: Barone R, editor. Anatomie comparé des mammifères domestiques. Tome 5 angiologie. Paris: Editions Vigot; 1996. p. 833–44.
2. L'Heureux M-C, Muinuddin A, Gaisano HY, et al. Feline lower oesophageal sphincter sling and circular muscles have different functional inhibitory responses. Am J Physiol Gastrointest Liver Physiol 2006;290:G23–9.
3. Lammers WJ, Slack JR, Stephen B, Pozzan O. The spatial behaviour of spike patches in the feline gastroduodenal junction *in vitro*. Neurogastroenterol Mot 2000;12: 467–73.
4. Gilbert SG. Pictorial anatomy of the cat. University of Washington Press; 1968. p. 49–55.
5. Kleinschmidt S, Nolte I, Hewicker-Trautwein M. Structural and functional

components of the feline enteric nervous system. Anat Histol Embryol 2011 (epub ahead of print).

6. Schreurs E, Vermote K, Barberet V, et al. Ultrasonographic anatomy of abdominal lymph nodes in the normal cat. Vet Radiol Ultrasound 2008;49:68–72.

7. Bebchuk TN. Feline gastrointestinal foreign bodies. Vet Clin Small Anim 2002;32:861–80.

8. Heng HG, Wrigley RH, Kraft SL, Powers BE. Fat is responsible for an intramural radiolucent band in the feline stomach wall. Vet Radiol Ultrasound 2005;46: 54–6.

9. Hall JA, Washbau RJ. Diagnosis and treatment of gastric motility disorders. Vet Clin Small Anim 1999;29:377–95.

10. Lamb CR. Recent developments in diagnostic imaging of the gastrointestinal tract of the dog. Vet Clin Small Anim 1999;29:307–42.

11. Evans SE, Bonczynski JJ, Broussard JD, et al. Comparison of endoscopic and full-thickness biopsy specimens for diagnosis of inflammatory bowel disease and alimentary lymphoma in cats. J Am Vet Med Assoc 2006;229:1447–50.

12. Felts JF, Fox PR, Burk RL. Thread and sewing needles as gastrointestinal foreign bodies in the cat: a review of 64 cases. J Am Vet Med Assoc 1984;184:56–9.

13. Evans KL, Smeak DD, Biller DS. Gastrointestinal linear foreign bodies in 32 dogs: a retrospective evaluation and feline comparison. J Am Anim Hosp Assoc 1994;30:445–50.

14. Anderson S, Lippincott CL, Gill PJ. Single enterotomy removal of gastrointestinal linear foreign bodies. J Am Anim Hosp Assoc 1992;28:487–90.

15. Basher AW, Fowler JD. Conservative versus surgical management of gastrointestinal linear foreign bodies in the cat. Vet Surg 1987;16:135–8.

16. Pearson H, Gaskell CJ, Gibbs C, Waterman A. Pyloric and oesophageal dysfunction in the cat. J Small Anim Pract 1974;15:487–501.

17. Bishop LM, Kelly DF, Gibbs C, Pearson H. Megaoesophagus and associated gastric heterotopic in the cat. Vet Pathol 1979;16: 444–9.

18. Liptak JM, Hunt GB, Barrs VR, et al. Gastroduodenal ulceration in cats: eight cases and a review of the literature. J Fel Med Surg 2002;4:27–42.

19. Mellanby RJ, Baines EA, Herrtage ME. Spontaneous pneumoperitoneum in two cats. Journal Small Anim Pract 2002;43: 543–6.

20. Lykken JD, Brisson BA, Etue SM. Pneumoperitoneum secondary to a perforated gastric ulcer in a cat. J Am Vet Med Assoc 2003;222:1713–16.

21. Cariou MP, Halfacree ZJ, Lee KC, Baines SJ. Successful surgical management of spontaneous gastric perforations in three cats. J Feline Med Surg 2010;12:36–41.

22. Boysen SR, Tidwell AS, Penninck DG. Ultrasonographic findings in dogs and cats with gastrointestinal perforation. Vet Radiol Ultrasound 2003;44:556–64.

23. Itoh T, Nibe K, Naganobu K. Tension pneumoperitoneum due to gastric perforation in a cat. J Vet Med Sci 2005;67:617–19.

24. Parsons KJ, Owen LJ, Lee K, et al. A retrospective study of surgically treated cases of septic peritonitis in the cat (2000-2007). Journal Small Anim Pract 2009;50:518–24.

25. Van Camp S, Love NE, Kumaresan S. Radiographic diagnosis – gastroesophageal intussusception in a cat. Vet Radiol Ultrasound 1998;39:190–2.

26. Martínez NI, Cook W, Troy GC, Waldron D. Intermittent gastroesophageal intussusception in a cat with idiopathic megaoesophagus. J Am Anim Hosp Assoc 2001;37:234–7.

27. Owen MC, Morris PJ, Bateman RS. Concurrent gastro-oesophageal intussusception, trichobezoar and hiatal hernia in a cat. N Z Vet J 2005;53:371–4.

28. van Geffen C, Saunders JH, Vandevelde B, et al. Idiopathic megaoesophagus and intermittent gastro-oesophageal intussusception in a cat. Journal Small Anim Pract 2006;47:471–5.

29. Graham KL, Buss MS, Dhein CR, et al. Gastroesophageal intussusception in a Labrador retriever. Can Vet J 1998;39: 709–11.

30. McGill SE, Lenard ZM, See AM, Irwin PJ. Nonsurgical treatment of a puppy with gastroesophageal intussusception. J Am Anim Hosp Assoc 2009;45:185–90.

31. Robotham GR. Congenital hiatal hernia in the cat. Fel Pract 1979;9:37–9.

32. Ellison GW, Lewis DD, Phillips L, et al. Esophageal hiatal hernia in small animals: literature review and a modified surgical technique. J Am Anim Hosp Assoc 1987;23:391–9.

33. Bright RM, Sackman JE, Denovo C, et al. Hiatal hernia in the dog and cat: a retrospective study of 16 cases. J Small Anim Pract 1990;31:244–50.

34. Hettlich BF, Hobson HP, Ducoté J, et al. Esophageal hiatal hernia in three exotic felines: *Lynx lynx, Puma concolore* and *Panthera leo.* J Zoo Wildl Med 2010;41: 90–4.

35. Zedan M, El-Ghazaly M, Fouda A, El-Bayoumi M. Tension gastrothorax: a case report and review of literature. J Pediatr Surg 2008;43:740–3.

36. Zarelli M, Carrillo JD, Soler M, et al. What is your diagnosis? Tension gastrothorax. J Am Vet Med Assoc 2010;236:733–4.

37. Bredal WP, Eggertsdóttir AV, Austefjord O. Acute gastric dilatation in cats: a case series. Acta Vet Scand 1996;37:445–51.

38. Formaggini L, Schmidt K, De Lorenzi D. Gastric dilatation-volvulus associated with diaphragmatic hernia in three cats: clinical presentation, surgical treatment and presumptive aetiology. J Fel Med Surg 2008;10:198–201.

39. Moore PF, Rodriguez-Bertos A, Kass PH. Feline gastrointestinal lymphoma: mucosal architecture, immunophenotype and molecular clonality. Vet Pathol 2011; epub ahead of print.

40. Briscoe KA, Krockenberger M, Beatty JA, et al. Histopathological and immunohistochemical evaluation of 53 cases if feline lymphoplasmacytic enteritis and low-grade alimentary lymphoma. J Comp Pathol 2011;145:187–98.

41. Page CP, Bohnen JM, Fletcher JR, et al. Antimicrobial prophylaxis for surgical wounds. Guidelines for clinical care. Arch Surg 1993;128:79–88.

42. Salinardi BJ, Harkin KR, Bulmer BJ, Roush JK. Comparison of complications of percutaneous endoscopic versus surgically placed gastrostomy tubes in 42 dogs and 52 cats. J Am Anim Hosp Assoc 2006;42: 51–6.

43. Ireland LM, Hohenhaus AE, Broussard JD, Weissman BL. A comparison of owner management and complications in 67 percutanesous esophagostomy and percutaneous endoscopic gastrostomy feeding tubes. J Am Anim Hosp Assoc 2003;39:241–6.

44. Bright RM, Burrows CF. Percutaneous endoscopic tube gastrostomy in dogs. Am J Vet Res 1988;49:629–33.

45. Washabau RJ. Gastrointestinal motility disorders and gastrointestinal prokinetic therapy. Vet Clin Small Anim 2003;33: 1007–28.

46. Nielsen C, Anderson GM. Metastasis of gastric adenocarcinoma to the abdominal wall following placement of a gastrostomy tube in a dog. Can Vet J 2005;46:641–3.

47. Boutilier P, Carr A. Fungal colonization and failure of a long-term gastrostomy tube in a cat. Can Vet J 2005;46:709–10.

Chapter | 29 |

Small intestines

G.W. Ellison

Surgery in the form of biopsy, enterotomy and enterectomy is required to diagnose or treat conditions of the small intestine in the cat such as neoplasia or foreign bodies. Surgery of the intestinal system is not without complications; dehiscence can result in life-threatening conditions such as peritonitis. This chapter will cover the principles of diagnosis and treatment of small intestinal problems in cats and give advice on how to perform intestinal surgery and how to minimize the chance of complications.

SURGICAL ANATOMY

The small intestine of the cat constitutes a simple continuation of the alimentary canal from the stomach to the large intestine, consisting of the duodenum, jejunum and ileum. The upper small intestine is primarily secretory and the lower small intestine primarily absorptive in function. Within the duodenum the location of the common bile duct and pancreatic ducts differs from the dog. The major duodenal papilla typically receives the common bile duct and major pancreatic duct, whereas a minor duodenal papilla is only present in cats, in which an accessory pancreatic duct persists. This reportedly occurs in approximately 20% of animals. Arterial supply to the small intestine is via branches of the cranial mesenteric artery and venous return is primarily by the cranial mesenteric vein, a major tributary of the hepatic portal vein. The intestinal wall consists of an outer serosa formed by visceral peritoneum, the tunica muscularis with its outer longitudinal, and inner circular layers. The submucosa, which is rich in collagen, also serves as the principal holding layer for sutures. The intestinal mucosa is lined by simple columns of epithelial cells mixed with variable population of mucus providing goblet cells. The cat's microvascular anatomy is similar to that of dogs, with the vasa recta perforating the outer longitudinal and inner circular muscularis layers and supplying a rich submucosal vascular plexus. One distinguishing factor in cats is the presence of prominent lymphatic nodules in the mucosa, mostly along the antimesenteric aspect of the small intestine.[1]

GENERAL CONSIDERATIONS

Clinical findings

In the cat (unlike the dog) it is as common to see anorexia and weight loss with intestinal obstruction as vomiting. It is essential to perform a thorough physical examination including abdominal palpation and oral examination. Cats are prone to ingestion of linear foreign bodies and sublingual examination will often lead to a quick diagnosis of yarn or fishing line entrapped at the glossal frenulum. One study of linear foreign bodies in cats reported a diagnosis rate of 75% using oral examination in combination with abdominal palpation (Fig. 29-1).[2]

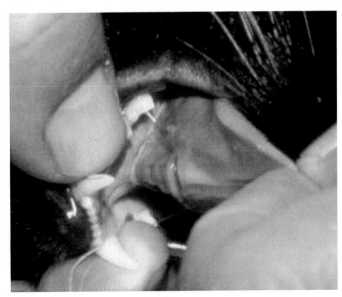

Figure 29-1 Photograph of a 6-week-old kitten with laceration of the lingual frenulum and sewing thread entrapped around base of tongue. *(Courtesy of Stephen Birchard, The Ohio State University.)*

© 2014 Elsevier Ltd
DOI: 10.1016/B978-0-7020-4336-9.00029-9

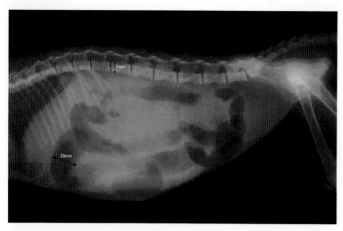

Figure 29-2 Lateral abdominal radiograph of a kitten with an intussusception. Black arrows indicate the ratio of the maximum diameter loop of small intestine (30 mm) divided by the dorsoventral height of the cranial endplate of L2 (9 mm) to be >3.0, making this suggestive of complete intestinal obstruction.[4]

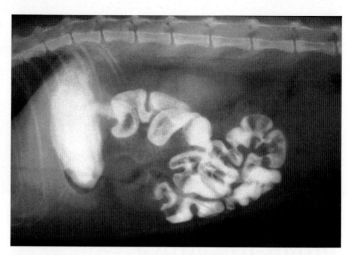

Figure 29-3 Contrast study of a cat with small intestinal pleating secondary to ingestion of linear foreign body. (Courtesy of Stephen Birchard, The Ohio State University.)

Physiology of obstruction

Distinguishing between simple mechanical and strangulated (ischemic) bowel obstruction is critical, because the latter condition requires early and rapid surgical intervention. Mechanical obstructions can be luminal (foreign bodies), intramural (neoplasia), or extramural (adhesions). With simple mechanical luminal obstruction, blood flow to the distended bowel is typically not completely obliterated, but increased bowel wall tension may cause both histologic and physiologic changes. Venous and lymphatic hydrostatic pressures are exceeded but arterial pressures are not, which results in vascular congestion. Reduced capillary flow, diminished tissue perfusion, and ultimate increase in vascular permeability result in extravasation of fluid into the interstitium. Mural edema further compromises blood flow causing hypoxia, tissue ischemia, and mucosal necrosis.

Strangulation obstruction often occurs secondarily to mesenteric vascular disruption caused by expansive foreign bodies, intussusception, mesenteric volvulus, a strangulated hernia, or trauma. With strangulation obstruction, the mucosa is sensitive to insufficient perfusion and anoxia and undergoes necrosis. After the mucosal barrier is destroyed, bacteria and endotoxins pass transmurally into the lymphatics and peritoneal cavity where they enter the systemic circulation and septic shock ensues. Eventually full thickness infarction and perforation may occur.

Diagnostic imaging

In cats with intestinal disease, abdominal radiographs may reveal a radiopaque foreign body, loss of visceral detail, or an obstructive gas pattern. Small intestinal distension of greater than 12–14 mm is suggestive of intestinal obstruction in this species.[3] Also, a quantitative index has been established in cats by calculating the ratio of the maximum small intestinal diameter/the dorsoventral cranial end plate measurement of the second lumbar vertebra. The probability of an intestinal obstructive is >70% if this ratio is greater than 3.0. (Fig. 29-2).[4] Linear foreign bodies will often cause pleating of the jejunum, which can be noted on palpation. Likewise, pleating of the small intestine can sometimes be seen on plain films. If contrast material is used the clinician should avoid the use of barium sulfate and instead use an iodine-containing contrast in order to avoid the potential for

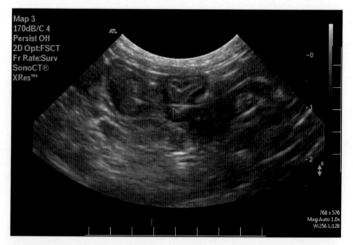

Figure 29-4 Ultrasound image of a linear foreign body (arrow) in a 10-month-old female cat. (Courtesy of the University of Cambridge.)

granulomatous peritonitis (Fig. 29-3). Ultrasonography is also a sensitive way of detecting foreign bodies and occasionally linear foreign bodies can be diagnosed using this non-invasive modality (Fig. 29-4). Ultrasonography may also be used to evaluate gastrointestinal motility, the presence of fluid distension, and diagnosing foreign bodies with characteristic acoustic signals.[5] Ultrasonography has been identified as a highly sensitive indicator of intussusception. On lateral views the intussusceptum is easily identified and on axial views a characteristic 'bull's eye' image is seen (Fig. 29-5). However, ultrasonography may not always accurately predict the presence of intestinal perforation.[6]

SURGICAL DISEASES OF THE SMALL INTESTINES

Diseases and conditions affecting the feline small intestine that may require surgery include foreign bodies, intussusception, mesenteric volvulus, trauma, and non-neoplastic lesions, such as feline infectious

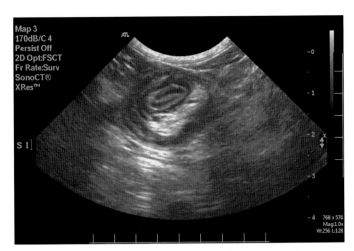

Figure 29-5 Axial ultrasonic image of an ileocolic intussusception showing the characteristic bull's eye sign. *(Courtesy of the University of Cambridge.)*

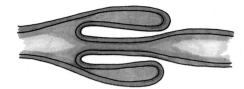

Figure 29-6 Illustration of typical anatomic configuration of a single intussusception with the inner invaginated intussusceptum and outer ensheathing intussuscipiens. *(Samantha J Elmhurst BA Hons/ www.livingart.org.uk from Stanley BR. The small intestine. In Williams JM and Niles JD. BSAVA Manual of Canine and Feline Abdominal Surgery. Gloucester 2005; p 107.)*

peritonitis, granulomas and adenomatous polyps, and neoplastic masses such as lymphoma.

Foreign bodies

Non-linear foreign bodies

Approximately half of the gastrointestinal foreign bodies in cats are caused by non-linear foreign bodies.[6] Non-linear foreign bodies commonly identified in the cat include coins, ear-plugs, small toys, almonds, or fishing tackle. Small intestinal obstruction by a foreign body can be complete or partial and the clinical signs vary in severity as a result of the level and degree of obstrucsion. The degree of obstruction also defines the variability in the presenting clinical signs. Abdominal palpation may identify intestinal distension, a palpable object, or abdominal pain. Cats commonly swallow coins but these usually do not exit the stomach. Rubber balls, cellophane, or chew toys tend to pass slowly or not at all and are more likely to cause complete mechanical obstruction requiring enterotomy or enterectomy. Opaque objects are easily identifiable on plain radiographs but many foreign bodies are radiolucent. Less dense foreign bodies are sometimes missed on ultrasound. If contrast radiography is needed for diagnosis aqueous iodine contrast should be used. Most proximal small intestinal obstructions are visible within six hours whereas a 24 hour study may be indicated for more distal obstructions. Surgical management of gastrointestinal foreign bodies varies depending on the type and location of the foreign body. Sharp foreign bodies such as straight pins, safety pins, bones, or glass will often pass through the gastrointestinal tract without creating intestinal perforation unless they are attached to thread or yarn.

Linear foreign body

Linear foreign bodies, caused by such items as fishing line, meat wrappers, or sewing yarn, present a difficult surgical problem. Some linear foreign bodies will pass spontaneously but the trailing end often catches over the base of the tongue or in the stomach and acts as an anchor.[7] Intestinal peristalsis moves the foreign body aborally resulting in bowel plication. Linear foreign bodies should be managed by initially identifying and releasing the anchor point, either from the tongue, or via a gastrotomy to free the wadded string or fishing line from its gastropyloric anchor (see Chapter 28). Multiple enterotomies are sometimes required to facilitate complete removal of the foreign body. If too few enterotomies are made, with too much traction placed on the string, the mesenteric border may be perforated in an area which is difficult to explore and suture. Occasionally the string has already cut through at several locations and peritonitis is evident. In 64 cases of linear foreign bodies in cats, most animals were less than four years old. Surgery and multiple enterotomies or enterectomy were used in 90% of the cases and 84% of the cases survived. However, the survival rate in cats that had concurrent bowel perforations was only 50%.[2] A single catheter technique for removal of linear foreign bodies can often be used successfully in cats, but survival rates for this technique are not known.[8] There have been failures associated with the single catheter technique for removal of linear foreign bodies. In one case report, passage of the catheter created tearing of the mesenteric border at the location where the linear foreign body was embedded, thus necessitating resection and anastomosis of 60% of the small intestine.[9] Likewise, in long-standing cases of intestinal linear foreign body, fibrosis may occur so that even after its removal the bowel retains its pleated configuration. In these cases, massive intestinal resection and anastomosis may be necessary.

Intussusception

The exact pathogenesis of the condition is unknown but theories include a local incongruency of the intestine caused by induration (secondary to neoplasia), or spasticity (intestinal parasitism), or anatomical diameter change occurs in which a proximal bowel segment invaginates (intussusceptum) into a distal section of bowel (intussuscipiens) (Fig. 29-6). Intussusceptions are also seen with increasing frequency after laparotomy on elective or non-elective intra-abdominal procedures. Clinical signs depend on the completeness and level of obstruction. In older cats intussusception is often associated with intestinal neoplasia (Fig. 29-7). The intussusception often becomes irreducible as a result of the congestion and outpouring of fibrinous exudate from the serosa. Although the invaginated bowel may become devitalized, perforation is rare because the outer ensheathing layer retains its viability and the adhesions seal the proximal border of the intussusception. Occasionally spontaneous recovery occurs when the non-viable intussusceptum is sloughed and patency of the lumen is recovered.

The outcome of 20 cats with gastrointestinal tract intussusception identified that this disease differs significantly from intussusception in dogs.[10] Intussusception in cats appears to be a biphasic disease, with one group of cats being less than one year of age and having concurrent intestinal endoparasitism. The second group was over six years of age and the majority of the older cats had either intestinal lymphoma or inflammatory bowel disease as the common etiology for their intussusception. Clinical signs included anorexia, lethargy, vomiting, dehydration, poor body condition, and signs of abdominal pain. Diagnosis was made using a combination of abdominal palpation, abdominal

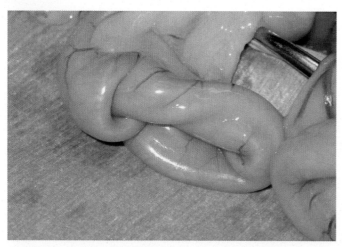

Figure 29-7 Intraoperative image of a mid-jejunal intussusception in a 13-year-old British short-haired cat.

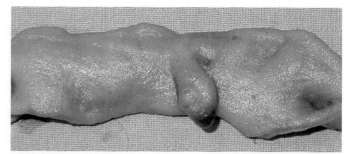

Figure 29-8 Benign adenomatous polyp located in mid-jejunum caused the intussusception in the cat described in Figure 29-7.

radiography, and abdominal ultrasonography. Most specific was abdominal ultrasonography, which was diagnostic in seven of seven cases in which it was performed. Jejunojejunal was the most common site of intussusception and no intussusceptions were found proximal to the duodenum. Thirteen cats were taken to surgery and 11 of these cats required intestinal resection and anastomosis.

The need for prophylactic bowel plication or enteropexy remains controversial. Bowel plication involves laying the bowel side by side in a series of gentle loops. The loops are sutured together on their antimesenteric border using simple interrupted sutures of non-absorbable 4/0 suture material that penetrate the seromuscular layers of bowel but do not enter the lumen.[11] However, a retrospective report in dogs indicated that intestinal plication might not be necessary since the risk of complications is higher after plication and there was only a slight reduction in the recurrence rate of intussusception.[12]

Mesenteric volvulus

Pathologic twisting of bowel on its mesenteric axis is termed intestinal or mesenteric volvulus. Mesenteric volvulus is rare in cats. There have been five cases reported in the literature with two survivors. Reported clinical signs included acute onset of abdominal distension in the presence of shock, anemia, air-filled loops of bowel, and vomiting or retching. Of the three non-survivors, two cases were diagnosed at necropsy and the third cat failed to survive surgery. Of the two successful surgical cases one was a 16-month-old domestic short hair and the other a five-year-old Bengal. Both animals had acute abdominal signs and presented in a very anemic state with packed cell volumes below 10%. Both animals received blood transfusions and had resection of the proximal jejunum and the ileum. The lengths of resected intestines were 35 and 40 cm, respectively. Postoperatively, both cats had chronic diarrhea for a period of time, which ultimately improved but did not completely resolve. Based on these two cases it appears that cats can survive mesenteric volvulus so long as surgery is performed promptly after appropriate stabilization of the cat, including blood transfusion (see Chapter 5) and some of the small intestine including the duodenum and upper jejunum is retained.[13]

Non-neoplastic lesions

Adenomatous polyps

Adenomatous polyps of the duodenum have been reported in cats. They were older cats with a median age of about 12 years and the

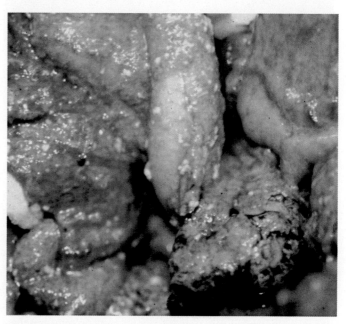

Figure 29-9 Feline infectious peritonitis-induced granulomatous change, which is widespread in the small intestine of an affected cat.

Siamese and Himalayan breeds were over represented. The polypoid mucosal masses were located in the upper duodenum and tended to cause vomiting and weight loss. When the lesions ulcerate hematemesis may occur. About half the cats became anemic secondary to chronic blood loss. Diagnosis was made on contrast radiography or endoscopically. This is a surgical disease and requires excision of the lesions through an enterotomy incision or via resection and anastomosis. The lesions are benign but regrowth is possible if inadequate submucosal resection occurs. In one case study, 13 of 18 cats were cured, four had recurring signs and one cat died following surgery.[14] The author has also seen benign adenomatous polyps located in the jejunum which caused a secondary intussusception (Fig. 29-8).

Feline infectious peritonitis (FIP) granulomas

A large case series of 26 cats with FIP had concurrent solitary mural intestinal lesions that mimicked intestinal neoplasia.[15] The majority of these cats had the lesions removed during exploratory laparotomy although some of the lesions were diagnosed at necropsy. The presumptive diagnosis in most of the cats was a solitary intestinal lesion most consistent with neoplasia. However, results of histologic examination revealed that the lesions were predominantly granulomatous, nodular, firm and white, and extended throughout the wall of the intestine on histologic examination (Fig. 29-9). Associated lymph

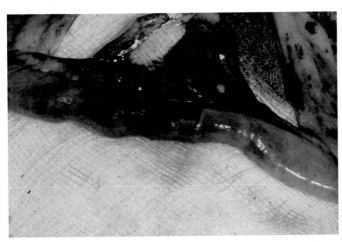

Figure 29-10 Small intestinal ischemia secondary to blunt abdominal trauma and avulsion of the mesenteric vessels in a five-month-old kitten.

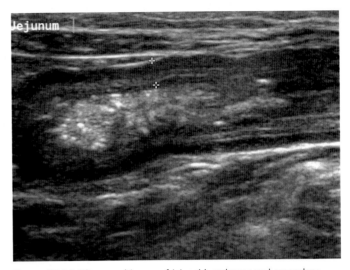

Figure 29-11 Ultrasound image of jejunal lymphoma and secondary intestinal obstruction in an 11-year-old domestic short-haired cat. Intestinal wall thickening (+) has caused accumulation of a radiodense foreign body in the intestinal lumen. *(Courtesy of Shona Reese.)*

nodes were enlarged and had evidence of inflammation. Serology was positive for the FIP virus in all 26 cats. The clinical outcome of these cats was poor. Many cats were euthanized at the time of surgery and all cats that were recovered from anesthesia died within nine months of the surgical procedure. Many of the cats also had signs of multi-systemic FIP. The clinical implications of this study are the focal nature of intestinal lesions with this type of FIP is easily confused with neo-plasia at the time of surgery and long-term prognosis is poor.

Trauma

Intestinal trauma may occur secondary to major abdominal trauma or incisional dehiscence and often involves evisceration (Fig. 29-10). With early surgical intervention and appropriate antibiosis the prognosis for these patients can be favorable.[16] A recent study reported on eight dogs and four cats with major abdominal evisceration. The evisceration was secondary to blunt abdominal trauma in four animals and secondary to spay wound dehiscence in eight animals. All cases had evisceration of the intestines and gross contamination with dirt, leaves or litter. The surgical procedure included lavage and replace-ment only in four cases, enterectomy in five cases, splenectomy in one case and primary colonic repair in another. All patients survived to discharge from the hospital, with a median duration of hospitaliza-tion of four days. Cultures were positive in all cases where they were taken, with three animals having single contaminants and nine animals having multiple contaminants. The most commonly used antimicrobial combinations were ampicillin, enrofloxacin, and met-ronidazole. Of the four cats, two required significant enterectomy needing resection of 60% and 100% of the jejunum, respectively. One of the cats with massive intestinal resection had long-term diarrhea up to three months after intestinal resection and anastomosis.

Neoplasia

Lymphosarcoma, adenocarcinoma and mast cell tumors are the three most common intestinal tumors in cats. Hemangiosarcoma, leiomyo-mas, and leiomyosarcomas are seen much less commonly. Ultrasono-graphic changes commonly seen with feline intestinal neoplasia include symmetrical hypoechoic changes seen with lymphosarcoma and/or asymmetric echogenicity seen with intestinal adenocarcinoma (Fig. 29-11). Intestinal lymphosarcoma in cats may occur as a diffuse infiltrative lesion or a distinct nodular mass. Extensive infiltration of the lamina propria and submucosa with neoplastic cells occurs.

Malabsorption, stearrhea, diarrhea, and weight loss are usually seen.[17] With immunohistochemistry typing it appears that both mucosal and transmural T-cell lymphoma are largely confined to the small intestine whereas the B-cell lymphoma is more likely to occur in the stomach, jejunum, and the ileocecal junction. If the lesion is confined to the mucosa survival times of up to 29 months are seen. However, with transmural extension survival times are short: T-cell tumors have a median survival rate of 1.5 months and B-cell tumors have a median survival rate of 3.5 months.[18] For lymphosarcoma, chemotherapy is sometimes effective in reducing tumor mass, but may 'melt' the tumor so that intestinal perforation results. For this reason it may be advis-able to resect obstructive lymphosarcoma lesions prior to instituting chemotherapy.

The *intestinal adenocarcinoma* neoplasm accounts for an estimated 20–35% of gastrointestinal neoplasia in the cat, with affected cats having an average age of greater than 10 years. The small intestine accounts for approximately 70% of the cases. Cats typically have a long history of non-specific gastrointestinal disease including weight loss and inappetence or vomiting. The sex distribution is approxi-mately 60% male and 40% female. Asian breeds such as Siamese and Persian are predisposed.[19] Intestinal adenocarcinoma usually causes a segmental intramural mass, which expands toward the lumen. This constricting ring, which is classically called a 'napkin ring lesion', usually undergoes very little external enlargement and may be mis-taken for a stricture (Fig. 29-12). Local invasion or seeding of the mesenteric omentum and regional lymph nodes is common. Surgical treatment involves wide resection of the tumor with a minimum of five and preferably ten centimeter margins and anastomosis of adja-cent segments of bowel. Survival times range from 0 to 24 months with some clinical studies showing mean survival times as low as 2.5 and others as long as 15 months. In one study tubular adenocarcino-mas had a mean survival time of almost 11 months whereas mucinous and undifferentiated carcinomas had a survival time of just four months.[19] In another study of 32 cats with intestinal adenocarcinoma, the tumors occurred in older animals with a mean age of about 12 years.[20] The lesions were typically located in the jejunum although duodenal or ileal lesions were also reported. Overt radiographic obstructive pattern was rare, 50% of the diagnoses were made on palpation and only 35% made radiographically. Although many of

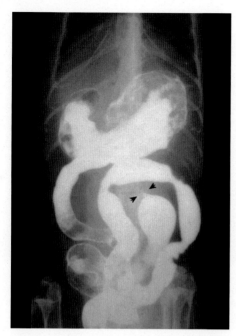

Figure 29-12 Contrast study showing mid-jejunal adenocarcinoma in a nine-year-old male Siamese cat. The lesion caused abrupt intraluminal narrowing and a radiographic 'cobra head' lesion (black arrows).

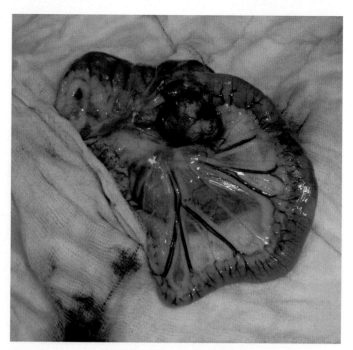

Figure 29-13 A 14-year-old female neutered Ragdoll had an intestinal mass detected on a routine physical examination prior to vaccination. Abdominal ultrasound revealed a 3 cm × 2 cm × 5 cm nodular mass at the ileocecocolic junction, with loss of layering of the intestinal wall. (Courtesy of Laura Owen.)

the cats in that study were euthanized intraoperatively those who underwent enterectomy did quite well, with a mean survival time greater than 15 months.

Intestinal mast cell tumor (MCT) is the third most common feline gastrointestinal tumor. It occurs in older cats with a mean age of 13 years and it is equally distributed between the duodenum, jejunum, and ileum. Peritoneal effusion is relatively common. The sonographic features of intestinal MCT were reviewed in 14 cats.[21] There were 16 focal intestinal tumors and one diffuse submucosal infiltrate. The most common pattern was focal, hypoechoic wall thickening that was non-circumferential and eccentric, or circumferential, asymmetric, and eccentric. The majority of the cats had enlarged abdominal lymph nodes, often due to MCT metastasis. Metastatic disease was not routinely detected in the liver or the spleen. Concurrent small cell (T-cell) lymphoma was present in four of 14 cats with intestinal MCT. A variant of feline intestinal MCT is also described in 50 cats.[22] These cats had a sclerosing variant of intestinal MCT (Fig. 29-13), which had a high propensity for metastasis and a guarded prognosis. Neoplastic cells formed a trabecular pattern admixed with moderate to abundant dense stromal collagen resulting in intestinal sclerosis. Neoplastic cells had poorly discernible intracytoplasmic granules that demonstrated metachromasia with special histochemical stains consistent with mast cell granules. Additionally, a subset of cases stained for mast cell-specific tryptase and c-kit demonstrated positive immunoreactivity. Eosinophilic infiltrates were moderate to marked in almost all cases. Lymph node and hepatic metastases were present in 66% of the cases. Prognosis was poor. Of 25 cases available for follow up, 23 patients died or were euthanized within two months of initial diagnosis.

PERIOPERATIVE CONSIDERATIONS

Preoperative complete blood count and clinical chemistries should be performed. Dehydration and electrolyte abnormalities should ideally be corrected prior to the induction of anesthesia, but in some emergency cases this may not be possible. Many cats with intestinal disease also suffer from anemia. Whole blood transfusion or packed red cells are an advisable addition to therapy in the perioperative period in patients with a packed cell volume (PCV) less than 20% (see Chapter 5). Cats with intestinal tumors are often aged and due process should be followed with respect to staging the disease using abdominal ultrasonography and thoracic radiography. Aged cats also need to have adequate cardiac workup to rule out cardiomyopathy.

Typically, cats are anorexic at the time of presentation so starving the patient prior to surgery is often unnecessary. Antibiotics should not be given preoperatively since in the case of intestinal perforation, samples for culture and sensitivity will be taken at the time of surgery. In the absence of pre-existing sepsis or spillage of ingesta during surgery antibiotic therapy is often given intravenously at the time of surgery and ceased within 24 hours. With intestinal perforations or pre-existing peritonitis the clinician should employ antibiotic therapy aimed at Gram positive and Gram negative aerobic as well as anaerobic bacteria for at least four to five days.

Intestinal healing

The inflammatory phase of intestinal healing lasts three to four days. Immediately after wounding, contraction of blood vessels occurs, the coagulation mechanism is activated, and fibrin clots are deposited to control hemorrhage. The fibrin clot offers minimal wound strength on the first postoperative day; the main wound support during the lag phase of healing comes from the sutures. Enterocyte replication and regeneration begins almost immediately after wounding; however, the epithelium offers little biomechanical support. The inflammatory phase is the most critical period during visceral wound healing, since most dehiscences take place within 72 to 96 hours after the wound has been created.

It is best to approximate the wound edges using 4/0 swaged on suture with a narrow tapered needle. Direct approximation of the wound edge allows for optimum rapid healing characterized by primary intestinal wound healing. Rapid mucosal re-epithelialization and early formation of young well-vascularized collagen between the submucosa, muscularis, and serosa occurs without compromising lumen diameter and minimizing the number of adhesions. Sutures should be snug but not overly tight. The crushing suture has been shown to cause more tissue ischemia directly at the suture line and its use is discouraged. Mucosal eversion or tissue overlap between sutures retards healing, increases the risk of leakage, and should be avoided. Inversion of the wound edge creates an internal cuff of tissue that reduces lumen diameter and should be avoided in cats.

SURGICAL MANAGEMENT AND TECHNIQUES FOR SMALL INTESTINAL SURGERY

With intestinal obstruction, varying degrees of intestinal distension are present and the distended loops of bowel may take on a cyanotic appearance. Intestinal viability is best evaluated after decompression of dilated loops of intestine. Decompression of fluid and gas from the proximal segment of the distended bowel is performed with a 20G needle and suction apparatus or a 60 mL syringe with a three-way stop cock. Standard clinical criteria for establishing intestinal viability are color, arterial pulsations, and the presence of peristalsis. Of these three parameters, peristalsis is the most dependable criterion of viability. In most cases of simple non-strangulated obstruction, bowel viability is maintained and the visual appearance of dark distended loops of bowel improves rapidly after decompression. Usually non-viable intestine is distended, blue, black, or gray in appearance and easily discernable from normal bowel. If intestinal wall ischemia and necrosis is present, then resection and anastomosis is performed.

Intestinal biopsy

Intestinal biopsy is indicated in all cases where neoplasia or inflammatory bowel disease (IBD) is suspected but there is no overt mass lesion present. In cases of suspected IBD it is advisable to biopsy the duodenum, jejunum, and ileum. The availability of transmural biopsies from all segments of the intestine and the collection of extraintestinal samples, especially mesenteric lymph nodes, is especially helpful for diagnosing intestinal tumors such as lymphomas and tumors of mast cell origin.[23] Biopsies can be taken using a number 15 blade and creating a transverse 2 mm wide × 3 mm long sample. The wound is then closed using two to three simple interrupted 4/0 monofilament absorbable sutures on a taper cut needle. Alternatively, the surgeon can use a 2 or 3 mm dermatologic skin punch to take a round sample. These small wounds are then closed using two simple interrupted sutures. Biopsy techniques are described in detail in Chapter 23 (open intestinal biopsy, Box 23-1) and Chapter 24 (laparoscopic-assisted intestinal biopsy, Box 24-5).

Enterotomy

The most common indication for enterotomy (Box 29-1) in cats is to remove intraluminal intestinal foreign bodies that cause obstruction. Enterotomy also is performed to examine the intestinal lumen for evidence of mucosal ulceration, strictures or neoplasia. Superficial ulcerations or intestinal polyps sometimes can be resected via enterotomy, but most intramural lesions require enterectomy.

Box 29-1 **Enterotomy**

The cat is positioned in dorsal recumbency and a midline celiotomy is performed (see Chapter 23). The entire intestinal tract should be evaluated by palpation, from stomach to colon, to determine the number of foreign bodies and assess the viability of the bowel wall. The affected bowel segment is isolated from the remainder of the viscera with saline-soaked laparotomy sponges. Intestinal contents are milked 10 cm to either side of the foreign body and the bowel is held between an assistant's fingers or with Doyen intestinal forceps. With a number 15 scalpel blade, a full thickness longitudinal incision is made in the antimesenteric border of the intestine in the viable tissue immediately proximal or distal to the foreign body. The length of the enterotomy approximates the diameter of the foreign body. Continuous suction is used to reduce spillage, and the surgeon pushes the foreign body gently through the enterotomy, taking care not to tear the incision margins. The bowel lumen is examined for evidence of perforations or strictures before closure.

Linear foreign bodies

These should be managed by identifying the proximal anchor point and releasing it during or just before laparotomy. Surgical management should be performed promptly following release at the base of the tongue, since loss of intestinal plication may expose areas of intestinal perforation and allow leakage of intestinal contents. Commonly, a gastrotomy (see Chapter 28) is necessary to free wadded string or fishing line from a gastropyloric anchor. The traditional way of linear foreign body removal requires multiple enterotomies to complete removal of the linear body. Occasionally, the intestinal foreign body perforates at several locations before surgery, and local peritonitis is evident; sometimes, enough fibrosis has occurred around the foreign body so, even after its removal, the bowel retains its plicated conformation. In both these groups of patients massive enterectomy may be necessary.

Linear foreign body removal using the urinary catheter technique

With this technique only one or two enterotomies are necessary. Once the foreign body is released from its proximal anchor point, it is tied or sutured to the tip of an eight to 12 French vinyl urinary catheter (Fig. 29-14A). As the catheter is pushed distally, the embedded linear foreign body disengages from the intestinal wall and the bowel unpleats itself (Fig. 29-14B). Once the foreign body is completely disengaged from the bowel wall, a second short enterotomy is made distally over the distal tip of the catheter and the remainder of the foreign body is retrieved (Fig. 29-14C). Alternatively, a longer catheter can be used and pushed down through the colon. The foreign body can then be retrieved from the anus. The author has found catheter-facilitated removal to be a very useful method for linear foreign body retrieval in cats.

Enterectomy (resection and anastomosis)

Enterectomy (Box 29-2) is indicated for removal of masses, both neoplastic and non-neoplastic, areas of devitalized intestine, non-reducible intussusceptions, eviscerated contaminated intestines, and after mesenteric volvulus. The procedure must be performed carefully to avoid intestinal spillage and with meticulous attention to closure to prevent postoperative leakage and peritonitis. Due consideration must also be given to the effects of enterectomy of a large percentage of the intestine and the consequences of short bowel syndrome.

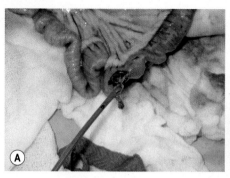 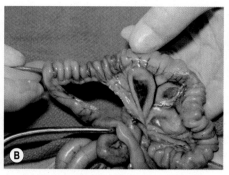 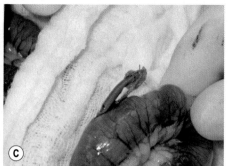

Figure 29-14 **(A)** A segment of yarn is sutured to the tip of a 12 French urinary catheter. **(B)** The catheter is pushed distally and the yarn is disengaged from the intestinal mucosa. **(C)** The yarn is retrieved through a small distal enterotomy incision.

Box 29-2 **Enterectomy**

The cat is positioned in dorsal recumbancy and a midline celiotomy is performed (see Chapter 23). The area to be resected is packed away from the abdomen with moistened laparotomy sponges. Intestinal contents are milked proximally and distally, and the bowel is held between an assistant's index fingers or with Doyen intestinal forceps 10 cm from the proposed resection site. A 1–2 cm margin of normal viable intestine is included in the proximal and distal boundaries of the area to be resected, which is clamped with Carmalt or Doyen forceps. If luminal disparity is present, the forceps are placed at a 75–90° angle on the dilated proximal segment and at a 45–60° angle on the contracted distal segment of bowel (Fig. 29-15). If angling the intestinal incision does not adequately correct for luminal disparity, the smaller stoma can be enlarged by incising the bowel section for a distance of 1–2 cm along the antimesenteric surface and then trimming off two triangular flaps. This procedure creates an ovoid larger stoma, which can be anastomosed to the larger diameter section of the bowel. Branches of the mesenteric artery and veins supplying the devitalized bowel are isolated with curved mosquito forceps and are double ligated. The arcadial vessels located within the mesenteric fat are double ligated at the area of proposed resection. A scalpel blade is used to excise the bowel along the outside of the intestinal forceps. With dissecting scissors, the vessels are divided, the mesentery is

transected, and the excised bowel is removed from the surgical field. After resection, the small intestinal mucosa has a tendency to evert and can be trimmed back with Metzenbaum scissors.

Suturing should be performed with 4/0 monofilament absorbable suture material using either simple interrupted or a modified Gambee suture pattern. The Gambee engages all layers except the mucosa, thus preventing mucosal protrusion between sutures (Fig. 29-16). When the anastomosis is closed with an interrupted suture technique, the first suture is placed at the mesenteric border because the presence of fat in this area makes suture placement most difficult, and this is where leakage is most likely to occur. The second suture is placed on the antimesenteric border, and the third and fourth sutures are placed laterally at 90° quadrants depending on bowel diameter; two to four more sutures are placed between each of the quadrant sutures. All sutures are placed 3 mm apart and 2–3 mm from the wound edge. Suture bites on the dilated side of the anastomosis are placed further apart than on the contracted side of the anastomosis to correct for luminal disparity. Once one side of the anastomosis is sutured, the bowel is flipped over, and the opposite side is completed. From 12 to 20 sutures are used to complete the anastomosis (Fig. 29-17). After the anastomosis has been completed, it is checked for leakage by infusing saline under low pressure into the bowel lumen and massaging the fluid past the anastomosis (Fig. 29-18). The anastomosis can also be checked by gently probing the spaces between sutures with mosquito hemostats for openings. The mesenteric defect is then closed with a simple continuous suture pattern, taking care not to include any mesenteric vessels within the suture line.

Alternatively, a simple continuous approximating technique can be used to create the anastomosis. This is performed with two lengths of suture. The first knot is tied at the mesenteric border and the second at the antimesenteric border. The sutures are then advanced around the perimeter approximately 3 mm from the cut edge, with the wound edges gently approximated.[24] The needles are advanced in opposite directions, so one knot is tied to the tag at the antimesenteric border. The final knot is tied to the tag on the mesenteric border. If the knot is tied too tightly, a purse-string effect will be produced, and stenosis of the anastomosis may occur. The completed anastomosis is tested for leakage, and the mesenteric defect is closed.

To help prevent anastomosis leakage, a pedicle of greater omentum is wrapped around the suture line. The omentum is critical to the successful healing of intestinal wounds because it can seal small anastomotic leaks and can prevent peritonitis. The omentum is tacked to the serosa with two simple interrupted sutures of 4/0 suture material placed on each side of the bowel wall (Fig. 29-19).

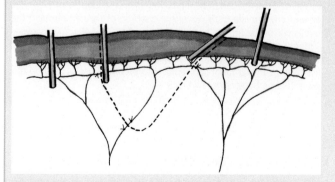

Figure 29-15 Enterectomy in a cat. After applying Doyen forceps the mesenteric vessels are ligated. Enterectomy incisions are made adjacent to straight forceps placed perpendicular to the intestine on the dilated segment and angled 45° on the contracted segment. *(Illustration by Samantha J. Elmhurst BA Hons/www.livingart.org.uk from Stanley BR. The small intestine. In Williams JM and Niles JD. BSAVA Manual of Canine and Feline Abdominal Surgery. Gloucester 2005; p 104.)*

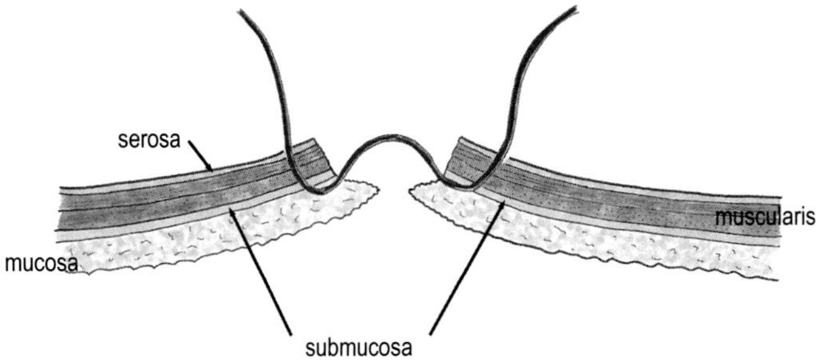

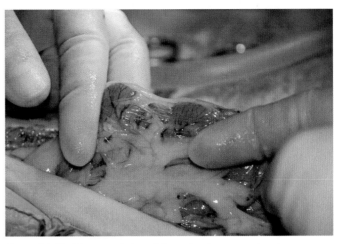

Figure 29-19 After completion of the enterotomy or enterectomy a segment of greater omentum is wrapped around the anastomosis. *(Courtesy of the University of Cambridge.)*

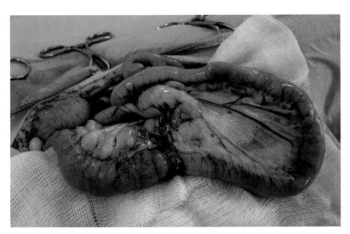

Figure 29-16 The modified Gambee suture pattern engages the serosa, muscularis and submucosa leaving an internal cuff of mucosa to help seal the intestinal lumen. *(Illustration by Samantha J. Elmhurst BA Hons/ www.livingart.org.uk from Stanley BR. The small intestine. In Williams JM and Niles JD. BSAVA Manual of Canine and Feline Abdominal Surgery. Gloucester 2005; p 103.)*

Figure 29-17 Intraoperative image of an end-to-end intestinal anastomosis after enterectomy with 4 cm margins for a sclerosing MCT (see Fig. 29-13). Repair was performed with 4/0 monofilament sutures of polydioxanone in a simple interrupted pattern. *(Courtesy of Laura Owen.)*

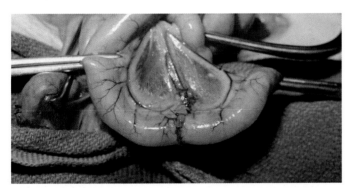

Figure 29-18 Intraoperative image of an intestinal anastomosis in a cat, performed with 4/0 monofilament sutures in an interrupted pattern. The mesentery has been closed to prevent strangulation and the anastomosis is leak tested with sterile saline.

POSTOPERATIVE CARE AFTER SMALL INTESTINAL SURGERY

Fluid and electrolyte deficits are corrected and antibiotic therapy is continued in the postoperative period. The author also uses metoclopramide 2.2 mg/kg IV every eight hours to reduce ileus and promote intestinal motility. Anorexia or vomiting in the presence of fever, abdominal tenderness, and leukocytosis suggests that anastomotic leakage and peritonitis may have occurred. If low glucose levels, degenerate neutrophils with engulfed bacteria, or free peritoneal bacteria are present on abdominocentesis, early re-exploration of the abdomen is warranted.

Nutrition after intestinal surgery

Early if not immediate postoperative enteral feeding has been shown to have a positive influence on the healing rate of intestinal anastomosis in dogs. Malnutrition induces intestinal mucosal atrophy, reduced motility, increased incidence of ileus, and the potential for bacterial translocation through the bowel wall, with resultant sepsis. Impaired wound healing due to nutritional causes may be ameliorated by feeding an enteral or parenteral diet that supplies energy needs in the form of fatty acids and sugars, and provides essential amino acids. Feeding high protein meals after injury can optimize conditions for normal visceral wound healing. Amino acids provided through enteral nutrition are utilized for the synthesis of structural proteins such as actin, myosin, collagen, and elastin. Bursting pressures and collagen levels of ileal and colorectal anastomosis were compared in Beagles fed elemental diets versus those fed only electrolytes and water for four days.[25] The dogs fed elemental diets had nearly twice the bursting strengths of the control group and nearly double the amount of both immature and mature collagen at the wound site. Conversely, total parenteral nutrition (TPN) does not appear to ameliorate the mucosal atrophy or increase collagen deposition as does enteral nutrition. In human studies, the incidence of septic complications was significantly lower in people fed between eight and 24 hours after surgery versus those maintained on TPN. Additionally, early fed patients had a reduced incidence of postoperative ileus and reduced hospital stay.

The effect of early feeding is unknown in cats but we advocate early postoperative feeding in our clinical setting based on studies in other species. Therefore feeding a bland diet such as canned I/D (Hills Pet Nutrition Inc., Topeka, KS), mixed with water to form a gruel, is initiated the evening of surgery. In uncomplicated cases, reasonable appetite usually resumes within 48 hours.

COMPLICATIONS AND PROGNOSIS

Feline intestinal surgery can generally be performed with a good result but any intestinal procedure is not without potential morbidity.

Dehiscence and peritonitis

Intestinal dehiscence and secondary peritonitis are the most significant complications. Intestinal leakage has been associated with a high mortality rate in dogs; as high as 74%. This compares with a mortality of only 7.2% in animals without intestinal dehiscence.[26] However, it appears that cats have fewer incidences of intestinal dehiscence and much higher survival rates than dogs.[27] In a study looking at leakage following intestinal anastomosis in 115 dogs and cats, there was a 16% anastomosis leakage rate in dogs (13 of 90 dogs) but there were no intestinal leakages in 25 cats.[28] It was suggested that the low incidence of intestinal dehiscence in cats and higher survival rates in that study were due to the fact that none of the cats had pre-existing peritonitis at the time of their initial surgery. On the other hand, cats with pre-existing peritonitis due to linear foreign body perforation had a 50% mortality rate in another study.[2] Preoperative factors significantly associated with development of anastomosis leakage include preoperative peritonitis, low serum albumin concentration, left shift, and the etiology of the obstruction. Enterotomy or enterectomy after intestinal foreign body removal is more likely to have leakage than cases with intestinal tumors. Because the risk of the dehiscence is multiplied according to the number of surgical wounds, reduction in the number of enterotomy wounds is desirable whenever possible.

Short bowel syndrome

Massive resection of part of the small intestine is sometimes indicated with ischemia secondary to intestinal volvulus or needed due to multiple perforations or continued pleating from linear foreign bodies. When large sections of the small intestine are resected short bowel syndrome may result. The propensity for short bowel syndrome after massive intestinal resection depends on the amount of tissue excised, the location of the resection, and the time allowed for adaptation. After resection of large portions of small intestine, maldigestion, malabsorption, diarrhea (induced by fatty acids or bile salts), bacterial overgrowth, and gastric hypersecretion may all occur. Location of the resection is important. High resection of the duodenum and upper jejunum may decrease pancreatic enzyme secretion because pancreatic-stimulating hormones such as secretin and cholecystokinin are produced in the mucosa of these sections. These reductions of pancreatic enzymes contribute to maldigestion of protein, carbohydrate, and fat with resultant catabolism, negative nitrogen balance, and steatorrhea. Unabsorbed sugars may also cause osmotic diarrhea. If the ileocecal valve is resected, bacteria may ascend, overgrow in the small bowel, and contribute to diarrhea.

After massive resection, the remaining small intestine adapts by increasing lumen diameter, microvilli height, and mucosal cell number. These compensatory changes may take several weeks and during this period parenteral fluids, electrolytes, and parenteral alimentation may be necessary for the survival of the animal. During this time, the cat ideally will be able to maintain weight even with diarrhea. Medical treatments for unresponsive diarrhea after massive resection include frequent small meals, low-fat diets, elemental diet supplements, medium-chain triglyceride oils, pancreatic enzyme supplements, B vitamins, kaolin antidiarrheal drugs, and poorly absorbed oral antibiotics such as neomycin.

In one clinical study involving seven cats with extensive (>50%) resection of small intestine all cats were discharged from the hospital and most had good outcomes, with mean survival times of two to three years.[29] However, in an experimental study in cats where 85% of the small intestine and all but 2 cm of the ileum were removed significant morbidity occurred in the form of moderate to severe diarrhea and weight loss. Administration of ursodeoxycholic acid was helpful in reducing the morbidity by reducing increasing intestinal transit time. However, these cats were all euthanized within a two-month period.[30]

REFERENCES

1. Hudson LC, Hamilton WP. Atlas of feline anatomy for veterinarians. Philadelphia: WB Saunders; 1993. p. 156–63.

2. Felts JF, Fox PR, Burk RL. Thread and sewing needles as gastrointestinal foreign bodies in the cat: a review of 64 cases. J Am Vet Med Assoc 1984;184:56–9.

3. Morgan JP. The upper gastrointestinal examination in the cat: Normal radiographic appearance using positive contrast medium. Vet Rad 1993;22: 148–91.

4. Adams WM, Sisterman LA, Klauer JM, et al. Association of intestinal disorders in cats with findings of abdominal radiography. J Am Vet Med Assoc 2010;236:880–6.

5. Larson MM, Biller DS. Ultrasound of the gastrointestinal tract. Vet Clin North Am: Small Anim Pract 2009;39: 747–59.

6. Bebchuck TN. Feline gastrointestinal foreign bodies. Vet Clin North Am: Small Anim Pract 2002;32:869–73.

7. Basher AWP, Fowler JD. Conservative vs surgical management of gastrointestinal linear foreign bodies in the cat. Vet Surg 1987;16:56–9.

8. Anderson SL, Lippincott CL, Gill PJ. Single enterotomy for removal of gastrointestinal linear foreign bodies. J Am Anim Hosp Assoc 1992;28:487–90.

9. Muir P, Rosen E. Failure of the single enterotomy technique to remove a linear intestinal foreign body from a cat. Vet Record 1995;136:75.

10. Burkitt JM, Drobatz KJ, Saunders HM, Washabau RJ. Signalment, history, and outcome of cats with gastrointestinal tract intussusception: 20 cases (1986–2000). J Am Vet Med Assoc 2009;234:771–6.

11. Oaks MC. Bowel plication for preventing recurrent intussusception. In: Bojrab MJ, editor. Current techniques in small animal surgery, 4th ed. Philadelphia: Williams and Wilkins; 1997. p. 254.

12. Applewhite AA, Hawthorne JC, Cornell KK. Complications of enteroplication for the prevention of intussusception recurrence in dogs: 35 cases (1989–1999). J Am Vet Med Assoc 2001;219: 1415–18.

13. Knell SC, Andreoni AA, Dennler M, Venzin CM. Successful treatment of small intestinal volvulus in two cats. J Feline Med Surg 2010;12:874–7.

14. MacDonald JM, Mullen HS, Moroff SD. Adenomatous polyps of the duodenum in cats: 18 cases (1985–1990). J Am Vet Med Assoc 1993;202:647–51.

15. Harvey CJ, Lopez JW, Hendrick MJ. An uncommon intestinal manifestation of feline infectious peritonitis: 26 cases (1986–1993). J Am Vet Med Assoc 1996;209:1117–20.

16. Gower SB, Weisse CW, Brown DC. Major abdominal evisceration injuries in dogs and cats: 12 cases (1998–2008). J Am Vet Med Assoc 2009;234: 1566–72.

17. Moore PF, Rodriguez-Bertos A, Kass PH. Feline gastrointestinal lymphoma:

Mucosal architecture, Immunophenotype and molecular clonality. Vet Path 2011, online April 11.

18. Pohlman LM, Higginbotham ML, Welles EG, Johnson CM. Immunophenotypic and histologic classification of 50 cases of feline gastrointestinal lymphoma. Vet Path 2009;46:259–68.

19. Cribb AE. Feline gastrointestinal adenocarcinoma: A review and retrospective study. Can Vet Journal 1988;29:709–12.

20. Kosovsky JE, Matthiesen DT, Patnaik AK. Small intestinal adenocarcinoma in cats: 32 cases (1978–1985). J Am Vet Med Assoc 1988;192:233–5.

21. Laurenson MP, Skorupski KA, Moore PF, Zwingenberger AL. Ultrasonography of intestinal mast cell tumors in the cat. Vet Radiol Ultrasound 2011;52:330–4.

22. Halsey CH, Powers BE, Kamstock DA. Feline intestinal sclerosing mast cell tumour: 50 cases (1997–2008). Vet Comp Oncol 2010;8:72–9.

23. Kleinschmidt S, Harder J, Nolte I, et al. Chronic inflammatory and non-inflammatory diseases of the gastrointestinal tract in cats: diagnostic advantages of full-thickness intestinal and extraintestinal biopsies. J Feline Med Surg 2010;12:97–103.

24. Weisman DL, Smeak DD, Birchard SJ, Zweigart SL. Comparison of a continuous suture pattern with a simple interrupted pattern for enteric closure in dogs and cats: 83 cases (1991–1997). J Am Vet Med Assoc 1999;214:1507–12.

25. Moss G, Greenstein A, Levy S, Bierenbaum A. Maintenance of bowel function after bowel surgery and immediate full nutrition. J Parent Enteral Nutrit 1980;4:535–8.

26. Allen DA, Smeak DD, Schertel ER. Prevalence of small intestinal dehiscence and associated clinical factors: a retrospective study of 121 dogs. J Am Anim Hosp Assoc 1992;28:70–6.

27. Wylie KB, Hosgood G. Mortality and morbidity of small intestinal surgery in dogs and cats 74 cases (1980–1992). J Am Anim Hosp Assoc 1994;30:469–74.

28. Ralphs SC, Jessen CR, Lipowitz AJ. Risk factors for leakage following intestinal anastomosis in dogs and cats: 115 cases (1991–2000). J Am Vet Med Assoc 2003;223:73–7.

29. Gorman SC, Freeman LM, Mitchell SL, Chan DL. Extensive small bowel resection in dogs and cats: 20 cases (1998–2004). J Am Vet Med Assoc 2006;228: 403–77.

30. Kouti V, Papazoglou LS, Laskos J, et al. Ursodeoxycholic acid promotes intestinal adaptation in a cat model of short bowel syndrome. Fundamental & Clinical Pharmacology. Online Jan 7th, 2011.

Chapter 30

Large intestine, rectum and anus

R.N. White

Colorectal disease is a common problem in cats. The term covers a wide range of conditions including congenital abnormalities such as atresia ani and rectovaginal fistulae, and acquired conditions such as megacolon and neoplasia. The surgical management of the majority of conditions encountered should not be considered routine as complications associated with both colonic and rectal surgery are reported commonly.

SURGICAL ANATOMY

The large intestine extends from the ileocecal valve to the anus. It is divided anatomically and functionally into the colon (ascending, transverse, and descending), rectum, and the anus. The walls of the colon and rectum comprise five distinct layers: mucosa, submucosa, inner circular muscle, outer longitudinal muscle, and serosa. The intraperitoneal colon and proximal part of the rectum are covered by serosa; much of the distal rectum is extraperitoneal and, therefore, lacks serosa.

The ascending colon communicates with the terminal small intestine (ileum) via the ileocolic orifice and with the cecum via the cecocolic orifice. The region of bowel containing these structures is often termed the ileocecocolic junction.

The short ascending colon turns towards the left side of the abdomen at the right colic (hepatic) flexure to become the transverse colon. The colon takes a further turn at the left colic (splenic) flexure to pass in a caudal direction, becoming the descending colon. There is no histological difference between the ascending, transverse, and descending colon; the sub-division is purely one of gross anatomical position. The descending colon with its associated mesocolon lies dorsal to the small intestine passing to the left side of the peritoneal cavity in a caudal direction towards the pelvic inlet. At the level of the pelvic inlet, the colon continues caudally as the rectum. The colorectal junction cannot be discerned grossly; it is positioned at the level of the pelvic brim, with the rectum continuing through the pelvic canal.

In the normal individual, the total colonic length as a percentage of the intestinal length is remarkably constant at $20.9 \pm 2.0\%$.[1] The layers of the colon are the mucosa, submucosa, muscularis, and serosa. Like the small bowel, it is the submucosal layer that is considered important in maintaining mechanical strength during the process of suturing or stapled closure and anastomosis.

The large intestine obtains its arterial blood supply from branches of both the cranial mesenteric and caudal mesenteric arteries (Fig. 30-1). The ileocolic artery, a branch of the cranial mesenteric artery, supplies the ileum, cecum, and ascending and transverse colon. The ileocolic artery gives rise to the middle colic and right colic arteries. The middle colic artery supplies part of the transverse colon and half of the descending colon. The right colic artery supplies the cecum, the ascending colon, and part of the transverse colon. The left colic and cranial rectal arteries arise from the caudal mesenteric artery. The left colic artery supplies the distal half of the descending colon before anastomosing with the right colic artery. Vessels arising from the caudal mesenteric artery and passing in a caudal direction are considered to be supplying the rectum. The cranial rectal artery primarily supplies the cranial and caudal rectum. The caudal rectum also receives a supply from vessels arising from the internal iliac artery via the prostatic or vaginal arteries.

The venous drainage follows similar anatomy to the arterial supply. The caudal mesenteric vein drains into the portal vein.

The paravertebral sympathetic trunk supplies the colon via the sympathetic ganglia. The parasympathetic innervation to the colon is supplied by the pelvic and vagus nerves.

DIAGNOSIS AND GENERAL CONSIDERATIONS

Cats need to have a complete history taken with specific attention paid to duration and onset of clinical signs, diet, and history of any trauma. A physical examination of the cat should be performed with a careful abdominal palpation, inspection of the anal and genital orifices and a rectal examination should be performed to check for narrowing or strictures; however, this is usually done with the cat sedated or anesthetized.

Definitions

Presenting signs of cats with colorectal disease will often typify the condition encountered such as the constipation associated with

© 2014 Elsevier Ltd
DOI: 10.1016/B978-0-7020-4336-9.00030-5

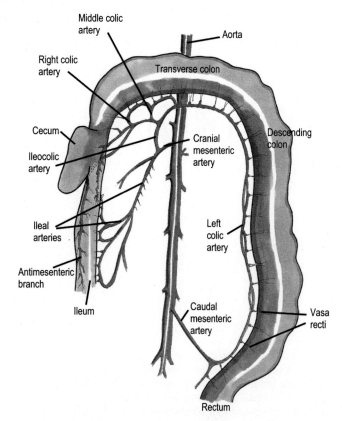

Figure 30-1 Blood supply to the large intestine.

megacolon and the complete lack of defecation in individuals suffering from atresia ani. Constipation has been defined as infrequent or difficult defecation associated with the retention of feces within the colon and rectum.[2] Obstipation is a condition of prolonged and intractable constipation resulting in severe fecal impaction throughout the rectum and colon. Obstipated animals are unable to eliminate the impacted fecal material. Dyschezia describes difficult or painful evacuation of feces from the rectum. This clinical sign is commonly associated with lesions in or near the anal region. Alimentary tenesmus is the clinical sign that characterizes an animal that strains to defecate. The straining is often painful and ineffectual. Alimentary tenesmus is commonly associated with disease of the large intestine and lower intestinal tract.

Diagnostic imaging for intestinal disease

Plain radiography and contrast radiography[3]

When examining the large intestine of the cat, orthogonal (lateral and ventrodorsal) survey radiographs including the pelvis and perianal region should be obtained. The normal colon will have a shape similar to a numeral '7' on the dorsoventral view. The cecum is generally not visible on plain radiography in the cat.

The content, position and size of the large intestine may be variable. The width of the normal feces-filled colon should not be greater than three times the width of the small intestines or the length of the seventh lumbar vertebra. Enlargement of the diameter of the colon beyond 1.5 times the length of the seventh lumbar vertebra is indicative of chronic large bowel dysfunction and megacolon.[4] The normal colonic wall may have a corrugated appearance (due to peristalsis) and this finding should not be interpreted as abnormal unless it is a consistent finding on subsequent, serial radiographs.

In cats without anal sac disease, gas (air) within one or both anal sacs should be considered an unusual but normal variant on survey radiographs that include the caudal aspects of the pelvis. This finding should not be mistaken for bony lysis of the ischial tuberosity on the ventrodorsal view.

Contrast radiography may be used to increase the radiographic contrast between the large bowel lumen and its mucosal surface. Some preparation of the patient is required to empty the large bowel of fecal material prior to performing a contrast procedure of the colon/rectum. Food should be withheld for at least 24 hours and some form of cleansing enema should be administered (see section on bowel preparation prior to surgery). Plain survey films should be obtained prior to performing the contrast studies.

Pneumocolonography describes the instillation of a negative contrast agent (most commonly air) into the rectum/colon via a catheter placed through the anus. In general, a volume of 8 mL/kg bodyweight will be sufficient and this should be instilled slowly to reduce the incidence of discomfort and increased peristaltic activity.

Positive contrast colonography describes the instillation of a positive contrast agent into the lumen of the large bowel via the anus. Positive contrast agents that are used include barium suspension and iodinated contrast media. A 20% w/v barium suspension (one part barium to two parts water) at a dose of 8 mL/kg should be instilled into the large bowel via a balloon tipped catheter (Foley catheter). Inflation of the balloon will discourage the leakage of contrast agent via the anus. The contrast should be instilled slowly to reduce the incidence of discomfort and peristaltic activity. The air can be removed at the end of the study.

Barium should not be used in any individual with suspected large bowel rupture or perforation. In such cases, diluted (20%) ionic or non-ionic iodinated contrast media should be used as an alternative (the use of an iodinated contrast media will result in a less well-defined mucosal surface since the agent is rapidly absorbed through the mucosal surface). The positive contrast should be gently aspirated at the end of the study.

Indications for positive contrast colonography include assessment of mucosal surface abnormalities, strictures, diverticula, and intussusception.

Double contrast colonography is performed by coating the mucosal surface of the large bowel with a positive contrast agent followed by the subsequent instillation of a negative contrast agent (air) to maximize the contrast interface. The technique is performed by instilling a positive contrast agent as described already. Once completely instilled, this agent is then removed and an equal volume of air is immediately instilled prior to obtaining orthogonal abdominal radiographs. The air can be removed at the end of the study.

Indications for double contrast colonography include assessment of space-occupying lesions of the wall of the large bowel and the location of strictures and intramural lesions.

Ultrasonography[5]

Although the entire colon is accessible for transabdominal ultrasonographic examination its gas and fecal contents often make it difficult to image the organ with clarity. Reverberation artifacts obscure the majority of the large bowel wall from observation; only the wall closest to the transducer can be clearly imaged in the majority of individuals.

Ultrasonography can be used to effectively assess lesions within the bowel wall (masses, strictures, intussusceptions, etc.). In certain cases the technique can be used to obtain ultrasound guided fine needle aspirates of a discrete lesion. High-resolution transducers can be used to visualize the regional lymph nodes (right colic, medial iliac, and hypogastric). Enlarged nodes may be amenable to fine needle aspiration under ultrasonographic guidance.

Ultrasonography can be useful for defining the presence and position of free peritoneal fluid. The technique should be performed in patients with suspected large bowel peritonitis and will allow pocketed fluid accumulations to be aspirated with the maximum degree of accuracy and safety.

Computed tomography

Computed tomography (CT) is a very useful modality for imaging the large bowel in the cat. Modern machines will provide high quality images that can be manipulated to show any cross-section view in all three dimensions. A CT scan is particular well suited for the investigation of intrapelvic disease. In addition, rapid staging of any neoplastic disease (pulmonary, liver, and local lymph node assessment) can be performed as necessary.

Colonoscopy/proctoscopy[6]

Colonoscopy and proctoscopy will, in general, be performed with a flexible endoscope in the cat. Such an endoscope should have a biopsy channel so that suitable lesions can be sampled at the time of the procedure. The importance of correct bowel preparation cannot be over-emphasized. Preparation will normally include a period of 24–48 hours of starvation with the administration of some form of enema (possibly on more than one occasion) prior to the study. To be performed safely, the procedure will require a full general anesthetic. Inadequate cleansing of the large bowel will produce unsatisfactory and meaningless findings at the time of the endoscopy. Difficulty in achieving adequate and safe cleansing of the bowel in the cat has led to a reluctance to perform the procedure in the species. This is unfortunate since the large bowel is very accessible for a complete endoscopic examination and the procedure will frequently provide a definitive diagnosis without recourse to surgery. Indications for colonoscopy include dyschezia, tenesmus, constipation, or chronic diarrhea containing mucus and/or fresh blood. For more information see Chapter 9.

SURGICAL CONDITIONS OF THE LARGE INTESTINE AND ANUS

Megacolon

Megacolon is a descriptive term only, and its use imparts no information regarding specific etiology or pathophysiology. The condition should be considered a disorder characterized by recurrent constipation and/or obstipation associated with dilatation and hypomotility of the colon. Often the underlying etiology for the condition remains unknown and in many cases it is more appropriate to define the mechanism by which the condition developed. The common two pathologic mechanisms are either dilatation or hypertrophy.[7]

Dilated megacolon is the end stage of colonic dysfunction. The underlying etiology for colonic dysfunction megacolon is nearly always idiopathic. Cats affected with idiopathic dilated megacolon have permanent loss of colonic structure and function although histologic assessment of the affected colon is normal in the majority of cases.

Hypertrophic megacolon develops as a consequence of an obstructive lesion such as malunion of a pelvic fracture or a distal large bowel tumor. Hypertrophic megacolon may be reversible if the site of obstruction is removed early in the course of the disease. With time, the changes within the colonic wall will become irreversible and removal of the site of obstruction will have little or no effect on the megacolon.

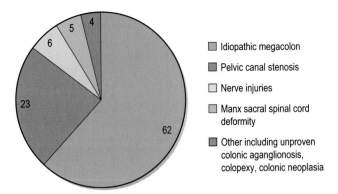

Figure 30-2 Causes of megacolon. *(From Washabau RJ, Hasler AH. Constipation, obstipation, and megacolon. In: August JR, editor. Consultations in Feline Internal Medicine. 3rd ed. Philadelphia: WB Saunders Company; 1997. p. 104–12.)*

In humans, a congenital form of megacolon (Hirshsprung disease) is well recognized. It occurs in neonates and is characterized by aganglionosis of a segment of colon, resulting in the persistent contraction of smooth muscle within the affected segment and the subsequent dilatation of the colon proximal to the constricted, affected site. This condition has been suggested to occur in cats,[8] although its true existence in this species has only been documented in one case.[9]

In a review of 120 cases of megacolon in cats, 62% were accounted for by idiopathic megacolon, 23% demonstrated pelvic canal stenosis, 6% demonstrated nerve injuries, 5% showed Manx sacral spinal cord deformity, and the remaining 4% included unproven colonic aganglionosis, complications of colopexy, and colonic neoplasia (Fig. 30-2).[10] It was concluded that although it remains true that megacolon may have an extensive list of differential diagnoses and may be associated with other disease processes including active colonic inflammation, dysautonomia, and metabolic disorders, the majority of cases are idiopathic, orthopedic, or neurologic in origin.

A diagnosis of megacolon is made by estimation of the colon size on radiography. Enlargement of the diameter of the colon beyond 1.5 times the length of the body of the seventh lumbar vertebra is indicative of chronic large bowel dysfunction and megacolon.[4]

Megacolon is most commonly observed in middle-aged (mean 5.8 years) male cats (70% male, 30% female) cats. The domestic shorthair (46%) followed by the domestic longhair (15%) and Siamese (12%) are the breeds most commonly affected.[10]

Specific therapy depends on the severity of the constipation and the underlying cause for the condition. A summary of non-surgical management and the drugs that can be used is listed in Box 30-1 and Table 30-1.

In the majority of cats with idiopathic megacolon, medical treatment using laxatives, enemas, and dietary management offers only a temporary relief of clinical signs. It is now widely accepted that colectomy should be considered in cats with the condition that is refractory to medical therapy. Several different surgical techniques for the management of the condition have been described and these include coloplasty,[11,12] a partial colectomy,[12–15] or the more complete or subtotal colectomy.[8,16–20] The surgical management of idiopathic megacolon and constipation has been reviewed comprehensively.[21]

Causes of outlet obstruction causing secondary megacolon in the cat are listed in Box 30-2. Of these, the most common cause of outlet obstruction causing secondary megacolon is pelvic fracture malunion.[22]

Outlet obstruction will initially result in the development of a hypertrophic megacolon.[32] Hypertrophic megacolon is often reversible with the early removal of the colonic outflow obstruction. If left

Box 30-1 Summary of non-surgical management of constipation in the cat

Removal of impacted feces

The removal of impacted feces may be accomplished using laxatives. The use of a suppository will require both a compliant patient and a compliant owner.

Alternatively, impacted fecal material can be removed with the aid of an enema in conjunction with manual extraction. Manual extraction will require the sedation or general anesthesia of the patient. Enema solution should be administered slowly via a well-lubricated 10–12 Fr feeding tube, or equivalent.

Administration of laxatives

Laxatives promote evacuation of the large bowel through stimulation of fluid and electrolyte transport and/or increase in propulsive motility. Bulk-forming laxatives are dietary fiber supplements of poorly digestible polysaccharides and celluloses. They should be used with care in cats with megacolon since if they fail to induce defecation their bulk-forming action may actually lead to a worsening of the fecal impaction. Lubricant laxatives such as mineral oil should also be used with caution;

they are likely to be most effective in mild cases of constipation and their administration should probably be limited to rectal administration as there is a significant risk of aspiration pneumonia with oral administration, especially in debilitated and depressed patients.[2] Of the stimulant laxative agents available, Bisacodyl is considered to be most effective. The drug brings about the production of diarrhea by the combined effect of increased mucosal secretion and colonic propulsive motility. Lastly, there are the hyperosmotic laxatives. Of these, the most effective is the polysaccharide, lactulose. The fermentation of the lactulose in the gastrointestinal tract leads to the production of organic acids, which stimulate colonic fluid secretion and propulsive motility.

Administration of colonic prokinetic agents

Unfortunately, the colonic prokinetic agent, Cisapride was withdrawn from sale in 2000 from Western Europe, North America, and Canada following reports of untoward cardiac effects in people. There is little or no data available at the present time regarding the use of other prokinetic agents in the management of constipation in the cat.

Table 30-1 Pharmaceutical products useful in the management of megacolon

Plan	Drugs and solutions	Administration	Comments
Laxatives	*Bulk-forming laxatives:* dietary fiber supplements of poorly digestible polysaccharides and celluloses	Orally mixed with food	Use with care since if fail to induce defecation may worsen the impaction
	Lubricant laxatives: mineral oil, glycerin	Best administered per rectum in debilitated animals as risk of aspiration[2]	Use with caution. Most effective in mild cases
	Stimulant laxatives: bisacodyl		Increases mucosal secretion and colonic propulsive motility
	Hyperosmotic laxatives: lactulose	Administer orally at a dose of 0.5 mL/kg body weight every 8–12 hours	Lactulose fermentation leads to production of organic acids, which stimulate colonic fluid secretion and propulsive motility. Overdose can lead to diarrhea
	Emollient laxatives: dioctyl sodium sulfosuccinate	Pediatric rectal suppository	Requires compliant cat and owner
Enema and manual extraction	Enema solutions include warm tap water, warm isotonic saline, dioctyl sodium sulfosuccinate, mineral oil, or lactulose	Administer slowly via lubricated 10–12 Fr feeding tube, or equivalent. Requires heavy sedation or general anesthesia	Sodium phosphate enemas are contraindicated in cats as high levels of sodium and phosphate might induce severe hypernatremia, hyperphosphatemia and hypocalcemia
Administration of colonic prokinetic agents	Cisapride	Oral	Withdrawn from sale in 2000 in many parts of the world due to cardiac effects in people

---

Box 30-2 Causes of outlet obstruction causing secondary megacolon in the cat

Pelvic fracture malunion[22]

Colonic and rectoanal tumors[19]

Extrapelvic extraluminal stricture formation following neutering surgery[23–27]

Intrapelvic extraluminal tumors or masses

Perineal herniation[28]

Intestinal foreign bodies[22]

Improper diet[22]

Anal, rectal or colonic atresia[29–31]

untreated, the obstruction will result in progression of the condition to an irreversible dilated megacolon. In general, therefore, prompt treatment of outlet obstruction will involve removal of the underlying cause of the obstruction. A major complication in cases that have already developed dilated megacolon is the continued dysfunction of the colon following the removal of the outlet obstruction. In such instances, continued problems with constipation/obstipation may be managed medically. In cases that are unresponsive to medical management, a subtotal colectomy should be considered.

Complications after surgery for megacolon include diarrhea from short bowel syndrome (see Chapter 29) and peritonitis from dehiscence of the anastomosis (see Chapter 26). In the long term, the most common complication is recurrence of the constipation. In the majority of such affected individuals, the constipation can be treated by dietary management, stool softeners, and the occasional manual removal of feces, until a satisfactory medical regime for the management of the constipation is developed.[7] Affected individuals should be carefully assessed to ensure that there is no evidence of either outlet obstruction or megarectum (see section below) that might cause ongoing issues with distal physical or functional bowel obstruction.

It might be expected that recurrent constipation would be a more common complication in individuals in which the ileocolic junction was retained at the time of colectomy. In these individuals, the retained colonic segment is likely to be larger than in those individuals in which the junction was resected and an enterocolostomy was performed. In fact, studies suggest that there is no significant difference in the rate of recurrent constipation between the two surgical procedures of colocolostomy and enterocolostomy.[20]

Colonic entrapment following ovariohysterectomy or castration

The development of constipation or obstipation is a rare complication following routine ovariohysterectomy or castration in the cat.[23-27] In all the reported cases the constipation/obstipation was associated with an extrapelvic, extraluminal stricture of the colon situated just cranial to the pelvic brim (Fig. 30-3).

In queens, the complication becomes manifest within ten weeks of the ovariohysterectomy. The cause of the stricture is either a collar of residual uterine horn tissue that forms adhesions with the mesocolon or a ring of non-adherent fibrous tissue, the origin of which remains unclear. Surgical resection of the offending tissues and fibrous adhesions appears to result in the long-term resolution of the obstructive

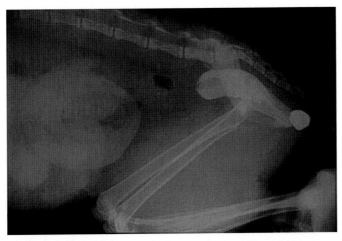

Figure 30-3 A 1-year-old cat presented with an inability to defecate eight weeks after ovariohysterectomy. Stenosis at the rectocolic junction is demonstrated after administering a barium enema.

clinical signs without the necessity to perform a subsequent subtotal colectomy.[24-26] It has been suggested that the risk of this complication may be reduced by ensuring that the uterus is amputated at, or as close to, the cervix as possible during the ovariohysterectomy procedure.[24,25]

A similar condition has been reported in the tom.[27] In this instance, an open castration had been performed and clinical signs of constipation and fecal tenesmus developed eight weeks after the surgery. The cause of the stricture was found to be a non-adherent fibrous ring encircling the distal descending colon. The origin of the fibrous band was unclear, but it was considered possible that retraction of the spermatic cord following an open castration may, especially if the procedure was performed without adequate asepsis, result in the formation of a fibrous ring around the descending colon. As with the female cats following ovariohysterectomy, removal of the offending tissue resulted in the long-term resolution of the clinical signs.

Constipation associated with perineal herniation

Perineal herniation is not as commonly diagnosed in the cat as in the dog, but in affected individuals the condition may induce fecal impaction, constipation, and obstipation.[28] Obstipated individuals may go on to develop a secondary dilated megacolon.

Surgical repair of the hernia or hernias (see Chapter 25) will alleviate the constipation in the majority of individuals. Cats with any degree of fecal colonic impaction should have the impacted feces removed prior to, or at the time of, hernia repair. In individuals in which fecal impaction recurs, a careful assessment of the repairs and/or assessment of a previously unaffected side should be performed to rule out the presence of further hernia development. If it is concluded that no further perineal herniation is present, but the animal is suffering from megacolon, a subtotal colectomy should be considered, since further straining associated with the fecal impaction/megacolon is likely to result in a breakdown of the herniorrhaphy repair. Therefore, the early removal of the diseased colon is to be recommended. In fact, it has been suggested that in individuals suffering from both perineal herniation and a secondary dilated megacolon, the removal of the megacolon alone may relieve the clinical signs, making concurrent perineal hernia repair unnecessary.[32]

Neoplasia of the colon

In cats, the most common large intestinal tumor is adenocarcinoma, followed by lymphoma and mast cell tumor.[33] In the largest case series of cats with tumors of the colon, the mean age at presentation was 12.5 years, 46% of the tumors were adenocarcinoma, 41% were lymphoma, and 9% were mast cell tumors.[34]

Clinical signs often include constipation, fecal tenesmus, diarrhea, anorexia, and weight loss.[35] Clinical examination will often confirm the presence of a caudal abdominal mass on abdominal palpation. Further investigations should include full blood analyses (including testing for feline leukemia and immunodeficiency viruses), imaging of the abdomen (survey radiographs, abdominal ultrasonography, contrast enhanced CT scan, etc.), and protoscopy/colonoscopy (to allow visualization and biopsy) (Fig. 30-4). In cases with cancer, the disease should be staged with thoracic radiography/CT and ultrasonography/CT imaging of the liver, spleen, and local lymph nodes.[36]

Treatment, in most instances, is the surgical excision of the mass followed by end-to-end anastomosis via a ventral midline celiotomy. Obtaining clean margins at the time of excision will, not surprisingly, increase survival time. Conversely, gross evidence of local or distant metastasis at the time of surgery will lead to a decrease in survival

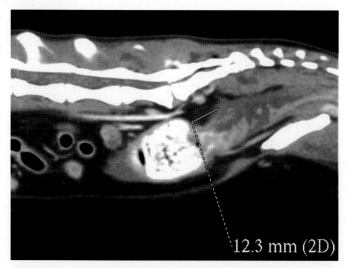

Figure 30-4 CT scan of a colorectal adenocarcinoma causing stenosis of the large bowel at the colorectal junction.

time. Margins of excision have been suggested to be at least 2.5 cm and, ideally, up to 5 cm from each end of the mass.[37] For tumors at the colorectal junction, it will often prove impossible to achieve such margins on the rectal side of the growth, making local recurrence at the site a real possibility. Access to the intrapelvic rectum can be improved by performing either a midline pubic symphysiotomy/symphysectomy with or without an ischial osteotomy.[38]

Cats suffering from adenocarcinoma are very likely to have metastatic disease at the time of presentation; in one study about 80% of cats with this colonic tumor had metastasis (local or distant) at the time of surgery.[34] Cats with negative lymph nodes at surgery lived a median of 259 days, versus 49 days if positive. Four cats with adenocarcinoma were treated with doxorubicin, and lived a median of 280 days, versus 56 days without.[34]

For cats with adenocarcinoma, there is some evidence to suggest that the excision of the mass should be combined with a subtotal colectomy. One study showed a mean survival time (MST) of 138 days in those cats undergoing mass excision and subtotal colectomy compared with a MST of 68 days in those in which only mass excision was performed.[34] The reason for this difference in survival time remains unclear but may reflect the increased possibility of obtaining 'clean' margins. No such advantage was seen with additional subtotal colectomy in cats surgically managed for lymphoma. Despite this, the current recommendation in cats suffering from an unidentified colonic mass is that, as part of their surgical management, they should receive a subtotal colectomy to increase survival time.

For large intestinal lymphoma, cats with surgery appear to fare equally poorly with or without adjunctive chemotherapy (MST of just over three months in both groups).[39]

There is little information available for the management of large intestinal mast cell tumor in the cat. In one study, in four cats with mast cell tumor, two had local metastasis; one distant and one local. All the cats were treated with surgery and prednisolone with a MST of 199 days.[34]

There is some evidence that cases with non-resectable colonic cancer might benefit from the placement of colonic stents as part of the management of their disease. Metal stents placed under fluoroscopy were palliative in two cats with colonic adenocarcinoma, one for 274 days (with good quality of life and euthanasia due to eventual distant metastasis) and one for only 19 days (euthanasia due to perceived reduction in quality of life).[40]

Cats with certain forms of colonic cancer may benefit from radiation therapy (see Chapter 15) of the local disease, but there are no reports describing its use for this disease at the present time.

Atresia coli

Atresia coli describes a segmental intestinal anomaly affecting a portion of the colon. The anomaly is characterized by the absence or closure of a segment of colon. Congenital atresia develops when areas of the intestine either fail to vascularize or the blood vessels degenerate early in development. Causes of the condition in domestic animals and humans include fetal enteritis, peritonitis, anomalies or diseases of the fetal blood vessels, and injuries sustained in utero by a previously normal fetus.[41,42] Although the condition is considered the most common segmental anomaly of the intestine in domestic animals, it has only rarely been described in the cat.[31,41]

Clinical signs include abdominal distension, abdominal discomfort, and an absence of defecation postpartum.

Although, in theory, the treatment for the condition involves the surgical excision of the affected portion of colon followed by colonic anastomosis, in reality the poor prognosis, very young age of affected individuals, and their poor body condition at presentation mean that euthanasia should be considered the most appropriate management in the majority of cases.

Should surgical intervention be performed, it may be more appropriate to perform a subtotal colectomy, thereby removing the proximal megacolon segment of colon at the same time as removing the underdeveloped atretic portion of large bowel. In some instances there is no gross evidence of the atretic portion of bowel and it is truly completely missing. Under such circumstances, the closed end of the distal portion of bowel will require excision to allow bowel anastomosis to be performed following proximal subtotal colectomy.

SURGICAL CONDITIONS OF THE RECTUM AND ANUS

Atresia ani

In the feline embryo, the gastrointestinal, urinary, and reproductive tracts communicate initially. At approximately seven weeks of development, the urorectal fold grows caudally, separating the urogenital and rectal tracts and their shared cloaca horizontally. The anal membrane eventually thins and ruptures, forming an anus. A failure of the cloacal membrane to resorb or rupture by the second month of embryological development will result in atresia ani.

Four types of atresia ani have been reported (Fig. 30-5 and Table 30-2).

Animals with type IV atresia ani may have normal development of the anus and terminal rectum including accessory structures such as the anal sacs and anal sphincter. Types III and IV have also been classified as rectal atresia or segmental rectal aplasia.

Clinical signs of atresia ani usually begin within a few weeks of birth. Cats with congenital stenosis (type I) will usually develop constipation and tenesmus soon after weaning. Cats with types II, III, and IV atresia ani usually have perineal swelling or anal membrane protrusion from accumulation of meconium and feces within the rectum. Other findings include abdominal distension, abdominal discomfort and an absence of defecation. If obstruction is longstanding, vomiting and dehydration can develop. Individuals with atresia ani may have multiple congenital anomalies and, therefore, should be fully examined with care before any form of surgical correction is considered. A number of concurrent congenital and acquired lesions have been

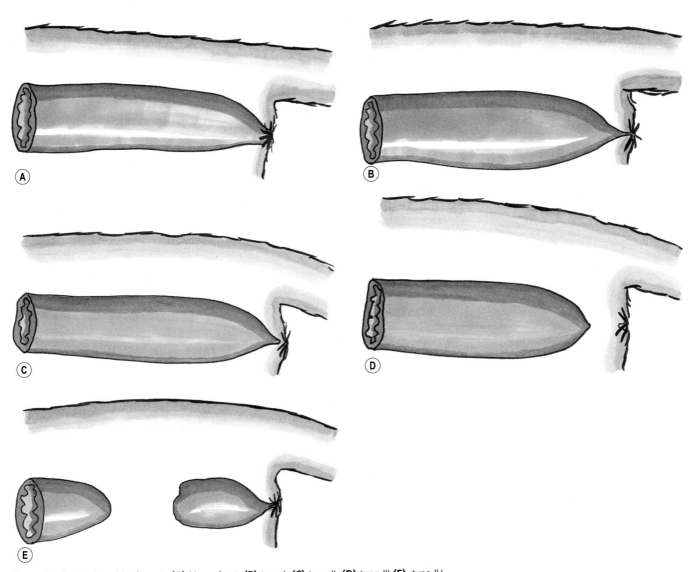

Figure 30-5 Atresia ani in the cat. **(A)** Normal cat, **(B)** type I, **(C)** type II, **(D)** type III **(E),** type IV.

Table 30-2 Types of atresia ani in the cat

Type I	Congenital stenosis of the anus
Type II	Imperforate anus; characterized by persistence of the anal membrane with the rectum ending blindly cranial to the imperforate anus
Type III	Imperforate anus combined with more cranial termination of the rectum as a blind pouch
Type IV	Discontinuity of the proximal rectum with normal anal and terminal rectal development

Box 30-3 Conditions seen in conjunction with atresia ani in the cat

Urethrorectal fistulae (congenital)
Rectovaginal fistulae (congenital)
Rectocutaneous fistulae (acquired)

reported in conjunction with atresia ani in the cat, the three most recognized are listed in Box 30-3.

Like atresia coli, the prognosis for atresia ani is poor. Affected individuals are young, small, and typically in poor body condition. Attempted surgical correction carries high rates of both morbidity and mortality. By the time surgical intervention is performed, chronic distension of the colon and rectum may have already led to irreversible damage. Repeated surgical procedures may be necessary as local dehiscence and stricture development at the site of surgery is a common complication.

Urethrorectal fistulae

Urethrorectal fistulae in association with atresia ani (commonly type II) has only rarely been reported in the cat.[29,43,44] This condition is described in Chapter 38.

Rectovaginal fistulae

Congenital rectovaginal fistulae in association with atresia ani (commonly type II) is reported rarely in the cat.[45] The condition is

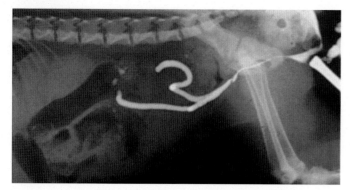

Figure 30-6 Positive contrast retrograde vestibule-vaginogram in a 12-week-old kitten showing the presence of a rectovaginal fistula.

characterized by a communication between the dorsal wall of the vagina and the ventral portion of the rectum, so that the vulva functions as a common opening to the urogenital and gastrointestinal tracts.

Clinical signs are similar to those seen with urethrorectal fistulae and include tenesmus, abdominal distension, megacolon, irritation of the vulva, and the passage of fluid fecal material through the vulva. Again, similar to urethrorectal fistulae, many of the signs will not be evident while the cat is on a liquid (milk) diet. Diagnosis is based on history, clinical signs, and physical examination. Radiographic examination with contrast medium infused through the vagina or fistula may be useful for determining the position of the fistula and terminal rectum (Fig. 30-6). Surgical management of this condition is described below.

Rectocutaneous fistulae

A rectocutaneous fistula represents an acquired communication between the rectum and the perirectal skin.[46] The condition may be the result of trauma, pelvic fracture, rectal foreign body, pararectal abscess, atresia ani, or surgery and has only been reported rarely in cats.[47] The defect will result in the discharge of fecal material through the skin wound.

Management of rectocutaneous fistulae is, in most instances, considered surgical. Very superficial fistulae (fistula-in-ano) may be 'laid open'. Deeper fistulae may require pararectal exploration, excision of the fistulous tract, and, most importantly, mucosal closure of the rectal wall opening. The cause of the fistula should be ascertained as part of the clinical investigation. Also, a full appreciation of the position and extent of the fistula/ae should be considered mandatory before embarking on the surgical management of the condition. This might require the use of proctoscopy and contrast radiography.

Dehiscence and local contamination of the pararectal tissues is considered a common complication of the surgery. In an attempt to minimize this complication, the use of a temporary incontinent end-in colostomy (see Box 30-7) has been described to divert fecal material from the rectum during the period of rectal wall healing.[47]

Anogenital clefts

Anogenital clefts are a rare congenital abnormality in the cat. In the female (anovulval cleft), the mucosa of the anus or rectum and the vestibule/vulva are continuous along the vertical perineal raphe. The anus may be incomplete ventrally or the anus may be atretic, in which case a rectal fistula may form part of the dorsal aspect of the cleft. In the male (anourethral cleft), the urethra is often incomplete ventrally, resulting in hypospadias. In such cases, the mucosa of the anus or rectum and the urethral mucosa are continuous along the

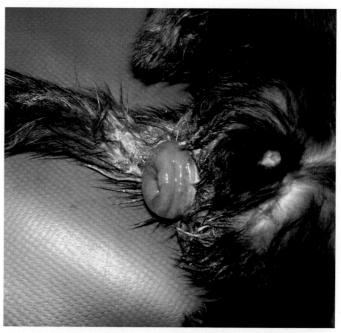

Figure 30-7 Rectal prolapse in a 10-week-old kitten that had a history of diarrhea.

vertical perineal raphe. Affected animals are usually both fecally and urinary continent. Surgical management is described below.

Colonic and rectal duplication cysts

Enteric duplication is a rare developmental malformation in the cat. The pathogenesis is not completely understood, but errors in normal embryological canalization or embryological connections between the developing intestines and the neural tube have been postulated. Confirmed diagnosis depends on the fulfillment of three anatomic criteria:[48] the cyst must be attached to the alimentary tract, it must be lined by mucous membrane similar to that part of the alimentary tract, and it must contain a smooth muscle layer. The condition has been described in both the colon and rectum in the cat.[49,50]

Presenting clinical signs include signs consistent with colonic/rectal obstruction: anorexia, obstipation, and straining to defecate. Abdominal palpation confirms the presence of a non-painful, smooth structure within the caudal abdomen and/or cranial pelvic canal. Imaging tests reveal a cystic mass associated with the descending colon (colonic duplication cyst) or rectum (rectal duplication cyst).

The treatment of choice for a duplication cyst is surgical excision. The approach is dependent on the site and position of the lesion and may be via the abdomen (caudal midline celiotomy), the pelvic canal (ventral pubic osteotomy or symphysectomy), or via the perineum. Complete removal of the cystic structure carries a good prognosis. Complications are related to difficulty in complete excision and intraoperative iatrogenic damage to local structures.

Rectal prolapse

Rectal prolapse most commonly occurs as a consequence of an underlying disorder that produces severe or persistent straining. It may be associated with intestinal diseases that cause diarrhea and tenesmus, anorectal diseases that produce constipation and dyschezia, or lower urinary tract diseases that cause stranguria and dysuria. The most common cause is severe enteritis/proctitis associated with endoparasites, most often affecting kittens under four months of age (Fig. 30-7).

Prolapses may be described as partial or complete, depending on whether they involve just mucosa, or all layers of the rectal wall. In most instances, the prolapsed mass will be cylindrical with a depression at its centre. In early cases, the prolapse might be intermittent, affecting only part of the circumference of the rectoanal junction. In general, the extent of the prolapse increases with continued straining, leading to the everted tissue becoming progressively more swollen and edematous. This makes spontaneous retraction of the prolapsed tissues less likely the longer the tissue has been prolapsed. With time, the prolapsed tissue may become traumatized, hemorrhagic, desiccated, and necrotic.

Management of rectal prolapse involves both repair of the prolapse and treatment/elimination of the underlying cause. It is important to differentiate rectal prolapse from ileocolic intussusception.[51] Grossly, they appear similar, but signs of partial or complete obstruction usually accompany intussusception. Confirmed differentiation of the two conditions can be achieved by probing the prolapse with a blunt probe; insertion of the probe lateral to the prolapsed mass is possible with an ileocolic intussusception but not possible in a case suffering from a rectal prolapse. Options for management of rectal prolapse have been well described[52] and are summarized in Box 30-4.

The prognosis for rectal prolapse is variable and depends on the severity and chronicity of the presenting condition and, subsequently,

on the complexity of the surgical intervention required to treat the condition.

A recent study has described the use of a silicone elastomer sling for the management of rectal prolapse in cats with less than adequate anal tone/musculature.[54] Although the procedure may prove effective in the management of the prolapse, it is associated with significant complications including the sling eroding through the perineal skin necessitating the removal of the device. As such, the technique cannot be recommended as any other than a 'last resort' procedure.

A further recent study has described performing a laparoscopic-assisted incisional colopexy.[55] The procedure was performed through two portals and was considered effective for the treatment of recurrent rectal prolapse, without postoperative complications or recurrences in both the short and long term.

SURGICAL CONDITIONS OF THE ANAL SACS

Anal sac impaction

Anal sac impaction is rare in the cat and is defined as the retention of anal sac secretions, often leading to inflammation and infection.[56]

The cause of anal sac impaction often remains unclear but possible causes are listed in Box 30-5.

Clinical signs of anal sac impaction are related to discomfort and include pain on defecation, licking and biting at the tail base, scooting, and fecal tenesmus. Examination of the glands may confirm the perianal region to be red and swollen but, in many cases, visual examination will reveal no apparent abnormalities. Gentle palpation of the perianal region will reveal the presence of a full anal sac (usually on both sides).

Treatment consists of expressing the anal sacs externally or with internal compression with a gloved finger in the rectum. It is likely that the cat will require sedation if adequate expression is to be achieved. Following expression, the sacs should be irrigated and flushed with an antiseptic solution. Expression and irrigation may need to be repeated intermittently into the longer term. The cat should be treated for possible tapeworm infection and any necessary changes made to the diet. If the condition becomes chronic and the sacs require frequent expression, it may become necessary to perform an anal sacculectomy (see Box 30-9).

Anal sacculitis

Anal sacculitis is a rare condition in the cat. Causes and clinical signs are similar to those for anal sac impaction.

Expression of an affected anal sac will produce a thin mucopurulent or serosanguineous discharge. Expressed sacs should be flushed and irrigated with an antiseptic solution and the flushed sac may then be filled with an antibiotic agent. Consideration should be given to the administration of a systemic broad-spectrum antibiotic.

Box 30-4 Treatment options for rectal prolapse in the cat

First minor prolapse

Treat the predisposing condition(s)

Warm water lavage, massage

Apply lubricant (e.g., water-soluble gel)

Sedation or general anesthesia, depending on the individual case. An epidural may be an important part of the treatment

Reduce the prolapse digitally and place a purse-string suture around a rectal probe

The cat should be fed a low residue diet and treated with a stool softener such as lactulose syrup

The purse-string suture should be left in place for three to five days

Moderate to massive prolapse with viable tissue, either first or recurrent episode

Treat the predisposing condition(s)

Sedation ± general anesthesia ± epidural

Warm water lavage, massage and apply lubricant. Reduce swelling with saline compresses

Reduce the prolapse and secure as described for first minor cases. If prolapse is recurrent, consider performing a colopexy[53]

Prolapse with devitalization and necrosis, either first or recurrent episode

Necrotic or irreducible prolapses must be resected and sutured in a circumferential manner, one quadrant at a time

Stay sutures should be placed before resection commences, to prevent retraction of healthy tissue

Correct alignment of margins must be maintained

A colopexy is advisable in severe or recurrent cases (in many cases, to reduce the risk of tension-related dehiscence, the colopexy should only be performed once the rectal resection and anastomosis surgery has completely healed)

(Modified from Pratschke K. Surgical diseases of the colon and rectum in small animals. In Pract 2005;27:354–62.)

Box 30-5 Possible causes of anal sac impaction in the cat[56]

Dietary (lack of roughage)

External anal sphincter dysfunction

Undersized anal sac ducts

Persistently loose feces

Tapeworm proglottids lodged in the anal sac duct orifice

Chronic or unresponsive anal sacculitis may progress to the formation of an anal sac abscess. Chronic anal sacculitis and anal sac abscessation will require anal sacculectomy (see Box 30-9).

Anal sac neoplasia

In the cat, the anal sacs are surrounded by tubular apocrine glands and sebaceous glands, whereas only apocrine glands are found in dogs.[57] Anal sac gland carcinoma (ASGC), also known as adenocarcinoma of the apocrine glands of the anal sac, is a malignant tumor arising within the apocrine secretory epithelium associated with the wall of the anal sac. The tumor has only rarely been reported in the cat and treatment options and prognosis remain unclear.

A recent retrospective study of 23 cases performed by the Veterinary Society of Surgical Oncology concluded that the domestic short-haired cat was the most common breed represented, with a mean age of 12.5 years.[58] Common clinical signs included rectal bleeding, perianal ulceration and tenesmus. Preoperative hypercalcemia was not observed in any cat. Surgical excision of the primary tumor was performed in all cases. Local recurrence was identified in 35% of cases and was the cause of death in the majority of these. Information regarding the use of adjunctive chemotherapy or radiation therapy remains unclear. The disease free interval and the median survival time following surgical excision of the primary tumor were 343 and 373 days, respectively. It was concluded that ASGC in the cat appears to be a locally invasive tumor with a low incidence of systemic metastasis and a lack of a hypercalcaemic paraneoplastic syndrome. Local recurrence was considered a significant issue (and probable cause of death) following the local excision of the tumor in the majority of cases.

PREOPERATIVE CONSIDERATIONS FOR LARGE INTESTINAL SURGERY

Preparation of the large intestine

Controversy remains with regards to the benefit and use of large bowel preparation in cats. In humans it is common to perform some form of mechanical cleaning of the large bowel prior to surgical intervention. The rationale for bowel preparation is that removing fecal material will decrease the bacterial load in the colon and rectum, thereby reducing the risk of contamination at the time of surgery and decreasing the incidence of postoperative infection.

Recent studies suggest that such mechanical cleansing of the large bowel actually produces only a transient reduction in overall colonic bacterial numbers, with any remaining fecal material containing high concentrations of both aerobic and anaerobic bacteria. Several studies in humans suggest that a mechanical bowel preparation does not decrease the risk of postoperative wound infection or anastomotic dehiscence.[59,60] There is little, or no, equivalent data available for cats but common sense would indicate that the use of an orally administered large bowel evacuant preparation would be dangerous and contraindicated in any individual suffering from large bowel obstructive disease such as neoplasia or chronic fecal impaction such as megacolon.

The use of enemas to promote fecal evacuation per rectum should also be viewed with caution. These products will commonly convert fecal material into a slurry which is much more likely to cause a local physical contamination at the time of colostomy/colectomy surgery when compared to the drier, impacted fecal material that was present originally. If enemas are to be used they should be administered a number of days before the date of the proposed surgery. Care should

---

Box 30-6 Perioperative administration of antibiotics before large intestinal surgery

Cefuroxime (second generation cephalosporin) at 20 mg/kg in combination with metronidazole at 10 mg/kg (given over at least 30 minutes)

Amoxicillin clavulanate at 20 mg/kg intravenously in combination with metronidazole at 10 mg/kg intravenously (given over at least 30 minutes)

---

also be taken to ensure that the enema does not contain soap as this is likely to induce mucosal irritation and colitis/proctitis. Enemas containing sodium phosphate are contraindicated in cats because of their potential to induce electrolyte disturbances. Safe enemas include warm tap water, warm isotonic saline, dioctyl sodium sulfosuccinate, mineral oil, or lactulose.

The potential complications associated with the use of enemas and their common failure to produce an empty and 'clean' large bowel at the time of surgery mean that the majority of surgeons perform no form of local bowel preparation prior to large bowel surgery in cats.

Perioperative administration of antibiotics

The use of perioperative prophylactic antibiotics should be considered mandatory in cats undergoing large intestinal surgery. The bacterial population within the colon and rectum is mixed and includes Gram positive and Gram negative aerobic and anaerobic bacteria. Prophylactic antibiotic coverage should, therefore, include the administration of agents that are effective across a wide range of both aerobic and anaerobic organisms. Practical and safe regimes are listed in Box 30-6.

The specific choice may be dictated by the specifics of the case and the personal preferences of the surgeon.

Antibiotics should be administered intravenously 30 minutes prior to surgery and, apart from metronidazole, should be repeated every 90 minutes for the duration of the surgery, unless otherwise indicated by the manufacturer's recommended dosing intervals.

Healing of the colon and rectum

As with all forms of intestinal surgery, the goal of colonic and rectal surgery is to achieve rapid healing without leakage, maintenance of normal luminal diameter without the development of stenosis, and a quick return to normal function. The consequences of colonic or rectal leakage or dehiscence are associated with both an increased morbidity and mortality due to the large numbers of pathogenic organisms present within the lumens of both structures (10^{10} to 10^{11} bacteria per gram of feces).

Although in humans many experiments have studied the mechanical properties and biochemical changes in the colon following anastomosis, there is a general consensus that the results of such studies should be interpreted with caution.[61] It is accepted that immediately following colonic anastomosis, as with small intestinal anastomosis, the site of anastomosis is sealed by fibrin. The breaking strength of the anastomosis is significantly less (up to 30%) than that of the intact colon, representing the holding strength of the sutures used to fashion the anastomosis.[62,63] Similar to the small intestine, the strongest suture-holding layer of the colon is the submucosa and, as such, great care should be taken to ensure that the sutures are anchored through this layer. Synthetic monofilament absorbable sutures should be used for large bowel closure; for example, polydioxanone, glycomer 631, or polyglyconate.

A prolonged lag phase in healing results in the rate of collagen lysis exceeding that of collagen synthesis for the first three to four days following bowel incision/anastomosis. The large bacterial population and high intraluminal pressures generated during the passage of fecal material, coupled with a prolonged lag phase in healing, mean that the risk of dehiscence is high for the first four days after surgery. In the healthy, well-sutured large bowel, bursting strength at the anastomosis is considered equal to, or greater than, control values by five to seven days postoperatively. To enhance colonic wound healing, the site of colostomy/anastomosis should be routinely wrapped in omentum prior to closure of the abdomen.

SURGICAL MANAGEMENT AND TECHNIQUES FOR LARGE INTESTINAL AND ANAL SURGERY

Coloplasty

Coloplasty is a technique for the reduction of the diameter of the affected bowel by the resection of a longitudinal elliptical section of the colon wall. It was first described in 1959,[11] but the procedure has not found long-term acceptance because further studies have indicated that the technique fails to resolve the clinical signs of megacolon.[12] Although the procedure may produce a narrower colonic segment, it has no effect on the smooth muscle function within the remaining colonic wall and thereby has no positive effect on colonic function.

Partial colectomy

Partial colectomy involves the removal of the segment of colon that demonstrates dilatation and atony at the time of surgical exploration. Colon that appears to be of normal shape and dimension is not resected, but is left in situ. The technique has been most commonly described in early veterinary literature relating to the management of megacolon.[12,13,15] Most authorities would now agree that differentiating diseased colon from normal colon is not possible at the time of surgery. In fact, it is likely that none of the colon remains unaffected in individuals with megacolon and it is, therefore, considered unwise to preserve a significant length of apparently unaffected colon at the time of colectomy.

Subtotal colectomy

The technique of subtotal colectomy (Box 30-7) involves the removal of the majority of the colon, whether it is grossly diseased or not. In essence, two techniques have been described and the main difference between the two is whether the resection procedure includes the removal of the ileocolic sphincter or not.

Preservation or resection of the ileocolic sphincter?

The ileocolic sphincter functions to allow small intestinal contents to enter the colon while preventing the reflux of colic contents into the ileum.[66] The removal of the sphincter is considered to allow the reflux of colonic microorganisms into the small intestine, with the subsequent development of small intestinal bacterial overgrowth and possible steatorrhea.[20,67,68] The rationale for preservation of the ileocolic junction is that it minimizes the development of postoperative diarrhea; the rationale for excision is that it minimizes recurrence of segmental megacolon and associated constipation.[10] Further studies have indicated that preservation of the ileocolic junction does not result in greater recurrences of constipation, but that excision of the ileocolic junction is associated with increased incidence and severity of diarrhea.[20,69] Such studies suggest that, if at all possible, the ileocolic junction containing the ileocolic sphincter should be preserved during colectomy. However, the issue of resection or preservation remains controversial.

The use of surgical staplers

Surgical stapling techniques have been described for performing the end-to-end colocolostomy following subtotal colectomy in the cat.[70-72] An end-to-end anastomosis stapling instrument is used to perform a colocolostomy following the resection of the diseased colon. In humans, when performing a colocolostomy, the access for the end-to-end stapling device would commonly be via the anus. In the cat, the anus is almost always too small to allow the passage of the end-to-end anastomosis stapler and the device is introduced via the dilatated and flaccid cecum instead. Safe introduction of a proprietary stapler (commonly with a working diameter of 21 mm) requires the cecum and proximal colon to be actively affected by the dilated megacolon condition. In many individuals with megacolon this is not the case, with the cecum and proximal colon still showing muscle tone with little or no evidence of flaccidity and/or dilatation. In such individuals, passage of a commercial available end-to-end stapler via the transcecal approach could be either unfeasible or very dangerous, carrying a high risk of cecal splitting. Advantages of stapled colocolostomies are reported to include formation of a mechanically stronger anastomosis, and a reduced surgical time with less potential for intraoperative contamination.[71]

Secondary hypertrophic megacolon associated with a malunion pelvic fracture

A malunion pelvic fracture in the cat will often result in the narrowing of the pelvic canal leading to the development of extraluminal obstruction to the distal descending colon. An outlet obstruction such as this will initially result in the development of hypertrophic megacolon. This form of megacolon is often reversible with the early removal of the outflow obstruction. Left untreated, the obstruction

---

Box 30-7 **Subtotal colectomy** (Fig. 30-8)

The cat is positioned in dorsal recumbency. The peritoneal cavity is approached via a routine ventral midline abdominal incision (see Chapter 23). This incision should extend from a point mid-way between the xiphoid process and umbilicus to the brim of the pubis. The enlarged colon, cecum and distal ileum are exteriorized and packed-off from the remaining peritoneal structures using moistened abdominal swabs.

Assuming that the ileocolic valve is to be preserved, the branches of the right colic, middle colic, and left colic arteries need to be identified, double ligated, and divided approximately 1–2 cm from the mesenteric side of the colon to be removed. Caudally, the blood supply to the distal colon requires ligation. Options include ligation of the left colic and caudal mesenteric arteries. Alternatively, only the vasa recta of the left colic and caudal mesenteric arteries may be

Box 30-7 **Continued**

ligated in an attempt to preserve as much blood supply as possible to the remaining distal segment of colon/rectum.

Colonic contents are milked manually into the segment of bowel to be removed. Atraumatic bowel clamps are applied to the bowel 2–3 cm proximal and distal to the proposed sites of proximal and distal resection, respectively. Further bowel clamps are applied to the proposed proximal and distal ends of the segment to be removed. The bowel is transected with the aid of a scalpel blade. Suitable samples of the excised bowel can be submitted for histopathology, if required. Everted mucosa at the ends of the bowel segments to be anastomosed should be trimmed using curved Metzenbaum scissors.

For healing of the bowel anastomosis to occur without complication and dehiscence, it is considered vital that minimal tension is applied to the site of anastomosis.[64] A trial apposition of the proximal and distal bowel segments should be performed to confirm the ability to perform the anastomosis in a tension-free manner. Should tension be an issue it may prove necessary to remove the ileocecocolic junction so that tension-free bowel continuity can be achieved by performing an ileocolic anastomosis.

Full thickness, simple interrupted appositional sutures of 3/0 or 4/0 monofilament absorbable material (for example, polydioxanone,

glycomer 631, or polyglyconate) are placed in the mesenteric and antimesenteric borders of the colocolostomy. These sutures are initially used as stay sutures. The intestine is then closed using either a simple interrupted or simple continuous suture pattern. The anastomosis may be achieved as a one- or a two-layer closure. There is no reported advantage to either of these techniques although single layer closure using a monofilament suture material is widely accepted as the preferred method.[19,20] There is no reported significant advantage between the use of a simple interrupted or a simple continuous suture pattern.[64]

When a luminal disparity exists between the two bowel segments to be anastomosed, one of two techniques is commonly used to achieve luminal parity; either the larger of the two lumens is sutured closed until its remaining lumen approximates the size of the lumen to which it is to be anastomosed,[65] or, the lumen of the smaller structure can be spatulated to achieve the luminal approximation.[20]

The finished anastomosis should be drape-wrapped with omentum prior to abdominal wall closure. It often proves impossible to close the rent in the mesentery following a subtotal colectomy in which the ileocolic valve has been preserved.

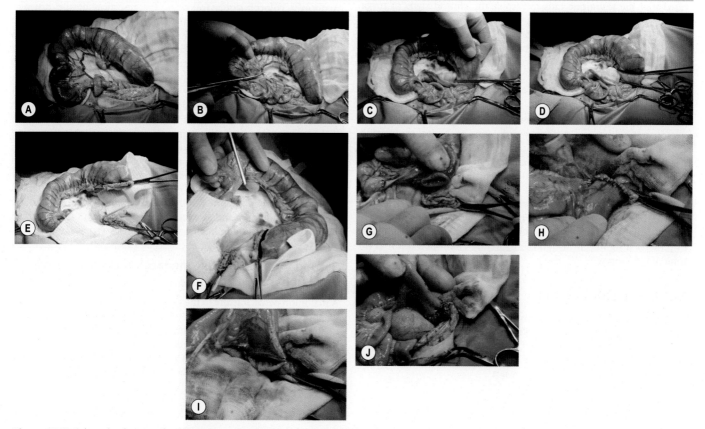

Figure 30-8 Subtotal colectomy for idiopathic megacolon in a five-year-old domestic short-haired cat. **(A)** The colon has been exteriorized and placed on a saline soaked laparotomy swab. **(B)** The local arterial supply to the colon is ligated and divided. In this case, the ileocecocolic junction is to be preserved. **(C)** A non-traumatic bowel clamp is placed near the colorectal junction. **(D)** An occlusion bowel clamp is placed proximal to the non-traumatic bowel clamp. Bowel contents have been 'milked' into the main body of the colon. **(E)** The colon is transected between the two bowel clamps using a scalpel blade. Note that the abdomen has been 'packed-off' using a number of sterile swabs to reduce the risk of contamination. **(F)** A non-traumatic bowel clamp is placed on the proximal colon near the ileocecocolic junction, which is to be preserved in this case. An occlusion clamp will then be placed distal to this allowing the affected part of the colon to be transected and excised. **(G)** The remaining two ends of colon are brought together to confirm that an end-to-end anastomosis can be performed without undue tension. The exposed mucosa may be trimmed using Metzenbaum scissors to ensure the formation of an adequate anastomosis. **(H)** One side of the anastomosis has been completed using a continuous suture pattern. Note the use of a single simple interrupted suture (mid closure) placed as a precaution in a portion of the closure that was considered inadequate. **(I)** The half-closed bowel has been turned revealing the remaining open side that is awaiting closure using a continuous suture pattern. **(J)** The appearance of the completed anastomosis. The site will be drape-omentalised prior to abdominal wall closure.

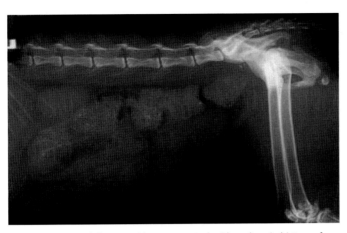

Figure 30-9 An eight-year-old cat presented with a chronic history of constipation and obstipation following conservative management of a pelvic fracture. The cat has a megacolon, and given the chronic history of problems, subtotal colectomy was deemed the most appropriate treatment for this cat.

will result in progression of the condition to an irreversible dilated megacolon (Fig. 30-9).

There remains some controversy with regards to the most appropriate treatment for cats with outlet obstruction associated with malunion pelvic fracture. Pelvic osteotomy without colectomy has been recommended for cats with pelvic fracture malunion and hypertrophic megacolon of less than six months, duration.[32,73,74] Although, in many instances, the early treatment of such cases with pelvic osteotomy will result in the relief of the clinical signs of constipation/obstipation, some authorities prefer to perform a colectomy because of the technical difficulty of performing an adequate osteotomy in many individuals.[30]

Surgical treatment is generally directed at widening the pelvic canal to relieve rectal impingement by removing the impinging bone (ostectomy), by redirecting the impinging bone (corrective osteotomy), or by separating and distracting the symphysis (symphyseal distraction osteotomy).[10,73–76]

Performing a subtotal colectomy (see Box 30-5) is recommended in cats with pelvic fractures if the colonic hypertrophy and clinical signs have persisted for longer than six months. Hypertrophy is superseded by neuromuscular degeneration and pathologic dilatation in these cases. Pelvic osteotomy alone will not provide relief from obstipation in such cases, whereas performing a colectomy without pelvic osteotomy will alleviate the clinical signs in the majority of affected individuals.[30]

Temporary colostomy for fecal diversion

Temporary colostomy (Box 30-8) is used to divert feces and facilitate rectal wall healing. This procedure results in an incontinent end-on colostomy requiring the use of an Elizabethan collar to prevent self-traumatization of the surgical site and owner compliance and commitment to minimize the formation of soiling and peristomal dermatitis.

Colopexy

Colopexy (Box 30-9) involves suturing the descending colon to the left ventrolateral abdominal wall in order to prevent recurrence of rectal prolapse.

Reconstruction of congenital rectovaginal and anal conditions

Rectovaginal fistulae

Two surgical techniques are described for the treatment of rectovaginal fistula and atresia ani: in one the fistula is isolated (via a horizontal incision between the anus and rectum), transected, and the rectum and vaginal defects are closed separately, followed by reconstruction of the anus (Fig. 30-11); in the other, the rectum is transected cranial to the fistulous opening, the affected segment is removed, and the terminal part of the rectum is sutured to the anus.[77–79]

Among the reported complications following surgery, fecal incontinence is one of the most important; it may be associated with lack of function, possible absence of the external anal sphincter, or nerve damage during the surgical procedure.[80] Other possible complications include obstipation and tenesmus, constipation, anal gland odor, edema of the anal area, rectal prolapse, urinary incontinence, anal stenosis, and wound dehiscence.[80]

Anogenital clefts

Surgical management of anogenital clefts in the female involves opening and/or reforming the anus, closure of the rectal fistula (see Fig. 30-11) if it is part of the condition, and reformation of the perineum (episioplasty) between the anus and vulva (Fig. 30-12).

Surgical management of the condition in the male involves the creation of a perineal urethrostomy (see Chapter 38) and reconstruction of the perineal skin.

Box 30-9 **Colopexy**

The cat is positioned in dorsal recumbency. A ventral midline celiotomy is performed. The descending colon is located, pulled cranially, and positioned adjacent to the left ventrolateral abdominal wall.

The colon may be anchored to the abdominal wall using either an incisional or a non-incisional technique. Regardless of the technique used, the colopexy should be formed on the left ventrolateral abdominal wall approximately 2–3 cm lateral to the linea alba.

Incisional technique: two adjacent seromuscular incisions are made, one in the antimesenteric colon and one in the adjacent abdominal wall. Each edge of the seromuscular layer of the colon is sutured to the corresponding edge of the incision in the abdominal wall (Fig. 30-10).

Non-incisional technique: a single row of five or six interrupted mattress sutures is placed between the antimesenteric colon and abdominal wall, making sure the colonic submucosa is incorporated in each suture.

With both techniques, care should be taken to avoid penetration of the colonic lumen. The site of colopexy may be 'drape' omentalized prior to closure of the linea alba. Suitable suture for the colopexy includes a non-absorbable monofilament material such as polypropylene, or an absorbable monofilament such as polydioxanone or polytrimethylene carbonate.

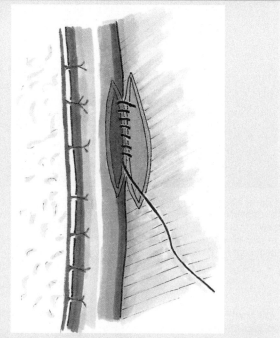

Figure 30-10 Diagram showing the formation of an incisional colopexy.

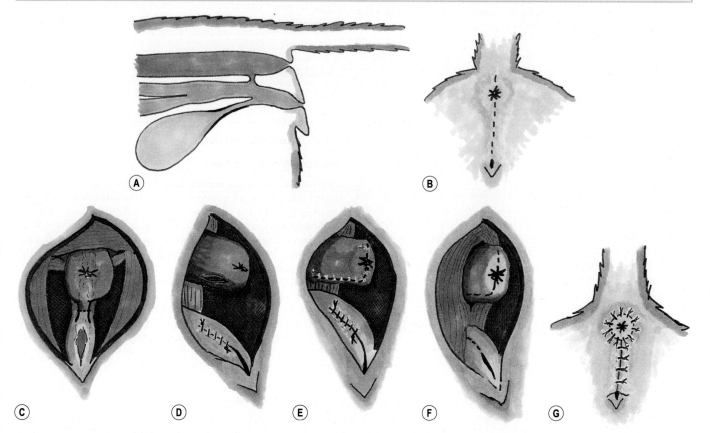

Figure 30-11 Diagrams illustrating the repair of rectovaginal fistula. **(A)** Fistula is shown between the rectum and vagina. **(B)** Site of incision on midline of perineum. **(C)** Incision is extended through dorsal wall of vagina and ventral wall of rectum to expose the fistula. This involves incising the ventral aspect of the anal sphincter. If a fistula is present, it is excised. If not, the incisions in the vagina and rectum are extended to expose the vaginorectal communication. **(D)** The rectum and vagina are separated and fibrous tissue is excised from the fistula's opening in both structures. The dorsal wall of the vagina and vulva is closed with continuous inverting or appositional sutures. **(E)** The rectal incision is closed in a similar manner. **(F)** Incised muscle of the anal sphincter is sutured and sutures are inserted around the anocutaneous junction. **(G)** The skin incision from vulva to anus is closed with simple interrupted sutures.

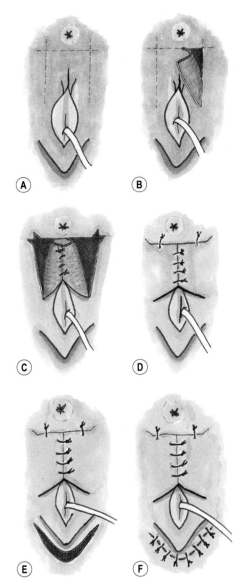

Figure 30-12 Repair of anovulval cleft. **(A)** An H-shaped incision is made between the anus and vulva. **(B)** Median and ventral edges of the incision are undermined. **(C)** Mucosal margins are apposed over the dorsal vagina using an absorbable suture. Lateral cutaneous edges of the wound are undermined. **(D)** Cutaneous edges are apposed with skin sutures. **(E,F)** Ventral episioplasty may be required to relieve tension on the wound.

Atresia ani

Cats with atresia ani (see Table 30-2) will usually need surgical treatment if they are to have any chance of survival, although as discussed (see above) mortality and morbidity is high and repeat surgery is often necessary. The surgical repair of imperforate anus and rectal agenesis is shown in Fig. 30-13.

Type I

The skin is incised over the anus with a cruciate incision. The resultant triangular flaps of skin are excised. The external anal sphincter is identified and bluntly dissected free from the rectal pouch. The rectal pouch is mobilized and incised with a cruciate pattern over the imperforate rectum. The resultant triangular flaps of rectum are excised and the rectum is sutured to the subcutaneous tissue and skin with a one-layer simple interrupted suture pattern using 4/0 or 5/0 monofilament suture material.

Type II

The skin is incised over the anus with a cruciate incision. The external anal sphincter should be identified and the underlying rectal pouch should be located adjacent to the anal sphincter. The rectum should be freed locally using blunt dissection so that it can be mobilized towards the skin (through the anal ring). The blind pouch is then incised and rectocutaneous apposition accomplished in a similar fashion to that described for the type I anomaly.

Type III

The skin is incised over the anus with a cruciate incision. The external anal sphincter should be identified. Blunt dissection is required to locate the caudal aspect of the distended rectal pouch. As with type II, the rectum should be freed locally using blunt dissection so that it can be mobilized towards the anal skin (through the anal ring). The blind pouch is then incised and rectocutaneous apposition accomplished in a similar fashion to that described for the type I anomaly.

Type IV

The normal anal opening is probed to assess the depth of the caudal blind pouch. The pouch is opened allowing the cranial segment of the rectum to be located, locally dissected and mobilized through and out of the caudal segment. Both portions of rectum are exteriorized (rectal pull out) allowing anastomosis using a one-layer simple interrupted suture pattern of 4/0 or 5/0 monofilament suture material.

Anal sacculectomy

Removal of anal sacs (Box 30-10) in cats may be indicated for chronic anal sacculitis that does not resolve after medical or dietary management, anal abscessation, or anal neoplasia.

POSTOPERATIVE CARE AFTER LARGE INTESTINAL AND ANAL SURGERY

Colonic surgery

Colonic surgery (colostomy, colectomy) will most commonly be performed via a ventral midline celiotomy. Postoperative analgesic requirements will be aimed at managing the discomfort associated with the celiotomy rather than the colonic surgery per se. As such, the administration of some form of systemic opioid will generally suffice. There is controversy regarding the use of non-steroidal anti-inflammatory drugs (NSAIDs) in small animals following colonic surgery; there is some evidence that these drugs might compromise the integrity and barrier function of the colonic mucosa in the postoperative period. In the clinical setting, the use of NSAIDs for analgesia in the postoperative period does not appear to be associated with significant compromise to healing of the surgical site.

Perioperative administration of antibiotics: An extended postoperative course (five to seven days) of oral broad-spectrum antibiotics will be a requirement in the majority of cases (see above).

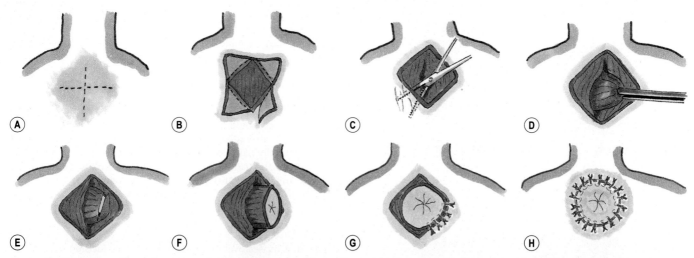

Figure 30-13 Diagrams illustrating surgery for imperforate anus. **(A)** Cruciate incision is made over the anal dimple. **(B)** The triangles of skin are excised and the ventral fibers of the external anal sphincter are severed. **(C)** The external sphincter is dissected free of its ventral attachments. **(D)** Dissection with forceps or blunt scissors will expose the blind end of the rectum, which can then be grasped and pulled caudally. **(E)** The blind end of the rectal pouch is excised. **(F)** The previously severed sections of the anal sphincter muscle are reunited at the ventral aspects of the rectal pouch. **(G)** The severed end of the rectum is sutured to the skin surrounding the orifice. **(H)** The completed procedure.

Box 30-10 Anal sacculectomy

Several techniques have been described for the removal of anal sacs. The techniques broadly can be classified as either 'open' or 'closed.

The 'open' technique

Once the cat has been anesthetized, both anal sacs are emptied and flushed with a dilute solution of chlorhexidine. The perianal fur (including ventral tail base) is clipped. A gauze swab may be placed in the rectum to reduce the incidence of fecal contamination during the procedure.

The cat is placed in sternal recumbency and the tail is held upright and forwards with ties or tapes. The orifice of the anal sac duct in cats opens on a pyramidal prominence approximately 0.25 cm lateral to the anus and not at the mucocutaneous junction as is seen in the dog. The anal sacs are located between the fibers of the external and internal anal sphincter at the 4 o'clock and 8 o'clock positions. A director (e.g. blunt-ended 1–2 mm diameter K-wire; Fig. 30-14A) is passed through the anal sac duct and positioned at the most lateroventral position within the sac. The tip of the director can then be angled towards the skin and an incision made directly over it using a scalpel blade. The incision should be started at the anal sac duct orifice and extended towards the lateroventral aspect of the sac using the director as a guide (Fig 30-14B). Once the anal sac has been opened its gray mucosal lining will be easily recognized (Fig. 30-14C). This may be grasped using Mosquito forceps. Gentle traction and the judicial use of blunt dissection using fine Metzenbaum scissors will allow the detachment of the sac from its surrounding tissues. Care should be taken to stay as close to the anal sac as possible, thereby minimizing trauma to the anal sphincter musculature. Once the sac has been freed it can be retracted, allowing the blunt dissection and complete removal of the associated anal sac duct. The external anal sphincter and subcutaneous tissues are apposed using an absorbable monofilament suture material placed in a simple interrupted or simple continuous suture pattern. The skin may be closed using subcuticular closure or skin sutures. The process is then repeated on the opposite side, if required.

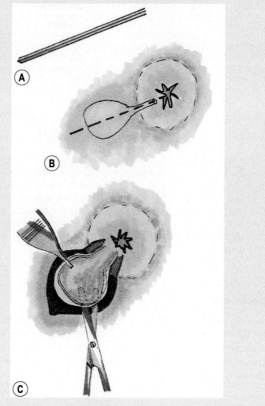

Figure 30-14 The open technique for anal sacculectomy. **(A)** Director. **(B)** The incisions are made over the director once placed in the anal gland. **(C)** The gland is cut open and the gray inner lining can be seen. This is dissected away from the surrounding tissue.

Box 30-10 **Continued**

The 'closed' technique

Once the cat has been anesthetized, both anal sacs are emptied and are subsequently filled with a proprietary bulking agent or wax. The perianal fur (including ventral tail base) is clipped. A gauze swab may be placed in the rectum to reduce the incidence of fecal contamination during the procedure.

The cat is placed in sternal recumbency and the tail is held upright and forwards with ties or tapes. The filled anal sac can be readily palpated and a curved incision is made directly over it (Fig. 30-15A) at the 4 o'clock position on the left side and 8 o'clock position on the right side). A combination of both sharp and blunt dissection can be used to locate the anal sac, which may then be grasped carefully with Mosquito forceps. Gentle traction and the judicial use of blunt dissection using fine Metzenbaum scissors will allow the detachment of the sac from its surrounding tissues (Fig. 30-15B). Care should be taken to stay as close to the anal sac as possible, thereby minimizing trauma to the anal sphincter musculature. Once the sac has been mobilized it can be retracted, allowing its associated duct to be freed from surrounding muscle fibers. The duct may then be ligated using a transfixion suture of an absorbable monofilament suture material. The external anal sphincter and subcutaneous tissues are apposed using an absorbable monofilament suture material placed in a simple interrupted or simple continuous suture pattern. The skin may be closed using subcuticular closure or skin sutures. The process is then repeated on the opposite side, if required.

The excised sac and duct may be submitted for histopathology, if considered appropriate.

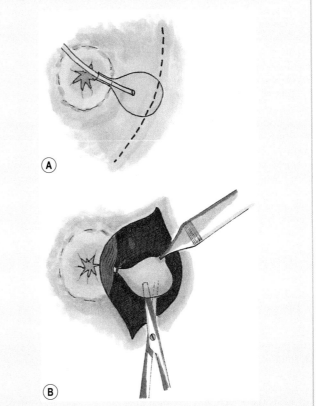

Figure 30-15 The closed technique for anal sacculectomy. **(A)** A tube is inserted into the anal duct and the gland filled and a curved incision made over the filled gland. **(B)** The intact gland is then dissected out trying to preserve the anal sphincter. The duct is ligated as close to the anus as possible.

In general, the patient can be fed their normal diet in the postoperative period. Straining associated with either diarrhea or constipation should be avoided if at all possible. Constipation may be treated by the judicial administration of an oral laxative.

An Elizabethan collar may be required to stop the patient self-traumatizing the abdominal skin wound.

The development of a raised rectal temperature, unexpected abdominal discomfort/guarding, abdominal distension, lethargy, anorexia, etc. should not be ignored as these signs might indicate the development of septic peritonitis (see Chapter 26). The development of any of these signs should prompt further investigations (abdominal radiography, abdominal ultrasonography, peritoneal paracentesis, etc.) to rule out the presence of peritonitis.

Rectal surgery

Rectal surgery at the level of the rectoanal junction is invariably associated with significant discomfort, especially during the process of defecation. Such a patient will often exhibit fecal tenesmus and dyschezia. In some instances, the discomfort will be sufficient to prevent defecation, leading to progressive constipation. This should be avoided since constipation will itself lead to straining and possible damage/dehiscence of the site of surgery. In the immediate postoperative period, such discomfort may be controlled with analgesics (for example, epidural analgesia, systemic opioids, systemic NSAIDs, local

suppository anti-inflammatory/analgesic drugs). In the longer term, the complication may be managed with the administration of an NSAID and the administration of an oral laxative to maintain a soft but formed fecal consistency.

The patient will commonly show fecal incontinence following rectoanal surgery. As a result, soiling of the perianal region is a common issue and should be managed be maintaining good hygiene of the area. This may best be achieved with gentle washing/showering rather than wiping. An Elizabethan collar should be used to prevent the patient excessively cleaning/grooming the perianal region. Local skin excoriation should be treated promptly with the application of some form of barrier cream/spray. In most instances, the postoperative fecal incontinence will be self-limiting but it is not uncommon for the issue to persist for a number of weeks following the surgery, necessitating a prolonged period of hospitalization.

An extended postoperative course (five to seven days) of oral broad-spectrum antibiotic (see above) will be a requirement in the majority of cases.

The development of a raised rectal temperature, unexpected abdominal discomfort/guarding, abdominal distension, lethargy, anorexia, etc. should not be ignored as these signs might indicate the development of septic peritonitis. The development of any of these signs should prompt further investigations (abdominal radiography, abdominal ultrasonography, peritoneal paracentesis, etc.) to rule out the presence of peritonitis.

Postoperative care after anal surgery

An Elizabethan collar should be placed prior to the patient's recovery from general anesthesia. In general, to stop the cat self-traumatizing the wounds, the collar should be left in place until the skin sutures are removed (approximately seven to ten days postoperatively). In many instances it will prove prudent to administer a five to seven day postoperative course of an oral broad-spectrum antibiotic such as clavulanate amoxicillin. A normal diet may be fed.

The owner should be warned that any form of anal surgery might lead to local swelling and/or temporary bruising of the sensory nerves at the anal mucocutaneous junction. This, in turn, may produce a degree of desensitization and short-term fecal incontinence. In general, no specific intervention is required for this self-limiting complication.

Surgery of the anus will often result in a degree of fecal tenesmus and dyschezia in the immediate postoperative period. Again, in most instances this complication will be self-limiting and may be controlled with the judicious use of an oral laxative and the oral administration of a NSAID.

COMPLICATIONS AFTER LARGE INTESTINAL SURGERY

The complications that can occur after large intestinal and anal surgery include wound dehiscence with peritoneal contamination and peritonitis and short bowel syndrome. Any intraoperative spillage of colonic contents is likely to result in bacterial contamination, with a localized or generalized peritonitis. Other than good surgical technique, the likely development of peritonitis may be reduced by not performing any form of preoperative bowel preparation and by the administration of perioperative broad-spectrum antibiotics (see above). The most common postoperative complication observed in cats following subtotal colectomy is the development of diarrhea or loose stools in the immediate period following the surgery. Other reported complications of subtotal colectomy include lethargy, depression, anorexia, weight loss, vomiting, diarrhea or the production of soft, unformed stools, increased defecatory frequency, tenesmus, hematochezia, and fecal incontinence.[21]

Short bowel syndrome

Removal of the majority of the colon will have obvious metabolic effects on the animal. In the normal individual, the role of the colon is to absorb water along an osmotic gradient created by the active absorption of sodium. Bicarbonate ions are secreted in exchange for chloride ions, and potassium is lost from the extracellular fluid and in mucus and cells shed from the colon. The distal colon stores the dehydrated fecal material.[22] All these functions will be affected to a greater or lesser degree following the subtotal colectomy procedure.

The enteric function of four cats that had undergone subtotal colectomy for idiopathic megacolon was compared to that of four normal cats.[17] It was concluded that, in general, enteric function in the operated cats was similar to that of the control cats. Bowel movements occurred slightly more frequently, with no significant differences in fecal volume or water content. In the operated cats, serum cobalamin concentrations and fecal water sodium concentrations were higher and fecal potassium concentrations were lower in comparison with unoperated cats. The results of the study demonstrated no significant clinical or subclinical evidence of abnormal bowel function in cats after subtotal colectomy. In the majority of individuals, stool consistency improves without further treatment so that within one to six weeks of the surgery a soft, formed stool is developed.

Dehiscence of the intestinal anastomosis

Incisional dehiscence at the site of bowel anastomosis is a rare but potentially life-threatening complication after colonic surgery.[64] The occurrence of dehiscence is most commonly associated with poor surgical technique, such as inaccurate suture placement or tension across the anastomosis.

Common signs of the development of dehiscence in the postoperative period include pyrexia, anorexia, decreased frequency or a failure to pass feces (associated with the development of ileus), and discomfort on palpation of the caudal abdomen. Plain radiography and/or abdominal ultrasound may be used to identify localized steatitis, free abdominal fluid, and ileus. Diagnostic peritoneal lavage may be used to confirm the presence of fecal material and free bacteria within the peritoneal cavity.

The frequency of leakage at the anastomosis site is considered similar when intestinal stapling techniques are compared to conventional suturing techniques.[71]

REFERENCES

1. Sturgess CP, Canfield PJ, Gruffydd-Jones TJ, Stokes CR. A gross and microscopical morphometric evaluation of feline large intestinal anatomy. J Comp Pathol 2001;124:255–64.

2. Foley P. Constipation, tenesmus, dyschezia, and fecal incontinence. In: Ettinger SJ, Feldman EC, editors. Textbook of veterinary internal medicine. 7th ed. St. Louis: Saunders Elsevier; 2010. p. 206–9.

3. Gaschen L. The large intestine and perianal region. In: R O'Brien, F Barr, editors. BSAVA manual of canine and feline abdominal imaging. Quedgeley: British Small Animal Veterinary Association; 2009. p. 132–43.

4. O'Brien TR. Large intestine. In: Radiographic diagnosis of abdominal disorders in the dog and cat. Philadelphia: WB Saunders Company; 1978. p. 352–95.

5. Gaschen L, Rodriguez D. Stomach, small and large intestines. In: Barr F, Gaschen L, editors. BSAVA manual of canine and feline ultrasonography. Quedgeley: British Small Animal Veterinary Association; 2011. p. 124–38.

6. Simpson JW. Gastrointestinal endoscopy. In: Hall EJ, Simpson JW, Williams DA, editors. BSAVA manual of canine and feline gastroenterology. Quedgeley: British Small Animal Veterinary Association; 2005. p. 34–49.

7. Rosin E. Megacolon in cats. The role of colectomy. Vet Clin North Am Small Anim Pract 1993;23:587–94.

8. Rosin E, Walshaw R, Mehlhaff C, et al. Subtotal colectomy for treatment of chronic constipation associated with idiopathic megacolon in cats: 38 cases (1979–1985). J Am Vet Med Assoc 1988;193:850–3.

9. Roe KA, Syme HM, Brooks HW. Congenital large intestinal hypoganglionosis in a domestic shorthair kitten. J Fel Med Surg 2010;12(5):418–20.

10. Washabau RJ, Hasler AH. Constipation, obstipation, and megacolon. In: August JR, editor. Consultations in feline internal

medicine. 3rd ed. Philadelphia: WB Saunders Company; 1997. p. 104–12.

11. Bruce RH. Operation for megacolon in cats. Mod Vet Pract 1959;40:66.

12. Leighton RL, Grain E. Partial colectomy for the treatment of feline megacolon. Fel Pract 1978;3:31–3.

13. Yoder JT, Dragstedt LR 2nd, Starch CJ. Partial colectomy for correction of megacolon in a cat. Vet Med Small Anim Clin 1968;63:1049–52.

14. Fellenbaum S. Partial colectomy in the treatment of recurrent obstipation/ megacolon in the cat. Vet Med Small Anim Clin 1978;73:737–42.

15. Webb SM. Surgical management of acquired megacolon in the cat. J Small Anim Pract 1985;26:399–405.

16. Bright RM, Burrows CF, Goring R, et al. Subtotal colectomy for treatment of acquired megacolon in the dog and cat. J Am Vet Med Assoc 1986;188:1412–16.

17. Gregory CR, Guilford WG, Berry CR, et al. Enteric function in cats after subtotal colectomy for treatment of megacolon. Vet Surg 1990;19:216–20.

18. Matthiesen DT, Scavelli TD, Whitney WO. Subtotal colectomy for the treatment of obstipation secondary to pelvic fracture malunion in cats. Vet Surg 1991;20: 113–17.

19. deHaan JJ, Ellison GW, Bellah JR. Surgical correction of idiopathic megacolon in cats. Feline Pract 1992;20:6–11.

20. Sweet DC, Hardie EM, Stone EA. Preservation versus excision of the ileocolic junction during colectomy for megacolon: a study of 22 cats. J Small Anim Pract 1994;35:358–63.

21. White RN. Surgical management of constipation. J Feline Med Surg 2002;4:129–38.

22. Bertoy RW. Megacolon. In: Bojrab MJ, editor. Disease mechanisms in small animal surgery. 2nd ed. Philadelphia: Lea & Febiger; 1993. p. 262–5.

23. Furneaux RW, Boysen BG, Mero KN. Complications of ovariohysterectomies. Can Vet J 1973;14:98–9.

24. Muir P, Goldsmid SE, Bellenger CR. Megacolon in a cat following ovariohysterectomy. Vet Rec 1991;129: 512–13.

25. Smith MC, Davies NL. Obstipation following ovariohysterectomy in a cat. Vet Rec 1996;138:163.

26. Coolman BR, Marretta SM, Dudley MB, Averill SM. Partial colonic obstruction following ovariohysterectomy: a report of three cases. J Am Anim Hosp Assoc 1999;35;169–72.

27. Demetriou JL, Welsh EM. Colonic obstruction in an adult cat following open castration. Vet Rec 2000;147;165–6.

28. Welches CD, Scavelli TD, Aronsohn MG, Matthiesen DT. Perineal hernia in the cat: a retrospective study of 40 cases. J Am Anim Hosp Assoc 1992;28:431–8.

29. van den Broek AHM, Else RW, Hunter MS. Atresia ani and urethrorectal fistula in a kitten. J Small Anim Pract 1988;29: 91–4.

30. Matthiesen DT, Marretta SM. Diseases of the anus and rectum. In: Slatter D, editor. Textbook of small animal surgery. 2nd ed. Philadelphia: WB Saunders Company; 1993. p. 627–45.

31. Bredal WP, Thoresen SI, Kvellestad A. Atresia coli in a nine-week-old kitten. J Small Anim Pract 1994;35:643–5.

32. Washabau RJ, Holt D. Pathogenesis, diagnosis, and therapy of feline idiopathic megacolon. Vet Clin North Am Small Anim Pract 1999;29:589–603.

33. North S, Banks T. Tumours of the gastrointestinal tract and associated structures. In: Small animal oncology: an introduction. Edinburgh: Saunders Elsevier; 2009. p. 129–43.

34. Slawienski MJ, Mauldin GE, Mauldin GN, Patnaik AK. Malignant colonic neoplasia in cats: 46 cases (1990–1996). J Am Vet Med Assoc 1997;211:878–81.

35. Bedford PN. Partial intestinal obstruction due to colonic adenocarcinoma in a cat. Can Vet J 1998;39(12):769–71.

36. Laurenson MP, Skorupski KA, Moore PF, Zwingenberger AL. Ultrasonography of intestinal mast cell tumors in the cat. Vet Radiol Ultrasound 2011;52: 330–4.

37. Carpenter JL, Andrews LK, Holzworth J. Tumors and tumor-like lesions. In: Holzworth J, editor. Diseases of the cat; medicine and surgery. Philadelphia: WB Saunders; 1987. p. 494–500.

38. Yoon HY, Mann FA. Bilateral pubic and ischial osteotomy for surgical management of caudal colonic and rectal masses in six dogs and a cat. J Am Vet Med Assoc 2008;232:1016–20.

39. Selting KA. Intestinal tumors. In: Withrow SJ, Vail DM, editors. Small animal clinical oncology. 4th ed. St Louis: Saunders Elsevier; 2007. p. 491–503.

40. Hume DZ, Solomon JA, Weisse CW. Palliative use of a stent for colonic obstruction caused by adenocarcinoma in two cats. J Am Vet Med Assoc 2006;228(3):392–6.

41. vanderGaag I, Tibboel D. Intestinal atresia and stenosis in animals: a report of 34 cases. Vet Path 1980;17:565–74.

42. Johnson R. Intestinal atresia and stenosis: a review comparing its etiopathogenesis. Veterinary Research Communications 1986;10:95–104.

43. Waknitz DW, Greer DH. Urethrorectal fistula in a cat. Vet Med Small Anim Clin 1983;78:1551–3.

44. Holt P. Anal and perianal surgery in dogs and cats. In Pract 1985;7:83–9.

45. Suess RP, Martin RA, Moon ML, Dallman MJ. Rectovaginal fistula with atresia in three kittens. Cornell Vet 1992;82: 141–53.

46. Fransson BA. Rectocutaneous fistulas. Compend Contin Educ Vet 2008;30(4): 224–7.

47. Tsioli V, Papazoglou LG, Anagnostou T, et al. Use of a temporary incontinent end-on colostomy in a cat for the management of rectocutaneous fistulas associated with atresia ani. J Feline Med Surg 2009;11:1011–14.

48. Gross RE, Holcomb GW Jr, Farber S. Duplications of the alimentary tract. Pediatrics 1952;9:449–68.

49. Kramer A, Kyles AE, Labelle P. Surgical correction of colonic duplication in a cat. J Am Anim Hosp Assoc 2007;43(2): 128–31.

50. Kook PH, Hagen R, Willi B, et al. Rectal duplication cyst in a cat. J Feline Med Surg 2010;12:978–81.

51. Bhandal J, Kuzma A, Head L. Cecal inversion followed by ileocolic intussusception in a cat. Can Vet J 2008;49:483–4.

52. Pratschke K. Surgical diseases of the colon and rectum in small animals. In Pract 2005;27:354–62.

53. Popovitch CA, Holt D, Bright R. Colopexy as a treatment for rectal prolapse in dogs and cats: a retrospective study of 14 cases. Vet Surg 1994;23:115–18.

54. Corgozinho KB, Belchior C, Moreira de Souza HJ, et al. Silicone elastomer sling for rectal prolapse in cats. Can Vet J 2010;51:506–10.

55. Secchi P, Filho HC, Scussel Feranti JP, et al. Laparoscopic-assisted incisional colopexy by two portals access in a domestic cat with recurrent rectal prolapse. J Feline Med Surg 2012;14(2): 169–70.

56. Bright RM, Bauer MS. Surgery of the digestive system. In: Sherding RG, editor. The cat: diseases and clinical management. 2nd ed. Philadelphia: WB Saunders Company; 1994. p. 1353–401.

57. Shoieb AM, Hanshaw DM. Anal sac gland carcinoma in 64 cats in the United Kingdom (1995–2007). Vet Path 2009;46: 677–83.

58. Cavanaugh R, Bacon NJ, Schallberger S, et al. Biologic behavior and clinical outcome of cats with anal sac adenocarcinoma: a veterinary society of surgical oncology retrospective study of 23 cats. Proceedings of the 28th Annual Conference of the Veterinary Cancer Society, Seattle, Washington, 2008. p. 63.

59. Fa-Si-Oen P, Roumen R, Buitenweg J, et al. Mechanical bowel preparation or not? Outcome of a multicenter, randomized trial in elective open colon surgery. Dis Colon Rectum 2005;48:1509–16.

60. Nicholson GA, Finlay IG, Diament RH, et al. Mechanical bowel preparation does not influence outcomes following colonic cancer resection. Br J Surg 2011;98: 866–71.

61. Holt DE, Brockman D. Large intestine. In: Slatter D, editor. Textbook of small animal surgery. 3rd ed. Philadelphia: Saunders; 1993. p. 665–82.

62. Bundy CA, Jacobs DM, Zera RT, Bubrick MP. Comparison of bursting pressure of sutured, stapled and BAR anastomoses. Int J Colorectal Dis 1993;8:1–3.

63. Schwab R, Wessendorf S, Gutcke A, Becker P. Early bursting strength of human colon anastomosis – an in vitro study comparing current anastomotic techniques. Langenbecks Arch Surg 2002;386:507–11.

64. Pavletic MM, Berg J. Gastrointestinal surgery. In: Lipowitz AJ, Caywood DD, Newton CD, Schwartz A, editors. Complications in small animal surgery. Baltimore: Williams & Wilkins; 1996. p. 365–98.

65. Bright RM. Subtotal colectomy in the cat. In: Bojrab MJ, editor. Current techniques in small animal surgery. 4th ed. Baltimore: Williams & Wilkins; 1990. p. 272–6.

66. Strombeck DR. Small and large intestine: normal structure and function. In: Guildford WG, Center SA, Strombeck DR, et al, editors. Strombeck's small animal gastroenterology. 3rd ed. Philadelphia: WB Saunders Company; 1986. p. 318–50.

67. Bright RM. A clinical, radiographic, histological and microbiological evaluation of subtotal colectomies in cats. Vet Surg 1986;15:115.

68. Holt DE, Johnston DE. Idiopathic megacolon in cats. Compendium on Continuing Education for the Practicing Veterinarian 1991;13:1411–16.

69. Bright RM. Idiopathic megacolon in the cat: subtotal colectomy with preservation of the ileocolic valve. Vet Med Rep 1991;3:183–7.

70. Kudisch M, Pavletic MM. Subtotal colectomy with surgical stapling instruments via a trans-cecal approach for treatment of acquired megacolon in cats. Vet Surg 1993;22:457–63.

71. Kudisch M. Surgical stapling of the large intestine. Vet Clin North Am Small Anim Pract 1994;24:323–33.

72. Banz WJ, Jackson DJ, Richter K, Launer DP. Transrectal stapling for colonic resection and anastomosis (10 cases). J Am Anim Hosp Assoc 2008;44:198–204.

73. Schrader SC. Pelvic osteotomy as a treatment for obstipation in cats with acquired stenosis of the pelvic canal: six cases (1978–1989). J Am Vet Med Assoc 1992;200:208–13.

74. McKee WM, Wong WT. Symphyseal distraction-osteotomy using an ulnar autograft for the treatment of pelvic canal stenosis in three cats. Vet Rec 1994;134:132–5.

75. Ferguson JF. Triple pelvic osteotomy for the treatment of pelvic canal stenosis in the cat. J Small Anim Pract 1997;37:495–8.

76. Prassinos NN, Adamama-Moraitou KK, Gouletsou PG, Rallis TS. Symphyseal distraction-osteotomy using a novel spacer of spirally fashioned orthopaedic wire for the management of obstipation. J Feline Med Surg 2007;9:23–8.

77. Aronson L. Rectum and anus. In: Slatter DH, editor. Textbook of small animal surgery. 3rd ed. Philadelphia: WB Saunders Company; 2003. p. 682–708.

78. Prassinos NN, Papazoglou LG, Adamama-Moraitou KK, et al. Congenital anorectal abnormalities in six dogs. Vet Rec 2003;153:81–5.

79. Wykes PM, Olson PN. Vagina, vestibule, and vulva. In: Slatter DH, editor. Textbook of small animal surgery. 3rd ed. Philadelphia: WB Saunders Company; 2003. p. 1502–10.

80. Rahal SC, Vicente CS, Mortari AC, et al. Rectovaginal fistula with anal atresia in 5 dogs. Can Vet J 2007;48:827–30.

Chapter **31**

Liver and biliary tract

J.K. McClaran, N.J. Buote

While hepatobiliary disease is quite common in feline patients, diseases requiring surgery are relatively limited. Metabolic functions of the liver include production and excretion of bile, detoxification of numerous substances, as well as synthesis of plasma proteins.[1] Diagnostic biopsy is most commonly performed as an isolated procedure or in conjunction with an abdominal exploration. Liver lobectomy (partial or complete) and diseases requiring biliary decompression, diversion, or cholecystectomy will be detailed. Anesthetic considerations and common complications following hepatic and biliary surgical procedures will be discussed.

SURGICAL ANATOMY

The feline liver consists of six lobes (Fig. 31-1). The liver may be further described by its visceral and parietal surfaces. The parietal surface is convex and abuts the diaphragm (Fig. 31-2) and the visceral surface is slightly concave and contacts the stomach, duodenum, and

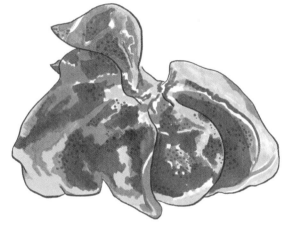

Figure 31-2 Parietal surface of the liver.

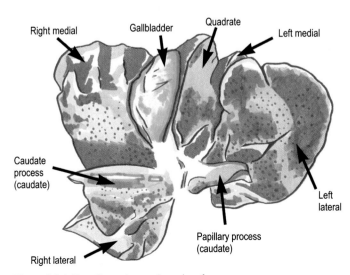

Figure 31-1 Hepatic anatomy, visceral surface.

Right medial — Gallbladder — Quadrate — Left medial — Caudate process (caudate) — Papillary process (caudate) — Right lateral — Left lateral

right kidney (Fig. 31-1). The gallbladder sits in the fossa between the right medial and quadrate lobes of the liver. The feline liver extends from the diaphragm into the xiphoid region between the left and right costal arches.[2] The afferent blood supply of the liver consists of the high pressure arterial system as well as the low pressure portal system. The portal system supplies 80% of the blood to the liver while the remaining 20% of the blood is supplied by branches of the proper hepatic arteries.[3] Efferent hepatic drainage is via the hepatic veins. Supporting ligaments of the liver include the right and left triangular ligaments (attaching to the muscular portion of the diaphragm), the right and left coronary ligaments (attaching to the central tendinous portion of the diaphragm), and the falciform ligament.[4] Nervous supply to the liver is from afferent and efferent fibers of the vagus nerve and by sympathetic fibers of the celiac plexus.[5]

BILIARY ANATOMY AND FLOW

The biliary system consists of a gallbladder, cystic duct, common bile duct (CBD), hepatic ducts, segmental, septal, and interlobular bile

DOI: 10.1016/B978-0-7020-4336-9.00031-7

ducts, bile ductules, and hepatic canaliculi.[6] The gallbladder is made up of the larger fundus toward the apex and the infundibulum, or neck, which empties into the cystic duct.[7] The gallbladder has four main functions: reservoir, absorptive, secretory and motor. Congenital biliary anomalies are seen commonly in cats (12.3%) and include partially divided gallbladders (bilobed, trilobed, or quadrupally divided gallbladder), double gallbladder, and a singular gallbladder with two or more ductular bladders.[8] Most of these cases are found incidentally at necropsy.

The cystic duct extends from the neck of the gallbladder to the junction with the first hepatic duct and continues distally as the CBD. The CBD continues to the duodenum, receiving more hepatic ducts along the way. In the dog, the CBD opens near the smaller of the two pancreatic ducts (the pancreatic duct). The larger duct is the accessory duct, which opens into the duodenum a few centimeters aboral on the minor duodenal papilla. In the cat, the CBD and the major pancreatic duct (which is the larger duct in this species) are usually fused prior to the entrance at the major duodenal papilla.[1] The major duodenal papilla is approximately 3–6 cm aboral from the pylorus or 2 cm aboral from the junction of the CBD and the duodenal serosa. Some cats have varied anatomy, with the major pancreatic duct opening separately but immediately adjacent to the CBD. Approximately 2 cm caudal to the major duodenal papilla, the accessory pancreatic duct enters the duodenum at the minor duodenal papilla. This duct is sometimes absent in the cat. Pancreatic and biliary disease are commonly seen together in the cat because of this highly integrated anatomy.[6,9]

The circulation to the gallbladder and CBD is derived from the left branch of the proper hepatic artery.[5] This circulation must be preserved during surgical procedures of the gallbladder in order to avoid necrotizing cholecystitis. The parasympathetic innervation of the gallbladder via the vagus nerve aids in contraction of the gallbladder and relaxation of the duodenal sphincter. The sympathetic innervation via the splanchnic nerves has the opposite effects.[10] Filling of the gallbladder occurs continuously and bile flow is driven by hepatic secretion and gallbladder contraction. This is a low-flow, low pressure system. The sphincter of Oddi is the functional sphincter located at the terminal portion of the CBD. This sphincter demonstrates both tonic and rhythmic contractions and acts as a one-way valve to regulate pressure within the biliary system. It also provides resistance against retrograde passage of duodenal contents into the biliary tree. Spontaneous contraction of the gallbladder is also known to occur, which explains why serum bile acid values may appear higher after a 12 hour fast than during a two hour postprandial period.[6]

GENERAL CONSIDERATIONS

Diagnostic tests

Diagnostics are usually initiated due to the presence of icterus or hyperbilirubinemia or clinical signs associated with hepatobiliary disease. Patients with extrahepatic biliary tract obstruction (EHBTO) are usually overtly icteric, have lost weight, and show symptoms of vague illness (anorexia, lethargy, etc.). Patients with clinical signs associated with necrotizing cholecystitis or septic bile peritonitis may present in shock, with diffuse abdominal pain or distension, icterus, and fever. Icterus is present when serum total bilirubin is greater than 2 mg/dL.[7] Serum biochemical profiles can indicate cholestasis by increased serum transaminases (alanine aminotransferase, ALT; aspartate aminotransferase, AST), alkaline phosphatase (ALP), and gamma-glutamyl transpeptidase (GGT), and increased total bilirubin. ALP lacks steroid induction in cats, therefore any increase in ALP is referable to cholecystic disease but does not distinguish extrahepatic and intrahepatic causes. Hypercholesterolemia and bilirubinuria may also be seen with EHBTO patients.[6,11]

Diagnostic imaging

Radiography can be of use in selected cases of hepatobiliary disease.[11] Liver size and configuration may be evaluated and hepatic masses can cause displacement of adjacent organs.[12] Mineralized densities within the gallbladder, or choleliths, can be seen in approximately 50% of cases. Identification of radiopaque choleliths is not diagnostic for biliary obstruction as these may be an incidental finding in some normal animals.[11] Dystrophic mineralization of the biliary tree can be seen in some cases of chronic cholangiohepatitis. Rarely, a mass or space-occupying lesion (pancreatitis, neoplasia, enlarged gallbladder) may be visible in the region of the CBD in cases of EHBTO. Diffuse peritoneal effusion seen on abdominal radiographs should encourage further diagnostics such as abdominocentesis to rule out bile peritonitis. Lastly, any presence of gas within the biliary structures or hepatic parenchyma indicates the presence of emphysematous cholecystitis or abscess, which should be surgically explored promptly.

Cholecystography is not commonly performed in small animals, but experimental studies with different contrast agents have been conducted in the past. This procedure can be performed using iodinated contrast agents given orally (ipodate sodium/calcium, 150–500 mg/kg) or intravenously (5.2% iodipamide meglumine, 0.3–1.0 mL/kg over 30 minutes); however, many variables affect the usefulness of this test and there is a potential for adverse reactions such as anaphylaxis and vomiting.[6,11] Cholecystography is best used for diagnosis of choleliths, polyps, or biliary sludge. Percutaneous transhepatic cholangiocystography (PTC) also allows for direct visualization of the gallbladder and biliary tract but requires ultrasound guidance. Approximately 25% of the bile should be withdrawn prior to injection of contrast media and radiographs should be taken immediately, 45 minutes, 120 minutes, and 24 hours after injection.[11]

Abdominal ultrasound is an excellent tool for assessing the structures of the biliary tree and hepatic parenchyma. Contrast-enhanced ultrasonography has been used to help differentiate between benign and malignant hepatic nodules in a series of canine patients.[13] Visualization of the normal gallbladder in cats can be difficult because the liver is oriented in a dorsoventral axis and displaced cranially under the ribs.[11] Distension of biliary ducts and increased wall thickness of the gallbladder can be seen easily as the anechoic oval shape of the gallbladder is well recognized. A healthy gallbladder wall is usually poorly visible, as are biliary and hepatic ducts when not distended by disease. The CBD lies ventral to the portal vein and has a diameter of less than 4 mm in healthy cats.[11] When thickening of the gallbladder wall is seen, many possibilities must be considered (Table 31-1). In one study an ultrasound measurement of the wall ≥1 mm was accurate in predicting gallbladder disease in cats.[14] Enlargement of the CBD can occur within 24–48 hours of acute bile duct obstruction, whereas intrahepatic biliary duct distension requires five to seven days of obstruction. Cholelithiasis can be diagnosed by ultrasonography because both radiodense and radiopaque stones can be imaged but stones within the cystic or CBD can be difficult to visualize as they are not surrounded by anechoic bile and there is the presence of interference by intestinal or gastric gas. When studying a cohort of cats with spontaneous EHBTO, ultrasound detected a CBD > 5 mm in 97% of cats but only 50% of cats had a dilated gallbladder.[15] Polyps, neoplastic masses such as adenomas or adenocarcinomas, or cysts within the gallbladder, cystic or CBD can be imaged via ultrasound although cystic hyperplasia with diffuse irregular wall thickening is more common.

Table 31-1 Diagnostic imaging techniques for hepatobiliary disease in cats

Ultrasound	Radiography	Cholecystography	Hepatic Scintigraphy	CT, ERCP
Thickened GB wall • partially empty • cholecystitis • wall edema (due to portal hypertension, hypoalbuminemia, or CHF) • ascites (spurious thickening) Enlarged GB size • anorexia • neoplasia • mucocele • EHBTO from CBD neoplasia, choleliths, pancreatitis Multifocal hyperechogenicity • cholangiohepatitis Distended bile ducts • EHBTO	Mineralized densities • choleliths • dystrophic mineralization Right quadrant mass effect: • pancreatitis • focal peritonitis • enlarged GB • neoplasia Emphysematous GB • cholecystitis • choledochitis Poor detail • effusion • peritonitis	Percutaneous transhepatic injection of contrast material: 25% of bile should be removed before injection; radiographs taken at 0, 45, 120 minutes, and 24 hours post injection	Intestinal transit should be seen within 3 hours of IV injection – if not EHBTO diagnosed	Only reported in experimental studies in dogs

CHF, congestive heart failure; CT, computed tomography; EHBTO, extrahepatic biliary tract obstruction; ERCP, endoscopic retrograde cholangio-pancreatography; GB, gallbladder.

Due to the close anatomic association between the biliary and pancreatic systems, the pancreas should always be imaged when using ultrasonography. Pancreatic enlargement, focal steatitis or masses can cause EHBTO and treatment depends upon an appropriate preoperative diagnosis. For cats with suspected cholangitis or cholangiohepatitis, ultrasonography also allows for diagnostic testing to be performed, such as cholecystocentesis if the biliary tree is not pathologically affected. Percutaneous ultrasound-guided cholecystocentesis can be performed in cats and in one experimental study performed in healthy cats the risks of this procedure appeared to be low.[16] Culture samples of bile yielded a significantly higher percentage of positive results when compared to hepatic cultures.[17] Cholecystocentesis of a diseased or distended gallbladder increases the risks of complications, therefore biochemical analysis of blood, including a coagulation panel, should be considered before performing this procedure. All patients should be monitored for any signs of peritonitis for 24 hours after the procedure.[18] In humans, severe vagal complications have been seen with diagnostic procedures of the gallbladder but this has not been reported in cats undergoing simple aspiration.

Hepatic scintigraphy has been reported in small animals and involves the use of radioisotopes such as technetium (^{99m}Tc) attached to organic anions (iminodiacetic analogs). In humans, this modality can diagnose CBD occlusion, acute and chronic cholecystitis, segmental biliary tree obstruction, and sphincter of Oddi dysfunction.[6] One study showed 83% sensitivity and 94% specificity for a diagnosis of biliary obstruction if no scintigraphic material was seen within the intestinal tract after passage of sufficient time for bile emptying (within three hours).[19] Another study reported scintigraphic criteria for partial biliary obstruction in small animals.[20] Disadvantages to this technique include limited availability, restrictions on patient handling, and the resultant delays to surgical intervention.

Future diagnostic imaging modalities for use in cats may include computed tomography (CT), magnetic resonance imaging (MRI), as well as endoscopic retrograde cholangio-pancreatography (ERCP). CT and MRI may be used to delineate the extent of hepatic masses and show promise in distinguishing between benign and malignant processes.[21] Three-dimensional spiral CT has been used in human studies of patients with suspected obstructive biliary disease.[22,23] These studies have shown excellent results in diagnosing EHBTO compared to other current techniques such as PTC but have not been reported in our small animal patients to date. ERCP has only been reported in dogs to date. This combination modality uses endoscopy and fluoroscopy to identify the CBD and major pancreatic duct.[24,25] This technique requires considerable training but is used commonly in humans to highlight masses, papillary stenosis, and choledocholiths.

PRESURGICAL CONSIDERATIONS

Thorough preoperative evaluation of patients undergoing hepatic or biliary surgery should include a complete blood count, biochemistry profile, urinalysis, and coagulation profile. Even though the liver has great regenerative capacity, the condition of the remaining liver determines how well removal of a portion of the liver may be tolerated. Diseases such as cirrhosis, prolonged biliary obstruction and hypoalbuminemia may result in reduced tolerance for removal of large amounts of liver tissue.[7,26] Patients may be anemic and preoperative blood typing and access to blood for transfusion (see Chapter 5) as needed during surgery is warranted. Hypoglycemia as well as hypoalbuminemia may be encountered in patients with hepatic insufficiency.[3] Animals with evidence of hepatic encephalopathy should be stabilized before proceeding with surgery. Decreased hepatic metabolism of drugs used to anesthetize patients should be taken into consideration (see Chapter 2). Doses of most drugs should be reduced and inhalant anesthetics are the preferred method of anesthetic maintenance.[3] Use of propofol for anesthesia in cats with primary hepatic lipidosis did not appear to increase morbidity or mortality in a study of feline patients undergoing feeding tube placement.[27] Prophylactic antibiotic usage is recommended for hepatic and biliary disease. Normally, the liver filters portal blood and bacteria may proliferate with hepatic ischemia or hypoxia.[3,7]

Cats with prolonged obstructive biliary disease are at risk for coagulopathies due to vitamin K malabsorption, which leads to deficiencies in factors II, VII, IX, and X.[3,7] Any evidence of clinical bleeding or increases in prothrombin or activated partial thromboplastin times should receive vitamin K1 (0.1–0.2 mg/kg SQ once daily) for 24 to 48 hours before surgery or a plasma transfusion.[3] Partial or complete biliary obstructions may allow ascending aerobic and anaerobic infection and subsequent bacteremia. The organisms most commonly isolated from biliary infections include *Escherichia coli*, *Klebsiella* spp., *Enterobacter* spp., *Proteus* spp., and *Pseudomonas* spp.[3,7] Antibiotics that are excreted in an active form in the bile are most effective for treatment (see Box 31-1).[3] Nutritional deficits should be considered (see Chapter 6), and placement of a feeding tube (see Chapter 12) either at surgery or preoperatively may be extremely important to aid in management of these cases.[28]

Anesthetic considerations (see Chapter 2) have been studied at length in animal models with regards to biliary surgery.[29,30] Most importantly, systemic hypotension has been repeatedly discovered as a complication with obstructive jaundice.[31,32] Loss of vascular responsiveness to sympathomimetic pressor agents with chronic bile duct obstruction is associated with systemic vasodilation and appears multifactorial.[33,34] This lack of responsiveness to pressor support may make intraoperative and postoperative management of these patients challenging and in many studies postoperative hypotension has been linked to a poor prognosis.[35,36]

The association between obstructive jaundice and renal failure has also been well established in the human population and is associated with a mortality rate of 70–80% in people who develop it.[37] Theories behind the cause of renal failure in this patient group include cardiovascular dysfunction (hypotension) leading to poor blood flow to the kidneys and acute renal tubular necrosis as a direct nephrotoxic effect of bile constituents. This functional hypovolemia may leave the kidneys more open to damage from endotoxemia and subsequent renal vasoconstriction as well.[33]

SURGICAL DISEASES OF THE LIVER

Hepatic trauma

Traumatic injury to the hepatic parenchyma may lead to hemorrhage. Isolated hepatic injury is uncommon and small lacerations or fractures of the parenchyma rarely require surgical intervention, but severe trauma leading to hemorrhage that cannot be controlled with conservative or medical management may require exploratory surgery.[7] Blunt trauma from automobiles is the most frequent cause of hepatic injury, although other rare causes such as hepatic rupture due to amyloidosis in six cats have been reported.[38] A surgical technique that may be used to control hemorrhage includes temporary occlusion of the hepatic artery and portal vein through the epiploic foramen via the Pringle maneuver to slow hemorrhage by using either a finger or an instrument to compress the vessels.[7] Other documented methods to control traumatic hemorrhage documented in human patients include direct suturing of intrahepatic vessels, resectional debridement, lobar resection, as well as perihepatic packing and replaparotomy.[39]

Hepatic cysts

Hepatic cysts are epithelium lined cystic cavities in cats and dogs that have been associated with liver tumors, polycystic kidney disease, liver hydatidosis and congenital hepatopathies.[40] Patients may be asymptomatic for cysts, present with abdominal pain, or a rare complication, seen in humans, may be biliary obstruction.[41] In a study reporting on nine cats with hepatic cysts, the common presenting clinical signs were anorexia, reduced activity, and vomiting. All patients had abdominal pain on palpation. Four out of nine cats had concurrent renal cysts. Ultrasound-guided drainage and alcoholization of the hepatic cysts was reported, with a low rate of complication and amelioration of clinical signs.[40] Other reported treatments include partial lobectomy, excision of the cystic membrane, as well as omentalization.[42,43] Hepatic cysts have also been reported in conjunction with peritoneopericardial diaphragmatic hernia in a cat.[44]

Hepatic abscess

Hepatic abscesses may form as isolated lesions, manifestations of systemic infections, or as diffuse microabscesses.[45] In human patients most abscesses are bacterial in nature and most commonly affect the right liver lobes. This may be due to its proximity to the biliary tree or the portal anatomy that permits translocation of intestinal flora.[46–48] In a study of 14 cats with reported hepatic abscesses, the overall mortality rate was high at 79%. Polymicrobial growth was cultured from 66% of the cats, with *E. coli* most frequently isolated.[45] Feline patients often present with non-specific clinical signs such as anorexia, lethargy and weight loss. Most affected cats were septic and many were hypothermic. In dogs with hepatic abscessation, 100% of patients were reported to have had an increase in serum ALP activity, while this study reported 50% of feline patients failed to have an increase in serum liver enzymes.[49] Most of the feline cases reported had multiple macroscopic abscesses, but the survival rate was higher (75%) in the cases where a solitary abscess was found which was surgically resected. Results were favorable in one cat treated with percutaneous ultrasound-assisted drainage and alcoholization of a focal hepatic abscess.[50]

Liver lobe torsion

Hepatic lobe torsion is exceptionally rare and has only been reported in one cat.[4] The left side of the liver is most commonly affected in dogs, with one study documenting a left lateral lobe torsion in 48% of animals[4] and the left medial lobe was most commonly affected in another study of 13 dogs.[51] The supposition is that the left lateral lobe is the largest, most well defined and most mobile of all hepatic lobes.[52,53] While an underlying cause for liver lobe torsion is often never found, one feline case report documented torsion of the right medial liver lobe, and the lobe contained a ruptured hepatocellular carcinoma.[4] This patient was presented to an emergency hospital in respiratory distress with dyspnea as well as anemia and hemoperitoneum. The patient was euthanized due to poor condition and the torsion was documented on postmortem examination. This is in contrast to dogs, where a good long-term outcome for dogs undergoing surgery for liver lobe torsion has been reported.[51] Other reported causes may include congenital absence or traumatic rupture of the supporting ligaments of the liver.[54,55]

Hepatobiliary neoplasia

Liver neoplasia may be primary or due to metastatic disease. Tumors may arise from hepatocytes, bile duct epithelium, neuroendocrine cells or stromal cells.[56] Tumors generally occur in older animals and

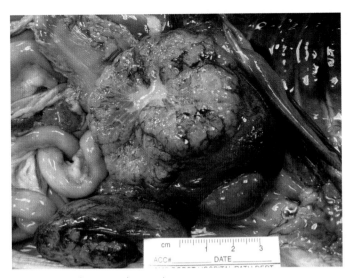

Figure 31-3 Biliary cystadenoma in a cat.

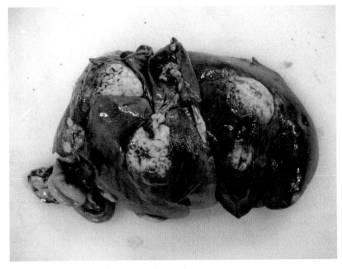

Figure 31-4 Metastatic pancreatic carcinoma.

presenting clinical signs are generally non-specific.[58] Cats with malignant tumors, though, are more likely to show clinical signs of illness than those with benign masses, and overall benign masses seem to be more common than malignant tumors.[58] In a study of 41 cases of cats with primary hepatobiliary masses, the most common malignant tumor type was found to be cholangiocellular carcinoma and the most common benign masses were cholangiocellular adenomas, hepatocellular adenomas, and biliary cysts (Fig. 31-3).[58] Cats with benign disease that underwent exploratory surgery had no complications or recurrence documented at two months following surgery, yet 86% of cats with malignant disease were euthanized or died during surgery.[58] Benign hepatic nodular myelolipomatosis has been reported in conjunction with a peritoneopericardial diaphragmatic hernia.[59] Reported survival following surgical excision of a solitary myelolipoma was favorable.[60] Carcinomas of the biliary system in cats behave aggressively and one report documented an 80% rate of metastasis.[61] Hepatobilliary neuroendocrine carcinoma has been studied in 17 cats, and was associated with a poor prognosis, with 14/17 cats being euthanized during or immediately after surgery.[57]

Treatment for solitary tumors is partial or complete liver lobectomy (see liver lobectomy information section below). Local lymph nodes should be evaluated for metastatic disease. In patients where diffuse neoplastic disease is present, liver biopsy is warranted (see liver biopsy information section below) (Fig. 31-4). In two reports, the liver was involved in 20–24% of cats with lymphocytic lymphoma (Fig. 31-5).[62,63]

Radiographic and ultrasound imaging can document the location and extent of hepatic tumors.[64] Additional imaging such as CT and MRI may be useful to determine resectability of a tumor and three-view thoracic radiographs should be taken to look for pulmonary metastatic disease.[56] Non-resectable and metastatic liver disease may be treated with novel techniques such as regional chemoembolization.[65]

SURGICAL PROCEDURES OF THE LIVER

Liver biopsy

Liver biopsy is commonly performed as a solitary procedure or in conjunction with an abdominal exploratory procedure (see

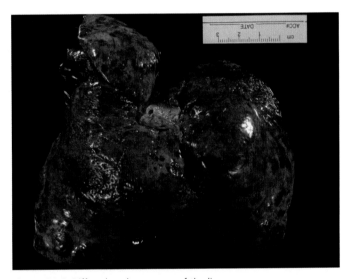

Figure 31-5 Diffuse lymphosarcoma of the liver.

Chapter 23). There are many indications for hepatic biopsy, including liver enzyme elevation for more than 30 days, ultrasonographic lesions, disease staging, and previous non-diagnostic cytologic study.[66] For diffuse hepatic disease, such as lipidosis (Fig. 31-6) or neoplasia, cytology may provide an adequate diagnosis, but fails to show architectural details that can only be obtained via histopathology. One study documented agreement between cytologic and histopathologic diagnosis of liver disease in only 51% of feline patients.[67] Another study documented several cats incorrectly diagnosed with only hepatic lipidosis instead of lymphosarcoma.[68] As cytology provides only a small sample size and does not detail parenchymal architecture, hepatic biopsy is generally favored.

Multiple techniques exist and each method has advantages and disadvantages. Less invasive methods are ideal but may provide only small tissue samples, yet general anesthesia may be needed to obtain larger specimens. Techniques reported for obtaining a liver biopsy including loop guillotine suture (Fig. 31-7), punch biopsy, ultrasonically activated scalpel (which can be used in both open and laparoscopic fashion), as well as stapling methods.[3,7,69] The loop suture method is adequate for sampling the margin of the liver, while a skin

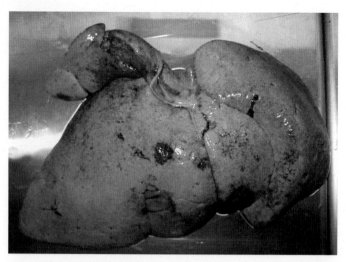

Figure 31-6 Hepatic lipidosis.

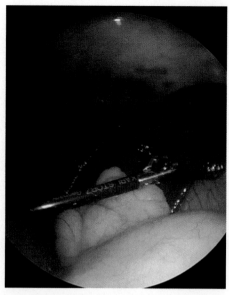

Figure 31-8 Laparoscopic biopsy of hepatic parenchyma.

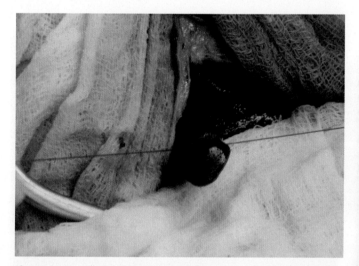

Figure 31-7 Guillotine (loop) biopsy of the liver.

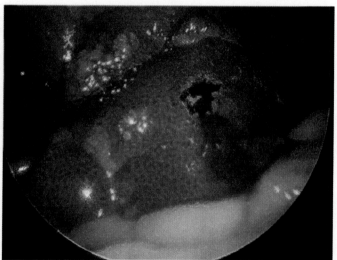

Figure 31-9 Appearance of biopsy site following laparoscopic biopsy.

punch biopsy is ideal for focal lesions within the central portions of the liver. Absorbable gelatin foam (Gelfoam Pfizer, New York), a mattress suture, or omental tissue may be used to control hemorrhage.[7] Use of tissue forceps is avoided in grasping the specimen to avoid creating a crushing artifact. Surgically obtained wedge samples should be at least 1 cm, preferably 2 cm deep, as subcapsular tissue contains more fibrous tissue and can be misleadingly interpreted as representing the entire liver.[70] An ideal liver biopsy should be of adequate size and taken from a location that is representative of the primary liver pathology. At least two to three samples should be obtained from separate liver lobes, including both peripheral and central locations, as well as grossly normal and abnormal-appearing tissue.[70] Human studies suggest that at least six to eight portal triads must be obtained for adequate histopathologic interpretation.[71]

Ultrasound-guided needle-core biopsy techniques are minimally invasive, but they require a skilled ultrasonographer, do not allow access to all areas of the peritoneal cavity, and have been shown to produce inferior samples in many cases when compared with open surgical or laparoscopic techniques.[72] In a study of 124 animals, the morphologic diagnosis assigned to needle biopsy specimens agreed with that of the wedge biopsy only 48% of the time.[73] Additionally, a high rate of complications using an automatic Tru-Cut biopsy device

in 26 cats has been reported. In that study, 19% of the cats developed fatality following biopsy, attributed to a pressure wave that may have caused a vagal mediated shock.[74]

Laparoscopic biopsy (see Chapter 24) is an ideal method for acquiring a larger sample size (Fig. 31-8). This technique allows for magnified visualization of hepatic pathology as well as permitting observation of the sites following biopsy to be monitored for hemorrhage (Fig. 31-9). In addition, laparoscopy has proven safe and effective for providing accurate specimens of hepatic parenchyma.[69,75] While laparoscopy is performed under general anesthesia, the time of the procedure is rapid, with a mean reported surgery time of 35 minutes.[75] Samples from laparoscopic biopsy forceps are usually about 5 mm in diameter, depending on surgeon technique and depth of penetration. Laparoscopic cup biopsies provide about 45 mg of tissue, a 14G Tru-Cut-type biopsy needle provides 15–20 mg, and an 18G needle biopsy provides only 3–5 mg of liver tissue.[70] Disadvantages of the laparoscopic biopsy include the expense of equipment and the expertise needed, but the advantages over open laparotomy are significant, including faster patient recovery, lower postoperative

Box 31-2 **Liver lobectomy and partial hepatectomy**

The cat is positioned in dorsal recumbency and a cranial midline abdominal approach is made. Additional surgical exposure can be provided via a paracostal incision or a caudal sternotomy. Thorough evaluation and palpation of both the parietal and visceral surfaces of all hepatic lobes should be performed.

Hand suturing

The liver is dissected around the hilus and individual vessels identified and ligated for complete lobectomy. A single encircling ligature at the base of the hilus is not recommended, as dislodging of the single suture may lead to postoperative hemorrhage. For a partial hepatectomy the parenchyma can be gently crushed by using the 'finger fracture' technique. After the parenchyma is separated the remaining vessels and biliary ducts may be individually ligated.

Stapling

The 2.0 mm and 3.5 mm devices are best suited for use in feline patients. The stapling device may be placed across the parenchyma, but placing the stapling device at the level of the hilus, where the parenchyma is less thick, may help ensure adequate hemostasis. More blood loss may occur using the suction and clip method compared to use of the SurgiTie, LigaSure, Ultracision Harmonic Scalpel or thoracoabdominal stapling devices.[77] Temporary inflow occlusion of the hepatic artery and portal vein with an atraumatic bulldog clamp may be used to minimize hemorrhage.[7]

Vascular occluding staples (hemoclips) or suturing may be used to reinforce staple lines. Minor bleeding may be controlled with electrocautery, absorbable gelatin foam (Gelfoam), oxidized regenerated cellulose (Surgicel), and by placing omentum along the remaining liver.

The abdomen is flushed with warm sterile saline and thoroughly inspected for hemorrhage (ensuring the patient is normotensive) before routine closure.

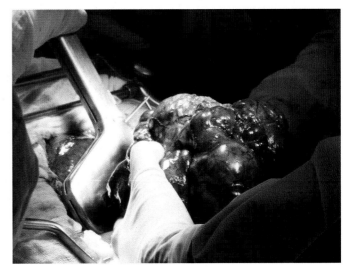

Figure 31-10 Use of the thoracoabdominal (TA) stapling device for liver lobectomy.

complete than suturing techniques.[79] Access to the central and right liver lobes is more difficult than access to the left liver lobe.[80] The thickness of the liver lobe is usually the limitation for lobectomy, and hepatic parenchyma can be more difficult to compress in a partial lobectomy, rather than stapling at the hilus for a complete lobectomy. The thoracoabdominal (TA) 3.5 mm or 4.8 mm stapling device has been used for a partial lobectomy in the dog, although the 2.0 mm (V3) vascular staples may be recommended for occlusion of hilar vessels (Fig. 31-10).[79,81] The 2.0 mm and 3.5 mm devices are best suited for use in feline patients. Vascular occluding staples (hemoclips) or suturing may be used to reinforce staple lines. A study comparing five surgical techniques for partial liver lobectomy in the dog found no difference in surgical time between techniques, but significantly more blood loss was encountered using the suction and clip method compared to use of the SurgiTie, LigaSure, Ultracision Harmonic Scalpel, or thoracoabdominal stapling devices.[77] Temporary inflow occlusion of the hepatic artery and portal vein with an atraumatic bulldog clamp may be used to minimize hemorrhage.[7]

DISEASES OF THE BILIARY SYSTEM

Cholecystitis

Cholecystitis, or inflammation of the gallbladder, can present acutely or be considered chronic in duration. Cholecystitis may be caused by bile stasis (EHBTO or choleliths), or blood-borne pathogens from hepatic circulation, or intestinal reflux into the biliary system. Clinical signs, as with many biliary diseases, can be quite vague, and include reduced appetite, anorexia, lethargy, vomiting, abdominal pain, and fever. The biochemical profile of affected animals includes elevated transferases, ALP, mildly elevated total bilirubin, and occasionally an elevated leukocyte count with a left shift.[7] In cats, a new classification scheme was proposed by the WSAVA Liver Disease Group: a neutrophilic, a lymphocytic, and a chronic cholangitis.[18] Diagnosis of cholecystitis relies most heavily on abdominal ultrasound as radiographs will only be helpful if the gallbladder rupture has led to diffuse peritoneal effusion or radiodense gallstones are visualized. The ultrasound results will vary according to the stage of the disease, ranging from a bright or thickened gallbladder wall, to distension of the gallbladder and associated ducts.

morbidity, decreased infection rate, less postoperative pain, and decreased hospitalization time.[70,72]

Open laparotomy (see Chapter 23) is generally not indicated for hepatic biopsy alone, but liver biopsy is often done in conjunction with an abdominal exploration. A keyhole incision may also be used, by making a 2–4 cm incision caudal to the xiphoid process and grasping a small portion of exposed liver.[76] Obviously, the increased morbidity associated with open laparotomy is necessary when a discrete mass of considerable size must be excised.

Lobectomy and hepatectomy

Partial lobectomy (Box 31-2) is defined as separation and removal of hepatic parenchyma at any location other than the hilus. Removal of a lobe at the level of the hilus is considered a complete liver lobectomy. A partial hepatectomy (see Box 31-2) involves removal of several hepatic lobes. Partial or complete liver lobectomy is generally performed through an open laparotomy via a cranial midline abdominal approach. Additional surgical exposure can be provided via a paracostal incision or a caudal sternotomy. Removal of up to 70% of the normal canine liver is tolerated, but no specific guidelines exist for feline patients.[7]

Partial or complete liver lobectomy may be performed with hand suturing or with stapling equipment. For tumors that encroach on the hilar region, a hilar liver lobectomy technique involving dissection of individual lobar vessels has been described in dogs.[78] Study of canine lobectomy found stapling techniques faster, simpler, and more

Treatment of cholecystitis also depends on the stage of the disease and the clinical picture of the patient. If caught early before the gallbladder wall becomes compromised, cholecystitis may respond to appropriate antibiotic and choloretic therapies. If cholecystocentesis can be performed safely, bile is collected for aerobic and anaerobic culture and sensitivity. The most commonly identified bacterial isolate was *E. coli* in one case series.[18] If gallbladder rupture is suspected, immediate exploratory surgery and probable cholecystectomy is warranted. As discussed later in this chapter, bile peritonitis causes a severe chemical peritonitis and if the bile is infected mortality rates in these patients can increase significantly. Gallbladder mucocoele, reported frequently in dogs, has only been reported once in a cat and did not have the characteristic stellate or striated pattern commonly described. In this case, concurrent hepatic lipidosis was present and a cholecystoenterostomy was performed to avoid the risk of EHBTO in the future.[82]

Cholelithiasis

Cholelithiasis, also known as gallstones, has been reported in the cat. Stone formation occurs due to multiple biliary variables including bile saturation, type and proportion of bile acids, protein, and mucin. Components in feline choleliths include bilirubin, and to varying degrees cholesterol and calcium. Even though calcium carbonate is the most common type of cholelith according to some studies, the calcium content in many stones is low enough that they remain radiolucent.[8,83–85] Cholestasis has been associated with cholelith formation due to the increase in mucin production and cholecystitis is lithogenic due to the associated inflammation, hemorrhage, and bacterial component.[6,7] Alterations of gallbladder motility associated with certain types of gastric surgery involving the antrum and pylorus may also cause gallstone formation. Co-ordination between gastric and gallbladder motor activity through extrinsic neural connections has been shown experimentally in dogs.[7]

Most choleliths remain asymptomatic unless they lead to biliary or pancreatic obstruction. With obstructive cholelithiasis, clinical signs include dehydration, vomiting, anorexia, icterus, and lethargy. Blood work abnormalities are consistent with extrahepatic biliary tract obstruction. The largest case series in cats reports on nine patients that underwent surgical treatment for obstructive cholelithiasis.[86] Five of the nine cats had a cholecystectomy, three cats had biliary diversion, and one had cholecystotomy. Concurrent hepatic lipidosis was associated with a higher mortality rate and cholecystectomy had the lowest postoperative morbidity. Treatment of choleliths is only undertaken if they are causing clinical signs or biochemical elevations. In human medicine, dissolution of gallstones by chenodeoxycholic acid is attempted as this decreases the hepatic synthesis and secretion of cholesterol. This is not usually attempted in small animals due to the low incidence of cholesterol stones. Surgical stone removal along with cholecystectomy is the treatment of choice in most cases. When a cholecystectomy is performed, patency of the CBD must be ensured. Cholecystotomy or choledochotomy alone can be performed to remove stones but most authors believe that leaving the gallbladder in situ may predispose to recurrence and leaves a nidus of disease.[7,87,88] Sample procurement for aerobic and anaerobic culture is always indicated.

Extrahepatic biliary tract obstruction

Extrahepatic biliary tract obstruction is associated with many different disease processes (Box 31-3).[8,85,89–94] Cholestasis leads to hepatic parenchymal injury, such as cell membrane and organelle damage within a few weeks. Over time, biliary stasis leads to inflammation, free radical formation, biliary epithelial hyperplasia, and eventually

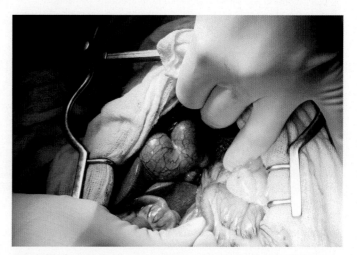

Figure 31-11 Torturous common bile duct from extrahepatic biliary tract obstruction.

necrosis and fibrosis of the bile ducts. Clinical signs associated with EHBTO are varied but include lethargy, jaundice, intermittent vomiting and inappetence. Gastroenteric ulceration at the pyloric-duodenal junction is common and can lead to substantial blood loss. Diagnosis of EHBTO includes increases in serum enzyme and total bilirubin concentrations. Coagulopathies can also appear due to vitamin K deficiency. Confirmation of EHBTO is made with ultrasound or exploratory surgery. Ultrasonographic features of bile duct obstruction include a distended and torturous CBD (Fig. 31-11), enlarged gallbladder, and enlarged intrahepatic bile ducts.[6,7] Hepatic scintigraphy could also be helpful in diagnosis of EHBTO but cholecystography is not recommended.

Certain causes of EHBTO such as parasitic infections with liver flukes may carry a poor prognosis in some cases due to severe damage to the biliary structures whereas congenital anomalies such as choledochal cysts may be managed quite successfully with palliative surgeries.[89,90,93,95] Although trauma-related (diaphragmatic herniation) or other extrabiliary causes (duodenal foreign body) of EHBTO are rare, they have been reported, and if addressed in a timely fashion may lead to successful outcomes for the patient.[94,96] Recently a case series of six cats presented data on obstructive sphincter of Oddi pathology.[97] In this report, three of the cats had dysfunction associated with pre-existing inflammatory bowel disease, two had inspissated bile causing an obstruction, and one cat was diagnosed with cholangiocellular carcinoma. All six cats were taken to surgery, where sphincterotomies as well as other procedures were performed. Four of the six cats did well postoperatively.

Not surprisingly, neoplasia of the gallbladder, CBD, or duodenal papilla holds a poor prognosis for most feline patients,[91,92] whereas pancreatitis or other inflammatory causes may respond to medical and surgical treatment much more readily.[10,98] Two large retrospective case series have been published reporting on prognostic factors and outcome in biliary diversion surgeries in cats.[36,37] In one, the mortality rate within 48 hours of surgery was 57%; in cats diagnosed with neoplasia it was 100% versus those with non-neoplastic causes, where it was 40%.[37] The second study looked at only cats undergoing cholecystoenterostomy procedures and identified risk factors associated with poor outcome in these patients. This study also found the majority of EHBTO was due to inflammatory causes (13/22) versus neoplastic (9/22). Only 27% of cats survived longer than six months after surgery, all of which had chronic inflammatory diseases.[36] This is in agreement with previous literature reviews.[99] The only variable associated with median survival time was the presence of neoplasia; 14 days for neoplasia versus 255 days with inflammatory disease.[36] Overall the prognosis of EHBTO in cats that require biliary diversion interventions is poor and the postoperative complication rate quite high.[36,37,99] The most common complications include postoperative hypotension, blood loss or anemia requiring transfusions, vomiting, anorexia, and cardiopulmonary arrest.

Bile peritonitis

Rupture of the biliary system occurs occasionally in cats with end-stage cholecystitis, EHBTO, cholelithiasis, blunt or sharp abdominal trauma, and iatrogenic injury from percutaneous cholecystocentesis. In the dog, the most common location for rupture is the gallbladder fundus and the CBD but this has not been determined in feline species.[6,7] Leakage of bile into the peritoneal cavity can be associated with clinical signs ranging from fever, anorexia, abdominal pain, icterus, lethargy, to shock. Abdominal effusion may take days to weeks to evolve depending on the amount and location of the leakage.[7,10] Blood work abnormalities can include increased liver transferases, ALP, GGT, and leukocytosis if there is chronic inflammation or sepsis. Abdominocentesis may illustrate bilirubin crystals and inflammatory cells in a brown-green fluid if the leakage is long-standing. Determination of bilirubin concentrations in fluid and serum will illustrate a disproportionate amount in the abdominal effusion (two times higher) and has been shown to be 100% effective in diagnosis.[100] With acute ruptures the effusion may be localized to directly surrounding the gallbladder and require ultrasound guidance to obtain samples. In these cases, omental adhesions may undergo an intense inflammatory reaction and derange the normal anatomy seen at ultrasound. Peritoneal reactions to bile leakage vary but eventually lead to large amounts of effusion. Unconjugated bile salts are cytotoxic and can induce tissue inflammation by altering the permeability of vascular structures within the peritoneal membranes. Small amounts of bile leakage may go undetected but if the bile is septic a life-threatening condition can quickly develop. Fluid shifts into the peritoneal cavity and translocation of bacteria from the liver and intestine can lead to systemic hypotension, endotoxemia, and shock. Other systemic effects of bile salts include red cell lysis, electrolyte imbalances, hypoproteinemia, anemia, and marked dehydration due to alkaline pH and hyperosmolality.[10]

Bile peritonitis has been reported in a retrospective case series on 24 dogs and two cats,[100] as well as in a case report of one cat

with a congenital duplex gallbladder and choledocholithiasis.[8] The most common cause of biliary leakage was trauma (blunt or penetrating or leakage from a previous surgical site) or necrotizing cholecystitis.

Treatment of bile peritonitis (see Chapter 26) almost always requires surgical exploration, especially in the case of suspected sepsis. At surgery, the abdomen should be lavaged until it is grossly free of bile-stained fluid. Many patients will need aggressive treatment for hypovolemic shock, endotoxemia, and hypoalbuminemia preoperatively. Culture samples should be collected to aid in postoperative antimicrobial selection and often there are multiple types of bacteria detected.[100] Overall survival with bile peritonitis is 50%, while septic peritonitis only carries a 27% survival rate. Patients with lower white blood cell counts (mean 20 608/μL) and lower neutrophil counts (mean 686/μL) had a significantly better survival rate.[100] If necrotizing cholecystitis is present, a cholecystectomy is required. If damage to the biliary ducts has occurred, biliary diversion is necessary but may be difficult depending on the condition of the tissue.

BILIARY PROCEDURES

Biliary decompression procedures

Much debate still remains regarding which patients may benefit from preoperative biliary drainage, but the procedure has been postulated to allow for normalization of liver enzymes, which may stabilize the patient before definitive surgery.[101–105] In some cases, percutaneous cholecystostomy may be used instead of open surgical techniques or endoscopic techniques. One experimental study in cats performed temporary biliary decompression after chronic CBD ligation and illustrated decreases in transaminases, total bilirubin and improved attitude and appetite; however, bacterial infections were common.[106] Self-retaining or pigtail catheters of sizes ranging from 8–10 French with 22G needles can be used in cats. Laparoscopic-assisted catheterization allowed for direct visualization to avoid penetrating the pleura.[107] If placed during laparotomy, the catheter is introduced through a right ventral abdominal wall stab incision and passed through omentum or hepatic tissue to decrease postoperative leakage. The potential for postoperative cholecystographic studies to determine CBD patency before tube removal is an advantage to this technique.

Biliary stenting as a primary treatment or adjunctive procedure for primary choledochal repairs has also been reported in small animals. This use is controversial but is commonplace in human medicine. The cited advantages include prevention of stricture formation in the early phase of healing, decompression of the gallbladder, and minimization of leakage. Potential complications associated with stent usage include stricture formation, ascending infections, and increased morbidity and hospitalization.[7] A more recent clinical study reported the use of choledochal stenting in seven cats for pancreatitis-associated EHBTO and found red rubber catheters placed surgically through the major duodenal papilla did allow for temporary biliary drainage without re-routing procedures. Five of the seven cats survived to discharge but there was a greater morbidity associated with this technique in cats than previously described in dogs, most likely due to differences in the pathogenesis of these diseases.[108,109]

Cholecystotomy/dochotomy

The most common indications for a cholecystotomy (Box 31-4) (incision into the gallbladder) or choledochotomy (Box 31-4) (incision into CBD) are inspissated bile, choleliths, or liver flukes.

Box 31-4 Cholecystotomy/dochotomy

The cat is positioned in dorsal recumbency and a cranial midline abdominal approach is made.

Cholecystotomy

The gallbladder may need to be mobilized from the hepatic fossa by gentle dissection. Dissection can usually be performed by a combination of electrocautery blunt dissection with cotton tipped applicators or hemostats and sharp dissection with scissors. Hepatic bleeding can usually be controlled by manual pressure or the application of hemostatic agents. Decompression of the gallbladder can be performed before dissection by cholecystocentesis but may make dissection more difficult.[7] Once emptied, an incision is made in the fundus of the gallbladder. Decompression is performed with a 22–20G needle attached to a syringe or extension set and syringe and gentle pressure is used to remove as much bile as possible. If the bile is inspissated, suction through a needle may be impossible and the cholecystotomy may have to be performed to empty the gallbladder. The gallbladder should be packed off with sterile lap sponges to ensure there is no contamination of the abdomen with bile. An incision is then made along the fundus of the gallbladder and the gallbladder is flushed. The cystic and CBDs can be cannulated with a red rubber catheter of the appropriate size to ensure patency. Cannulating from this direction (normograde) may be difficult because of the sharp turn the cystic duct usually makes entering the CBD. If there is any question of patency, the duodenum should be opened on the antimesenteric border to allow retrograde cannulation through the major duodenal papilla (Fig. 31-12). The gallbladder should be closed in one layer in a simple continuous inverting (Lembert or Cushing) or simple interrupted pattern using absorbable suture (4/0 to 5/0).[7,28,110] The abdomen is flushed with warm sterile saline and thoroughly inspected before routine closure.

Choledochotomy

The area surrounding the CBD is packed with moist gauze to avoid leakage of any material into the abdomen. A longitudinal incision is made along the grossly dilated bile duct. After the material has been removed, a catheter is passed in a normograde and retrograde fashion to ensure patency and to flush out any residual debris. This incision is closed with 4/0 to 6/0 absorbable sutures in a simple interrupted or simple continuous pattern.[7] If there are concerns regarding the diameter of the duct, the incision can be closed transversely. A stent can also be placed to divert bile across this incision. This is accomplished by performing a duodenotomy, placing a red rubber catheter through the major duodenal papilla and suturing it in place at the papilla with one to two 4/0 to 5/0 absorbable simple interrupted sutures. The abdomen is flushed with warm sterile saline and thoroughly inspected before routine closure.

Box 31-5 Cholecystectomy

The cat is positioned in dorsal recumbency and a cranial midline abdominal approach is made.

The gallbladder can be mobilized from the hepatic fossa by gentle dissection accomplished with a combination of electrocautery, manual traction with cotton tipped applicators and blunt dissection with hemostats. The cystic duct and artery are then identified. Special care must be taken not to ligate or damage any of the hepatic lobar ducts (especially those of the central division that enter the CBD near the cystic duct) emptying into the CBD.[7] It is important to determine that the CBD is patent before performing a cholecystectomy. A small duodenotomy should be made to catheterize the major duodenal papilla and a red rubber catheter (3.5–5 French) used to flush the duct. Once that has been performed, the cystic duct and artery are double ligated with non-absorbable suture (3/0 to 4/0) or hemostatic clips. The cystic duct is then transected distal to ligatures and the gallbladder is submitted for histopathologic analysis and bile is submitted for culture.[3]

The abdomen is flushed with warm sterile saline and thoroughly inspected before routine closure.

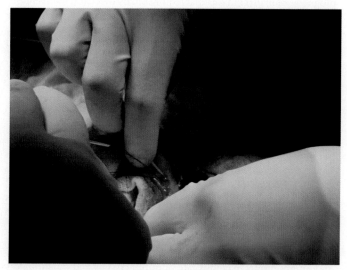

Figure 31-12 Catheterization of the major duodenal papilla after duodenotomy.

Cholecystectomy

Removal of the gallbladder (cholecystectomy) (Box 31-5) in cats is most commonly performed for trauma, neoplasia, necrotizing cholecystitis, EHBTO, and cholelithiasis. Laparoscopic cholecystectomy has been reported in one case series for dogs afflicted with mucoceles.[111] This technique has not been reported in cats and care must be taken that the surgeon be absolutely convinced the major duodenal papilla and CBD are patent before performing this procedure because this technique does not allow for catheterization of these structures.

Biliary diversion

Biliary diversion techniques (Box 31-6) include cholecystoduodenosotomy (CCD), cholecystojejunostomy, and choledochoenterostomy. These techniques are used most commonly for EHBTO, neoplasia of the CBD, and trauma. CCD is a more physiologic technique as it empties bile into the duodenum where it usually is released. Cultures of bile and biopsies of any masses and liver should be obtained at surgery. Liver histology will help predict future hepatobiliary compromise. Complications of these procedures include bile or intestinal content leakage from the stoma, ascending cholangiohepatitis from intestinal reflux, stoma obstruction, and pancreatic exocrine insufficiency if the pancreatic duct is sacrificed.[28,110,112] Pancreatic insufficiency can be treated by supplementation with pancreatic enzymes. The most important factor for success when performing these techniques is to create an appropriate sized stoma between the gallbladder and the intestine. Contraction of approximately 50% should be

Box 31-6 **Biliary diversion techniques**

The cat is positioned in dorsal recumbency and a cranial midline abdominal approach is made.

Cholecystoduodenostomy

CCD is performed by positioning the duodenum next to the gallbladder. The gallbladder is completely dissected from the hepatic fossa as described previously to decrease the tension along the suture line.[7] The gallbladder and duodenum are packed off with moistened lap sponges or gauze to minimize leakage of bile and intestinal contents. An incision of approximately 2.5–3 cm in length is made in the duodenum and an attempt is usually made to cannulate the major duodenal papilla to confirm that an obstruction is present. If neoplasia is the suspected cause of an obstruction, biopsies of the papilla or CBD are performed. Then an incision of the same length is made in the gallbladder to lie parallel to the duodenal incision. Stay sutures placed at the cranial and caudal aspects of these incisions can aid in stabilization and manipulation during suturing. The cranial dorsal incision line is closed with 4/0 synthetic absorbable suture from within the lumen in a simple continuous or simple interrupted pattern. The caudal ventral incision lines are closed to complete the anastomosis (Fig. 31-13). Special attention is paid to the knot security at both ends of the anastomosis in continuous patterns as this is the most likely area for leakage.

Cholecystojejunostomy

CCJ is performed by positioning the jejunum next to the gallbladder. It is not usually necessary to mobilize the gallbladder with this technique as the jejunum is not tethered by the duodenocolic ligament and therefore the incision will not be under tension. Two incisions approximately 2.5–3 cm in length are made parallel to each other in the gallbladder and jejunum. Once again, an obstruction at the major duodenal papilla is usually confirmed prior to the gallbladder incision and all necessary biopsies are performed. The cranial dorsal incision line is closed with 4/0 synthetic absorbable suture from within the lumen

in a simple continuous or simple interrupted pattern. The caudal ventral incision lines are closed to complete the anastomosis. Special attention is paid to the knot security at both ends of the anastomosis in continuous patterns as this is the most likely area for leakage.

An alternative technique is to use the Roux-en-Y loop.[7,110] A segment of jejunum is anastomosed to the gallbladder as previously described but the oral aspect of the jejunal loops is transected and sutured closed. The jejunum just caudal to the duodenum is then anastomosed to this segment of jejunum approximately 40 cm aboral to the gallbladder anastomosis.

Choledochoenterostomy

Choledochoenterostomy should only be performed if the CBD is dilated to at least 1 cm and a stoma of approximately 2.5 cm can be created.[7] The CBD is isolated as described previously and transected at the area of greatest dilation. Then a longitudinal incision of 5–10 mm is made in the CBD at the end of the duct. A piece of the proximal duodenum or jejunum is positioned to allow for as little tension as possible and a transverse incision is made into the lumen. The length of the incision should be approximately half the diameter of the CBD. The anastomosis is performed using 3/0 to 5/0 synthetic absorbable or monofilament non-absorbable sutures in a simple interrupted pattern. Care should be taken if the CBD must be resected to try to preserve the major pancreatic duct and all hepatic lobar ducts emptying into it. If the pancreatic duct must be ligated, pancreatitis and pancreatic exocrine insufficiency should be anticipated. If neoplasia of the CBD or the major duodenal papilla is suspected, biopsies should be procured. This procedure does not allow for extensive margins so other procedures should be performed if the mass is large.

After all the procedures described, the abdomen is flushed with warm sterile saline and thoroughly inspected before routine closure.

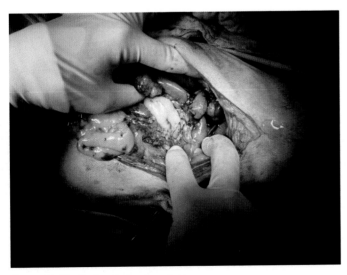

Figure 31-13 Cholecystoduodenostomy.

expected after healing.[7] An incision of at least 2.5 cm, approximating the length of the fundus to the infundibulum, must be created to take into account the inevitable fibrosis that occurs during healing. This opening size not only allows for drainage of bile but also of any refluxed intestinal contents that could lead to severe ascending cholangiohepatitis. Cholangiohepatitis must be treated with antibiotics and usually responds as long as the stoma is not obstructed.

CCD is usually performed by making two parallel incisions in the gallbladder and duodenum and then suturing the two resultant apertures together (Box 31-6). Other authors have reported a technique in which the gallbladder is first sutured to the duodenum and then the incisions are made into the lumens for stoma creation.[3,28] This creates a two-layer closure but there has been no evidence that this technique is preferable and it adds to surgical trauma as well as potentially decreases the size of the stoma.[7,28,110] A newer technique recently reported the use of a 30 mm endoscopic gastrointestinal anastomosis (GIA) stapling device to perform a CCD in 28 dogs.[113] The overall survival rate in this study was 64%, which is similar to other studies but this technique has not been reported in cats.

Cholecystojejunostomy (CCJ) can be performed in a similar manner to CCD but leads to bile being emptied into the jejunum, which is less physiologic. Maldigestion of lipids and an increased incidence in duodenal ulceration have been described with this technique.[3,7] An alternative technique in which an isoperistaltic antireflux (Roux-en-Y) loop is utilized have also been described (Box 31-6).[7,110] This technique is performed to decrease or prevent intestinal reflux into the biliary system but may lead to overgrowth of bacteria due to stagnant intestinal contents or short bowel syndrome, as the resected segment is usually more than half the length of the jejunum.[7]

Choledochoenterostomy (Box 31-6) is best performed if the CBD is dilated to at least 1 cm and a stoma of approximately 2.5 cm can be created.[7] The size of the CBD in small animals makes choledochoenterotomies difficult. Care should be taken if the CBD must be resected to try to preserve the major pancreatic duct and all hepatic lobar ducts emptying into it. If the pancreatic duct must be ligated, pancreatitis and pancreatic exocrine insufficiency should be anticipated.

Repair of common bile duct trauma

The techniques to repair the CBD are dependent on the location and severity of the injury. If the injury is severe and distal to the hepatic ducts, the duct should be ligated and a biliary diversion procedure is recommended (Box 31-6).[3,7] Incidence of leakage and dehiscence is reportedly high for primary repairs, and placement of stents (as described above) across the incision line is recommended by one reference.[7] The ends of the CBD are identified, the edges debrided if necessary and reapposed, paying close attention to avoid tension as this will lead to an increased risk of stricture. The ends are sutured in a simple interrupted pattern using absorbable suture (5/0 to 6/0).

Sphincterotomy/plasty

Sphincterotomy is a procedure performed through a duodenotomy in which the duodenal surface of the major duodenal papilla is enlarged.[7] The sphincter mechanism is destroyed by this procedure and intestinal reflux is expected. Indications are limited to causes of intraluminal obstructions (partial or complete), which are rare (choledocholithiasis, inflammatory bowel disease, neoplasia).[97] After a routine duodenotomy, the major duodenal papilla is identified and cannulated. The catheter is then removed and one blade of a Metzenbaum or Iris scissor is placed within the intraluminal bile duct and incised through the sphincter and duodenal mucosa. This incision is not full thickness through the wall of the bile duct or duodenum and careful attention should be paid to try to avoid the pancreatic duct, which enters at the same location. Sphincteroplasty utilizes the same technique as above except that the incised mucosa of the bile duct is sutured to the incised mucosa of the duodenum with fine (6/0) absorbable suture. This technique has not been reported in cats but does carry the potential advantage of maintaining the stoma for longer periods of time.[7]

HEPATOBILIARY SURGICAL COMPLICATIONS

Hemorrhage is the most common complication reported in both human and canine patients following liver lobectomy.[114,115] Following liver biopsy or lobectomy, patients should be monitored closely for bleeding and serial measurement of packed cell volume is warranted. Intraoperative techniques to control acute hemorrhage, such as temporary occlusion of the hepatic artery and portal vein are detailed in Box 31-2. At the time of surgery, several techniques can be used to reinforce biopsy or staple lines. Minor bleeding may be controlled with electrocautery, hemostatic clips or suture material. A small piece of absorbable gelatin foam (Gelfoam) can also be used to control hemorrhage. Alternatively, oxidized regenerated cellulose (Surgicel) may be used and has an antibacterial effect due to its lower pH.[79] Hepatic abscessation in conjunction with the use of gelatin sponges has been reported.[79,116] A study of coagulation abnormalities in 22 cats with liver disease found that at least one coagulation abnormality was present in 82% of feline patients, including prolongation of prothrombin time, diminished factor VII activity, and vitamin K deficiency. Cats that had marked increases in alkaline phosphatase activity were more likely to have coagulation abnormalities.[117] There is no indication, however, that cats have more complications with bleeding following hepatic surgery than dogs. Overall rate of complication in dogs following hepatic lobectomies is low, with only three of 18 dogs requiring blood transfusions following surgery.[115] No similar data for feline patients is available.

Other postoperative considerations include close monitoring following anesthetic recovery due to the increased half-life of many drugs in animals with hepatic dysfunction.[3] Additionally, transient hypoglycemia may occur within 48 hours of partial hepatectomy.[7] Postoperative glucose supplementation should be considered with large resections. Other reported postoperative metabolic alterations following hepatectomy include glucagon elevation, hypoalbuminemia and an increase in ALP and ALT concentrations following removal of 70% of the liver in dogs.[7]

Following hepatobiliary procedures, patients should be kept on intravenous fluid support, with close monitoring of protein levels and blood pressure. As mentioned previously, many of these patients have difficulty maintaining normal blood pressure and will require interventions such as vasopressor support. Some patients will require critical care postoperatively involving blood or plasma transfusions and enteral or parenteral nutrition. Broad-spectrum antibiotics are of special importance to animals undergoing biliary diversion surgeries due to the potential for ascending infections. Administration of gastroprotectants such as sucralfate and pepcid are recommended due to the high incidence of gastrointestinal ulceration.

REFERENCES

1. Zawie DA, Shaker E. Diseases of the liver. In: Sherding RG, editor. The cat disease and clinical management, 1st ed, vol. 2. New York: Churchill Livingston; 1989. p. 1015–36.

2. Done SH, Goody PC, Evans AE, Stickland NC. The cat. In: Done SH, Goody PC, Evans AE, Stickland NC, editors. Veterinary anatomy of the dog and cat, 1st ed, vol. 3. London: Mosby-Wolfe; 1996. p. 10.22–10.23.

3. Fossum TW. Surgery of the liver. In: Fossum TW, editor. Small animal surgery, 3rd ed, vol. 1. St Louis: Mosby; 2007. p. 531–59.

4. Swann HM, Brown DC. Hepatic lobe torsion in 3 dogs and a cat. Vet Surg 2001;30:482–6.

5. Evans HE. The digestive apparatus and abdomen. In: Evans HE, editor. Miller's anatomy of the dog, 3rd ed, vol. 1. Philadelphia: WB Saunders; 1993. p. 451–8.

6. Center S. Diseases of the gallbladder and biliary tree. In: Guillford WA, Center SA, Williams DA, Meyer DJ, editors. Strombeck's small animal gastroenterology. 3rd ed. Philadelphia: WB Saunders; 1996. p. 860–88.

7. Martin RA, Lanz OI, Tobias KM. Liver and biliary system. In: Slatter D, editor. Textbook of small animal surgery, 3rd ed, vol. 1. Philadelphia: Saunders; 2003. p. 708–26.

8. Moores AL, Gregory SP. Duplex gallbladder associated with choledocholithiasis, cholecystitis, gallbladder rupture and septic peritonitis in a cat. J Small Anim Pract 2007;48: 404–9.

9. Zawie DA, Garvey MS. Feline hepatic disease. Vet Clin North Am Small Anim Pract 1984;14:1201–30.

10. Neer TM. A review of disorders of the gallbladder and extrahepatic biliary tract in the dog and cat. J Vet Int Med 1992;6:186–92.

11. Smith SA, Biller DS, Kraft SL, et al. Diagnostic imaging of biliary obstruction. Compend Cont Educ Pract Vet 1998;20:1225–34.

12. Wrigley RH. Radiographic and ultrasonographic diagnosis of liver diseases in dogs and cats. Vet Clin North Am Small Anim Pract 1985;15: 21–38.

13. Nakamura K, Takagi S, Sasaki N, et al. Contrast-enhanced ultrasonography for characterization of canine focal liver lesions. Vet Radiol Ultrasound 2010;51: 79–85.

14. Hittmair KM, Vielgrader HD, Loupal G. Ultrasonographic evaluation of gallbladder wall thickness in cats. Vet Rad Ultrasound 2001;42:149–55.

15. Gaillot HA, Penninck DG, Webster CR, Crawford S. Ultrasonographic features of extrahepatic biliary obstruction in 30 cats. Vet Radiol Ultrasound 2007;48: 439–47.

16. Savary-Bataille KCM, Bunch SE, Spaulding KA, et al. Percutaneous ultrasound-guided cholecystocentesis in healthy cats. J Vet Intern Med 2003;17: 298–303.

17. Wagner KA, Hartmann FA, Trepanier LA. Bacterial culture results from liver, gallbladder, or bile in 248 dogs and cats evaluated for hepatobiliary disease: 1998–2003. J Vet Intern Med 2007;21: 417–24.

18. Brain PH, Barrs VR, Martin P, et al. Feline cholecystitis and acute neutrophilic cholangitis: clinical findings, bacterial isolates and response to treatment in six cases. J Feline Med Surg 2006;8:91–103.

19. Boothe HW, Boothe DM, Komkov A, Hightower D. Use of hepatobiliary scintigraphy in the diagnosis of extrahepatic biliary obstruction in dogs and cats: 25 cases (1982–1989). J Am Vet Med Assoc 1992;201: 134–41.

20. Head LL, Daniel GB. Correlation between hepatobiliary scintigraphy and surgery or postmortem examination findings in dogs and cats with extrahepatic biliary obstruction, partial obstruction, or patency of the biliary system: 18 cases (1995–2004). J Am Vet Med Assoc 2005;227:1618–24.

21. Gaschen L. Update on hepatobiliary imaging. Vet Clin North Am Small Anim Pract 2009;39:439–67.

22. Park SJ, Han JK, Kim TK, Choi BI. Three-dimensional spiral CT cholangiography with minimum intensity projection in patients with suspected obstructive biliary disease: comparison with percutaneous transhepatic cholangiography. Abdom Imaging 2001;26:281–6.

23. Fleischmann D, Ringl H, Schöfl R, et al. Three-dimensional spiral CT cholangiography in patients with suspected obstructive biliary disease: comparison with endoscopic retrograde cholangiography. Radiology 1996;198: 861–68.

24. Spillmann T, Happonen I, Kähkönen T, et al. Endoscopic retrograde cholangio-pancreatography in healthy beagles. Vet Radiol Ultrasound 2005;46:97–104.

25. Spillman T, Schnell-Kretschmer H, Dick M, et al. Endoscopic retrograde cholangio-pancreatography in dogs with chronic gastrointestinal problems. Vet Radiol Ultrasound 2005;46:293–9.

26. Bjorling DE, Prasse KW, Holmes RA. Partial hepatectomy in dogs. Compend Cont Educ Pract Vet 1985;7: 257–63.

27. Posner LP, Asakawa M, Erb HN. Use of propofol for anesthesia in cats with primary hepatic lipidosis: 44 cases (1995–2004). J Am Vet Med Assoc 2008;232:1841–3.

28. Bjorling DE. Surgical management of hepatic and biliary disease in cats. Compend North Am Small Anim 1991;9:1419–25.

29. Utkan ZN, Utkan T, Sarioglu Y, Gönüllü NN. Effects of experimental obstructive jaundice on contractile responses of dog isolated blood vessels: role of endothelium and duration of bile duct ligation. Clin Exp Pharmacol Physiol 2000;27:339–44.

30. Schafer J, d'Almeida MS, Weisman H, Lautt WW. Hepatic blood volume responses and compliance in cats with long-term bile duct ligation. Hepatology 1993;8:969–77.

31. Friedman LS. The risk of surgery in patients with liver disease. Hepatology 1999;29:1617–23.

32. Green J, Beyar R, Sideman S, et al. The jaundiced heart: a possible explanation for postoperative shock in obstructive jaundice. Surgery 1986;100:14–20.

33. Rege RV. Adverse effects of biliary obstruction: implications for treatment of patients with obstructive jaundice. Am J Roentol 1995;164:287–93.

34. Bomzon A, Rosenberg M, Gali D, et al. Systemic hypotension and decreased pressor response in dogs with chronic bile duct ligation. Hepatology 1986;6: 595–600.

35. Buote NJ, Mitchell SL, Penninck D, et al. Cholecystoenterostomy for treatment of extrahepatic biliary tract obstruction in cats: 22 cases (1994–2003). J Am Vet Med Assoc 2006;228:1376–82.

36. Mayhew PD, Holt DE, McLear RC, Washabau RJ. Pathogenesis and outcome of extrahepatic biliary obstruction in cats. J Small Anim Pract 2002;43: 247–53.

37. Green J, Better O. Systemic hypotension and renal failure in obstructive jaundice – mechanistic and therapeutic aspects. J Am Soc Nephrol 1995;5:1853–71.

38. Beatty JA, Barrs VR, Martin PA, et al. Spontaneous hepatic rupture in six cats with systemic amyloidosis. J Small Anim Pract 2002;43:355–63.

39. Krige JE, Bornman PC, Terblanche J. Liver trauma in 446 patients. S Afr J Surg 1997;35:10–15.

40. Zatelli A, D'Ippolito P, Bonfanti U, Zini E. Ultrasound-assisted drainage and alcoholization of hepatic and renal cysts: 22 cases. J Am Anim Hosp Assoc 2007;43:112–16.

41. Terada N, Shimizu T, Imai Y, et al. Benign, non-parasitic hepatic cyst causing obstructive jaundice. Intern Med 1993;32:857–60.

42. Washizu M, Kobayashi K, Misaka K, et al. Surgery of hepatic cysts in a cat. J Vet Med Sci 1992;54:1051–3.

43. Friend EJ, Niles JD, Williams JM. Omentalisation of congenital liver cysts in a cat. Vet Rec 2001;149:275–6.

44. Liptak JM, Bissett SA, Allan GS, et al. Hepatic cysts incarcerated in a peritoneopericardial diaphragmatic hernia. J Feline Med Surg 2002;4:123–5.

45. Sergeeff JS, Armstrong PJ, Bunch SE. Hepatic abscesses in cats: 14 cases (1985–2002). J Vet Intern Med 2004;18: 295–300.

46. Balint TD, Bailey BM, Mendelson KG, Pofahl W. Hepatic abscess: Current concepts in diagnosis and treatment. Curr Surg 2001;58:381–4.

47. Perez B, Velasco RN, Marine RE. Solitary pyogenic abscess of the left lobe of the liver. Rev Sanid Milit Argent 1953;52: 5–8.

48. Klatchko BA, Schwartz SI. Diagnostic and therapeutic approaches to pyogenic abscess of the liver. Surg Gynecol Obstet 1989;168:332–6.

49. Farrar ET, Washabau RJ, Saunders HM. Hepatic abscesses in dogs: 14 cases (1982–1994). J Am Vet Med Assoc 1996;208:243–7.

50. Zatelli A, Bonfanti U, Zini E, et al. Percutaneous drainage and alcoholization of hepatic abscesses in five dogs and a cat. J Am Anim Hosp Assoc 2005;41:34–8.

51. Schwartz SG, Mitchell SL, Keating JH, Chan DL. Liver lobe torsion in dogs: 13

cases (1995–2004). J Am Vet Med Assoc 2006;228:242–7.

52. Morin M, Sauvageau R, Phaneuf JB, et al. Torsion of abdominal organs in sows: a report of 36 cases. Can Vet J 1984;25: 440–2.

53. Turner TA, Brown CA, Wilson JH, et al. Hepatic lobe torsion as a cause of colic in a horse. Vet Surg 1993;22:301–4.

54. Tate PS. Hepatic torsion and dislocation with hypotension and colonic obstruction. Am Surg 1993;59:455–8.

55. McConkey S, Briggs C, Solano M, Illanes O. Liver torsion and associated bacterial peritonitis in a dog. Can Vet J 1997;38: 438–9.

56. Balkman C. Hepatobiliary neoplasia in dogs and cats. Vet Clin North Am Small Anim Pract 2009;39:617–25.

57. Patnaik AK, Lieberman PH, Erlandson RA, Antonescu C. Hepatobiliary neuroendocrine carcinoma in cats: a clinicopathologic, immunohistochemical, and ultrastructural study of 17 cases. Vet Pathol 2005;42:331–7.

58. Lawrence HJ, Erb HN, Harvey HJ. Nonlymphomatous hepatobiliary masses in cats: 41 cases (1972 to 1991). Vet Surg 1994;23:365–8.

59. Schuh JC. Hepatic nodular myelolipomatosis (myelolipomas) associated with a peritoneo-pericardial diaphragmatic hernia in a cat. J Comp Pathol 1987;97:231–5.

60. McCaw DL, da Silva Curiel JM, Shaw DP. Hepatic myelolipomas in a cat. J Am Vet Med Assoc 1990;197:243–4.

61. Patnaik AK. A morphologic and immunocytochemical study of hepatic neoplasms in cats. Vet Pathol 1992;29: 405–15.

62. Gabor LJ, Malik R, Canfield PJ. Clinical and anatomical features of lymphosarcoma in 118 cats. Aust Vet J 1998;76:725–32.

63. Kiselow MA, Rassnick KM, McDonough SP, et al. Outcome of cats with low-grade lymphocytic lymphoma: 41 cases (1995–2005). J Am Vet Med Assoc 2008;232:405–10.

64. Whiteley MB, Feeney DA, Whiteley LO, Hardy RM. Ultrasonographic appearance of primary and metastatic canine hepatic tumors A review of 48 cases. J Ultrasound Med 1989;8:621–30.

65. Weisse C. Hepatic chemoembolization: a novel regional therapy. Vet Clin North Am Small Anim Pract 2009;39:627–30.

66. Rawlings CA, Howerth EW. Obtaining quality biopsies of the liver and kidney. J Am Anim Hosp Assoc 2004;40:352–8.

67. Wang KY, Panciera DL, Al-Rukibat RK, Radi ZA. Accuracy of ultrasound-guided fine-needle aspiration of the liver and cytologic findings in dogs and cats: 97 cases (1990–2000). J Am Vet Med Assoc 2004;224:75–8.

68. Willard MD, Weeks BR, Johnson M. Fine-needle aspirate cytology suggesting hepatic lipidosis in four cats with infiltrative hepatic disease. J Feline Med Surg 1999;1:215–20.

69. Vasanjee SC, Bubenik LJ, Hosgood G, Bauer R. Evaluation of hemorrhage, sample size, and collateral damage for five hepatic biopsy methods in dogs. Vet Surg 2006;35:86–93.

70. Rothuizen J, Twedt DC. Liver biopsy techniques. Vet Clin North Am Small Anim Pract 2009;39:469–80.

71. Bravo AA, Sheth SG, Chopra S. Liver biopsy. N Engl J Med 2001;344: 495–500.

72. Mayhew P. Surgical views: techniques for laparoscopic and laparoscopic assisted biopsy of abdominal organs. Compend Contin Educ Vet 2009;31:170–6.

73. Cole TL, Center SA, Flood SN, et al. Diagnostic comparison of needle and wedge biopsy specimens of the liver in dogs and cats. J Am Vet Med Assoc 2002;220:1483–90.

74. Proot SJ, Rothuizen J. High complication rate of an automatic Tru-Cut biopsy gun device for liver biopsy in cats. J Vet Intern Med 2006;20:1327–33.

75. Petre SP, McClaran JK, Bergman PJ, Monette S. Safety and efficacy of laparoscopic hepatic biopsy. J Am Vet Med Assoc 2012;240:181–5.

76. Tobias KM. Liver biopsy. In: Tobias KM, editor. Manual of small animal soft tissue surgery, 1st ed, vol. 1. Ames: Wiley–Blackwell; 2010. p. 131–2.

77. Risselada M, Ellison GW, Bacon NJ, et al. Comparison of 5 surgical techniques for partial liver lobectomy in the dog for intraoperative blood loss and surgical time. Vet Surg 2010;39:856–62.

78. Covey JL, Degner DA, Jackson AH, et al. Hilar liver resection in dogs. Vet Surg 2009;38:104–11.

79. Lewis DD, Bellenger CR, Lewis DT, Latter MR. Hepatic lobectomy in the dog A comparison of stapling and ligation techniques. Vet Surg 1990;19:221–5.

80. Bellah JR. Surgical stapling of the spleen, pancreas, liver, and urogenital tract. Vet Clin North Am Small Anim Pract 1994;24:375–94.

81. Lewis DD, Ellison GW, Bellah JR. Partial hepatectomy using stapling instruments. J Am Anim Hosp Assoc 1987;23: 597–602.

82. Bennett SL, Milne M, Slocombe RF, Landon BP. Gallbladder mucocoele and concurrent hepatic lipidosis in a cat. Aust Vet J 2007;85:397–400.

83. van Geffen C, Savary-Bataille K, Chiers K, et al. Bilirubin cholelithiasis and haemosiderosis in an anaemic pyruvate kinase-deficient Somali cat. J Small Anim Pract 2008;49:479–82.

84. Elwood CM, White RN, Freeman K, White M. Cholelithiasis and hyperthyroidism in a cat. J Feline Med Surg 2001;3:247–52.

85. Harvey AM, Holt PE, Barr FJ, et al. Treatment and long-term follow-up of extrahepatic biliary obstruction with bilirubin cholelithiasis in a Somali cat with pyruvate kinase deficiency. J Fel Med Surg 2007;9:424–31.

86. Eich CS, Ludwig LL. The surgical treatment of cholelithiasis in cats: a study of nine cases. J Am Anim Hosp Assoc 2002;38:290–5.

87. Naus MJA, Jones BR. Cholelithiasis and choledocholithiasis in a cat. NZ Vet J 1978;26:160–1.

88. Jorgensen LS, Pentlarge VW, Flanders JA, Harvey HJ. Recurrent cholelithiasis in a cat. Comp Cont Educ Pract Vet 1987;9: 265–70.

89. Best EJ, Bush DJ, Dye C. Suspected choledochal cyst in a domestic shorthair cat. J Fel Med Surg 2010;12:814–17.

90. Grand JG, Doucet M, Albaric O, Bureau S. Cyst of the common bile duct in a cat. Aust Vet J 2010;88:268–71.

91. Stimson EL, Cook WT, Smith MM, et al. Extraskeletal osteosarcoma in the duodenum of a cat. J Am Anim Hosp Assoc 2000;36:332–6.

92. Geigy CA, Dandrieux J, Miclard J, et al. Extranodal B-cell lymphoma in urinary bladder with cytological evidence of concurrent involvement of the gall bladder in a cat. J Small Anim Pract 2010;51:280–7.

93. Haney DR, Christiansen JS, Toll J. Severe cholestatic liver disease secondary to liver fluke (Platynosomum concinnum) infection in three cats. J Am Anim Hosp Assoc 2006;42:234–37.

94. Della Santa D, Schweighauser A, Forterre F, Lang J. Extrahepatic biliary tract obstruction secondary to a duodenal foreign body in a cat. Vet Radiol Ultrasound 2007;48:448–50.

95. Jenkins CC, Lewis DD, Brock KA, et al. Extrahepatic biliary obstruction associated with Platynosomum concinnum in a cat. Compend Contin Educ Pract Vet 1988;10:628–32.

96. Cornell KK, Jakovljevic S, Waters DJ, et al. Extrahepatic Biliary Obstruction secondary to diaphragmatic hernia in two cats. J Am Anim Hosp Assoc 1993;29:502–7.

97. Furneaux RW. A series of six cases of sphincter of Oddi pathology in the cat (2008–2009). J Feline Med and Surg 2010;12:794–801.

98. Herman BA, Brawer RS, Murtaugh RJ, Hackner SG. Therapeutic percutaneous ultrasound-guided cholecystocentesis in three dogs with extrahepatic biliary obstruction and pancreatitis. J Am Vet Med Assoc 2005;227:1782–86.

99. Bacon NJ, White RS. Extrahepatic biliary tract surgery in the cat: a case series and review. J Small Anim Pract 2003;44: 231–35.

100. Ludwig LL, McLoughlin MA, Graves TK, Crisp MS. Surgical treatment of bile peritonitis in 24 dogs and 2 cats: a retrospective study (1987–1994). Vet Surg 1997;26:90–8.

101. Aly EAH, Johnson CD. Preoperative biliary drainage before resection in obstructive jaundice. Dig Surg 2000;18: 84–9.

102. van Sonnenberg E, D'Agostino HB, Casola G, et al. The benefits of percutaneous cholecystostomy for decompression of selected cases of obstructive jaundice. Radiology 1990;176:15–18.

103. Pitt HA, Cameron JL, Postier RG, Gadacz TR. Factors affecting mortality in biliary tract surgery. Am J Surg 1981;141: 66–72.

104. Kawarada Y, Higashiguchi T, Yokoi H, et al. Preoperative biliary drainage in obstructive jaundice. Hepatogastroenterology 1995;42: 300–7.

105. Sewnath ME, Karsten TM, Prins MH, et al. A meta-analysis on the efficacy of preoperative biliary drainage for tumors causing obstructive jaundice. Ann Surg 2002;236:17–27.

106. Lawrence D, Bellah JR, Meyer DJ, Roth L. Temporary bile diversion in cats with experimental extrahepatic bile duct obstruction. Vet Surg 1992;21:446–51.

107. Murphy SM, Rodríguez JD, McAnulty JF. Minimally invasive cholecystostomy in the dog: evaluation of placement techniques and use in extrahepatic biliary obstruction. Vet Surg 2007;36: 675–83.

108. Mayhew PD, Weisse CW. Treatment of pancreatitis-associated extrahepatic biliary tract obstruction by choledochal stenting in seven cats. J Small Anim Pract 2008;49:133–8.

109. Mayhew PD, Richardson RW, Mehler SJ, et al. Choledochal tube stenting for decompression of the extrahepatic portion of the biliary tract in dogs: 13 cases (2002–2005). J Am Vet Med Assoc 2006;228:1209–14.

110. Blass CE. Surgery of the extrahepatic biliary tract. Compend Contin Educ 1983;10:801–9.

111. Mayhew PD, Mehler SJ, Radhakrishnan A. Laparoscopic cholecystectomy for management of uncomplicated gall bladder mucocele in six dogs. Vet Surg 2008;37:625–30.

112. Tanger CH, Turrell JM, Hobson HP. Complications associated with proximal duodenal resection and cholecystoduodenostomy in two cats. Vet Surg 1982;11:60–4.

113. Morrison S, Prostredny J, Roa D. Retrospective study of 28 cases of cholecystoduodenostomy performed using endoscopic gastrointestinal anastomosis stapling equipment. J Am Anim Hosp Assoc 2008;44: 10–18.

114. Voyles CR, Vogel SB. Hepatic resection using stapling devices to control the hepatic veins. Am J Surg 1989;158: 459–60.

115. Kosovsky JE, Manfra-Marretta S, Matthiesen DT, et al. Results of partial hepatectomy in 18 dogs with hepatocellular carcinoma. J Am Anim Hosp Assoc 1989;25:203–6.

116. Lipowitz AJ, Blue J. Spleen. In: Slatter DH, editor. Textbook of small animal surgery, 2nd ed, vol. 1. Philadelphia: WB Saunders; 1993. p. 948–61.

117. Lisciandro SC, Hohenhaus A, Brooks M. Coagulation abnormalities in 22 cats with naturally occurring liver disease. J Vet Intern Med 1998;12:71–5.

Chapter |32|

Portosystemic shunts

V. Lipscomb, M.S. Tivers

'Portosystemic shunting' is a broad term that has several possible underlying causes. In cats the main cause of portosystemic shunting is a congenital portosystemic shunt (CPSS), although even this is seen uncommonly, with a reported incidence of 2.5 per 10 000 cats treated in referral practice.[1] This chapter provides a comprehensive summary of feline shunts, their diagnosis and surgical management.

SURGICAL ANATOMY

A CPSS is an abnormal communicating vessel between the portal vasculature (draining the stomach, intestines, spleen, and pancreas) and the systemic vasculature. The abnormal vessel results in the diversion of blood away from the portal blood system into the systemic system, thus bypassing the liver and resulting in high levels of waste products (such as ammonia) being present in the systemic circulation which manifest clinically as signs of hepatic encephalopathy. Cats with CPSS also have reduced blood supply to the liver via the portal vein and therefore the liver is not stimulated to develop in a normal fashion. This results in a small, underdeveloped liver and functional hepatic insufficiency.

Normal feline portal vein and caudal vena cava anatomy is depicted in Fig. 32-1. CPSS can take the form of an extrahepatic (outside the hepatic parenchyma) or an intrahepatic (lying partly or wholly within the hepatic parenchyma) vessel. Extrahepatic CPSSs are the most common form, accounting for 73–100% of CPSSs in cats.[1-11] The most commonly reported extrahepatic CPSS in cats is an abnormal vessel connecting the left gastric vein to the caudal vena cava[6,9,12,13] (Fig. 32-1B). Other extrahepatic shunt morphologies described in cats include porto-azygous, portocaval and shunting vessels between the colonic vein or gastrosplenic vein and caudal vena cava.[7,8,10,12,14,15] The majority of intrahepatic CPSSs in cats are due to a patent ductus venosus (PDV), which results from failure of this normal embryonic vessel, on the left side of the liver, to close after birth[16,17] (Fig. 32-1C). Right-sided and centrally located intrahepatic shunts have also been reported in cats.

DIAGNOSIS AND GENERAL CONSIDERATIONS

Signalment and clinical signs

Cats with a CPSS are typically young (under six months of age) but the condition is also recognized in mature animals which may not have exhibited clinical signs for months or years.[1,6,7,10,12,14,15,17-20] Although the majority of affected cats are domestic short-haired breeds, a number of pedigree breeds have been suggested as being predisposed, including the Persian, Himalayan, and Siamese.[1,6,8,10-12,17,20,21]

The clinical signs associated with a CPSS can be variable and non-specific. Signs often wax and wane and can be intermittent. Some cats can essentially appear 'normal' and the condition may only be identified as a result of abnormalities seen on routine blood tests in older cats. However, the vast majority of cats (93–100%) present with some degree of neurologic abnormality due to hepatic encephalopathy: including seizures, ataxia, central blindness, behavioral changes, aggression, lethargy, head pressing, and tremors.[5-7,12,20] These neurological signs are typically intermittent and can be triggered by or worsen following feeding, gastrointestinal bleeding, or azotemia.[1,5,18]

The pathogenesis of hepatic encephalopathy (HE) is poorly understood and it is likely that multiple factors are involved. HE results from the failure of the liver to remove toxic products of gut metabolism from the portal blood and also from the failure of the liver to produce factors important for normal brain function. One of the major factors contributing to HE is ammonia but several other factors have been implicated including aromatic amino acids (phenylalanine, tyrosine, tryptophan, and methionine), central nervous system inhibitors (gamma-aminobutyric acid [GABA] and GABA receptors), mercaptans, and increased short chain fatty acids. It is believed that several of these factors act synergistically in a given animal with HE and this may partly explain the variation in clinical signs between individuals.

Another hallmark of CPSS is ptyalism (hypersalivation), which is reported in 67–84% of cats.[5,7,10,12] Cats may be small or stunted with

© 2014 Elsevier Ltd
DOI: 10.1016/B978-0-7020-4336-9.00032-9

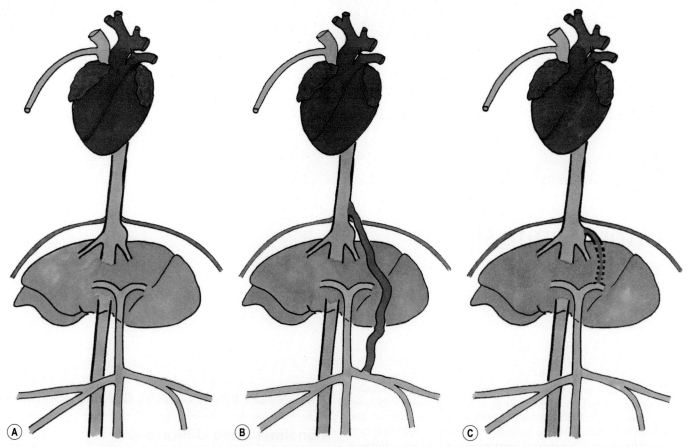

Figure 32-1 Feline portal vein anatomy and congenital portosystemic shunts. **(A)** Normal feline portal vein and caudal vena cava anatomy. **(B)** The most common extrahepatic CPSS in cats is an abnormal vessel between the left gastric vein and the caudal vena cava. **(C)** The most common intrahepatic CPSS in cats is a PDV, which empties into a venous dilatation (ampulla) just prior to entering the caudal vena cava in a post-hepatic location in front of the diaphragm.

a low body condition score, have copper-colored irises (13–64%) (Fig. 32-2), or intolerance to anesthetics or sedatives.[1,6,7,10,12,13,18,20] Other clinical signs include gastrointestinal signs (vomiting and diarrhea), urinary tract signs (dysuria, hematuria or stranguria relating to urate urolithaisis), and polyuria/polydipsia, but these signs are not as commonly seen in cats as in dogs.[1,6,7,12]

Biochemical and hematological investigations

Biochemical and hematological changes are typically mild and non-specific and may be largely unremarkable in cats with CPSS. Performing routine hematological and biochemical analysis of blood may be most useful to rule out other differential diagnoses in the investigation of cats with suspected CPSS. The most common abnormality is low urea due to reduced synthesis of urea in the liver as the product of ammonia metabolism (Krebs–Henseleit urea cycle).[10,12,13,22] Hypoalbuminemia, hypoproteinemia, hypoglycemia and anemia are less frequently reported compared with dogs with CPSS.[1,10,12,13] There have not been any studies examining clotting abnormalities in cats with CPSS but these have been reported in affected dogs.[23,24] The presence of ammonium biurate crystals in urine sediment increases the suspicion of CPSS.

A bile acid stimulation test is the most accurate test available to measure liver function for the diagnosis of hepatobiliary disease. It is very reliable for the diagnosis of portosystemic shunting in cats, with

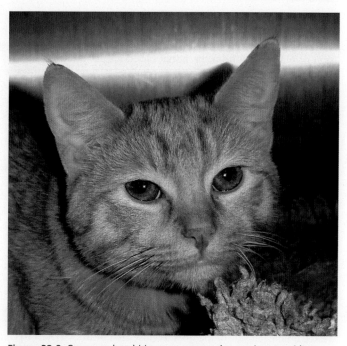

Figure 32-2 Copper-colored irises are commonly seen in cats with a CPSS.

a sensitivity of 58–100% (preprandial) and 100% (postprandial), and a specificity of 84% (fasting).[1,10,12,25,26] Fasting ammonia is increased in the majority of cats with CPSS but can occasionally be normal.[6,10,12,14,18,22,25] The sensitivity and specificity of ammonia for the diagnosis of CPSS in cats has been reported as 83% and 86%, respectively.[25] Ammonia is very labile so samples must be analyzed very quickly e.g., using a 'point of care' ammonia analyzer, which has been shown to have potential in cats.[27]

Differential diagnoses

The most likely diagnosis for portosystemic shunting is a CPSS; other very rare differentials include multiple acquired portosystemic shunts (secondary to severe liver disease and portal hypertension), primary portal vein hypoplasia, and arteriovenous fistula.[2,3,4] Management of multiple acquired shunts involves treatment of the underlying liver disease if possible and medical management of HE (Table 32-1). Primary portal vein hypoplasia was previously called microvascular dysplasia and is described as microscopic portosystemic shunting within the liver which results in similar clinical signs to animals with a gross CPSS and is managed using medical therapy for HE (Table 32-1). In some animals, primary portal vein hypoplasia is associated with hepatic fibrosis and portal hypertension and this can also lead to the development of multiple acquired shunts. Primary portal vein hypoplasia is a specific disease that should not be confused with underdevelopment (unfortunately also referred to as hypoplasia) of the portal vein. Cats with an extrahepatic CPSS often have an underdeveloped/small portal vein secondary to diversion of blood flow away from the portal vein into the shunt. Hepatic arteriovenous fistula is a communication between the arterial and venous systems e.g., hepatic artery to portal vein, and treatment is by removal of the liver lobe(s) containing the abnormal vascular structures.

Diagnostic imaging

Although surgery often allows the direct diagnosis of a CPSS, in most instances some form of preoperative imaging is performed to both confirm the diagnosis before electing to proceed with surgery and to acquire information regarding the nature of the shunt to help with surgical planning.

Plain abdominal radiographs may be performed as part of a diagnostic workup but cannot be used alone to diagnose a CPSS. Abdominal ultrasonography can be extremely useful, particularly as it is relatively inexpensive and non-invasive, but unfortunately it is highly operator dependent. Ultrasonography (Fig. 32-3) has been reported to have a sensitivity and specificity of 100% for shunt diagnosis and type in one study,[20] whereas other studies have only identified approximately 47–50% of CPSS in cats.[1,10] Per rectum portal scintigraphy with technetium pertechnetate ($^{99}Tc^mO_4-$) can be very reliable in the diagnosis of CPSS in cats, with good sensitivity and specificity[1,12,28,29] (see Chapter 8). However, this is not readily available and its use may be limited in some countries by radiation safety guidelines and availability. Scintigraphy does not provide anatomical information regarding the shunt for preoperative surgical planning, although it may have a role in the follow up of surgically treated cats to assess for continued shunting.[29]

Many different techniques involving contrast imaging have been described, including cranial mesenteric angiography, splenoportography, and mesenteric portovenography.[21,30,31] For intraoperative mesenteric portovenography, contrast is injected through a catheter into a jejunal vein and imaged using a mobile fluoroscopy unit or a mobile radiography unit (Fig. 32-4). Intraoperative portography allows the imaging and surgical attenuation of the shunt to be performed concurrently and avoids the necessity to move the cat into radiography for the imaging or the requirement for two procedures.[17] While intraoperative mesenteric portovenography is not essential for every case, it is a quick procedure (approximately ten minutes) and easy to perform with the right equipment.

Confirmation of the presence of a shunt and its morphology using portovenography is particularly useful if a CPSS could not be identified preoperatively and/or if the shunt is not easily identified at surgery (more likely if the shunt is intrahepatic). Additionally, portovenography rules out the presence of a second congenital shunt (very rare) or multiple acquired shunts (these may be mistaken for a CPSS

Table 32-1 Recommendations for medical therapy in cats with a CPSS

Medical treatment	Recommendations
Dietary modification (there are a variety of commercially available hepatic diets which may be suitable for cats with CPSS)	Highly digestible, highly palatable Carbohydrate as prime source of calories Protein of high biological value that meets the cat's needs without being excessive High levels of branched chain amino acids and arginine (low levels of aromatic amino acids and methionine)
Lactulose	0.5–2 mL orally two to three times a day (ideally cat produces two to three soft stools daily)
Antibiotics, choose from: Ampicillin Amoxicillin-clavulanate Metronidazole	10–20 mg/kg orally three times daily 12.5 mg/kg orally twice daily 10 mg/kg orally twice daily
Anti-seizure medication (if needed): Phenobarbitone	1.5–3 mg/kg orally twice daily (serum phenobarbitone levels should be measured two to three weeks after starting therapy and the dose adjusted accordingly. Dose may be tapered following prolonged period without seizures (e.g., three to six months)
Levetiracetam	20 mg/kg orally three times daily

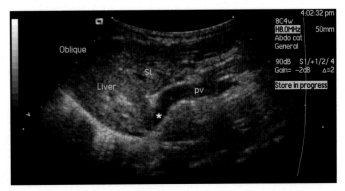

Figure 32-3 Abdominal ultrasound image of a cat with an extrahepatic CPSS. St, stomach; pv, portal vein; *, shunt branching from portal vein and bypassing the liver. *(Courtesy of Chris Lamb.)*

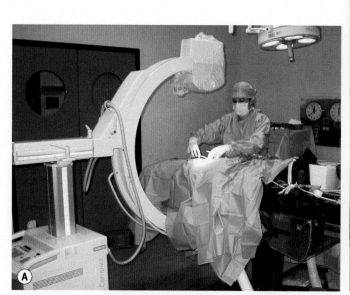
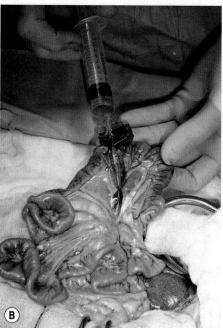

Figure 32-4 (A) The 'C-arm' of a mobile digital fluoroscopy unit has been positioned around the operating table over the region of the shunt. **(B)** Intraoperative portovenograms are then obtained by injecting contrast through a catheter into a jejunal vein.

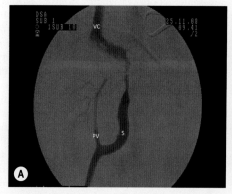
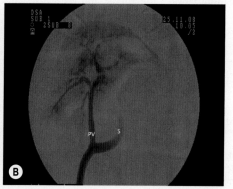

Figure 32-5 Ventrodorsal portovenograms from a cat with a left gastric extrahepatic CPSS. Contrast has been injected through a jejunal vein under fluoroscopic guidance with digital subtraction. The images are orientated so that cranial is at the top. VC, vena cava; PV, portal vein; S, shunt. **(A)** The majority of the contrast flows through the large shunt vessel (S). The portal vein (PV) and its intrahepatic branches are faint (less contrast opacifying them compared to the shunt). There is minimal intrahepatic portal vein branching. **(B)** Repeat portovenogram following temporary intraoperative occlusion of the shunt demonstrates increased contrast opacification of the liver and a vast increase in intrahepatic portal vein branching. There is no contrast progressing beyond the point of temporary shunt attenuation.

if one is much larger than the others). Repeating portovenography after temporary intraoperative occlusion of the shunt confirms the correct vessel has been identified as the shunt and provides an assessment of the degree of intrahepatic portal vascular branching, which may be used to help decide if a CPSS will tolerate complete permanent attenuation (Fig. 32-5). One study examined the extent of intrahepatic vasculature development as assessed on portovenography in cats with CPSS and found it was useful as a prognostic indicator.[6]

There have been reports of the use of computed tomography (CT) angiography or magnetic resonance angiography (MRA) for diagnosing CPSS in dogs.[32,33] Although only one report of the use of CT angiography in a cat with CPSS has been published it is likely that both techniques will be used increasingly to provide a definitive diagnosis

and detailed information regarding shunt morphology and intrahepatic vasculature development prior to surgery.[34]

PREOPERATIVE STABILIZATION

Surgery involving some form of shunt attenuation is the recommended treatment for most cats with a CPSS. The purpose of surgery is to identify the shunting vessel and to attenuate it in order to redirect blood flow to the liver and improve hepatic function. Thus surgical treatment should theoretically offer the best long-term outcome for the individual. There have not been any studies comparing surgical

Table 32-2 Treatment protocol for the collapsed/seizuring cat with a suspected CPSS

1. Physical examination and minimum database	• Check for other causes of neurological signs, not related to CPSS: in particular electrolyte abnormalities or hypoglycemia • Give IV fluid therapy to correct acid–base deficits, dehydration and/or hypovolemia • Supplement with glucose and potassium as necessary
2. If the cat is conscious give oral medication	• Lactulose: 0.5–2 mL two to three times daily • Antibiotics: ampicillin (10–20 mg/kg three times daily), amoxicillin-clavulanate (12.5 mg/kg twice daily) or metronidazole (10 mg/kg twice daily)
3. If the cat is not conscious or unable to take oral medication provide parenteral/rectal drugs	• Cleansing warm water enema: 10 mL/kg • Lactulose: retention enema 20 mL/kg of a 3:7 dilution with water for 30 minutes every six to eight hours • Antibiotics: Intravenous (recommended) amoxicillin-clavulanate 20 mg/kg every eight hours, or a retention enema of neomycin 15 mg/kg diluted with water every six hours • Mannitol: 0.25–0.5 g/kg intravenously over 30 minutes (severe cases with cerebral edema)
4. If the cat is seizuring	• [Diazepam: 0.5–1.0 mg/kg intravenously, repeated up to three times]* • Phenobarbitone: A loading dose of up to a maximum of 8–12 mg/kg should be given as 2–3 mg/kg boluses intravenously as necessary to control the seizures (allow at least 20–30 minutes between doses and reassess the cat prior to dosing). Once loaded, phenobarbitone should be continued at 1.5–3 mg/kg every 12 hours • Propofol: 0.5–1 mg/kg bolus intravenously followed by 0.05–0.4 mg/kg/min infusion titrated to effect • Levetiracetam: 20 mg/kg intravenously or as a retention enema every eight hours followed by same dose orally once recovered

*Note: The use of diazepam in cats with a CPSS is controversial. See the text for a full explanation.

and medical treatment in the cat. However, a study comparing surgical and medical treatment of CPSS in dogs concluded that in terms of overall survival time surgical treatment was preferable.[35]

Stabilization and medical management

Many cats with a CPSS show relatively severe clinical signs at the time of diagnosis and medical management is recommended to stabilize their condition prior to definitive surgical treatment. In one study of 25 cats managed medically prior to surgery there was no response to medical treatment in 12%, a partial response in 56%, and 32% of cats had complete resolution of their clinical signs.[6] Medical management of cats with CPSS treats the signs of HE but does not correct the underlying portosystemic shunting. Medical therapy (see Table 32-1) aims to reduce ammonia (and other toxin) levels, which usually significantly improves the clinical signs of HE.

In some instances cats can be presented collapsed, comatose, or in status epilepticus due to severe HE and in these cats additional investigations and therapies are required (Table 32-2). A minimum database (including blood glucose and serum electrolytes) should be performed to rule out other potential causes of seizure or collapse such as electrolyte abnormalities or hypoglycemia and to identify any complicating factors. Cats should be given intravenous fluid therapy with appropriate supplementation to correct any hypoperfusion, dehydration, or metabolic abnormalities, which may be potentiating the problem. In a comatose or seizuring cat it will not be possible to administer drugs orally and parenteral antibiotics are given, although they are likely to be less efficacious than oral antibiotics. The authors recommend intravenous amoxicillin-clavulanate but neomycin can be given rectally as an alternative. Lactulose can be administered as a retention enema. A warm water cleansing enema is administered prior to medicated enemas. The cleansing enema will remove feces and hence reduce ammonia absorption from the colon. If there is evidence of gastrointestinal hemorrhage then omeprazole (a proton pump inhibitor) is recommended.

Preoperative seizure management

Cats can suffer seizures for a variety of reasons and will often receive diazepam as a first-line treatment. However, there is some controversy over the use of diazepam in cats with CPSS due to concerns over increased GABA and GABA receptors in cats with HE. Cats that do not respond to diazepam and aggressive treatment of HE should be treated with phenobarbitone intravenously. Once the cat is stabilized oral phenobarbitone can be started. If seizures are not controlled by intravenous phenobarbitone administration then it may be necessary to treat the cat with propofol either by bolus or infusion to control the seizures for 24–48 hours before attempting downstaging back to phenobarbitone alone. Propofol infusions should be used with care in cats as prolonged use is associated with delayed recoveries and may in rare cases cause Heinz body anemia. Cats treated with phenobarbitone and propofol infusions should be closely monitored, with regular measurement of pulse rate, respiratory rate, temperature and blood pressure. Endotracheal intubation may be necessary in some instances. Levetiracetam is a relatively new antiseizure medication that has been used in cats, although there are no published reports of its use in cats with HE.[36] In cats with severe HE, cerebral edema can develop and may contribute to neurologic signs. In these situations a single bolus of mannitol can be administered to see if this improves the clinical signs. Mannitol should not be used in severely dehydrated or hypoperfused animals. Monitoring progression and response to therapy of severely encephalopathic cats may be facilitated by use of a modified Glasgow coma scale described in dogs.[37]

PREPARATION FOR SURGERY

Surgical management of CPSS typically requires advanced surgical and critical care facilities: advice on anesthetizing cats with a CPSS is given in Box 32-1. Careful, meticulous planning is required prior to surgery. Shunt attenuation is generally not performed as an emergency

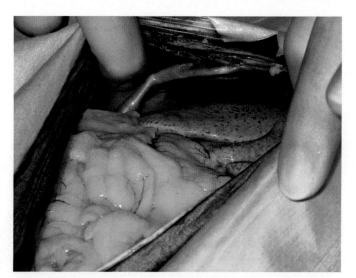

Figure 32-6 Grossly, the liver of a cat with a CPSS is usually small and may demonstrate abnormal color. This picture shows a very pale-colored liver in a cat with a CPSS.

procedure so all the necessary preoperative investigations, blood tests, imaging, and stabilization should have been conducted, and a comprehensive plan made both for surgery and for the postoperative care.

The most important intraoperative considerations should include how to identify the shunt, decide if it is possible to complete or partially attenuate it, and how to assess portal pressure before and after attenuation.

Concurrent procedures during shunt attenuation

Concurrent procedures such as removal of calculi, neutering, and hepatic biopsy may need to be performed. Liver biopsy is recommended at the same time as surgical correction of CPSS in cats. This allows assessment of the underlying pathology and identification of any additional pathology. Grossly, the liver of a cat with a CPSS is usually smaller in size and may have abnormal coloration (Fig. 32-6).

Typical histopathologic changes associated with CPSS include lobular atrophy, hepatocyte degeneration, reduced or absent portal veins, arteriole hyperplasia, biliary hyperplasia, dilated lymphatics, and occasionally mild portal fibrosis.[7,10,22,29] No studies in cats have investigated the relationship, if any, between the histopathologic changes and outcome, although none has been identified in dogs with CPSS.[38,39]

A cat with a CPSS should not be used for breeding and neutering of affected cats should be considered at the same time as shunt attenuation. Cystic calculi can be removed from affected cats at the same time as surgical correction of the CPSS. If the surgery is prolonged or complicated then both neutering and the removal of calculi may be postponed until the cat has recovered sufficiently for a second procedure.

Portal hypertension

Normal portal pressure in cats is between 6 and 10 mmHg. Cats with a CPSS usually have normal or low portal pressure. Low portal pressure in a cat with a CPSS is a result of the majority of the splanchnic circulation being diverted through the shunt, bypassing the portal vein. Portal hypertension is an excessive increase in portal pressure caused by obstruction of the portal vein. Some cats with a CPSS tolerate complete occlusion (obstruction) of the portal vein whereas in others the portal vein is poorly developed (hypoplastic) and unable to accommodate the increased hepatic blood flow resulting from acute occlusion of the CPSS. This causes portal hypertension, which is rapidly fatal if the vessel is left occluded. Portal hypertension can be assessed by direct measurement of portal pressures using a catheter placed in a mesenteric vessel and connected to a manometer or pressure transducer. There is little published information on acceptable increases in portal pressures in the cat. The authors use a combination of values extrapolated from the information available in the cat and those reported for clinical use in dogs[5,17,19,21,40–42] (Box 32-2). It is also recommended to monitor arterial blood pressure (ideally directly via an arterial catheter) and central venous pressure (via a jugular catheter) because excessive portal hypertension should cause a significant drop in both of these measurements. Portal hypertension can also be assessed subjectively by observing the intestines and pancreas, and this is reported to be as reliable as objective measurements.[17,45] Intestinal hypermotility, pulsation in jejunal vessels, and cyanosis of the intestine and pancreas are all associated with portal hypertension. Portal pressure and other objective measurements are influenced by a variety of factors and may not be accurate so they should always be interpreted together with subjective changes and, if available, the appearance of the hepatic vasculature on portovenography.[17]

Development of the portal vein

Some reports have described cats with portal atresia where the portal vein was apparently underdeveloped or absent.[1,8,14] Some of these cats were euthanized due to a perceived poor prognosis. Cats with CPSS are likely to have a degree of underdevelopment (hypoplasia) of the portal vein as a consequence of the shunting vessel. This will vary in severity and in extreme instances the portal vein may appear absent. The authors believe that true portal vein aplasia is extremely uncommon in cats. A very underdeveloped portal vein may not be visible on gross inspection at laparotomy but may become obvious after temporary occlusion of the CPSS. Similarly, studies have shown that although there may be no opacification of the intrahepatic vasculature on portovenography before attenuation there is a significant improvement following temporary occlusion of the CPSS.[6,9]

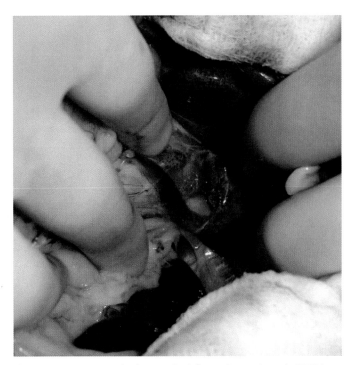

Figure 32-7 Intraoperative image of a left gastric extrahepatic CPSS in a cat. The stomach has been retracted caudally to reveal the large shunt vessel. This shunt is easiest to dissect around surgically cranial to the stomach but caudal to the liver (see also Fig. 32-1B).

SURGICAL MANAGEMENT AND TECHNIQUES

There are a variety of surgical techniques described for the management of CPSS in cats. Making a decision between different techniques is made more difficult by the limited availability of evidence supporting one technique over another. Ideally, a CPSS is attenuated at its point of drainage into the systemic circulation to ensure that any branches to it are also attenuated. However, this is not practical for all types of shunt configuration and in some cats the shunt is attenuated as far cranially as possible, but at least beyond any branches to the shunt (this is very simple to assess if access to intraoperative portovenography is available). Left gastric shunts in cats are usually attenuated cranial to the stomach but caudal to the drainage site in the caudal vena cava, which is relatively inaccessible due to the surrounding liver (Figs 32-1B and 32-7). Conversely, it is possible to attenuate a PDV in cats in a posthepatic location, just in front of the diaphragm, as it enters a venous dilatation/ampulla just prior to entering the caudal vena cava[46] (Fig. 32-1C). The key points in the surgical management of CPSSs in cats are listed in Box 32-3.

Intraoperative complications are not common, but hemorrhage from the shunt is occasionally reported.[6,8,9,12] Surgical dissection around a CPSS (whichever method is chosen for attenuation) must be carefully performed. The dissection is usually uncomplicated for an extrahepatic CPSS (Fig. 32-8) but is more challenging when the CPSS is less accessible (see 'intrahepatic shunts' below).

Partial vs complete attenuation

Several studies have shown that cats with complete CPSS attenuation have a better long-term outcome than those treated with partial attenuation. Cats treated with partial attenuation had a high frequency of relapse of clinical signs which are usually attributable to persistent shunting but may also be due to the development of multiple acquired shunts.[1,5,8,14,19,47] Nevertheless, some cats can have a good outcome following partial attenuation.[14,17,47] It is unclear whether these animals achieve full attenuation with time or whether they cope with a small amount of residual shunting. A second surgery is recommended at a later date to achieve full vessel occlusion, if possible.

Box 32-3 Key points in the surgical management of congenital portosystemic shunts in cats

- Surgical CPSS attenuation is the recommended treatment but the method of choice remains controversial. Cats with a simple extrahepatic CPSS that cannot tolerate complete attenuation at surgery have the option of having a staged suture attenuation (two surgeries), placement of an ameroid constrictor, or placement of a cellophane band. Substantial long-term data that directly compares these techniques is lacking

- Intrahepatic shunts are more challenging to treat surgically. In some instances where space around the CPSS is restricted, attenuation may only be achieved by placement of a suture ligature. A cellophane band is more likely to fit around an intrahepatic shunt than an ameroid constrictor

---

Suture ligation of CPSSs

The surgical technique originally described for cats with CPSS was attenuation of the shunting vessel using a ligature[1,14,18,19,22] (Box 32-4). However, in some cats the hepatic vasculature is poorly developed (hypoplastic) and is unable to accommodate the increased hepatic blood flow resulting from acute occlusion of the CPSS. This causes portal hypertension, which is rapidly fatal if the vessel is left occluded. Consequently complete, acute attenuation of the CPSS is only possible in a proportion of cats. It is therefore important to temporarily occlude the shunting vessel to assess for evidence of portal hypertension prior to deciding whether complete attenuation will be possible (Box 32-5 and Fig. 32-9).

In cats with portal hypertension (either objectively or subjectively) a partial attenuation is performed, which causes an acceptable increase in portal pressure and has no or a minimal effect on the pancreas and

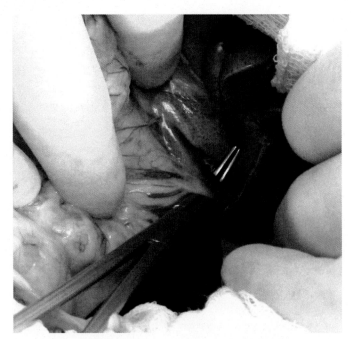

Figure 32-8 Mixter forceps have been used to carefully dissect around the left gastric extrahepatic shunt in this cat.

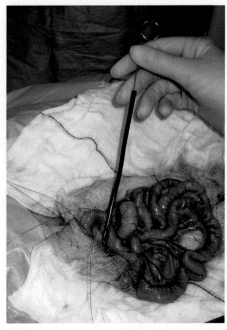

Figure 32-9 Suture material that has been placed around a shunt has been passed through a piece of tubing (Rummel tourniquet) to enable temporary, atraumatic occlusion of the shunting vessel during surgery.

Box 32-4 Surgical attenuation of a single extrahepatic congenital portosystemic shunt

The cat is placed in dorsal recumbency, clipped and prepared for aseptic surgery. A midline laparotomy is made extending from the pubic brim to the xiphisternum. The abdomen is explored for the shunting vessel. An accurate knowledge of normal anatomy is required to be able to identify the abnormal vessel. The descending duodenum is elevated to examine the caudal vena cava at the level of the epiploic foramen for presence of a portocaval shunt entering the caudal vena cava cranial to the right kidney/adrenal gland. The double leaf of greater omentum is perforated and the stomach is retracted caudally to permit visualization of a left gastric portosystemic shunt coursing cranially in front of the stomach to insert on the caudal vena cava in front of the diaphragm (insertion site is not visualized). Intraoperative portovenography may be performed to identify/confirm the shunting vessel by injection of contrast through a catheter placed into a jejunal vein and imaged using a mobile fluoroscopy unit or a mobile radiography unit (Fig. 32-4). Dependent on the protocol adopted once the shunting vessel is identified, it is attenuated by placement of a suture (ligature), an ameroid constrictor, or cellophane band.

The abdomen is inspected for signs of portal hypertension prior to closure.

A liver biopsy is taken (see Chapter 31). If appropriate, removal of cystic calculi or ovariohysterectomy may be performed at this stage. Abdominal closure is routine (see Chapter 23).

Suture ligation

Ligation is achieved by placement of a prolene suture. Whether to go for total occlusion or partial is dependent on several factors. Acute occlusion can be rapidly fatal if it results in portal hypertension. It is important to temporarily occlude the shunting vessel to assess for evidence of portal hypertension prior to deciding whether complete attenuation will be possible (see section on portal hypertension). In cats with portal hypertension (either objectively or subjectively) a partial attenuation is performed, which causes an acceptable increase in portal pressure and has no or a minimal effect on the pancreas and intestines. In cats that only have partial ligation performed a second piece of suture material can be left around the shunting vessel. This can then be tied at a second surgery and preplacement avoids the need for further dissection around the shunt.

Ameroid constrictor (AR) and cellophane banding (CB)

The aim with ameroid constrictors or CB is that they will cause gradual occlusion of the shunt over time, thus potentially avoiding the negative effects of acute occlusion and allowing a gradual development in hepatic vasculature. Some surgeons simply place an AR or CB around a CPSS without measuring portal pressure and without any initial shunt attenuation, others recommend measuring portal pressure and performing temporary complete CPSS occlusion regardless in all cases. Any cat that can tolerate complete shunt occlusion will have a better prognosis than with gradual shunt occlusion, thus temporary intraoperative shunt occlusion is recommended in all cats for the reasons outlined in Box 32-5. A 5 mm constrictor is most commonly used (although sizes used in cats range from 2–6.5mm)[10] – placement can be tricky and it is important to limit dissection around the vessel so there is less chance for the constrictor to move and acutely occlude the shunt. Excess cellophane is cut approximately a centimeter distal to the surgical clips.

For CB a three-layer strip of cellophane approximately 10 cm long and 4 mm wide is placed around the shunt and secured with surgical clips to achieve a degree of partial attenuation, depending on evidence of portal hypertension.

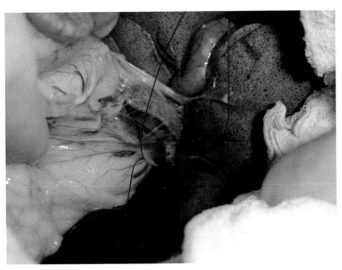

Figure 32-10 Two lengths of polypropylene suture have been passed around the shunting vessel to allow temporary occlusion and subsequent ligation.

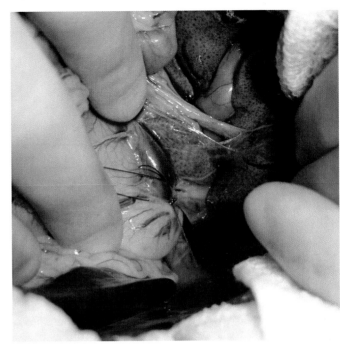

Figure 32-11 Complete occlusion of the abnormal vessel was tolerated in this cat so the suture has been tied tightly. The other length of suture will be removed prior to routine abdominal closure.

Box 32-5 Temporary complete CPSS occlusion in cats

The advantages of measuring portal pressure and performing temporary complete CPSS occlusion in cats are:

- Any cat that can tolerate a complete acute CPSS attenuation (using suture or a CB) can benefit from this, instead of receiving a gradual, possibly incomplete, CPSS attenuation
- A cat with a very high initial portal pressure (e.g., >25 mmHg) following temporary CPSS occlusion may not be a good candidate for an AC due to the risk of development of multiple acquired shunts if the rate of shunt attenuation exceeds the capacity of the intrahepatic portal vasculature to accommodate the increased blood flow[30]
- A CB can be placed to provide initial partial attenuation of the CPSS to an acceptable level (similarly to partial suture attenuation), with the expectation of further attenuation with time

Ameroid constrictor and cellophane banding of portosystemic shunts

Ameroid constrictors (AR) and cellophane banding (CB) have been used for the surgical treatment of CPSS in cats with the aim of gradually attenuating the shunt over a period of weeks. This approach is intended to produce complete shunt attenuation gradually without causing portal hypertension, therefore avoiding the need for multiple surgeries in cats that cannot tolerate complete attenuation at the first attempt. Long-term residual shunting is common with both techniques and the exact rate of attenuation is unknown.

Although some surgeons simply place an AR or CB around a CPSS without measuring portal pressure and without any initial shunt attenuation, others recommend measuring portal pressure and performing temporary complete CPSS occlusion regardless in all cases with several potential advantages (Box 32-5).

Whichever technique is used it is still important to perform close postoperative monitoring in all cats as it is possible for acute portal hypertension to develop if an AC suddenly moves and occludes the CPSS, if a CB is applied too tightly, or with either method if acute thrombus formation in the CPSS occurs.

Ameroid constrictors

Ameroid constrictors (Fig. 32-12; see Chapter 12) have been shown experimentally to cause vessel occlusion primarily by thrombus formation. This occlusion may be more rapid than desired and re-canalization is possible.[48,49]

Cellophane banding

'Normal' cellophane (e.g., from a florist) is used (Fig. 32-13). The cellophane is cut and folded to form a three-layer strip approximately 10 cm long and 4 mm wide. The cellophane is placed around the

intestines. In the original publications silk is used for the ligatures,[1,14,18,19,22] but the authors recommend the use of prolene suture material for shunt ligation as it has superior strength and knot security (Fig. 32-10). Conversely, silk loses tensile strength and is slowly absorbed over the course of two years (there is a report of recurrence of shunting following dissolution of a silk ligature in a dog[47]). Complete ligation of the CPSS has been reported in 29–43% of cats[1,5,6,7,9,19] (Fig. 32-11).

A second surgery performed two to three months later allows a second attempt at complete attenuation in cats treated initially with partial suture attenuation.[30,47] During this time the hepatic vasculature will have developed, allowing full attenuation in the majority of cats.[1,6,7,19] This is supported by the findings of a study comparing portovenography at first and second surgery, which showed that the degree of opacification of intrahepatic vessels increased significantly between surgeries.[6] The authors routinely perform follow-up surgery in cats that have had partial attenuation and leave a length of suture material around the shunt to be tied at the second surgery, thus avoiding further dissection around the shunt. Repeat surgery has a negligible postoperative complication rate.[6]

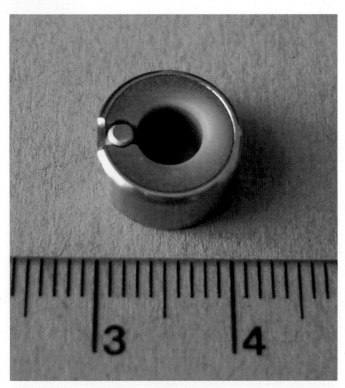

Figure 32-12 An ameroid constrictor.

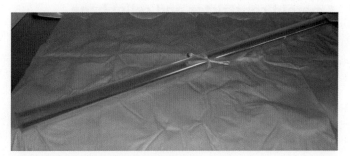

Figure 32-13 Roll of cellophane used for attenuation of CPSS.

shunt and secured with surgical clips to provide a degree of partial attenuation, depending on evidence of portal hypertension. The cellophane causes fibrosis of the vessel, resulting in gradual occlusion over a period of weeks.

SURGICAL MANAGEMENT OF INTRAHEPATIC CPSS

Intrahepatic CPSSs are more challenging to treat surgically than extrahepatic shunts due to their location within the hepatic parenchyma. Intraoperative mesenteric portovenography is particularly useful to aid correct identification of a shunt that is mostly obscured by hepatic parenchyma at surgery. It is usually possible to attenuate an intrahepatic shunt directly with suture material either posthepatically in cats with left divisional CPSS or via intrahepatic dissection in right or central divisional CPSS, without the need for more complicated intravascular techniques.[7,17] Note that when a PDV is attenuated, the left

hepatic vein is not included in the ligation[46] (Fig. 32-1C). One report described the successful use of an ameroid constrictor in a Siamese cat with a right divisional intrahepatic CPSS but it is usually more difficult to apply either an AC or CB to an intrahepatic shunt because there is generally restricted space around the shunt following dissection compared to an extrahepatic shunt.[50] Intraoperative hemorrhage is much more of a concern for intrahepatic shunts and ideally these cats should be cross-matched to a blood donor cat prior to surgery. An alternative to surgical management is coil embolization using interventional radiology, which has been described in one cat with an intrahepatic CPSS.[51]

POSTOPERATIVE CARE AND COMPLICATIONS

Postoperative monitoring is critically important in feline patients following surgical attenuation of a CPSS. Temperature should be monitored and cats kept warm (ideally in an incubator) until normal body temperature is restored. Glucose is monitored and intravenous fluid therapy is continued (with additional glucose if necessary) at 2–4 mL/kg/hour until the cat is eating and drinking normal quantities. The most serious complication is development of neurologic signs, which can develop with any of the methods of attenuation. It is best treated promptly and aggressively, and occurs more frequently in cats compared to dogs. Other postoperative complications include mild to moderate ascites (likely due to subclinical portal hypertension which is an expected sequel to CPSS attenuation), seroma formation, a clinical coagulopathy, a transfusion reaction, and pyrexia.[7,10]

Portal hypertension

Heart rate, respiratory rate, arterial blood pressure, central venous pressure (if a jugular catheter was placed), and signs of abdominal pain or distension should be monitored to assess for progressive shock that could indicate development of portal hypertension. Portal hypertension is characterized by ascites, abdominal pain, hypovolemic shock, and hemorrhagic diarrhea. Significant portal hypertension that requires re-operation to remove a ligature or gradual occlusion device is indicated by progressive hypovolemic shock that is not responsive to initial stabilization measures such as increased fluid therapy and appropriate analgesia. Historically, the development of postoperative portal hypertension, which can be fatal, was a major concern following CPSS surgery. However, with improvements in anesthesia and surgery and more familiarity with the risk of portal hypertension, overall surgical mortality has decreased and the risk of serious portal hypertension is very rare. Recent studies of treatment with suture ligation or ameroid constrictors report mortality rates of 0–4.5%, with mortality in these studies being due to neurologic complications, *not* portal hypertension.[7,10,12]

Neurologic complications

Neurologic problems are the most common postoperative complication in cats and are reported in 13.3–37%.[7,8,12,52] It has been shown that these complications do not seem to relate to HE or hypoglycemia as ammonia has been normal or dramatically reduced postsurgery compared with the situation before surgery and glucose and electrolytes are normal.[6,7,53] Neurologic signs are variable and include mild tremors or ataxia, central blindness, depression and weakness, hyperesthesia, seizures, and status epilepticus. Seizures are a particularly severe complication and are reported in 6.5–22.4% of cats treated with suture attenuation.[1,7,8,17] Seizures usually occur within 72 hours of surgery and it is recommended that cats are monitored closely during this time.[6,7,10,53] In cats treated with ameroid constrictors it might be expected that neurologic signs present before surgery would persist for a period of time and no new neurologic signs would occur, as attenuation of the CPSS should be gradual. However, neurologic complications still occur following placement of gradual occlusion devices.[10,12] Two studies have reported the outcome for cats with extrahepatic CPSS treated with ameroid constrictors with mixed results: one study did not identify any postoperative complications,[12] whereas the other study found a high rate of primarily neurologic complications (77%) during the immediate postoperative period.[10]

Phenobarbitone is the first line of treatment for cats with neurologic complications. However, cats with severe or refractory seizures may also need boluses of propofol or an infusion to manage their signs during the initial 24–48 hours[6,7,51] (see Table 32-2). Levetiracetam could be used in addition or as an alternative to phenobarbitone but there is no published information regarding its postoperative use in cats with seizures following shunt surgery. Although treatment for HE should be continued in animals that have had a partial or gradual attenuation this is rarely effective in cats with postoperative neurologic complications and antiseizure medication should be given as early as possible. Any confounding factors such as hypoglycemia or gastrointestinal hemorrhage should also be treated. Unfortunately, a number of cats (4–13.3%) die or are euthanized due to the severity of neurologic complications.[7,8,10] Other cats never fully recover or require long-term antiseizure medication. One study identified that cats with poor development of their intrahepatic vasculature (as assessed on portovenography) had an increased risk of developing postoperative neurologic complications.[6] However, no other risk factors have been identified for the occurrence of postoperative neurologic signs and there does not seem to be a difference between intrahepatic and extrahepatic CPSS, full or partial ligation, the age of the cat, or the presence of seizures preoperatively.[7] Despite postoperative neurologic problems cats can still make a full recovery, with 56% having complete resolution of neurologic signs and 22% having a good quality of life with medical management of their neurologic signs in one study.[7]

The origin of postoperative neurologic complications is unclear because seizures can occur in cats following surgery despite a postoperative return to normal shunt fractions on scintigraphy and normal bile acid stimulation results.[12] Thus, continued neurologic signs may be related to primary alterations in the central nervous system. In addition, HE has a profound effect on cerebral metabolism and it is suggested that this chronic abnormal metabolism affects the brain so that it is unable to function normally immediately after the shunt has been corrected.[54] Postsurgical decreases in endogenous inhibitory central nervous system benzodiazepine agonist levels or an imbalance of excitatory and inhibitory neurotransmitters are possible explanations for these neurologic signs.[55] It is also possible that in some cats preoperative seizures result in a degree of irreversible damage to the nervous system that persists after surgical correction of the CPSS (although this clearly does not account for cats without seizures prior to surgery).

Prophylactic treatment of cats with phenobarbitone has been suggested in order to reduce the likelihood of postoperative seizures. Little information is available to support this concept in the cat. Seizures or neurologic complications occurred despite preoperative antiseizure medication in 83–100% of cats.[10,12] Phenobarbitone is metabolized in the liver and must be used carefully in animals with hepatic insufficiency. For these reasons the authors do not routinely give preoperative phenobarbitone to cats, but do closely monitor cats for development of neurologic signs in the postoperative period so that these can be detected and treated as soon as possible, even if relatively mild.

PROGNOSIS

Recent data suggests that most cats have a good outcome following surgery, which is comparable to outcomes reported for dogs[7]. However, all long-term outcome data are based on subjective owner assessment. Although objective measures such as bile acid testing and scintigraphy have been used in some studies, these have assessed short-term outcome (six months or less).[7,10,12,52] It therefore remains unclear whether all cats achieve full shunt attenuation following surgery and what proportion develops multiple acquired shunts. Although it has been shown that cats have a better outcome with full attenuation compared with partial attenuation, in some instances partial attenuation may be associated with a good outcome as assessed by the owner. The authors still recommend complete attenuation in all instances if possible.

The degree of vascular development at first surgery has been shown to be significantly associated with age, duration of and response to medical treatment, the probability of neurologic complications, the clinical response, the existence of neurologic signs at follow up and decrease in bile acids at follow up.[6] Thus, portovenography can also be used as a prognostic indicator. Logically, cats with well-developed intrahepatic vasculature are likely to have a better response to treatment, with fewer complications.

Follow-up bile acids can be used to assess cats after surgery. However, in some cats bile acids may still be mild to moderately increased, despite a good clinical outcome.[7] Scintigraphy has also been used to monitor response to treatment.[10] In instances when cats have had a less than excellent outcome scintigraphy has shown persistent shunting, presumably due to failure to achieve complete attenuation or due to the formation of multiple acquired shunts.[10] However, in one study using ameroid constrictors 57% of cats had persistent shunting at eight to ten weeks following surgery but 75% went on to have an excellent outcome.[10]

In the largest case series which reported cats treated with suture ligation 30/36 cats were still alive after a median of 47 months, with only two having been euthanized due to development of postoperative neurologic complications/seizures.[7] Of the 36 cats, 56% were considered to be normal, 19% exhibited very minor clinical signs, 8% had a good quality of life with continued medical management for HE, 11% were treated medically for intermittent seizures, and 6% had been euthanized due to persistent seizures.[7] This suggests that surgical treatment is associated with a good long-term outcome.

Two case series described the outcome of cats treated with ameroid constrictors.[10,12] In one study, four of nine (45%) cats with long-term follow up were euthanized at a median of 11.5 months after surgery because of progression or persistence of seizures or neurologic signs.[12] Three cats (33%) were clinically normal ten months to five years after surgery and the remaining two cats (22%) had progression or recurrence of clinical signs six months after surgery. In the other study follow up was available for 20/21 cats at a mean of 26 months.[10] Three cats (15%) had been euthanized or died due to persistent neurologic signs, two cats (10%) had intermittent clinical signs (one was on medical treatment) and 15 cats (75%) were considered to be normal. Studies have also shown persistent portosystemic shunting (as measured with scintigraphy) in a significant proportion of cats treated with ameroid constrictors, suggesting failure of the ameroid to fully occlude the CPSS or the development of multiple acquired shunts.[10,12,56]

One study described the outcome of CB in five cats.[50] The cellophane was applied so that it partially attenuated the shunt. All of the cats survived the postoperative period although one developed mild neurologic signs, which resolved after seven days. Three cats had normal liver function assessed by ammonia or bile acid testing and two cats had persistent abnormal liver function. Repeat surgery revealed that one cat had developed multiple acquired shunts and the other cat had persistent shunting due to failure of the cellophane to produce fibrosis. Another study described CB in nine cats but in contrast to the earlier study the cellophane band was applied without any initial portosystemic shunt attenuation.[57] Two cats died in the postoperative period due to refractory seizures. Another cat was euthanized three months after surgery due to recurrence of clinical signs refractory to medical therapy. Five cats were clinically well with normal serum bile acid concentrations three months postoperatively. In the longer term, two cats were lost to follow up at five and eight months, two cats were alive and clinically normal after one year, one cat was alive after three years with persistent ptyalism but normal serum bile acid concentration, and one cat was alive after three years but required a cystotomy for removal of urate calculi.

REFERENCES

1. Levy JK, Bunch SE, Komtebedde J. Feline portosystemic vascular shunts. In: Bonagura JD, editor. Kirk's current veterinary therapy XII small animal practice. Philadelphia: WB Saunders; 1995. p. 743–9.

2. Van den Ingh TS, Rothuizen J, Meyer HP. Circulatory disorders of the liver in dogs and cats. Vet Quart 1995;17(2):70–6.

3. Legendre AM, Krahwinkel DJ, Carrig CB, et al. Ascites associated with intrahepatic arteriovenous-fistula in a cat. J Am Vet Med Assoc 1976;168(7):589–91.

4. d'Anjou MA, Penninck D, Cornejo L, et al. Ultrasonographic diagnosis of portosystemic shunting in dogs and cats. Vet Radiol Ultrasound 2004;45(5):424–37.

5. Birchard SJ, Sherding RG. Feline portosystemic shunts. Comp Cont Ed Prac Vet 1992;14(10):1295–301.

6. Lipscomb VJ, Lee KC, Lamb CR, et al. Association of mesenteric portovenographic findings with outcome in cats receiving surgical treatment for single congenital portosystemic shunts. J Am Vet Med Assoc 2009;234(2):221–8.

7. Lipscomb V, Jones HJ, Brockman DJ. Complications and long-term outcomes of the ligation of congenital portosystemic shunts in 49 cats. Vet Rec 2007;160(14):465–70.

8. Wolschrijn CF, Mahapokai W, Rothuizen J, et al. Gauged attenuation of congenital portosystemic shunts: results in 160 dogs and 15 cats. Vet Quart 2000;22(2):94–8.

9. White RN, Macdonald NJ, Burton CA. Use of intraoperative mesenteric portovenography in congenital portosystemic shunt surgery. Vet Radiol Ultrasound 2003;44(5):514–21.

10. Kyles AE, Hardie EM, Mehl M, et al. Evaluation of ameroid ring constrictors for the management of single extrahepatic portosystemic shunts in cats: 23 cases (1996–2001). J Am Vet Med Assoc 2002;220(9):1341–7.

11. Hunt GB. Effect of breed on anatomy of portosystemic shunts resulting from congenital diseases in dogs and cats: a review of 242 cases. Austr Vet J 2004;82(12):746–9.

12. Havig M, Tobias KM. Outcome of ameroid constrictor occlusion of single

13. Center SA, Magne ML. Historical, physical-examination, and clinicopathological features of portosystemic vascular anomalies in the dog and cat. SeminVet Med Surg Small Anim 1990;5(2):83–93.

14. Blaxter AC, Holt PE, Pearson GR, et al. Congenital portosystemic shunts in the cat – a report of 9 cases. J Small Anim Pract 1988;29(10):631–45.

15. Rothuizen J, Vandeningh TS, Voorhout G, et al. Congenital porto-systemic shunts in 16 dogs and 3 cats. J Small Anim Pract 1982;23(2):67–81.

16. Lamb CR, White RN. Morphology of congenital intrahepatic portacaval shunts in dogs and cats. Vet Rec 1998;142(3):55–60.

17. White RN, ForstervanHijfte MA, Petrie G, et al. Surgical treatment of intrahepatic portosystemic shunts in six cats. Vet Rec 1996;139(13):314–17.

18. Scavelli TD, Hornbuckle WE, Roth L, et al. Portosystemic shunts in cats – 7 cases (1976–1984). J Am Vet Med Assoc 1986;189(3):317–25.

19. VanGundy TE, Boothe HW, Wolf A. Results of surgical management of feline portosystemic shunts. J Am Anim Hosp Assoc 1990;26(1):55–62.

20. Lamb CR, ForstervanHijfte MA, White RN, et al. Ultrasonographic diagnosis of congenital portosystemic shunt in 14 cats. J Small Anim Pract 1996;37(5):205–9.

21. Schunk CM. Feline portosystemic shunts. Semin Vet Med Surg Small Anim 1997;12(1):45–50.

22. Berger B, Whiting PG, Breznock EM, et al. Congenital feline portosystemic shunts. J Am Vet Med Assoc 1986;188(5):517–21.

23. Kummeling A, Teske E, Rothuizen J, et al. Coagulation profiles in dogs with congenital portosystemic shunts before and after surgical attenuation. J Vet Int Med 2006;20(6):1319–26.

24. Niles JD, Williams JM, Cripps PJ. Hemostatic profiles in 39 dogs with congenital portosystemic shunts. Vet Surg 2001;30(1):97–104.

25. Ruland K, Fischer A, Hartmann K. Sensitivity and specificity of fasting ammonia and serum bile acids in the diagnosis of portosystemic shunts in dogs and cats. Vet Clin Pathol 2010;39(1):57–64.

26. Center SA, Baldwin BH, Erb H, et al. Bile-acid concentrations in the diagnosis of hepatobiliary disease in the cat. J Am Vet Med Assoc 1986;189(8):891–6.

27. Goggs R, Serrano S, Szladovits B, et al. Clinical investigation of a point-of-care blood ammonia analyzer. Vet Clin Pathol 2008;37(2):198–206.

28. Koblik PD, Hornof WJ. Transcolonic sodium pertechnetate Tc-99m scintigraphy for diagnosis of macrovascular portosystemic shunts in dogs, cats, and potbellied pigs – 176 Cases (1988–1992). J Am Vet Med Assoc 1995;207(6):729–33.

29. Forster-van Hijfte MA, McEvoy FJ, White RN. Per rectal portal scintigraphy in the diagnosis and management of feline congenital portosystemic shunts. J Small Anim Pract 1996;37(1):7–11.

30. Tillson DM, Winkler JT. Diagnosis and treatment of portosystemic shunts in the cat. Vet Clin N Am Small Anim Pract 2002;32(4):881–999.

31. Moon ML. Diagnostic imaging of portosystemic shunts. Semin Vet Med Surg Small Anim 1990;5(2):120–6.

32. Zwingenberger A. CT diagnosis of portosystemic shunts. Vet Clin N Am Small Anim Pract 2009;39(4):783–92.

33. Seguin B, Tobias KM, Gavin PR, et al. Use of magnetic resonance angiography for diagnosis of portosystemic shunts in dogs. Vet Radiol Ultrasound 2009;40(3):251–8.

34. Brown JC Jr, Chanoit G, Reeder J. Complex extrahepatic portocaval shunt with unusual caval features in a cat: computed tomographic characterisation. J Small Anim Pract 2010;51(4):227–30.

35. Greenhalgh SN, Dunning MD, McKinley TJ, et al. Comparison of survival after surgical or medical treatment in dogs with a congenital portosystemic shunt. J Am Vet Med Assoc 2010;236(11):1215–20.

36. Smith Bailey K, Dewey CW. The seizuring cat. Diagnostic work-up and therapy. J Feline Med Surg 2009;11(5):385–94.

37. Platt SR, Radaelli ST, McDonnell JJ. The prognostic value of the modified Glasgow

coma scale in head trauma in dogs. J Vet Int Med 2001;15(6):581–4.

38. Baade S, Aupperle H, Grevel V, et al. Histopathological and immunohistochemical investigations of hepatic lesions associated with congenital portosystemic shunt in dogs. J Comp Pathol 2006;134(1):80–90.

39. Parker JS, Monnet E, Powers BE, et al. Histologic examination of hepatic biopsy samples as a prognostic indicator in dogs undergoing surgical correction of congenital portosystemic shunts: 64 cases (1997–2005). J Am Vet Med Assoc 2008;232(10):1511–14.

40. Martin RA, Freeman LE. Identification and surgical management of portosystemic shunts in the dog and cat. Semin Vet Med Surg Small Anim 1987;2(4):302–6.

41. Birchard SJ. Surgical management of portosystemic shunts in dogs and cats. Compendium of continuing education for the practicing veterinarian 1984;6(9):795–801.

42. Butler LM, Fossum TW, Boothe HW. Surgical management of extrahepatic portosystemic shunts in the dog and cat. Semin Vet Med Surg Small Anim 1990;5(2):127–33.

43. Mathews K, Gofton N. Congenital extrahepatic portosystemic shunt occlusion in the dog – gross observations during surgical correction. J Am Anim Hosp Assoc 1988;24(4):387–94.

44. White RN, Burton CA. Anatomy of the patent ductus venosus in the cat. J Feline Med Surg 2001;3(4):229–33.

45. Burton CA, White RN. Portovenogram findings in cases of elevated bile acid concentrations following correction of portosystemic shunts. J Small Anim Pract 2001;42(11):536–40.

46. Besancon MF, Kyles AE, Griffey SM, et al. Evaluation of the characteristics of venous occlusion after placement of an ameroid constrictor in dogs. Vet Surg 2004;33(6):597–605.

47. Adin CA, Gregory CR, Kyles AE, et al. Effect of petrolatum coating on the rate of occlusion of ameroid constrictors in the peritoneal cavity. Vet Surg 2004;33(1):11–16.

48. Bright SR, Williams JM, Niles JD. Outcomes of intrahepatic portosystemic shunts occluded with ameroid constrictors in nine dogs and one cat. Vet Surg 2006;35(3):300–9.

49. Weisse C, Schwartz K, Stronger R, et al. Transjugular coil embolization of an intrahepatic portosystemic shunt in a cat. J Am Vet Med Assoc 2002;221(9):1287–91, 1266–7.

50. Hunt GB, Kummeling A, Tisdall PL, et al. Outcomes of cellophane banding for congenital portosystemic shunts in 106 dogs and 5 cats. Vet Surg 2004;33(1):25–31.

51. Heldmann E, Holt DE, Brockman DJ, et al. Use of propofol to manage seizure activity after surgical treatment of portosystemic shunts. J Small Anim Pract 1999;40(12):590–4.

52. Matushek KJ, Bjorling D, Mathews K. Generalized motor seizures after portosystemic shunt ligation in dogs – 5 cases (1981–1988). J Am Vet Med Assoc 1990;196(12):2014–17.

53. Hardie EM, Kornegay JN, Cullen JM. Status epilepticus after ligation of portosystemic shunts. Vet Surg 1990;19(6):412–17.

54. Vogt JC, Krahwinkel DJ, Bright RM, et al. Gradual occlusion of extrahepatic portosystemic shunts in dogs and cats using the ameroid constrictor. Vet Surg 1996;25(6):495–502.

55. Hunt GB, Bellenger CR, Pearson MRB. Transportal approach for attenuating intrahepatic portosystemic shunts in dogs. Vet Surg 1996;25(4):300–8.

56. Swalec KM, Smeak DD. Partial versus complete attenuation of single portosystemic shunts. Vet Surg 1990;19(6):406–11.

57. Cabassu J, Seim HB III, MacPhail CM, et al. Outcomes of cats undergoing surgical attenuation of congenital extrahepatic portosystemic shunts through cellophane banding: 9 cases (2000–2007). J Am Vet Med Assoc 2011;238(1):89–93.

Pancreas

L.M. Liehmann

Cats are susceptible to a wide range of exocrine pancreatic diseases: acute and chronic pancreatitis, pancreatic abscess, pancreatic pseudocyst and cyst, exocrine pancreatic insufficiency, and neoplasia. This chapter will review the anatomy of the pancreas, investigations for and the diseases of the pancreas, and their surgical management where applicable.

SURGICAL ANATOMY

The pancreas develops from the dorsal and ventral primordium in the hepatopancreatic ring of the duodenum and grows into the dorsal omentum. It has a long and slender configuration in the cat, taking the shape of a wide V or boomerang. The right or duodenal lobe is located in the mesoduodenum and often takes a hook-like shape at the end.[1] It is best accessed surgically by gentle traction on the descending duodenum ventrally and medially. The left or splenic lobe runs in the dorsal mesogastrium towards the dorsal extremity of the spleen and has an omental connection to the mesocolon. For surgical visualization the omentum and stomach need to be retracted ventrally, or alternatively the omental pouch can be opened by tearing the ventral leaf. Both pancreatic lobes unite in the pancreatic body close to the cranial part of the duodenum and pylorus (Fig. 33-1).

The normal pancreas has a pale pink color and is finely lobulated. The exocrine portion of the pancreas is a compound tubuloacinar gland whose ducts are totally concealed within the substance of the organ.[2] Interlobular and interlobar ducts unite to form the main pancreatic duct that opens into the duodenum on the major duodenal papilla together with the common bile duct. In about 20% of cats, a second smaller duct, the accessory pancreatic duct, opens approximately 10 mm aboral on the minor duodenal papilla (Fig. 33-1).[3] A pancreatic bladder consisting of aberrant pancreatic tissue with a dilated pancreatic duct is described in 0.2% of cats.[4] It lies beside the gall bladder with which it can communicate. It is regarded as a pathologic variant without clinical significance. Rarely, accessory nodular pancreatic lobes are found along the feline gut, especially in the area of the duodenum, and in the portal mesentery. These often extend towards the hepatic fossa.[4]

The endocrine part of the pancreas consists of several thousand pancreatic islets of Langerhans and accounts for approximately 2% of the gland's weight.[5] Pancreatic α- and β-cells produce glucagon and insulin, respectively, which regulate carbohydrate homeostasis. δ-Cells secrete the growth inhibiting hormone somatostatin and PP cells produce pancreatic polypeptide that self regulates pancreas secretion activities and affects hepatic glycogen levels and gastrointestinal secretions.

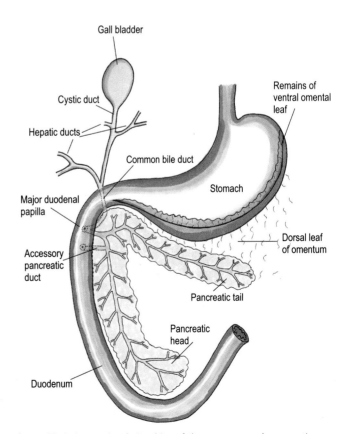

Figure 33-1 Anatomic relationships of the pancreas and pancreatic ducts.

DOI: 10.1016/B978-0-7020-4336-9.00033-0

The exocrine portion of the gland consists of acinar and ductal cells. Acinar cells are arranged in clusters around the terminal pancreatic ductules.[6] They primarily secrete digestive enzymes: proteases (trypsinogen, chymotrypsinogen, proelastase, procarboxypeptidase, ribonucleases, and deoxyribonucleases), which cleave polypeptide chains; amylase and lipase, which hydrolyze carbohydrates and fat; and trypsin inhibitors. To prevent pancreatic autodigestion, enzymes are either synthesized, stored and secreted as inactive zymogens (proteases) and activated within the intestinal tract,[7] or an inactive form is directly secreted and activated within the duodenum (pro-phospholipase A_2) and/or they need cofactors like bile salts and coli-pase for function (phospholipase A_2, lipase, carboxylesterase). Amylase is secreted intact and active.[8]

Ductal cell secretions contain bicarbonate and water that serve to neutralize pH in the duodenum, intrinsic factor that facilitates cobalamin (vitamin B_{12}) absorption in the distal ileum, and antibacterial proteins that regulate small intestinal bacterial flora.[7] In cats, the pancreas is the only source of intrinsic factor, whereas in dogs intrinsic factor is also secreted by the stomach.

The pancreatic arterial supply derives mainly from the celiac artery: the splenic artery contributes branches to the left pancreatic limb and the cranial pancreaticoduodenal artery and right gastric artery give radicles to the cranial part of the right pancreatic limb. The caudal pancreaticoduodenal artery originates from the cranial mesenteric artery and supplies the caudal half of the right pancreatic limb (Fig. 33-2).[9] Anastomoses between these various vessels occur within the gland.[10] Venous drainage is via portal tributaries.

Lymphatic drainage is into the pancreaticoduodenal and hepatic lymph nodes; however, there are lymph vessels draining from the pancreas to the jejunal and splenic lymph nodes.[11]

Innervation is via vagal afferents that increase pancreatic secretions, and sympathetic fibers from the celiac and mesenteric ganglia that decrease pancreatic secretions.

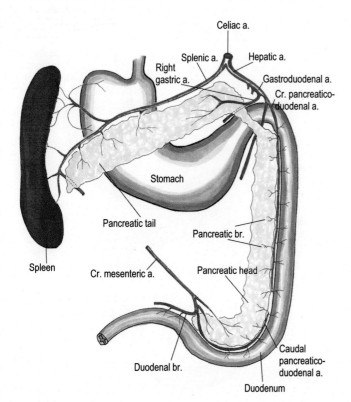

Figure 33-2 Blood supply of the feline pancreas and proximal duodenum.

DIAGNOSIS AND GENERAL CONSIDERATIONS

Cats seem to be susceptible to a wide range of exocrine pancreatic diseases: acute and chronic pancreatitis, pancreatic abscess, pancreatic cyst/pseudocyst, exocrine pancreatic insufficiency, and neoplasia. Middle-aged to older cats are most often affected with pancreatitis; cats with pancreatic mass lesions such as neoplasia, cyst/pseudocysts, and abscesses tend to be older (mean 12.8 years, range 4–20 years). Clinical signs are often non-specific, and additionally could be easily attributable to concurrent hepatic and intestinal disease. Hence the level of suspicion of the attending clinician is often low and the disease prevalence seems to be underestimated. Nevertheless, even with an insidious onset the disease can quite dramatically progress to a life-threatening state of acute pancreatic necrosis. Pancreatic disease in the cat is difficult to diagnose, and a careful integration of collected historical data, physical examination results, laboratory, and imaging findings is mandatory in order to establish a preliminary diagnosis. It is not recommended to rely on a single diagnostic modality to diagnose pancreatic disease; furthermore, histopathology might be necessary to support a definitive conclusion. Diagnosis and treatment of the most common pancreatic disorders are described in the following section.

History and clinical examination

Historical data usually includes lethargy, anorexia and, in more chronic cases, weight loss. In acute pancreatitis, cats suddenly deteriorate or clinical signs worsen in spite of aggressive therapy. Vomiting is only present in about 35% of cats.

A complete physical examination including a thorough evaluation of the cat's abdomen is mandatory. Cranial abdominal masses and cranial abdominal discomfort are easily overlooked as the clinical response of the cat can be very subtle. Jaundice is a common finding and is usually a sign of complicating cholangiohepatitis, hepatic lipidosis, or biliary obstructions secondary to pancreatic disease. Lethargy, anorexia, dehydration, and hypothermia are the most prevalent clinical signs (Tables 33-1 and 33-2). The cat can dramatically deteriorate with development of shock and progression to a moribund state despite aggressive fluid therapy.[12]

Clinicopathologic tests

A minimum database should consist of a complete blood cell count, serum bilirubin, cholesterol, glucose, total protein, albumin, and

Table 33-1 Common clinical findings in cats with acute pancreatitis[78]

Clinical finding	Occurrence	Clinical finding	Occurrence
Anorexia	97%	Jaundice	37%
Lethargy	81%	Fever	25%
Dehydration	54%	Abdominal pain	19%
Weight loss	47%	Diarrhea	12%
Hypothermia	46%	Abdominal mass	11%
Vomiting	46%		

Table 33-2 Typical clinical findings in cats with pancreatic neoplasia[48,60,66]

Exocrine pancreatic adenocarcinoma		Gastrinoma	Insulinoma
Anorexia	75%	Vomiting ±	Seizures
Vomiting	63%	hematemesis	Depression
Abdominal pain	38%	Abdominal pain	Disorientation
Palpable cranial		Hematochezia	Weakness
abdominal mass		Anorexia	Hypothermia
Jaundice			Bradycardia
Paraneoplastic alopecia			
Abdominal effusion			
Depression			

serum activity of liver enzymes (serum alanine aminotransferase and alkaline phosphatase), calcium, urea, creatinine, and potassium. Common clinicopathologic findings in cats with pancreatic disease are listed in Tables 33-3 and 33-4. Ionized hypocalcemia was found to be a negative prognostic indicator in cats.[13]

The measurements of serum lipase and amylase activities do not seem to be of clinical value in the diagnosis of feline pancreatic disease. Several different lipase isoenzymes originate from various cells in the body and circulate in the blood; they are all detected by catalytic lipase assays, thus the tissue of origin cannot be determined. Species-specific immunoassays for the measurement of feline trypsin-like immunoreactivity (fTLI) and feline pancreatic lipase immunoreactivity (fPLI) have therefore been developed and validated. Feline pancreatitis is best detected by the measurement of elevated fPLI.[14,15] A summary of specific tests for pancreatic disease is given in Table 33-5.

Abdominal effusion is sometimes encountered during physical examination, abdominal ultrasound, or on radiographs. Abdominocentesis typically reveals serosanguineous fluid characteristic of a sterile exudate or a modified transudate. Cytological evaluation can be helpful in the diagnosis of pancreatic neoplasia.

Table 33-3 Common clinicopathologic abnormalities in cats with acute pancreatitis[78]

Abnormality	Occurrence	Abnormality	Occurrence
Anemia	38%	Total bilirubin ↑	58%
Leukocytosis	46%	Cholesterol ↑	72%
Leukopenia	15%	Hyperglycemia	45%
Hemoconcentration	17%	Hypokalemia	56%
ALT ↑	57%	Hypocalcemia	65%
ALP ↑	49%	Albumin ↓	36%

ALP, Alkaline phosphatase; ALT, Alanine aminotransferase.

Table 33-4 Clinicopathologic abnormalities in cats with pancreatic neoplasia[48,60,66]

Exocrine pancreatic adenocarcinoma	Gastrinoma	Insulinoma
Leukocytosis	Regenerative anemia	Hypoglycemia
Hyperglycemia	Leukocytosis	<3.3 mmol/L
ALT ↑	Neutrophilia	Normal or high
	ALP ↑	insulin level
	Albumin ↓	(reference range
	Electrolyte abnormalities	72–583 pmol/L)
	due to vomiting	

ALP, Alkaline phosphatase; ALT, Alanine aminotransferase.

Table 33-5 Pancreas-specific serum tests and their availability

Substrate tested	Application	Reference range	Availability
Serum lipase activity assay	Serum test not recommended for the diagnosis of feline pancreatitis because of very low sensitivity and specificity	25–250 U/L	Routine
fTLI	Diagnosis of exocrine pancreatic insufficiency (if low). Elevation may be indicative of pancreatitis, but sensitivity is low and specificity is less than in dogs	12–82 µg/dL	Texas A+M University, gastrointestinal laboratory SCL Bioscience Services, UK
fPLI	Sensitivity 82% Specificity up to 100% for the detection of pancreatitis in cats[15]	2.0–6.8 µg/L, 6.8–12 µg/L mild or resolving pancreatitis, >12 µg/L diagnostic for pancreatitis	IDEXX laboratories, SNAP test
Glucose, insulin	Diagnosis of insulinoma	Glucose <3.3 mmol/L Insulin 72–583 pmol/L diagnostic if insulin is normal or high	Specialist endocrine laboratories UK: Cambridge Specialist Labs

fPLI, feline pancreatic lipase immunoreactivity; fTLI, feline trypsin-like immunoreactivity.

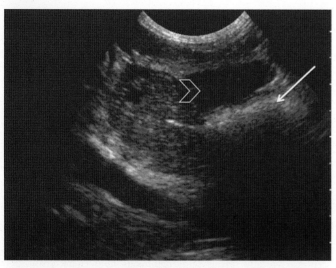

Figure 33-3 Abdominal ultrasound of a cat with severe pancreatitis. Note the hypoechogenic pancreas (arrowhead) and hyperechogenic peripancreatic tissue (arrow). *(Courtesy of Katharina M. Hittmair.)*

Diagnostic imaging

Radiography

Lateral and ventrodorsal projections are evaluated for loss of peritoneal detail suggestive of peritoneal effusion or a cranial abdominal mass and subsequent displacement of internal organs into the upper right quadrant of the abdomen. The duodenum often appears displaced and corrugated in traumatic pancreatitis; rarely, calcification in the pancreatic and peripancreatic area is visible.[16] In acute cases, radiographs are also useful to rule out other causes of acute abdomen.

Ultrasonography

Ultrasonography is the most useful imaging modality to support the diagnosis of feline pancreatic disease (Fig. 33-3).[14,17,18] Soft tissue masses located in the cranial abdomen can be caused by pancreatitis, cysts/pseudocysts, abscesses, or neoplasia. Concurrent abdominal effusions can be readily identified. Acute feline pancreatic disease is associated with a hypoechoic pancreas with hyperechoic peripancreatic fat and thickening of gastric and duodenal walls. More chronic cases with acute flare-ups usually show mixed echogenicity of the peripancreatic tissues. Cats with chronic disease can have a dilatation of the gall bladder and common bile duct.[17–19] The use of Doppler ultrasonography has shown promise in preliminary studies.[20] Although specificity is high, the overall sensitivity of abdominal ultrasound to detect feline pancreatitis is low (24–35%).[17,18] While acute pancreatitis can be identified as described above, chronic pancreatitis does not often produce ultrasonographically visible changes.

Computed tomography (CT)

The feline pancreas can be visualized using CT scans, and CT imaging might be useful in the identification of pancreatic mass lesions. However, it is not a useful diagnostic test for feline pancreatitis.[14]

SURGICAL DISEASES

Conditions of the feline pancreas can often be treated successfully with therapeutic intervention and nutritional manipulation. In

non-responsive cases, severely affected animals or those with malignant disease, surgical intervention by celiotomy or laparoscopy may be required to obtain biopsy specimens and thus a definitive diagnosis for specific therapy. In cases with mass lesions, surgery may be required for definitive treatment.

Pancreatitis

Depending on the presence of permanent histopathologic changes after resolution of the disease, pancreatitis is classified as acute (no permanent changes) or chronic (irreversible morphological change).[21]

Acute necrotizing pancreatitis (ANP) is characterized by a predominance of pancreatic acinar cell necrosis and peripancreatic fat necrosis.[12] Various amounts of inflammation, hemorrhage, and mineralization can be present.[7] Some fibrosis is possible if there is chronic underlying disease with an acute flare-up. The etiopathogenesis of ANP is unknown and it is mostly considered idiopathic; however, various diseases and conditions have known associations with cats developing ANP (Box 33-1).

Pancreatitis may be caused by a reduction in pancreatic blood flow due to hypotension under general anesthesia, or due to temporary venous outflow occlusion during surgery.[22] It rarely develops secondary to pancreatic biopsy or excision of pancreatic neoplasia.[23,24]

In *acute suppurative pancreatitis*, neutrophilic inflammation is the predominant histologic feature. The condition is less common than ANP and appears to affect younger animals.[12,13,25,26]

Chronic non-suppurative pancreatitis (CP) is a continuous and usually progressive inflammatory process of the pancreas, where the predominant feature are lymphocytic inflammation, fibrosis, and acinar atrophy.

There is significant overlap in the various forms of pancreatitis, and ultimately histopathology is needed to distinguish the conditions.[25]

Pancreatic atrophy is believed to be the consequence and end stage of CP in most feline cases and it may or may not affect the endocrine portion of the gland as well.[7] Many cats develop exocrine pancreatic insufficiency, resulting in severe nutrient maldigestion, acid injury to the duodenal mucosa, cobalamin and fat-soluble vitamin malabsorption, and bacterial proliferation in the gut.[27]

Pathophysiology

In pancreatitis, it is generally believed that premature trypsin activation of digestive zymogens within pancreatic acinar cells is followed by pancreatic autodigestion and inflammation: acinar cell necrosis, hemorrhage, and fat necrosis and saponification take place.[7] Systemic consequences of intracellular enzyme activation are mast cell degranulation, leukocyte chemotaxis, platelet aggregation, vasodilation, surfactant degradation within the lungs and, in severe cases, initiation of disseminated intravascular coagulation (DIC). Under normal conditions, circulating proteolytic enzymes are bound by α-macroglobulins and rapidly cleared. When circulating α-macroglobulins are depleted, proteases activate the kinin, coagulation, fibrinolytic and complement cascades, resulting in the development of acute DIC and death.[5]

Therapy

Supportive and symptomatic care is central to the treatment of cats with pancreatitis. Aggressive therapy is critical in order to improve the chance for survival. Underlying causes for pancreatitis should be diagnosed and treated if possible.

Fluid, acid–base and electrolyte deficits should be corrected. Pancreatitic cats can be hypokalemic and hypocalcemic. Calcium gluconate should be given at a dose of 50–150 mg/kg IV over 12–24 hours if necessary and serum total or ionized calcium concentration should be monitored during therapy. Anemic cats with a packed cell volume below 15–20% are transfused with whole blood or packed red blood cells after blood typing and cross-matching (see Chapter 5). Plasma transfusion may be beneficial to increase available α-macroglobulins that bind circulating active proteases, and to combat DIC. Increased concentrations of albumin will help to maintain plasma oncotic pressure and blood volume and reduce pancreatic edema.

A short period of fasting has been recommended in the past especially for dogs with pancreatitis. This should only be extrapolated to the cat in cases of severe vomiting at risk for aspiration pneumonia. With their predilection for the development of fat mobilization and hepatic lipidosis, it is extremely important to feed cats through their bouts of pancreatitis. Esophagostomy, gastrostomy, gastroduodenostomy, or jejunostomy feeding tubes may be placed to provide enteral support in anorexic animals (see Chapter 12). Ideally, small frequent portions of a diet high in carbohydrate and low in fat are given.

Aggressive analgesic therapy based on systemic opioids should be provided (Table 33-6). Pain in cats is not easily detected as they tend to exhibit pain by withdrawal (being quiet, purring, hiding), thus severe pain should be suspected in any animal with pancreatitis. Nausea and vomiting in affected cats can be severe and there is a variety of anti-emetics available for use in cats; these are listed in Table 33-6.

Septic complications of acute pancreatitis are rare in cats, but broad-spectrum antibiotics should be given if toxic changes are present in the blood or if the patient is febrile. Necrosis and inflammation predispose to colonic bacterial translocation and colonization of the pancreas, mainly with *E. coli* and other coliforms.[28,29]

Indications for surgery for pancreatitis include an enlarging or persistent pancreatic mass in a patient unresponsive to medical treatment, and sepsis non-responsive to aggressive medical treatment and extraluminal bile duct obstruction. Abscesses and large necrotic areas are debrided (see Box 33-3), and omentectomy (see Chapter 19) with

---

Table 33-6 Therapeutics for pancreatitis cases

Drug	Dose rate and interval	Comments
Analgesia		
Methadone	0.1–0.3 mg/kg slowly IV, IM, SQ every 3–4 hours up to 0.6 mg/kg oral transmucosal[76] every 3–4 hours	Suitable to treat moderate to severe pain, may produce euphoria[29] Monitor analgesic effect
Morphine	0.1–0.4 mg/kg slowly IV, IM every 3–4 hours or continuous rate infusion 0.1–0.2 mg/kg/hour IV	Monitor analgesic effect
Fentanyl	2–5 µg/kg as an IV loading dose, followed by a continuous rate infusion of 1–5 µg/kg/hour	Very potent analgesic, suitable for the treatment of severe pain Causes respiratory depression
Buprenorphine	20–30 µg/kg IV, IM, SQ or oral transmucosal every 6 hours	Provides visceral and somatic analgesia, has a longer duration of action compared to other opioids[80]
Pethidine	3–5 mg/kg IM or SQ every 2–4 hours	Requires frequent dosing to be effective[81,82]
Butorphanol	0.2–0.4 mg/kg SQ every 90 minutes	
Ketamine	Continuous rate infusion of 2–10 µg/kg/min. IV preceded by loading dose of 0.25 mg/kg	Used as supplements to opioids in patients with more severe pain[83]
Lidocaine	Continuous rate infusion of 20 µg/kg/min. IV preceded by a slowly administered loading dose of 0.25–1.0 mg/kg	Used as supplements to opioids in patients with more severe pain[83] Cats tend to be more sensitive to CNS side effects
Anti-emetics		
Maropitant	0.5–1 mg/kg PO or SQ every 24 hours	
α$_2$-Adrenergic antagonist, e.g., chlorpromazine	0.2–0.4 mg/kg IM or SQ every 8 hours	
5-HT$_3$ antagonists: Ondansetron Granisetron Dolasetron	0.1–1.0 mg/kg 0.1–0.5 mg/kg 0.5–1.0 mg/kg PO or IV every 12 to 24 hours	
Dopaminergic antagonists, e.g., metoclopramide		Less effective anti-emetic agents in cats[84]

or without splenectomy (see Chapter 34) is performed if necessary. The abdomen is lavaged with warm sterile saline to remove activated proteases from the abdomen. Hyperbilirubinemia due to extrahepatic bile duct obstruction can occur as a consequence to pancreatitis or pancreatic fibrosis and needs to be addressed surgically if non-responsive to medical treatment. In those instances, a biliary diversion technique such as cholecystoduodenostomy or cholecystojejunostomy (see Chapter 31) can be used. Alternatively, biliary diversion is facilitated by tube cholecystostomy. Recently, choledochal stenting has been advocated in cats to achieve biliary decompression.[30] Numbers of operated cats are low and prognosis seems to be less favorable than in the dog. Two of seven cats died directly postoperatively, three more within seven to 24 months and only two survived long term following stenting. An overall mortality rate of 50% for biliary diversion techniques in the cat has been reported,[31] so it seems prudent to be very cautious not to operate prematurely.

Samples for culture (aerobic and anaerobic) and sensitivity should be taken from the pancreas and the liver. Open or closed abdominal drainage might be required, depending on the severity of intra-abdominal changes.

Pancreatic abscess

Pancreatic abscess is a rare complication of acute pancreatitis in cats,[32] it consists of a circumscribed collection of purulent and necrotic material in the pancreatic parenchyma. It may extend into adjacent tissue and organs. In most feline and canine cases the abscesses are sterile, but in one of the three reported cats, cultures positive for *Escherichia coli* were obtained. Typically, a hypoechoic mass can be found on ultrasound adjacent to the pancreas, as well as signs of generalized severe pancreatitis.

Preoperative fine needle aspiration cytology should be performed to differentiate pancreatic abscess from other pancreatic mass lesions and to assess the severity of pancreatic changes. Surgery is recommended in the face of a persisting or enlarging pancreatic mass non-responsive to aggressive medical treatment. It consists of debridement of the abscess(es) and necrotic tissue. Alternatively, drainage and omentalization of the abscess is helpful in cases where complete excision would compromise the main pancreatic duct (Fig. 33-4). Patency of the common bile duct is ensured or biliary decompression

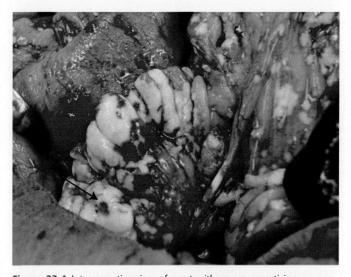

Figure 33-4 Intraoperative view of a cat with severe necrotizing pancreatitis and a pancreatic abscess (arrow). The location of the abscess in the pancreatic angle prohibited complete excision and necrotic material was carefully debrided and omentalized.

provided if necessary. Ultrasound-guided percutaneous or endoscopic drainage of pancreatic abscesses has been reported in human beings; however, experience in veterinary medicine is rare. Antibiotic treatment should be based on culture and sensitivity results.

Two of the three cats with pancreatic abscess that were treated surgically, survived. Survival of dogs with pancreatic abscesses treated surgically is 29–40%.[33-37]

Pancreatic pseudocyst and pancreatic cyst

Pancreatic pseudocysts are non-epithelial lined cavity lesions filled with fluid containing pancreatic cells and/or pancreatic enzymes. They are a common complication of acute or chronic pancreatitis in humans, and are seen less frequently in dogs and cats.[38,39] Clinical signs are those associated with pancreatitis. There seems to be a predilection for the left pancreatic limb;[39,40] large lesions can promote vomiting by indentation of the stomach. True pancreatic cysts are lined by a layer of cuboidal epithelium and typically do not communicate with the pancreatic duct. There are three reports of feline cases that were either associated with polycystic disease in the liver and kidneys,[41] pancreatitis alone,[42] or pancreatitis, pancreatic atrophy, and the development of diabetes mellitus.[43]

A large fluid-filled lesion might be felt on a thorough abdominal palpation, but it is usually diagnosed by ultrasonography, CT scan, during surgery, or at necropsy.[39] In ultrasound, a cystic structure adjacent to the pancreas is noted, which can be solitary or multiple. Definitive diagnosis is via aspiration and evaluation of the fluid. Pseudocysts usually consist of modified transudate with a higher concentration of pancreatic enzymes than in the serum.

Medical treatment consists of supportive treatment of pancreatitis, percutaneous ultrasound-guided aspiration of the cyst/pseudocyst and close monitoring of the size of the lesion. If clinical signs do not improve, the lesion enlarges or fails to resolve, or if percutaneous drainage is not possible, *surgical intervention* is considered. The lesion is either drained internally or externally or completely excised. Three cats with pancreatic pseudocysts are reported in the veterinary literature. Two cats were treated medically and they died ten days and two months after diagnosis, the other cat had surgery including complete excision of the pseudocyst. This cat survived. Unfortunately, necropsies were not performed that could explain the two cats' deterioration. True pancreatic cysts have been reported in three cats; two of them underwent surgical resection. In one case multiple cysts recurred one month after surgery, and the cat was euthanized because of the lack of clinical improvement. Internal drainage techniques including cysto-gastrostomy, cystoduodenostomy, or cystojejunostomy are preferred in human medicine.

Pancreatic trauma

Blunt abdominal trauma such as automobile accidents or high-rise syndrome has been associated with ANP,[44,45] and pancreatic rupture has been described following high-rise syndrome in the cat in 1% and 0.6% of cases.[16,46] The incidence of traumatic pancreatitis might be underestimated because of the vague clinical signs and being masked by other, more obvious diseases. The incidence of pancreatic injury and subsequent pancreatitis seems to increase with the height of the fall. Time to diagnosis and surgery is often protracted and ranges from one to 17 days.[16,46]

Pancreatic rupture leads to leakage and activation of pancreatic enzymes in the abdominal cavity and rapid progression to severe generalized pancreatitis and peripancreatic fat necrosis. The condition is likely to result in multiorgan failure and death if not diagnosed and treated aggressively early in the course of the disease. Abdominal pain seems to be very prevalent in cats after pancreatic rupture. Abdominal

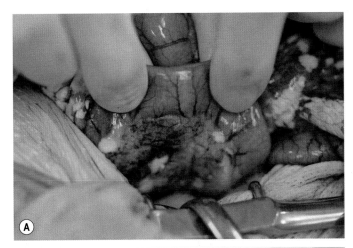

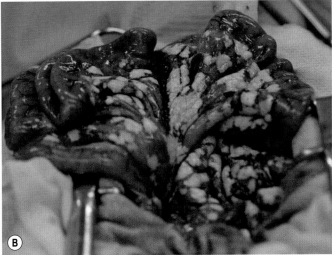

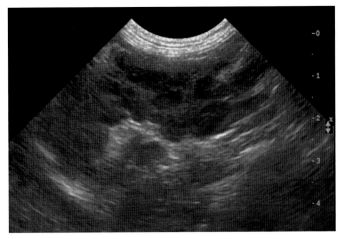

Figure 33-6 Abdominal ultrasound scan of a cat with a cystic pancreatic neoplasia in the right pancreatic limb. On histopathology, adenocarcinoma was diagnosed. *(Courtesy of Katharina M. Hittmair.)*

Figure 33-5 **(A)** Intraoperative view of the severely inflamed right pancreatic limb of a cat after a trauma from a high-rise syndrome. **(B)** Severe fat necrosis and saponification are seen as yellow-whitish areas within the mesentery.

effusion might be detected on ultrasound and typically consists of a sterile modified transudate. Lipase activity in the peritoneal fluid seems to be elevated compared to serum lipase activity in cats with traumatic pancreatitis and pancreatic rupture.[46,47] Otherwise, clinical signs and diagnosis resemble those of severe acute pancreatitis.

In cats with deteriorating clinical signs and worsening ascites, surgical exploration is indicated. Treatment is partial pancreatectomy (see Box 33-3) of the ruptured pancreas, performed in a similar manner as for severe pancreatitis (Fig. 33-5).

Prognosis for cats with pancreatic rupture is very guarded. In the two studies reported, only one cat out of ten and two out of four cats survived; the others were either euthanized or died during the perioperative period.

Pancreatic neoplasia

Pancreatic neoplasia can be exocrine or endocrine (hormone secreting). Most exocrine pancreatic neoplasia is adenocarcinoma or adenoma with acinar or ductular origin. Nodular hyperplasia is a common finding in older cats during ultrasonography or surgery and is a differential diagnosis of pancreatic masses; however, there are no

associated clinical signs. Likewise, inflammatory masses of chronic pancreatitis can resemble neoplasia and need to be considered as differentials. Gastrinoma and insulinoma are the most common endocrine tumors of the feline pancreas, and *glucagonomas* have been described in the dog, but not in cats. Pancreatic endocrine tumors originate from specialized neuroendocrine cells, the amine precursor uptake, and decarboxylation cells, and are also called APUDomas.

Adenocarcinoma and adenoma

Feline exocrine pancreatic tumors are uncommon, with an incidence ranging from 0.013% to 0.6% in various reports.[48–50] Cats suffering from diabetes mellitus seem to be at higher risk.[51,52] History and clinical signs mostly resemble those of pancreatitis. Anorexia, vomiting, abdominal pain, a palpable mass, and icterus from biliary obstruction are the most prevalent findings. Abdominal effusion might be secondary to tumor seeding into the peritoneum or to vena cava compression. Paraneoplastic alopecia may be seen, which usually is a non-pruritic, symmetrical alopecia affecting the face, ventral body, and medial aspects of the limbs. Crusty lesions sometimes present on the footpads.[53,54]

Alterations of echogenicity and mass effects can be seen ultrasonographically in many pancreatitis cases (Fig. 33-6), so further evaluation via ultrasound-guided fine needle aspiration or biopsy is warranted. Alternatively, abdominal effusion can be examined cytologically, but sensitivity is much lower.[55]

Therapy of exocrine pancreatic carcinoma should be directed at surgical excision since the tumor is uniformly resistant to chemotherapy and radiation therapy. Pancreaticoduodenectomy (Whipple procedure) has been advocated for humans and carries an intraoperative morbidity of 5–10%. Unfortunately, mortality and morbidity in diseased animals is much higher. Also, invasive growth and metastasis are present in most cases at the time of diagnosis. Metastases occur to the liver, to the lung (frequently producing pleural effusion), to the small intestine, and regional and distant lymph nodes. Lesions have also been found in the heart and diaphragm. Palliative surgical bypass such as gastrojejunostomy for relief of bowel obstruction is recommended for metastatic disease in humans, but yields only short-lived success. There is a single case report of a cat with an exocrine pancreatic adenocarcinoma that was completely excised from the left pancreatic lobe, but metastasis occurred 18 weeks after surgery and the cat was euthanized.[54] Prognosis is generally grave.

Gastrinoma

Gastrinomas are islet cell tumors that secrete excessive amounts of gastrin. They have been identified in the pancreas, but also in the peripancreatic lymph nodes and mesentery. Gastrinomas are part of the Zollinger–Ellison syndrome consisting of a non-B-cell neuroendothelial pancreatic tumor, hypergastrinemia and gastrointestinal ulceration. They are highly metastatic; up to 75% of patients show involvement of the liver, lymph nodes, spleen, and mesentery at the time of surgery.[56,57] The clinical signs are related to the severe gastric acid hypersecretion, with gastrointestinal ulceration occurring in 80% of cases and often consist of vomiting with or without hematemesis, abdominal pain, hematochezia, and anorexia. Endoscopically, esophagitis, gastritis, and upper gastrointestinal ulceration might be noted.

Laboratory findings show a regenerative anemia due to gastrointestinal bleeding and leukocytosis and neutrophilia caused by gastrointestinal inflammation. Biochemical abnormalities include hypoalbuminemia and elevated alkaline phosphatase and electrolyte abnormalities consistent with chronic vomiting. Diagnosis is made by measurement of elevated fasted serum gastrin levels, but should be suspected in any animal with severe gastrointestinal signs. Somatostatin receptor scintigraphy with pentreotide has been reported in a dog[58] and might be helpful to diagnose suspected gastrinoma in cats.

Treatment is directed at surgical excision if possible and a reduction of tumor burden, even if complete removal of the gastrinoma is not possible. This will reduce gastrin secretory capacity and thus improve the efficacy of medical therapy. Gastrointestinal ulcerations can be removed during exploratory surgery. Medical therapy consists of oral proton pump inhibitors (e.g., omeprazole), H_2-blockers, and sucralfate. Prognosis is poor, and survival times in animals undergoing surgery followed by medical treatment range from one week to 18 months.[57]

Insulinoma

Insulinomas are functional B-cell tumors arising from insulin-producing pancreatic islet cells. They are rare in cats, and have been reported in six cats older than 12 years. Three of the cats were Siamese, two were domestic short-hair cats and one was a Persian cat. Insulinomas have multihormonal productivity independent of negative feedback mechanisms.[59] Clinical signs associated with insulinomas are typically secondary to hypoglycemia and result from neuroglycopenia and hypoglycemia-mediated stimulation of the sympathoadrenal system. Intermittent periods of normoglycemia do occur, caused by the effect of those counter-regulatory hormones, mainly catecholamines and glucagon, cortisol, and growth hormone.

Clinical signs include seizures, weakness, ataxia, mental dullness, disorientation and collapse, staggering with muscle fasciculations, and weight loss with polydipsia. Prolonged neuroglycopenia can lead to irreversible neurologic complications.[60] In dogs and ferrets, insulin-secreting B-cell tumors are malignant with a high likelihood of metastasis at the time of diagnosis[56] and the same probably holds true for feline insulinomas. Metastasis in cats is reported to the pancreatic lymph nodes and liver. In the dog, insulinomas also metastasize to the mesentery, omentum, duodenum, spleen, kidney, and spinal cord.[61]

Diagnosis normally requires detection of hypoglycemia (blood glucose <3.3 mmol/L) and the presence of a normal to high insulin level in a cat with seizure-like symptoms. Some cats need to be fasted to show hypoglycemia. Hematology, blood biochemistry, and urinalysis results typically are normal or reflect those of other, concurrent disease. Ultrasound can be helpful to find pancreatic nodules and hypoechoic hepatic lesions suspicious of metastases. Nuclear scintigraphy with radiolabeled somatostatin analogs has been used in

humans and dogs to diagnose insulinomas and metastasis successfully. As this modality becomes more widely available, it might prove useful for the diagnosis, presurgical planning, and prognostic assessment in the feline species as well.

Surgical resection is the treatment recommended for insulinomas. Existing hypoglycemia should be corrected with dextrose infusions. In hypoglycemic crisis 0.25–0.5 g dextrose per kilogram can be given as a 25% solution as a bolus over three to five minutes. Treatment should be continued with a continuous rate infusion of a maintenance solution with added 2.5% dextrose. Blood glucose levels are monitored during and after surgery. During surgery, the pancreas is carefully inspected and palpated to detect abnormalities. Intravenous infusion of methylene blue to stain insulinomas intraoperatively has been recommended in dogs; the procedure is not recommended in the cat because of possible adverse effects of hemolytic anemia due to Heinz body formation and acute renal failure secondary to hemoglobinuric nephrosis.

Partial pancreatectomy (see Box 33-3) is the method of choice and can be undertaken easily if the tumor involves the extremity of the left pancreatic limb. Great care has to be taken not to destroy the duodenal blood supply when part of the right pancreatic limb is resected. The procedure has a better prognosis than enucleation alone.[62] In three out of five cats reported in the veterinary literature, insulinomas were located in the left pancreatic limb, one in the right pancreatic limb and one in the body between the portal vein and the pancreatic duct.[60,63-66] If the tumor location precludes partial pancreatectomy or if multiple lesions are present, careful enucleation of the tumor and metastases is recommended. Metastases of the lymph nodes and liver are resected if possible to achieve cytoreduction. It is important not to euthanize the animal because of an abnormal gross hepatic appearance as there is little correlation between visual inspection and histology of hepatic biopsies.[67] Large masses in the area of the pancreatic head can be very difficult to excise, and excessive manipulation can lead to severe postoperative pancreatitis. Debulking for cytoreduction and, in severe cases, a conservative approach including medical therapy should be considered. If no primary tumor can be detected, a surgical biopsy is taken to rule out diffuse pancreatic disease. Postoperative hypoglycemia is usually a sign of remaining tumor cells. Repeat surgery or medical treatment can be considered. If cats are normoglycemic after surgery, continued monitoring of glucose levels is recommended. Hyperglycemia occurs if islet cell insulin production is suppressed by the tumor and in severe cases, insulin can be given until normal function of islet cells is restored.

Medical treatment is aimed at prevention of hypoglycemia by a variety of approaches: small frequent meals of a diet high in fat, protein, and complex carbohydrates should be fed. Glucocorticoids stimulate hepatic glycogenolysis and gluconeogenesis and antagonize the effect of insulin production at a cellular level. Prednisolone is started at a dose of 0.5–1 mg/kg PO twice daily; increasing doses may be necessary.[56] If hypoglycemia is not controlled adequately, diazoxide (5–20 mg/kg PO twice daily), the somatostatin-uptake inhibitor octreotide (1–2 μg/kg SQ q8–12h), and propanolol (0.2–1.0 mg/kg PO q8h) have been recommended.[56,68]

Prognosis in the few reported cases seems to be poor to guarded. Recurrence of clinical signs is described at five days, six days, seven months and 18 months postoperatively. One cat was euthanized because of persistence of neurologic signs 1 month after surgery; however, one cat was still alive and clinically normal 32 months after surgery. In dogs, median survival without metastasis at the time of surgery is about 18 months and seven to nine months for those with metastasis.[69] In a more recent study, dogs undergoing surgery for insulinoma survived for a median of 785 days, while dogs that received additional medical treatment after relapse of hypoglycemia lived for a median of 1316 days.[70]

SURGICAL MANAGEMENT AND TECHNIQUES

Pancreatic biopsy (Box 33-2)

Biopsy is indicated for tissue diagnosis of pancreatic disease. Cytology from an ultrasound-guided fine needle aspiration is the first step to establish a diagnosis and often yields reliable results.[55] Should the diagnosis not be conclusive, histopathology from pancreatic biopsies is indicated. Biopsies can be taken laparoscopically or surgically. Laparoscopy (see Chapter 24) offers a minimally invasive and safe modality to obtain high quality pancreatic biopsies.[5,71,72] Laparoscopic biopsy results in local reactions, but neovascularization and adhesions are less pronounced than after surgical biopsy.[73,74]

Partial pancreatectomy (Box 33-3)

Partial pancreatectomy is indicated for focal lesions like neoplasms, abscesses or pseudocysts.

Total pancreatectomy

Therapeutic total pancreatectomy is rarely performed in cats and dogs since it bears a high preoperative morbidity and mortality.[5] Possible indications are intractable pancreatitis or trauma. Total pancreatectomy for exocrine pancreatic neoplasia is not recommended because of the high metastatic rate and poor prognosis. Experimentally, total pancreatectomy is described for the dog only.[76,77]

The critical part in total pancreatectomy surgery is the removal of the right pancreatic limb and pancreatic head. Because of extensive

---

Box 33-2 Pancreatic biopsy

The cat is placed in dorsal recumbency, clipped and prepared for aseptic abdominal surgery.

Laparoscopic pancreatic biopsy

The cat is placed in dorsal recumbency and after establishment of a pneumoperitoneum and routine camera and instrumental portal insertion (typically a three-port technique is used) (see Chapter 24), the left and right pancreatic limbs are inspected. The left limb can be manipulated by lifting and retracting the spleen to the right. A punch type biopsy instrument should be used, as it has been shown to help obtain biopsy specimens with minimal crush or traction artifacts.[55] Special care has to be taken to avoid damage to the pancreatic blood supply and duct system when tissue is excised from the pancreatic body or the right lobe.

Open surgical pancreatic biopsy

A cranial midline abdominal incision is made. A TruCut needle is used or a small tissue wedge is taken using a scalpel blade from abnormal pancreatic tissue after incising the mesoduodenum or dorsal omental

leaf. Alternatively, small tissue samples can be retrieved via suture fracture technique or blunt dissection and ligation technique. For the suture fracture technique, the mesoduodenum or dorsal omental leaf is opened and non-absorbable suture material is passed around the tissue to be removed. By tightening the suture, pancreatic parenchyma is crushed, thereby ligating small pancreatic ducts and blood vessels. The tissue distal to the suture is cut with a scalpel blade and submitted for histopathology (Fig. 33-7).

For the dissection and ligation technique, sterile cotton buds or Halstead mosquito forceps are used to dissect the pancreatic parenchyma (Fig. 33-8). Pancreatic ducts and blood vessels remain and are ligated and transected. Alternatively, careful bipolar cautery can be used for transection and ligation. The mesoduodenum is closed with fine absorbable suture material. The abdomen is thoroughly lavaged with warm sterile saline solution to reduce the concentration of activated digestive enzymes and toxins. If the cat has been anorexic or not eating well, establishment of an esophagostomy, gastroduodenostomy, or jejunostomy tube should be considered (see Chapter 12).

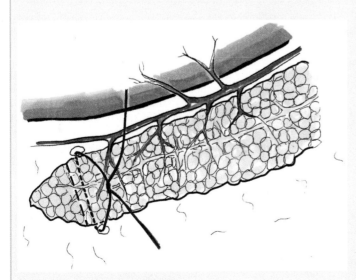

Figure 33-7 Suture fracture technique.

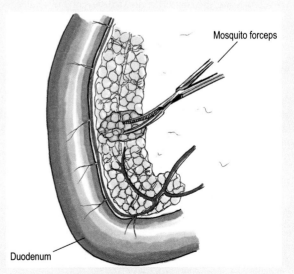

Mosquito forceps

Duodenum

Figure 33-8 Blunt dissection and ligation technique.

Box 33-3 Partial pancreatectomy

The cat is placed in dorsal recumbency, clipped and prepared for aseptic abdominal surgery. A cranial midline incision is made to enable entry into the abdomen.

A suture fracture or dissection and ligation technique can be employed. For the suture fracture technique, the mesoduodenum or dorsal omental leaf is opened and non-absorbable suture material is passed around the tissue to be removed. By tightening the suture, pancreatic parenchyma is crushed, thereby ligating small pancreatic ducts and blood vessels. The tissue distal to the suture is cut with a scalpel blade and submitted for histopathology (Fig. 33-7).

For the dissection and ligation technique, sterile cotton buds or Halstead mosquito forceps are used to dissect the pancreatic parenchyma (Fig 33-8). Pancreatic ducts and blood vessels remain and are ligated and transected. Alternatively, careful bipolar cautery can be used for transection and ligation.

For dissection of the left pancreatic limb, blood supply coming from the splenic artery is ligated and transected, or cauterized if vessels are small; care is taken to preserve integrity of the splenic artery. In disease with severe peripancreatic involvement this might not prove feasible, then splenectomy is required. For excision of the distal part of the right pancreatic limb, great care has to be taken not to obstruct the caudal pancreaticoduodenal artery, because of the particular blood supply in the cat.[9] Because of the strong regenerative capacity of the pancreas, up to 80% of the pancreas can be resected without impairment of the exocrine or endocrine function.[75] Non-resectable abscesses in the pancreatic body should be drained and omentalized.

The mesoduodenum or dorsal omental leaf are closed with fine absorbable suture material.

In cats with severe peritonitis or pancreatic abscess, closed abdominal drainage with a Jackson-Pratt drain should be considered to provide ongoing evacuation of fluid from the abdomen. Routinely, two drains are used: one is placed cranial to the liver and the second one should lie in the area of the pathology (i.e., pancreas) to optimize drainage. An esophagostomy, gastrostomy, gastroduodenostomy, or jejunostomy feeding tube is placed.

intake should be restricted for 12–24 hours; however, longer periods of anorexia should be avoided. Food is mostly provided via a surgically placed gastroduodenostomy or jejunostomy tube. As obligate carnivores, cats have a predilection for the development of fat mobilization and hepatic lipidosis if protein intake is not adequate. If the cat is vomiting in spite of anti-emetic treatment, parenteral nutrition should be instituted to meet nutritional requirements. Even in these cases, minimal amounts of oral food intake will be beneficial to maintain enterocyte integrity. Fluid and electrolyte balance is monitored and maintained as necessary.

Glucose levels should be monitored at least twice daily and, if hypoglycemia is present, 2.5% dextrose in balanced electrolyte solution is administered. Persistent hypoglycemia after removal of insulinoma is typically a sign of remaining tumor cells. Insulin is used to treat hyperglycemia.

Cats with peritonitis are closely monitored for the development of sepsis and DIC. It is critical to treat hypoalbuminemia by administration of synthetic colloids, human albumin, or plasma transfusions. Broad-spectrum antibiotics are administered in those patients until culture and sensitivity results are available.

COMPLICATIONS

Pancreatitis is a possible complication after pancreatic surgery. Fortunately, the incidence after surgical biopsy of the pancreas or resection of pancreatic neoplasia is low when atraumatic tissue handling is strictly executed.[23,24,73]

Hepatic lipidosis is a well-recognized complication after ANP and is a poor prognostic sign. This underlines the necessity for adequate nutritional intake in cats with pancreatitis. Cats with necrotizing and suppurative or septic conditions of the pancreas need to be monitored carefully for the development of septic peritonitis, pneumonia, and thoracic effusion.

Pre-existing diabetes mellitus might worsen after a further bout of pancreatitis or after pancreatic surgery. Diabetes mellitus is a rare complication of chronic pancreatitis.

inflammatory changes it is most often not feasible to excise the pancreatic tissue without traumatizing the shared pancreatic and duodenal vasculature, so pancreaticoduodenectomy and cholecystojejunostomy are necessary.

POSTOPERATIVE CARE

Postoperative care is dependent on the underlying disease. Analgesia is provided as necessary. Opioid agonists-antagonists like buprenorphine 10–30 μg/kg IV q6–8h were historically preferred over pure agonists, since they were thought not to increase pressure of the sphincter of Oddi and are not associated with gastrointestinal hypomotility. However, pain relief is paramount so clinicians should not be afraid to administer pure opioid agonists to the painful cat. Oral

PROGNOSIS

Generally, prognosis for surgical inflammatory pancreatic disease in cats is guarded to poor. Non-specific clinical signs require high levels of suspicion by the attending clinician, and diagnosis is often delayed. Many cats with severe necrotizing pancreatitis or pancreatic rupture are only diagnosed during exploratory laparotomy or at postmortem examination. New diagnostic developments such as the radioimmunoassay for detection of serum fPLI might help to diagnose conditions earlier, but still the systemic effects of pancreatitis can be severe. Aggressive treatment must be started immediately in order to improve survival and stop the vicious circle of intra-abdominal pancreatic enzyme activation and necrosis. Pancreatic tumors are mostly malignant and highly metastatic and, with the exception of resectable insulinomas, bear a poor to grave prognosis.

REFERENCES

1. Vollmerhaus B, Habermehl KH. Bauchspeicheldrüse. In: Frewein J, Vollmerhaus B, editors. Anatomie von Hund und Katze. Berlin: Blackwell-Wissenschafts-Verlag; 1994. p. 163–5.
2. Motta PM, Macchiarelli G, Nottola SA, Correr S. Histology of the exocrine pancreas. Microsc Res Tech 1997;37:384–98.
3. Schummer A, Vollmerhaus B. Bauchspeicheldrüse, Pankreas. In:

Nickel R, Schummer A, Seiferle E, editors. Lehrbuch der Anatomie der Haustiere. Berlin, Hamburg: Verlag Paul Parey; 1987. p. 128–31.

4. Boyden EA. The problem of the pancreatic bladder – A critical survey of six new cases, based on new histological and embryological observations. American Journal of Anatomy 1925;36(1):151–83.

5. Cornell K, Fischer J. Surgery of the exocrine pancreas. In: Slatter D, editor. Textbook of small animal surgery. Philadelphia: Saunders; 2003. p. 752–62.

6. Brobst DF. Pancreatic function. In: Kaneko JJ, Harvey JW, Bruss M, editors. Clinical biochemistry of domestic animals. San Diego, California: Academic Press; 1997. p. 353.

7. Washabau RJ. Feline pancreatic disease. In: Ettinger SJ, Feldman EC, editors. Textbook of veterinary internal medicine: diseases of the dog and the cat. St. Louis, Mo: Elsevier Saunders; 2010. p. 1704–9.

8. Cornell K. Pancreas. In: Tobias KM, Johnston SA, editors. Veterinary surgery: small animal. Elsevier, Saunders; 2012. p. 1659–73.

9. Pott G. Die arterielle Blutversorgung des Magendarmkanals, seiner Anhangsdruesen (Leber, Pankreas) und der Milz bei der Katze. Hannover, Germany: Veterinary Medical Dissertation; 1949.

10. Egerbacher M, Böck P. Morphology of the pancreatic duct system in mammals. Microsc Res Tech 1997;37(5–6):407–17.

11. Baum H. Das Lymphgefässystem des Hundes. Archiv der wissenschaftlichen und praktischen Tierheilkunde 1918;44:521–650.

12. Hill RC, Van Winkle TJ. Acute necrotizing pancreatitis and acute suppurative pancreatitis in the cat. A retrospective study of 40 cases (1976–1989). J Vet Intern Med 1993;7(1):25–33.

13. Kimmel SE, Washabau RJ, Drobatz KJ. Incidence and prognostic value of low plasma ionized calcium concentration in cats with acute pancreatitis: 46 cases (1996–1998). J Am Vet Med Assoc 2001;219(8):1105–9.

14. Forman MA, Marks SL, De Cock HE, et al. Evaluation of serum feline pancreatic lipase immunoreactivity and helical computed tomography versus conventional testing for the diagnosis of feline pancreatitis. J Vet Intern Med 2004;18(6):807–15.

15. Steiner JM, Wilson BG, Williams DA. Development and analytical validation of a radioimmunoassay for the measurement of feline pancreatic lipase immunoreactivity in serum. Can J Vet Res 2004;68(4):309–14.

16. Lettow E, Kabisch D, Arnold U. Pankreasruptur nach Fenstersturz bei der Katze. Kleintierpraxis 1989;31:191–6.

17. Gerhardt A, Steiner JM, Williams DA, et al. Comparison of the sensitivity of different diagnostic tests for pancreatitis in cats. J Vet Intern Med 2001;15(4):329–33.

18. Saunders HM, VanWinkle TJ, Drobatz K, et al. Ultrasonographic findings in cats with clinical, gross pathologic, and histologic evidence of acute pancreatic necrosis: 20 cases (1994–2001). J Am Vet Med Assoc 2002;221(12):1724–30.

19. Hittmair KM, Vielgrader HD, Loupal G. Ultrasonographic evaluation of gallbladder wall thickness in cats. Vet Radiol Ultrasound 2001;42(2):149–55.

20. Rademacher N, Ohlerth S, Scharf G, et al. Contrast-enhanced power and color Doppler ultrasonography of the pancreas in healthy and diseased cats. J Vet Intern Med 2008;22(6):1310–16.

21. De Cock HE, Forman MA, Farver TB, Marks SL. Prevalence and histopathologic characteristics of pancreatitis in cats. Vet Pathol 2007;44(1):39–49.

22. Yotsumoto F, Manabe T, Ohshio G, et al. Role of pancreatic blood flow and vasoactive substances in the development of canine acute pancreatitis. J Surg Res 1993;55(5):531–6.

23. Lightwood R, Reber HA, Way LW. The risk and accuracy of pancreatic biopsy. Am J Surg 1976;132(2):189–94.

24. Wilson JW, Maywood DD. Functional tumors of the pancreatic beta cells. Am J Surg 1981;3:458.

25. Ferreri JA, Hardam E, Kimmel SE, et al. Clinical differentiation of acute necrotizing from chronic nonsuppurative pancreatitis in cats: 63 cases (1996–2001). J Am Vet Med Assoc 2003;223:469–74.

26. Swift NC, Marks SL, MacLachlan NJ, Norris CR. Evaluation of serum feline trypsin-like immunoreactivity for the diagnosis of pancreatitis in cats. J Am Vet Med Assoc 2000;217(1):37–42.

27. Washabau RJ, Holt DE. Pathophysiology of gastrointestinal disease. In: Slatter D, editor. Textbook of Small Animal Surgery. 3rd ed. vol 1. Philadelphia: Saunders; 2003. p. 530–52.

28. Widdison AL, Alvarez C, Chang YB, et al. Sources of pancreatic pathogens in acute pancreatitis in cats. Pancreas 1994;9(4):536–41.

29. Widdison AL, Karanjia ND, Reber HA. Antimicrobial treatment of pancreatic infection in cats. Br J Surg 1994;81(6):886–9.

30. Mayhew PD, Weisse CW. Treatment of pancreatitis-associated extrahepatic biliary tract obstruction by choledochal stenting in seven cats. J Small Anim Pract 2008;49(3):133–8.

31. Bacon NJ, White RA. Extrahepatic biliary tract surgery in the cat: A case series and review. J Small Anim Pract 2003;44(5):231–5.

32. Son TT, Thompson L, Serrano S, Seshadri R. Surgical intervention in the management of severe acute pancreatitis in cats: 8 cases (2003–2007). J Vet Emerg Crit Care (San Antonio) 2010;20(4):426–35.

33. Salisbury SK, Lantz GC, Nelson RW, Kazacos EA. Pancreatic abscess in dogs: six cases (1978–1986). J Am Vet Med Assoc 1988;193(9):1104–8.

34. Thompson LJ, Seshadri R, Raffe MR. Characteristics and outcomes in surgical management of severe acute pancreatitis: 37 dogs (2001–2007). J Vet Emerg Crit Care (San Antonio) 2009;19(2):165–73.

35. Anderson JR, Cornell KK, Parnell NK, Salisbury SK. Pancreatic abscess in 36 dogs: A retrospective analysis of prognostic indicators. J Am Anim Hosp Assoc 2008;44(4):171–9.

36. Johnson MD, Mann FA. Treatment for pancreatic abscesses via omentalization with abdominal closure versus open peritoneal drainage in dogs: 15 cases (1994–2004). J Am Vet Med Assoc 2006;228(3):397–402.

37. Bellenger CR, Ilkiw JE, Malik R. Cystogastrostomy in the treatment of pancreatic pseudocyst/abscess in two dogs. Vet Rec 1989;125(8):181–4.

38. Hess RS, Saunders HM, Van Winkle TJ, et al. Clinical, clinicopathologic, radiographic, and ultrasonographic abnormalities in dogs with fatal acute pancreatitis: 70 cases (1986–1995). J Am Vet Med Assoc 1998;213(5):665–70.

39. VanEnkevort BA, O'Brien RT, Young KM. Pancreatic pseudocysts in 4 dogs and 2 cats: Ultrasonographic and clinicopathologic findings. J Vet Intern Med 1999;13(4):309–13.

40. Hines BL, Salisbury SK, Jakovljevic S, DeNicola DB. Pancreatic pseudocyst associated with chronic-active necrotizing pancreatitis in a cat. J Am Anim Hosp Assoc 1996;32(2):147–52.

41. Bosje JT, van den Ingh TS, van der Linde-Sipman JS. Polycystic kidney and liver disease in cats. Vet Q 1998;20(4):136–9.

42. Coleman MG, Robson MC, Harvey C. Pancreatic cyst in a cat. N Z Vet J 2005;53(2):157–9.

43. Branter EM, Viviano KR. Multiple recurrent pancreatic cysts with associated pancreatic inflammation and atrophy in a cat. J Feline Med Surg 2010;12(10):822–7.

44. Suter PF, Olsson SE. Traumatic hemorrhagic pancreatitis in the cat: A report with emphasis on the radiological diagnosis. J Am Vet Rad Soc 1969;10:4–11.

45. Westermarck E, Saario E. Traumatic pancreatic injury in a cat – a case history. Acta Vet Scand 1989;30(3):359–62.

46. Liehmann LM, Dörner J, Hittmair KM, et al. Pancreatic rupture in four cats with high-rise syndrome. J Feline Med Surg 2012;14(2):131–7.

47. Guija de Arespacochaga A, Hittmair KM, Schwendenwein I. Lipase activity in

peritoneal fluid in cats – a complimentary diagnostic tool? Vet Clin Pathol 2007;36(4):392–3.

48. Seaman RL. Exocrine pancreatic neoplasia in the cat: A case series. J Am Anim Hosp Assoc 2004;40(3):238–45.

49. Priester WA. Data from eleven United States and Canadian colleges of veterinary medicine on pancreatic carcinoma in domestic animals. Cancer Res 1974;34(6):1372.

50. Owens JM, Drazner FH, Gilbertson SR. Pancreatic disease in the cat. J Am Anim Hosp Assoc 1975;11:83–9.

51. Goossens MM, Nelson RW, Feldman EC, Griffey SM. Response to insulin treatment and survival in 104 cats with diabetes mellitus (1985–1995). J Vet Intern Med 1998;12(1):1–6.

52. Kipperman BS, Nelson RW, Griffey SM, Feldman EC. Diabetes mellitus and exocrine pancreatic neoplasia in two cats with hyperadrenocorticism. J Am Anim Hosp Assoc 1992;28(5):415–18.

53. Brooks DG, Campbell KL, Dennis JS, Dunstan RW. Pancreatic paraneoplastic alopecia in three cats. J Am Anim Hosp Assoc 1994;30(6):557–63.

54. Tasker S, Griffon DJ, Nuttall TJ, Hill PB. Resolution of paraneoplastic alopecia following surgical removal of a pancreatic carcinoma in a cat. J Small Anim Pract 1999;40(1):16–19.

55. Bennett PF, Hahn KA, Toal RL, Legendre AM. Ultrasonographic and cytopathological diagnosis of exocrine pancreatic carcinoma in the dog and cat. J Am Anim Hosp Assoc 2001;37(5):466–73.

56. Nelson RW. Beta-Cell neoplasia: Insulinoma. In: Feldman EC, Nelson RW, editors. Canine and feline endocrinology and reproduction. St. Louis, Mo: Saunders; 2004. p. 616–44.

57. Ward CR. Gastrointestinal endocrine disease. In: Ettinger SJ, Feldman EC, editors. Textbook of veterinary internal medicine: diseases of the dog and the cat. St. Louis, Mo, Elsevier Saunders; 2010. p. 1857–65.

58. Altschul M, Simpson KW, Dykes NL, et al. Evaluation of somatostatin analogues for the detection and treatment of gastrinoma in a dog. J Small Anim Pract 1997;38(7):286–91.

59. Jackson TC, Debey B, Lindbloom-Hawley S, et al. Cellular and molecular characterization of a feline insulinoma. J Vet Intern Med 2009;23(2):383–7.

60. Kraje AC. Hypoglycemia and irreversible neurologic complications in a cat with insulinoma. J Am Vet Med Assoc 2003;223(6):812–14.

61. Kyles A. Endocrine pancreas. In: Slatter D, editor. Textbook of Small Animal Surgery. 3rd ed. vol 2. Philadelphia: Saunders; 2003. p. 1724–36.

62. Mehlhaff CJ, Peterson ME, Patnaik AK, Carillo JM. Insulin-producing islet cell neoplasms: surgical considerations and general management in 35 dogs. J Am Anim Hosp Assoc 1985;21:607–12.

63. Hawks D, Peterson ME, Hawkins KL, Rosebury WS. Insulin-secreting pancreatic (islet cell) carcinoma in a cat. J Vet Intern Med 1992;6(3):193–6.

64. O'Brien TD, Norton F, Turner TM, Johnson KH. Pancreatic endocrine tumor in a cat: Clinical, pathological, and immunohistochemical evaluation. J Am Anim Hosp Assoc 1990;26(5):453–7.

65. McMillan FD, Barr B, Feldman EC. Functional pancreatic islet cell tumor in a cat. J Am Anim Hosp Assoc 1985;21(6):741–6.

66. Greene SN, Bright RM. Insulinoma in a cat. J Small Anim Pract 2008;49(1):38–40.

67. Tobin RL, Nelson RW, Lucroy MD, et al. Outcome of surgical versus medical treatment of dogs with beta cell neoplasia: 39 cases (1990–1997). J Am Vet Med Assoc 1999;215(2):226–30.

68. Bergman PJ. Paraneoplastic syndromes. In: Withrow SJ, Vail DM, editors. Withrow & MacEwen's small animal clinical oncology. St. Louis, Mo: Saunders Elsevier; 2007. p. 77–94.

69. Caywood DD, Johnston SD, Norris AM, et al. Pancreatic insulin-secreting neoplasma: Clinical, diagnostic, and prognostic features in 73 dogs. J Am Anim Hosp Assoc 1988;24:577–84.

70. Polton GA, White RN, Brearley MJ, Eastwood JM. Improved survival in a retrospective cohort of 28 dogs with insulinoma. J Small Anim Pract 2007;48(3):151–6.

71. Harmoinen J, Saari S, Rinkinen M, Westermarck E. Evaluation of pancreatic forceps biopsy by laparoscopy in healthy beagles. Vet Ther 2002;3(1):31–6.

72. Webb CB, Trott C. Laparoscopic diagnosis of pancreatic disease in dogs and cats. J Vet Intern Med 2008;22(6):1263–6.

73. Cosford KL, Shmon CL, Myers SL, et al. Prospective evaluation of laparoscopic pancreatic biopsies in 11 healthy cats. J Vet Intern Med 2010;24(1):104–13.

74. Lutz TA, Rand JS, Watt P, Galloway A. Pancreatic biopsy in normal cats. Aust Vet J 1994;71(7):223–5.

75. Mizumoto R, Yano T, Sekoguchi T, Kawarada Y. Resectability of the pancreas without producing diabetes, with special reference to pancreatic regeneration. Int J Pancreatol 1986;1(3–4):185–93.

76. Cobb LF, Merrell RC. Total pancreatectomy in dogs. J Surg Res 1984;37(3):235–40.

77. Papachristou DN, Fortner JG. A simple method of pancreatic transplantation in the dog. Am J Surg 1980;139(3):344–7.

78. Washabau RJ. Acute necrotizing pancreatitis. In: August JR, editor. Consultations in feline internal medicine, vol 5. St. Louis, Mo: Elsevier Saunders; 2006. p. 109–19.

79. Ferreira TH, Rezende ML, Mama KR, et al. Plasma concentrations and behavioral, antinociceptive, and physiologic effects of methadone after intravenous and oral transmucosal administration in cats. Am J Vet Res 2011;72:764–71.

80. Jakobs R, Adamek MU, von Bubnoff AC, Riemann JF. Buprenorphine or procaine for pain relief in acute pancreatitis. A prospective randomized study. Scand J Gastroenterol 2000;35(12):1319–23.

81. Lascelles BD, Robertson SA. Use of thermal threshold response to evaluate the antinociceptive effects of butorphanol in cats. Am J Vet Res 2004;65(8):1085–9.

82. Steiner JM, Williams DA. Feline exocrine pancreatic disorders. Vet Clin North Am Small Anim Pract 1999;29(2):551–75.

83. Gaynor AR. Acute pancreatitis. In: Silverstein DC, Hopper K, editors. Small animal critical care medicine. St. Louis, Mo: Saunders/Elsevier; 2009. p. 537–41.

84. Allenspach K, Chan DL. Antiemetic therapy. In: August JR, editor. Consultations in Feline Internal Medicine, vol. 6. St. Louis: Saunders Elsevier; 2010. p. 232–9.

Chapter |34|

Spleen

N.J. Bacon, D.A. Kamstock

Disease of the feline spleen is not common. Splenic lesions in feline necropsy specimens range from 0.3–5.9%[1,2] and so veterinary surgeons can go many years without ever knowingly encountering feline splenic disease. Splenomegaly, or splenic enlargement, may be diffuse (symmetric) or focal (asymmetric) and feline splenic disease is more likely to be neoplastic than canine splenic disease[2] with up to 73% of splenic changes being neoplastic.[3] Despite this, however, the feline spleen is less frequently removed than its canine counterpart. This chapter outlines broad principles involved with splenic disease, with attention paid to the spectrum of conditions encountered in the cat.

SURGICAL ANATOMY

The spleen is often not immediately visible on opening the abdomen, where it is located in the left cranial quadrant. The head of the spleen is closely associated with the fundus of the stomach and the body and tail can be entirely on the left or move more towards the midline. The blood supply comes from the celiac artery; branches are sent off to the left lobe of the pancreas, and then the splenic artery divides into dorsal and ventral branches a centimeter or so from the spleen. The ventral branch arborizes with the left gastroepiploic artery after supplying the main body of the spleen. The dorsal branch gives rise to the short gastric arteries after supplying the dorsal extremity of the spleen. Venous drainage is via the splenic vein, which drains into the portal vein via the gastrosplenic vein (Fig. 34-1).

There are unique ultrastructural properties of the non-sinusoidal feline spleen which make it unable to remove non-deformable erythrocytes containing Heinz bodies from the circulation,[4] resulting in the high incidence of Heinz bodies in clinically normal cats.[5]

GENERAL CONSIDERATIONS

History and clinical signs

Cats presenting with splenic disease are typically older, with a median age of 12 years, and with no sex predilection.[6] Presenting signs of

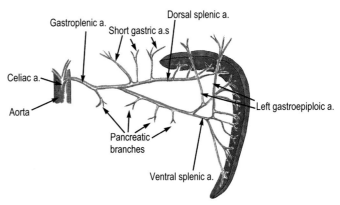

Figure 34-1 Blood supply of the spleen.

splenic disease in cats are typically non-specific, and the history usually includes weight loss, anorexia, lethargy and vomiting.[3] A palpable abdominal mass or splenomegaly is found in approximately 50% of cases,[3,6,7] although the spleen is usually enlarged in over 80% of cats with lymphoma. It is typical to find splenomegaly when the spleen is infiltrated with mast cells, and the spleen is often irregular in contour.[3] These patients also often present with anorexia and vomiting due to gastric and duodenal ulcers from paraneoplastic histamine release.[8]

Hemoperitoneum

Most cases of hemoperitoneum in cats are traumatic in nature and evidence of abdominal effusion or a palpable abdominal mass is often absent.[7] Following blunt trauma, the spleen and liver are the most likely sources of severe ongoing hemorrhage.[9] The clinical signs tend to be non-specific and include lethargy, anorexia, vomiting, abdominal distension, generalized weakness, pale mucous membranes, hemoglobinuria, and sometimes syncope and overt signs of shock.

Cats rarely present with spontaneous hemoperitoneum, with only four cats out of 19 undergoing splenectomy having free abdominal blood in one study.[6] In spontaneous hemoperitoneum cases bleeding occurs most commonly from the liver, with the spleen only accounting for 17% of cases.

© 2014 Elsevier Ltd
DOI: 10.1016/B978-0-7020-4336-9.00034-2

A ruptured spleen from hemangiosarcoma is the most common neoplastic cause although neoplasia only accounted for 46% of cases. Splenic lymphoma is a rare cause of spontaneous hemoperitoneum.[7,10]

Blood analysis

Cats with spontaneous hemoabdomen are often anemic, with many having a packed cell volume of 20% or lower. An increased reticulocyte count and thrombocytopenia are also frequently found.[6,7] Decreases in total protein, often through hypoalbuminemia, are common. Cats with hemoabdomen also often have high serum lactate levels, indicative of their low circulating blood volume and poor blood pressure. Elevations in serum urea and creatinine may also be present, typically with a pre-renal cause. With primary visceral mast cell disease involving the spleen, it is common to see a circulating eosinophilia and up to 40% of cats have a buffy coat layer that is positive for mast cells.[11] Erythrocytosis due to catecholamine release as seen in dogs is not expected in cats, as they lack the muscular component to the spleen and sinusoid splenic blood.[12]

Common abnormalities in the coagulation profile of cats with hemoabdomen include prolongation in prothrombin time (PT) and partial thromboplastin time (PTT).

Imaging

Ultrasound is the most useful imaging modality for examination of the spleen though inflated thoracic radiographs or computer tomography[13] are used to screen for metastatic disease. The normal feline spleen is diffusely homogenous, has a finer echotexture than the liver (like the dog), and is more echogenic than the liver or renal cortex.

Splenic masses can appear both hypoechoic and hyperechoic on ultrasound.[7] The spleen in cats with lymphoma is reportedly diffusely hypoechoic, mottled in texture and may contain small hypoechoic foci, although the foci can be up to 1–2 cm in diameter.[3,14] Abdominal effusion and at least one enlarged abdominal lymph node are also found. Myeloproliferative disease involving the spleen is also diffusely hypoechoic. Mast cell disease often results in a subjectively larger spleen, with a diffusely hypoechoic or nodular/mottled texture although it might present as single or multiple nodules.[15] Liver involvement is also present in approximately 30% of cases. No characteristics allowing differentiation of cats with lymphosarcoma from cats with mast cell tumor have been described, although the former are more likely to have abdominal effusion or lymphadenopathy.[3] Common incidental findings in feline spleens include myelolipomas which are well-defined, hyperechoic foci.[16]

Rarely, the splenic vein will thrombose, normally in association with feline liver disease or portal vein thrombosis; in this situation color flow Doppler will reveal no flow within the spleen.[17]

Computed tomography is increasingly being explored for staging of neoplasia involving intra-abdominal organs such as the spleen, or for identifying the origin of an abdominal mass.[18] It is likely this practice will increase with growing availability of these scanners.

Magnetic resonance imaging (MRI) is not widely used at this time for imaging the feline cranial abdomen although the appearance of normal liver, spleen, kidneys, and pancreas has been published as a reference guide.[19]

Cytology

Ultrasound-guided fine needle aspirates can be used to distinguish causes of splenomegaly, and they provided a diagnostic sample in 81 of 101 cats,[3] although in another study fine needle aspirates could not identify an underlying cause of splenomegaly in two of five cats[20] and in another study cytology only corresponded to the histologic diagnosis in 61% of splenic aspirates, although this included cats and dogs.[21] The cat is sedated and positioned in right lateral or dorsal recumbency and a 23G or 25G 1–1.5 inch needle is used. Samples should be collected with a non-aspiration technique (needle pushed into spleen and retracted and redirected several times), as this has been shown in the feline spleen to provide higher cellularity and less blood yet the same cell morphology compared to samples obtained by aspiration techniques (applying suction through a syringe).[22]

There is no evidence to suggest that bleeding is common or important after splenic aspiration in cats, even in the face of thrombocytopenia.[23] There is also no evidence in the cat or dog to suggest splenic aspiration has resulted in tumor-seeding to the needle tract in the body wall.

SURGICAL DISEASES

Surgery is not always indicated in splenic disease. The proper diagnostic tests (along with signalment, history, and clinical signs) should be pursued to obtain the most accurate diagnosis. These tests may include hematology, imaging, and cytology as addressed above, as well as biochemical analysis, bone marrow aspirate to rule out myeloproliferative diseases or leukemia (acute myeloid leukemia or chronic myeloid leukemia),[24–27] polymerase chain reaction to rule out specific infectious agents,[28–30] culture for fungal[30] or bacterial splenitis or possibly bacteremia inducing immune-responsive splenomegaly/hyperplasia. Also, while these diseases are less common, genetic tests are available to rule out specific hemolytic (e.g., pyruvate kinase deficiency)[31,32] or storage diseases, which can also result in splenomegaly. Special stains on cytological samples may also be of benefit.[26,27,33]

Surgical conditions of the feline spleen include laceration, torsion, some neoplasia (benign and malignant), and occasionally other causes such as foreign bodies and abscesses, as listed in Box 34-1. Abscesses within the spleen are uncommon in the cat and usually found in association with hepatic abscesses.[39] Many neoplastic conditions, when limited to the spleen, warrant surgical intervention (e.g., splenic mast cell tumor, hemangiosarcoma, leiomyosarcoma, fibrosarcoma), but many do not (Box 34-1). Conditions of the spleen may be generalized or localized, but the decision about whether a patient requires surgery is more dependent on the overall clinical situation rather than the exact distribution of lesions within the spleen.

Splenic laceration, trauma and torsion

Laceration of the splenic capsule, splenic hematoma, and avulsion of the splenic vessels are all possible sequelae to abdominal trauma. Iatrogenic laceration of the spleen with a scalpel or scissors is also possible when entering the abdomen during a laparotomy, especially if the abdomen is already distended. Following blunt trauma, the spleen and liver are the most likely sources of severe ongoing hemorrhage.[9] Many smaller tears or lacerations will spontaneously seal and do not require further treatment. If small tears are encountered during surgery, the capsule can be carefully sutured with a simple continuous pattern of monofilament absorbable material, such as poliglecaprone. Larger lacerations might require topical hemostatic agents, for example Gelfoam (gelatin) or Surgicel (cellulose). For large lacerations or fractures, or if a large section of the spleen has had the blood supply avulsed, a partial or total splenectomy may be required.

Occasionally following trauma, the spleen can herniate into the thorax through a diaphragmatic tear, along with other organs such as stomach, liver, or intestines. Splenic infarction is a possible outcome

Box 34-1 **Conditions of the feline spleen**

Traumatic*
  Laceration (Fig. 34-2)
  Torsion/vascular occlusion
Infectious/inflammatory (generalized)
  Visceral leishmaniasis, histoplasmosis, cryptococcosis, mycobacteriosis
  Cytauxzoonosis (typically granulomatous)
  FIP, Sporotrichosis, Blastomycosis (typically pyogranulomatous)
  Bacterial splenitis, Toxoplasmosis (typically suppurative)
  Hypereosinophilic syndrome (eosinophilic)
  Hemotropic mycoplasmosis (lymphoplasmacytic)
Benign neoplasia (localized/multifocal)*
  Hemangioma,[34] myelolipoma[15] (Fig. 34-3), lipoma, leiomyoma
Malignant neoplasia (localized)*
  Hemangiosarcoma,[35] fibrosarcoma, liposarcoma, leiomyosarcoma, chondrosarcoma, myxosarcoma, rhabdomyosarcoma and extraskeletal osteosarcoma,[36] histiocytic sarcoma[37]
Malignant neoplasia (generalized/multifocal)
  Lymphoma, mast cell neoplasia*, myeloproliferative disease, acute myeloid leukemia (AML), chronic myeloid leukemia (CML)
Metastatic neoplasia (localized or multifocal)
  Pancreatic adenocarcinoma, cholangiocellular adenocarcinoma, colonic carcinoma, thyroid carcinoma, transitional cell carcinoma (Fig. 34-4)
Other
  Foreign body*[38]
  Nodular hyperplasia
  Hematoma*
  Splenic abscess*
  Lymphoplasmacytic splenitis (secondary to antigenic stimulus)
  Hemolytic diseases
  Storage diseases

*Potential surgical disease (taking into consideration the entire clinical picture).

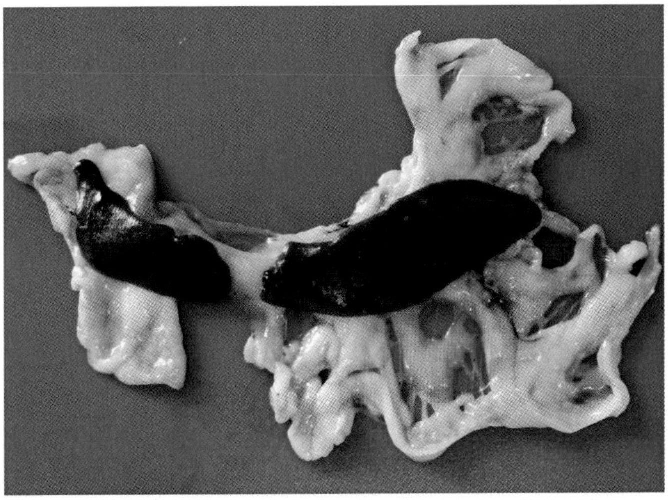

that can be diagnosed with ultrasound.[40] Rarely, the spleen is found amongst other abdominal viscera in a pericardioperitoneal diaphragmatic hernia.[41]

Torsion

Splenic torsion is rare, but an affected cat might present with abdominal pain, splenomegaly and cardiovascular shock. Some cats may have a more insidious onset, with clinical signs of anorexia, vomiting, ascites, anemia, and progressive neutrophilia.

After splenic torsion acute venous obstruction occurs initially, without arterial occlusion, resulting in splenic distension, sequestration of blood in the spleen, and ultimately hemolysis. Following thrombosis of the splenic artery, the spleen becomes necrotic, leading to bacterial proliferation. It would be unusual for splenic torsion to present with hemabdomen. Diagnosis is made by ultrasound examination and this is confirmed at exploratory celiotomy once the patient is stable following intravenous crystalloids or even blood products. It is not recommended to untwist the splenic pedicle at time of surgery for fear of releasing bacteria and associated toxins into the circulation. Either the hilar splenectomy or pedicle splenectomy approach as outlined below can be used. It should be noted that the short gastric vessels are often already avulsed.

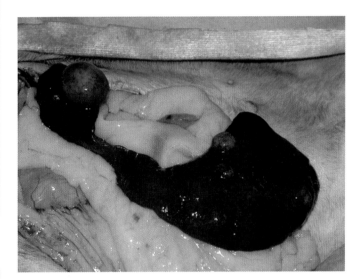

Figure 34-3 Multifocal myelolipoma in a 10-year-old cat.

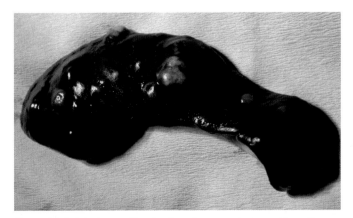

Figure 34-4 Splenic transitional cell carcinoma metastasized from the bladder in a 15-year-old cat.

Figure 34-2 A stray cat presumed to have died from a road traffic accident had a small blood clot adjacent to a fractured spleen presumed to be due to traumatic rupture. *(Courtesy of University of Cambridge.)*

Neoplasia

Primary neoplasia of the spleen includes lymphoma, mast cell neoplasia, hemangiosarcoma,[35] fibrosarcoma, liposarcoma, leiomyosarcoma, chondrosarcoma, myxosarcoma, rhabdomyosarcoma, and extraskeletal osteosarcoma.[36] Benign diseases include hemangioma,[34] myelolipoma,[15] lipoma, leiomyoma, and hematoma. The spleen can also be a site of metastatic, or secondary tumors, such as thyroid,[14] spleen,[42] colonic adenocarcinoma,[43,44] pancreatic carcinoma,[45] and cholangiocarcinoma[46] (see Box 34-1).

Splenic neoplasia is generally found in middle-aged to older cats. In a recent review of neoplasia in cats less than 12 months of age, only two of 233 submissions were from the spleen, so in young cats splenic neoplasia is rare.[34]

Mast cell neoplasia is the most common splenic disorder in cats, accounting for 15–53% of splenic lesions,[2,6] although primary splenic mast cell disease in cats is rare in real terms. The splenic and more common cutaneous forms appear to arise independently, rarely being present simultaneously,[47] with only one out of 30 cats being diagnosed with both splenic and cutaneous forms concurrently.[8,48] Patients are typically older cats with a median age of 10–12 years.

Hemangiosarcoma of the spleen is rare in the cat compared to the dog, with the disease affecting an estimated 2–21% of abnormal spleens.[2,6] In one study only two of 53 cases of feline hemangiosarcoma occur red in the spleen, the majority were cutaneous or subcutaneous[35] (see Box 34-1). Hemangiosarcoma in the cat is similar to the dog, with affected animals having abdominal effusion and anechoic foci seen on ultrasound.[3]

PREOPERATIVE PREPARATION FOR SURGERY

Cats with splenic disease need stabilization prior to surgery. Many are dehydrated and inappetent and have a history of weight loss. A thorough investigation should have been performed prior to surgery, including imaging and cytology of any mass or splenomegaly.

Antibiotic therapy prior to surgery is rarely indicated unless clearly directed by the findings of physical examination and cytology of any abdominal mass.

Crystalloid fluid therapy preoperatively is usually indicated. If the cat has a hemoperitoneum then a blood transfusion may be required preoperatively (see Chapter 5). It is worth noting that in one study 73% cats undergoing splenectomy required a blood transfusion, most of which did not have free abdominal blood,[6] and steps to prepare for this prior to surgery should be taken.

SURGICAL TECHNIQUES

The two main surgical techniques that are performed on the spleen are partial or total splenectomy.

Splenectomy

Removal of a bleeding spleen provides relief of clinical signs and a chance to stabilize an otherwise critical patient. The majority of splenic surgery in the cat, however, will differ from the dog in that the spleen is unlikely to be bleeding at the time of surgery.

In one study the average surgical time for a total splenectomy in a cat was 90 minutes[6] and the entire surgical team should be prepared for a procedure of this duration. This surgical time also included the

---

Box 34-2 Splenectomy

Following induction of anesthesia, the patient is surgically prepared for a midline celiotomy and an incision made from midway between the umbilicus and the xiphoid, extending approximately 10 cm caudally. The spleen is identified and exteriorized from the abdomen, placing it onto moistened gauze swabs at the incision site. The spleen should be handled very gently to avoid rupture and unnecessary hemorrhage or tumor spread.

Total splenectomy

Techniques of splenectomy vary, but the simplest involve double-ligating the line of splenic hilar vessels with 2M (3/0) absorbable material (e.g., poliglecaprone or polyglactin) and incising between the knots. This approach will keep the surgeon away from dissecting near the splenic vein, or the blood supply to the left side of the stomach, although splenectomy is also possible by ligating the major splenic vessels and short gastric arteries. Electrothermal bipolar vessel sealing devices (e.g., Ligasure) have been used for canine splenectomies[49] and will become increasingly used for feline splenic surgery as they become more available.

Hemisplenectomy

The hilar vessels feeding the abnormal section are ligated, and then large gauge silk (e.g. 3.5M [0]) is used to circumferentially ligate the spleen, crushing and encircling the pulp vessels as the loop tightens. The isolated section of spleen can be excised leaving a 5 mm cuff of normal spleen adjacent to the ligature. There is no need to oversew the exposed splenic tissue, although the omentum could be brought in to cover the raw surface.

Any suspicious lesions within the omentum and liver should also be biopsied and submitted for analysis (see Chapters 23 and 31).

Before the abdomen is closed, the peritoneal cavity should be gently lavaged with warm saline to dislodge any remaining blood clots. The splenic pedicle should be inspected for bleeding.

Following surgery, the entire spleen should be sliced as a loaf of bread to help tissue fixation in formalin or to find abnormal areas of different tissue and texture within the spleen if the whole organ cannot be submitted.[50]

---

need in many cats for additional surgical procedures, including biopsy of suspected metastatic lesions, for example in the liver or lymph nodes, or placement of an esophageal or gastric feeding tube in anorexic patients.

Partial splenectomy

Although uncommonly performed, partial splenectomy can salvage some splenic tissue when non-neoplastic disease is considered to be localized to the tail or the head of the spleen. It is usually a hemisplenectomy procedure (Box 34-2), with care being taken to identify the major splenic vessels to be preserved.

POSTOPERATIVE CARE AND COMPLICATIONS

Following removal of large splenic masses, there is a risk of postoperative hypotension due to pooling of blood in the mesenteric vessels following the rapid decrease in intra-abdominal pressure. This is complicated by the possibility of hemorrhage, either ongoing if the splenic pedicle was not securely ligated, or delayed if the ligatures on the pedicle come loose. The patient should be monitored for signs of hypoperfusion, including lethargy, weakness, pale mucous membranes, and collapse. Fluid volume needs to be maintained with crystalloids, and potentially even cross-matched blood transfusions if packed cell volume is low (see Chapter 5). Diagnosis of hemoabdomen post splenectomy is not an immediate indication for re-exploration as long as the facilities and resources exist to closely monitor and support the patient. Free fluid obtained by abdominocentesis should have the hematocrit measured. If the value closely approximates peripheral hematocrit then ongoing bleeding is likely. Any indication that the patient is worsening clinically, or is failing to respond to supportive measures, should be an indication to review the case management and decide whether surgical re-exploration is now sensible.

Complications arising from splenectomy include vascular damage to the left lobe of the pancreas or the gastric fundus. These will manifest themselves as pancreatitis, pancreatic abscess formation, or gastric injury or necrosis. In people there are concerns about immunologic impairment following splenectomy, but the reality of this has not been determined in the cat or the dog. It is known, however, that blood-borne diseases such as hemobartonellosis and babesiosis are more common in splenectomized dogs.

The most severe complication following splenectomy in the cat is sudden death, which may occur within 24 hours of surgery. The exact cause may differ between patients, but common causes include sudden catastrophic internal hemorrhage from one or more bleeding vessels, respiratory failure from pulmonary thromboembolism, and ventricular tachycardia of unknown origin post splenectomy.

For further general information on postoperative care after abdominal surgery see Chapters 3 and 4.

PROGNOSIS

The prognosis following splenectomy is dependent on whether the cat has neoplastic or non-neoplastic disease, with reported survival times of 197 versus 339 days, respectively.[6]

Splenic mast cell disease typically carries a significantly worse prognosis than cutaneous/subcutaneous mast cell disease in the cat. Historically, splenectomy has been described to result in the spontaneous regression of metastatic mast cell lesions and survival is reported to be 132–365 days,[6,51] although survival times ranging from 1–80 days were reported in one paper.[8,48] Death is typically due to euthanasia after return of clinical signs. A variety of chemotherapeutic agents including prednisolone, dexamethasone, vinblastine, CCNU, and cyclophosphamide have all been used to treat mast cell disease in cats, but the relative benefit is unclear.[8,48] Anorexia, significant weight loss, and male gender are considered negative prognostic indicators for cats with splenic mast cell disease.

Median survival time for hemangiosarcoma in cats post splenectomy is reportedly 77–197 days.[6,24,52] Chemotherapy for hemangiosarcoma has not been extensively studied in cats but doxorubicin-based protocols are a sensible choice. In one study of 65 cats with hemoperitoneum, most were euthanized and only 12% survived to discharge. There were no details of whether this number included any cats with splenic disease.[7]

The prognosis following surgery for splenic lymphoma is largely unknown, with only two cases described; one cat lived for three days and one lived 415 days.[6]

REFERENCES

1. Ishmael J, Howell J. Observations on the pathology of the spleen of the cat. J Small Anim Pract 1968;9:7–13.

2. Spangler W, Culbertson M. Prevalence and type of splenic disease in cats; 455 cases (1985–1991). J Am Vet Med Assoc 1992;201:773–6.

3. Hanson JA, Papageorges M, Girard E, et al. Ultrasonographic appearance of splenic disease in 101 cats. Vet Radiol Ultrasound 2001;42:441–5.

4. Christopher MM, White JG, Eaton JW. Erythrocyte pathology and mechanisms of Heinz body-mediated hemolysis in cats. Vet Pathol 1990;27:299–310.

5. Beritic T. Studies on Schmauch Bodies. I. the incidence in normal cats (felis domestica) and the morphologic relationship to Heinz bodies. Blood 1965;25:999–1008.

6. Gordon SSN, McClaran JK, Bergman PJ, et al. Outcome following splenectomy in cats. J Feline Med Surg 2010;12:256–61.

7. Culp WTN, Weisse C, Kellogg ME, et al. Spontaneous hemoperitoneum in cats: 65 cases (1994–2006). J Am Vet Med Assoc 2010;236:978–82.

8. Litster AL, Sorenmo KU. Characterisation of the signalment, clinical and survival characteristics of 41 cats with mast cell neoplasia. J Feline Med Surg 2006;8: 177–83.

9. Crowe DT. The Steps to Arresting Abdominal Hemorrhage. Vet Med 1988;83:676.

10. Ottenjann M, Kohn B, Weingart C. Rupturiertes Hamangiosarkom der Milz als Ursache eines Hamoperitoneums bei 4 Katzen. Kleintierpraxis 2003;48:345–52.

11. Murphy S. Skin neoplasia in small animals 2. Common feline tumours. In Practice 2006;28:320–5.

12. Stockham SL, Keeton KS, Szladovits B. Clinical assessment of leukocytosis: distinguishing leukocytoses caused by inflammatory, glucocorticoid, physiologic, and leukemic disorders or conditions. Vet Clin North Am Small Anim Pract 2003;33:1335–57.

13. Pastore GE, Lamb CR, Lipscomb V. Comparison of the results of abdominal ultrasonography and exploratory laparotomy in the dog and cat. J Am Anim Hosp Assoc 2007;43:264–9.

14. Marioni-Henry K, Van Winkle TJ, Smith SH, et al. Tumors affecting the spinal cord of cats: 85 cases (1980–2005). J Am Vet Med Assoc 2008;232:237–43.

15. Sato A, Solano M. Ultrasonographic findings in abdominal mast cell disease: a retrospective study of 19 patients. Vet Radiol Ultrasound 2004;45:51–7.

16. Hanson JA, Papageorges M, Girard E, et al. Ultrasonographic appearance of splenic disease in 101 cats. Vet Radiol Ultrasound 2001;42:441–5.

17. Rogers C, O'Toole T, Keating J, et al. Portal Vein Thrombosis in Cats: 6 Cases (2001–2006). J Vet Int Med 2008;22: 282–7.

18. LeBlanc A, Daniel G. Advanced Imaging for Veterinary Cancer Patients. Veterinary Clinics of North America: Small Animal Practice 2007;37:1059–77.

19. Newell SM, Graham JP, Roberts GD, et al. Quantitative magnetic resonance imaging of the normal feline cranial abdomen. Vet Radiol Ultrasound 2000;41:27–34.

20. O'Keefe DA, Couto CG. Fine-needle aspiration of the spleen as an aid in the diagnosis of splenomegaly. J Vet Int Med 1987;1:102–9.

21. Ballegeer EA, Forrest LJ, Dickinson RM, et al. Correlation of ultrasonographic appearance of lesions and cytologic and histologic diagnoses in splenic aspirates from dogs and cats: 32 cases (2002–2005). J Am Vet Med Assoc 2007;230: 690–6.

22. LeBlanc C, Head L. Comparison of aspiration and nonaspiration techniques for obtaining cytologic samples from the canine and feline spleen. Vet Clin Pathol 2009;38:242–6.

23. O'Keefe DA, Couto CG. Fine-needle aspiration of the spleen as an aid in the

diagnosis of splenomegaly. J Vet Int Med 1987;1:102–9.

24. Yates RW, Weller RE, Feldman BF. Myeloproliferative disease in a cat. Mod Vet Pract 1984;65:753–7.

25. Blue JT, French TW, Kranz JS. Non-lymphoid hematopoietic neoplasia in cats: a retrospective study of 60 cases. Cornell Vet 1988;78:21–42.

26. Sharifi H, Nassiri SM, Esmaelli H, et al. Eosinophilic leukaemia in a cat. J Feline Med Surg 2007;9:514–17.

27. Mylonakis ME, Petanides TA, Valli VE, et al. Acute myelomonocytic leukaemia with short-term spontaneous remission in a cat. Aust Vet J 2008;86:224–8.

28. Carli E, Trotta M, Chinelli R, et al. Cytauxzoon sp. infection in the first endemic focus described in domestic cats in Europe. Vet Parasitol 2012;183:343–52.

29. Sukasi P. Development of multiplex polymerase chain reaction for detection of feline hemotropic mycoplasma in blood and tissue specimens. SE Asian J Trop Med Public Health 2010;41:1447–53.

30. Bromel C, Sykes JE. Histoplasmosis in dogs and cats. Clin Tech Small Anim Pract 2005;20:227–32.

31. Mansfield CS, Clark P. Pyruvate kinase deficiency in a Somali cat in Australia. Aust Vet J 2005;83:483–5.

32. Kohn B, Goldschmidt MH, Hohenhaus AE, et al. Anemia, splenomegaly, and increased osmotic fragility of erythrocytes in Abyssinian and Somali cats. J Am Vet Med Assoc 2000;217:1483–91.

33. Jordan HL, Cohn LA, Armstrong PJ. Disseminated *Mycobacterium avium complex* infection in three Siamese cats. J Am Vet Med Assoc 1994;204:90–3.

34. Schmidt J, North S, Freeman K, et al. Feline paediatric oncology: retrospective assessment of 233 tumours from cats up to one year (1993 to 2008). J Small Anim Pract 2010;51:306–11.

35. Johannes CM, Henry CJ, Turnquist SE, et al. Hemangiosarcoma in cats: 53 cases (1992–2002). J Am Vet Med Assoc 2007;231:1851–6.

36. Dimopoulou M, Kirpensteijn J, Moens H, et al. Histologic Prognosticators in Feline Osteosarcoma: A Comparison with Phenotypically Similar Canine Osteosarcoma. Vet Surg 2008;37:466–71.

37. Ide K, Setoguchi-Mukai A, Nakagawa T, et al. Disseminated Histiocytic Sarcoma with Excessive Hemophagocytosis in a Cat. J Vet Med Sci 2009;71:817–20.

38. Culp WTN, Drobatz KJ, Glassman MM, et al. Feline visceral hemangiosarcoma. J Vet Int Med 2008;22:148–52.

39. Sergeeff J, Armstrong P, Bunch S. Hepatic abscesses in cats: 14 cases (1985–2002). J Vet Int Med 2004;18:295–300.

40. Baker T, Davidson A. Pediatric abdominal ultrasonography. Vet Clin NAm: Small Anim Prac 2006;36:641–55.

41. Reimer SB, Kyles AE, Filipowicz DE, et al. Long-term outcome of cats treated conservatively or surgically for peritoneopericardial diaphragmatic hernia: 66 cases (1987–2002). J Am Vet Med Assoc 2004;224:728–32.

42. Novosad CA, Bergman PJ, O'Brien MG, et al. Retrospective evaluation of adjunctive doxorubicin for the treatment of feline mammary gland adenocarcinoma: 67 cases. J Am Anim Hosp Assoc 2006;42:110.

43. Hume DZ, Solomon JA, Weisse CW. Palliative use of a stent for colonic obstruction caused by adenocarcinoma in two cats. J Am Vet Med Assoc 2006;228:392–6.

44. Cribb A. Feline gastrointestinal adenocarcinoma: a review and retrospective study. Can Vet J 1988.

45. Seaman RL. Exocrine pancreatic neoplasia in the cat: a case series. J Am Anim Hosp Assoc 2004;40:238.

46. Feldman B, Strafuss A, Gabbert N. Bile duct carcinoma in the cat: three case reports. Feline Prac 1976;1:33–9.

47. Liska WD, Macewen EG, Zaki FA, et al. Feline Systemic Mastocytosis – Review and Results of Splenectomy in 7 Cases. J Am Anim Hosp Assoc 1979;15:589–97.

48. Litster AL, Sorenmo KU. Characterisation of the signalment, clinical and survival characteristics of 41 cats with mast cell neoplasia. J Feline Med Surg 2006;8(3):177–83.

49. Rivier P, Monnet E. Use of a vessel sealant device for splenectomy in dogs. Vet Surg 2011;40:102–5.

50. Smith AN. Hemangiosarcoma in dogs and cats. Vet Clinics NAm Small Anim Prac 2003;33:533.

51. Carpenter J, Andrews L, Holzworth J. Tumors and tumor-like lesions In: Holzworth J, editor. Diseases of the cat medicine and surgery. Philadelphia: WB Saunders; 1987. p. 406–596.

52. Scavelli TD, Patnaik AK, Mehlhaff CJ, et al. Hemangiosarcoma in the Cat – Retrospective Evaluation of 31 Surgical Cases. J Am Vet Med Ass 1985;187:817–19.

Chapter |35|

Adrenal gland

A. Harvey, E.J. Friend

Adrenal gland problems in the cat are recognized with increasing frequency. They are most commonly identified in cats presenting for investigation of clinical signs attributed to excessive aldosterone, cortisol, or progesterone secretion. Surgery can be performed in selected cases of neoplasia, but first thorough investigation and stabilization are paramount. Adrenal surgery in cats is certainly not without risk, and is a technically challenging surgery that requires thorough planning, together with intensive perioperative care.

SURGICAL ANATOMY

The adrenal glands are found cranial to each kidney. They are cream colored as they are rich in lipids, and on ultrasound examination they have been reported to be 0.29–0.53 cm in size along their short axis.[1] At surgery, the duodenal maneuver is used to identify the right side and the colonic maneuver the left.

The right adrenal gland is harder to visualize than the left gland, because it is situated more cranially and it sits slightly dorsal to the vena cava; the caudate lobe of the liver may also partly cover it. The phrenico-abdominal veins cross over both adrenal glands.

The arterial blood is supplied by branches of the renal artery, directly from the aorta and from the phrenico-abdominal and lumbar arteries. Venous drainage is into the vena cava, phrenico-abdominal or lumbar veins. Neoplastic disease will often disrupt this and make an understanding of this supply rather academic.

Disease of the adrenal gland may affect surrounding structures, including the vena cava medially (and possibly the aorta), the kidneys caudally, and the sublumbar musculature dorsally.

DIAGNOSIS AND GENERAL CONSIDERATIONS

It is important for the surgeon to have knowledge of the disease processes involved, to ensure that surgical management is appropriate, and that the patient has been optimally stabilized preoperatively, with medical management where appropriate. Adrenal disorders predominantly affect older cats, and so concurrent disease may be common, and this is important to consider as it may significantly influence management. For the adrenal conditions reported there does not appear to be breed predisposition; most cases have been described in domestic short-hair cats. No sex predisposition exists; all reported cases have affected neutered animals, with roughly equal proportions of female and male cats.

Diagnostic imaging

Imaging is essential both for diagnostics and patient assessment before surgery. Currently, ultrasonography is the best imaging modality for detecting adrenal masses in dogs and cats. Inflated thoracic radiographs and/or computed tomography are used to rule out metastatic disease. Abdominal ultrasound, preferably combined with CT or MRI, should be performed to look for evidence of metastatic disease within the abdominal cavity (liver, spleen, lymph nodes), but also to assess local invasion or thrombosis within the vena cava. This information can make a great difference to surgical planning and treatment advice. Invasion into the adjacent vena cava, or renal vessels, renal or liver parenchyma is possible with more aggressive neoplasms and may be a contraindication for surgery if invasion is extensive. There are few reports in the literature about surgical management of caval invasion in the cat[2] and so guidelines are not available for when surgery should be undertaken, but this may be largely dictated by surgeon experience.

SURGICAL DISEASES

Hyperaldosteronism (Conn syndrome)

Hyperaldosteronism or Conn syndrome is a condition caused by increased secretion of aldosterone from the adrenal glands. It has become increasingly recognized in cats, but whether this is due to an increased awareness and testing for the condition, or a true increase in frequency is not known.

© 2014 Elsevier Ltd
DOI: 10.1016/B978-0-7020-4336-9.00035-4

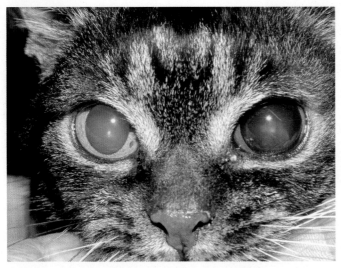

Figure 35-1 A cat with retinal detachment and vitreal hemorrhage, as a result of systemic hypertension associated with hyperaldosteronism. *(Photo courtesy of Tim Knott, Rowe Veterinary Group, UK. Reprinted from August, JR. 2010 Consultations in Feline Internal Medicine 6e, W.B. Saunders, with permission from Elsevier.)*

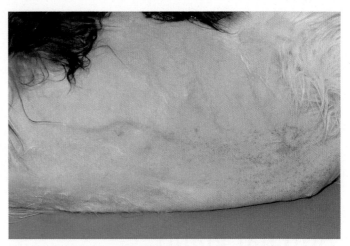

Figure 35-2 The ventral abdomen of a cat with concurrent hyperaldosteronism and hyperprogesteronism. Note the failure of hair regrowth and the thin skin with prominent subcutaneous blood vessels.

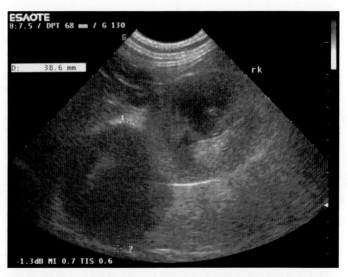

Figure 35-3 Ultrasound image demonstrating the typical hypoechoic appearance of an adrenal mass cranial to the right kidney. This was an adrenocortical carcinoma. *(Reprinted from August JR. (2010) Consultations in Feline Internal Medicine, 6, W.B. Saunders, with permission from Elsevier.)*

Etiology

Hyperaldosteronism may be of primary or secondary etiology. Secondary hyperaldosteronism occurs as a response to stimulation of the renin–angiotensin–aldosterone system (RAAS) and therefore may occur in any disease that stimulates the RAAS, such as dehydration, hypotension, reduced renal perfusion (most commonly secondary to renal disease), or sodium deficiency (reduced intake or increased loss). In primary hyperaldosteronism (PHA) there is an inappropriate increase in aldosterone secretion, independent of the RAAS. Unilateral adrenocortical neoplasia is the most commonly described cause of PHA in cats, with unilateral adrenal adenomas and carcinomas appearing to have approximately equal incidence. Although rare, bilateral adrenal neoplasms have also been described. Bilateral adrenal hyperplasia[3] is also recognized, and in these cases medical management is advised.

Clinical features

The major clinical signs of primary hyperaldosteronism are similar, whether it results from adrenal adenoma, carcinoma or hyperplasia, and they can be divided into two main groups:

- Hypokalemic polymyopathy
- Intraocular hemorrhage or acute onset blindness resulting from retinal detachment (Fig. 35-1) as a result of systemic hypertension.

Additional clinical signs such as polyuria, polydipsia, and polyphagia have also been reported

Concurrent hyperaldosteronism and hyperprogesteronism has also been reported in some cases of adrenal neoplasia.[4,5] In these cases the signs of hyperprogesteronism usually predominate, resulting in very similar clinical signs to those encountered with hypercortisolemia (Fig. 35-2).

Diagnosis

On serum biochemistry, hypokalemia is most often present; however, the degree is variable and normokalemia does not exclude the possibility of primary hyperaldosteronism. Serum sodium concentrations are usually normal or only mildly increased. Creatine kinase is usually elevated in cats with polymyopathy, with the degree of elevation being highly variable. Urea and creatinine may be elevated secondary to hyperaldosteronism, and so the presence of azotemia should not lead the clinician to conclude that hypokalemia and/or hypertension is a consequence of the renal disease itself.

Adrenal masses are rarely visible on radiographs, but if the mass is seen it is more likely to be an adrenocortical carcinoma than an adenoma. Pulmonary metastases can occur, albeit infrequently. In all reported feline cases of primary hyperaldosteronism in which adrenal ultrasonography was performed, unilateral adrenal enlargement with evidence of an adrenal mass was identified, ranging in size from 10–46 mm in diameter (Fig. 35-3). The contralateral adrenal gland may appear normal in appearance or may be unidentifiable. It is, however, vital that the contralateral gland be assessed, because bilateral adrenal neoplasms have been reported. Ultrasonography should also be used to identify the presence and degree of invasion of the caudal vena cava by the tumor or related thrombus, and the presence of metastasis to other organs. Close association of the tumor with the

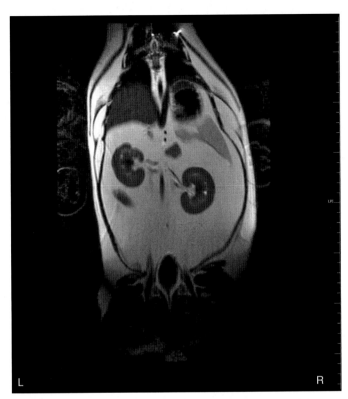

Figure 35-4 T2-weighted sagittal MRI scan of the abdomen demonstrating significantly enlarged right adrenal gland.

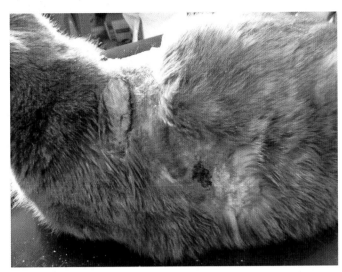

Figure 35-5 A cat with hyperadrenocorticism, illustrating skin tears as a result of skin fragility syndrome.

caudal vena cava is usually evident. Other imaging modalities, including MRI (Fig. 35-4), CT, and saphenous venography, have been used in a small number of cases in an attempt to establish the extent of the adrenal mass before undertaking surgery.

Confirmation of diagnosis relies mainly on demonstrating an elevated plasma aldosterone concentration. The assay is widely available at commercial endocrine laboratories and requirements for collection and handling of serum or plasma are routine. Ideally, plasma aldosterone concentration needs to be interpreted together with plasma renin activity, which would be expected to be elevated in cases of secondary hyperaldosteronism. There are difficulties with measuring plasma renin activity and as a consequence demonstration of the presence of adrenocortical neoplasia concurrently with a markedly elevated plasma aldosterone concentration is considered to be sufficient to make a diagnosis of aldosterone-secreting adrenocortical tumor in cats, especially in conjunction with persistent hypokalemia and hypertension. Histopathologic confirmation of the neoplasm together with resolution of clinical signs and plasma aldosterone measurements postoperatively assist in confirming the diagnosis.

If no adrenal mass is present, then non-neoplastic primary hyperaldosteronism should be considered, and this is more difficult to diagnose without assessment of plasma renin activity. Surgical treatment would not be indicated in these cases.

Medical management

Initial treatment of primary hyperaldosteronism is directed at controlling hypokalemia and/or hypertension. Potassium supplementation using potassium gluconate at doses of 2–6 mmol PO q12h has been used; intravenous potassium chloride may be required in more severely hypokalemic cases. Amlodipine besylate (0.625–1.25 mg PO q24h) is the initial treatment of choice for hypertension. Most hypertensive cats become normotensive with the aforementioned

amlodipine treatment, but higher doses are sometimes required. Spironolactone, a competitive aldosterone receptor antagonist, is also recommended (2–4 mg/kg PO q24h), for the control of both hypokalemia and hypertension.

Hyperadrenocorticism (Cushing's syndrome)

Hyperadrenocorticism or Cushing's syndrome is rare in cats and usually associated with pituitary neoplasia rather than primary disease of the adrenal glands.

Etiology

Hyperadrenocorticism results from chronic cortisol excess, and may occur secondary to iatrogenic cortisol administration, or with naturally occurring disease. Naturally occurring disease can be pituitary dependent, whereby a pituitary neoplasm secretes excessive ACTH with subsequent bilateral adrenocortical hyperplasia and increased cortisol secretion, or it may be adrenal dependent, as a result of a cortisol secreting adrenal neoplasm. Hyperadrenocorticism is rare in cats, but when it does occur the majority of cases (~80%) are pituitary dependent, most commonly as a result of a pituitary adenoma. About 50% are microadenomas (<3 mm diameter) and 50% are macroadenomas (>3 mm diameter). Pituitary carcinoma has only been rarely reported. In reported cases of adrenal-dependent disease, about 50% have been adrenocortical adenomas, and 50% adrenocortical carcinomas.

Clinical features

The major clinical signs are similar, whether hyperadrenocorticism results from adrenal adenoma, carcinoma or hyperplasia. Approximately 75% of cats with hyperadrenocorticism develop secondary diabetes mellitus, and the signs of uncontrolled diabetes mellitus usually predominate, namely polyuria, polydipsia, and polyphagia. Other clinical signs include lethargy, weight loss, an unkempt coat, and abdominal enlargement/pot belly appearance, although this is usually less appreciable than it is in dogs. Failure of hair regrowth, thin skin, and poor wound healing are common dermatologic features. Cushingoid cats may also exhibit severe skin fragility where the skin is so thin that it easily tears (Fig. 35-5). This is a serious complication as resultant wounds heal poorly, and it can also result in life-threatening sepsis.

Diagnosis

There are no striking hematological and biochemical abnormalities in cats with hyperadrenocorticism. Of particular note is that the classical biochemical abnormalities seen in dogs with hyperadrenocorticism are not observed in cats. Cats lack the steroid-induced isoenzyme of alkaline phosphatase (ALP) so the marked elevation in serum ALP frequently seen in dogs does not occur in cats. There may be mild to moderate elevations in liver enzymes, often secondary to diabetes mellitus, but this is not a consistent feature. Hyperglycemia may be present as a result of secondary diabetes mellitus in many cases. In dogs the urine is often isosthenuric; in cats very few have urine specific gravity of less than 1.025, and urinary tract infections have been uncommon in the reported cases.

Urine cortisol to creatinine ratio performed on a home collected sample can be used to exclude hyperadrenocorticism if it is normal. However, although not thoroughly evaluated in cats, it is likely to be very non-specific as in dogs, and so an elevated result is difficult to interpret. In cats, the adrenocortical trophic hormone (ACTH) stimulation test has not been as widely evaluated as it has in dogs, and its sensitivity and specificity has been questioned. Nevertheless, it is often the first endocrine function test to be performed since it is relatively straightforward and inexpensive to perform, and can distinguish iatrogenic from naturally occurring disease. The test (Box 35-1) is performed slightly differently to that in dogs, because the peak cortisol response following ACTH administration is variable, and so the optimum timing for blood sampling differs. The best time for blood sampling following ACTH administration remains controversial, with different studies suggesting different times for peak cortisol. The authors' protocol is shown in Box 35-1.

The low dose dexamethasone suppression test appears to be a very sensitive test for hyperadrenocorticism in cats and so is recommended as the test of choice for screening. The protocol for this test (Box 35-2) also differs to that used in dogs, with a higher per kilogram dose of dexamethasone given to cats.

In a normal cat, cortisol levels should be low at both four and eight hours, whereas in a cat with hyperadrenocorticism cortisol levels should remain high at four and eight hours, or can be suppressed at four hours, and high again by eight hours. This test, however, is not very sensitive for differentiating adrenal versus pituitary-dependent disease, and for this either a high-dose dexamethasone suppression test (using 1 mg/kg dexamethasone), or a combination of endogenous ACTH measurement and adrenal ultrasound is recommended. Plasma ACTH levels are expected to be undetectable with adrenal-dependent disease, and high with pituitary-dependent disease. The disadvantages of measuring endogenous ACTH are that it is expensive, blood must be collected in plastic or silicone lined EDTA tubes, collected and kept on ice, and it needs to be immediately centrifuged and frozen. Incorrect handling will lead to falsely low results.

On abdominal radiography, hepatomegaly, increased intra-abdominal fat, and a pot-bellied appearance may be evident. Abdominal ultrasonography may reveal bilaterally enlarged adrenal glands in the case of pituitary-dependent hyperadrenocorticism, but this is, highly operator dependent and is not sensitive or specific for diagnosing pituitary-dependent hyperadrenocorticism. Ultrasound is, however, very useful for discriminating between adrenal and pituitary-dependent disease, since in cases of adrenal-dependent disease, a unilateral adrenal mass should be evident, with the contralateral adrenal gland being either normal in appearance or unidentifiable.

Advanced imaging, such as MRI and CT scanning may be of use for adrenal-dependent disease to assist in surgical planning. For pituitary-dependent disease, MRI/CT of the brain can detect macroadenomas (>3 mm in diameter), and may be useful for preoperative (hypophysectomy) or preradiotherapy assessment.

Medical management

If surgery is being considered, then medical stabilization should be attempted first, with the aim of reducing risks of sepsis, wound dehiscence, and thromboembolic disease. Any concurrent diabetes mellitus should also be partially stabilized. There is, however, no ideal medical treatment for feline hyperadrenocorticism. A few reports exist of treatment using mitotane, ketoconazole, and metyrapone, with variable success. The most promising treatment is trilostane, which has been reported to be efficacious in some cats with hyperadrenocorticism.[6] Unilateral adrenalectomy is the treatment of choice in adrenal-dependent cases that are suitable surgical candidates. Bilateral adrenalectomy used to be recommended for pituitary-dependent disease, but has probably been largely replaced by the use of external beam radiotherapy of the pituitary gland, which has shown some promising results,[7] medical treatment with trilostane, or trans-sphenoidal hypophysectomy (see Chapter 58).

Other endocrinologically active adrenal neoplasms

Hyperprogesteronism can occur alone, or in combination with hyperaldosteronism. Reported cases have been due to unilateral[4,5] or bilateral[8] adrenocortical carcinomas. Clinical features are very similar to those seen in hyperadrenocorticism, and so the diagnosis is most often considered in a cat with clinical signs suggestive of hyperadrenocorticism, but where low dose dexamethasone suppression and ACTH stimulation tests yield normal results. Definitive diagnosis is based on demonstrating an elevated serum progesterone concentration, together with identification of an adrenal mass. The particular significance of these cases in relation to performing surgery is that there are more potential complications that could occur. The potential complications are similar to those seen in cats with hyperadrenocorticism. Effective medical management of hyperprogesteronism has not been reported. One of the authors (A.H.) has used trilostane in one cat with concurrent hyperaldosteronism and hyperprogesteronism. Treatment was only attempted for a short period of time when the clinical signs were quite advanced, and was not successful in suppressing progesterone concentrations. Use of aminoglutethimide has also been reported

---

Box 35-1 Protocol for the adrenocorticotrophic hormone (ACTH) stimulation test for cats

1. Take blood sample for base-line cortisol
2. Administer 125 µg of synthetic ACTH intravenously
3. Take blood samples for cortisol measurement one and three hours later (ensure cat is kept quiet and calm throughout this time)
4. Place 1 mL blood in plain/serum tubes
5. Submit to endocrine laboratory (there are no special sample handling or storage requirements)

Box 35-2 The low dose dexamethasone suppression test for cats

1. Take blood sample for base-line cortisol
2. Administer 0.1 mg/kg of dexamethasone intravenously
3. Take blood samples for cortisol measurement four and eight hours later (ensure cat is kept quiet and calm throughout this time)
4. Place 1 mL blood in plain/serum tubes
5. Submit to endocrine laboratory (there are no special sample handling or storage requirements)

for preoperative stabilization in one case[4] but was of questionable benefit.

Cases of excessive production of androstenedione, testosterone, and estradiol have also been reported, either due to an adrenocortical adenoma[9] or bilateral adrenal gland enlargement.[10] These cases presented with aggressive male-type behavior and urine spraying. Elevated serum concentrations of sex hormones were demonstrated. A good outcome was achieved with unilateral adrenalectomy in the cat with a unilateral adrenal adenoma. A moderate improvement in clinical signs was seen with trilostane treatment in the cat with bilateral adrenal enlargement.

PREOPERATIVE CONSIDERATIONS

Indications and contraindications for surgery

The primary indication for surgery is presence of unilateral adrenal gland neoplasia, secreting excessive aldosterone, progesterone, cortisol, or sex hormones. Bilateral adrenalectomy has been described for treatment of pituitary-dependent hyperadrenocorticism.

The main contraindications for surgery are the presence of bilateral adrenal disease with hyperaldosteronism, a poorly medically stabilized patient, presence of metastatic disease (rare, but can occur with adrenal carcinomas), extensive invasion of the caudal vena cava by the adrenal neoplasm, and the presence of significant concurrent disease.

Preoperative assessment

It is important that thorough investigations are performed to establish a diagnosis so that the patient can be optimally stabilized preoperatively. Intraoperative hemorrhage can be profuse with adrenalectomy

and blood typing/cross-matching (see Chapter 5) is recommended to prepare for blood transfusion should it be required during surgery. Packed cell volume and platelet count, as well as coagulation profiles, should be collected within 48 hours prior to surgery. Careful attention to electrolyte status should be paid, and monitoring should be continued during the perioperative period.

Anesthesia and medication for adrenalectomy

Premedication is routine; an induction agent such as propofol or alphaxalan should be used followed by intubation and maintenance with gaseous anesthesia. Muscle relaxant anesthesia may aid exposure of the abdominal organs. Perioperative antibiotics are recommended as the surgery will often be prolonged and the patient may be systemically unwell even after preoperative stabilization. For further information on anesthesia see Chapter 2.

For cortisol-producing adrenal tumors intravenous soluble corticosteroid (e.g., hydrocortisone 0.6 mg/kg/hour) should be started at the time of anesthetic induction (it takes about an hour to reach effective levels). This produces blood cortisol levels of the order of 500 nmol/L, which is equivalent to the hematogenous levels that would be expected in cats subjected to major trauma and surgery.

SURGICAL MANAGEMENT AND TECHNIQUES

Adrenalectomy

The surgical technique is similar whether the indication is resection of neoplastic tissue or bilateral adrenalectomy for primary hyperaldosteronism. The affected adrenal gland(s) are usually removed through a midline laparotomy (Box 35-3). Laparoscopic adrenalectomy has

---

Box 35-3 Adrenalectomy

The animal is placed in dorsal recumbency and the ventral abdomen and caudal thorax are clipped and prepared for aseptic surgery. An incision from the xiphisternum to the pubis is recommended, as a long incision will improve access to the craniodorsal abdomen. Although a combined ventral midline and paracostal incision is recommended in canine patients by some surgeons, this is unnecessary in the cat due to its smaller size and more flexible abdominal wall.

Careful hemostasis using electrocautery should be maintained at all times. A thorough exploration should be made, in particular looking for evidence of metastatic disease in other abdominal organs. If this is suspected, fine needle aspirate samples or Tru-Cut biopsies should be taken.

The affected side should be exposed with the aid of an assistant by performing the duodenal or colonic maneuver, and abdominal retractors (Fig. 35-6A). Laparotomy swabs moistened with sterile saline should then be used to pack around the adrenal gland if neoplasia is suspected, in order to reduce contamination of surrounding structures during the surgical excision.

Dissection is best started laterally or abaxially, away from the great vessels that are more axial or medial, by incising the peritoneum followed by blunt dissection using sterile cotton-tipped swabs (Fig. 35-6B). The tumor is usually contained within a capsule and care is taken to avoid entering this (Fig. 35-6C). The phrenico-abdominal vein is ligated with vascular clips, divided, and blunt dissected free from the underlying gland.

On the right side, the caudate lobe of the liver is freed, by incising the peritoneal fold that holds it caudally, and then retracted cranially with a malleable retractor. Partial liver lobectomy using a thoracoabdominal stapling device can be used if the tumor is involving

this lobe. Nephrectomy may be required if extensive invasion of the adjacent kidney has occurred (see Chapter 36).

Blunt dissection continues dorsally around the gland, maintaining hemostasis with electrocautery. Intermittent compression of the vena cava is inevitable during dissection and so monitoring of arterial blood pressure is important. Dissection should be intermittently halted to allow periods of normal caval blood flow to occur. As the dissection progresses great care should be taken to ensure the tumor is removed from the great vessels without entering their lumen.

If preoperative imaging suggests caval invasion or thrombosis has occurred, then Rummel tourniquets should be placed around the cava cranial and caudal to the tumor. Occlusion time should be as short as possible and so planning and thought are required before surgery. Once dissection has freed up the lateral parts of the tumor, the Rummel tourniquets are tightened and the cava incised; any thrombus can be removed and the portion of caval wall invaded by tumor excised with sharp dissection if appropriate. Closure of the cava wall is performed with 1.5M polypropylene in a simple continuous pattern. Air is removed from the lumen using a 20 mL syringe, three-way tap and intravenous over-the-needle catheter, and the tourniquets are then released.

If there is no caval invasion, dissection continues bluntly around the tumor until it is free. The laparotomy swabs should be removed and gloves and instruments should be changed. The site of excision should be checked for bleeding and hemostasis achieved using electrocautery. The author often packs the site with hemostatic gel (such as collagen sponge) and closure of the peritoneum is performed with absorbable suture if the tumor was relatively small and this is possible. Swabs are counted and abdominal closure is routine.

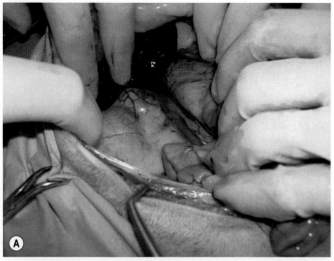

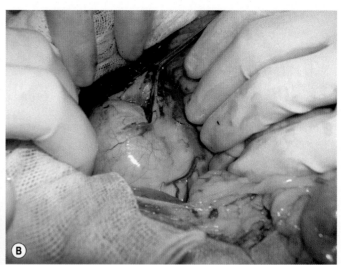

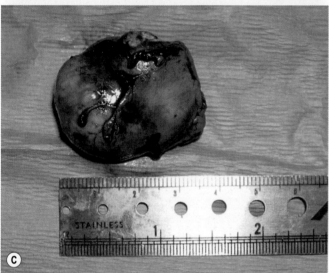

Figure 35-6 A ten year old female neutered cat with hyperadrenocorticism is having adrenalectomy for a unilateral adrenal tumor. **(A)** Exposure of right kidney and adrenal gland. The caudate lobe has been retracted cranially, and the duodenal maneuver performed. The adrenal mass is craniomedial to the kidney and lateral to the vena cava. **(B)** The peritoneum has been incised over the kidney on the lateral side of the adrenal mass. Dissection can now progress with blunt dissection, particularly dorsomedially. **(C)** The excised mass proved to be an adenoma on histopathology. Note the capsule has not been disrupted during excision.

been described in the dog for cases of adrenocortical carcinoma in which there was no caval invasion detected on MRI scan.[11] This technique is not yet reported in the feline but is likely to be applicable if caval involvement is ruled out. See Chapter 25 for information on laparoscopy.

Trans-sphenoidal hypophysectomy (see Chapter 58) has been described as a treatment for pituitary-dependent hyperadrenocorticism[12] and for acromegaly.[13] Specialized equipment and surgical technique are required for this procedure.

POSTOPERATIVE CARE

Supplementation with intravenous soluble corticosteroid is recommended in patients with active cortisol-producing tumors until the contralateral gland becomes functional. Intravenous soluble corticosteroid (e.g., hydrocortisone) infusion should be continued at the same rate as started preoperatively (e.g., hydrocortisone 0.6 mg/kg/hour) for approximately 12 hours post surgery, and then the rate arbitrarily weaned down 24 hours later (e.g., reduce to 0.3 mg/kg/hour hydrocortisone). From day 3 onwards there should only be a need for maintenance cortisol therapy, which can be given orally at

1 mg/kg cortisone acetate twice daily for several weeks, to allow the contralateral adrenal gland to recover from atrophy, and then arbitrarily weaned off. Dexamethasone or prednisolone can be used instead of cortisol but the advantages of using cortisol are that it is replicating the endogenous hormone, it has both mineralocorticoid and glucocorticoid activity, and if necessary both blood and urinary corticoid levels can be measured to assess whether the dose being used is appropriate.

Blood products may be required if hemorrhage has been extensive, and are usually given immediately post recovery whilst adequate monitoring for a transfusion reaction can occur. Analgesia should be maintained until the cat is comfortable postoperatively, the mainstay being opioid analgesia. These are usually maintained for at least 48 hours after surgery. Fluid therapy is continued to ensure good circulatory function, and regular monitoring of electrolytes should be continued (every eight hours for the first 24 hours). Mineralocorticoids are indicated if persistent hyponatremia or hyperkalemia is documented, or post bilateral adrenalectomy.[14] Postoperative antibiotics are continued for seven days, as these cats are systemically compromised and sepsis has been reported postoperatively.[14,15] Food should be offered as soon as the cat can safely swallow, and fluid therapy continues until the patient is eating a normal amount and regulating its own fluid intake. Small room confinement is recommended for four weeks postoperatively to ensure the abdominal wall has adequate time to heal.

COMPLICATIONS AND PROGNOSIS

Surgery for adrenal masses is challenging, and in the dog, perioperative mortality rates of 19 to 22% have been reported.[16,17] In the largest case series of adrenal tumor surgery in the cat, four cases out of ten did not survive beyond 14 days post surgery, in most cases due to severe hemorrhage from the caudal vena cava immediately following surgery.[15] Survival appeared unrelated to histologic type of adenoma versus carcinoma;[15] there is a similar finding in the dog.[16] Survival times in the cats that survived the perioperative period,

however, were often prolonged with follow-up periods of 240 to 1803 days.

The impact of invasion of the caudal vena cava is difficult to assess, as in most studies surgery has been ruled out in cases where this has occurred. In one case report of surgery involving caval venotomy survival was prolonged postoperatively,[2] but instinctively one would imagine postoperative complications would be more likely.

Cats with hyperprogesteronism or hypercortisolemia pose additional surgical risks, including wound dehiscence, sepsis, pancreatitis, and thromboembolic disease. The prognosis for these cases remains guarded, with affected cats rarely surviving longer than one year even when they have survived the postoperative period. Hypoadrenocorticism is an additional complication for cats undergoing bilateral adrenalectomy, and life-long mineralocorticoid and glucocorticoid supplementation is required in these cases.

REFERENCES

1. Zimmer C, Hörauf A, Reusch C. 2000 Ultrasonographic examination of the adrenal gland and evaluation of the hypophyseal-adrenal axis in 20 cats. J Small Anim Pract 2000;41:156–60.

2. Rose SA, Kyles AE, Labelle P, et al. Adrenalectomy and caval thrombectomy in a cat with primary hyperaldosteronism. J Am Anim Hosp Assoc 2007;43:209–14.

3. Javadi S, Djajadiningrat-Laanen SC, Kooistra HS, et al. Primary hyperaldosteronism, a mediator of progressive renal disease in cats. Domest Anim Endocrinol 2005;28:85–104.

4. DeClue AE, Breshears LA, Pardo ID, et al. Hyperaldosteronism and hyperprogesteronism in a cat with an adrenal cortical carcinoma. J Vet Int Med 2005;19:355–8.

5. Briscoe K, Barrs VR, Foster DF, Beatty JA. Hyperaldosteronism and hyperprogesteronism in a cat. J Feline Med Surg 2009;1:758–62.

6. Neiger R, Witt AL, Noble A, German AJ. Trilostane therapy for treatment of pituitary-dependent hyperadrenocorticism in 5 cats. J Vet Intern Med 2004;18: 160–4.

7. Mayer MN, Greco DS, LaRue SM. Outcomes of pituitary tumor irradiation in cats. J Vet Intern Med 2006;20:1151–4.

8. Quante S, Sieber-Ruckstuhl N, Wilhelm S, et al. Hyperprogesteronism due to bilateral adrenal carcinomas in a cat with diabetes mellitus. Schweiz Arch Tierheilkd 2009;151:437–42.

9. Millard RP, Pickens EH, Wells KL. Excessive production of sex hormones in a cat with an adrenocortical tumor. J Am Vet Med Assoc 2009;234:505–8.

10. Boag AK, Neiger R, Church DB. Trilostane treatment of bilateral adrenal enlargement and excessive sex steroid hormone production in a cat. J Small Anim Pract 2004;45:263–6.

11. Jiménez Peláez M, Bouvy BM, Dupré GP. Laparoscopic adrenalectomy for treatment of unilateral adrenocortical carcinomas: technique, complications and results in seven dogs. Vet Surg 2008;37:444–53.

12. Meij BP, Voorhout G, Van Den Ingh TS, Rijnberk A. Transsphenoidal hypophysectomy for treatment of pituitary-dependent hyperadrenocorticism in 7 cats. Vet Surg 2001;30:72–86.

13. Meij BP, Auriemma E, Grinwis G, et al. Successful treatment of acromegaly in a diabetic cat with transsphenoidal hypophysectomy. J Fel Med Surg 2010;12:406–10.

14. Feldman EC, Nelson RW Acromegaly and hyperadrenocorticism in cats: A clinical perspective. Proceedings of ESFM Study Day, WSAVA 2000. J Feline Med Surg 2000;2:153–8.

15. Ash RA, Harvey AM, Tasker S. Primary hyperaldosteronism in the cat: a series of 13 cases. J Feline Med Surg 2005;7: 173–82.

16. Anderson CR, Birchard SJ, Powers BE, et al. Surgical treatment of adrenocortical tumors: 21 cases (1990–1996). J Am Anim Hosp Assoc 2001;37:93–7.

17. Schwartz P, Kovak JR, Koprowski A, et al. Evaluation of prognostic factors in the surgical treatment of adrenal gland tumors in dogs: 41 cases (1999–2005). J Am Vet Med Assoc 2008;232:77–84.

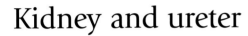

Chapter | 36 |

Kidney and ureter

L.R. Aronson

Many conditions affecting the upper urinary tract of cats require surgical intervention. The most common conditions currently identified in the author's practice are partial and complete ureteral obstructions secondary to calcium oxalate urolithiasis and cases of urinary tract trauma.

SURGICAL ANATOMY

Kidney

The kidneys are retroperitoneal organs that lie adjacent to the sublumbar musculature on either side of the abdominal aorta and caudal vena cava. The right kidney lies more cranial than the left, lying within the renal fossa of the caudate lobe of the liver attached by the hepatorenal ligament. Although the right kidney is located at the L1–L4 vertebrae and the left kidney is located at L2–L5, the kidneys are not rigidly fixed to the surrounding tissues and are equally mobile. The entire left kidney can often be easily palpated on physical examination; the cranial pole of the right kidney may be harder to palpate because of its location adjacent to the ribs and liver. Normal renal size in the cat has been determined radiographically by calculating the ratio of kidney length to the second lumbar vertebral body length. Based on multiple studies, a normal renal size ratio of 2.0–3.0 has been reported.[1-5] Additionally, there is a significant difference in the ratios between neutered and intact cats. Neutering of cats resulted in a ratio of 1.9–2.6 compared with 2.1–3.2 for intact cats and should be taken into consideration when evaluating kidney size, particularly in the diseased state.[6]

The renal hilus, located medially, is the opening into the renal sinus and transmits the renal artery, vein, nerves and is the location of the renal pelvis (Fig. 36-1). Because the aorta is normally located to the left of the caudal vena cava, the left kidney has a long renal vein and the right kidney has a long renal artery. The renal artery in the cat typically lies dorsal and sometimes slightly cranial to the renal vein. Upon entering the kidney, the renal artery divides into interlobar arteries. These vessels radiate through the medulla to the corticomedullary junction, where arcuate arteries are formed.[7] These arteries then give rise to other interlobar arteries that run perpendicular through the cortex and eventually give rise to the afferent arterioles of the glomerulus.[7,8] The surface of the feline kidney is grooved because of the presence of large subcapsular veins that eventually join the renal vein at the renal hilus.[8] The left testicular or ovarian vein typically drains into the left renal vein. Normal renal vascular anatomy was evaluated in a group of 114 healthy feline kidney donors using helical computed tomography angiography (CTA). Similar to humans, multiple renal veins were more common on the right (45/114) compared to the left (3/114) and multiple renal arteries were more common on the left (8/114) compared to the right (0/114).[9] Additionally, a split vena cava was occasionally identified.

Ureter

The ureter, which is retroperitoneal for the proximal two-thirds and intraperitoneal for the distal third, courses adjacent to the sublumbar musculature from the renal hilus, travels through the two layers of peritoneum which form the lateral ligaments of the bladder and terminates on the dorsal surface at the bladder neck.[10] It courses in a 'J' shape, looping around the ductus deferens in the male, eventually

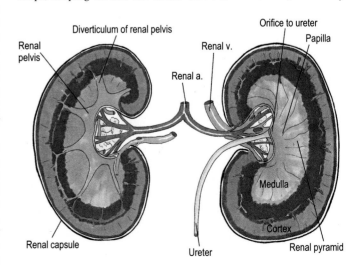

Figure 36-1 Anatomy of the feline kidney.

© 2014 Elsevier Ltd
DOI: 10.1016/B978-0-7020-4336-9.00036-6

passing obliquely through the bladder wall to empty into the lumen just cranial and lateral to the vesicourethral juncture. The oblique passage of the distal ureter is important in preventing reflux from the bladder into the ureter. As the bladder expands, the terminal ureter becomes compressed. Enough pressure generated by a peristaltic wave is necessary to force urine through the compressed distal ureter.[11] The blood supply of the feline ureter is derived from multiple sources including a cranial supply from the renal artery, a caudal supply from the vaginal or prostatic artery, and additional branches that join the ureteral artery from surrounding sources.[12,13] The cranial and caudal arteries anastomose along the length of the ureter within the outer layers of the adventitia.[14] Venous drainage follows the arterial supply.[4]

The ureter is composed of smooth muscle with an inner longitudinal layer and middle circular layers. An outer longitudinal layer is also present and is best developed adjacent to the bladder.[11] The normal pacemaker for this muscle is located within the kidney[15] and when the muscle contracts, urine is propelled from cranial to caudal in peristaltic waves. Surrounding the smooth muscle is a layer of adventitia containing the ureteral vessels, lymphatics, and fat. Innervation of the ureter is derived from sympathetic, parasympathetic, and sensory nerves. This innervation is not necessary for normal ureteric function; however, sympathetic tone may affect the frequency and force of an individual peristaltic wave.[16]

DIAGNOSIS AND GENERAL CONSIDERATIONS

The clinical approach to evaluating a patient with renal and/or ureteral disease that may require surgical intervention begins with a thorough history and physical examination. Historical information including the onset and progression of clinical signs, previous response to therapy as well as any history of trauma, toxin exposure, previous surgery or illness, and dietary history is important. Specific clinical signs that may suggest a disorder of the upper urinary tract include the presence of polyuria/polydipsia and/or hematuria, particularly hematuria at the end of urination. Anuria may be identified in patients with bilateral ureteral obstructions and is life threatening if not addressed immediately. It is important to note that patients with disorders of the upper urinary tract may have no clinical signs present. In patients with a known history of trauma, pain on palpation in the sublumbar region or evidence of bruising may be suggestive of a primary renal and or ureteral injury. A complete physical examination should include a fundic examination to evaluate the retina for any evidence of hemorrhage or detachment that may be an indication of hypertension. The patient is evaluated for evidence of weight loss and dehydration and the kidneys are evaluated for size, shape, evidence of discomfort on palpation, and location. Patients that have sustained trauma to the kidney and/or ureter may have varying degrees of retroperitoneal and/or peritoneal effusion depending on the integrity of the peritoneal lining.

In addition to taking a history and performing a physical examination, a complete blood count, serum chemistry profile, and urinalysis should be performed. Blood work may reveal varying degrees of azotemia and anemia or may be unremarkable in patients with unilateral disease. Neither the cause nor the reversibility of renal dysfunction can be determined from the degree of azotemia.[17] A routine urinalysis should be performed to evaluate the physical and chemical properties of the urine as well as evaluate the urine sediment. If the patient has a history of urinary tract infections or if there is evidence of bacteria, pyuria, and/or hematuria on sediment evaluation, then a urine culture should be performed on aseptically collected urine.

Determining the cause as well as the extent of the renal disease, chronicity, reversibility as well as progression, and the presence of

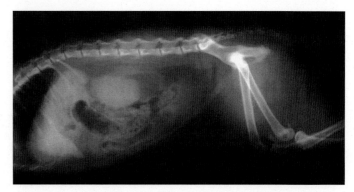

Figure 36-2 Lateral abdominal radiograph of a four-year-old male (castrated) domestic short-haired cat that was hit by a car and had a partial avulsion of the renal pelvis. There is an increase in density as well as a widening of the retroperitoneal space secondary to urine leakage. Additionally, displacement of the kidneys is identified.

complicating factors such as the identification of an obstruction or infection, and prognosis are important questions that should be answered prior to recommending surgical treatment.

Diagnostic imaging

Common imaging modalities used to evaluate the upper urinary tract in the cat include survey radiography, ultrasonography, and intravenous urography (IVU). Depending on the underlying condition, other techniques that may be employed include antegrade pyelography, computed tomography, angiography, and magnetic resonance imaging.

Radiography

Plain abdominal radiography provides information on renal size, shape, and position. The right kidney is positioned slightly cranial to the left kidney although it can be superimposed, and renal size can be assessed by comparing renal length with the length of vertebra L2. Although plain abdominal radiography does not often provide additional information when evaluating a normal ureter, the technique can be very informative for patients with radiopaque renal and/or ureteral calculi. Additionally, this technique can be helpful in the assessment of the retroperitoneal space. Urine leakage or hemorrhage in the retroperitoneal space can result in widening of the space, displacement of the kidneys from their normal position, as well as an increased heterogeneous opacity that can be visualized (Fig. 36-2).

Ultrasonography

Ultrasonography is often performed in conjunction with plain radiography and provides information regarding the size, shape, internal architecture and location, information on surrounding tissues and allows for the differentiation of solid from fluid-filled lesions. Normal ureters are typically not visible, but the distal portion of the ureter as well as the vesicoureteral junction may be seen using a high resolution transducer.[16,17] Diseases of the upper urinary tract identified with ultrasonography that may require surgical intervention include neoplastic disease, hydronephrosis and/or hydroureter secondary to urolithiasis, blood clots, mural fibrosis or extramural compression, perinephric pseudocysts, ectopic ureter, and a ureterocele.[17] It is important to note that the presence of urinary dilation does not definitely diagnose an obstruction and the presence of a surgically correctable disorder.[18,19] The presence of retroperitoneal fluid in conjunction with renal pelvic and ureteral dilation may be visualized in a patient with a ruptured ureter.[20] Additionally, patients that are candidates for renal transplantation may have changes suggestive of end stage or polycystic kidney disease.

Contrast radiographic studies

Intravenous urography

Baseline films should be taken first to make sure that the colon is empty. General anesthesia is necessary to ensure accurate positioning and minimize adverse reactions associated with contrast administration. IVU can be performed using a bolus technique or an infusion technique. The bolus technique is useful for assessing the renal vasculature as well as identifying any parenchymal lesions during the angiographic, nephrographic, and pyelographic phases. The infusion technique optimizes visualization of the ureters and any pathology that may exist.[10] The technique can provide detailed information regarding the location, size, morphology, and integrity of the kidneys and ureters. Contrast seen outside of the kidneys or ureters is indicative of rupture (Fig. 36-3).

Antegrade pyelography

In patients with a complete ureteral obstruction, the pyelographic phase of an IVU may be inadequate and percutaneous antegrade pyelography may be the preferred technique (Fig. 36-4). The technique can be performed under ultrasonographic and/or fluoroscopic guidance. To perform this technique, a 22G spinal needle is placed percutaneously into the renal cortex perpendicular to the capsule and

into the renal pelvis. Nephropyelocentesis is performed until the diameter of the pelvis is reduced by about one-half and a small bolus of a non-ionic contrast media such as iohexol is administered. A urinalysis and culture should be performed. If ultrasound guidance is used, abdominal radiographs should be taken immediately after injection to visualize the ureters and then repeated in 15 minutes.[10,21]

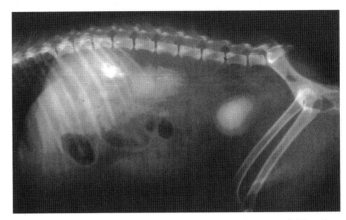

Figure 36-3 Intravenous urography performed in a five-year-old female (spayed) domestic short-haired cat that was attacked by a dog. Note the extravasation of contrast from the renal pelvis. The urine leakage was confined to the retroperitoneal space and the patient was not azotemic on presentation. A ureteronephrectomy was performed.

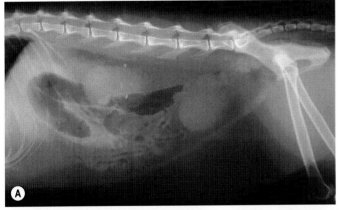

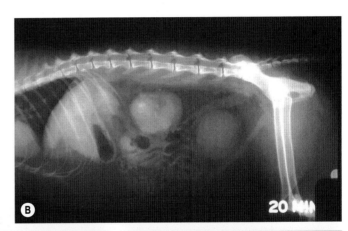

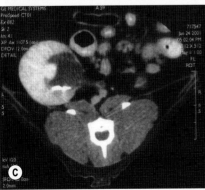

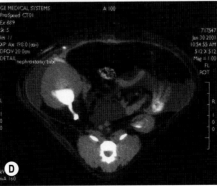

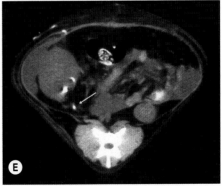

Figure 36-4 A five-year-old male (castrated) domestic short-haired cat that presented acutely azotemic. **(A)** Note the small right kidney and the compensatory hypertrophy of the left kidney. Multiple nephroliths are present in the left kidney as well as a proximal ureterolith obstructing the left kidney. **(B)** Intravenous urography was performed. Although the pyelographic phase of the unobstructed right kidney is easily visible, the pyelographic phase of the obstructed left kidney is inadequate. **(C–E)** CT angiography was performed in conjunction with antegrade pyelography to determine the location of the ureteral obstruction. Additionally, CT angiography was able to identify a more distal ureteral calculus (yellow arrow) not identified on plain survey radiographs.

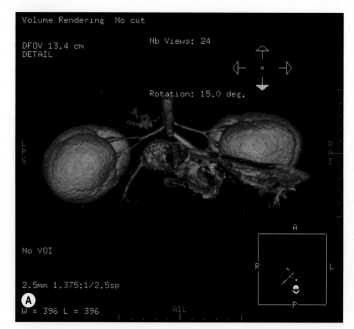

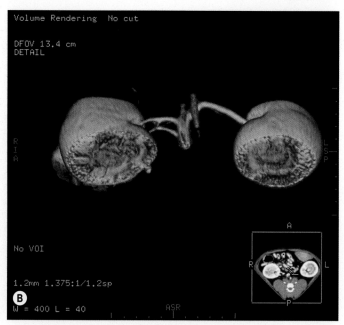

Figure 36-5 (A) Arterial phase of CT angiography. Note the single renal artery with a split close to the kidney arising from the aorta on both the right and left side. **(B)** Venous phase of CT angiography. Note the double renal vein on the right side.

Potential risks include renal injury and bleeding, clot formation resulting in a ureteral obstruction, laceration of the renal pelvis, and contrast ± urine leakage from the pyelocentesis site.[22] In a study of antegrade pyelography for suspected ureteral obstruction in 11 cats (18 kidneys), leakage of contrast developed in 8/18 cases and prevented interpretation in five of those cases.[23] For the 13 cases that did not have leakage of contrast material, the technique allowed for correct identification of the anatomical location of the ureteral obstruction.

Computed tomographic angiography (Fig. 36-5)

Helical computed tomographic angiography is a non-invasive technique that has been used extensively to evaluate the renal vasculature of cats selected for renal donation in feline renal transplantation. In addition to providing a three-dimensional image of the renal vasculature, detailed information regarding renal anatomy as well as the identification of pathology can be obtained.

SURGICAL DISEASES

Diseases of the kidney and ureter that may benefit from surgery include uroliths that can cause blockage and affect function, trauma, neoplasia, and ectopic ureters.

Urolithiasis in cats

Calcium oxalate (CaOx)-containing uroliths are the predominant stone type identified in the kidney and ureter of cats (Fig. 36-6).[24,25] The increase in occurrence of CaOx urolithiasis in cats over the past 20 years has paralleled the increase in identification of these stones in the kidneys and ureters.[26] In fact, information collected from nine different veterinary teaching hospitals during this time period found a tenfold increase in frequency of upper urinary tract uroliths, with calcium oxalate emerging as the predominant mineral type.[26] Seventy

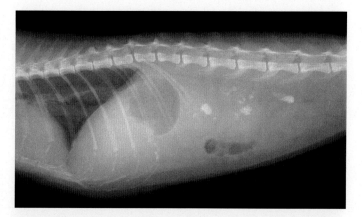

Figure 36-6 A seven-year-old female (spayed) domestic long-haired cat with multiple renal and ureteral uroliths.

per cent of nephro-ureteroliths evaluated from 1599 cats between 1981 and 2003 were composed of CaOx; only 8% were composed of magnesium ammonium phosphate.[26]

In addition to urolithiasis, dried solidified blood (DSB) calculi have also been identified in the upper urinary tract of cats associated with ureteral obstructions (Fig. 36-7). These DSB calculi are firm and feel like stones, but typically do not contain crystalline material.[27] These stones present a diagnostic challenge since they are not typically radiopaque and often not identified on ultrasonographic examination. Although uncommon, fibrosis, congenital stenosis, stricture, circumcaval ureter, neoplasia, blood clots, surgical trauma, and retroperitoneal infarction have all been associated with ureteral obstruction in cats.[28-35]

Medical and minimally invasive management

It is not clear if CaOx uroliths lodged in the kidney or ureter will migrate into the bladder. Anecdotal evidence suggests that some stones will eventually pass into the bladder without therapy. In one

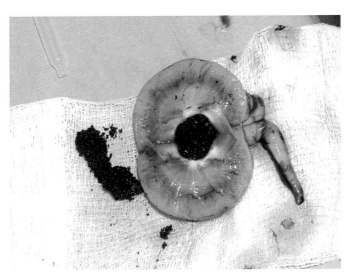

Figure 36-7 Dried solidified blood calculi within the renal pelvis and ureter of a cat. *(Courtesy of Dr Allyson Berent.)*

report of 11 cats with ureteral CaOx uroliths, however, imaging studies were performed over periods of 11 to 42 days and no stone migrated in any of the cats over these time periods.[36] Patients diagnosed with ureteroliths are often treated initially with a period of medical management, including the parenteral administration of fluids alone or in combination with diuretic therapy (mannitol) to determine if passage of ureteral calculi will occur. Additional therapies with anecdotal efficacy include the administration of various smooth muscle relaxants including prazosin, the tricyclic antidepressant amitryptilline, and other alpha antagonists such as tamsulosin. There are no reported studies as to the efficacy of any of these drugs in cats with ureterolithiasis. Unfortunately, these uroliths are less susceptible to fragmentation using shock wave lithotripsy compared to those in dogs. Because of the high number of shock waves that may be necessary in cats in order to fragment a nephrolith or ureterolith, significant renal injury may occur.[37]

Clinical presentation and investigation

Cats with uroliths affecting the kidney and ureter can appear asymptomatic on presentation, or with non-specific clinical signs including lethargy, weight loss, anorexia, vomiting, fever, and polydipsia and polyuria.[36,38] Hematuria may or may not be present, but was the most commonly reported sign in one study on feline nephrolithiasis.[39] Patients may also present with abdominal pain and splinting or renomegaly.[36] A complete physical examination is performed, as many affected cats are older and may have concurrent disease(s). A urinalysis and urine culture, complete blood count, biochemical profile, and plain abdominal radiographs are usually recommended as initial investigative steps. In a study of 163 cases of ureteral calculi, azotemia (83%; 134/162) and hyperphosphatemia (54%; 84/156) were commonly identified; hypercalcemia (14%;22/152) was less commonly reported.[38] A urinary tract infection was documented in 8% of cases (10/119).[38] Uroliths are often visualized on plain radiographs, although small ureteroliths, radiolucent ureteroliths or those calculi overlying colonic contents are occasionally missed. Further imaging studies including ultrasonography, excretory urography, antegrade pyelography, and computed tomography are often helpful in identifying small ureteroliths, the presence of hydronephrosis and hydroureter, as well as delineating the level of a ureteral obstruction. In one report, a combination of survey radiography and abdominal ultrasonography revealed ureteroliths in 90% (63/73) of cats.[38] In cats with unilateral

obstructions, 76% (58/76) were azotemic and ultrasonographic evaluation of the contralateral kidney revealed changes suggestive of parenchymal disease. It is important to note that using these modalities, the end point of the ureteral obstruction is not always identified.

Surgical management of uroliths

As medical dissolution of CaOx uroliths is not available, surgical removal is often recommended if the stones are causing clinical disease. The presence of nephrolithiasis in normal cats and those with naturally occurring stage 2 or 3 chronic kidney disease is not necessarily an indication for surgical removal. In a recent study in cats with nephrolithiasis and mild or moderate chronic kidney disease, the presence of nephrolithiasis was not associated with disease progression or an increase in mortality rate.[40] If surgical intervention is necessary, it is not always clear how long one should wait to address either renal or ureteral uroliths. The degree of dilatation of the renal pelvis does not correlate with the amount of functional damage.[36] In the author's experience, if medical management does not appear to be effective within 24–48 hours and a partial or complete ureteral obstruction is present, or the ureterolith is associated with an infection that does not respond to medical therapy, surgical removal is recommended. Factors that also need to be considered with regards to prognosis include the function of the contralateral kidney and the overall health of the patient. The ability of the feline kidney to recover from partial or complete outflow obstruction is unknown. Recovery of renal function depends on the severity and duration of the obstruction and the presence of pre-existing renal disease. Unfortunately, in cases of unilateral ureteral obstruction, a diagnosis may go undetected if function in the opposite kidney is normal.

There are two options for removing nephroliths, a nephrotomy or pyelithotomy (see Box 36-3). Pyelithotomy may be performed if the renal calculi have created dilation of the renal pelvis and avoids occlusion of the renal vasculature. Stones lodged in the proximal ureter may be removed by ureterotomy (see Box 36-6). This technique can also be used for the mid to distal ureter or the affected area of the ureter may be removed in toto and ureteral re-implantation or a ureteroneocystostomy performed (Fig. 36-8; see Box 36-8).

Ureteral stenting

Ureteral stenting is a novel technique currently being performed in cats. The author has used this technique for patients with multiple ureteroliths located unilaterally or bilaterally with or without the presence of nephroliths (Fig. 36-9). Nephroliths do have the potential to pass into a ureter that was recently unobstructed, but the exact occurrence of this complication is unknown in cats.[41] As the majority of stent cases are performed surgically (in some female cats they can be placed cystoscopically), knowing the incidence of re-obstruction in cases with nephroliths but only a few ureteroliths would be important when making a decision regarding the appropriate treatment option (ureterotomy vs stenting). Patients that have had a ureterotomy performed should be evaluated periodically following surgery since nephroliths have the ability to migrate into the ureter and cause subsequent obstructions.

Renal and ureteral trauma

Trauma to the upper urinary tract can be associated with automobile accidents or falls, penetrating wounds secondary to bites, gunshot wounds and penetrating foreign bodies, iatrogenic injury secondary to surgical trauma, and trauma related to the presence of obstructive or irritating calculi. Because of their retroperitoneal location, the kidneys and ureters are less commonly damaged when compared to

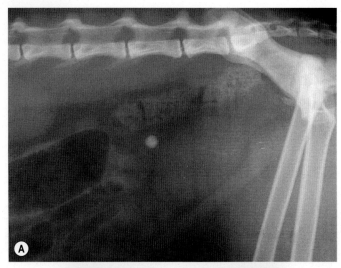

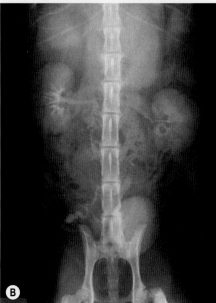

Figure 36-8 **(A)** A 10-year-old female (spayed) domestic short-haired cat with a large stone in the distal ureter. **(B)** An IVU reveals that the stone is causing a partial obstruction of the right ureter. The left ureter is normal and the cat was not azotemic. A neoureterostomy was performed.

the bladder and urethra. If the peritoneal lining remains intact following a traumatic event and only one kidney and/or ureter is affected, the cat's clinical presentation may be subtle and not reflect the severity of the injury. If the retroperitoneal space has been disrupted resulting in urine leakage into the peritoneal cavity, the patient's clinical signs will be more representative of the injury. In patients in hypovolemic shock, body fluids may redistribute and minimize the presence of abdominal effusion.

A diagnosis of renal and/or ureteral trauma is based on history, physical examination, clinical pathological findings, evaluation of peritoneal or retroperitoneal fluid (if present), abdominal radiographs, abdominal ultrasound, and contrast studies. Advanced diagnostic imaging including fluoroscopy and CT may also be beneficial in some cases of urinary tract trauma. Not only is it important to make a diagnosis, but the aim is also to determine the location of urinary injury and/or leakage.

Patients should also be evaluated carefully for other systemic injuries. Along with trauma to the upper urinary tract, patients may

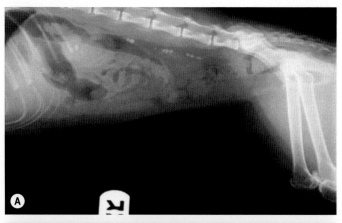

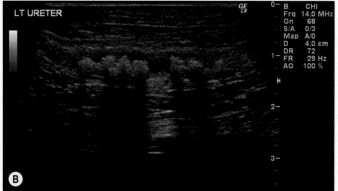

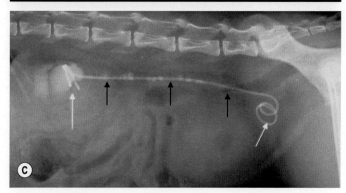

Figure 36-9 **(A)** Abdominal radiograph of a four-year-old female (spayed) Himalayan cat with multiple ureteroliths bilaterally. **(B)** Abdominal ultrasound revealing extensive shadowing from the multiple ureteroliths along the length of the left ureter. **(C)** Post ureteral stent placement. Stent is bypassing the ureteroliths in the right ureter. Black arrows identify the shaft of the stent, yellow arrows are the double pigtails curled in the renal pelvis and bladder.

present with a life-threatening bleed associated with splenic or hepatic trauma, neurological deficiencies, as well as respiratory distress associated with thoracic trauma. Thoracic radiographs should be performed on any trauma patient to rule out pneumothorax, pulmonary contusions, rib fractures, as well as a possible diaphragmatic hernia. Although not life threatening, fractures and superficial skin wounds should also receive appropriate first aid following resuscitation and patient stabilization.

Initial stabilization

Depending on the time delay until diagnosis, many patients will have electrolyte and acid–base abnormalities that need to be corrected as much as possible prior to surgery, since these changes can make them poor anesthetic candidates. Urinary leakage into the peritoneal cavity from a renal or ureteral injury can result in dehydration, azotemia, hyperkalemia, hyponatremia, hypochloremia, acidosis, and hypovolemic shock; however, these electrolyte abnormalities are not always a consistent finding in the cat. The rate of fluid administration as well as the type of fluid therapy should be based on a patient's specific needs. Although potassium-free solutions such as 0.9% saline are recommended, a balanced electrolyte solution such as Normosol-R will correct hypovolemia and not contribute substantially to the serum potassium on an acute basis. Cats are typically started at a rate of 40–60 mL/kg/hour. The patient is then reassessed after approximately 30 minutes and the rate and supplementation adjusted accordingly.

An ECG trace should be recorded and if hyperkalemia is present, it should be treated (see Chapter 2). In some severely unstable patients that present with a uroperitoneum, temporary peritoneal dialysis (see Box 36-3), hemodialysis or urinary diversion may be necessary to more completely resolve azotemia and fluid, electrolyte, and acid-base imbalances prior to definitive surgery.

Clinicopathological evaluation

A complete blood count, serum biochemical analysis and urinalysis should be performed. Depending on the time to presentation, degree of trauma, and concurrent abnormalities, the complete blood count may reveal a regenerative or non-regenerative anemia and if significant hemorrhage has occurred, the platelet count may be low due to consumption. A neutrophilia with or without a left shift may be indicative of inflammation or sepsis, particularly if there was a urinary tract infection present prior to the injury. Serum biochemistry may reveal azotemia, hyperkalemia, hyperphosphatemia, hypochloremia, and hyponatremia. A venous blood gas may reveal a metabolic acidosis due to lactic acidosis in hypoperfused patients, uremia, or renal tubular acidosis. If peritoneal effusion is present, a sample should be obtained by abdominocentesis with or without ultrasound guidance or from a peritoneal dialysis catheter if one had been previously placed. The concentration of the creatinine and potassium in the fluid retrieved on abdominocentesis should be compared with that of the peripheral blood (see Chapter 37). Cytological evaluation of the abdominal fluid should also be performed to evaluate for signs of inflammation, sepsis or evidence of damage to other intra-abdominal organs.

Kidney

Isolated renal trauma is often difficult to diagnose since clinical signs are often non-specific. Historical information in conjunction with the presence of gross or microscopic hematuria and pain on palpation in the sublumbar region may be suggestive of a primary renal injury, but are not pathognomonic for the condition.[42,43] It is important to note that the degree of hematuria does not necessarily correlate with the severity of the injury.[44] Survey radiographs may reveal loss of detail and the inability to visualize one or both kidneys, displacement or asymmetry of the kidneys, and an increase in density as well as widening of the retroperitoneal space secondary to fluid accumulation. Fluid evaluation is important to determine if uroretroperitoneum or hemorrhage in the retroperitoneal space is present. If the peritoneal lining has been compromised, fluid accumulation within the peritoneal cavity will result in loss of normal abdominal detail. Occasionally, renal injury can be confirmed by excretory urography and abdominal ultrasound; however, if the renal vascular pedicle has been damaged, CT and MR angiography or exploratory surgery may be necessary in order to make a diagnosis. If excretory urography is performed, it is important that a patient be hemodynamically stable ensuring adequate renal perfusion prior to the administration of contrast material.

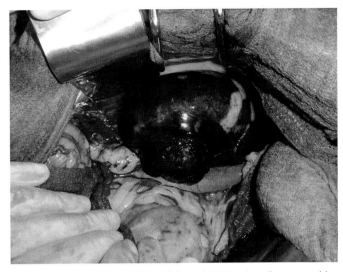

Figure 36-10 Complete avulsion of the right kidney in a three-year-old male (castrated) domestic short-haired cat after being hit by a car. The vascular pedicle was identified and was not bleeding. It appeared to have twisted and clotted.

An increased risk of toxicity exists when contrast material is administered to azotemic animals.[45]

Treatment of renal trauma is dictated by the extent of injury. Many patients that are azotemic secondary to renal contusions are treated with supportive care to address their renal failure. Simple lacerations as well as the presence of a subcapsular hematoma may be successfully managed conservatively; some lacerations of the kidney need to be sutured. This can be performed using a fine, absorbable suture material such as Polydioxanone (3/0 or 4/0) in a continuous, interrupted or mattress suture pattern. Additionally, depending on the extent of the injury, the laceration can be augmented with a transversus abdominis muscle flap or omentum. In some cases in which significant damage has occurred to the renal pelvis resulting in urine extravasation, surgical repair can be augmented with the placement of an ipsilateral nephrostomy tube (see below) with or without a ureteral stent (see below). Both of these techniques can be performed at the time of surgical repair or percutaneously with intraoperative fluoroscopic guidance. If severe injury has occurred resulting in persistent hemorrhage, urine extravasation, or the presence of non-viable tissue, a ureteronephrectomy (see below) is often necessary, provided the remaining kidney is thought to be functional. Although not common, complete avulsion of the kidney can occur, potentially resulting in severe and often fatal hemorrhage in the patient (Fig. 36-10).

Ureter

Similar to unilateral renal injury, unilateral ureteral tears can be difficult to diagnose if urine accumulation is confined to the retroperitoneal space. Clinical signs in these patients are often vague and may include lethargy, dehydration, weak peripheral pulses, pale mucous membranes, prolonged capillary refill time, sublumbar pain, vomiting, anorexia, and pyrexia.[46] Clinicopathological findings in these patients may be normal. Similar to renal trauma, abdominal radiographs often reveal a loss of retroperitoneal detail and an increased size of the retroperitoneal space. Ultrasound may identify fluid accumulation. If both ureters are disrupted, signs of acute azotemia will occur. If urine leakage enters the peritoneal cavity secondary to traumatic disruption of the parietal peritoneum, uroperitoneum will develop. Excretory urography, antegrade pyelography or contrast enhanced CT is beneficial in cases of both unilateral and bilateral ureteral abnormalities. Similar to patients that have sustained renal injury, it is imperative that the patient be hemodynamically stable prior to performing the study.

Treatment options for ureteral trauma are often dictated by patient stability, function of the contralateral kidney and integrity of the contralateral ureter, damage to the ipsilateral kidney, and location of the injury. Options include primary repair, end-to-end anastomosis (ureteroureterostomy), ureteral re-implantation (neoureterocystostomy), ureteral stenting or ureteronephrectomy. Ureteral stenting can be used alone or in conjunction with primary repair or end-to-end anastomosis to allow for urinary diversion while the incision sites are healing. A nephrostomy tube can also be placed in these cases to divert urine away from the primary surgical site.

Ureteral pelvic disruption

In cases of ureteral pelvic disruption or avulsion, repair of the injury should be performed in conjunction with a nephrostomy tube and a ureteral stent for urinary diversion as well as to promote healing and prevent stricture.[42] Anastomosis of the ureter to the renal pelvis is performed with 5/0 or smaller synthetic absorbable monofilament suture in an interrupted pattern. If the contralateral kidney function is normal, ureteronephrectomy is considered because of the technical difficulty in performing this type of repair and associated complications.

Proximal ureter injuries

In many cases of trauma involving the proximal ureter, a ureteronephrectomy is performed in cats with normal contralateral renal function. Although rarely identified, small lesions resulting in urine extravasation can be repaired primarily using 8/0 nylon or 8/0 vicryl in a single interrupted or single continuous suture pattern. More often, injuries to the proximal ureter are repaired using an end-to-end anastomosis. This technique is particularly difficult in cats and should only be performed using appropriate magnification and by someone with experience in microvascular surgery.

Injuries to the middle and distal ureter

Although primary repair as well as uretero-ureterostomy can be performed for injuries to the middle and distal ureter, more often ureteral re-implantation is performed. In the author's experience, because of the mobility of the feline kidney, particularly following dissection from its retroperitoneal attachments, ureteral re-implantation can also be performed for some proximal ureteral injuries. In these cases, ureteral re-implantation is always performed in conjunction with a renal descensus and a cystonephropexy.

Devascularization or crushing injuries

The effect of devascularization or crushing of the feline ureter has not been previously evaluated. In dogs, damage to the ureteral vascular supply and the duration and extent of the obstruction dictate the severity of injury to the ureter and associated kidney. In dogs, devascularization injuries were more devastating than crush injuries.[47] In one canine research study, approximately 50% of ureters that were devascularized by removing 2–3 cm of proximal adventitia developed persistent strictures and obstruction.[47] In contrast, crushing injuries lasting up to 60 minutes did not result in permanent renal damage and radiographic evaluation demonstrated that 90% of the strictures returned to normal within 12 weeks. Crushing of the ureter iatrogenically during surgery by grasping or ligation (e.g., inadvertently during ovariohysterectomy) may not require treatment following release of the ureter.[48] If a ligature can be removed from the ureter within one week of placement, normal function of the kidney and ureter should be regained.[49] In humans, obstruction of the ureter for greater than or equal to four weeks results in complete loss of function.[50,51] The effect of a partial obstruction of the feline ureter on long-term function is unknown.

Para-ureteral and perinephric pseudocysts and urinomas

Although rare, *urinomas (para-ureteral pseudocysts)* have been described in cats secondary to trauma.[52,53] These pseudocysts contain extravasated urine following disruption of the proximal urinary tract. Physical examination might reveal a palpable dorsal abdominal mass and imaging confirms the presence of a fluid-filled mass in the retroperitoneal space with evidence of ureteral obstruction. A diagnosis is confirmed with exploratory laparotomy. Ureteronephrectomy with or without omentalization of the cavity has been performed to treat the condition.[54] If contralateral renal function is normal the prognosis for these patients is very good.

Perinephric pseudocysts are fluid-filled cavities in a perirenal location, usually a subcapsular accumulation of a transudate, which lack a true epithelial lining. Pseudocysts can be unilateral or bilateral and patients often present with renomegaly and abdominal distension (Fig. 36-11). These occur most commonly in older male cats, with clinical signs of renal dysfunction, but no history of trauma.[55,56] In these cases, underlying renal pathology often dictates the prognosis. Percutaneous drainage is not effective in controlling recurrence of fluid accumulation. Resection of the pseudocyst wall can relieve clinical signs, but is not likely to provide long-term benefit unless the underlying disease is reversible (Fig. 36-12).[57] If surgical resection is performed, omentalization may be helpful to resolve continued transudation.[58] Survival in these patients is dictated by the degree of azotemia at presentation.

A *perirenal urinoma* has been grouped under the term perinephric pseudocyst; however, these contain urine and are thought to be acquired secondary to trauma, surgical injury, or rupture associated with urolithiasis.[59–61] A diagnosis is confirmed using excretory urography demonstrating a communication between the urinary tract and the pseudocyst. Additionally, fluid analysis from the fluid-filled cavity will demonstrate a high blood urea nitrogen (BUN) and creatinine concentration compared to peripheral blood. The azotemia resolves after fluid drainage and removal of the source of extravasation. Treatment options include nephrectomy, ureteral anastomosis or

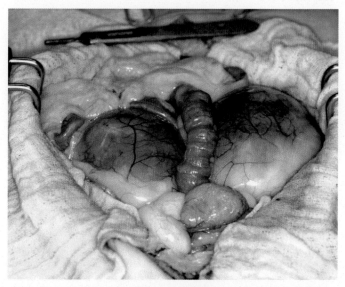

Figure 36-11 Bilateral pseudocysts in an eight-year-old male (castrated) Persian cat. The cat presented with renomegaly and abdominal distension.

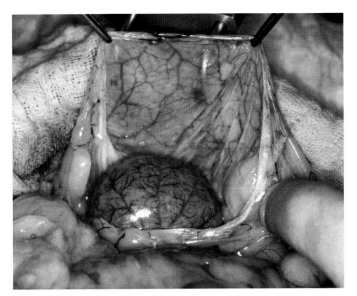

Figure 36-12 Surgical resection of the pseudocyst wall in the cat in Figure 36-11. Resection can relieve clinical signs, but will likely not provide long-term benefit unless the underlying disease is reversible.

ureteral re-implantation, depending on the extent and location of the damage.

Renal and ureteral neoplasia

Renal tumors in cats are uncommon, comprising 1.6–2.5% of all neoplasia identified.[61] Primary ureteral neoplasia has not been reported. The most common renal tumor in the cat is lymphoma, with the kidney often being the site of metastasis rather than a primary site of disease.[62–65] Lymphoma confined to the kidneys occurs in approximately 40% of documented cases and is usually bilateral.[63] In the largest retrospective study to date on primary renal tumors in cats, carcinomas (tubular and tubulopapillary) were the most common, followed by transitional cell carcinomas.[66] Adenoma, hemangiosarcoma, and nephroblastoma were also identified.[66]

Presenting clinical signs in cats with primary renal tumors are non-specific, with signs of anorexia, weight loss, depression, and lethargy being the most common.[66] Hematuria was identified in six of nine patients for which urine was evaluated and may be an indication of the presence of primary renal neoplasia.[66] Other signs including neurological signs, abdominal pain and distension, blindness, and dyspnea have also been reported. Polycythemia, possibly secondary to an increase in erythropoietin production, has been reported in one cat.[66]

Diagnostic evaluation should include a complete blood count, biochemical panel, urinalysis, three-view thoracic radiographs, and an abdominal ultrasound examination. Contrast enhanced computed tomography may also be useful in differentiating tumoral from non-tumoral regions.[67] Blood work may reveal anemia with varying degrees of azotemia, hypo- or hyperphosphatemia, hyperkalemia, hypoalbuminemia, hypocalcemia, hypernatremia and increased creatinine phosphokinase activity.[66,68] Hematuria and/or proteinuria may be present. If renal lymphoma is suspected, a fine needle aspirate and/or biopsy is recommended for cytological evaluation and diagnosis confirmation.[63]

Treatment

If lymphoma is diagnosed, the cancer should be clinically staged and, if appropriate, the patient treated with chemotherapy. For patients

diagnosed with primary renal neoplasia, if the disease is unilateral and the remaining kidney is functional, the treatment is ureteronephrectomy (see Box 36-4).[61,69]

Ureteral ectopia

Ureteral ectopia is a rare congenital condition identified in the cat and usually associated with urinary incontinence. To date, less than 30 cases have been reported in the veterinary literature.[70–81] Unilateral and bilateral cases appear with equal frequency, with the urethra being the most common site of ureteral termination. Intravenous urography in conjunction with retrograde urethrography in males and vaginourethrography in females are used to make the diagnosis. Concomitant abnormalities can include hydroureter and hydronephrosis (most common), cystitis, pyelonephritis, urinary tract infection, and renal and bladder hypoplasia and aplasia. Extramural ectopia is common in the cat, with the ureters completely bypassing the bladder. Surgical treatment is often curative and may include ureteronephrectomy (see below) or ureteral re-implantation (see below).

SURGICAL MANAGEMENT AND TECHNIQUES

Renal biopsy

Renal biopsy is indicated in order to determine a histologic diagnosis of the cause of renal failure as well as establish progression of a condition and response to therapy. A renal biopsy can be performed using a blind percutaneous technique, percutaneously under ultrasound guidance or surgically. Because cat kidneys are readily palpable and easy to immobilize, the blind percutaneous technique works well. Prior to performing a biopsy, a hematocrit, plasma protein, and clotting ability should be evaluated. When performing the technique percutaneously, care should be taken when directing the biopsy needle so as not to damage the renal vasculature or pelvis. Because of the larger vessels present in the renal medulla, which can result in infarction and fibrosis following biopsy, the biopsy needle should be directed so that only cortical tissue is obtained (Fig. 36-13). This can be challenging because of the small renal size in cats. For a sample collected percutaneously, the most commonly employed biopsy instrument is the Tru-Cut biopsy needle (Box 36-1). Following biopsy, a brisk fluid diuresis should be performed to prevent clot formation within the renal pelvis.[17]

In a large multi-institutional study on the methods and complications of renal biopsy, complications were reported in 18.5% of feline cases.[82] The most common complication reported was hemorrhage. If the biopsy is performed percutaneously, following the biopsy the perirenal area should be assessed under ultrasound guidance for any evidence of hemorrhage. Subcapsular hemorrhage may occur at the biopsy site and there may be evidence of microscopic hematuria during the first two days following the procedure. Macroscopic hematuria is much less common. The patient's hematocrit and total protein should be monitored regularly over the first 24 hours and if concerns of severe hemorrhage into the peritoneal cavity exist, the patient should be treated aggressively with whole blood transfusions, a compression bandage of the abdomen and possibly exploratory surgery. Care must also be taken when performing biopsies to avoid penetration of the renal pelvis. Although rare, bleeding into the renal pelvis with subsequent clot formation may result in a ureteral obstruction and hydronephrosis. The author has identified one case of ureteral obstruction secondary to clot formation from a biopsy that resulted in leakage of urine from the biopsy site.

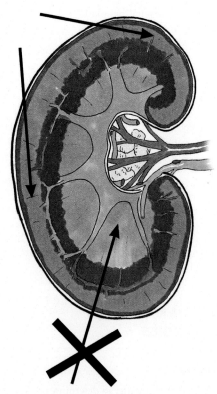

Figure 36-13 A Tru-Cut biopsy needle can be used percutaneously or surgically. The biopsy needle should be inserted in the direction of the plain black arrows so that only cortical tissue is obtained, and not into the medulla (crossed black arrow).

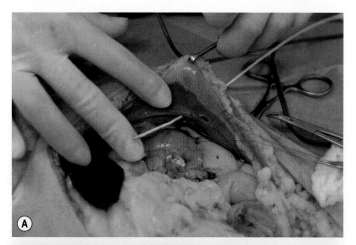

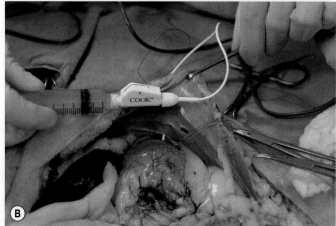

Figure 36-14 (A) Placement of a temporary nephrostomy tube for a cat that had a proximal ureterotomy to remove a ureterolith. A 5 French gauge locking loop catheter has been passed through the body wall. Prolene sutures are being preplaced to pexy the kidney to the body wall. **(B)** The sharp trocar tip of the catheter allows for placement of the catheter into the renal pelvis. The catheter can then be attached to an external drainage system. Note the proximal ureterotomy.

Box 36-1 **Renal biopsy**

To perform a renal biopsy surgically, a similar technique using the Tru-Cut biopsy needle can be performed during a standard laparotomy. Alternatively, a wedge of cortical tissue (2–5 mm thick) can be obtained. To perform this technique, retroperitoneal fat is dissected from the kidney to mobilize it and provide access to the convex lateral surface. In many cases in the cat, however, minimal to no dissection is necessary. Using finger pressure, an assistant can temporarily occlude the renal artery and vein. A preplaced mattress suture using 3/0 to 4/0 synthetic absorbable suture material is placed, but not tied, on the convex surface through cortical tissue. A number 11 blade is then used to cut a wedge of cortical tissue from within the limits of the mattress suture. Once the wedge is removed, the mattress suture is tied to appose the cortical parenchyma and capsule. The site is assessed for any evidence of hemorrhage. Renal biopsy can also be performed laparoscopically (see Chapter 24).

Nephrostomy

In some patients that are severely azotemic and unstable, hemodialysis or the placement of an emergency nephrostomy tube may be beneficial in stabilizing the patient prior to surgery. Because of the mobility of the feline kidney and the risk of leakage, some clinicians recommend that feline nephrostomy tubes be placed surgically. The placement of a nephrostomy tube can allow for the preoperative assessment of renal function in the obstructed kidney as well as determining whether a ureterolith will pass on its own with time.[83]

In cats, a 5 or 6 French locking loop catheter is used (Fig. 36-14). The tube can be secured on the skin with a purse-string and Chinese finger trap suture.

Complications that have been reported with nephrostomy tubes include the development of uroabdomen (25%; 6/24), tube dislodgement, and poor drainage (21%; 5/24).[41]

Peritoneal dialysis

Peritoneal dialysis may be useful for severely unstable patients that present with a uroperitoneum, to more completely resolve azotemia and fluid, electrolyte, and acid-base imbalances prior to definitive surgery. The technique of peritoneal dialysis (Box 36-2) should be performed using aseptic technique under general anesthesia or with the use of a local anesthetic

Maintenance of sterility is critical to the success of peritoneal dialysis. The most common complications reported with peritoneal dialysis in cats are dialysate retention and sequestration of dialysate under the skin.[85] Other reported complications include catheter obstruction, leakage of fluid from the catheter site, abdominal pain, septic peritonitis and pleural effusion.[85] Laboratory abnormalities may include hypoproteinemia, hyponatremia, hypochloremia, and hyperglycemia.[85,86]

A small stab incision is made 2–3 cm caudal to the umbilicus and just off midline and the peritoneal catheter introduced.[84] A wide variety of peritoneal dialysis catheters have been used for the cat, most being made out of Silicon with multiple fenestrations and one or two Dacron cuffs (see Chapter 11).[85,86] The fenestrated portion of the catheter is positioned into the peritoneal cavity and the cuffs are placed within the subcutaneous tissue. Ideally, the catheter should not be used for approximately 24 hours following placement to allow a fibrin seal to form; however, often the animal's condition dictates immediate use. The dialysate should be similar to plasma and contain physiologic concentrations of calcium, magnesium, sodium, and chloride. Additionally, the dialysate should be mildly to moderately hyperosmolar depending on the needs of the patient. Dextrose is the most commonly used osmotic agent in cats. The exchange procedure initially occurs frequently (every 45–60 minutes) and then is gradually decreased (four times a day) as the uremia improves. At each exchange, the volume infused is 40 mL/kg.

Nephrotomy and pyelolithotomy

A nephrotomy (Box 36-3) provides the greatest exposure of the renal pelvis and collecting duct system, but entails temporary interruption of the affected kidney's blood supply. Alternatively, pyelolithotomy (Box 36-3) may be performed if the renal calculi have created dilation of the renal pelvis. This approach does not provide as good an exposure of the pelvis as a nephrotomy, but does not necessitate occlusion of the renal vasculature.

Two separate studies have evaluated the effect of nephrotomy on renal function in clinically normal cats. In the first study, bisection nephrotomy did not adversely affect renal function during the 12 week study period.[87] In the second study, nephrotomy resulted in a 10–20% reduction in mean single kidney glomerular filtration rate (GFR) compared with the contralateral control kidney, but no significant difference from cats that underwent a sham surgical procedure. This difference may reflect the ability of the non-operated contralateral kidney to undergo compensatory hypertrophy in response to the decrease in GFR in the kidney that had the nephrotomy performed.[88]

Ureteronephrectomy

Ureteronephrectomy is commonly performed in cats with normal contralateral renal function, if severe renal injury has occurred resulting in persistent hemorrhage, urine extravasation, or the presence of non-viable tissue in cases of severe trauma involving the proximal ureter, and for para-ureteral and perirenal urinomas. Additionally, ureteronephrectomy is also used for patients diagnosed with primary renal neoplasia, if the disease is unilateral and the remaining kidney is functional.[62,70,73,81]

To perform a nephrectomy and ureterectomy (Box 36-4), the kidneys are exposed through a ventral midline incision. The author prefers this technique over a retroperitoneal flank incision since the entire abdomen can be explored including examination of both kidneys. Alternatively, based on the surgeon's experience, the kidneys can be removed laparoscopically (see Chapter 24).

Ureteroureterostomy

Although rarely identified, small lesions resulting in urine extravasation can be repaired primarily using 8/0 nylon or 8/0 vicryl in a single

Nephrotomy

The kidney is partially dissected from its retroperitoneal location. The renal artery and vein are isolated and temporarily occluded with Rommel tourniquets. A longitudinal incision is made with a scalpel through the convex lateral surface of the kidney (Fig. 36-16). The blunt end of the scalpel handle can then be used to extend the incision through the renal parenchyma. Calculi are removed from the renal pelvis and the collecting duct system, both of which are flushed with sterile saline. The nephrotomy incision is closed by approximating the two 'halves' of the kidney and the renal capsule is sewn with 4/0 PDS in a simple continuous pattern. The Rommel tourniquets are released and the two 'halves' of the kidney are held firmly opposed for five minutes.

Pyelolithotomy

To expose the pelvis, the kidney is dissected free of its peritoneal attachments and folded medially. An incision is made over the proximal ureter and pelvis and the stones are removed (Fig. 36-15A). A suture (5/0 prolene) can be passed distally to ensure that there is no obstruction of the more distal ureter. The proximal ureter and pelvis are closed with either a continuous suture pattern or single interrupted, appositional sutures using polydioxanone, polyglactin, polypropylene, or nylon (Fig. 36-15B).

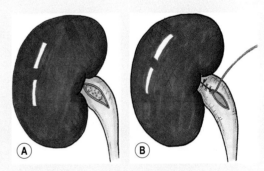

Figure 36-15 Pyelolithotomy. **(A)** An incision is made on the dorsal surface of the dilated renal pelvis and proximal ureter and calculi removed. **(B)** After flushing and catheterization of the ureter to ensure patency, the incision is closed with a simple continuous suture pattern.

The cat is positioned in dorsal recumbency and a midline celiotomy performed. To expose the left kidney for nephrectomy, the mesentery of the descending colon can be used to reflect away some of the abdominal viscera. The right kidney can be exposed using the mesoduodenum in a similar manner. The kidney can then be dissected from its retroperitoneal attachments to expose the renal artery and vein (Fig. 36-17). Care should be taken to identify all vessels supplying the kidney since multiple renal arteries can be identified on the left and multiple renal veins can be identified on both the right and left side.[9] The left testicular or ovarian vein should also be identified as it often drains into the renal vein rather than the caudal vena cava. The renal artery and vein are ligated separately with 2/0 to 3/0 silk or synthetic absorbable suture such as polydioxanone. Both vessels are ligated twice and one of those sutures can be a transfixation suture. The ureter is then isolated by dissecting down to the urinary bladder and ligating close to the vesicoureteral junction with one or two sutures of 2/0 or 3/0 synthetic absorbable suture. A transfixation suture is not necessary.

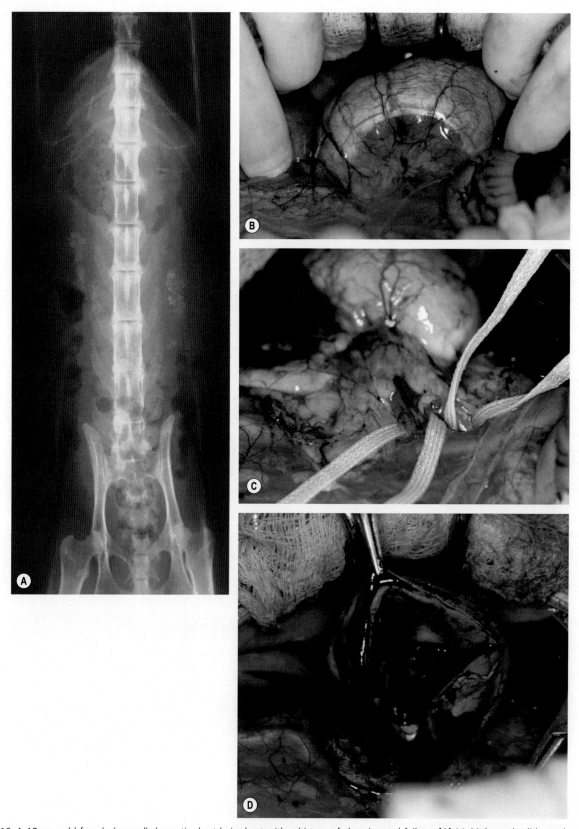

Figure 36-16 A 12-year-old female (spayed) domestic short-haired cat with a history of chronic renal failure. **(A)** Multiple nephroliths and ureteroliths are identified bilaterally. **(B)** The right kidney at surgery. The kidney was turgid and retroperitoneal effusion was present. **(C)** The renal artery and vein are isolated with Rommel tourniquets. Note the multiple renal veins (three) that are present. **(D)**. Following temporary occlusion of the Rommel tourniquets, a nephrotomy was performed. Significant loss of renal cortex is noted.

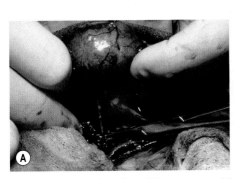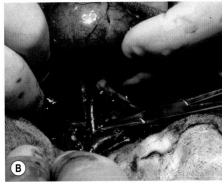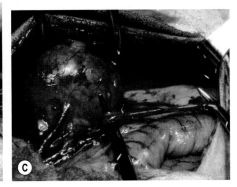

Figure 36-17 Isolation of the **(A)** renal artery, **(B)** vein, and **(C)** ureter for nephrectomy.

Box 36-5 **End-to-end anastomosis (ureteroureterostomy)**

To perform this technique, both ends of the ureter should be mobilized, taking care not to disrupt the blood supply or inadvertently traumatize the ureter. Debridement of the disrupted edges should be performed. Because of the small size of the ureteral lumen in a cat, a ureteral guidewire or stent can be placed retrograde from the ureterovesicular junction across the two ends to aid in suture placement. The ends of the ureter can also be spatulated with microvascular scissors prior to anastomosis to aid in closure (Figs 36-18 and 19). The author prefers to use 8/0 nylon or 8/0 polyglactin in an interrupted suture pattern. The ureteral stent can be left in place to prevent stricture formation and allow for urinary diversion. The stent can be removed at a later date, cystoscopically in a female and with a limited surgical approach to the bladder in a male, if indicated. Following complete ureteral transection and repair, normal peristalsis was reported to return from seven to ten days to three weeks post anastomosis.[89]

Boari flap

The Boari flap or a modification of the flap could theoretically be used if a significant loss of ureteral length exists. To perform this technique, a full thickness bladder flap is created with the base located at the apex of the bladder. The bladder defect is closed routinely and the edges of the flap are sutured together to create a tube, which can then be sutured to the distal end of the ureter. To minimize tension, a cystopexy can be performed. In a modification of this technique, following creation of the flap, the ureter could be placed through the flap, spatulated and then ureteral mucosa sutured to bladder mucosa. The edges of the bladder flap are then sutured together to create a tube and the top of the tube sutured closed.

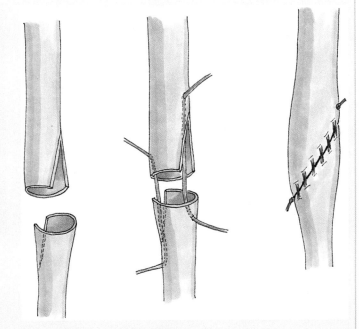

Figure 36-18 Ureteroureterostomy.

---

interrupted or single continuous suture pattern. More often, injuries to the proximal ureter are repaired using an end-to-end anastomosis (Box 36-5). This technique is particularly difficult in cats and should only be performed using appropriate magnification and by someone with experience in microvascular surgery.

Ureterotomy (Box 36-6)

Indications for ureterotomy include urolith removal from the proximal, middle and distal ureter.

Ureterotomy performed by a surgeon experienced with microsurgical technique does not require the placement of a nephrostomy tube. The most common complications associated with ureterotomy are leakage and stricture formation.[36,92] In a large multicenter study

evaluating 153 cases, the prevalence of complications in cats following surgical removal of ureteral calculi was 31%, with the most common complication being urine leakage, followed by persistence of ureteral obstruction. The 12 month survival rate following medical and surgical management was 66% and 91%, respectively.[41]

Surgical stenting of the ureter

Ureteral stenting (Box 36-7) is a novel technique currently being performed in cats. The author has used this technique for patients with multiple ureteroliths located unilaterally or bilaterally with or without the presence of nephroliths (see Fig. 36-9). Surgical stents can be placed retrograde via a cystotomy, antegrade via pyelocentesis, or through a ureterotomy site (antegrade or retrograde).[93]

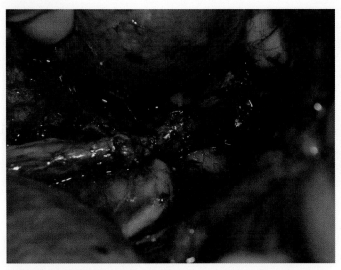

Figure 36-19 Ureteroureterostomy performed after surgical transection and resection of the proximal ureter during an ovariohysterectomy. Mobilization of both ends of the ureter was performed, debrided and a double pigtail ureteral stent was placed to aid in suture placement and allow for urinary diversion during healing. Stent not visible.

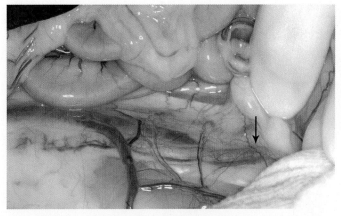

Figure 36-20 A seven-year-old female (spayed) domestic short-haired cat with a partial obstruction of the distal ureter. Two small stones can be identified on visualization and palpation (black arrow).

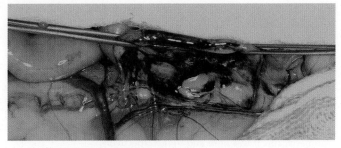

Figure 36-21 The affected segment of ureter is isolated using silastic material proximally and distally.

Ureteral re-implantation (neoureterocystostomy)

Neoureterocystostomy (Boxs 36-8–36-11) is indicated for extramural ectopic ureters (see Chapter 37), ureteral calculi, strictures, cystectomy involving the trigone or ureteral papilla, and renal transplantation.

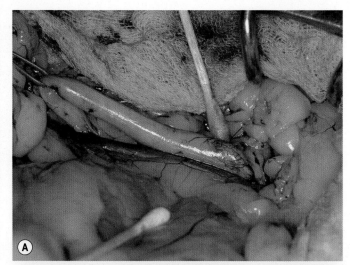

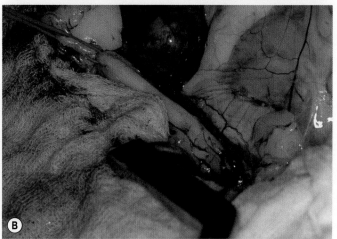

Figure 36-22 (A) A 13-year-old male (castrated) domestic short-haired cat with a distal ureteral stone causing a partial ureteral obstruction. **(B)** The stone was embedded into the wall of the ureter and so the ureterotomy was made directly over the stone.

For injuries to the middle and distal ureter, ureteral re-implantation is the most common technique performed. Ureteral re-implantation can also be performed for some proximal ureteral injuries, because of the mobility of the feline kidney, particularly following dissection from its retroperitoneal attachments. In these cases, ureteral re-implantation is always performed in conjunction with a renal descensus and a cystonephropexy.

Various neoureterocystostomy techniques including intravesicular, extravesicular, and ureteral papilla implantation techniques have been described in the cat, all attempting to reduce the complications that can occur when re-implanting the ureter due to its very small luminal diameter (see Box 36-4).[94,95]

The normal ureter in a cat measures approximately 0.4 mm in diameter at the level of insertion in the bladder, making an operating microscope essential when working with normal-sized ureters. However, cats with ectopic ureters or any degree of chronic obstruction often have hydroureter, making ureterovesicular anastomosis less technically demanding in some cases.

For conditions that require the distal end of the ureter to be transected from the bladder and then re-implanted in a different location, such as extramural ectopic ureters or tumors involving the trigone or ureteral papilla, either an extravesicular or intravesicular

Box 36-6 **Ureterotomy**

The cat is positioned in dorsal recumbency and a midline celiotomy is performed. Ureteral surgery in cats generally requires substantial magnification. The author recommends 8 to 10 times magnification provided by an operating microscope. Ureteral calculi may be visible on inspection of the ureter or palpable along the length of the ureter (Fig. 36-20). Once the location of the calculus is identified, the affected segment of ureter is isolated using silastic material proximally and distally (Fig. 36-21). In addition to decreasing urine flow into the surgical field, this preparation prevents spontaneous retrograde movement of ureteroliths.[90] Care is taken when manipulating the ureter so as not to disrupt the blood supply or inadvertently traumatize the ureter. A longitudinal incision is made in the dilated ureter just proximal to the obstruction. In some cases, because the calculus is embedded within the ureteral wall, the incision is made directly over the calculus (Figs 36-22A,B and Fig. 36-23A). Following removal, a piece of suture material can be passed proximally and distally from the ureterotomy site to ensure ureteral patency. The ureterotomy incision is closed with either simple interrupted sutures or a continuous suture pattern using monofilament suture material (Fig. 36-23B). Absorbable material is preferred so that the suture does not act as a nidus for new stone formation. Recently, a novel approach using endoscopic assistance to retrieve a ureteral calculus lodged 4 cm distal to the renal pelvis was described.[91] Removal of the calculus through a hole made in the renal capsule avoided complications identified following ureteral surgery including leakage from the ureterotomy site and stricture.

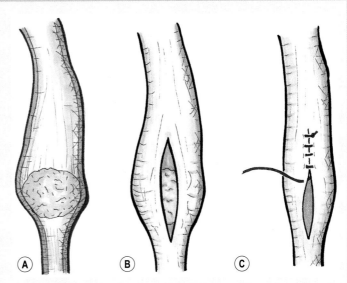

Figure 36-23 (A) Diagram of obstructive ureteral calculi. **(B)** Longitudinal incision to remove calculi. **(C)** Closure of the longitudinal ureterotomy using a simple continuous suture pattern.

Box 36-7 **Ureteral surgical stenting**

Retrograde technique

To perform the retrograde technique, a ventral cystotomy is performed and the ureteral orifices are located. An angled hydrophilic guidewire is advanced through the ureterovesicular junction (UVJ) and up the distal ureter. An open ended ureteral catheter is then advanced over the wire into the ureter and the hydrophilic guidewire temporarily removed. Fluoroscopy can be used to identify the location of the catheter within the ureter. A retrograde ureteropyelogram is then performed under fluoroscopic guidance to identify any stones, filling defects or other lesions. The catheter is left in place for 5 minutes to allow for passive ureteral dilation. Following the ureteropyelogram, the guidewire is then readvanced up the ureter and two loops of the guidewire are placed in the renal pelvis. The catheter is removed and an indwelling double pigtail ureteral stent is passed over the guidewire until one curl is in the renal pelvis. The other curl is pushed into the urinary bladder.

Antegrade technique

To perform the antegrade technique, a renal access needle or 22G IV catheter is used in conjunction with ultrasound or fluoroscopy to perform a percutaneous or surgical pyelocentesis. A contrast study is performed and a hydrophilic guidewire passed into the urinary bladder and then out the urethra. This wire acts as a safety wire so that access is not lost.[93] A catheter is then placed retrograde over the wire into the ureter. A second guidewire is then placed in a retrograde fashion up the catheter and the catheter removed. The stent is then placed in a retrograde fashion over the second wire.

neoureterocystostomy technique may be used, depending upon the specific circumstances. A specific disadvantage of the intravesicular technique is the excessive swelling of the bladder wall that occurs as a result of everting the lumen of the bladder to facilitate the anastomosis.[94]

For cats with an intact ureteral papilla that can be preserved for re-implantation, neoureterocystostomy can be performed using the ureteral papilla implantation technique.[96] This technique has been described for cats undergoing renal transplantation. Advantages of this technique include the technical ease of suturing the ureteral papilla since it is larger than the transected distal ureter alone, and sutures can be placed several millimeters away from the ureteral stoma. The risk of granulation tissue formation and subsequent stricture is potentially less since sutures do not directly enter the ureteral lumen, and the risk of ureteral avulsion is reduced with a complete two-layer closure. Finally, there is less potential for vesicoureteral reflux since the normal anatomy of the ureteral papilla is preserved.

Following neoureterocystostomy, cats should be monitored closely for potential complications including obstruction of the ureter from swelling or inflammation, torsion, or stricture, leakage of urine from dehiscence of the anastomosis site, cystolith formation due to the presence of intraluminal sutures, pyelonephritis due to ascending infection, and vesicoureteral reflux due to loss of an effective valve mechanism at the implantation site. Diagnostic tests including serum creatinine levels, renal and bladder ultrasonography, intravenous or percutaneous pyelography, and cystography should be performed as necessary if any of the above complications are suspected. Some degree of renal pelvic or ureteral dilation is commonly observed after ureteroneocystostomy, but should resolve within several weeks.

Box 36-8 Neoureterocystotomy – Intravesicular technique

To perform the intravesicular technique, a ventral midline cystotomy is performed. A mosquito hemostat is placed through the apex of the bladder and then the end of the ureter is grasped and brought into the bladder lumen. Some surgeons prefer to remove a 3–4 mm diameter section of mucosa from the desired area on the internal surface of the bladder prior to placing the hemostat. The bladder is everted and the distal end of the ureter is excised. If necessary, excessive periureteral fat is removed. The end of the ureter is then spatulated a distance of 0.5–0.75 cm using straight microvascular scissors (Fig. 36-24). The ureteral mucosa is sutured to the bladder mucosa using either 8/0 nylon or 8/0 polyglactin in a simple interrupted pattern (Fig. 36-25). The first and most important suture is placed at the proximal end of the ureteral incision (point of the 'V'). It is important that no periureteral fat is exposed once suturing is complete as this can lead to adhesions and granuloma formation, potentially resulting in a ureteral obstruction. To aid in identifying and maintaining the lumen of the ureter during suturing, a piece of 5/0 nylon or polypropylene suture can be placed in the lumen to serve as a stent and to check for ureteral patency. Following completion of the anastomosis, the bladder is inverted and closed routinely.

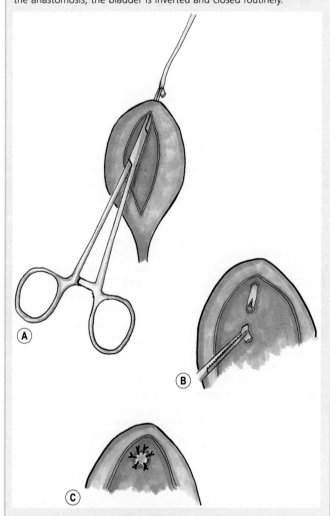

Figure 36-24 (A) A ventral cystotomy is performed. A mosquito hemostat is used to make a hole at the apex of the bladder and then the end of the ureter is grasped and brought directly into the bladder lumen. Tunneling of the ureter through the bladder wall is not performed. **(B)** The crushed end of the ureter is excised and the end of the ureter spatulated using straight microvascular scissors. **(C)** Simple interrupted sutures are placed between bladder mucosa and the ureteral wall.

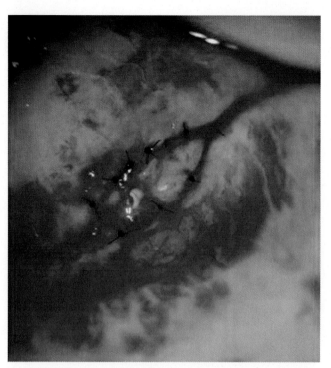

Figure 36-25 The ureteral mucosa is sutured in an interrupted pattern to the bladder mucosa using simple interrupted sutures of either 8/0 nylon or 8/0 vicryl. It is important that no periureteral fat is exposed once suturing is complete as this can lead to adhesions and granuloma formation, potentially resulting in a ureteral obstruction. Once completed, the bladder is then closed routinely. *(Courtesy of Dr Dan Degner.)*

POSTOPERATIVE CARE

Postoperative care

Postoperative care is tailored for each individual patient, but typically includes the administration of a balanced electrolyte solution until the patient is eating and drinking. Fluid diuresis is advocated after surgery of the upper urinary tract to prevent clot formation. Analgesia is usually provided by opioids and with the judicious use of non-steroidals only in patients with normal renal function. Urination should be carefully monitored and urine samples assessed for macro- and microscopic hematuria (see Chapter 4).

Patients that have had a ureterotomy performed should be evaluated periodically following surgery since nephroliths have the ability to migrate into the ureter and cause subsequent obstructions. For further information see Chapters 3 and 4.

COMPLICATIONS

Complications seen after upper urinary tract surgery include microscopic and macroscopic hematuria which can result in ureteral or urethral obstruction from blood clots. Ureteral surgery carries the risk of urinary leakage from the surgical site resulting in uroabdomen or subsequent stricture formation which may not be recognized if unilateral. Surgery on the kidney, though not detrimental in experimental studies, may cause further renal compromise in clinical cases which

Box 36-9 **Neoureterocystotomy – Extravesicular technique**

In the extravesicular technique, a 1 cm incision is made on the ventral surface of the bladder through the seromuscular layer allowing the mucosa to bulge through the incision.[56] A smaller incision (3–4 mm) is made through the mucosal layer of the bladder at the caudal aspect of the seromuscular incision (Fig. 36-26). The distal end of the ureter is prepared as previously described for the intravesicular technique. Using 8/0 nylon or 8/0 vicryl, ureteral mucosa is sutured to bladder mucosa. The proximal and distal sutures are placed first. Once the ureteral anastomosis is complete, the seromuscular layer is apposed in a simple interrupted pattern over the ureter with 4/0 absorbable suture.

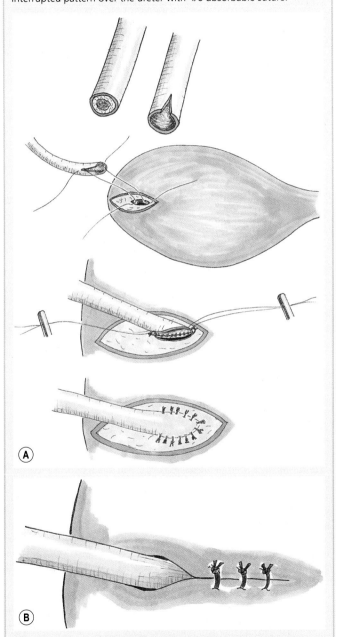

Figure 36-26 Extravesicular technique for ureteroneocystostomy.
(A) A 1 cm incision is made on the ventral surface of the bladder through the seromuscular layer allowing the mucosa to bulge through the incision. A smaller incision (3–4 mm) is made through the mucosal layer of the bladder at the caudal aspect of the seromuscular incision. The distal end of the ureter is spatulated and the ureteral mucosa is sutured to bladder mucosa using 8/0 nylon. The proximal and distal sutures are placed first. **(B)** The seromuscular layer is closed over the ureter in a simple interrupted suture pattern.

Box 36-10 **Neoureterocystotomy – Ureteral papilla implantation technique**

Using an operating microscope, the ureter is dissected from retroperitoneal attachments. The seromuscularis around the ureteral papilla including a 1–2 mm cuff of bladder wall is incised with microdissecting scissors until the mucosa begins to bulge from the lumen (Fig. 36-27A). The mucosa is then incised around the papilla, taking care not to injure the ipsilateral or contralateral ureteral stoma. After resecting the ureteral papilla, the defect in the bladder is closed in either one or two layers or dealt with as appropriate if the surrounding bladder is to be included in a partial cystectomy or other procedure (Fig. 36-27B). A 4 mm full thickness, circular incision is made in the desired area on the external surface of the bladder for re-implantation of the ureter. The ureteral papilla and cuff of bladder wall is then re-implanted using an extravesicular technique (Fig. 36-27C). The papilla is sutured to the bladder in 2 layers (mucosa to mucosa and seromuscularis to seromuscularis) using a simple continuous suture pattern with 8/0 absorbable suture material (Fig. 36-27D).

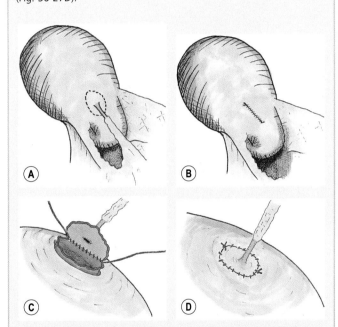

Figure 36-27 Ureteral papilla implantation technique. **(A)** Isolation of the distal ureter and ureteral papilla including a 2–3 mm cuff of bladder wall (dashed line). **(B)** Closure of the seromuscularis layer of the bladder using a simple continuous pattern. **(C)** Anastomosis of the ureteral papilla to the apex of the bladder. The mucosa of the ureteral papilla is being sutured to the mucosa of the bladder using a simple continuous pattern, and **(D)** completed anastomosis of the ureteral papilla. *(Redrawn from Hardie RJ, et al. Ureteral papilla implantation as a technique for neoureterocystostomy in cats. Vet Surg 2005;34:393–398. With permission from John Wiley & Sons.)*

Box 36-11 Neoureterocystotomy – Renal descensus and cystonephropexy

Although uncommon, ureteroneocystostomy can be performed when only the proximal third of the ureter is available for anastomosis. If tension along the suture line remains a concern, a renal descensus and a cystonephropexy can be performed (Fig. 36-28). To perform this technique, the kidney is mobilized from its retroperitoneal attachments and moved caudally. The renal capsule can then be sutured to an incision made in the adjacent body wall using four to six interrupted sutures of 4/0 polypropylene. The bladder can be fixed cranially to the body wall or to the tendon of the psoas muscle (psoas hitch) and a nephrocystopexy performed using 3/0 to 4/0 absorbable or non-absorbable sutures to relieve tension on the ureteral anastomosis or re-implantation site.[97]

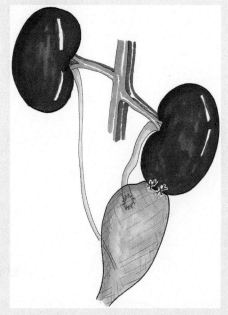

Figure 36-28 Renal descensus and cystonephropexy.

have pre-existing renal damage. Careful postoperative monitoring of renal function is advocated in these cases.

RENAL TRANSPLANTATION

Renal transplantation continues to remain a viable treatment option for cats in both acute and chronic renal failure. It is not performed throughout the world for a variety of reasons including: ethical concerns relating to the donor, the requirement for a specialized transplant team and the necessity for specialized equipment and experience in microsurgery. Success has been attributable to a number of factors including the development of microsurgical techniques for the feline patient, the ability to use an allograft from an unrelated or related donor, and a better understanding of the immune response to foreign tissue and the introduction of the drug ciclosporin for immunosuppressive therapy.[98–100] Although there are those that question renal transplantation as a treatment option for renal failure in cats, the procedure appears to prolong survival time as well as quality of life compared to the medical management of the disease.[101]

Evaluation of a potential recipient

Appropriate screening is performed by the referring veterinarian in conjunction with the transplant surgeon to decrease the incidence of morbidity and mortality that can occur following the procedure. Surgical intervention is recommended in cats with early decompensated chronic kidney disease or irreversible acute renal failure.[102,103] Indications of decompensation may include continued weight loss and worsening of the azotemia and anemia in the face of medical management. It is important to note that some candidates that are clinically stable can rapidly deteriorate and die without prior evidence that decompensation was present.

Both physical and biochemical parameters need to be evaluated carefully in order to determine if a cat is suitable for transplantation. The degree of azotemia, anemia, urine specific gravity, and age do not determine, by themselves, a suitable patient for transplantation, but both age and the degree of azotemia have been associated with survival. In one study, cats older than 10 years of age were found to have an increase in mortality, particularly during the first six months following surgery.[104] In a second study, median survival decreased when comparing cats less than five years of age (median 1423 days) with cats between the ages of five and 10 (613 days) and those greater than 10 years of age (150 days). Additionally, the degree of azotemia prior to surgery was found to be a risk factor. In one study, cats with a Cr >10 and an increased BUN were more likely to suffer mortality prior to discharge.[101] In a second study, the level of azotemia significantly increased the risk of neurologic complications in the perioperative period.[104] Finally, weight and preoperative blood pressure (BP) have also been shown to influence overall survival.[101]

Current evaluation involves a complete blood count/chemistry/blood type and cross-match/thyroid evaluation, evaluation of the urinary tract (urinalysis, urine culture, urine protein:Cr ratio, abdominal radiographs, abdominal ultrasound), evaluation for cardiovascular disease (thoracic radiography, electrocardiography, echocardiography, BP), and screening for infectious disease (feline leukemia virus (FeLV)/feline immunodeficiency virus (FIV), *Toxoplasma* titer (IgG and IgM)).

Evaluation of a potential donor

Donor cats accepted into the program are between one and three years of age and in excellent health. Standard evaluation includes a serum chemistry profile, complete blood count and blood type, urinalysis and culture, FeLV and FIV testing, and a toxoplasmosis titer (IgG and IgM).

Additionally, CT angiography is performed on all donors to evaluate the renal vasculature as well as evaluate the renal parenchyma for any abnormalities. This technique has allowed us to identify patients unsuitable for donation prior to surgery including patients with multiple renal arteries bilaterally as well as renal infarcts. A suitable home is found for any donor that fails the screening process. Donors that pass the screening process are adopted by the family of the recipient and followed for the rest of their lives. In a study of 16 donors that were followed between 24 and 67 months postoperatively to evaluate the long-term effects of performing a unilateral nephrectomy in healthy cats, 15/16 cats were clinically normal and serum creatinine concentrations for these cats remained within the reference range. One cat was diagnosed with chronic renal insufficiency 52 months following surgery.[105]

Preoperative treatment

Preoperative medical management will vary depending on the stability of the patient. The recipient is typically placed on intravenous fluid therapy at 1.5–2 times the daily maintenance requirements. Depending on the stability of the cat, an attempt is made to correct the anemia using either packed red cells or whole blood transfusions prior to or at the time of surgery. The first unit that is administered is a unit that had been previously collected from the cross-match compatible donor cat (see Chapter 5). Additionally, if the cat is hypertensive, the calcium channel blocker amlodipine (0.625 mg/cat PO q24h) may be indicated prior to surgery. Gastrointestinal protectants and phosphate binders are given if deemed necessary and if the patient is anorectic, a nasogastric or esophagostomy tube may be placed to administer nutritional support.

Two protocols currently exist for immunosuppression of the feline renal transplant recipient. The protocol currently used by the author includes a combination of the calcineurin inhibitor, ciclosporin (CsA) and the glucocorticoid, prednisolone. These drugs are used together for their synergistic effects. Because of the small dose of ciclosporin often required in cats, an oral liquid formulation Neoral (100 mg/mL) is used so that the dose can be titrated for each individual cat. Ciclosporin is started 24–96 hours prior to transplantation and is administered at a dose of 1–4 mg/kg PO q12h depending on the patient's appetite. A 12-hour whole blood trough concentration is obtained the day before surgery to adjust the oral dose for surgery. A target 12-hour trough concentration of 300–500 ng/mL prior to surgery using the technique of high-pressure liquid chromatography (HPLC) is the goal.[106] This level is maintained for one to three months following surgery and is then tapered to approximately 250 ng/mL for maintenance therapy. Prednisolone administration is begun the morning of surgery and started at a dose range of 0.5–1 mg/kg q12h orally for the first three months and then tapered to q24h. Another option for immunosuppression allows for once a day administration of medication. With this protocol, ketoconazole (10 mg/kg PO q24h) is administered in addition to the CsA and prednisolone.[105,107] Once ketoconazole is added to the immunosuppressive protocol, CsA and prednisolone are administered once a day and CsA doses are adjusted into the therapeutic range by measuring 24 hour whole blood trough levels.

Renal transplantation surgery

The donor cat is brought into the surgical suite approximately 30–45 minutes prior to the recipient so that the donor kidney can be prepared for the nephrectomy. At the time of the incision, the donor cat is given a dose of mannitol (0.25 g/kg IV over 15 minutes). Mannitol helps to minimize renal arterial spasms, improve renal blood flow and protect against injury during the warm ischemia period.

The CT angiography that was performed on the donor prior to anesthesia provides important information regarding the renal vasculature. Although many renal arteries bifurcate close to the kidney, a minimal length of 0.5 cm of single artery is necessary for the arterial anastomosis. Because of the longer renal vein, the left kidney is preferred over the right kidney. If two renal veins are present, the smaller vein can be sacrificed. It is important to identify where the ureteral vein drains to make sure that the renal vein that it drains into is not being sacrificed. The renal artery and vein are cleared of as much fat and adventitia as possible and the ureter is dissected free to the point where it joins the bladder. Templates are made of both the artery and vein to determine the size of the venotomy and aortotomy to be performed in the recipient's aorta and vena cava. The nephrectomy will be performed when the recipient is prepared to receive the kidney. An additional dose of mannitol (1.0 g/kg IV) is given to the donor cat fifteen minutes prior to nephrectomy.

An operating microscope is used for the majority of the recipient surgery. Following a full abdominal exploratory, the colon and ileum are tacked to the body wall using 3/0 chromic gut to aid in surgical

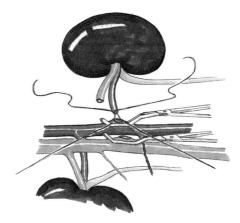

Figure 36-29 Transplantation of the renal allograft onto the recipient's abdominal aorta and vena cava. The renal artery in anastomosed end-to-side to the aorta using 8/0 nylon and the renal vein is anastomosed end-to-side to the vena cava using 7/0 silk. *(Redrawn from Slatter D. Textbook of small animal surgery. 3rd ed. W.B. Saunders, with permission from Elsevier, 2003.)*

exposure. In the current surgical technique used by the author, the renal artery is anastomosed end-to-side to the caudal aorta (proximal to the caudal mesenteric artery), and the renal vein is anastomosed end-to-side to the caudal vena cava (Fig. 36-29).[108] Partial occlusion clamps are used to obstruct blood flow in both the aorta and the caudal vena cava. Using the previously made templates from the donor vessels, windows are created in both the aorta and vena cava that match the size of the renal artery and vein, respectively. An aortotomy clamp is used to create the hole in the aorta and adventitial scissors are used to create an oval defect in the vena cava. Both aorta and vena cava are flushed with a heparinized saline solution. Two sutures of 8/0 nylon are placed at the cranial and caudal aspect of the aortotomy site. Following the second mannitol infusion in the donor, the graft is harvested and flushed with a phosphate-buffered sucrose preservation solution. The end of the renal artery is dilated and any excess adventitia that is present on the end of the renal artery is excised.

The renal artery is anastomosed to the aorta using 8/0 nylon in two rows of simple continuous sutures; one on the medial aspect and one on the lateral aspect of the artery. The renal vein is anastomosed to the vena cava using 7/0 silk. A back wall technique is used first to suture the portion of the renal vein closest to the renal artery. The anastomosis is completed once the second side of the vein is sutured using a continuous pattern. The venous clamp is removed first and then the arterial clamp. A small amount of hemorrhage often occurs and is controlled with pressure. Any significant leaks may need to be repaired with the placement of additional single interrupted sutures. Occasionally, renal arterial spasming can occur following release of the vascular clamps. The application of topical lidocaine, chlorpromazine or acepromazine has been advocated to address this problem.[109] Once the arterial and venous anastomoses are complete, a ureteroneocystostomy is performed (see Box 36-8).

Prior to closure, if not previously performed, a biopsy of one of the native kidneys is taken. An esophagostomy tube is placed if nutritional support is deemed necessary. Finally, the allograft is pexied to the abdominal wall. This is performed by incising the adjacent body wall and then the incised edge is sutured to the renal capsule using six interrupted sutures of 4/0 polypropylene. The native kidneys are usually left in situ to act as a reserve if graft function is delayed (Fig. 36-30). If necessary, one or both of the native kidneys can be removed at the time of surgery (in cases of severe polycystic kidney disease) or at a later time if warranted.

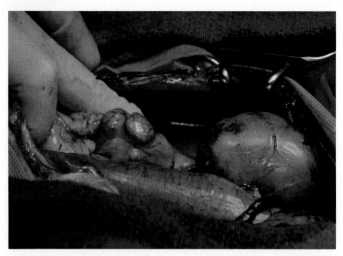

Figure 36-30 Image of the allograft and the native kidney. The native kidneys are usually left in situ to act as a reserve if graft function is delayed.

Postoperative care

Postoperative care is tailored for each individual patient, but typically includes the administration of a balanced electrolyte solution until the patient is eating and drinking, blood products as needed, and antibiotic therapy (cefazolin, 22 mg/kg IV q8h), which is continued as oral antibiotic therapy following discharge (clavamox, 62.5 mg PO q12h) until the feeding tube is removed. If the cat is *T. gondii* positive, clindamycin (25 mg PO q12h) is administered and continued for the lifetime of the cat. Postoperative pain has been controlled successfully at our facility using either hydromorphone (0.1–0.2 mg/kg IM or SQ q4-6h), buprenorphine (0.005–0.02 mg/kg IV q4-6h), methadone (0.15–0.3 mg/kg IV q4-6h), or a constant rate infusion of butorphanol (0.1–0.5 mg/kg/h). The packed cell volume, total protein, electrolytes, blood glucose and acid-base status is initially evaluated two to three times daily and then depending on the stability of the cat. A renal panel is checked every 24–48 hrs and a ciclosporin level checked every three to four days and adjusted accordingly. The prednisolone dose is continued as previously described (0.5–1 mg/kg PO q12h). Voided urine is collected daily to assess urine specific gravity. If surgery is successful, azotemia typically resolves and the cat clinically improves within the first 24–72 hours following surgery. Cats are discharged from the hospital when graft function appears adequate and ciclosporin blood levels are stable.

Long-term management and complications

Patients should be evaluated by their veterinarian once a week for the first six to eight weeks initially, and then extended to monthly intervals depending on the animal's stability. During each exam, clinical pathological evaluation including a renal panel, packed cell volume, total protein, a ciclosporin level and a urinalysis if a free-catch urine sample is available is performed. Body weight and BP are also monitored regularly. A complete blood count and serum chemistry panel is performed every three to four months and an echocardiography performed every six to 12 months if the patient had been diagnosed with underlying cardiac disease prior to transplantation.

Postoperative care and perioperative complications

Complications include those related to the allograft and those associated with chronic immunosuppressive therapy. Renal complications following transplantation have included vascular pedical complications, acute and chronic rejection, CaOx nephrosis, ureteral complications including retroperitoneal fibrosis, delayed graft function, hemolytic uremic syndrome, and allograft rupture. Complications secondary to chronic immunosuppressive therapy include the development of infections (including opportunistic infections), diabetes mellitus (DM), and neoplasia. Based on both published and unpublished reports, 70–92% of cats have been discharged following surgery, with median survival times ranging from 360–613 days.[95,101,110] Current information suggests that survival times continue to improve. Continued clinical experience with short and long-term management as well as the ability to identify specific risk factors both pre and postoperatively will hopefully continue to improve long-term outcome in these patients.

REFERENCES

1. Barrett R, Kneller S. Feline kidney mensuration. Acta Radiol Supp 1972;319:279–380.

2. Lee R, Leowijuk C. Normal parameters in abdominal radiology of the dog and cat. J Small Anim Pract 1982;23:251–69.

3. Walter P, Feeney D, Johnston G, et al. Feline renal ultrasonography: quantitative analysis of imaged anatomy. Am J Vet Res 1987;48:596–9.

4. Owens J. The genitourinary system. In: Biery D, editor. Radiographic interpretation for the small animal clinician. St. Louis: Ralston Purina Co.; 1982. p. 185–92.

5. Biers D. Upper urinary tract. In: O'Brien T, editor. Radiographic diagnosis of abdominal disorders in the dog and cat: radiographic interpretation, clinical signs, pathophysiology. Davis: Covel Park Vet. Co.; 1981. p. 484.

6. Shiroma JT, Gabriel JK, Carter RL, et al. Effect of reproductive status on feline renal size. Vet Radiol Ultrasound 1999;40:242–5.

7. Marais J. Cortical microvasculature of the feline kidney. Acta Anat 1987;130: 127–31.

8. Christie BA. Anatomy of the urinary system. In: Slatter D, editor. Textbook of small animal surgery. vol. 2. 3rd ed. Philadelphia, PA: Saunders; 2003. p. 1558–74.

9. Caceres AV, Zwingenberger AL, Aronson LR, et al. Characterization of normal feline vascular anatomy with dual phase CT angiography. Vet Radiol Ultrasound 2008;49:350–6.

10. Baines E. Practical contrast radiography-Urogenital studies. In Pract 2005;27: 466–73.

11. Fletcher TF. Applied anatomy and physiology of the lower urinary tract. Vet Clin North Am Small Anim Pract 1996;26:181–95.

12. Christie BA. Collateral arterial blood supply to the normal and ischemic canine kidney. Am J Vet Res 1980;41: 1519–25.

13. Bjorling DE. Traumatic injuries of the urogenital system. Symposium on urogenital surgery. Vet Clin North Am Small Anim Pract 1984;14:6161–76.

14. Mingledorff WE. Experimental study of the blood supply of the distal ureter with reference to cutaneous ureterostomy. J Urol 1964;92:424–8.

15. Hardie EM, Kyles AE. Management of ureteral obstruction. Vet Clin North Am Small Anim Pract 2004;34:989–1010.

16. Elbadawi A, Schenk EA. Innervation of the abdominopelvic ureter in the cat. Am J Anat 1969;126:103–20.

17. DiBartola SP. Clinical approach and laboratory evaluation of renal disease. In: Ettinger SJ, Feldman EC, editors. Textbook of veterinary internal medicine. vol. 2. 7th ed. St Louis, MO: WB Saunders; 2010. p. 1955–69.

18. Jaffe RB, Middleton AW. Whitaker test: differentiation of obstructive from non-obstructive uropathy. AJR Am J Roentgenol 1980;134:9–15.

19. Pfister RC, Papanicolaou N, Yoder IC. The dilated ureter. Semin Roentgenol 1986;21:224–35.

20. Nyland TG, Mattoon JS, Wisner ER. Ultrasonography of the urinary tract. In: Nyland TG, Mattoon JS, editors. Veterinary diagnostic ultrasound. Philadelphia, PA: WB Saunders; 1995. p. 95–125.

21. Rivers BJ, Walter PA, Polzin DJ. Ultrasonographic-guided, percutaneous antegrade pyelography: technique and clinical application in the dog and cat. J Am Anim Hosp Assoc 1997;33:61–8.

22. Heuter KJ. Excretory Urography. Clin Tech Small Anim Pract 2005;20: 39–45.

23. Adin CA, Herrgesell EJ, Nyland TG, et al. Antegrade pyelography for suspected ureteral obstruction in cats: 11 cases (1995–2001). J Am Vet Med Assoc 2003;222:1576–81.

24. Cannon AB, Westropp JL, Ruby AL, Kass PH. Evaluation of trends in urolith composition in cats: 5,230 cases (1985–2004). J Am Vet Med Assoc 2007;231(4):570–6.

25. Thumchai R, Lulich J, Osborne C, et al. Epizootiologic evaluation of urolithiasis in cats: 3,498 cases (1982–1992). J Am Vet Med Assoc 1996;208:547–9.

26. Westropp JL. Current trends in feline urolithiasis: what do we see and where do we see them? In: The North American veterinary conference, Orlando, FL, USA; 2007. p. 714–16.

27. Westropp JL, Ruby AL, Bailiff N, et al. Dried solidified blood calculi in cats. J Vet Intern Med 2005;20:828–34.

28. North DC. Hydronephrosis and hydroureter in a kitten – a case report. J Small Anim Pract 1978;19:237–40.

29. Prasad MC, Mohan K. Hydronephrosis in the cat. Indian Vet J 1968;45:107–8.

30. Speakman CF, Pechman RD, D'Andrea GH. Aortic thrombosis and unilateral hydronephrosis associated with leiomyosarcoma in a cat. J Am Vet Med Assoc 1983;182:62–3.

31. Nwadike BS, Wilson LP, Stone EA. Use of bilateral temporary nephrostomy catheters for emergency treatment of bilateral ureter transection in a cat. J Am Vet Med Assoc 2000;217:1862–5.

32. Zaid MS, Berent AC, Weisse C, et al. Feline ureteral strictures: 10 cases (2007–2009). J Vet Intern Med 2011;25: 222–9.

33. Ragni RA, Fews D. Ureteral obstruction and hydronephrosis in a cat associated with retroperitoneal infarction. J Feline Med Surg 2007;10:259–63.

34. Zotti A, Poser H, Chiavegato D. Asymptomatic double ureteral stricture in an 8-month-old Maine Coon cat: an imaging-based case report. J Feline Med Surg 2004;6:371–5.

35. Leib MS, Allen TA, Konde LJ, et al. Bilateral hydronephrosis attributable to bilateral ureteral fibrosis in a cat. J Am Vet Med Assoc 1988;192:795–7.

36. Kyles AE, Stone EA, Gookin J, et al. Diagnosis and surgical management of obstructive ureteral calculi in cats:11 cases (1993–1996). J Am Vet Med Assoc 1998;213:1150–6.

37. Adams LG, Williams Jr JC, McAteer JA, et al. In vitro evaluation of canine and feline calcium oxalate urolith fragility via shock wave lithotripsy. J Am Vet Med Assoc 2005;66:1651–4.

38. Kyles AE, Hardie EM, Wooden BG, et al. Clinical, clinicopathologic, radiographic, and ultrasonography abnormalities in cats with ureteral calculi:163 cases (1984–2002). J Am Vet Med Assoc 2005;226:932–6.

39. Carter WO, Hawkins EC, Morrison WB. Feline nephrolithiasis: eight cases (1984–1989). J Am Anim Hosp Assoc 1993;247–56.

40. Ross SJ, Osborne CA, Lekcharoensuk C, et al. A case-control study of the effects of nephrolithiasis in cats with chronic kidney disease. J Am Vet Med Assoc 2007;230:1854–9.

41. Kyles AE, Hardie EM, Wooden BG, et al. Management and outcome of cats with ureteral calculi:153 cases (1984–2002). J Am Vet Med Assoc 2005;226:937–44.

42. Coburn M. Genitourinary trauma. In: Feliciano DV, Mattox KL, Moore EE, editors. Trauma. 6th ed. New York, NY: McGraw-Hill; 2008. p. 789–825.

43. Thornhill JA, Cechner PE. Traumatic injuries to the kidney, ureter, bladder and urethra. Symposium on emergency medicine. Vet Clin North Am Small Anim Pract 1981;11:157–69.

44. Aumann M, Worth LT, Drobatz KJ. Uroperitoneum in cats: 26 cases (1986–1995). J Am Anim Hosp Assoc 1998;34:315–24.

45. Selcer, BA. Urinary tract trauma associated with pelvic trauma. J Am Anim Hosp Assoc 1982;19:785–93.

46. Weisse C, Aronson LR, Drobatz K. Traumatic rupture of the ureter: 10 cases. J Am Anim Hosp Assoc 2002;38: 188–92.

47. Brodsky SL, Zimskind PD, Dure-Smith P, Lewis PL. Effects of crush and devascularizing injuries to the proximal ureter. An experimental study. Invest Urol 1977;14:361–5.

48. Bellah JR. Diagnosis and management of urinary tract trauma. Symposium on Soft Tissue Surgery, Palmerton North, Christ Church, New Zealand, 30th–31st October 1999.

49. Bjorling DE, Christie BA. Ureters. In: Slatter D, editor. Textbook of small animal surgery. vol. 2. 2nd ed. Philadelphia, PA: Saunders; 1995. p. 1443–50.

50. Wilson DR. Renal function during and following obstruction. Annu Rev Med 1977;28:329–39.

51. Wilson DR. Nephron functional heterogeneity in the postobstructive kidney. Kidney Int 1975;7:19–26.

52. Worth AJ, Tomlin SC. Post-traumatic paraureteral urinoma in a cat. J Small Anim Pract 2004;45:413–16.

53. Moores AP, Bell AM, Costello M. Urinoma (para-ureteral pseudocyst) as a consequence of trauma in a cat. J Small Anim Pract 2002;43:213–16.

54. Bacon NJ, Anderson DM, Baines EA, White RAS. Post-traumatic para-ureteral urinoma (uriniferous pseudocyst) in a cat. Vet Comp Orthot Traumatol 2002;15:123–6.

55. Ochoa VB, DiBartola SP, Chew DJ, et al. Perinephric pseudocysts in the cat: a retrospective study and review of the literature. J Vet Intern Med 1999;13: 47–55.

56. Beck JA, Bellenger CR, Lamb WA, et al. Perirenal pseudocysts in 26 cats. Aust Vet J 2000;78:166–71.

57. Inns JH. Treatment of perinephric pseudocyst by omental drainage. Aust Vet Pract 1997;27:174–7.

58. Worth AJ, Tomlin SC. Post-traumatic paraureteral urinoma in a cat. J Small Anim Pract 2004;45:413–16.

59. Geel JK. Perinephric extravasation of urine with pseudocyst formation in a cat. J S Afr Vet Assoc 1986;57:33–4.

60. Lemire TD, Read WK. Macroscopic and microscopic characterization of a uriniferous perirenal pseudocyst in a domestic short hair cat. Vet Path 1998;35:68–70.

61. Crow SE. Urinary tract neoplasms in dogs and cats. Comp Cont Educ Pract Vet 1985;7:607–18.

62. Hammer AS, Larue S. In: Ettinger SJ, editor. Textbook of veterinary internal medicine. Philadelphia, PA: WB Saunders; 1995. p. 1788–96.

63. Mooney SC, Hayes AA, Matus RE, MacEwen EG. Renal lymphoma in cats: 28 cases (1977–1984). J Am Vet Med Assoc 1987;191:1473–7.

64. Wellman ML, Hammer AS, DiBartola SP, et al. Lymphoma involving large

granular lymphocytes in cats: 11 cases (1982–1991). J Am Vet Med Assoc 1992;201:1265–9.

65. Osborne CA, Johnson KH, Kurtz HJ, Hanlon GF. Renal lymphoma in the dog and cat. J Am Vet Med Assoc 1971;158: 2058–70.

66. Henry CJ, Turnquist SE, Smith A, et al. Primary renal tumours in cats: 19 cases (1992–1998). J Feline Med Surg 1999;1:165–70.

67. Yamazoe KJ, Ohashi F, Kadosawa T, et al. Computed tomography on renal masses in dogs and cats. J Vet Med Sci 1994;56: 813–16.

68. Gabor LJ, Malik R, Canfield PJ. Clinical and anatomical features of lymphosarcoma in 118 cats. Aust Vet J 1998;76:725–32.

69. Klein MK, Cockerell GL, Harris CK, et al. Canine primary renal neoplasms: a retrospective review of 54 cases. J Am Anim Hosp Assoc 1988;24:443–52.

70. Ghantous SN, Crawford J. Double ureters with ureteral ectopia in a domestic shorthair cat. J Am Anim Hosp Assoc 2006;42:462–6.

71. D'Ippoloti P, Nicoli S, Zatelli A. Proximal ureteral ectopia causing hydronephrosis in a kitten. J Feline Med and Surg 2006;8:420–3.

72. Steffey MA, Brockman DJ. Congenital ectopic ureters in a continent male dog and cat. J Am Vet Med Assoc 2004;224: 1607–10.

73. Rutgers C, Chew DJ, Burt JK. Bilateral ectopic ureters in a female cat without urinary incontinence. J Am Vet Med Assoc 1984;184:1394–5.

74. Smith CW, Burke TJ, Froehlich P, Wright WH. Bilateral ureteral ectopia in a male cat with urinary incontinence. J Am Vet Med Assoc 1983;182:172–3.

75. Biewnega WJ, Rothuizen J, Voorhout G. Ectopic ureters in the cat – a report of two cases. J Small Anim Pract 1978;19: 531–7.

76. Bebko RL, Prier JE, Biery DN. Ectopic ureters in a male cat. J Am Vet Med Assoc 1977;171:738–40.

77. Grauer GF, Freeman LF, Nelson AW. Urinary incontinence associated with an ectopic ureter in a female cat. J Am Vet Med Assoc 1983;182:707–8.

78. Burbidge HM, Jones BR, Mora MT. Ectopic ureter in a male cat. N Z Vet J 1989;37:123–5.

79. Lawler DF, Evans RH. Urinary tract disease in cats. Water balance studies, urolith and crystal analyses, and necropsy findings.Vet Clin North Am Small Anim Pract 1984;14:537–53.

80. Lulich JP, Osborne CA, Lawler DF, et al. Urologic disorders of immature cats.

Vet Clin North America small animal practice 1987;17:663–96.

81. Holt PE, Gibbs C. Congenital urinary incontinence in cats: a review of 19 cases. Vet Rec 1992;130:437–42.

82. Vaden SL, Levine JF, Lees GE. Renal biopsy: a retrospective study of methods and complications in 283 dogs and 65 cats. J Vet Intern Med 2005;19: 794–801.

83. Nwadike BS, Wilson LP, Stone EA. Use of bilateral temporary nephrostomy catheters for emergency treatment of bilateral ureter transection in a cat. J Am Vet Med Assoc 2000;217:1862–5.

84. Labato MA. Peritoneal dialysis in emergency and critical care medicine. Clin Tech Small Anim Pract 2000; 15:126–35.

85. Cooper RL, Labato MA. Peritoneal dialysis in cats with acute kidney injury: 22 cases (2001–2006). J Vet Intern Med 2011;25:14–19.

86. Dorval P, Boysen SR. Management of acute failure in cats using peritoneal dialysis: a retrospective study of six cases (2003–2007). J Feline Med Surg 2009;11:107–15.

87. King MD, Waldron DR, Barber DL, et al. Effect of nephrotomy on renal function and morphology in normal cats. Vet Surg 2006;35:749–58.

88. Bolliger C, Walshaw R, Kruger JM, et al. Evaluation of the effects of nephrotomy on renal function in clinically normal cats. Am J Vet Res 2005;66:1400–7.

89. Bellah JR. Wound healing in the urinary tract. Sem Vet Med Surg (Small Anim) 1989;4:294–303.

90. Dalby AM, Adams LG, Salisbury SK, et al. Spontaneous retrograde movement of ureteroliths in two dogs and five cats. J Am Vet Med Assoc 2006;229:1118–21.

91. Kuntz CA. Retrieval of ureteral calculus using a new method of endoscopic assistance in a cat. Aust Vet J 2005;83: 480–2.

92. Fossum TW. Surgery of the kidney and ureter. In: Fossum TW, editor. Small animal surgery. 2nd ed. St. Louis, MO: Mosby; 2002. p. 549–71.

93. Berent AC. Ureteral obstructions in dogs and cats: a review of traditional and new interventional diagnostic and therapeutic options. J Vet Emerg Crit Care 2011;21: 86–103.

94. Mehl ML, Kyles AE, Pollard R, et al. Comparison of 3 techniques for ureteroneocystostomy in cats. Vet Surg 2005;34:114–19.

95. Hardie RJ, Schmiedt C, Phillips L, et al. Ureteral papilla implantation as a technique for neoureterocystostomy in cats. Vet Surg 2005;34:393–8.

96. Rawlings CA, Bjorling DE, Christie BA. Kidneys. In: Slatter D, editor. Textbook of small animal surgery, 3rd ed. vol. 2. Philadelphia, PA: Saunders; 2003. p. 1606–19.

97. Gregory CR, Gourley IM, Taylor NJ, et al. Preliminary results of clinical renal allograft transplantation in the dog and cat. J Vet Intern Med 1987;1:53–60.

98. Gregory CR, Gourley IM. Organ transplantation in clinical veterinary practice. In: Slatter DH, editor. Textbook of small animal surgery. Philadelphia PA: WB Saunders; 1993. p. 95–100.

99. Gregory CR. Renal transplantation. In: Bojrab MJ, editor. Current techniques in small animal surgery. 4th ed. Baltimore: Williams and Wilkins; 1998. p. 434–43.

100. Schmiedt CW, Holzman G, Schwarz T, et al. Survival, complications and analysis of risk factors after renal transplantation in cats. Vet Surg 2008;37:683–95.

101. Gregory CR, Bernsteen L. Organ transplantation in clinical veterinary practice. In: Slatter DH, editor. Textbook of small animal surgery. Philadelphia: WB Saunders; 2000. p. 122–36.

102. Mathews KG. Renal transplantation in the management of chronic renal failure. In: August J, editor. Consultation in feline internal medicine. 4th ed. Philadelphia: WB Saunders; 2001. p. 319–27.

103. Adin CA, Gregory CR, Kyles AE, Cowgill L. Diagnostic predictors and survival after renal transplantation in cats. Vet Surg 2001;30:515–21.

104. Lirtzman RA, Gregory CR. Long-term renal and hematologic effects of uninephrectomy in healthy feline kidney donors. J Am Vet Med Assoc 1995;207: 1044–7.

105. Bernsteen L, Gregory CR, Kyles AE, et al. Renal transplantation in cats. Clin Tech Small Anim Pract 2000;15:40–5.

106. Katayama M, McAnulty JF. Renal transplantation in cats: techniques, complications, and immunosuppression. Compend 2002;24:874.

107. McAnulty JF, Lensmeyer GL. The effects of ketoconazole on the pharmacokinetics of cyclosporine A in cats. Vet Surg 1999;28:448–55.

108. Bernsteen L, Gregory CR, Pollard RE, et al. Comparison of two surgical techniques for renal transplantation in cats. Vet Surg 1999;28:417–20.

109. Aronson LR. Renal transplantation, unpublished manuscript, 2011.

110. Mathews KG, Gregory CR. Renal transplants in cats: 66 cases (1987–1996). J Am Vet Med Assoc 1997;211:1432–6.

Chapter |37|

Bladder

J.P. Little, R.J. Hardie

Bladder surgery is commonly performed in the cat for many conditions, the most common being cystic calculi. Other indications for bladder surgery include trauma, neoplasia, urachal diverticula, and ectopic ureters. The bladder generally heals rapidly, but knowledge of anatomy and adherence to meticulous surgical technique are important to reduce morbidity, particularly when the bladder is compromised from disease. This chapter covers the fundamental aspects of bladder surgery including anatomy, general surgical considerations, diagnostic procedures, surgical diseases, surgical techniques, postoperative care, and complications.

SURGICAL ANATOMY

The feline urinary bladder is a hollow, distensible organ that may be ovoid or teardrop-shaped, depending on the volume of urine it contains. The layers of the bladder wall include the mucosa, submucosa, muscularis, and serosa. The mucosal layer is made up of transitional epithelium that is irregularly folded when the bladder is empty, but capable of significant expansion as the bladder distends with urine. The submucosa serves as the holding layer of the bladder and is composed of loose connective tissue and collagen. The muscular layer is comprised of irregularly shaped, interwoven bundles of smooth muscle, and the serosa is made up of a thin layer of fibrous connective tissue.

Unlike the canine bladder, the feline bladder remains consistently craniad to the pubis regardless of its degree of distension.[1] The bladder is located ventral to the descending colon, with the ductus deferens or uterine body contacting the dorsal surface in intact males and females, respectively. The bladder is attached to the caudal abdominal body wall by three serosal folds. In the female, two lateral vesical folds are continuous with the uterine broad ligaments and contain the round ligaments of the bladder, which are fetal remnants of the umbilical arteries. A third median vesical fold arises from the ventral abdominal wall and contains the vestigial fetal urachus. The bladder consists of two distinct anatomic areas, the neck and the body. The body comprises the majority of the bladder, and its most cranial aspect is the apex. The neck contains the trigone, which is a triangular area on the dorsal aspect of the bladder bound by the urethral orifice caudally and the ureteral openings cranially (Fig. 37-1). The main vascular supply arises from the caudal vesicle artery which originates from the vaginal or prostatic artery, which are branches of the internal pudendal artery. The paired caudal vesicle arteries enter the bladder at the neck and course both ventrally and dorsally to anastomose with the contralateral vessels. The nervous supply to the bladder consists of both autonomic and somatic innervation. Autonomic control is mediated via the sympathetic (hypogastric nerve) and parasympathetic (pelvic nerve) nervous systems and the somatic control is mediated via the pudendal nerves. The lymphatics of the feline bladder drain into the hypogastric and lumbar lymph nodes.

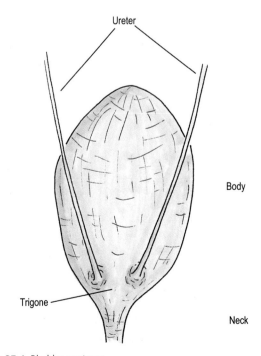

Figure 37-1 Bladder anatomy.

© 2014 Elsevier Ltd
DOI: 10.1016/B978-0-7020-4336-9.00037-8

GENERAL CONSIDERATIONS

Diagnostic procedures

Evaluation of suspected bladder disease generally starts with a minimum database, including urinalysis, complete blood count, serum chemistry panel, and aerobic culture and sensitivity of a urine sample.

Radiography

Survey radiography of the bladder is useful for general evaluation of the size, shape, presence of radiopaque calculi, or other abnormalities of the bladder (Fig. 37-2). If additional information is required following survey radiographs, contrast procedures may be indicated. If contrast radiography is performed on an elective basis, overnight fasting and a cleansing enema should be performed to aid in the detection of subtle urinary tract abnormalities by limiting the amount of ingesta and gas in the small intestine and colon that may obscure the bladder and urethra. The following contrast procedures complement each other, and they should be done in the order outlined below if it is likely that multiple procedures will be performed as part of the diagnostic workup. However, all of these contrast procedures are rarely indicated for a single case.

Pneumocystography can be useful for evaluating the bladder for wall thickness, radiopaque calculi, and diverticula. Pneumocystography can be performed with infusion of air or CO_2 into the bladder via a urethral catheter after the bladder has been emptied to prevent any residual urine from creating the appearance of an artificially thickened bladder wall. Full distension of the feline bladder is generally achieved with 15–45 mL, and can be detected with digital palpation. In many cases, partial distension of the bladder is sufficient for evaluation and may be more useful for demonstrating small urachal diverticula that are not apparent with full distension.[2]

Double contrast cystography aids in detection of bladder wall lesions and radiolucent calculi, which appear as intraluminal filling defects when outlined by the contrast material (Fig. 37-3). It is performed by infusing 1 mL of aqueous organic iodinated contrast solution through a urethral catheter, followed by infusion of air or CO_2 to further distend the bladder. If a positive contrast cystogram is to be performed, the bladder should be emptied before moderately distending it with contrast solution. Positive contrast cystography is useful for detecting bladder location, rupture or leaks, and urachal diverticula (Fig. 37-4).

Ultrasonography

Ultrasonography is a valuable tool for diagnosing various diseases or conditions of the bladder including wall thickening or inflammation, masses or neoplasia, and cystoliths (Fig. 37-5). Both radiopaque and radiolucent calculi as small as 2 mm in diameter can routinely be diagnosed with ultrasound.[3] The ability to detect calculi or assess the size and location of a mass is influenced by the degree of bladder distension, and accuracy can be improved by infusing physiologic saline into the bladder to separate the walls and better isolate specific lesions. However, ultrasonography is not as sensitive as survey radiography for determining the exact size, number, and possible composition of radiopaque calculi.

Cystoscopy

Cystoscopy is an excellent diagnostic tool that allows for direct visualization of various lesions, as well as sampling, using a biopsy instrument or basket (see Chapter 9). Transurethral cystoscopy can be performed in male and female cats using small diameter flexible or rigid cystoscopes, respectively.[4] Examination of the lumen of the urethra and bladder can be accomplished for diagnosis of lesions such as tumors, polyps, inflammation, mucosal tears, calculi, and ectopic ureters. In many cats, it can be difficult or impossible to pass a biopsy

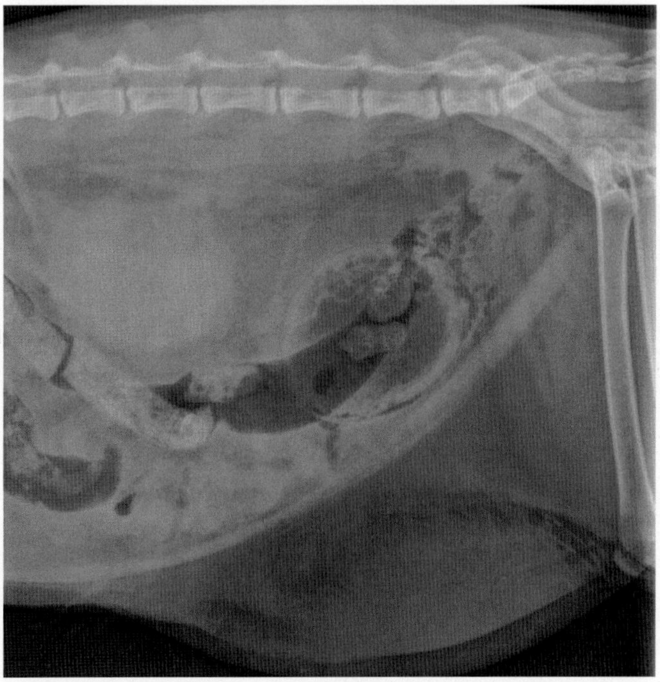

Figure 37-2 Lateral abdominal radiograph of a cat with emphysematous cystitis.

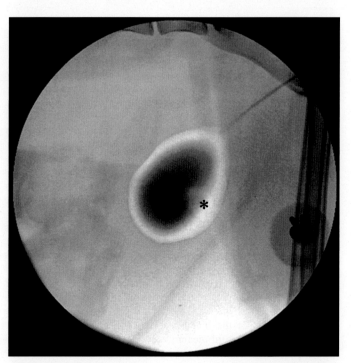

Figure 37-3 Lateral fluoroscopic image of a double contrast cystogram of a cat. Note the subtle filling defect on the ventral aspect of the bladder lumen as indicated by the asterisk.

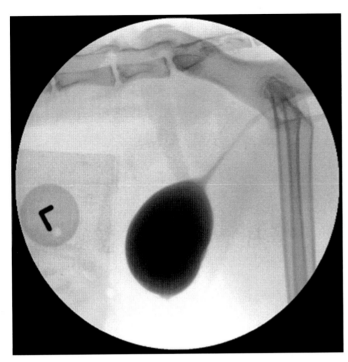

Figure 37-4 Lateral fluoroscopic image of a positive contrast cystogram of a cat.

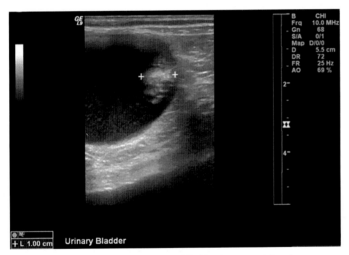

Figure 37-5 Ultrasound image of the bladder in a cat with a 1 cm diameter intraluminal mass as indicated by the crosses.

instrument simultaneously with the cystoscope and, therefore, if samples of the bladder are desired, the cystoscope can be used to guide percutaneous fine needle aspiration of specific lesions.[5]

SURGICAL DISEASES

Calculi

The composition of feline uroliths has evolved during the past thirty years (Fig. 37-6). Struvite uroliths were very common in the early 1980s, while calcium oxalate was much more rare, comprising only 2% of uroliths submitted to the University of Minnesota Urolith Center.[6] Since that time, reformulation of commercial diets is thought to have altered the distribution of urolith composition and by 2002

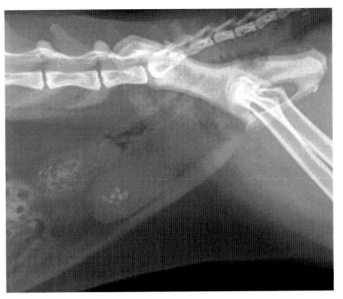

Figure 37-6 Lateral abdominal radiograph of a cat with multiple radiopaque cystic calculi.

calcium oxalate comprised 55% of feline uroliths, whereas struvite made up 33%.[6] Since 2002, struvite uroliths have increased again and are now more common than calcium oxalate in the US, with the more recent decrease in calcium oxalate being most likely due to further reformulation of commercial diets.[6] In Canada, analyses of over 11 000 cystoliths submitted from 1998–2008 revealed a different distribution, with calcium oxalate being slightly more prevalent than struvite.[7] Overall, struvite and calcium oxalate comprised 92% of feline cystolith submissions. Male domestic cats were 1.4 times more likely to develop calcium oxalate versus struvite cystoliths, whereas females were 1.3 times more likely to develop struvite versus calcium oxalate cystoliths.[7] Other cystoliths that have been reported in cats include calcium phosphate, xanthine, silica, cysteine, sodium pyrophosphate, and dried solidified blood calculi. Interestingly, 85% of cystoliths from Egyptian Mau cats were urate.[7]

While there is currently no effective method to dissolve calcium oxalate cystoliths, dietary management is instrumental in preventing or reducing recurrence. Administering oral citrate and feeding a non-acidifying, high-moisture diet formulated to avoid excessive protein, calcium, oxalate, and sodium minimizes cystolith formation.[8] In contrast, medical dissolution of struvite cystoliths in cats can be very effective. Most sterile struvite cystoliths will dissolve within four weeks when feeding an acidifying, high-moisture diet with reduced magnesium.[9] Because sterile struvite cystoliths can be successfully managed with medical therapy, it is important to determine cystolith composition prior to instituting therapy. Urine sediment examination for crystalluria, urine pH, and radiographic appearance of cystoliths provides valuable information for predicting the composition. Dissolution diets should be fed for one month past radiographic resolution of cystoliths. Infected struvite cystoliths require substantially longer dietary and antimicrobial therapy for dissolution. Once dissolution is achieved, cats should remain on a urolith preventative diet for life.

Physical removal of cystoliths leads to a rapid resolution of clinical signs, definitive diagnosis of cystolith composition, and reduced risk of urethral obstruction. Removal options include voiding hydropulsion, cystoscopic basket retrieval, laser lithotripsy, cystotomy (see Box 37-1), laparoscopic-assisted cystotomy, and laparoscopic-assisted cystoscopy. Regardless of the removal method, postoperative imaging should be performed to document removal of all cystoliths. Voiding urohydropulsion is generally effective for stones with diameters

<3 mm in females and <1 mm in males.[10] It is also more likely to be effective for smooth, rather than irregularly marginated stones. General anesthesia is recommended for hydropulsion, with the main contraindications being stones that are too large to pass through the urethra, recent bladder surgery, and active urinary tract infections. If infection is present, the increased pressure on the bladder wall can potentially lead to vesicoureteral reflux of urine and pyelonephritis. For this reason, prophylactic antibiotics are recommended for five days following the procedure.

Cystoscopic basket retrieval can be used to remove cystoliths smaller than the diameter of the distended urethra. This technique is generally limited to females, or males with a perineal urethrostomy. When cystoliths larger than the diameter of the urethra are present, cystoscopic laser lithotripsy with a holmium:yttrium-aluminum-garnet laser can be used to fragment the cystoliths.[11] Laser lithotripsy has been shown to be safe and effective in cats;[11] however, when large numbers or sizes of cystoliths are present, the time necessary to remove all cystoliths makes surgical intervention a more efficient method of removal. Complications with cystotomy are rare, and several minimally invasive approaches to surgical removal are available and are discussed later.

Trauma

Bladder rupture most commonly occurs following blunt trauma, but can also result from other types of penetrating trauma, unalleviated urethral obstruction, or iatrogenically from catheterization or bladder expression.[12] Traumatic ruptures occur most frequently at the apex and may be associated with pelvic fractures, although the condition is not recognized to the same extent as in dogs. A ruptured bladder does not necessarily prevent normal urination, thus making it difficult to diagnose based on clinical signs alone. Similarly, the presence of a palpable bladder does not eliminate the possibility of rupture since 20% of cats with a ruptured bladder had a palpable bladder on abdominal palpation.[12] Peritoneal fluid from cats with a ruptured bladder is usually serosanguinous, and does not always resemble urine. Consequently, biochemical analysis of fluid for creatinine and potassium levels, in addition to routine cytology, protein level, and cell counts, are essential. In a study of 26 cats with uroperitoneum, the mean serum-to-abdominal fluid ratio for creatinine was 1 : 2 (range, 1 : 1.1 to 1 : 4.1). Similarly, the mean serum-to-abdominal fluid ratio for potassium was 1 : 1.9 (range, 1 : 1.2 to 1 : 2.4).[12] While the serum-to-abdominal fluid creatinine and potassium ratios may be lower in cats than dogs, they remain clinically useful for diagnosis of uroperitoneum. The location of a suspected urinary tract rupture should be confirmed with contrast imaging such as an excretory urogram, positive contrast cystourethrogram, or cystoscopy (Fig. 37-7). Surgical correction of bladder rupture is rarely an emergency, and care should be taken to stabilize concurrent injuries and correct any azotemia or hyperkalemia prior to anesthesia. For small tears or punctures, maintaining the bladder in a decompressed state with an indwelling catheter for seven to ten days is generally sufficient time for small defects in the bladder wall to heal and has been used successfully in both cats and humans.[13,14] However, most tears require visual assessment and debridement, and surgical exploration and repair is indicated if any doubt exists as to the extent of the injury.

Neoplasia

Neoplasia of the bladder is relatively rare in cats and is nearly always primary in origin. Males are markedly overrepresented, accounting for 65–75% of all cases,[15,16] and a predisposition for older cats exists, with a median age of 15.2 years in a retrospective study of 20 cats.[15] Hematuria is the most common clinical sign associated with bladder

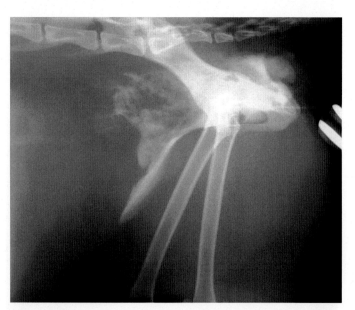

Figure 37-7 Lateral positive contrast cystogram of a cat demonstrating intra-abdominal leakage of contrast media due to a ruptured bladder. *(Courtesy of the University of Cambridge.)*

neoplasia, although any lower urinary tract sign may be encountered. Between 57 and 75% of cats have positive urine cultures at the time of diagnosis;[15,16] therefore, urine culture should be performed in cats suspected of having bladder neoplasia, and therapy instituted based on antimicrobial susceptibility testing. No correlation has been shown between feline bladder cancer and positive feline leukemia status.[16]

Definitive diagnosis can occasionally be made from cytologic examination of samples obtained from urine sediment, traumatic catheterization, or percutaneous fine needle aspirates. However, cytologic diagnosis is often complicated by the presence of reactive transitional epithelial cells, which can be impossible to differentiate from neoplastic cells, making cytologic examination of urine sediment diagnostic only 30% of the time.[17] Percutaneous aspiration of bladder masses is controversial and should be done with caution due to the risk of seeding the abdomen or body wall with neoplastic cells. Other diagnostic techniques should be attempted first, since implantation of neoplastic cells following needle aspirate of the bladder has been reported in the cat. In humans, it is reported to occur in 1 in 10 000 cases.[15,18] Approximately 20% of cats have evidence of metastatic disease at the time of diagnosis of transitional cell carcinoma.[15] Therefore, staging for both local and distant metastasis with ultrasound, thoracic radiography, or CT is important prior to surgical intervention. Rectal examination should also be performed to detect evidence of urethral extension or sublumbar lymph node involvement. To obtain a definitive diagnosis, histologic examination of cystoscopic or surgical biopsy samples of the tumor (and regional lymph nodes) is recommended.

Carcinoma is the most common urinary bladder cancer. In a review of 27 cats with bladder neoplasia, 15 were diagnosed as carcinoma, five were sarcoma, five were benign leiomyomas or fibromas, and two were lymphoma. Transitional cell carcinoma accounted for 30% of all neoplasms.[16] In a study of 23 cats with bladder neoplasia examined at two American universities between 1990 and 2004, 20 were diagnosed with transitional cell carcinoma.[15] Over 50% of these tumors were located in an area other than the trigone (Fig. 37-8). Similarly, in another study, tumors were more commonly located on the ventral aspect or apex.[19]

Treatment of bladder neoplasia depends upon the location, the extent of involvement, the histopathologic diagnosis, and the presence

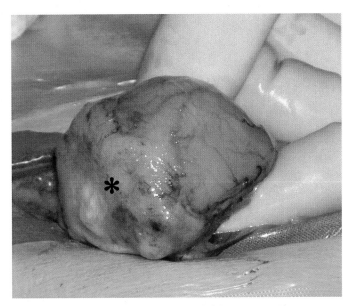

Figure 37-8 Intraoperative photo of the bladder in a cat with a transitional cell carcinoma involving the cranioventral aspect of the apex as indicated by the asterisk.

of metastasis. When the trigone is not involved and metastases are not detected, partial cystectomy (see Box 37-3) can be considered. Prior to partial cystectomy, the ureters and urethra should be carefully examined for evidence of adjacent neoplastic growth, and local lymph nodes should be biopsied to rule out regional metastasis. During surgical removal, a 1–2 cm tumor-free margin should be attempted whenever possible. The maximum amount of bladder that can be resected and still maintain normal bladder function postoperatively is approximately 75%. With extensive bladder resection, an indwelling urethral catheter may be necessary postoperatively to minimize distention of the bladder during healing. With the trigone preserved, the bladder wall will stretch over several months until normal function is regained. When the tumor involves the trigone, total cystectomy with ureteral transplantation may be considered; however, due to the overall poor prognosis and quality of life, urinary diversion is generally not recommended. With any surgical manipulation of the bladder, iatrogenic metastasis is possible; therefore instruments and gloves should be changed prior to closure. Early diagnosis and surgical treatment of neoplasia may lead to an improved prognosis, but an overall guarded prognosis should be given due to high metastatic and local recurrence rates. The median progression-free interval in one study of eight cats surviving the immediate postoperative period was documented to be 89 days, with a range of 61 to 1545 days, following partial cystectomy and adjunctive therapy for transitional cell carcinoma.[15]

Urachal diverticula

Urachal diverticula occur when the urachus located at the bladder apex fails to close after birth, creating an area for possible urine accumulation. Urachal diverticula can be congenital or more commonly, acquired. Congenital macroscopic diverticula allow urine and bacteria to persist in the lumen of the diverticulum and predispose cats to recurrent urinary tract infection. If urinary tract infection persists or recurs in the face of appropriate antibiotic therapy, diverticulectomy should be considered.[20] Acquired diverticula occur in older adult cats with inflammation of the lower urinary tract in response to persistent increased intraluminal bladder pressure, where microscopic urachal diverticula are thought to develop into macroscopic diverticula.[21]

Macroscopic diverticula may be entirely intramural or may extend beyond the bladder serosa and be extramural. Contrast radiography revealed evidence of diverticula in 22% of cats with feline lower urinary tract disease.[21] Interestingly, serial contrast radiography demonstrated resolution of some diverticula as quickly as 19 days after successful treatment of feline lower urinary tract disease. This supports the theory that diverticula are a sequela to, and not the cause of, lower urinary tract disease. Additionally, the majority of young cats with lower urinary tract disease do not have positive urine cultures, indicating that acquired urachal diverticula are not important predisposing causes to infection. In cats with lower urinary tract disease and urachal diverticula, efforts should focus on eliminating the cause of inflammation, obstruction, or cystoliths. Urachal diverticula should be reassessed two to four weeks after resolution of the lower urinary tract disease for evidence of persistence. It is postulated that macroscopic diverticula may resolve with production of connective tissue at the site of previous inflammation.[21] However, diverticula may prevent eradication of infection-associated cystoliths, and in such cases cystotomy with diverticulectomy should be considered. Furthermore, diverticulectomy may be indicated in cats that have undergone perineal urethrostomy to eliminate a potential source of recurrent urinary tract infections.

Ectopic ureters

Ectopic ureter is a congenital condition where one or both ureters fail to migrate normally in utero and thus do not empty into the trigone of the bladder, often resulting in urinary incontinence and persistent urinary tract infection. Suspicion for ectopic ureters should be high if urinary incontinence has been present since birth. Ectopic ureters can be either extramural or intramural depending upon the course the ureter takes when bypassing the trigone. With extramural ectopic ureters, the ureter completely bypasses the bladder before opening distally into the urethra or vagina. With intramural ectopic ureters, the ureter enters the bladder wall in the normal location, but then tunnels distally within the bladder wall before opening into the urethra or vagina. To the author's knowledge, intramural ectopic ureters have not been reported in the cat. In a review of 31 feline ectopic ureters, all were extramural, with 28 emptying into the urethra, and three into the vagina.[22] Diagnosis is made with intravenous urography, intravenous urography combined with CT, or cystoscopy. In 23 cats with ectopic ureters, no breed or sex predilection was reported, with 13 having unilateral and ten having bilateral ectopia.[22] As ectopic ureters are usually extramural in the cat, treatment generally involves transection and re-implantation rather than intramural diversion. If minimal ureteral dilation is present, an operating microscope is recommended for ureteral re-implantation. Surgery is generally curative, and the prognosis is good following ureteral re-implantation, although concurrent pyelonephritis and hydroureter may be present and require additional treatment. Potential complications after ureteral implantation include urine leakage, stricture of the neoureterocystostomy site, persistent incontinence, or cystolith formation. A single case of urinary incontinence secondary to double ectopic ureters has been described in the cat.[23] Double ureters are a rare congenital anomaly that occurs when two ureteric buds originate from the mesonephric duct of a duplex kidney. Neoureterocystostomy is described in Chapter 36.

GENERAL SURGICAL CONSIDERATIONS

The bladder is an organ that heals rapidly and is capable of regaining 100% of normal tensile strength within 21 days. However, despite this biologic advantage, a key principle of bladder surgery is gentle tissue handling to minimize swelling and inflammation that could delay healing or compromise the integrity of the closure. Whenever possible, stay sutures should be used to manipulate the bladder to minimize unnecessary direct handling of the tissues. Due to its vascular supply, the bladder tends to bleed liberally when incised; however, most hemorrhage arises from the capillary level and therefore decreases significantly after several minutes. For more substantial bleeders, hemorrhage can be controlled with judicious use of electrocautery. When suturing the bladder, it is important to use absorbable suture material to reduce the risk of the suture acting as a nidus for cystolith formation. Analysis of 303 recurrent cystoliths in cats revealed that 4% were suture associated.[24] Bacterial cystitis is common with many urinary tract diseases including cystoliths, diverticula, ectopic ureters, and neoplasia, and therefore should be ruled out with urine culture and sensitivity as part of the diagnostic workup.

SURGICAL TECHNIQUES

Cystotomy

Cystotomy (Box 37-1) may be indicated for cystic calculi removal, bladder wall or mass biopsy (Fig. 37-9), bladder mucosa culture, and ureteral catheterization or stent placement.

The popularity of minimally invasive surgical techniques for cystolith removal is increasing. Laparoscopic-assisted cystotomy, also called percutaneous cystolithotomy, is performed through an incision just large enough for cystolith removal. Briefly, a laparoscopic port is placed on the caudal ventral abdominal midline just cranial to the umbilicus. A second port is placed over the ventral aspect of the bladder with laparoscopic guidance. Using the second port, the bladder is grasped with laparoscopic Babcock forceps, the port incision is lengthened, the bladder is exteriorized, and stay sutures are placed in the bladder wall. A stab incision is made into the bladder, and cystoliths are removed with graspers. Once all the cystoliths are removed, the bladder is flushed and closed as previously described.

Laparoscopic-assisted cystoscopy, similar to laparoscopic-assisted cystotomy, is a minimally invasive surgical technique that may also be applicable for cystolith retrieval in cats and is done with smaller incisions in the bladder.[27] Laparoscopic ports are placed as previously described and the bladder is grasped, exteriorized, and stabilized with stay sutures. A 30° 2.7 mm cystoscope is placed through a small cystotomy incision in the cranioventral aspect of the bladder. The cystoscope is used to remove urine and instill saline before inspecting the bladder and urethra for calculi. Once identified, calculi are immobilized with the cystoscope, and then a second stab incision is made in the bladder for introduction of a grasping instrument for cystolith retrieval. Following retrieval, the bladder and urethra can be cystoscopically explored to ensure removal of all cystoliths.

Tube cystostomy

Tube cystostomy (Box 37-2) is an effective option for temporary or permanent diversion of urine for management of lower urinary tract injury or obstruction. Temporary cystostomy is indicated for the management of urethral obstruction from trauma, urolithiasis, inflammation, or strictures. Urinary diversion via tube cystostomy has been demonstrated to permit rapid healing of the urethra within 7–14 days and is an alternative to indwelling urethral catheterization.[28] Permanent cystostomy may be indicated for neurogenic bladder dysfunction or lower urinary tract obstruction secondary to tumors. It is a viable alternative for urinary tract drainage in cats that might otherwise require extensive surgery or euthanasia.

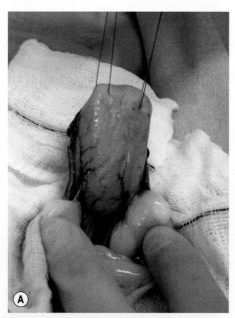

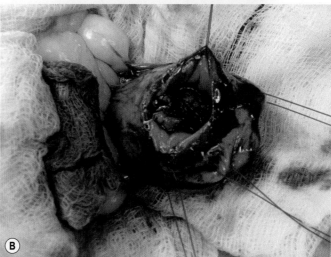

Figure 37-9 A 10-year-old female domestic short-haired cat with a bladder tumor. **(A)** Sponges are packed around the bladder and stay sutures are placed in the ventral bladder apex. **(B)** A cystotomy was performed in order to obtain tissue for histopathological analysis. *(Courtesy of the University of Cambridge.)*

Use of a low-profile cystostomy tube has been reported in one cat and is an option to reduce the risk of tube dislodgement, eliminate the need for cumbersome bandages, improve mobility, and improve aseptic care of the distal tube.[29] There are several commercially available low-profile gastrostomy tubes that have been used as cystostomy tubes in small animals.[29] Alternatively, a mushroom-tipped catheter can be used as described above, but then trimmed so that only 1–3 cm extends beyond the skin surface. An anti-reflux valve is then placed on the tube and attached by a hinged clip. Low-profile cystostomy tubes may also be placed through a mature stoma created by a previously placed tube and may be a good option if long-term use is deemed necessary.

A less invasive inguinal approach for tube cystostomy placement has been reported in six cats.[30] The procedure is performed with the cat in lateral recumbency, which is particularly useful for obstructed cats that are poor anesthetic candidates due to metabolic derangements from postrenal azotemia. The bladder is palpated, and an

Box 37-1 **Cystotomy**

The cat is placed in dorsal recumbency and the ventral abdomen is clipped and aseptically prepared. If intraoperative placement or manipulation of a urethral catheter is anticipated, the perineal region should also be prepared and draped accordingly. If bacterial cultures are to be obtained during surgery, prophylactic antibiotics should be withheld until urine or tissue samples are collected. A caudal ventral midline laparotomy is made starting 1–2 cm caudal to the umbilicus and extending to the pubis. The bladder is gently exteriorized, and packed off from abdominal contents with moistened laparotomy sponges. Full thickness stay sutures of 3/0 monofilament suture on a taper needle are placed on either side of the proposed longitudinal cystotomy site (Fig. 37-10). The cystotomy incision should be made in a relatively avascular area on the ventral aspect of the bladder apex. A stab incision is made into the bladder with a number 11 or number 15 scalpel blade and the bladder contents are suctioned with a Poole

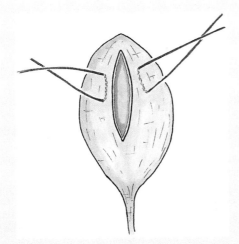

Figure 37-10 Stay sutures are placed in the bladder prior to making the cystostomy incision in the ventral bladder wall.

suction tip. Metzenbaum scissors are then used to extend the bladder incision for approximately 3–4 cm until adequate exposure is achieved. During cystolith removal, careful palpation of the bladder neck and proximal urethra is helpful to prevent calculi from being accidentally forced into the urethra. In addition, catheterization (antegrade and ideally retrograde) and flushing of the urethra is essential to ensure all calculi and sediment are removed or flushed through the urethra (Fig. 37-11).

There are many options for closing the bladder depending on the thickness and integrity of the wall and the location of the cystotomy incision relative to the urethra. A one or two-layer closure using a rapidly absorbable 3/0 or 4/0 monofilament suture (poliglecaprone 25, Glycomer 631) on a fine taper needle is generally acceptable. If the bladder wall is normal, a single layer closure using a simple continuous or inverting suture pattern incorporating the submucosa as the holding layer is generally sufficient. A simple continuous appositional pattern, if properly performed, does not usually require additional support.[25] If the bladder wall is inflamed or thickened, a two-layer closure may be necessary to achieve an adequate seal; however, inverting sutures can be difficult to place when the bladder wall is thickened and less compliant. The first layer is completed using a simple continuous pattern in the mucosa/submucosa, followed by a simple continuous or continuous inverting (Cushing or Lembert) pattern in the seromuscularis layer. Alternatively, the inverting layer can be performed in an interrupted fashion to allow for more variability in the spacing of the 'bites' and the degree of inversion.

Following closure, the bladder may be leak tested by instilling sterile saline into the lumen and applying gentle pressure. The stay sutures are then removed and the abdomen is closed routinely. For cats with radiopaque cystoliths, postoperative radiographs should be made to document the removal of all calculi. Residual cystoliths were detected in the lower urinary tract of 20% of cats following cystotomy in one veterinary teaching hospital.[26] After surgery, cats should be monitored closely to determine that they are able to adequately pass urine. Hematuria is common for the first 24–48 hours; however, urethral catheterization is usually unnecessary.

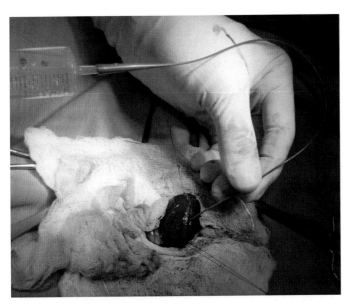

Figure 37-11 Intraoperative photo of a ventral cystotomy in a cat, demonstrating antegrade flushing of the bladder and urethra using a 3.5 French red rubber catheter and syringe.

oblique 2–3 cm skin incision is made in the inguinal region directly over the bladder. The subcutaneous tissue and aponeurosis of the external abdominal oblique are incised, and a grid approach through the internal abdominal oblique and transversus abdominus muscles is performed. Once the abdomen is entered, the bladder is stabilized with stay sutures and the tube is placed through a purse-string suture. The technique is performed as described (see Box 37-2), with the exception that the tube exits the abdomen through the same incision used for the approach and the cystopexy is performed by incorporating bladder wall into the closure of the abdominal musculature.

The cystostomy tube should be drained every six to eight hours, or attached to a closed collection system. Gloves should be worn when handling the tube and antiseptic cleaning of the tube and exit site with dilute chlorhexidine or tris-EDTA is recommended. Tubes should be left in place for a minimum of 14 days to ensure adequate adhesion formation between the bladder and body wall to minimize the risk of uroperitoneum after removal.[31] Removal of a Foley catheter is accomplished by deflating the balloon and then applying gentle traction until the tube is pulled through the body wall. Removal of a mushroom-tipped catheter requires more persistent traction while simultaneously stabilizing the abdominal wall with the opposite hand. If necessary, a blunt stylette can be placed through the lumen of the tube to extend and narrow the mushroom tip, decreasing the force required to pull the tube through the abdominal wall. Following

Box 37-2 Tube cystostomy

A caudal ventral midline laparotomy is performed. The bladder is exteriorized and packed-off with sterile laparotomy sponges. A suitable location for the cystostomy tube placement is chosen on the ventrolateral abdominal wall. A hemostat is used to bluntly tunnel through the abdominal musculature and subcutaneous tissue, exiting the skin lateral to the laparotomy incision. A Foley or mushroom-tipped catheter is then drawn into the abdomen through the tunnel with the hemostats. A purse-string suture is preplaced in the ventrolateral apex of the bladder wall with monofilament absorbable suture. A stab incision is made in the bladder wall in the center of the purse-string suture. The catheter is then placed in the bladder, inflated if applicable, and the purse-string suture is tightened around the tube (Fig. 37-12A). The bladder is then filled with saline via the tube and assessed for leakage around the purse-string suture. A cystopexy is then performed by placing four simple interrupted sutures adjacent to the tube (Fig. 37-12B). The sutures incorporate partial thickness 'bites' of the bladder wall and transversus abdominus muscle. Omentum may be wrapped around the cystopexy site. The laparotomy incision is closed routinely and the cystostomy tube is fixed to the skin with a finger trap suture.

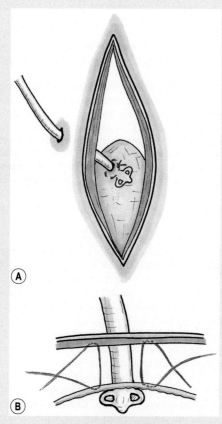

Figure 37-12 Tube cystostomy. **(A)** The tube is shown after being passed through the abdominal wall and the purse-string suture into the bladder lumen. **(B)** Two of the four cystopexy sutures are shown between the bladder wall and abdominal wall.

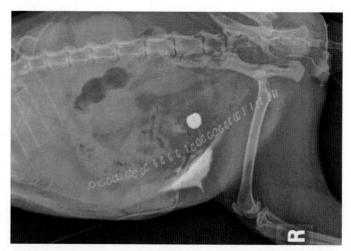

Figure 37-13 Oblique abdominal radiograph of a cat demonstrating subcutaneous leakage of contrast media after being injected through the cystostomy tube.

tube) can generally be replaced through the existing stoma. The tube should be replaced immediately to avoid interference from granulation tissue that rapidly fills the stoma once the tube is no longer present. The prevalence of urinary tract infection is high, with nearly all animals having evidence of nosocomial infection after cystostomy tube removal.[28,31] Urine culture is recommended after tube removal and administration of antibiotic therapy instituted based on culture and susceptibility results. Fecal contaminants are the most commonly isolated organisms and may form a biofilm on the tube, increasing the risk of recurrent infections. However, prophylactic antibiotics are generally contraindicated due to the potential for development of multi-drug resistant bacteria, and antimicrobials should only be used to treat documented infections. Other less significant complications may include fistula formation, irritation or inflammation around the tube, and intermittent hematuria. The use of silicone catheters may reduce the incidence of stoma irritation. Cystostomy tubes have been maintained in some cats for several years, although deterioration of the tube usually requires replacement through the established stoma approximately every six months,[30] which in most cases can be accomplished under heavy sedation or a short general anesthetic.

Partial cystectomy

Partial cystectomy (Box 37-3) may be indicated in cats with bladder tumors or trauma that does not extensively involve the bladder neck or trigone region. If uncertainty exists regarding the extent of trigone involvement, an excretory urogram, contrast cystogram, ultrasound, contrast CT, or cystoscopy should be performed to better assess the extent of the lesion and to screen for secondary hydroureter.

POSTOPERATIVE CARE

After most urinary bladder procedures, urination should be monitored closely to ensure the cat is able to void without excessive stranguria, dysuria, or signs of complete obstruction. Intravenous fluids are generally recommended postoperatively to promote diuresis and aid in flushing residual blood clots from the bladder. Hematuria, stranguria, and dysuria may occur after surgery, but should gradually improve over several days. If bladder decompression is critical or if there are concerns for outflow obstruction due to excessive swelling

cystostomy tube removal, the stoma may leak for one to four days until granulation tissue gradually closes the stoma.

The most common complications with cystostomy tubes include urine leakage, urinary tract infection, and tube dislodgement (Fig. 37-13). In cases of tube dislodgement, a new (but possibly smaller

Box 37-3 **Partial cystectomy**

A ventral midline laparotomy is performed. Prior to partial cystectomy, thorough examination of the abdomen should be performed to assess for regional lymph node metastasis, ureteral involvement, or bladder vasculature compromise. The bladder is then packed off from the abdominal cavity with moist laparotomy sponges to prevent contamination and tumor seeding of the abdomen. The tumor location is identified by gentle palpation, and a stab incision is made into the bladder wall 1–2 cm away from the mass, taking care to avoid the ureteral papilla. To increase the likelihood of complete excision a 1–2 cm margin around the entire mass should be attempted (Fig. 37-14). If the mass extends to one or both ureteral papilla, resection of the ureter(s) can be performed and the ureter re-implanted (see Chapter 36) in the remaining healthy portion of the bladder. The bladder is closed as described previously; however, inverting patterns should be performed with care near ureteral orifices or the urethra to minimize the risk of mechanical obstruction. Prior to closure of the abdominal wall, instruments and gloves should be changed to minimize the risk of iatrogenic metastasis. If more than 50% of the bladder is resected, an indwelling catheter is recommended to keep the bladder decompressed. Up to 75% of the bladder may be resected, with return to near normal function within three months.[20]

Patching of large defects

During radical cystectomy, serosal patching utilizing the antimesenteric surface of a loop of jejunum can be implemented to augment closure of the bladder defect. The jejunum is sutured to the bladder wall in a simple interrupted pattern using non-absorbable 3/0 or 4/0 suture material. The sutures are placed through the submucosa of the jejunum and bladder, avoiding knots that enter the bladder lumen. The serosa of the jejunum provides a surface for migrating urothelium to fill the defect and has been reported to occur within 30 days.[20] The use of porcine small intestine and urinary bladder submucosa in sheet form has also been described for replacement of portions of the bladder wall after partial cystectomy in dogs, pigs, and rabbits with relative success and may have merit as an option for cats.[32–35] For this technique, a sheet of submucosa material is cut to the appropriate size and then sutured to the bladder wall using a simple continuous pattern to create a watertight seal. In an experimental study involving rabbits, gross and histologic examination of the bladder augmented with porcine small intestine submucosa revealed it to be almost indistinguishable from the normal bladder after 12 months.[36]

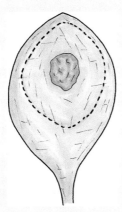

Figure 37-14 A 1–2 cm margin of normal bladder around the entire mass is removed if possible to increase the likelihood of complete excision.

or inflammation of the urethra, an indwelling urinary catheter attached to a closed collection system can be placed at the time of surgery and maintained until it is anticipated that the cat is able to void normally. If necessary, empirical antibiotic therapy can be continued after surgery and then changed if necessary, based upon the bacterial culture and sensitivity taken at the time of surgery.

COMPLICATIONS

The complications associated with bladder surgery vary depending upon the specific procedure performed but generally include dehiscence and leakage, persistent hematuria, pollakiuria, or stranguria, transient incontinence due to reduced bladder capacity, outflow obstruction due to excessive swelling or blood clots, persistent or recurrent cystoliths, local recurrence or metastasis of tumors, and stricture or obstruction of the ureters or urethra if involved.

Hematuria, pollakiuria, stranguria, and dysuria are not uncommon after surgical manipulation of the bladder, but should improve or resolve after several days. Persistence of any or all of these signs would be an indication of a potential complication that should be further investigated to rule out problems such as persistent cystic calculi, hematomas, urethral swelling, or active urinary tract infection. Outflow obstruction of the bladder may occur due to excessive swelling or inversion of the wall during closure requiring temporary urethral catheterization. To minimize the risk for these complications, use of an inverting pattern when closing the bladder near the urethra or ureteral papilla should be avoided. To reduce the likelihood of suture-induced cystolith formation, use of rapidly absorbable, synthetic suture material is recommended and ideally sutures should not penetrate the lumen of the bladder. Finally, although not an immediate postoperative complication, seeding of the abdominal wall has been reported after percutaneous fine needle aspiration or direct surgical manipulation of bladder tumors and the risk of such an event should be considered during diagnostic and treatment procedures.

REFERENCES

1. Johnston GR, Osborne CA, Jessen CR, et al. Effects of urinary bladder distension on location of the urinary bladder and urethra of healthy dogs and cats. Am J Vet Research 1986;47:404–15.

2. Johnston GR, Feeney DA, Osborne CA. Urethrography and cystography in cats

Part I. Techniques, normal radiographic anatomy, and artifacts. Compend Continuing Educ 1982;4:823–35.

3. Vörös K, Wladár S, Marsi A, et al. Ultrasonographic study of feline lower urinary tract diseases: 32 cases. Acta Vet Hung 1997;45:387–95.

4. Messer JS, Chew DJ, McLoughlin MA. Cystoscopy: Techniques and clinical applications. Clin Tech Small Anim Pract 2005;20:52–64.

5. McCarthy T. Veterinary endoscopy for the small animal practitioner. St Louis: Elsevier; 2005.

6. Osborne CA, Lulich JP, Kruger JM, et al. Analysis of 451,891 canine uroliths, feline uroliths, and feline urethral plugs from 1981 to 2007: perspectives from the Minnesota urolith center. Vet Clin Small Anim 2008;39:183–97.

7. Houston DM, Moore AEP. Canine and feline urolithiasis: examination of over 50,000 urolith submissions to the Canadian Veterinary Urolith Centre from 1998 to 2008. Can Vet J 2009;50: 1263–8.

8. Lekcharoensuk C, Osborne CA, Lulich JP, et al. Association between dietary factors and calcium oxalate and magnesium ammonium phosphate urolithiasis in cats. J Am Vet Med Assoc 2001;219: 1228–37.

9. Osborne CA, Lulich JP, Forrester D, et al. Paradigm changes in the role of nutrition for the management of canine and feline urolithiasis. Vet Clin Small Anim 2008;39:127–41.

10. Langston C, Gisselman K, Palma D, et al. Methods of urolith removal. Compend Continuing Educ 2010;32(6):E1–7.

11. Adams LG. Lithotripsy using shock waves and lasers. 24th Annu ACVIM Forum 2006:439–41.

12. Aumann M, Worth LT, Drobatz KJ. Uroperitoneum in cats: 26 cases (1986–1995). J Am Anim Hosp Assoc 1998;34:315–24.

13. Osborne CA, Sanderson SL, Lulich JP, Medical management of iatrogenic rents in the wall of the feline urinary bladder. Vet Clin Small Anim 1996;26:551.

14. Gomez RG, Ceballos L, Coburn M, et al. Consensus statement on bladder injuries. BJU Int 2004;94:27–32.

15. Wilson HM, Chun R, Larson VS, et al. Clinical signs, treatments, and outcome in cats with transitional cell carcinoma of the urinary bladder: 20 cases (1990–2004). J Am Vet Med Assoc 2007;231:101–6.

16. Schwartz PD, Greene RW, Patnaik RK. Urinary bladder tumors in the cat: a review of 27 cases. J Am Anim Hosp Assoc 1985;21:237–45.

17. Henry CJ. Management of transitional cell carcinoma. Vet Clin Small Anim 2003;33:597–613.

18. Smith EH. Complications of percutaneous abdominal fine-needle biopsy, review. Radiology 1991;178:253–8.

19. Schwartz PD, Willer PD. Urinary bladder neoplasia in the dog and cat. Prob Vet Med 1989;1:128–40.

20. Wilson GP, Dill RS, Goodman RZ. The relationship of urachal defects in the feline urinary bladder to feline urologic syndrome. In Proceedings 7th Kal Kan Symposium. Vernon, California: Kal Kan Foods Inc.; 1983. p. 125–9.

21. Osborne CA, Johnston GR, Kruger JM, et al. Etiopathogenesis and biological behavior of feline vesicourachal diverticula: Don't just do something – stand there. Vet Clin Small Anim 1987;17:697–733.

22. Holt PE, Gibbs C. Congenital urinary incontinence in cats: a review of 19 cases. Vet Rec 1992;130:437–42.

23. Ghantous SN, Crawford J. Double ureters with ureteral ectopia in a domestic shorthair cat. J Am Anim Hosp Assoc 2006;42:462–6.

24. Appel SL, Lefebvre SL, Houston DM, et al. Evaluation of risk factors associated with suture-nidus cystoliths in dogs and cats: 176 cases (1999–2006). J Am Vet Med Assoc 2008;233:1889–95.

25. Thieman-Mankin KM, Ellison GW, Jeyapaul CJ, et al. Comparison of short-term complication rates between dogs and cats undergoing appositional single-layer or inverting double-layer cystotomy closure: 144 Cases (1993–2010). J Am Vet Med Assoc 2012;240: 65–8.

26. Lulich JP, Osborne CA. Changing paradigms in the diagnosis of urolithiasis. Vet Clin Small Anim 2008;39:79–91.

27. Rawlings CA. Resection of inflammatory polyps in dogs using laparoscopic-assisted cystoscopy. J Am Anim Hosp Assoc 2007;43:342–6.

28. Williams JM, White RAS. Tube cystostomy in the dog and cat. J Small Anim Pract 1991;32:598–602.

29. Stiffler KS, Stevenson MM, Cornell KK, et al. Clinical use of low-profile cystostomy tubes in four dogs and a cat. J Am Vet Med Assoc 2003;223: 325–9.

30. Bray JP, Doyle RS, Burton CA. Minimally invasive inguinal approach for tube cystostomy. Vet Surg 2009;38:411–16.

31. Beck AL, Grierson JM, Ogden DM, et al. Outcome of and complications associated with tube cystostomy in dogs and cats: 76 cases (1995–2006). J Am Vet Med Assoc 2007;230:1184–9.

32. Record RD, Hillegonds D, Simmons C, et al. In vivo degradation of 14C-labeled small intestinal submucosa (SIS) when used for urinary bladder repair. Biomaterials 2001;19:2653–9.

33. Caione P, Capozza N, Zavaglia D, et al. In vivo bladder regeneration using small intestinal submucosa: experimental study. Pediatric Surg Int 2008;7:593–9.

34. Badylak SF, Kropp B, McPherson T, et al. Small intestine submucosa: a rapidly resorbed bioscaffolds for augmentation cystoplasty in a dog model. Tissue Eng 1998;4:379–87.

35. Boruch AV, Nieponice A, Qureshi IR, et al. Constructive remodeling of biologic scaffolds is dependent on early exposure to physiologic bladder filling in a canine model. J of Surg Research 2010;161: 217–25.

36. Ayyildiz A, Akgül KT, Huri E, et al. Use of porcine small intestine submucosa in bladder augmentation in rabbit: Long-term histological outcome. ANZ J Surg. 2008;78:82–6.

Chapter 38

Urethra

J.F. Ladlow

Feline lower urinary tract disease is common and in male cats can result in urethral obstruction. Relief of obstruction and repair of iatrogenic ruptures or strictures resulting from urinary catheterization are two of the most common causes for urethral surgery in the cat. Trauma and neoplasia are other less common conditions that are treated surgically. Surgical options for the urethra consist of urinary diversion with secondary intention healing, proximal urethrostomy, and primary repair.

SURGICAL ANATOMY

The urethra extends from the trigone of the bladder to the urethral meatus or orifice.

Female urethra

Embryologically the female urethra is formed from an elongation between the bladder and the urogenital sinus. The urethra is positioned between the pelvic floor and the vagina and it empties into a groove on the ventral floor of the vestibule at the external urethral orifice.

The cranial two-thirds of the female urethra is covered by detrusor fibers, connective tissue, and smooth muscle which comprises the internal urethral sphincter; the caudal third of the urethra is initially encircled by striated urethralis muscle, which comprises the external urethral sphincter. In the caudal urethra, the urethralis muscle expands dorsally and encircles both the vagina and urethra. The urethral smooth muscle contains circular fibers which act as a sphincter and longitudinal fibers that contract to dilate the urethra. The epithelium changes from transitional to stratified squamous in the caudal quarter of the urethra.[1]

Male urethra

The male cat has an elongated bladder neck or preprostatic urethra, a short wider prostatic section, a postprostatic or pelvic section, and the distal penile urethra that narrows significantly at the glans (Fig. 38-1).

Embryologically, the prostatic urethra is equivalent to the female urethra, the pelvic portion of the urogenital sinus forms the membranous portion, and the penile urethra is derived from the phallic portion of the sinus.

The prostate and the bulbourethral glands are accessory sex glands that are situated dorsolaterally to the urethra. The prostate is located at the level of the acetabulae and the bulbourethral glands empty dorsally into the postprostatic urethra at the ischial arch; their entry marks the start of the penile urethra.

The preprostatic urethra consists of epithelium, submucosa, and three layers of smooth muscle, which are continuous with the detrusor muscle at the vesicourethral junction. At the prostate, the muscle changes from smooth to striated fibers. The postprostatic urethra has circumferentially orientated striated muscle fibers, the urethralis muscle, which corresponds to the external urethral sphincter. This contributes to resting urethral tone but also contains fast twitch fibers that are capable of responding to sudden changes in vesicular pressure and thus maintaining continence during coughing or sudden movement.[2] The muscle mass increases just caudally to the bulbourethral glands with the insertion of the ischiocavernosus muscles ventrally and the bulbocavernosus muscles dorsally. The penile urethra has longitudinally orientated muscle fibers ventrally but not dorsally; however, in this area the urethra is surrounded by highly vascular collagenous connective tissue and the corpus cavernosus dorsally.[3] The epithelium of the male urethra is mainly transitional with stratified squamous epithelium near the urethral orifice.[4]

The male urethra is approximately 8.5–10.5 cm long[3] and the dimensions of each part are shown in Figure 38-1. The urethral circumference is not affected by castration although fibrocyte density increases with castration.[4]

Blood supply

In the female, the urethral blood supply is via the vaginal arteries from the urogenital artery.

In the male, the prostatic artery (from the internal pudendal artery) supplies the prostatic and membranous urethra along with branches from the urethral artery, which extends to the cavernous tissue and distal urethra.

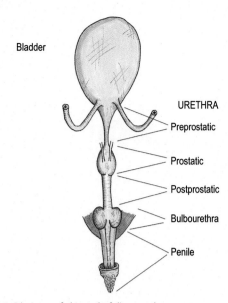

Bladder

URETHRA

Preprostatic

Prostatic

Postprostatic

Bulbourethra

Penile

Figure 38-1 Diagram of the male feline urethra.

Innervation

Normal micturition requires a brainstem reflex and can be initiated or suppressed consciously. The striated urethralis muscle is innervated by the pudendal nerve, arising from segments S1–S3. The pelvic plexus is located bilaterally on the lateral surface of the parietal peritoneum lining the pelvic cavity and this has sympathetic input via the hypogastric plexus and parasympathetic input via the pelvic nerve. The hypogastric nerve originates from L2–L5 and stimulation of the sympathetic input inhibits detrusor contraction, stimulates the internal urethral sphincter, and inhibits parasympathetic synapses in the pelvic plexus. The pelvic nerve originates from S1–S3 and stimulates detrusor contraction.

Functional anatomy

The functional anatomy of the feline urethra has been studied experimentally by urethral pressure profile measurements.[3,5,6] Urethral tone results from the interaction of the smooth muscle, striated skeletal muscle, fibroelastic and vascular tissue. The smooth muscle offers most resistance to urine leakage in the non-voiding animal. The external urethral sphincter is maintained at a low tone but activates with sudden increases in intra-abdominal or intravesicular pressure rises. The external urethral sphincter tone increases in response to fluid flow along the urethra or distension of the urethra.

In the female, the maximal urethral closure pressure is predominantly in the distal third of the urethra at the level of the urethralis muscle[6] (Fig. 38-2A). Interestingly, unlike in the dog, there have been no significant differences found in the urethral pressure profiles of intact and ovariectomized females.[6]

In the male, the urethral pressure profiles reveal a pressure peak at the prostatic and early postprostatic urethra followed by high-pressure peaks in the bulbourethral and penile areas that usually have the maximal urethral closure pressure (Fig. 38-2B). The prostatic and postprostatic pressure peaks arise at the level of the urethralis muscle and the external urethral sphincter whilst the penile increase in urethral pressure results from the small diameter of the penile urethra.

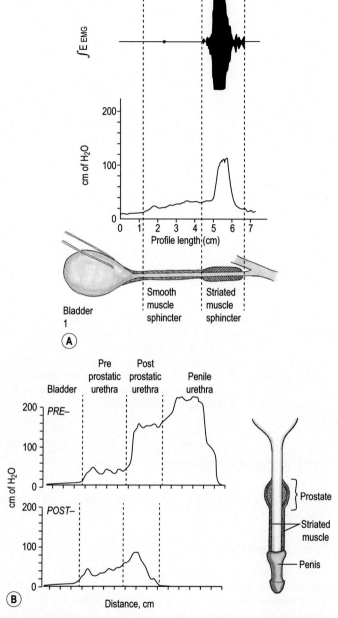

Figure 38-2 (A) Urethral pressure profile of the female cat. **(B)** Urethral pressure profile of the male cat. ([A] From Gregory CR, Willits NH. Electromyographic and urethral pressure evaluations: Assessment of urethral function in female and ovariohysterectomized female cats. American Journal of Veterinary Research 1986;47:1472, with permission; [B] from Gregory CR, et al, Electromyographic and urethral pressure profilometry: Assessment of urethral function before and after perineal urethrostomy in cats. American Journal of Veterinary Research 1984;45:2062–5, 1984. http://avmajournals.avma.org/loi.ajvr with permission.)

GENERAL CONSIDERATIONS

The details regarding whether the cat has been urinating normally are not always easy to ascertain in a cat, particularly if it has access to the outdoors. Early signs of urinary tract disease and obstruction may be missed and veterinary attention only sought when the cat is showing

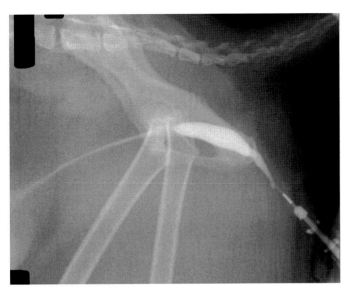

Figure 38-3 A four-year-old male neutered domestic short-hair cat presented with recurrent lower urinary tract obstruction. A retrograde urethrocystogram is performed to ensure there is no narrowing proximal to the penile urethra that would contraindicate perineal urethrostomy. No narrowing is present in this cat.

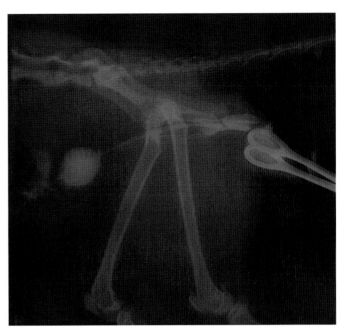

Figure 38-4 Retrograde vaginourethrogram in a female cat with a normal urethra and ruptured bladder.

systemic signs. A careful physical examination including gentle abdominal palpation for the urinary bladder and inspection of the penis and vulva should be performed as routine.

Diagnostic imaging

A combination of imaging modalities are used to evaluate the urethra.

Radiography

Urogenital radiographic studies, including contrast studies, are used to evaluate the integrity and diameter of the urethra. Prior to performing these radiographic studies, it is desirable that large intestinal content is minimal, which can be difficult to achieve in cats. Sodium citrate micro-enemas (Micralax, Micolette, Relaxit) should be used both on the evening prior to the investigation and on the morning of the investigation. The cat should be fasted overnight. If the colon is still impacted with feces, it is worth performing a warm water cleansing enema under anesthesia prior to radiography in order to achieve optimal results. For good quality radiographs, deep sedation or anesthesia is required. A positive contrast urethrogram or urethrocystogram is the best radiographic technique for evaluation of the urethra (Fig. 38-3). Urogenital radiographic studies, including contrast studies are described in chapter 8.

Female urethral catheterization is usually easier than the male and is aided by pulling the vulval lips caudally and then advancing a well lubricated 4 or 5 French balloon catheter along the ventral wall of the vagina (Fig. 38-4).

In the male cat, a 3.5 or 4 French catheter is appropriate. The urethra should initially be gently extended caudally and dorsally during catheterization to avoid traumatizing the distal penile urethra, which has a natural V-shaped configuration (see Fig. 9-19A,B). The catheter should be well lubricated with sterile petroleum jelly and advanced gently 1–2 cm into the urethra. If difficulties are encountered during

catheterization, stay sutures placed in the prepuce allow an assistant to gently extend the penile urethra. If urine leakage occurs prior to distension of the urethra a balloon catheter can be used with the balloon gently inflated until resistance is felt.

It is not necessary to distend the bladder prior to urethrography and prior bladder distension may actually obscure normal anatomy.

The urethral crest is a midline dorsal ridge of tissue that protrudes into the urethra. It is seen as a linear midline radiopacity after contrast studies. In the bladder the urethral crest branches into two columns that lead into one of the two ureteric papillae.

In the male urethra, particularly in cats with feline lower urinary disease, a narrowing of the pelvic urethra is sometimes seen (Fig. 38-5). This is a symmetrical, smooth tapering and may be a result of prostatic compression, urethritis, or muscular spasm. It can be eliminated by antegrade urethrography or higher volume retrograde urethrography and should not be confused with a urethral stricture.[7]

Ultrasound

Although not traditionally thought of as a useful imaging modality for the urethra, the integrity of the proximal urethra can be assessed ultrasonographically. It is also useful for evaluating periurethral urine leakage and intra- and extraluminal urethral masses.

Cystoscopy

This is a useful technique in the cat that can aid in diagnosing urethral masses, calculi, strictures, and tears. In the female (or male following perineal urethrostomy) biopsies can be taken using an endoscope with an instrument channel. Transurethral cystoscopy can be performed in the male cat using a flexible endoscope or prepubic percutaneous cystoscopy and urethroscopy. In cases with lower urinary tract disease, inflammation of the urethra and bladder wall can result in microtears of the mucosa and hemorrhage, which can obscure the examination. Cystoscopy is described in detail in Chapter 8.

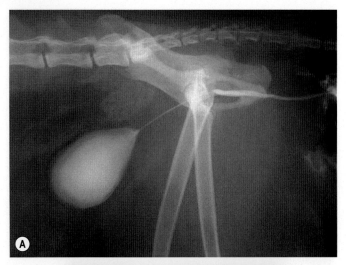

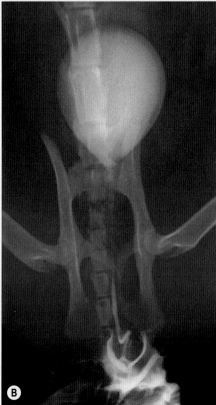

Figure 38-5 **(A)** Lateral and **(B)** ventrodorsal retrograde urethrogram of a male cat following relief of feline lower urinary tract disease (FLUTD) obstruction showing a gradual symmetrical narrowing of the pelvic urethra due to urethritis.

SURGICAL DISEASES

Most surgical diseases of the urethra in cats are related to feline lower urinary tract obstruction or trauma.

Feline lower urinary tract obstruction

Feline lower urinary tract disease (FLUTD) encompasses urethral plugs (20–50%), feline interstitial cystitis (20–50%), bacterial cystitis

(10–20%), and urolithiasis (10–20%).[8-11] Cats at most risk of FLUTD are kept indoors, male, overweight, and fed on dried diets.[12] Bacterial cystitis is more commonly seen in elderly cats with renal compromise which prevents concentration of the urine.[13] Clinical signs of FLUTD include inappropriate urination, stranguria, hematuria, dysuria, and pollakiuria progressing to include various systemic signs (pain, bradycardia, depression, and vomiting) with complete obstruction. Males have a much higher risk of blocking. The diagnostic approach depends on the frequency and severity of episodes but should include urine analysis and culture even on first presentation. Obstructed cats require serum biochemistry profiles with electrolytes to allow stabilization of cases with hyperkalemia or marked azotemia prior to sedation or anesthesia. Risk factors for mortality include hypocalcemia and hyperkalemia.[12]

Many cases of FLUTD can be treated medically without resorting to surgery; however, recurrence rates after an episode of urethral obstruction are in the range of 30–40%, with obstruction rates being higher for urethral plugs.[12] A 2002 multiple center study in North America reported a 70% reduction in perineal urethrostomy in a 20-year period from 1980–1999.[13] This decrease in surgical management of FLUTD may reflect an improvement in medical treatment of the condition. However, if a cat has regular recurrence of urethral obstruction despite appropriate medical management, a perineal obstruction should be considered. In certain cases (e.g., if the owner is regularly away overnight) surgery can be considered earlier.

In cats with urolithiasis it is preferable to retropulse calculi into the bladder and perform a cystotomy rather than operate on the urethra. If the calculus is firmly lodged, and a retrograde urethrogram confirms the obstruction, a temporary cystostomy tube can be placed to allow urinary diversion or repeat cystocentesis can be used. Retropulsion can be attempted again after a few days of treatment with anti-inflammatory medication and urethral relaxants. Alternatively, a perineal urethrostomy can be performed to relieve the obstruction once the cat is systemically stable.

In a study of 43 cats with urethral obstruction, 26% died or were euthanized because of their disease. Perineal urethrostomy was performed in 22% of cats and resulted in resolution of clinical signs in 50% of cases.[14] Cats that had a perineal urethrostomy were half as likely to be euthanized due to their disease although this was a relatively small study. It is important to counsel owners, however, that if surgery is performed for obstructive cases of FLUTD the disease will still be present and further medical treatment may be required although re-obstruction is less likely to occur.

Other complications reported following perineal urethrostomy include urinary tract infection, stricture formation, periurethral urine extravasation, and stoma dehiscence. The incidence of postoperative urinary tract infection is reported to be from 23–50%.[15-18] The range in results may be due to the fact that the infections are often asymptomatic and self-limiting, though in chronic cases struvite urolithiasis can result.[19]

Urethral trauma

Urethral trauma may occur after blunt or penetrating injuries but is most commonly seen in males after traumatic urethral catheterization in cases of obstructed FLUTD.[20,21] With iatrogenic catheter damage the frequent sites for damage are the distal penile urethra and the ischial arch. Damage at the level of the distal penile urethra (Fig. 38-6) is due to inadequate caudal straightening of the penile urethra prior to catheterization or an inadequately sedated or anesthetized cat. Damage at the ischial arch (Fig. 38-7) is likely due to a combination of the caudal traction on the penile urethra being maintained whilst the catheter is entering the postprostatic pelvic urethra and traumatic catheters, particularly those with a stylet still in place. With an obstructed cat

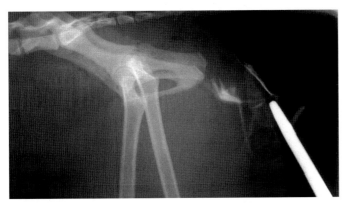

Figure 38-6 Retrograde urethrogram showing rupture of the distal penile urethra secondary to traumatic urethral catheterization in a four-year-old domestic short-haired cat with obstructive FLUTD.

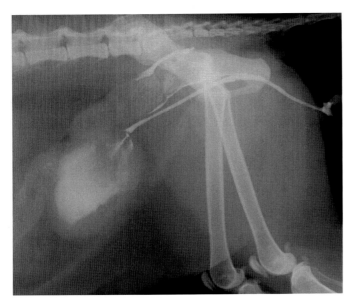

Figure 38-7 Retrograde urethrogram of a ruptured urethra at the ischial arch demonstrating perforation of the colon by the catheter and subsequent colonogram in a six-year-old domestic long-haired cat with obstructive FLUTD.

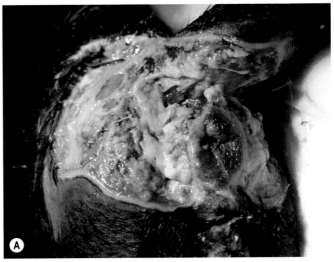

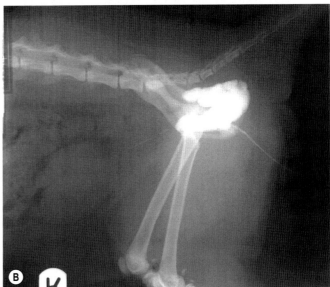

Figure 38-8 **(A)** Skin slough secondary to a caudal urethral rupture and extravasation of urine around the tail base in a 10-month-old domestic short-haired cat that had a road traffic accident. **(B)** Retrograde urethrogram demonstrating this urethral rupture, with the contrast spreading around the tail base.

hydropulsion via a urethral catheter rather than the catheter itself should be used to relieve the obstruction. Clinical signs of urethral rupture are listed in Box 38-1.

Cases of penile or postprostatic urethral rupture will often have urine leakage into the perineum and the dorsum around the tail base. If a fluctuant swelling is evident in these areas in a cat where there is a possibility of urethral rupture, the fluid should be drained with aspiration or placement of a small closed suction drain to prevent skin necrosis[22,23] (Fig. 38-8). If the urethral rupture is further proximal, the urine will leak into the abdomen, resulting in uroabdomen and a chemical peritonitis, which will be septic if there was a pre-existing urinary tract infection present.

The ability to urinate normally or pass a urinary catheter into the bladder does not exclude a urethral tear. Diagnosis is confirmed by imaging, including positive contrast urethrocystography. If contrast is seen both in the bladder and extravasating from the urethra a partial rupture is present. If no contrast agent is seen in the bladder the rupture can be partial or complete.[24] Ultrasound examination may be useful to determine disruption of the proximal urethra and bladder neck. Biochemical analysis of blood, including electrolytes, should be

---

Box 38-1 Clinical signs of urethral rupture

Dysuria or anuria

Hematuria

Perineal swelling and bruising

Skin necrosis, sloughing and cellulitis due to extravasation of urine in the subcutaneous tissue which is extremely irritating

Dehydration

Uremia

Depressed mentation

---

checked prior to sedation or anesthesia to rule out hyperkalemia, hyponatremia, hypochloremia, metabolic acidosis, or azotemia. If uroabdomen is present, abdominocentesis with biochemical analysis of the peritoneal fluid will support the diagnosis if the peritoneal creatinine, urea or potassium levels are higher than serum levels.[25]

Treatment options for urethral rupture include urinary diversion, primary repair, or proximal urethrostomy. Small lacerations will generally heal in three to five days with urinary diversion using an indwelling urethral catheter or cystostomy tube. Larger lacerations will heal if a strip of uroepithelium remains intact but strictures may result. In cases where catheterization is difficult, normograde placement of a catheter via a small cystostomy followed by placement of a guidewire aids retrograde placement of the urethral catheter.[24] An indwelling catheter is required for up to three weeks depending on the size of the tear.

The extent of damage may be difficult to assess by a retrograde urethrogram and surgical exploration of the urethra is sometimes advisable to gauge the size of the deficit, particularly if there is excessive contrast leakage on a urethrogram. In cases that have suffered a road traffic accident, the urethra can be damaged ventrally, presumably by crushing against the pubis. In these cases the urethral damage can be considerable and stricture is likely with conservative management.

Most lesions of the penile urethra in cats are treated by a perineal urethrostomy.[20] Complete transection of the more proximal urethra is treated by urethral resection and anastomosis, which carries the risk of stricture formation, or a prepubic urethrostomy if the damage is severe. A vaginourethoplasty has recently been reported in a female cat after primary repair of a pelvic urethra rupture resulted in a stricture.[26] Prognosis is worse for cats with multiple traumatic injuries.[20] Complications which may occur after urethral rupture include strictures, incontinence, and urethrocutaneous fistulas.

Urethral tumors

Urethral tumors are rare and more commonly seen in males than females. Affected cats tend to present later in life than those affected with FLUTD and often have a lean body condition. Presenting clinical signs include dysuria, hematuria, inappetence, constipation, and weight loss. Cases reported in the literature include a transitional cell carcinoma of the preprostatic urethra and a cat with leiomyoma.[27,28] Prostatic tumors (usually carcinomas) are rare in the cat but can cause extramural obstruction.[29] Urethral tumors generally carry a poor prognosis and due to their rarity effectiveness of treatment protocols is difficult to assess. Chemotherapeutic protocols including piroxicam, doxorubicin, and cyclophosphamide have been reported for urethral transitional cell carcinomas,[30] but the few cases reported have had poor survival times. A case report of surgical excision of a transitional cell carcinoma followed by radiotherapy on recurrence had a survival time of over a year.[27] Self-expanding metallic stents have been used in cases of urethral carcinoma but the survival times have been disappointing due to tumor occlusion of the stents.[31,32]

Urethrorectal fistulas

Urethrorectal fistulas are rarely reported, usually congenital and may be associated with atresia ani (see Chapter 30).[33] Clinical signs include simultaneous urination from the urethra and anus, dribbling of feces from the vagina, and recurrent urinary tract infection. Traumatic urethrorectal and vaginorectal fistulas can occur after trauma, including urethral catheterization. Diagnosis is made via a positive contrast retrograde urethrogram.

Treatment is by identification and ligation of the fistula followed by removal of the tract. If possible, the tract should be visualized and catheterized to aid dissection. If perforation of the rectum occurs during urethral catheterization, conservative treatment with an indwelling urethral catheter and antibiotic cover can be a successful management regime.

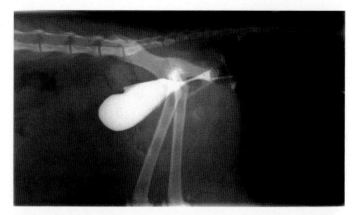

Figure 38-9 Hypoplastic urethra in a four-month-old British short-hair kitten with vaginal aplasia and entry of the uterine horns into the dorsal bladder wall.

Hypoplastic urethra

Hypoplastic urethra is seen in female cats that usually have a history of incontinence from birth. Diagnosis is by retrograde urethrogram; the urethra is exceptionally short, with the bladder neck seeming to extend to the external urethral meatus (Fig. 38-9). Most reported cases also have vaginal aplasia, with termination of the uterine horns in the dorsal bladder wall.[34]

Treatment consists of elongating the urethra using a cystoplasty, formed by making two V-shaped flaps in the ventral aspect of the bladder, with the point of the V at the caudal extent of an incision in the proximal urethra. The two flaps are sutured together, forming a pouch whilst the remaining ventral bladder wall is closed to make a tube. In this manner the bladder neck is tubed into a pseudo urethra. The bladder flaps are created to preserve bladder volume and are optional, as bladder volume will return to a normal value in three to four months following partial cystectomy. Any uterine remnants and ovaries should be resected during the surgery to avoid bladder diverticuli.

In a case series of eight cats with urethral hypoplasia that were treated surgically, clinical signs resolved in three cats and improved in the remaining five cats.[35] Medical treatment in the form of phenylpropanolamine has not been evaluated in cats.

PREOPERATIVE CONSIDERATIONS AND PREPARATION FOR SURGERY

Systemic effects

In cats with obstructive disease, possible urine leakage or chronic disease, routine hematology and biochemistry blood profiles should be performed to rule out azotemia, electrolyte abnormalities, dehydration, or anemia which requires correction prior to general anesthesia (see Chapter 1). Urinary diversion may be required to allow stabilization, which depending on the status of the patient, may consist of cystocentesis, cystostomy tube (see Chapter 37), or urethral catheterization.

Healing

Superficial mucosal defects heal rapidly in about seven days with an initial urothelial proliferation during the lag phase, although the deeper layers and corpus spongiosum can take three to five weeks to

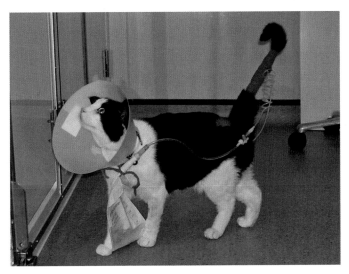

Figure 38-10 A urethral catheter is maintained comfortably in this cat with a urethral rupture with the use of a spiral extension set attached to the tail.

regenerate.[36] Continuous exposure of the wound to urine slows healing and results in fibrosis and contracture leading to stricture formation. If the urethra is more severely damaged, regeneration is possible providing a strip of urothelium one-third of the diameter remains.[36] In cases with complete urethral transection, the severed mucosa retracts due to muscular contraction of the edges, and periurethral tissues can cover the urothelium, resulting in fibrous tissue and strictures.[37] To prevent stricture, urinary diversion should be used, either in the form of a urethral catheter or a cystostomy tube. The catheter can be maintained up to three weeks if required. Polyvinyl or silicon catheters are preferred to polypropylene catheters, which have been shown to cause a microscopically detectable urethritis, which may be severe.[38] Both cystostomy and urethral catheters should be connected to closed collection urine systems to avoid nosocomial infections. In the rare cat that does not tolerate a closed collection system the catheters can be bunged and emptied every four to six hours via the bung, using an aseptic technique. The manipulation of the perineal area this requires is often resented more than the closed collection urine bag. An alternative is to attach the urethral catheter to a curly giving set (Fig. 38-10). This is then wrapped around the tail before being connected to the urine collection bag, which prevents any pressure being applied to the perineum on movement. After primary repair or resection and anastomosis, a positive contrast urethrogram at seven days is indicated to evaluate the integrity of the repair.

Handling and suture material

The urothelium is delicate and tissue handling should be gentle, with the use of stay sutures where possible for manipulation and non-traumatic DeBakey forceps. The urethra bleeds readily, though this can usually be controlled with gentle pressure from swabs and cold saline.

Due to the rapidity of healing of the mucosa it is only necessary to use a monofilament suture material that retains tensile strength for two to three weeks. This is preferable so rapid resorption of the suture material occurs and avoids the suture material forming a calculytic nidus. Suitable suture materials include polydiaxanone, glycomer 631, polyglycolic acid, polyglyconate and poliglecaprone (for smaller defects). A suitable sized suture for most urethral surgery is 1.0–1.5 M.

Antibiotics

Another consideration prior to surgery is the presence of urinary tract infection (UTI). Urine samples (preferably obtained via cystocentesis) should be submitted for routine analysis and culture prior to any elective surgery and any infection pretreated with an appropriate antibiotic for two to four weeks. To ensure the UTI has resolved, a cystocentesis culture should be repeated a week after antibiotic treatment has finished. Often urethral surgery is not elective. If the urine has not been cultured prior to surgery a sample should be obtained and submitted at surgery to determine if postoperative antibiotics are required. Urethral surgery is considered 'clean-contaminated' so perioperative antibiotics are indicated. The antibiotic chosen should be effective against the usual feline UTIs, which are often fecal contaminants, such as *Escherichia coli*, *Streptococcus* spp., *Staphylococcus* spp. and *Enterobacter faecalis*. First-line antibiotics that are often recommended include amoxicillin and trimethoprim/sulfonamide.

In cases of urinary diversion with a cystostomy or urethral catheter, the cat should not be placed on antibiotics whilst the catheter is in situ (unless there is a separate nidus of infection or risk of sepsis) and the tip of the catheter should be cultured after removal. At this stage any UTI can be treated appropriately without the risk of favoring resistant microbes.

SURGICAL TECHNIQUES

The most frequently performed urethral surgery is the perineal urethrostomy. Other urethral surgical procedures, including more proximal urethrostomies, resection anastomosis, and primary repair, are performed less frequently.

In cats, the preferred place for a urethrostomy is at the perineum, which involves suturing the wider postprostatic pelvic urethra to the skin or preputial mucosa. Prepubic (also sometimes termed antepubic), transpubic or subpubic urethrostomy are salvage procedures.

Perineal urethrostomy

Perineal urethrostomy is performed for rare cases of FLUTD in which the obstructed calculi cannot be moved or in recurrent severe cases of obstructive FLUTD that have had appropriate medical treatment. Other indications for perineal urethrostomy include stricture or trauma of the penile urethra (often post catheterization) or, uncommonly, for neoplasia in this region. As cats with LUTD may have trauma after repeated catheterization it is advisable to perform a retrograde urethrogram and ensure the lesion is caudal to the bulbourethral glands prior to surgery. The rationale of the surgery is to remove the narrow penile urethra and create a stoma in the wider postprostatic/pelvic urethra.

In the modified perineal urethrostomy the urethral mucosa is sutured to the preputial mucosa. This technique was first described by Christensen in 1964[39] and more recently modified slightly by Yeh & Chin in 2000.[40] In the author's experience, it results in less postoperative discomfort and a better cosmetic appearance (Fig. 38-11). This technique may also decrease UTIs as the mucosal barrier is preserved. As the anastomosis site is within the subcutaneous tissue, any self-traumatization of the wound is not as damaging as with the traditional technique and thus the cats can be safely discharged once they are urinating well. The traditional technique was described by Wilson & Harris in 1971[41] and it differs in that the urethral mucosa is sutured directly to the skin (Box 38-2).

Postoperative care includes the use of shredded paper rather than cat litter and a buster collar that should be left in place until the stoma

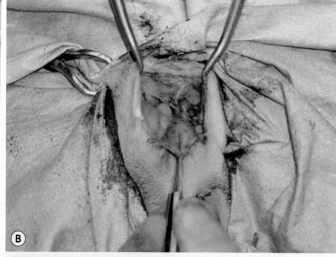

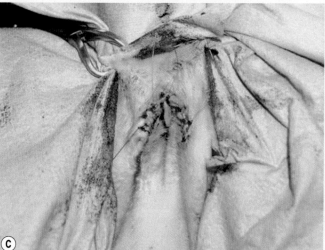

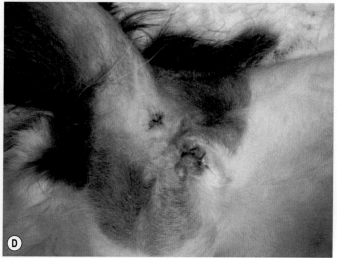

Figure 38-11 Modified perineal urethrostomy in a six-year-male neutered domestic short-haired cat. **(A)** Prepuce inverted after removal of penile urethra. **(B)** Preputial mucosa anastomosed to pelvic urethra. **(C)** Immediate postoperative appearance of modified perineal urethrostomy. **(D)** Four months post modified perineal urethrostomy surgery

---

Box 38-2 **Perineal urethrostomy**

The cat is positioned in sternal recumbency with the hind limbs extended over the edge of the table and the tail tied over the body. The perineum and caudal proximal hind limbs are clipped and aseptically prepared. A purse-string suture is placed in the anus, carefully avoiding the anal sacs. A urinary catheter is placed if possible to aid manipulation of the penis.

Modified technique using preputial mucosa[39,40]

A triangular-shaped section of skin is removed from between the anus and prepuce (if the cat is entire a castration is performed at this stage) (Fig. 38-12A). Identify the penis and dissect it free from the connective tissue. Carefully separate the preputial mucosa from the penis at the fornix using iris scissors or a number 11 blade (Fig. 38-12B). The fornix is identified by placing a hemostat into the prepuce. Pull the penis out of the prepuce leaving a tube of preputial mucosa (Fig. 38-12C).

Reflect the penis dorsolaterally and dissect the subcutaneous tissue ventrally and laterally, towards the ischial arch. Sever the ventral penile ligament. Transect the ischiocavernosus muscles and ischiourethralis

muscles (these can be ligated or transected by using electrosurgery). Transect the muscles near the ischium to avoid damaging the branches of the pudendal nerves and to decrease hemorrhage.

So to avoid damaging these structures dissection in this area should be maintained close to the urethra.

Expose the bulbourethral glands (paired pea-like structures on the dorsal aspect of the urethra) proximal and cranial to the severed muscles. Elevate and remove the retractor penis muscle to the level of the bulbourethral glands. Make a longitudinal incision into the urethra using a number 11 blade, which is aided by the placement of a urethral catheter, and extend the incision with scissors to the bulbourethral glands. Curve the incision around the ventral wall of the urethra and resect the distal half of the penile urethra. The diameter of the urethra at this point should be such that the boxlock of a pair of Kelly hemostat forceps can pass through.

Incise the ventral wall of the preputial tube in order to spatulate the mucosa (Fig. 38-12D). Suture the dorsal aspect of the preputial mucosa to the dorsal edge of the incised penile urethral mucosa and

Box 38-2 **Continued**

anastomose the preputial mucosa to the pelvic urethra using 4/0 or 1.5 M monofilament suture material (Fig. 38-12E). Use simple interrupted sutures or two simple continuous sutures. Close the subcutaneous tissues routinely and place skin sutures or an intradermal suture to close the wound (Fig. 38-12F).

Traditional Wilson and Harris technique[41]

Make an elliptical incision around the scrotum, prepuce and penis, leaving at least 1 cm of skin between the anus and the proximal extent of the incision. Follow the above technique to dissect the urethra to the level of the bulbourethral glands.

Make a longitudinal incision into the urethra using a number 11 blade, which is aided by the placement of a urethral catheter, and extend the incision with iris scissors. Extend the incision to approximately 1 cm beyond the bulbourethral glands. The diameter of the urethra at this point should be such that the boxlock of a pair of Kelly hemostat forceps will pass through (Fig. 38-13).

Suture the urethral mucosa to skin with 4/0 1.5 M monofilament suture; these can be simple interrupted or simple continuous sutures. Place the most proximal sutures first at a 45° angle. Suture the proximal two-thirds of the urethra to the skin and resect the distal third (Fig. 38-14).

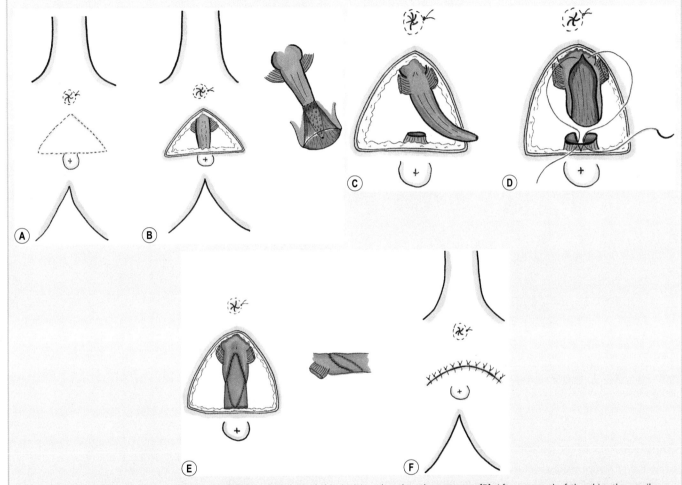

Figure 38-12 Modified perineal urethrostomy. **(A)** Crescent-shaped skin incision dorsal to the prepuce. **(B)** After removal of the skin, the penile urethra is revealed by blunt dissection through the fat and gently elevated to invert the prepuce. **(C)** Dissection of the penile urethra from the prepuce, leaving a tube of preputial mucosa. **(D)** Resection of the distal penile urethra and spatulation of the dorsal aspect of the urethra to the level of the bulbourethral glands and of the ventral aspect of the preputial tube in order to increase the diameter of the anastomosis. **(E)** Urethropreputial anastomosis that will be positioned in the subcutaneous tissue. **(F)** Postoperative appearance.

has healed. Non-absorbable sutures should be removed around 14 days postoperatively; this usually requires sedation.

A urethral catheter should be avoided as it may result in more stricture formation.

In the case of the modified perineal urethrostomy, the long-term cosmetic result is similar to a normal cat (Fig. 38-11C). The owner should be advised that all future veterinary surgeons should be informed that the cat has had surgery (give the owner discharge instructions with the technique clearly described) to avoid the unfortunate scenario of a veterinary surgeon attempting to prolapse the penis after this surgery.

If a UTI has been diagnosed, appropriate antibiotics should be used for two to four weeks post surgery. A cystocentesis culture is indicated a week after finishing the antibiotics to ensure the infection has resolved.

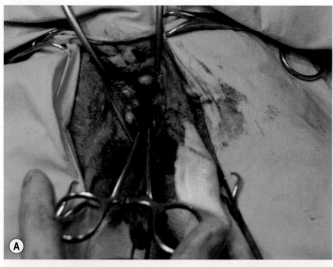

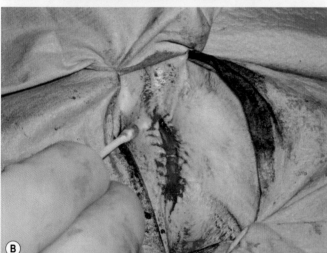

Figure 38-13 Traditional perineal urethrostomy. **(A)** Urethra at the resection site proximal to the level of the bulbourethral glands; it should be possible to gently insert the boxlock of a small pair of hemostats. **(B)** Immediate postoperative appearance after traditional perineal urethrostomy.

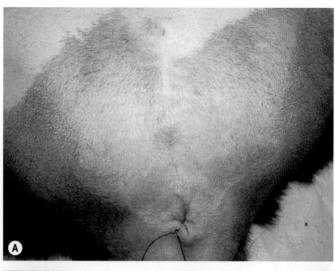

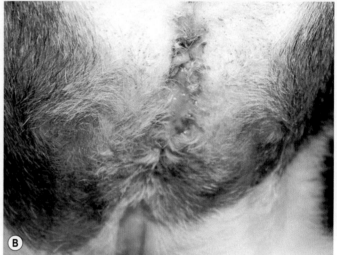

Figure 38-14 **(A)** Stricture six months after a traditional perineal urethrostomy in a six-year-old domestic short-haired cat. **(B)** Two days after revision of the perineal urethrostomy; sufficient urethra was available to create a washboard.

Complications after perineal urethrostomy

A number of complications are reported post perineal urethrostomy and these should be discussed with the owner prior to surgery.

Urinary tract infection

A number of factors may contribute to an increased incidence of UTI post perineal urethrostomy. The anatomical alteration of the urethral meatus decreases the distance between the anus and the urethral stoma and compromises the urethral mucosal barrier. The underlying uropathy present may also increase the risk of infection. Many cats have reduced striated urethral sphincter function post surgery, which decreases urethral closure pressures, although this can be temporary.[16] This decrease in urethral pressure occurs whether minimal sharp or extensive blunt ventral pelvic dissection is used,[42] reinforcing the importance of avoiding trauma dorsal to the urethra during the surgery.[43] In cats that maintained low urethral pressures post surgery, the infection rate was over 50% compared to less than 20% in cats where the urethral pressures returned to the normal ranges.[44] There is generally about a 25–50% incidence of UTI after traditional perineal urethrostomy.[12,14,45]

Stricture formation

This usually results from the stoma being positioned in the proximal penile rather than distal postprostatic pelvic urethra; this is due to inadequate mobilization of the penile urethra, often with failure to transect the ischiocavernosus and ischiourethralis muscles. Other causes of stricture include: tension on the mucosa and skin; postoperative subcutaneous urine leakage and subsequent granulation tissue formation; traumatization of the stoma; and the use of indwelling urethral catheters post surgery.[46]

In cases of stricture formation, the perineal urethrostomy should be revised (Fig. 38-14). An elliptical incision is used to remove the strictured stoma and the urethra is further mobilized by careful dissection, which is primarily ventral. The dorsal urethra is then incised in order to create a new stoma. The surgeon should be prepared to perform a transpubic/subpubic urethrostomy if required, though revision surgeries are usually successful.[47]

Postoperative urine leakage

Postoperative urine leakage into the subcutaneous tissue can result from poor skin–mucosal apposition, excessive tension at the surgical site due to inadequate ventral dissection, or pre-existing mucosal damage. Clinical signs include severe bruising and sensitivity of the perineal area and hind limbs and marked pain during and after urination. The urine extravasation can result in excessive granulation tissue at the stoma site with risk of stricture, or in severe cases, dehiscence of the stoma and sloughing of the surrounding skin. In severe cases urinary diversion with a cystostomy tube may be warranted whilst the stoma heals. In cases where inadequate dissection was performed in the first surgery, the perineal urethrostomy should be revised.

The author has seen two cats with damaged, friable urethral tissue develop urine leakage in the subcutaneous tissue after modified perineal urethrostomy. This urine leakage resolved after an indwelling Foley urethral catheter was used for three days and no further complications were reported.

Hemorrhage

Hemorrhage during the surgery results from sectioning of the ischiocavernosus muscles or when the cavernosus tissue is cut on the incision into the urethra. This can usually be controlled with pressure and abates as the mucosa is sutured. Postoperative hemorrhage is usually mild unless there is traumatization of the wound. Any clots that appear to occlude the stoma should be gently removed under sedation.

Urinary incontinence

Urinary incontinence is occasionally seen postoperatively but is usually temporary.[16] This may be due to excessive dorsal dissection of the pelvic plexus and pudendal nerve during the surgery or due to bladder damage during an obstructive episode. Rectal prolapse, perineal hernia, and urethrorectal fistulas are rarely reported complications.[15,48]

Although the list of potential complications following perineal urethrostomies is extensive, the majority of cats have a good quality of life postoperatively and owners who are satisfied with the technique.[18,21] If performed by a competent surgeon the incidence of complications is generally low.

Prepubic urethrostomy

The prepubic urethrostomy is a salvage procedure used mainly in cats after urethral trauma/stricture or failed perineal urethrostomy (Fig. 38-15). In the prepubic urethrostomy (Box 38-3) the urethra is exposed through the abdominal wall cranial to the pubis. It is important to ensure that the urethra is not kinked or twisted during the surgery and to maintain as much urethral length as possible to avoid incontinence.

The improved continence seen when longer lengths of urethra are retained has led to the subpubic/transpubic modification of the prepubic urethrostomy, where the urethral stoma is positioned at the level of the postprostatic pelvic urethra, either by removing a section of the ischial bone or performing a pubic osteotomy.

Results after prepubic urethrostomy are unpredictable with a number of complications seen, including urinary incontinence, subcutaneous leakage of urine, stricture of the urethrostomy, recurrent UTIs, and urine-scald dermatitis. In two case series of 32 and 16 cats that underwent prepubic urethrostomy, around one-third underwent euthanasia due to urinary incontinence or stomal complications[49,50] and owner satisfaction in the remaining cats was not high.

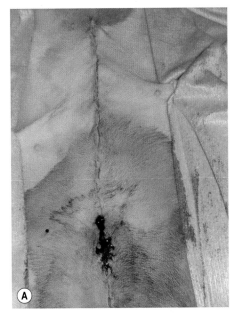

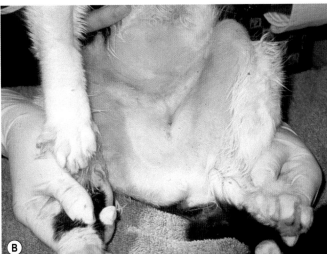

Figure 38-15 (A) Immediate postoperative appearance of prepubic urethrostomy in a six-year-old male neutered cat. **(B)** Two months postoperative appearance.

Transpelvic urethrostomy

The transpelvic urethrostomy uses the postprostatic pelvic urethra, which is exteriorized caudally after removing a section of the ischial bone (Box 38-4).[51]

In a series of 19 male cats that underwent transpelvic urethrostomy there was one case of temporary urinary incontinence and one case of stricture although the presence of UTI was not assessed for all cases and three cats had peristomal or leg urine staining.[51]

The subpubic urethrostomy was devised as a solution for a failed perineal urethrostomy and designed so that the urethrostomy is sufficiently caudal to avoid the inguinal fat pads and the increased length avoids incontinence. In this technique, the postprostatic urethra is visualized by a pubic osteotomy and after transection cranial to the stricture, tunneled into a subpubic subcutaneous position where the

The cat is placed in dorsal recumbency and clipped and aseptically prepared for a caudal celiotomy.

A ventral celiotomy is made from the umbilicus to the pubis. Using blunt dissection the urethra is mobilized (using as little dissection as possible) as far as the pelvic canal. The most distal part of the healthy urethra is ligated and the urethra transected just cranial to the ligature. A urinary catheter is placed. The urethra is exteriorized through the caudal celiotomy incision using stay sutures or umbilical tape for manipulation, ensuring the urethra is not kinked as it passes through the linea alba.

A partial thickness suture is placed through the urethra as it exits the linea alba. This is to secure the urethra in place and protect the urethral stoma.

The celiotomy is closed routinely (see Chapter 25). The end of the urethra is spatulated prior to suturing to increase the diameter of the stoma (Fig. 38-16). The urethral mucosa is sutured to the skin with 1.5–1 M monofilament suture material using either a simple interrupted or simple continuous suture pattern. The subcutaneous tissue and skin is closed in a routine manner.

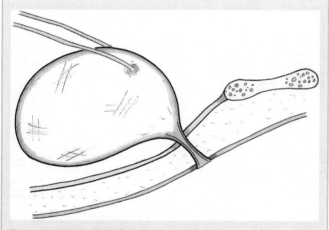

Figure 38-16 Diagram of a prepubic urethrostomy.

The cat is placed in dorsal recumbency. The ventral abdomen and pelvis is clipped from the umbilicus to the perineum and aseptically prepared.

An elliptical incision is made around the scrotum and prepuce and continued up to the cranial border of the pubis. If the cat is an entire male a routine castration should be performed at this stage.

The penis is undermined ventrally and the caudal and ventral pubis exposed by blunt dissection.

The adductor, gracilis and external obturator muscles are elevated bilaterally to expose a 1.2–1.5 cm by 1.4–1.6 cm section of the ventral pubis. This section of the pubis is removed with rongeurs to expose the postprostatic urethra.

The urethra is transected at the level of the bulbourethral glands and a urinary catheter placed (this can be placed at the start of the procedure if preferred via a cystostomy). The ventral wall of the urethra is incised to create a urethrotomy which is 10–12 mm long and the urethral mucosa everted and sutured to the skin to create a new stoma. The skin incision around the stoma site is closed routinely.

The cat is positioned in dorsal recumbency and a midline celiotomy performed.

Intrapelvic damage requires either a pubic symphysiotomy or bilateral pubic and ischial osteotomies, which create a pubic flap, that is replaced after the repair. Pubic symphysiotomy usually provides adequate exposure (2–3 cm) with the use of self-retaining retractors such as pediatric Finochietto rib retractors or Gelpi retractors and is a simple procedure with low morbidity (Fig. 38-17).

After exposure of the damaged urethra, the urethral ends require identification. In cases with marked trauma where this may be difficult, normograde catheterization from the bladder can be useful after a limited cystostomy. The urethral ends should be debrided for at least 1–2 mm to expose the mucosa but debridement may need to be more extensive and should continue until the tissue appears viable. Incising the urethral ends at an angle increases the diameter of the anastomosis. The urethra is repaired using simple interrupted or continuous monofilament full thickness sutures over a urethral catheter, being careful to appose mucosa to mucosa. It is important to avoid tension on the anastomosis and thus the urethra should be mobilized if necessary. If there is concern about the repair, a supporting muscle flap such as the internal obturator or rectus abdominis can be used to augment the repair.

A urethral catheter or cystostomy tube should be used for urinary diversion for five to seven days postoperatively after resection anastomosis to decrease stricture formation.[53]

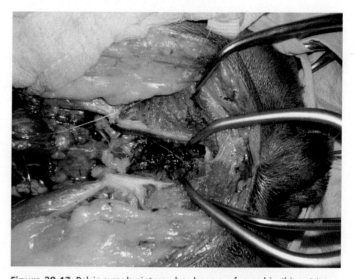

Figure 38-17 Pelvic symphysiotomy has been performed in this cat to allow access to the pelvic urethra.

stoma is made. The pubic flap is then repositioned. This technique was reported with success in a case report.[52]

Urethral resection/anastomosis

Urethral resection and anastomosis (Box 38-5) is indicated for cases of trauma, stricture, and rarely for neoplasia.

In a canine study, there were no significant differences in urethral healing after urethral resection and anastomosis whether urine diversion was performed via a urethrostomy catheter, cystostomy catheter, or both.[54] In a rat study, however, prepubic catheterization markedly decreased the inflammation following urethral injury.[55] After removal

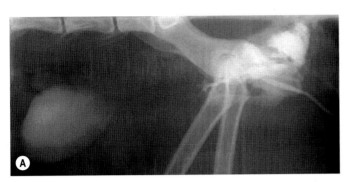
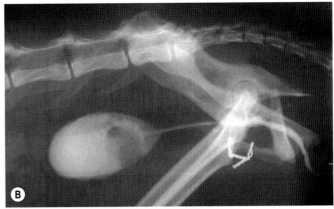

Figure 38-18 (A) Ruptured postprostatic pelvic urethra in a four-year-old male (neutered) domestic short-haired cat following a road traffic accident. **(B)** Six week postoperative check after primary repair. *(Courtesy of Sue Gregory.)*

of the catheter, the tip should be submitted for bacterial culture and any UTIs treated according to the results.

Primary repair

Primary repair of the urethra (Fig. 38-18) is possible in some cases of urethral rupture or partial rupture though it is challenging due to the small size of the feline urethra, and its benefit over alignment and secondary healing with a urethral catheter is uncertain.[24] Urinary diversion should be used after primary repair for five to 21 days depending on the extent of the defect and the quality of the repair.[20] Repeat positive contrast urethrography can be used at weekly intervals to assess the integrity of the repair. The most serious complication that is seen after primary repair is stricture formation. Strictures will cause clinical signs in dogs once they occlude over 60% of the urethral lumen.[55] Due to the decreased luminal wall ratio in the cat, dysuria is likely to be seen with less severe strictures. Fascia lata autografts have been used successfully experimentally in dogs to repair urethral defects[56] and in human surgery acellular matrix and buccal and bladder mucosal grafts are used. There are no reports of grafts being used in the cat.

Urethral stents

Urethral stents have been used in cases of neoplastic obstruction and inflammatory stricture.[30,31,55] The stents used were self-expandable or balloon-expandable nitinol or platinol stents. In the case reports of neoplastic obstruction (urothelial carcinoma) the stents were palliative with one and two month survival times, respectively.[30,31] In the inflammatory case report the stricture was situated in the postprostatic pelvic urethra and responded well to placement of a 5 mm nitinol stent under fluoroscopic guidance with a seven month follow up.[57] Complications seen in dogs after stent placement include luminal re-stenosis by epithelial hyperplasia, re-obstruction due to mucosal swelling or blood clots, and urinary incontinence.[58,59] There is little information on urethral stents in cats.

POSTOPERATIVE CARE

Postoperative urination often causes discomfort due to the exposure of tissues to acidic urine and analgesia, usually in the form of opiates, can ease this pain. Epidural injections of local anesthetics plus or minus preservative-free morphine can also produce excellent

analgesia for many of the techniques described. Diuresis is advisable to flush the urinary tract and dilute macroscopic hemorrhage. Urination should be carefully monitored and any dysuria and stranguria noted. If a urinary catheter is in place it should be emptied using an aseptic technique and the volume of urine recorded. It is preferable not to give antibiotics whilst a urinary catheter is in place as this may encourage bacterial resistance. Instead, the end of the catheter should be cultured after removal and an appropriate course of antibiotics prescribed depending on the culture results. As a common complication with urethral catheters and cystostomy catheters is accidental dislodgement, the catheters should be securely attached to the cat and a buster collar used if necessary.

After perineal, transpubic, and prepubic urethrostomies, shredded paper should be used in the litter tray rather than cat litter and a buster collar should be used until the stoma has healed. The stoma should be inspected daily and any blood clots that could cause obstruction gently dislodged with a moist sterile cotton bud.

COMPLICATIONS AND PROGNOSIS

Complications which may occur after urethral surgery include urine leakage from the surgical site, strictures, incontinence, infection, and urethrocutaneous fistulas.

Postoperative urine leakage into the subcutaneous tissue or abdomen can result from poor skin–mucosal or mucosal–mucosal apposition, excessive tension at the surgical site, or pre-existing mucosal damage. Clinical signs may include severe bruising and sensitivity of the perineal area and hind limbs, marked pain during and after urination, or development of a uroabdomen. The urine extravasation can result in excessive granulation tissue at a stoma site with risk of stricture or, in severe cases, dehiscence of the stoma and sloughing of the surrounding skin. In severe cases, urinary diversion with a cystostomy tube may be warranted whilst the stoma heals. Stricture formation results from excessive tension on an anastomosis, pre-existing mucosal damage, failure to appose mucosa to mucosa, or poor surgical technique. Chronic strictures which cause obstruction may require revision or stenting.

Urinary incontinence occurs from excessive dorsal dissection around the urethra or too short a length of urethra being retained. Most cases due to dissection are temporary and resolve within a matter of days. The incidence of UTI after urethral surgery in cats is unclear as many cats are asymptomatic whilst others have recurrent episodes of FLUTD which may mask a UTI. In male cats, decreasing the length of the urethra and creating proximal stomas will compromise the urethral defense mechanisms and is likely to result in an increased incidence of UTIs. It is sensible to routinely monitor cats that have undergone urethrostomy and submit urine cultures yearly even if asymptomatic.

The most commonly performed urethral surgery is the perineal urethrostomy. Though a number of complications are reported following this surgery, the majority of cats have a good quality of life postoperatively and owners that are satisfied with the technique's result.[21,24]

REFERENCES

1. Cullen WC, Fletcher TF, Bradley WF. Morphometry of the female feline urethra. J Urol 1983;129:190–2.
2. Cullen WC, Fletcher TF, Bradley WF. Morphometry of the male feline pelvic urethra. J Urol 1983;129:186–9.
3. Wang B, Bhadra N, Grill WM. Functional anatomy of the male feline urethra: morphological and physiological correlations. J Urol 1999;161:654–9.
4. Herron MA. The effect of prepubertal castration on the penile urethra of the cat. J Am Vet Med Assoc 1972;160:208–11.
5. Sackman JE, Sims MH. Use of fine-wire electrodes for electromyographic evaluation of the external urethral sphincter during urethral pressure profilometry in male cats. Am J Vet Res 1991;52:314–16.
6. Gregory CR, Willits NH. Electromyographic and urethral pressure evaluations: assessment of urethral function in female and ovariohysterectomized female cats. Am J Vet Res 1986;47:1472–5.
7. Johnston GR, Feeney DA, Osborne CA. Urethrography and cystography in cats. Part 1. Techniques, normal radiographic anatomy, and artefacts. Compend Contin Educ Pract Vet 1982;4:823–35.
8. Saevic BK, Trangerud C, Ottesen N, et al. Causes of lower urinary tract disease in Norwegian cats. J Feline Med Surg 2011;13:410–17.
9. Kruger JM, Osborne CA, Goyal SM, et al. Clinical evaluation of cats with lower urinary tract disease. J Am Vet Med Assoc 1991;199:211–16.
10. Gerber B, Boretti FS, Kley S, et al. Evaluation of clinical signs and causes of lower urinary tract disease in European cats. J Small Anim Pract 2005;46:571–7.
11. Eggertsdottir AV, Lund HS, Krontveit R, Sørum H. Bacteriuria in cats with feline lower urinary tract disease: a clinical study of 134 cases in Norway. J Feline Med Surg 2007;9:458–65.
12. Segev G, Livne H, Ranen E, Lavy E. Urethral obstruction in cats: predisposing factors, clinical, clinicopathological characteristics and prognosis. J Feline Med Surg 2011;13:101–8.
13. Lekcharoensuk C, Osborne CA, Lulich JP. Evaluation of trends in frequency of urethrostomy for treatment of urethral obstruction in cats. J Am Vet Med Assoc 2002;221(4):502–5.

14. Gerber B, Eichenberger S, Reusch CE. Guarded long-term prognosis in male cats with urethral obstruction. J Feline Med Surg 2008;10:16–23.
15. Gregory CR, Vasseur PB. Long term examination of cats with perineal urethrostomy. Vet Surg 1983;12:210–12.
16. Gregory CR, Holliday TA, Vasseur PB, et al. Electromyographic and urethral pressure profilometry: Assessment of urethral function before and after perineal urethrostomy in cats. Am J Vet Res 1984;45:2062–5.
17. Osborne CA, Caywood DD, Johnston GR, et al. Perineal urethrostomy versus dietary management in prevention of recurrent lower urinary tract disease. J Small Anim Pract 1991;32:296–305.
18. Bass M, Howard J, Gerber B, Messmer M. Retrospective study of indications for and outcome of perineal urethrostomy in cats. J Small Anim Pract 2005;46:227–31.
19. Osborne CA, Caywood DD, Johnston GR, et al. Feline perineal urethrostomy: a potential cause of feline lower urinary tract disease. Vet Clin North Am Small Anim Pract 1996;26:535–49.
20. Anderson RB, Aronson LR, Drobatz KJ, Atilla A. Prognostic factors for successful outcome following urethral rupture in dogs and cats. J Am Anim Hosp Assoc 2006;42:136–46.
21. Corgozinho KB, de Souza HJ, Pereira AN, et al. Catheter-induced urethral trauma in cats with urethral obstruction. J Feline Med Surg 2007;9:481–6.
22. Holt PE. Hindlimb skin loss associated with urethral rupture in two cats. J Small Anim Pract 1989;30:406–9.
23. Clarke BS, Findji L. Bilateral caudal superficial epigastric skin flap and perineal urethrostomy for wound reconstruction secondary to traumatic urethral rupture in a cat. Vet Comp Orthop Traumatol 2011;24:142–5.
24. Meige F, Sarrau S, Autefage A. Management of traumatic urethral rupture in 11 cats using primary alignment with a urethral catheter. Veterinary Comparative Orthopaedics and Traumatology 2008;21:76–84.
25. Aumann M, Worth LT, Drobatz KJ. Uroperitoneum in cats: 26 cases (1986–1995). J Am Anim Hosp Assoc 1998;34:315–24.
26. Halfacree ZJ, Tivers MS, Brockman DJ. Vaginourethroplasty as a salvage

procedure for management of traumatic urethral rupture in a cat. J Feline Med Surg 2011;13:768–71.
27. Takagi S, Kadosawa T, Ishiguro T, et al. Urethral transitional cell carcinoma in a cat. J Small Anim Pract 2005;46:504–6.
28. Swalec KM, Smeak DD, Baker AL. Urethral leiomyoma in a cat. J Am Vet Med Assoc 1989;195(7):961–2.
29. Caney SMA, Holt PE, Day MJ, et al. Prostatic carcinoma in two cats. J Small Anim Pract 1998;39:140–3.
30. Wilson HM, Chun R, Larson VS, et al. Clinical signs, treatments, and outcome in cats with transitional cell carcinoma of the urinary bladder: 20 cases (1990–2004). J Am Vet Med Assoc 2007;231:101–6.
31. Newman RG, Mehler SJ, Kitchell BE, Beal MW. Use of a balloon-expandable metallic stent to relieve malignant urethral obstruction in a cat. J Am Vet Med Assoc 2009;234:236–9.
32. Christensen NI, Culvenor J, Langova V. Fluoroscopic stent placement for the relief of malignant urethral obstruction in a cat. Aust Vet J 2010;88:478–82.
33. Van den Broek AHM, Else RW, Hunter MS. Atresia ani and urethrorectal fistula in a kitten. J Small Anim Pract 1988;29:91–4.
34. Holt PE, Gibbs C. Congenital urinary incontinence in cats: a review of 19 cases. Vet Rec 1992;130:437–42.
35. Holt PE. Surgical management of congenital urethral sphincter mechanism incompetence in eight female cats and a bitch. Vet Surg 1993;22:98–104.
36. McRoberts JW, Ragde H. The severed canine posterior urethra: a study of two distinct methods of repair. J Urol 1970;104:724–9.
37. Weaver RG, Schulte JW. Experimental and clinical studies of urethral regeneration. Surg Gynecol Obstet 1962;115:729–36.
38. Lees GE, Osborne CA, Stevens JB, Ward GE. Adverse effects caused by polypropylene and polyvinyl feline urinary catheters. Am J Vet Res 1980;41(11):1836–40.
39. Christensen NR. Preputial urethrostomy in the male cat. J Am Vet Med Assoc 1964;145:903–8.
40. Yeh LH, Chin SC. Modified perineal urethrostomy using preputial mucosa in cats. J Am Vet Med Assoc 2000;216(7):1092–5.

41. Wilson GP, Harrison JW. Perineal urethrostomy in cats. J Am Vet Med Assoc 1971;159:1789–93.

42. Sackman JE, Sims MH, Krahwinkel DJ. Urodynamic evaluation of lower urinary tract function in cats after perineal urethrostomy with minimal and extensive dissection. Vet Surg 1991;20:55–60.

43. Gregory CR, Vasseur PB. Electromyographic and urethral pressure profilometry: long-term assessment of urethral function after perineal urethrostomy in cats. Am J Vet Res 1984;45:1318–21.

44. Griffon DW, Gregory CR, Kitchell RL. Preservation of striated-muscle urethral sphincter function with use of a surgical technique for perineal urethrostomy in cats. J Am Vet Med Assoc 1989;194(8):1057–60.

45. Griffon DW, Gregory CR. Prevalence of bacterial urinary tract infection after perineal urethrostomy in cats. J Am Vet Med Assoc 1992;200:681–4.

46. Smith CW, Schiller AG, Smith AR, et al. Effects of indwelling urinary catheters in male cats. J Am Anim Hosp 1981;17:427–33.

47. Phillips H, Holt DE. Surgical revision of the urethal stoma following perineal urethrostomy in 11 cats (1998–2004). J Am Anim Hosp Assoc 2006;42:218–22.

48. Welches CS, Scavelli TD, Aronsohn MG, Matthiesen DT. Perineal hernia in the cat: a retrospective study of 40 cases. J Am Anim Hosp Assoc 1992;28:431–8.

49. Mendham JH. A description and evaluation of antepubic urethrostomy in the male cat. J Small Anim Pract 1970;11:709–21.

50. Baines SJ, Rennie S, White RS. Prepubic urethrostomy: A long-term study in 16 cats. Vet Surg 2001;30:107–14.

51. Bernarde A, Viguier E. Transpelvic urethrostomy in 11 cats using an ischial ostectomy. Vet Surg. 2004;33:246–52.

52. Ellison GW, Lewis DBF. Subpubic urethrostomy to salvage a failed perineal urethrostomy in a cat. Comp Cont Educ Pract Vet 1989;11:946–51.

53. Layton CE, Ferguson HR, Cook JE, Guffy MM. Intrapelvic urethral anastomosis. A comparison of three techniques. Vet Surg 1987;16:175–82.

54. Cooley AJ, Waldron DR, Smith MM, et al. The effects of indwelling transurethral catheterization and tube cystostomy on urethral anastomoses in dogs. J Am Anim Hosp Assoc 1999;35:341–7.

55. Singh M, Blandy JP. The pathology of urethral stricture. J Urol 1976;115:673–6.

56. Atalan G, Cihan M, Sozmen M, Ozaydin I. Repair of urethral defects using fascia lata autografts in dogs. Vet Surg 2005;34:514–18.

57. Choi R, Lee S, Hyun C. Urethral stenting in a cat with refractory obstructive feline lower urinary tract disease. J Vet Med Sci 2009;71(9):1255–9.

58. Weisse C, Berent A, Todd K, et al. Evaluation of palliative stenting for management of malignant urethral obstructions in dogs. J Am Vet Med Assoc 2006;229:226–34.

59. Latal D, Mraz J, Zerhau P, et al. Nitinol urethral stents: long-term results in dogs. Urol Res 1994;22:295–300.

Chapter |39|

Male genital tract

E.J. Friend

Conditions of the male feline genital tract are rare, but include crypt-orchidism and neoplasia of the testicles, intersex abnormalities of the penis, and rare reports of neoplasia of the testes. Urethral conditions by contrast are very common in the cat and these are covered in detail in Chapter 38.

SURGICAL ANATOMY

The male genital tract of the cat is comprised of similar components to the canine genital tract,[1] but with some specific differences. The scrotum is covered with hair and situated just ventral to the anus, and the penis is directed caudally and the preputial orifice is positioned more dorsally than it is in the dog. The prepuce is comparatively short, and with a narrow preputial orifice that makes extrusion of the penis very difficult in the conscious cat.

The urethral orifice is small and present on the tapered tip of the glans. It can become obscured in some clinical situations that cause inflammation (such as obstructive disorders associated with feline lower urinary tract disease). The entire adult cat has numerous short horny spines on the glans part of the penis that are often noted but have no clinical significance (Fig. 39-1).

The vas deferens from each testis courses caudally and ventrally after leaving the scrotum and enters the abdominal cavity via the inguinal ring on the ipsilateral side. Once inside the abdomen, the vas loops around and enters the urethra in the region of the prostate.

In the cat, there is a short length (3–5 cm) of preprostatic urethra.[2] The prostatic urethra is 1.5–1.9 cm in length; the postprostatic urethra in the region of the caudal pubis is the widest (and longest) part of the feline male urethra.

As it passes further caudally and courses over the end of the pubis, the urethra bends ventrally, before leveling off at the tip of the penis. This bend means that catheterization is best performed while pulling the penis gently caudally and dorsally, which tends to straighten the urethra. The distal urethra is the narrowest part and is therefore a common site for obstruction.

The preprostatic urethral wall contains three layers of smooth muscle, which gradually disappear in the prostatic urethra to be replaced further caudally by increasing amounts of striated muscle.[2] This has significance when pharmacologic control of urethral relaxation is required. There is a delicate urethral mucosa (with transitional cell epithelium) that is more easily traumatized than in the dog because of the narrow urethral lumen.

The bulbourethral glands are paired, pea-size pale yellow glands situated dorsolateral to the postprostatic urethra (Fig. 39-2). Paired ischiocavernosus/ischiourethralis muscles are present just distal to these glands and are highly vascular. Running along the dorsal surface of the penis at this level is the retractor penis muscle (Fig. 39-3), which is sometimes firmly attached to the penis, and on the ventral surface there is the ventral penile ligament (Fig. 39-4).

GENERAL CONSIDERATIONS

Clinical signs of genital tract disorders in the male cat commonly include dysuria and/or hematuria, or they are related to testosterone and include inappropriate urination and malodorous urine. Investigations include taking a complete history from the owner; a thorough

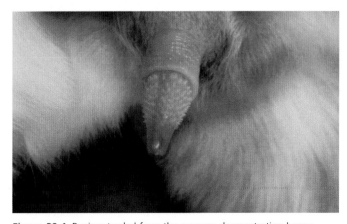

Figure 39-1 Penis extruded from the prepuce demonstrating horny spines of the intact male cat.

© 2014 Elsevier Ltd
DOI: 10.1016/B978-0-7020-4336-9.00039-1

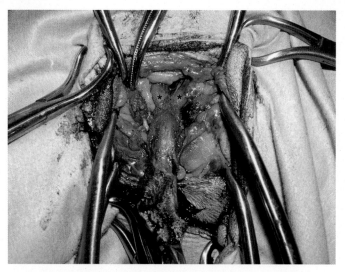

Figure 39-2 Dissection of the urethra during perineal urethrostomy. The paired bulbourethral glands are visible just proximal to the incised ischiocavernosus muscles.

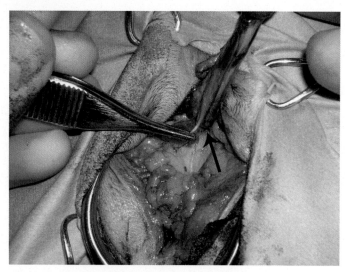

Figure 39-4 Penis reflected dorsally to expose the ventral penile ligament (arrow).

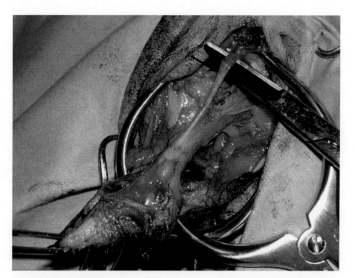

Figure 39-3 Retractor penis muscle identified (arrow) during perineal urethrostomy dissection.

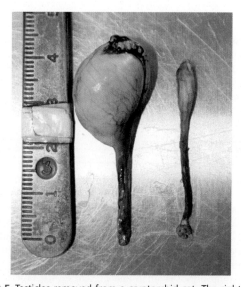

Figure 39-5 Testicles removed from a cryptorchid cat. The right testicle in the picture was inguinal; it is small and poorly developed. If there is any doubt it should be submitted for histopathologic evaluation for definitive confirmation that it is a testicle. *(Courtesy of Jon Hall.)*

physical examination; hormone assay after gonadotrophin stimulation; and diagnostic imaging (in particular abdominal ultrasound and contrast urethrography). A diagnosis should ideally be made before exploratory surgery.

SURGICAL DISORDERS OF THE SCROTUM AND TESTIS

Congenital disorders of the scrotum and testis are uncommon, and if present are often associated with disorders of other parts of the urogenital tract. Aplasia of the testes has been described,[3] along with other anomalies such as a urethral-scrotal fistula[4] and non-fused scrotal pouches.[5] Monorchism occurred in 0.1% of cats presenting for routine neutering in one case series.[6] Acquired conditions of the testis are uncommon in clinical practice because most cats are castrated at a young age. There are a few reports of neoplasia in the literature.[7-9]

Cryptorchidism

This is the most common congenital disorder, that accounted for 1.7% of male cats presenting for neutering in one case series,[5] and 1.3% of cats in another.[6] The testicle may be located anywhere along its embryonic pathway, from the region of the kidney to the internal inguinal ring (abdominal) or from the external inguinal ring to the base of the scrotum (inguinal). If both testes are affected, one study suggested an abdominal location was more likely,[5] but an inguinal location would appear to be more common overall.[6]

Clinical signs may be related to ongoing hormonal influence from the testicle (mainly inappropriate urination and malodorous urine), but may be related to neoplastic transformation.[3] Diagnosis is usually by history taking and physical examination. Identifying the location, however, can be difficult. In some cases, the testicle can be easily palpated in the inguinal area in the anesthetized cat.

If the individual has a large inguinal fat reserve, however, this can be difficult, especially as the testicle is sometimes small and poorly developed (Fig. 39-5).[11]

Further diagnostic tests can be performed, but represent something of a dilemma, as an experienced surgeon is usually able to locate the retained testis using good surgical principles alone. Ultrasound examination by an experienced operator, both of the abdomen and the inguinal area, may be helpful to locate the testicle. Testosterone assay following stimulation by human chorionic gonadotrophin (hCG) may be useful in some cases to confirm the presence of testicular tissue; reference ranges are not applicable as there is so much variation over time and between individuals, but generally a two- to fourfold increase post-stimulation is expected if active testicular tissue is present. The presence of spines on the glans penis is often highly suggestive of the presence of active testicular tissue.

Neoplasia

Neoplasia of the testis is rare in the cat and there are few examples in the literature. Tumor types reported include interstitial cell tumor,[7] Sertoli cell tumor[8] and teratoma,[9] although it would be reasonable to assume that malignant transformation of any cell type present in the testis could occur. Two of the reports are of neoplasia occurring in retained testicles, which may suggest this predisposes to malignancy, as it does in the dog. Thorough evaluation of the patient should be made when a testicular tumor is suspected, with staging of the tumor being of paramount importance. Left and right lateral chest radiographs should be taken, and abdominal ultrasound used to examine the sublumbar lymph nodes, liver, and spleen. The surgery required for most histological types is simple castration (i.e., excisional biopsy) although removing the scrotal skin is recommended if the testicle is adherent to the overlying tissue. It is impossible to assess prognosis given the few cases reported.

SURGICAL DISORDERS OF THE PENIS AND PREPUCE

Congenital conditions of the penis and prepuce are occasionally seen in the cat. There are reports in the literature of hypospadias,[12] phimosis,[13] and intersex disorders.[5]

Hypospadia is a failure of embryonic fusion of the embryonic folds, leaving a defect in the ventral tissue of the penis and urethra; it has been reported as a cause of chronic cystitis in a pure breed cat.[12] Phimosis is the inability to extrude the penis beyond the preputial orifice, and has been reported as a congenital defect causing hematuria and pollakiuria in a domestic short-hair cat;[13] stranguria and pollakiuria were reported as the most common clinical signs in a series of ten cats with phimosis. Clinical signs resolved when surgery was performed to widen the preputial orifice.[14] Intersex diseases have also been uncommonly reported: in one case a pure breed cat showing no clinical signs had a genital cleft rather than a true prepuce or vulva, with a large clitoris with horny spines similar to those on a normal penis. There were no chromosomal abnormalities found and so a diagnosis of pseudohermaphroditism was made.[4] In any congenital disease of the urogenital tract, surgical intervention is indicated only if functional disease results, such as dysuria or predisposition to urinary tract infections. The extent of the disease often means that surgical intervention is difficult and may not bring much benefit for the animal.

Balanoposthitis was reported in an entire male cat that presented with incontinence and preputial swelling; postmortem examination revealed the presence of chronic pyelonephritis and prostatitis.[15]

Acquired diseases of the penis are uncommon, and more often relate to diseases of the urethra rather than being specific to the penis (see Chapter 38). Management is mainly aimed at maintaining or restoring urethral function to allow urination. Preputial skin can develop neoplasms of the same type as any area of skin.

SURGICAL DISORDERS OF THE PROSTATE

Diseases of the accessory sex glands are very rarely seen, probably due to routine early castration in this species. There are several single case reports of prostatic diseases. Neoplastic transformation of a retained testis led to prostatic squamous metaplasia and prostatitis in one reported case, causing signs of obstructive dysuria.[7] An entire cat with chronic prostatitis presented with urinary incontinence and a palpable caudal abdominal mass in another case report.[15] The author has heard of an anecdotal report of prostatitis in a middle-aged pure breed stud cat, which responded to prolonged antibiotic therapy and orchiectomy. A prostatic abscess has been described in a neutered six-year-old cat that presented with vomiting and constipation which resolved with surgical drainage and omentalization.[16] A five-year-old Ragdoll cat was affected with a prostatic cyst. The cat presented with a history of frequent urination, cystitis, and a large caudal abdominal fluid-filled mass. A retrograde urethrogram demonstrated a small communication of the urethra with a cyst at the colliculus seminalis. Exploratory surgery found the cyst to be prostatic in origin and it was resected. The urethral communication at the colliculus seminalis was oversewn and the cat made a full recovery with only temporary incontinence in the immediate postoperative period (Fig. 39-6).

There are occasional reports in the literature of primary neoplasia of the prostate gland in the cat, again causing clinical signs of obstructive dysuria and hematuria.[17-18] Prostatectomy and prepubic urethrostomy has been successfully performed in one cat for a primary prostatic tumor.[19] The outcome was poor in all the other cases, suggesting the prognosis may be the same as it is in the dog.[19]

SURGICAL TECHNIQUES

The commonest surgical procedure performed on the male genital tract is castration, which is often an elective procedure in a healthy

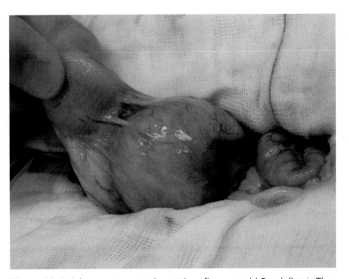

Figure 39-6 A large paraprostatic cyst in a five-year-old Ragdoll cat. The bladder is on the left in the surgeon's fingers. *(Courtesy of Davina Anderson.)*

animal. Surgery procedures for penile problems are covered in Chapter 38.

Castration

Population control is an obvious reason for neutering, but many owners elect to have their cats castrated in order to avoid the undesirable characteristics of fighting, roaming, and urine malodor/spraying. Behavioral modification after castration is reliable and swift in cats, with an 80% decrease in fighting, roaming, and urine spraying within three weeks.[20] It may also reduce the likelihood of acquiring feline immunodeficiency virus (FIV).

Castration (Box 39-1) is usually performed before the onset of sexual maturity, at approximately 6 months of age. There seems to be no adverse effect on general development, with the possible exception of delayed closure of growth plates. In a series of non-traumatic femoral capital physeal fractures in adult cats, 14 of 16 cats had been neutered at less than 6 months of age.[10] Looking at the whole population, however, castration probably prevents more diseases than it causes, as well as improving welfare by population control.

Box 39-1 **Castration**

The cat is anesthetized and placed in right lateral recumbency (for right-handed surgeons). The scrotum is clipped or plucked to remove hair and aseptically prepared. Surgical drapes are not required. The right testicle may be preferable to remove first, so if there is hemorrhage it does not interfere with visualization of the left. The testicle is tensed up against the scrotal skin, which is incised dorsoventrally with a number 15 scalpel blade (Fig. 39-7A).

The skin is thin and there is minimal subcutaneous tissue. The testicle can then be exteriorized by further gentle squeezing of the scrotum (Fig. 39-7B).

An 'open' technique is used by most, and so the scalpel is used to gently incise (also dorsoventrally) through the vaginal tunic (Fig. 39-7C). The vaginal tunic has been incised to the left of the picture and the testicle is being extruded.

Care is taken not to incise the tunica albuginea, the tough covering of the testicle itself, as minor hemorrhage results. The ligament of the tail of the epididymis should then be separated by tearing it from the overlying tunica (Fig. 39-7D). The vas and vascular supply are seen to the left of the figure.

The epididymis, vas deferens (right of picture) and testicular vascular supply (left of picture) can now be seen (Fig. 39-7E).

Three different techniques can now be used to ligate the blood vessels:

i. The vas and blood vessels can be ligated either all together or separately, preferably using synthetic multifilament absorbable suture material

ii. The vas deferens can be separated from the testicle, usually at the level of the tail of the epididymis (Fig. 39-7F). A square knot can then be tied between the vas deferens and the vascular supply (still attached to the testicle) (Fig. 39-7G)

iii. A knot can be created using forceps. The combined vascular supply and vas deferens is looped around a pair of curved mosquito forceps (Fig. 39-7H). The tips of the forceps are then turned to point distally, and the vascular supply/vas is grasped in the tips of the forceps next to the testicle (Fig. 39-7I,J). The testicle is removed, and the knot lying over the forceps is pushed proximally up the vascular supply/vas (Fig 39-6K) until it is separate from the forceps (Fig. 39-7L)

The knot is then allowed to retract back into the scrotum.

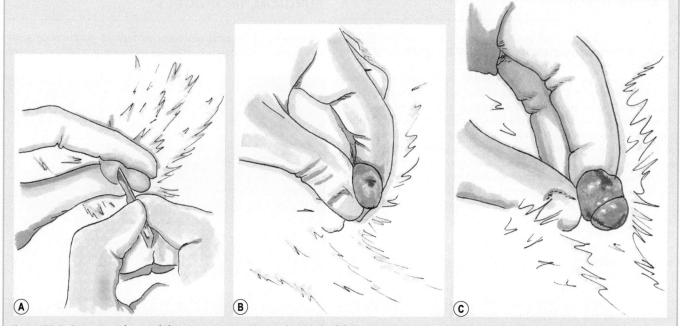

Figure 39-7 Castration of a cat. **(A)** Incise scrotum with a scalpel blade. **(B)** The testicle is exteriorized by squeezing scrotum. **(C)** Vaginal tunic carefully excised and testicle extruded.

Box 39-1 **Continued**

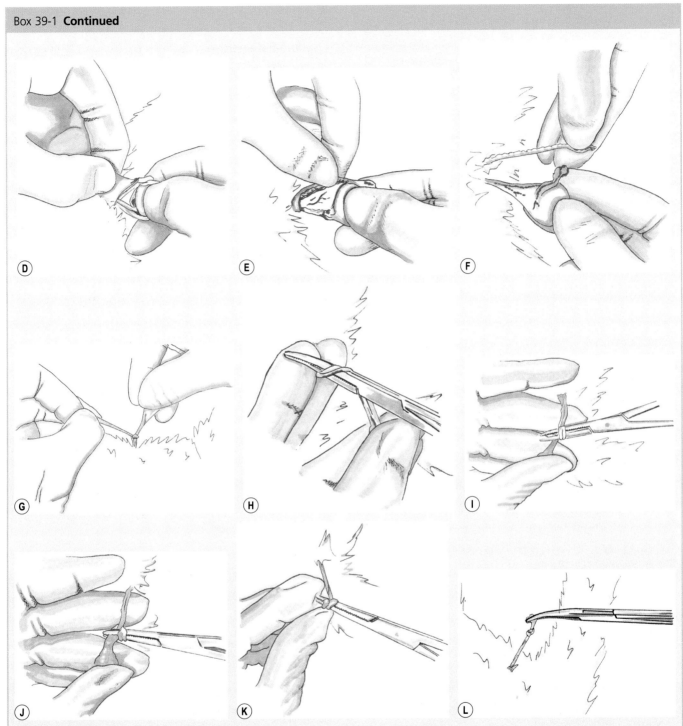

Figure 39-7, Continued (D) The ligament of the tail of epididymis separated from tunic. **(E)** The epididymis, vas deferens (right of picture) and testicular vascular supply (left of picture) can now be seen. **(F)** The vas deferens can be separated from the testicle, usually at the level of the tail of the epididymis. **(G)** A square knot can then be tied between the vas deferens and the vascular supply (still attached to the testicle), **(H)** or a knot can be created using forceps. The combined vascular supply and vas deferens is looped around a pair of curved mosquito forceps. **(I)** The tips of the forceps are then turned to point distally (towards the testicle). **(J)** The vascular supply/vas is grasped in the tips of the forceps next to the testicle. **(K)** The testicle is removed, and the knot lying over the forceps is pushed proximally up the vascular supply/vas. **(L)** The knot is separated from the forceps and allowed to retract back into the scrotum.

Box 39-2 **Surgical technique for cryptorchidism**

The animal is placed in dorsal recumbency and the ventral abdomen is clipped and prepared for aseptic surgery from the xiphisternum to the prepuce.

Inguinal testicle

If the testicle can be palpated in the inguinal area, or it has been found to be inguinal on ultrasound examination, a parasagittal incision can be made over the ipsilateral inguinum. It is worth noting that in cases of unilateral cryptorchidism, it is not always possible to decide whether the descended testicle is on the left or right side. In these cases, a longer midline skin incision can be made and the wound retracted to examine first one side and then the other (Fig. 39-8). Blunt dissection through the commonly large inguinal fat pad is used to identify the testicle; gentle surgical technique is recommended as wound complications such as seroma are common. Care should be taken to avoid traumatizing the large caudal superficial epigastric artery and vein that emerge through the inguinal ring and head cranially. If the testicle cannot be found, the external inguinal ring should be identified and the vas deferens followed as it emerges from the ring. Once the testicle is identified, the vas and testicular vessels can be ligated with 3/0 absorbable multifilament suture material (such as polyglactin 910) and removed. Dead space should be minimized and the skin closed routinely.

Abdominal testicle

If the testicle cannot be palpated in the inguinum, or ultrasound demonstrates the testicle is intra-abdominal, a caudal exploratory celiotomy should be performed. Abdominally retained testicles can also be removed using minimally invasive surgical techniques,[11,21] but the principles of finding the testicle remain the same. If a celiotomy is performed, a single stay suture of 3/0 monofilament suture (e.g., polypropylene) should be placed in the cranial pole of the bladder and the bladder should be retracted cranially. Cotton-tipped swabs can be used to carefully dissect any fat away from the ventral and lateral bladder neck, if required. As the bladder is retracted ventrally and cranially, the vasa can be identified as they enter the region of the prostate (Fig. 39-9). These can then be followed to where they originate from the testicle(s). If the vas is found to leave the abdomen via the inguinal ring, the inguinum can be explored via an extension of the celiotomy skin incision or through a small separate inguinal incision (Fig. 39-10). Gentle traction on the intra-abdominal portion of the vas will help locate the testicle. Once found, the testicle can be removed as described earlier.

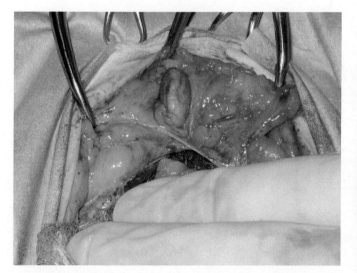

Figure 39-8 Cryptorchid cat. An inguinal testicle was identified through the midline approach. Note the extensive inguinal fat pad that makes palpating the testicle challenging.

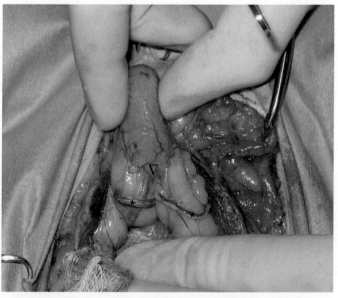

Figure 39-9 Both vasa deferens (*) can be found as they enter the urethra in the region of the prostate. Note the ureters as they enter the bladder in the region of the trigone (∇) and the large deposit of fat in the periurethral region.

If the testicle has not descended and the animal is cryptorchid then further investigations may be required and a thorough examination must be performed preoperatively. The surgeon should be prepared to do inguinal or abdominal surgery as necessary (Box 39-2).

COMPLICATIONS AND PROGNOSIS

Complications after castration are very rare, and are usually non-specific (anesthetic related, hemorrhage, infection). Hemorrhage is probably the most common complication and is most likely related to a loose ligature or knot in the tissues when performing castration, particularly when performed by inexperienced surgeons or on older cats. If hemorrhage does occur, most cases can be managed conservatively with direct pressure of the surgical site with cold compresses. Sedation is usually required to perform this. A clotting disorder should be considered, and laboratory tests for clotting function performed

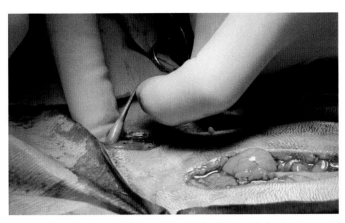

Figure 39-10 A cryptorchid cat with no palpable testicle in the inguinum. An abdominal approach was made and the vas deferens was traced back from the urethra into the inguinal canal. A very small inguinal testicle was then located through a separate inguinal incision (both testicles are shown in Fig. 39-5). *(Courtesy of Jon Hall.)*

where appropriate (see Chapter 3). If the hemorrhage persists, then surgical exploration of the site should be considered, the vessels should be clamped and ligated with absorbable suture material. Colonic obstruction was reported several weeks after castration in one cat, and was thought to be due to fibrosis around the vas deferens after it retracted into the abdomen post surgery. The area of scarring was successfully excised in this case.[22]

Anecdotally, cats appear to have a tendency to gain weight after castration, and this is consistent with experimental evidence. The weight gain after castration was associated with decreased energy expenditure in one preliminary study,[23] and with increased food intake in another.[24] Estradiol declines after castration and if it is then supplemented by injection, there is a reduction in the expected increase in food intake.[25]

REFERENCES

1. Ellenport CR. Urogenital system. In: Getty R, Editor. Sisson and Grossman's the anatomy of the domestic animals. 5th ed. Chapter 53, 1975. p. 1580–4.

2. Wang B, Bhadra N, Grill WM. Functional anatomy of the male feline urethra: morphological and physiological correlations. J Urol 1999;161:654–9.

3. Hakala JE. Reproductive tract anomalies in 2 male cats. Mod Vet Pract 1984;65:629.

4. Foster SE. Congenital urethral anomaly in a kitten. J Feline Med Surg 1999;1:61–4.

5. Bredal WP, Thoresen SI, Kvellestad A, Lindblad K. Male pseudohermaphroditism in a cat. J Small Anim Pract 1997;38:21–4.

6. Millis DL, Hauptman JG, Johnson CA. Cryptorchidism and monorchism in cats: 25 cases (1980–1989). J Am Vet Med Assoc 1992;200:1128–30.

7. Tucker AR, Smith JR. Prostatic squamous metaplasia in a cat with interstitial cell neoplasia in a retained testis. Vet Pathol 2008;45:905–9.

8. Miller MA, Hartnett SE, Ramos-Vara JA. Interstitial cell tumour and Sertoli cell tumour in the testis of a cat. Vet Pathol 2007;44:394–7.

9. Miyoshi N, Yasuda N, Kamimura Y, et al. Teratoma in a feline unilateral cryptorchid testis. Vet Pathol 2001;38:729–30.

10. McNicholas WT. Spontaneous femoral capital physeal fractures in adult cats: 26 cases (1996–2001). J Am Vet Med Assoc 2002;221:1731–6.

11. Birchard SJ, Nappier M. Cryptorchidism. Compend Contin Educ Vet 2008;30:325–36.

12. King GJ, Johnson EH. Hypospadias in a Himalayan cat. J Small Anim Pract 2000;41:508–10.

13. Bright SR, Mellanby RJ. Congenital phimosis in a cat. J Feline Med Surg 2004;6:367–70.

14. May LR, Hauptman JG. Phimosis in cats: 10 cases (2000–2008). J Am Anim Hosp Assoc 2009;45:277–83.

15. Pointer E, Murray C. Chronic prostatitis, cystitis, pyelonephritis and balanoposthitis in a cat. J Am Anim Hosp Assoc 2011;47(4):258–61.

16. Mordecai A, Liptak JM, Hofstede T, et al. Prostatic abscess in a neutered cat. J Am Anim Hosp Assoc 2008;44:90–4.

17. Caney SM, Holt PE, Day MJ, et al. Prostatic carcinoma in two cats. J Small Animal Pract 1998;39:140–3.

18. Zambelli D, Cunto M, Raccagni R, et al. Successful surgical treatment of a prostatic biphasic tumour (sarcomatoid carcinoma) in a cat. J Feline Med Surg 2010;12(2):161–5.

19. Tursi M, Costa T, Valenza F, Aresu L. Adenocarcinoma of the disseminated prostate in a cat. J Feline Med Surg 2008;10:600–2.

20. Hart BL, Barrett RE. Effects of castration in fighting, roaming and urine spraying in adult male cats. J Am Vet Med Assoc 1963;163:290–2.

21. Vannozzi I, Benetti C, Rota A. Laparoscopic cryptorchidectomy in a cat. J Feline Med Surg 2002;4:201–3.

22. Demetriou JL, Welsh EM. Colonic obstruction in an adult cat following open castration. Vet Rec 2000;147:165–6.

23. Martin L, Siliart B, Dumon H, et al. Leptin, body fat content and energy expenditure in intact and gonadectomized adult cats: a preliminary study. J Anim Physiol Anim Nutr 2001;85:195–9.

24. Kanchuk ML, Backus RC, Calvert CC, et al. Weight gain in gonadectomized normal and lipoprotein lipase-deficient male domestic cats results from increased food intake and not decreased energy expenditure. J Nutr 2003;133:1866–74.

25. Backus R. Plasma oestrogen changes in adult male cats after orchiectomy, body-weight gain and low-dosage oestradiol administration. Brit J Nutr 2011;106(Suppl 1):S15–8.

Chapter |40|

Female genital tract

S.J. Langley-Hobbs

The most common surgical procedure performed on the female genital tract is ovariohysterectomy. The high prevalence of this surgery in some countries ensures a low number of unwanted pregnancies and diseases associated with the female reproductive tract such as pyometra and mammary gland neoplasia. In breeding queens and entire females conditions of the uterus such as uterine torsion and cesarean may require surgery.

SURGICAL ANATOMY

The female reproductive tract consists of the ovaries, oviducts, uterus, vagina, urogenital sinus, and vulva (Fig. 40-1). The ovaries lie caudal to the kidneys. They are small oval bodies about 1 cm in length.[1] The left ovary is usually more caudal than the right one, in keeping with the position of the kidneys. The ovaries are supported by a part of the broad ligament, the mesovarium. A narrow tube, the oviduct, with a funnel shape infundibulum, encircles the ovary. The oviduct ascends along the infundibular side of the ovary, bends over its cranial end and descends along the opposite side where at the caudal end of the ovary it joins the uterus. The ovary is held to the horn of the uterus by the proper ligament, a part of the broad ligament that extends cranially as the suspensory ligament to insert on the middle part of the last one or two ribs. The horn of the uterus is supported by a part of the broad ligament known as the mesometrium. There is also a round ligament, a thickening in the edge of a peritoneal fold, which derives from the broad ligament. The round ligament extends from the cranial end of the uterine horn and runs caudally to the internal inguinal ring. The right and left horns of the uterus join medially to form the body of the uterus. This lies ventral to the colon and rectum and dorsal to the bladder. It extends into the cranial end of the pelvis where it projects into the vagina forming a prominent papilla, the cervix.

The vagina extends dorsal to the pelvic symphysis to just cranial to the caudal border of the ischiatic symphysis where it receives the urethra from the urinary bladder. The remainder of the tube from this point caudally is the vestibule or urogenital sinus. It extends to the external opening, which lies just ventral to the anus. The external opening of the urogenital sinus forms the vulva.

The ovarian blood supply is from the ovarian artery, which branches directly off the aorta. The right ovarian vein drains into the caudal vena cava and the left ovarian vein drains into the left renal vein. The ovarian lymphatics drain into the lumbar lymph nodes. The uterus is supplied by anastomosing branches of the ovarian artery and the

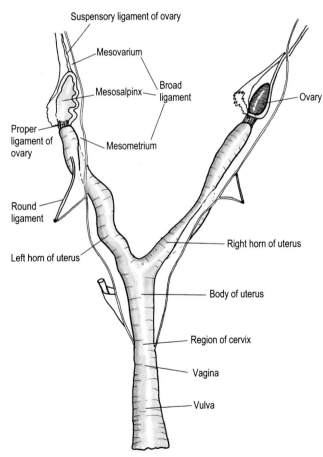

Figure 40-1 The feline reproductive tract. *(From Crouch JE. (1969) Text Atlas of Cat Anatomy. Philadelphia: Lea & Febiger.)*

DOI: 10.1016/B978-0-7020-4336-9.00040-8

uterine artery; the latter is a branch of the vaginal artery which arises from the internal pudendal artery. Uterine lymphatics drain to the hypogastric and lumbar lymph nodes. The blood supply to the vagina, urethra, and vestibule is provided by the vaginal artery, which arises from the internal pudendal artery. The vulval blood supply is provided by branches of the external pudendal artery. The lymphatics of the vagina and vestibule drain into the internal iliac lymph nodes and the vulval lymphatics drain to the superficial iliac lymph nodes.

REPRODUCTIVE CYCLE

Cats are a seasonal polyestrus species and induced ovulators. The average age of puberty is variable, but usually starts when the cat reaches 2.3–2.5 kg in weight and is between six and nine months of age.[2] Breeds like the Siamese or Burmese appear to be more precocious, reaching puberty at lower weights and younger ages than breeds like the Persian, which may not have their first estrous cycle until 18 months of age. However, the main influencing factor is day length: increasing hours of daylight usually stimulate estrous cycles. In the absence of pregnancy or false pregnancy cats will show repeated estrous cycles every two to three weeks throughout the spring, summer, and autumn.[2]

GENERAL CONSIDERATIONS

A full history should be taken with particular focus on neuter status, stage of cycling, hormonal treatment received, history of pregnancies and evidence of abnormal behavior.

The physical examination should look for signs of vulval abnormalities such as enlargement or discharge and abdominal palpation is performed for uterine enlargement. Mammary glands are examined for general enlargement or focal masses (see Chapter 21). Vaginal smear evaluation is less useful in queens for determining stage of estrus for breeding management, particularly as the act of carrying out the procedure can affect the cycle. Hematological and biochemical analysis of blood for evidence of sepsis or other systemic abnormalities with conditions such as pyometra is indicated and hormone levels are assayed in cases of retained ovarian remnant syndrome and potentially cystic ovaries.

Diagnostic imaging

Radiography is of fairly limited value for the female genital tract investigation, but it may show uterine enlargement. Occasionally, sutures at ovarian vessels or the uterine body may mineralize and therefore be radiopaque. Fetuses are visible between 36 and 45 days and a skull count will give the fetal number (Fig. 40-2).

Ultrasonography is of more use for investigation of organ size, tissue texture, and the presence of fluid. It can be used to investigate the ovaries and uterus for masses or fluid accumulation. It is also useful to confirm pregnancy, but is less helpful in differentiating between hydrometra, mucometra, pyometra, and hemometra.[3] Ultrasound analysis of uterine fluid is unreliable in determining cellular make up, and differentiation is best made on the basis of clinical signs, results of examination, and laboratory analyses.

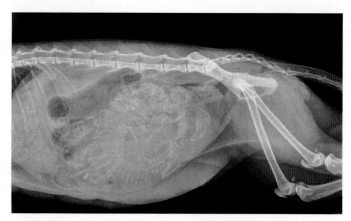

Figure 40-2 Two fetal feline skulls are visible on the abdominal radiograph of this pregnant cat, which therefore must be at least 36–45 days into gestation.

SURGICAL DISEASES OF THE OVARIES

Disease of the ovary is uncommon in the cat. Conditions include agenesis or hypoplasia, cysts, neoplasia, and retained ovarian remnants; the latter are likely to be due to surgical error. Some conditions are detected incidentally at laparotomy for ovariectomy or ovariohysterectomy.

Congenital ovarian abnormalities

Ovarian agenesis is rare and results in permanent anestrus and infertility. Small ovarian remnants containing fibrous tissue may be identified at laparotomy or laparoscopy.[4]

Ovarian hypoplasia has been reported in the queen[5] and phenotypically normal queens may have non-functional ovaries secondary to chromosomal abnormalities.[6]

Ovarian cysts

Ovarian cysts are common and their frequency increases with age.[6] There are two main types: follicular cysts that arise from mature or atretic follicles,[7] and other cysts not of ovarian origin. True follicular cysts are associated with hyperestrogenism if cells lining the cyst secrete estrogen[5] and may be associated with exaggerated sexual behavior and prolonged estrus. Administration of progestagen may inhibit the luteinizing hormone surge necessary to induce ovulation and may cause formation of follicular cysts.[7] Other cysts, not of ovarian origin, are remnants of mesonephric and rete tubules.[8] These cysts are endocrinologically inactive and do not produce clinical signs.

The cysts may be detected incidentally at ovariectomy (Fig. 40-3). In animals exhibiting hyperestrogenism, the diagnosis is made on the basis of clinical signs, measurement of plasma estrogen concentrations or demonstration of persistent cornification of vaginal epithelial cells.[8] Large cysts may be detected by ultrasound. Human chorionic gonadotrophin (hCG) may be administered to induce ovulation and thereby treat the cyst but in most cases ovariectomy or the use of progestagens to suppress the clinical signs is necessary.[8]

Ovarian tumors

Tumors of the ovary are classified on the basis of their cell of origin as epithelial, germ cell, or sex cord stromal and all types have been seen in the cat. The most frequent types seen in queens are granulosa

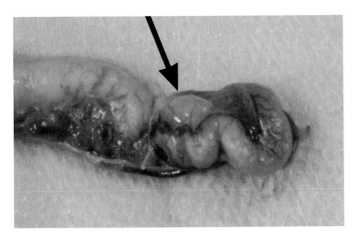

Figure 40-3 An ovarian follicle (arrow) identified as an incidental finding at ovariohysterectomy.

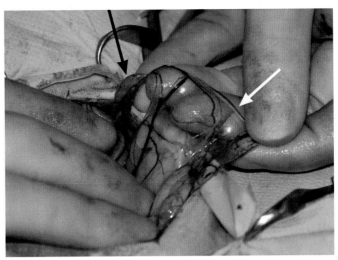

Figure 40-4 Unicornuate uterus in a stray female cat. An ovariohysterectomy performed through a flank incision had to be converted to a midline incision due to failure to locate the contralateral uterine horn. The ovary is arrowed (black) and there is a structure resembling a round ligament (white arrow) in the mesometrium but no uterine horn identifiable.

cell tumors, which can metastasise.[9] In the largest review of 22 ovarian tumors, a single cat had bilateral cystadenomas of epithelial origin, seven animals had dysgerminomas or teratomas that are germ cell tumors, and 14 animals had granulosa cell tumors and interstitial gland tumors, which are neoplasms of sex cord stromal origin.[9] Four of the cats with granulosa cell tumors had clinical evidence of hormonal disturbance. Cats may have signs of persistent estrus, cystic endometrial hyperplasia, and bilaterally symmetrical alopecia.[10]

Ovarian remnant syndrome

Onset of estrus (lordosis, rolling, posturing, excessive vocalization) after gonadectomy is a complication related to a retained ovarian remnant. It is more common after ovariohysterectomy than ovariectomy as the incision made for the former technique is more caudal and access to the ovaries is more difficult. One unproven theory is that there are accessory ovaries that may be small and located in the proper ligament of the ovary; once the normal ovary has been removed these accessory structures may become functional.[11] It is also possible for dropped ovarian tissue to become functional,[12] although all the cases reported in the literature have had residual ovarian tissue at one or both pedicles.[13] Ultrasound is useful for diagnosis and may reveal a cystic structure caudal to the kidney. The diagnosis is also supported by hormonal assays. In the queen, resting serum progesterone values are of little value unless the queen has been bred or induced to ovulate after showing signs of estrus.[14] An alternative method of diagnosis is to perform a hormonal stimulation test. In the queen during the breeding season cyclical activity occurs every two to three weeks, and at this time the queen can be readily stimulated to ovulate by the administration of exogenous gonadotrophin-releasing hormone (GnRH) or hCG. Elevated plasma progesterone concentrations one week after such treatment should confirm the presence of ovarian tissue.[15] At surgery, a thorough exploration of the peritoneal cavity is essential, checking the caudal poles of the kidneys, the omentum, and the peritoneal walls. The ovarian remnants are usually found adjacent to the previously ligated pedicle.[16]

SURGICAL DISEASES OF THE UTERUS

Congenital anomalies of the uterus

Suspected congenital anomalies of the uterus were identified in 0.09% (49/53 258) of female cats.[17] Uterine anomalies identified included

unicornuate uterus (33 cats) (Fig. 40-4), segmental agenesis of one uterine horn (15 cats), and uterine horn hypoplasia (one cat). These lesions are often only identified at exploratory laparotomy as they rarely cause clinical signs. Queens may still be fertile if the lesion is unilateral.

Ipsilateral renal agenesis was present in 29.4% (10/34) of the affected cats in which the kidneys were also evaluated. Identification of uterine developmental anomalies in dogs and cats should trigger evaluation of both kidneys and both ovaries because ipsilateral renal agenesis is common, but both ovaries are likely to be present and should be removed during ovariohysterectomy.

Uterine tumors

Most cats affected with uterine neoplasia are intact and are middle aged or older.[18]

Malignant endometrial adenocarcinoma is the most common endometrial uterine tumor; mixed Müllerian tumors (adenosarcoma) have also been reported.[18] Myometrial tumors include benign tumors such as leiomyomas and malignant leiomyosarcomas. Other more unusual uterine neoplasms or neoplastic-like lesions include lymphosarcoma, adenomyosis (refers to the presence of endometrium within the myometrium) and endometrial polyps.

Uterine neoplasia may be associated with infertility, pyometra, a persistent hemorrhagic vulvar discharge and straining, and abdominal or pelvic masses. Ovariohysterectomy (see Box 40-1) is the treatment of choice. Prognosis for endometrial adenocarcinoma is guarded. In one retrospective study 50% of adenocarcinomas had metastasized at presentation and only two out of the eight cats survived for longer than five months.[18]

Cystic endometrial hyperplasia and pyometra

Cystic endometrial hyperplasia and pyometra (CEH-P) complex is the most frequent and important endometrial disorder in cats and is a sequel to progesterone simulation of the endometrium, and ascending uterine infection by vaginal bacteria[19,20] or anogenital

Box 40-1 **Ovariohysterectomy**

Midline ovariohysterectomy

The cat is positioned in dorsal recumbency and hair is clipped from cranial to the xiphoid to caudal to the pubis between the nipples. The bladder should be expressed to make locating the uterus easier and to decrease the chance of iatrogenic bladder damage.

The distance between the umbilicus and the pubis is divided into three and a 2–2.5 cm midline incision through the skin and subcutaneous tissue is made in the middle third. In kittens less than 12 weeks of age the incision is situated more caudally, approximately two-thirds the distance from the umbilicus to the pubis.

The linea alba is tented with Adson rat-toothed forceps and a small incision made with a scalpel blade, which is extended cranially and caudally keeping to the midline. The uterus is found either by digital palpation of the dorsal abdominal wall or by reflecting the urinary bladder and locating the uterine horns and body, which lie dorsal to this. The uterus is gently exteriorized with fingers or an oophorectomy hook. One horn of the uterus is then followed cranially to locate the ovary. The suspensory ligament is broken down or stretched as necessary by blunt dissection or by tearing between thumb and first finger. A hole is made in the mesovarium and two hemostats are placed across the ovarian pedicle approximately 1 cm dorsal to the ovary (Fig. 40-5A). Alternatively, a three-hemostat technique can be used, with the most proximal ligature placed in the crush of the most proximal clamp (furthest from the ovary) but this is not usually necessary in cats. A ligature of 1.5–2M absorbable suture material (polyglactin 910 or polysorb) is placed proximal to the hemostats (or in the crush if using a third hemostat) across the ovarian artery and vein (Fig. 40-5A). One or two encircling ligatures are placed; two may be preferable in an older, larger cat or one in estrus. The ovarian pedicle is divided between the hemostats by cutting with a scalpel or twisting and pulling on the distal hemostat (the one closest to the ovary). The ovary is exteriorized and the ovarian pedicle gently released and checked for bleeding. It is important that the ovarian stump is checked for bleeding after tension has been released as tension on ovarian vessels will often prevent hemorrhage, and ligatures that appear tight while the stump is under tension may slip after tension is released. The procedure is repeated for the opposite ovary.

The broad ligaments and round ligaments are bluntly dissected and separated to exteriorize the uterine horns. Two hemostats are placed across the uterine horns at the level of or just proximal to the cervix. Alternatively, a three-hemostat technique can be used (Fig. 40-5B) with the most proximal ligature placed in the crush of the most distal clamp (closest to the cervix). Clamps may cut rather than crush a friable or engorged uterus and cause transection before ligature placement so ligatures can be placed directly without the use of clamps if preferred.

One or two ligatures are placed encircling the whole uterine body, just proximal to the cervix. Alternatively, one encircling and one transfixing ligature can be used;[69] use of a transfixing ligature (Fig. 40-5C) is particularly recommended in larger cats or in a cat with a very vascular uterus. The uterus is transected between the hemostats by use of a scalpel. The uterus and ovaries are now free and can be laid aside after opening the ovarian bursa and checking the entire ovary has been removed. The uterine body is carefully released and checked for hemorrhage. The abdomen is examined for bleeding prior to closure. The ventral linea alba is closed using an absorbable suture material of 2M gauge (polydioxanone, polyglactin 910, polysorb, maxon or poliglecaprone) in a simple continuous pattern. The subcutaneous tissue may be closed with a simple continuous suture of absorbable suture material such as 2M poliglecaprone or caprosyn and the skin with 2M nylon simple interrupted sutures or an intradermal suture.

Alternatively, an ultrasonic scalpel, vascular sealer, or hemostatic clips or staples can be used for vessel ligation.

Flank ovariohysterectomy

The cat is placed in right lateral recumbency and legs extended caudally with ties. The position for the incision is identified by visualizing an equilateral triangle with vertices at the greater trochanter, wing of the ilium, and the centre point of the incision[70] (Fig. 40-6). The skin, subcutaneous fat, external aponeuroses, internal and transverse abdominal oblique muscles, and peritoneum are incised in a dorsal to ventral direction along the muscle fibers. The uterus is identified and exteriorized (the incision may need to be extended if this is difficult) and ligatures placed as above. The muscle layers can be sutured individually or in a single layer for maximum strength of closure.

Ovariectomy

The technique for ovariohysterectomy is initially followed but the incision is made more cranially at the umbilicus. After ligation of the ovarian pedicle two clamps are placed on the proximal uterine horn close to the ovary (Fig. 40-7) and a ligature placed distal to this. The ovary is removed after cutting between the hemostats. Closure continues as described above.

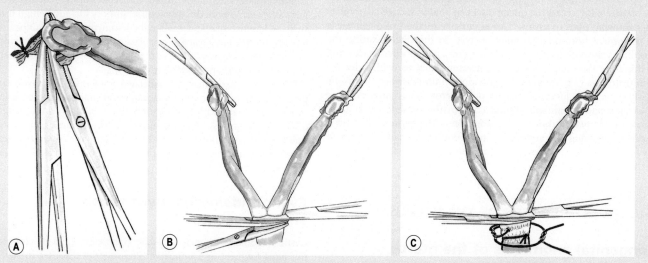

(A)   (B)   (C)

Figure 40-5 (A) The ovarian pedicle is double clamped and the vascular pedicle ligated proximal to the proximal clamp. **(B)** The uterine body is triple clamped. **(C)** The distal clamp on the uterine body is removed and a transfixation ligature placed in the crush created by the temporary clamp placement. A second encircling ligature is placed around the uterine body.

Box 40-1 **Continued**

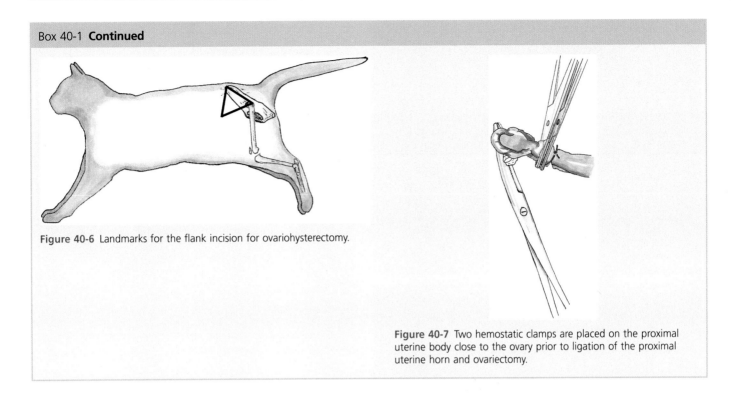

Figure 40-6 Landmarks for the flank incision for ovariohysterectomy.

Figure 40-7 Two hemostatic clamps are placed on the proximal uterine body close to the ovary prior to ligation of the proximal uterine horn and ovariectomy.

contamination. It is more common in older cats[21,22] and is uncommon in winter when queens are acyclic. Approximately half the cases are seen in unmated queens, which is unusual as there should be no luteal phase in these animals, but queens may ovulate spontaneously without mating.[8] In one study of 20 queens presenting with CEH-P, all affected cats were in diestrus.[23] The prevalence of CEH-P in entire female cats increases with age, and most cases of pyometra or endometritis in cats are associated with retained corpora lutea.[22]

Endogenous ovarian steroid hormones and their derivatives, especially progestogens used to control or suppress estrus, may enhance CEH-P and mammary tumor genesis in cats. The risk of CEH-P is variable and related to the particular progestogen administered, route of administration, amount, frequency and duration of treatment. Megestrol acetate tablets were used as an estrus suppressing agent in 244 cats in Norway in 1974. A weekly dose of 2.5 mg megestrol acetate was given for at least 30 weeks. One cat developed pyometra after three years of treatment with the preparation.[24] One queen developed CEH-P, ovarian cysts, mammary adenoma, fibrosarcoma and cystic-papillary adenocarcinoma after continual administration of medroxyprogesterone acetate (MPA) for nine years.[25] Experimentally, uterine changes were seen in prepubertally ovariectomized cats after administration of only six weeks of oral megestrol acetate.[26] In another ovariectomized cat, pyometra developed at three years of age, the cat had been treated with proligestone for a dermatologic condition for two years prior to this disease developing.[27]

Clinical signs and investigations

The most common signs noted by owners include vaginal discharge, anorexia, and lethargy.[28] The malodorous vaginal discharge usually makes diagnosis easy, although the queen will often fastidiously clean her perineum.[8] Estrus may have occurred within four weeks of the discharge appearing.

Physical examination in early cases may just reveal thickening of the uterine wall, due to endometrial hyperplasia with glandular dilatation, and no or minimal clinical signs. In later cases vaginal discharge

(Fig. 40-8), abdominal distension, dehydration, a palpable uterus, and pyrexia are the commonest findings.[28] Great care must be exercised when palpating the abdomen in order not to rupture the uterus.

Animals should be assessed for dehydration, electrolyte imbalance, anemia, azotemia, hypo- or hyperglycemia, sepsis, hepatic damage, cardiac dysrhythmias, and clotting abnormalities. Intravenous fluids are mandatory and since the commonest acid-base abnormality is metabolic acidosis then Lactated Ringers is the most appropriate choice. The most common bacteria isolated are *Escherichia coli*, with staphylococci and streptococci other common isolates; cephalosporins are good first choice antimicrobials.

Imaging

A combination of ultrasonography, radiography, hematology, and clinical examination is used to confirm the diagnosis. An enlarged uterus was seen in 138/169 affected cats.[28] A stump pyometra appears as a fluid-filled mass between the bladder or urethra and colon and is always associated with a retained ovarian remnant, which may be identified on ultrasonography as a small cystic structure caudal to one or both kidneys.

Treatment

In general, a closed pyometra should be treated as soon as possible with antibiosis and fluid therapy, and ovariohysterectomy once stable (see Box 40-1). Both medical management and flushing the uterus via a laparotomy have been tried with some success.[29,30]

Prognosis

In one study 8% of cats died or were euthanized due to a variety of causes including sepsis and bacterial peritonitis secondary to rupture of the uterus, liver disease, non-regenerative anemia, and anorexia. A ruptured uterus carries a poor prognosis, with more than 50% of cases (four of seven cats) dying in one series.[28]

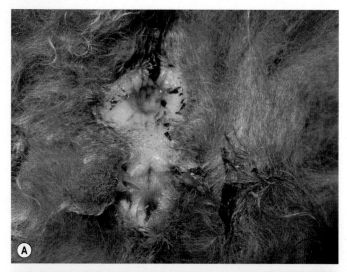

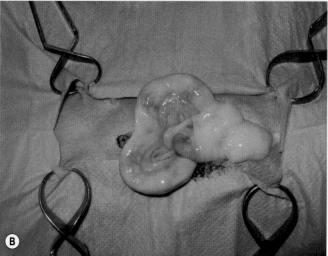

Figure 40-8 (A) Vulval discharge in a 6-year-old cat with an open pyometra. **(B)** The uterus is found to be enlarged with thickened uterine walls at surgery.

Uterine torsion

Uterine torsion is defined as a twisting of the uterus or uterine horn perpendicular to its long axis.[31] There are several reports of uterine torsion in pregnant cats in the literature[31-42] and torsion of a uterine horn has also been reported in three cats with pyometra[28,43,44] (Fig. 40-9). Torsion can vary from 90–900°, usually involving one horn of the uterine body in near-full term pregnancies.[31,32]

Affected cats range in age from 18 months to four years and not all of these are multiparous queens. A history of normal delivery 24–48 hours earlier is a common finding. Clinical signs vary with duration and degree of torsion and include acute depression, restlessness, anorexia, vomiting, and vaginal discharge (bloody, mucoid or serosanguineous). Cats may crouch and strain as if in labor or as if trying to urinate or defecate. Uterine torsions of 180° may persist for days or weeks without clinical signs until labor ensues.[31]

A precise diagnosis of uterine torsion as a cause of an obstructive dystocia is difficult, even with good quality imaging techniques. Affected cats can require intensive pre- and postoperative care; biochemical abnormalities can include hyperkalemia, hyponatremia, anemia, and azotemia.[41,43] Fatal hemorrhage as a complication

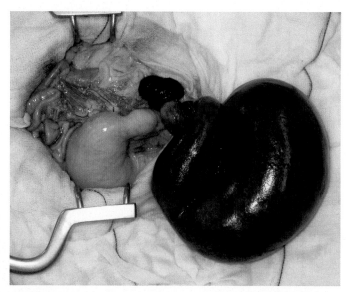

Figure 40-9 Uterine horn torsion in an 11-year-old cat with pyometra. There was a 900° torsion of the left uterine horn along the longitudinal axis. Ovariohysterectomy was performed without correction of the torsion. *(Courtesy of Benito De La Puerta.)*

of uterine torsion in a cat has been reported[35] and disseminated intravascular coagulation was suspected in one case due to marked prolongation of activated partial thromboplastin time.[41] Intensive supportive care is recommended for affected cats (see Chapter 3). Often the diagnosis is only made at laparotomy, in which case a prompt hysterotomy, for rapid removal of fetuses when present, followed by ovariohysterectomy (see Box 40-1), should be performed. The torsion should not be corrected, as release of toxins can be fatal.

Uterine prolapse or eversion

Postparturient prolapse or eversion of the uterus can occur in cats.[45] The everted uterus can be removed in situ by exposure and ligation of blood vessels through a vaginal incision. But unless tissues are grossly oedematous or traumatized then it is better performed at laparatomy after the eversion is reduced by gentle traction.

Dystocia

The average gestation length in the cat is 63–65 days but it can vary from 59–70 days. Dystocia has been reported in 5.8% of 2928 litters involving 735 queens.[46] Pedigree cats were at a significantly higher risk than cats of mixed breeding and dolichocephalic and brachycephalic breeds were found to have a significantly higher level of dystocia than mesocephalic breeds.

Dystocia can be due to maternal factors such as inadequacies of the birth canal or uterine torsion or a deficiency of expulsive force[47] (Table 40-1). Expulsive deficiency such as primary uterine inertia[48] is a common cause of dystocia in polytocous species. It is thought to be responsible for 37.8% of dystocia in queens.[49] Secondary inertia is the inertia of exhaustion and is essentially a result rather than a cause of dystocia; for example, it may be secondary to obstruction by a very large fetus. Sometimes in the queen, normal parturition will commence, but after the birth of a few kittens it will then cease even if there is no obstruction. This has been referred to as primary partial inertia and is responsible for about 23% of dystocia cases in the cat.[47] The differentiation of this from secondary inertia can be difficult. The

Table 40-1 Frequency of causes of dystocia in queens[47]

Cause of dystocia	Number of cases	Percentage
Maternal		
Uterine prolapse	1	0.6
Uterine strangulation	1	0.6
Narrow birth canal (fetomaternal disproportion)	8	5.2
Uterine inertia	94	60.6
Subtotal	104	67.0
Fetal		
Faulty disposition	24	15.5
Fetal congenital defects	12	7.7
Fetomaternal disproportion	3	1.9
Fetal death	7	4.5
Subtotal	46	29.6
Other causes	5	3.2
Total	**155**	**99.8**

underlying cause should be corrected, such as removal of a fetus, and normal parturition may then commence. Calcium borogluconate and oxytocin can also be tried.[48]

Only about a quarter of dystocia cases can be managed successfully non-surgically.[46,49]

If calcium borogluconate or oxytocin therapy is not successful, or if the litter is very large or small (a single kitten), or there is an identifiable obstruction or uterine torsion then a cesarean operation is indicated. An early decision to perform a cesarean or hysterotomy should be made as the fetuses will soon die, or may already be dead.[48]

Extrauterine fetuses

Occasional instances of extrauterine fetuses have been recorded.[50,51] These probably result from uterine rupture during pregnancy, possibly associated with uterine torsion rather than from an ectopic pregnancy. The presence of fetuses in the peritoneal cavity as a result of uterine rupture is usually of little consequence and affected animals can survive indefinitely without surgery, the fetal remnants becoming encapsulated by the omentum or mesentery.[51]

SURGICAL DISEASES OF THE VAGINA AND VULVA

Vaginal hypoplasia/atresia

In vaginal hypoplasia there is abnormal development of the vagina, which may result in retention of uterine fluid and cause endometrial changes and infertility. The uterus may dilate so much that it is palpable or abnormalities are visible on ultrasound. In rare cases, simple vaginal bands or strictures can be broken down, allowing normal coitus.

Atresia or aplasia is the absence or closure of an organ and vulvar and vaginal atresia may occur separately or simultaneously. Small labia with or without stenosis of the vestibule are observed in the former, while stenosis of the vagina is also observed in the latter.[52,53]

Neoplasia of the vagina and vulva

Neoplasia of the vagina or vulva in the cat is rare. A case of lymphosarcoma and a vulvar leiomyosarcoma have been reported. The cat with a vulvar leiomyosarcoma had a history of vulvar swelling, bleeding, and stranguria. The mass was located at the ventral commissure of the vulva; it was resected but recurred two months later when the cat was euthanized shortly after a second surgery.[54]

PREOPERATIVE CONSIDERATIONS FOR SURGERY

Neutering

Age to neuter

There are three age categories that are usually considered when deciding when to neuter a cat. These are early age prepubertal cats, traditional age prepubertal cats, or after puberty. The main advantages of prepubertal neutering are prevention of unwanted pregnancy and a marked reduction in the risk of mammary neoplasia.

Early age prepubertal gonadectomy (6–14 weeks)

Early age prepubertal gonadectomy is defined as surgical sterilization of immature animals aged from 6–14 weeks. Several studies have looked at early age versus traditional age prepubertal neutering,[55,56] and the results of these studies are summarized in Table 40-2. The main advantage of early age prepubertal gonadectomy for charitable organization or shelters is that it can be done before rehoming, ensuring that cats are neutered and thereby reducing pet overpopulation.

Traditional age prepubertal neutering (5–7 months)

With prepubertal gonadectomy at a more traditional age (5–7 months), cats are more mature so the potential for anesthetic complications such as hypoglycemia, hypothermia, or delayed recovery due to slow metabolism of drugs is less. As cats have completed the majority of the long bone growth, effects on bones will be less. Behavior is less likely to be affected in the older cat with a more established character. The disadvantage is that the cat may already have started cycling, pregnancy is already possible, and the uterus is more active and hemorrhage is more likely during surgery.

Effect of neutering on mammary neoplasia

The age of spaying has been shown to have an effect on the development of mammary gland carcinoma in cats. Queens gonadectomized prior to six months of age had a 91% reduction in risk of developing mammary neoplasia compared with intact cats. Those spayed prior to one year had an 86% reduction in risk.[61] Spaying cats after two years of age had minimal effect on mammary tumor development. Another study showed that intact cats were seven times overrepresented in a population of cats diagnosed with mammary tumors.[62]

Timing of surgery

The ideal stage of the estrous cycle at which to perform gonadectomy is anestrous in dogs, but the queen is not known to experience any

Table 40-2 Advantages and disadvantages of early age (6–14 week) prepubertal ovariohysterectomy

Advantages	Disadvantages
Can be done before adoption, ensuring that adopted animals do get neutered	A 30% decrease in basal metabolic rate
Less invasive and less traumatic surgery as uterus very small and inactive[55,56]	Minor swelling of abdominal incision[55,56]
No increase in incidence of physical or behavioral problems for at least a three year period following neutering[57]	Delay in closure of growth plates[58]
	Mild decrease in diameter of prepubic urethra in the female cat[a][59]
Reduced risk of asthma, gingivitis and hyperactivity if neutered before 5.5 months of age[58]	Cats 'neutered' prior to 5 months have an increase in shyness to strangers[60]

[a]No clinical significance was found to be associated with this.

Table 40-3 Advantages and disadvantages of neutering female cats

Advantages	Disadvantages
Decrease or absence of: Pregnancy, Pregnancy-related diseases, Parturition-related diseases, Mammary gland disease, Uterine disease, Progesterone-related disease, Estrogen-related disease, Ovarian disease	Irreversible if owners change their mind
	Generic risks of surgery: Hemorrhage
	Retained ovarian remnant
	Ureteral obstruction resulting from inadvertent ligation
Decreased roaming	Ureterovaginal fistula
Less hypervocalization and a more relaxed attitude	Granuloma of ovarian or uterine pedicle – non-absorbable suture material
	Behavioral abnormalities, e.g. laziness
	Obesity with its inherent risks

specific problems in relation to the stage of the estrous cycle in which she is gonadectomized.[63]

Anesthesia

Ovariohysterectomy and ovariectomy are usually elective procedures and routine anesthesia is employed; special care with regards to hypoglycemia, hypothermia, and anesthesia must be taken if neutering at a young age (e.g. 6–14 week old kittens).[64] See Chapter 2 for more information.

Cesarean

In animals being prepared for cesarean there are special considerations prior to surgery. The queens should be oxygenated prior to induction, and it is recommended to use rapidly metabolized or reversible agents for anesthesia so the fetuses are not unduly affected by the anesthetic agents. For information on anesthesia for cesareans see Chapter 2.

When positioning for surgery the head should be elevated slightly to reduce pressure on the diaphragm by the enlarged abdominal contents and also tilted slightly to one side but not so much to make surgery and localization of the linea alba more difficult.

SURGICAL TECHNIQUES

Surgical gonadectomy refers to the removal of the gonads under general anesthesia. In the female, gonadectomy (spaying) is generally performed by removing both ovaries (ovariectomy) or both ovaries and uterus (ovariohysterectomy) by a midline or flank abdominal approach. Laparoscopy has also been used for ovariectomy and ovariohysterectomy[65] (see Chapter 24). Whether to remove the ovary and uterus or just the ovaries is a dilemma for many veterinarians. By removing both ovaries and uterus all reproductive tissue is removed and no further problems can be encountered. It may not, however, be necessary to remove the uterus as once the ovaries are removed the uterus will quickly atrophy. Pyometra or endometrial hyperplasia should not occur in an ovariectomized animal. In dogs, the

complication rates of ovariectomy and ovariectomy were no different, although similar studies have not been reported in cats. Hysterectomy alone should not be performed as ovaries may become cystic and animals are still attractive to males.[63]

Feline ovariohysterectomy

The most common indication for feline ovariohysterectomy (Box 40-1) is as an elective procedure in a healthy animal to prevent pregnancy. There are potential advantages and disadvantages to neutering female cats (Table 40-3). Other indications for ovariohysterectomy include pyometra, cesarean, uterine prolapse, neoplasia, trauma, rupture, infarction and neutering during pregnancy.

In cats, the ovaries are relatively easy to retract from the abdomen but the uterine body is harder to exteriorize and the cervix is not clearly visible. The uterus can be located with an oophorectomy or spay hook (see Chapter 13) or finger. Some find that the omentum can be easier to engage with a spay hook than the broad ligament so use of a spay hook in the cat can be frustrating. Spay hooks should not be used if the animal has a pyometra or gravid uterus as they can cause damage to the friable tissues, and can also damage the spleen or omentum. The ureters may be located in the broad ligament near the cervical region, therefore to avoid damaging the ureters the uterine body should be ligated just below the bifurcation. When performing surgery in early age prepubertal animals (6–14 week old kittens), any bleeding during surgery should be meticulously controlled; fragile pediatric tissues require gentle handling as they are liable to tear.

Cats can be neutered or spayed via a midline or flank approach. Complications with the two techniques are similar[66] except more swelling, wound tenderness, and drainage may occur after flank spay.[67] Flank ovariohysterectomy (Box 40-1) may be preferable in cats with mammary fibroadenomatous hyperplasia or lactating cats. Possible advantages of the flank approach are avoidance of evisceration, less surgical trauma and shorter surgical time. Complications include discoloration or darkening of oriental cats' fur when it regrows after clipping[68] and more difficulty in locating the uterus, particularly for the inexperienced surgeons. It is more problematic to neuter a pregnant animal through a flank laparatomy and more traumatic to enlarge the incision if an ovarian or uterine pedicle is dropped, if there are congenital anomalies, or there is bleeding to control.

In preparation for surgery the abdomen should be clipped from cranial to the xiphoid to caudal to the pubis to enable removal of the enlarged uterus. Great care should be exercized when entering the abdomen through the linea alba not to perforate the uterus. The uterus is more friable than normal, with an increased risk of rupture; thus a long incision is made so the uterus can be lifted out carefully without the need for pulling which could cause rupture.

After exteriorizing the uterus, it is packed off from the remainder of the abdomen with laparotomy swabs to avoid spillage of contents into the abdomen if inadvertent rupturing occurs. An ovariohysterectomy is performed as described in Box 40-1. The suspensory ligaments are often stretched and do not need breaking down. The broad ligament is likely to be far more vascular and should be bunch ligated. The uterine pedicle is transected at the level of the proximal vagina with absorbable suture material. The uterine body should not be oversewn, which may increase the chance of granuloma formation, but if it is thought to be contaminated then omentum can be placed over it after flushing. The abdomen should be lavaged with copious volumes of warm saline prior to routine abdominal closure.

Ovariectomy

Ovariectomy (Box 40-1) is potentially a quicker surgery requiring a shorted anesthetic, shorter surgical incision, and is less invasive overall. As long as both ovaries are removed in entirety then the uterus should atrophy and hormonally related disease such as pyometra should not occur. Contraindications are older animals with uterine disease such as pyometra or tumors.

Cystic endometrial hyperplasia and pyometra

The uterus is often enlarged, friable, and vascular so some additional care and precautions should be taken when performing an ovariohysterectomy for a cat with cystic endometrial hyperplasia and pyometra (Box 40-2; see Fig. 40-5).

Ovarian remnants and stump pyometra

Surgery should be performed through a midline celiotomy and the abdomen explored for ovarian remnants near the caudal poles of kidneys, by reflecting the mesoduodenum or mesocolon, respectively. If the remnants are not easily located then the omentum and the peritoneal walls should be inspected, as these are also commonly affected sites, and any thick residual tissue around previously ligated pedicle sites resected.[16]

Excised ovarian tissue should be submitted for microscopic examination. If a stump pyometra is also present then it requires resection after removal of the ovarian remnant. The ureters should be identified prior to resection of the pyometra as these are often located immediately dorsal to the stump. The uterine stump is dissected free from surrounding tissues, ligated, transected, and removed. Non-resectable stumps can be opened and omentalized (see Chapter 19).

Cesarean

Precise indications for hysterotomy or cesarean are not well documented and gravid ovariohysterectomy through a midline incision

Speed of surgery is important to prevent fetal hypoxia.

In preparation for surgery the abdomen should be clipped and prepped from cranial to the xiphoid to caudal to the pubis. The cat is positioned in dorsal recumbency with the table tilted so the abdominal contents are not compressing the diaphragm (Fig. 40-10A). A long celiotomy incision is made to expose the whole uterus. The linea alba is often thin and stretched so great care is needed not to damage the gravid uterus. One or both uterine horns are exteriorized (Fig. 40-10B) and packed off to prevent contamination of the abdomen with fetal fluid. The uterus is incised in a relatively avascular area on the ventral surface of the uterine body, taking care not to lacerate the fetuses. The incision is extended with scissors. The fetuses within the uterine body are removed first and then remaining fetuses are 'milked-down' to the same incision. The kittens are best handled by the head or pelvis. Umbilical vessels are clamped 2 cm from the ventral abdominal wall of the kitten and the cord severed distally. The kittens are then passed to an assistant for resuscitation. If there are two remaining kittens within tips of opposite uterine horns, bilateral cornual incisions are indicated rather than a single uterine body incision.

After each kitten is delivered the associated placenta should be removed by gentle traction or by gentle squeezing of the uterine wall and twisting of the cord. Those that are firmly adherent should be left in position since forceful removal will result in hemorrhage. Such placentas will be expelled by uterine involution supplemented by exogenous oxytocin administration after termination of the procedure. Both uterine horns up to the ovaries and the uterine body are carefully inspected to ensure all kittens have been removed. Any gross damage to the uterus is repaired. The uterus should rapidly begin to contract and involute.

The uterine incision is closed using either an inverting continuous pattern such as a Cushing or Lembert or an appositional pattern with absorbable suture material such as 2M poliglecaprone, caprosyn, polyglactin 910 or polysorb.

The celiotomy is closed routinely. An intradermal suture may be preferable for skin closure to avoid interference of skin sutures by suckling kittens.

Gravid (en bloc) ovariohysterectomy

If elective ovariohysterectomy is planned then an en bloc removal of the ovaries and uterus can be done first. After the uterus and ovaries are exposed the broad ligament is broken down. The ovarian pedicles and uterine body are double or triple clamped and transected. The whole gravid uterus is then passed in an aseptic manner to a team of assistants who will open the uterus and revive the kittens.

(Box 40-3) is performed more frequently than hysterotomy except in pedigree cats. Unless the cat is intended for further breeding, gravid ovariohysterectomy (Box 40-1) may be preferable to hysterotomy and is well tolerated. Gravid or en bloc ovariohysterectomy involves ovariohysterectomy before hysterotomy and removal of the neonates. In one study 26 cats had this procedure performed.[71] Intraoperative complications were limited to one cat that bled excessively during surgery and was later found to have a clotting disorder. Postoperative complications included anemia that required blood transfusion in three cats, and death in one cat. The rate of neonatal survival was 42% for cats, which was similar to that documented by previous studies of medical and surgical management of dystocia.[71]

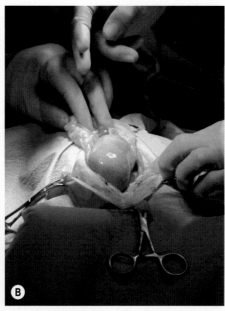

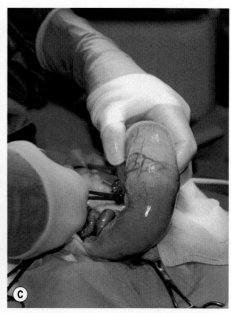

Figure 40-10 Cesarean in a cat with one large dead fetus. **(A)** The cat is positioned with the head and thorax elevated above the abdomen to relieve pressure on the diaphragm and therefore limit lung compression. **(B)** Care must be taken on entering the abdomen not to damage the uterine wall. **(C)** An en bloc ovariohysterectomy is being performed with the first ovarian pedicle being clamped prior to being cut.

POSTOPERATIVE CARE

After elective ovariohysterectomy routine postoperative care is performed including provision of analgesia, and keeping the animal in a warm quiet environment where it can be monitored for any postoperative complications. The use of a Buster collar may be indicated to prevent self-trauma and interference or premature suture removal.

For early age neutering in particular, kittens should be offered food shortly after standing to minimize hypoglycemia. Dextrose administration can be considered if recovery is slow or prolonged.[55]

Cesarean

After retrieval, the kittens are briskly rubbed to stimulate respiration, and amniotic fluid suctioned from nares and nasopharynx. Naloxone drops under the tongue will reverse opioids. Dopram may stimulate respiration in apneic neonates. The umbilical vein can be used for injections if required.

After completion of the surgery the abdominal skin should be cleaned to remove antiseptics and debris before neonates are allowed with the queen. The mother and kittens are placed in an incubator to keep them warm. Neonates should be allowed to nurse as soon as possible to ensure colostrum intake. If the queen is not yet lactating then the kittens may need to be given a proprietary milk replacement product.

The queen should be monitored postoperatively for hypothermia, hypotension, hypocalcemia, neonatal rejection, and agalactia. Any vulval hemorrhage is also monitored as delayed uterine involution can result in severe life-threatening hemorrhage.

Pyometra

Following ovariohysterectomy for pyometra cats will need intensive supportive care, ensuring adequate hydration, treatment for sepsis, and monitoring for deterioration. See Chapter 3 for further information on postoperative management.

COMPLICATIONS AND PROGNOSIS

Inclusion of a ureter in the vaginal stump ligature or ovarian pedicle ligature is a serious though rare complication. It is usually unilateral and results in renal enlargement and hydronephrosis. If diagnosis is rapid and the ligature removed then some recovery of renal function may occur. Otherwise, function in that kidney will be lost and ureteronephrectomy is usually recommended (see Chapter 36).

If a stump pyometra is diagnosed in an animal following neutering, an ovarian remnant has been left behind and should be identified and removed. In one report the main presenting sign of a cat with a stump pyometra was abdominal straining.[72] The enlarged uterine stump had caused rectal compression. The stump was drained and removed and a small ovarian fragment was removed from the right side. Intestinal strangulation has been reported when intestines passed through a mesenteric tear following an elective ovariohysterectomy.[73]

After pyometra or cesarean section peritonitis is a possible complication, particularly if the uterus ruptures or if there are necrotic or decaying fetuses present. Adhesions may occur after cesareans, which may interfere with subsequent exteriorization of the uterus if future cesareans are required.

Hemorrhage

One of the commonest complications after ovariohysterectomy is hemorrhage due to ligature failure. This is more likely to occur if the surgeon is inexperienced, the animal is obese, and the uterus is vascular. If ovarian pedicles or the uterine body are inadvertently dropped during a midline approach the incision can be extended to allow

After hysterotomy hemorrhage may occur after forcible separation of placentae. This hemorrhage can be life threatening and should not be ignored. Oxytocin injection should be repeated or administered if not already given. Animals may need blood transfusion or hysterectomy if severe anemia occurs or the bleeding due to subinvolution of the uterus does not abate within 8-10 weeks.

Weight gain

Neutering is a commonly associated risk factor for obesity.[73-78] Cats were found to increase body weight due to an approximately 25% lower maintenance energy requirement after ovariohysterectomy.[60] Thus, $313.6 \times$ ideal body weight (kg) (0.67) kJ is proposed for the maintenance energy requirement of spayed adult cats.[60] In practice this means that ad libitum feeding of cats once neutered is not recommended, portion size should be reduced, and regular weighing recommended.[78] Many adverse sequelae of obesity exist, including diabetes, where obesity and neutering have been found to be predisposing factors for the disease.[79]

retrieval and ligation (Boxes 40-4 and 40-5). If surgery was performed through a flank incision, it may be possible to retrieve bleeding vessels for ligation through the same incision or after enlargement of the incision, particularly in thin cats. Alternatively, consideration should be given to closing the abdominal flank incision and performing a midline incision if abdominal hemorrhage is evident. If bleeding occurs due to a loose ligature and this is not recognized or addressed at surgery then affected animals will be slow to recover, with signs of hypovolemic shock such as tachycardia, tachypnoea, pale mucous membranes, a weak pulse, and a prolonged CRT. Ultrasound examination can be useful to determine if there is a build-up of abdominal fluid. If the cat is showing signs of hypovolemic shock, repeat surgery through a midline incision should be performed after stabilization. A blood transfusion may be required (see Chapter 5).

REFERENCES

1. Crouch JE. Text-Atlas of cat anatomy. Philadelphia: Lea & Febiger; 1969. p. 177.

2. Verstegen JP. Physiology and endocrinology of reproduction in female cats. In: England G, Von Heimendahl A, editors. BSAVA manual of canine and feline reproduction and neonatology. 2nd ed. Gloucs: BSAVA Publications; 2010. p. 11–16.

3. Matton JS, Nyland TG. Ovaries and uterus. In: Small animal diagnostic ultrasound. 2nd ed. Philadelphia Saunders Co; 2002. p. 231–49.

4. Schmidt PM. Feline breeding management. Vet Clin North Am Small Anim Pract 1986;16:435–51.

5. Herron MA. Infertility from noninfectious causes. In: Morrow DA, editor. Current veterinary therapy in theriogenology. 2nd ed. Philadelphia: WB Saunders; 1986. p. 829–34.

6. Johnston SD, Kustritz MVR, Olson PN. Disorders of the mammary glands of Queens. Canine and feline theriogenology. Philadelphia: WB Saunders; 2001. p. 474–6.

7. Keskin A, Yilmazbas G, Yilmaz R, et al. Pathological abnormalities after long-term administration of medroxyprogesterone acetate in a queen. J Feline Med Surg 2009;11:518–21.

8. England G. Genital surgery in the bitch and queen. In: Noakes DE, Parkinson TJ, England GCW, editors. Veterinary reproduction and obstetrics. Edinburgh: Saunders Elsevier; 2009. p. 367–80.

9. Gelberg HB, McEntee K. Feline ovarian neoplasms. Vet Pathol 1985;22:572–6.

10. Barrett RE, Theilen GH. Neoplasms of the canine and feline reproductive tracts. In: Kirk RW, editor. Current veterinary therapy: small animal practice. 6th ed. WB Saunders Philadelphia; 1977. p. 1263–7.

11. Ball RL, Birchard SJ, May LR, et al. Ovarian remnant syndrome in dogs and cats: 21 cases (2000–2007). J Am Vet Med Assoc 2010;236:548–53.

12. DeNardo GA, Becker K, Brown NO, Dobbins S. Ovarian remnant syndrome: revascularization of free-floating ovarian tissue in the feline abdominal cavity. J Am Anim Hosp Assoc 2001;37:290–6.

13. Miller DM. Ovarian remnant syndrome in dogs and cats: 46 cases (1988–1992). J Vet Diagn Invest 1995;7:572–4.

14. Wallace MS. The ovarian remnant syndrome in the bitch and queen. Vet Clin North Am Small Anim Pract 1991;21:501–7.

15. England GC. Confirmation of ovarian remnant syndrome in the queen using hCG administration. Vet Rec 1997;141(12):309–10.

16. Heffelfinger DJ. Ovarian remnant in a 2-year-old queen. Can Vet J 2006;47: 165–7.

17. McIntyre RL, Levy JK, Roberts JF, Reep RL. Developmental uterine anomalies in cats and dogs undergoing elective ovariohysterectomy. J Am Vet Med Assoc 2010;237:542–6.

18. Miller MA, Ramos-Vara JA, Dickerson MF, et al. Uterine neoplasia in 13 cats. J Vet Diagn Invest 2003;15:515–22.

19. Dow C. Experimental uterine infection in the domestic cat. J Comp Path 1962a;72: 303–7.

20. Dow C. The cystic hyperplasia- pyometra complex in the cat. Vet Rec 1962;74: 141–6.

21. Lein DH, Concannon PW. Infertility and fertility treatments and management in the queen and tomcat. In: Kirk RW, editor. Current veterinary therapy: small animal practice. 8th ed. Philadelphia: WB Saunders; 1983. p. 936–42.

22. Potter K, Hancock DH, Gallina AM. Clinical and pathologic features of endometrial hyperplasia, pyometra, and endometritis in cats: 79 cases (1980–5). J Am Vet Med Assoc 1991;198:1427–31.

23. Misirlioglu D, Nak D, Ozyigit MO, et al. HER-2/neu (c-erbB-2) oncoprotein in hyperplastic endometrial polyps detected in two cats. J Feline Med Surg 2009;11: 885–8.

24. Oen EO. The oral administration of megestrol acetate to postpone oestrus in cats. Nord Vet Med 1977;29:287–91.

25. Keskin A, Yilmazbas G, Yilmaz R, et al. Pathological abnormalities after long-term administration of medroxyprogesterone acetate in a queen. J Feline Med Surg 2009;11:518–21.

26. Bellenger CR, Chen JC. Effect of megestrol acetate on the endometrium of the prepubertally ovariectomised kitten. Res Vet Sci 1990;48:112–18.

27. van Haaften B. Pyometra in an ovariectomized cat following treatment with proligestone. Tijdschr Diergeneeskd 1989;114:383–7.

28. Kenney KJ, Matthiesen DT, Brown NO, Bradley RL. Pyometra in cats: 183 cases (1979–1984). J Am Vet Med Assoc 1987;191:1130–2.

29. Nak D, Nak Y, Tuna B. Follow-up examinations after medical treatment of pyometra in cats with the progesterone-antagonist aglepristone. J Feline Med Surg 2009;11:499–502.

30. Davidson AP, Feldman EC, Nelson RW. Treatment of pyometra in cats, using prostaglandin F2 alpha: 21 cases (1982–1990). J Am Vet Med Assoc 1992;200:825–8.

31. Biller DS, Haibel GK. Torsion of the uterus in a cat. J Am Vet Med Assoc 1987;191:1128–9.

32. Young RC, Hiscock RH. Torsion of the uterus in a cat. Vet Rec 1963;75:872.

33. Sharma HN. Uterine torsion in a cat. Indian Vet J 1964;41:421–5.

34. Singer A. Torsion of the uterus in a cat. J Am Vet Med Assoc 1960;137:290.

35. Pankhurst JW. A case of torsion of the uterus in the pregnant cat with fatal hemorrhage. Vet Rec 1961;73:1269.

36. Kudale ML, Wadia DS, Jambagi SN. Torsion of uterus in a cat: a case report. Indian Vet J 1972;49:1148–9.

37. Jolivet MR. Uterine torsion in a pregnant cat. Mod Vet Pract 1987;68:240.

38. McIntire JW, Waugh SL. Uterine torsion in a cat. Fel Pract 1987;11:41–2.

39. Freeman L. Feline uterine torsion. Compend Contin Educ Pract Vet 1988;10:1078–82.

40. Montgomery RD, Saidla JE, Milton JL. Feline uterine horn torsion: a case report and literature review. J Am Anim Hosp Assoc 1989;25:189–90.

41. Ridyard AE, Welsh EA, Gunn-Moore DA. Successful treatment of uterine torsion in a cat with severe metabolic and haemostatic complications. J Feline Med Surg 2000;2:115–19.

42. Thilagar S, Yew YC, Dhaliwal GK, et al. Uterine horn torsion in a pregnant cat. Vet Rec 2005;157:558–60.

43. Stanley SW, Pacchiana PD. Uterine torsion and metabolic abnormalities in a cat with a pyometra. Can Vet J 2008;49: 398–400.

44. De La Puerta B, McMahon LA, Moores A. Uterine horn torsion in a non-gravid cat. J Feline Med Surg 2008;10:395–7.

45. England G. Infertility and subfertility in the bitch and queen. In: Noakes DE, Parkinson TJ, England GCW, editors. Veterinary reproduction and obstetrics. Edinburgh: Saunders Elsevier; 2009. p. 639–70.

46. Gunn-Moore DA, Thrusfield MV. Feline dystocia: prevalence and association with cranial conformation and breed. Vet Rec 1995;136:350–3.

47. Ekstrand C, Linde-Forsberg C. Causes of dystocia in queens. J Small Anim Pract 1994;35:459–64.

48. Noakes D. Maternal dystocia: causes and treatment. In: Noakes DE, Parkinson TJ, England GCW, editors. Veterinary reproduction and obstetrics. Edinburgh: Saunders Elsevier; 2009. p. 232–46.

49. Linde-Forsberg C, Eneroth A. Parturition. In: Simpson GM, England GCW, Harvey M, editors. Manual of small animal reproduction and neonatology. Cheltenham: BSAVA Publications; 1998. p. 127–42.

50. Linzell JL. An extra-uterine foetus in the cat. Vet Rec 1951;63:223–5.

51. Rosset E, Galet C, Buff S. A case report of an ectopic fetus in a cat. J Feline Med Surg 2011;13:610–13.

52. Saperstein G, Harris S, Leipold HW. Congenital defects in domestic cats. Feline Pract 1976;6:18–43.

53. Nomura K, Koreeda T, Kawata M, Shiraishi Y. Vaginal atresia with transverse septum in a cat. J Vet Med Sci 1997;59: 1045–8.

54. Firat I, Haktanir-Yatkin D, Sontas BH, Ekici H. Vulvar leiomyosarcoma in a cat. J Feline Med Surg 2007;9:435–8.

55. Aronsohn MG, Fagella AM. Surgical technique for neutering 6- to 14-week-old kittens. J Am Vet Med Assoc 1993;202: 53–5.

56. Howe LM. Short term results and complications of prepubertal gonadectomy in cats and dogs. J Am Vet Med Assoc 1997;211:57–62.

57. Howe LM, Slater MR, Boothe HW, et al. Long-term outcome of gonadectomy performed at an early age or traditional age in cats. J Am Vet Med Assoc 2000;217:1661–5.

58. Root MV, Johnston SD, Olson PN. The effect of prepuberal and postpuberal gonadectomy on radial physeal closure in male and female domestic cats. Vet Radiol Ultrasound 1997;38:42–7.

59. Root MV, Johnston SD, Johnston GR, Olson PN. The effect of prepubertal and postpubertal gonadectomy on penile extrusion and urethral diameter in the domestic cat. Vet Radiol Ultrasound 1996;37:363–6.

60. Spain CV, Scarlett JM, Houpt KA. Long-term risks and benefits of early age gonadectomy in cats. J Am Vet Med Assoc 2004;224:372–9.

61. Overley B, Shofer FS, Goldschmidt MH, et al. Association between ovarihysterectomy and feline mammary carcinoma. J Vet Int Med 2005;19:560–3.

62. Misdorp W, Romijn A, Hart AA. Feline mammary tumors: a case-control study of hormonal factors. Anticancer Res 1991;11:1793–8.

63. Romagnoli S, Sontas H. Prevention of breeding in the female. In: England G, Von Heimendahl A, editors. BSAVA manual of canine and feline reproduction and neonatology. 2nd ed. Gloucs: BSAVA Publications; 2010. p. 23–33.

64. Joyce A, Yates D. Help stop teenage pregnancy. Early-age neutering in cats. J Feline Med Surg 2011;13:3–10.

65. Van Nimwegen SA, Kirpensteijn J. Laparoscopic ovariectomy in cats: comparison of laser and bipolar electrocoagulation. J Feline Med Surg 2007;9:397–403.

66. Coe RJ, Grint NJ, Tivers MS, et al. Comparison of flank and midline approaches to the ovariohysterectomy of cats. Vet Rec 2006;159:309–13.

67. Grint N J, Murison PJ, Coe RJ, Waterman Pearson AE. Assessment of the influence of surgical technique on postoperative pain and wound tenderness in cats following ovariohysterectomy. J Feline Med Surg 2006;8:15–21.

68. Gorelick J. Discoloration of exotic cats hair following flank ovariohysterectomy. Vet Med Small Anim Clin 1974;69:943–6.

69. Hedlund CS. Mammary neoplasia. In: Fossum T, editor. Small animal surgery 3e. St Louis: Mosby Elsevier; 2007. p. 729–47.

70. Feathers DJ. Locating site of incision for flank approach to feline OVH. Vet Med Small Anim Clin 1974;69:1069.

71. Robbins MA, Mullen HS. En bloc ovariohysterectomy as a treatment for dystocia in dogs and cats. Vet Surg 1994;23:48–52.

72. Rota A, Pregel P, Cannizzo FT, et al. Unusual case of uterine stump pyometra in a cat. J Feline Med Surg 2011;13: 448–50.

73. Kuan SY, Ticehurst K, Hoffmann KL, et al. Intestinal strangulation after elective

ovariohysterectomy. J Feline Med Surg 2010;12:325–9.

74. Mitsuhashi Y, Chamberlin AJ, Bigley KE, Bauer JE. Maintenance energy requirement determination of cats after spaying. Br J Nutr 2011;106:S135–8.

75. Alexander LG, Salt C, Thomas G, Butterwick R. Effects of neutering on food intake, body weight and body composition in growing female kittens. B J Nutr 2011;106:S19–23.

76. Belsito KR, Vester BM, Keel T, et al. Impact of ovariohysterectomy and food intake on body composition, physical activity, and adipose gene expression in cats. J Anim Sci 2009;87;594–602.

77. Flynn MF, Hardie EM, Armstrong PJ. Effect of ovariohysterectomy on maintenance energy requirement in cats. J Am Vet Med Assoc 1996;209:1572–81.

78. Harper EJ, Stack DM, Watson TD, Moxham G. Effects of feeding regimens on bodyweight, composition and condition score in cats following ovariohysterectomy. J Small Anim Pract 2001;42:433–8.

79. Rand JS, Fleeman LM, Farrow HA, et al. Canine and feline diabetes mellitus: nature or nurture? J Nutr 2004;134: S2072–80.

Section | 6 |

J.L. Demetriou, S.J. Langley-Hobbs

Thorax

Thoracic surgery in the cat is considered to be advanced surgery. Practices should have resources and personnel confident in performing intermittent positive pressure ventilation in cats when considering a thoracotomy, in addition to the capability of providing appropriate pre- and postoperative care. Cats are prone to pleural conditions, many of which may be managed medically after drainage and placement of a thoracic drain, but in some instances surgical intervention is required, e.g., in cases of chylothorax or pyothorax that are unresponsive to medical management.

In the first section of this part of the book the chapters cover the region of the pleural cavity, with the first two chapters covering the basics of thoracotomy and thoracoscopy in the cat. In subsequent chapters specific conditions of the pleural cavity and thoracic wall are discussed and their surgical management described. Trauma to the thoracic wall in cats (from vehicles, dog bites or gunshot) is common and resulting wounds may necessitate thoracic wall reconstruction. In the final chapter, conditions of the diaphragm are covered, the most common of which is diaphragmatic rupture. The management of this condition usually involves a celiotomy but as the thoracic cavity is effectively open during surgery then aspects of thoracic surgery,

particularly the anesthestic management, are important additional considerations.

In the second section of this part of the book the chapters focus on cardiorespiratory surgery. In the first chapter, surgical management of tracheal and bronchial conditions is described. Cats with respiratory disease are often not diagnosed until the condition is far advanced as some of the clinical signs such as exercise intolerance can be overlooked or may not be clearly evident. Tracheal avulsion or rupture is a condition seen in cats that can cause overt clinical signs several weeks after its occurrence. Surgical correction is usually successful with good technique if careful attention is paid to the anesthetic management. The surgeon performing lung lobectomy is advised to read the chapter on thoracotomy first, prior to the chapter specifically related to conditions of the lung. The final chapter in the book describes diseases and surgical management of conditions of the heart. Although surgical management is not commonly indicated for disease of this organ, descriptions of some of the more frequently encountered cardiac conditions are included e.g., management of a patent ductus arteriosus, pericardectomy, and placement of an epicardial pacemaker.

Chapter 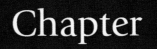 |41|

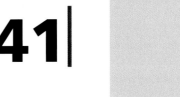

Thoracotomy

A.L. Moores

Cats with thoracic disease may present with a range of clinical signs, depending upon the organ system involved and the pathophysiology of the disease. Individual disease processes are covered in subsequent chapters.

Surgical intervention may be necessary for the management of a number of thoracic diseases in cats. Access to gas and fluid can be obtained by thoracocentesis or thoracostomy drain placement. Intercostal thoracotomy allows access to a limited area of one hemithorax and is well tolerated. Median sternotomy is more invasive but allows surgical access to the entire thoracic cavity.

DIAGNOSTIC APPROACH TO THE CAT WITH IMPAIRED RESPIRATORY FUNCTION

A careful physical examination is imperative for animals presenting with clinical signs attributable to thoracic disease. Hyperpnea and tachypnea (Table 41-1) are common physical examination findings.

Cats may often compensate for impaired respiratory function by becoming less active and owners may not notice clinical signs until they are severe. Cats are therefore more likely to be severely affected at first presentation than dogs with the same disease. Observation of the cat prior to physical examination should recognize those cats that are at risk of respiratory embarrassment during physical examination. When necessary, measures to prevent a respiratory crisis (such as providing oxygen support, but also interventions such as

thoracocentesis) should never be delayed but should be undertaken in such a way as to minimize handling or restraint. Indicators of impending respiratory crisis are listed in Box 41-1.

Careful observation of the pattern of respiration may help determine the type of thoracic disease present (Table 41-2). For example, pleural disease may result in short shallow respiration, whereas upper respiratory obstruction is more likely to result in a long deep inspiratory pattern. Thoracic auscultation also provides highly valuable additional information. Firstly, a basic assessment of whether or not there are audible breath sounds needs to be made and if breath sounds are absent, locating where the sounds are missing can rapidly help in identifying the type of pathology present. The use of gentle percussion must also always accompany auscultation to help identify fluid lines in cases of, for example, pyothorax. If breath sounds are auscultatable, then assessing whether they are appropriate for the respiratory effort of the patient is the next step. In a normal cat, breath sounds are quiet but audible, and they naturally become louder as respiratory rate increases e.g., with stress, exertion. However, increased respiratory rate does not normally generate abnormal breath sounds, so the identification of crackles or wheezes indicates the presence of pulmonary pathology and should always be investigated. It is also important to distinguish abnormal lower respiratory tract sounds from referred upper airway noise caused by upper respiratory tract disease.

Prior to any diagnostic or therapeutic intervention, and certainly prior to anesthesia, pre-oxygenation is recommended to improve oxygen delivery to tissues in patients with compromised respiratory function (Fig. 41-1). Whilst an oxygen cage or incubator provides the greatest fractional inspired concentration of oxygen, they are rarely available and do not allow concurrent physical examination. The

Table 41-1 Definitions of common terms used to describe changes in breathing patterns

Term	Definition
Dyspnea	Subjective experience of breathing discomfort
Hyperpnea	Fast and/or deep breathing
Tachypnea	Increased breathing rate, usually shallow
Hyperventilation	Increased breathing that causes CO_2 loss

Box 41-1 Indicators of an impending respiratory crisis in cats

Failure to find a comfortable position
Paradoxical abdominal movement
Open mouth breathing
Cyanosis

© 2014 Elsevier Ltd
DOI: 10.1016/B978-0-7020-4336-9.00041-X

Table 41-2 Classification pathologic respiratory patterns

Respiratory pattern	Disease examples
Prolonged inspiratory phase ± stridor	Upper respiratory tract disease, e.g., laryngeal obstruction, tracheal obstruction/stenosis
Expiratory effort, crackles on auscultation	Pulmonary disease, e.g., inhalation pneumonia
Short shallow respiration, decreased lung sounds on auscultation, hyporesonant percussion	Pleural disease with effusion, e.g., pyothorax
Wheezing on auscultation	Lower airway disease, e.g., feline bronchial disease

Box 41-2 **Thoracocentesis**

In most cats, thoracocentesis can be performed with the cat sitting or in sternal recumbency with minimal restraint. Following clipping and aseptic preparation of the lateral thoracic wall, a 19–22G butterfly needle attached to a syringe via a three-way tap is introduced at a 45° angle in the seventh or eighth intercostal space. The needle should be positioned immediately adjacent to the cranial aspect of the rib to avoid the intercostal neurovascular bundle on the caudal aspect of the rib. If a butterfly needle is not available then an intravenous catheter or a hypodermic needle can be used. If the presence of air is suspected the needle can be inserted in the dorsal third of the thoracic cavity; if fluid is suspected the needle can be inserted in the ventral third, but care must be taken to avoid the internal thoracic artery which lies ventral and deep to the costochondral junctions. If the nature of pleural disease is unknown the needle is generally placed halfway down the thoracic cavity. It is preferable to have three people present; one to monitor the cat and administer oxygen, a second to drain the chest via an extension tube, whilst the third holds the needle to assess the point at which the lungs are felt on the needle tip, thereby signaling the time to stop drainage. In practice it is possible for one person to drain the chest with just a single assistant, especially in cats, where the needle is less likely to be displaced from the thorax during respiratory excursions than in dogs. The absence of a complete mediastinum in most cats means that drainage of air or fluid from both hemithoraces can usually be achieved with unilateral thoracocentesis. However, trial thoracocentesis on the contralateral side is warranted if clinical signs do not improve significantly following unilateral drainage, particularly in cases where loculation of fluid may be present (e.g., pyothorax). Any pleural fluid should be placed into an EDTA tube in addition to direct smears being made for cytology, and into a plain tube for bacteriologic culture and sensitivity testing (Fig. 41-3).

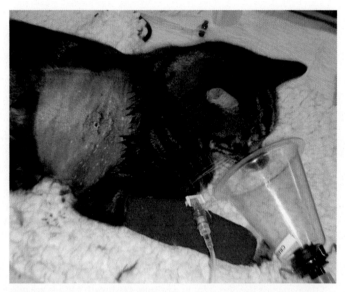

Figure 41-1 Cat with an air gun pellet injury to the thorax. The cat is receiving supplemental oxygenation via a mask during clipping and cleaning of the wound. (© *Alison Moores.*)

practitioner may have to rely on mask or flow-by techniques, which only provide a minimal increase in fractional inspired oxygen compared to room air. Cats may find restraint, supplemental oxygenation, and diagnostic techniques distressing, leading to an increase in oxygen consumption and risk of further respiratory distress. Careful, continual assessment is therefore vital to ensure that attempted stabilization methods do not worsen the clinical status of the patient.

The choice of diagnostic test is determined by history and physical examination findings. If a pleural effusion is suspected, thoracocentesis should be performed, preferably after a brief ultrasound scan to confirm the presence of pleural fluid (Box 41-2, Fig. 41-2). Thoracocentesis can be both diagnostic and therapeutic and is often safer to perform than radiography, which may require manual or chemical restraint.

Diagnostic imaging for thoracic disease

Thoracic radiography can provide extremely useful information on the causal pathology of thoracic diseases (see Chapter 8), and should be

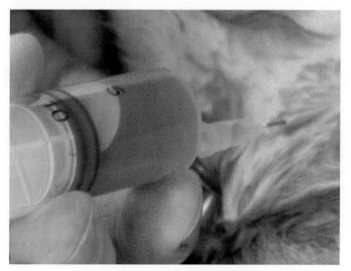

Figure 41-2 Thoracocentesis being performed in a kitten with pleural fluid. (© *Davina Anderson.*)

undertaken following evacuation of pleural fluid or air and with minimal stress. In many circumstances a single dorsoventral radiograph may be sufficient to make a preliminary diagnosis, and it can be followed by a complete imaging study under sedation or anesthesia when the cat is more stable (Fig. 41-4). Thoracic radiography will

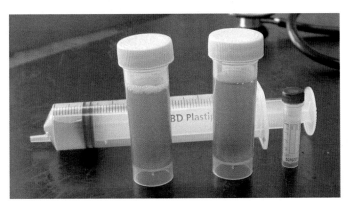

Figure 41-3 Pleural fluid from the kitten in Figure 41-2 has been placed into EDTA for cytology and a plain tube for bacteriologic culture and sensitivity. (© Davina Anderson.)

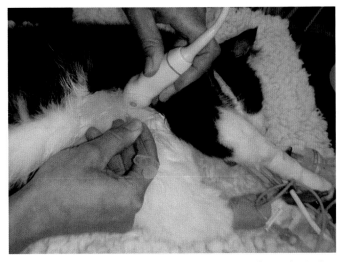

Figure 41-5 Ultrasound-guided fine needle aspiration of a mediastinal mass in an anesthetized cat. Note the use of a heat/moisture exchanger (Thermovent). (© Alison Moores.)

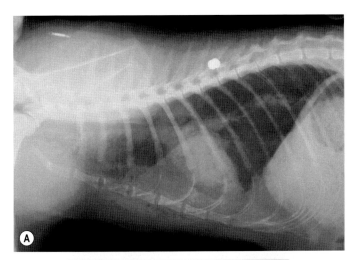

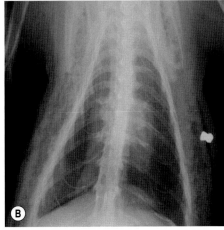

Figure 41-4 **(A)** Lateral and **(B)** dorsoventral radiographs of the cat shown in Figure 41-1. A radiolucent tract is seen where the air gun pellet has entered on the right and it has stopped under the skin on the left side of the thorax. There is massive heterogenous subcutaneous emphysema in the soft tissues circumferentially around the thoracic cavity. Small air bubbles suggest associated subcutaneous hemorrhage. Interpretation of the lung parenchyma is difficult due to superimposition of subcutaneous emphysema. Cystic lesions in the right caudal lobe are consistent with penetration by the pellet; these lesions usually heal rapidly and were not seen on subsequent radiographs. (© Alison Moores.)

indicate the presence or absence of pathology within the thoracic wall, lungs, and mediastinum, but it may be difficult to differentiate soft tissue structures and determine the exact location of disease. Ultrasonography is extremely useful for imaging patients that have pleural effusions, mediastinal disease, and lung lobe consolidation and in patients with mass lesions. Both ultrasound and computed tomography (CT) can be used to obtain fine needle aspirates and needle core biopsies, which can be submitted for cytology, histopathology, and bacteriologic/fungal culture and sensitivity (Fig. 41-5). The three-dimensional imaging techniques, especially CT, have made a significant impact on managing feline thoracic disease (Figs 41-6 and 41-7). CT is more sensitive in detecting metastatic pulmonary disease than radiography and localization of thoracic disease makes surgical planning and choice of thoracotomy approach easier. Due to the more accurate lesion localization afforded, more animals are likely to undergo lateral thoracotomy than median sternotomy if CT is available.

PREPARATION FOR THORACIC SURGERY

Before surgery is ever undertaken, it is vital to recognize the cases in which appropriate medical management of the disease before surgery is likely to improve clinical parameters (e.g., allowing time for pulmonary contusions to improve following trauma) and in such cases this should always be performed. Likewise, the attending clinician should also recognize cases in which rapid surgical intervention is required as soon as the cat is cardiovascularly stable or as stable as can be achieved (e.g., clinically significant intrathoracic hemorrhage following trauma).

Depending upon the disease process for which thoracotomy is being performed, cats may have an American Society of Anesthesiologists (ASA) score varying from ASA 2–3 (a patient with mild to severe systemic disease, e.g., patent ductus arteriosus) to ASA 5 (a moribund patient in whom surgery is performed in desperation due to the life-threatening nature of their disease). Extreme care must be taken to try to prevent deterioration of clinical parameters during induction and maintenance of anesthesia. As previously described, a period of pre-oxygenation (e.g., five minutes) can be beneficial in most cases.

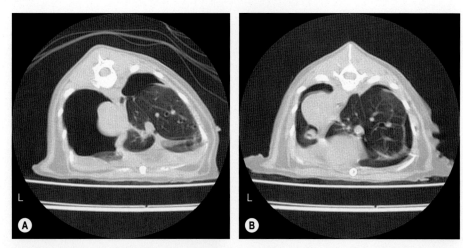

Figure 41-6 CT images of a cat that had presented with increased respiratory sounds and coughing. Two CT studies are shown **(A)** before and **(B)** after drainage of pneumothorax and these demonstrate the importance of thoracocentesis for improving lung expansion. (A) Bilateral pneumothorax. It is more marked on the left, with a collapsed lung lobe ventrally and air surrounding a left caudal lung lobe mass. There is moderate air present in the dorsal right hemithorax. (B) After drainage there is significant reduction in pleural air present, with increased expansion of the right middle, accessory and left cranial lung lobes. There is mediastinal shift of the left caudal lung lobe containing the mass and no air within this lung lobe. *(© Alison Moores.)*

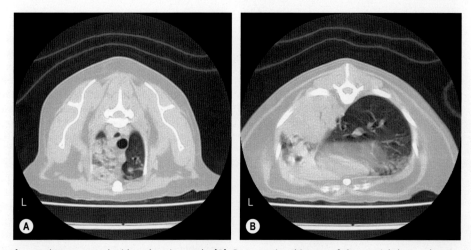

Figure 41-7 CT images of a cat that presented with a chronic cough. **(A)** Cross-sectional image of the cranial thorax showing a generalized, heterogenous, alveolar/bronchial infiltrate of the cranial part of the left cranial lung lobe, with a concurrent ill-defined nodular soft tissue infiltrate. On the right there is a nodular soft tissue lesion ventrally. **(B)** Cross-sectional image of the caudal thorax showing an ill-defined left caudal lung lobe soft tissue mass with the same ill-defined margin of heterogenous alveolar/bronchial infiltrate and nodular soft tissue infiltrate as seen in the previous CT image. Differential diagnoses include pulmonary neoplasia with pulmonary metastasis or severe inflammatory disease, which can be evaluated further by cytology or histopathology. *(© Alison Moores.)*

The correct choice of which premedicant and induction agent to use is vital, to allow the induction of anesthesia with minimum stress, whilst avoiding excessive respiratory or cardiac depression.[1] Intravenous induction, establishing a patent airway, and being able to ventilate if necessary, are all instrumental to safe induction of anesthesia. Intraoperative monitoring is also extremely important and should include serial monitoring of heart and respiratory rate, pulse oximetry, capnography, ECG, and core body temperature. Mechanical ventilation is required during thoracotomy, and also in laparotomies where the diaphragm is not intact, as opening the pleural space very significantly restricts effective natural ventilation. Mechanical ventilation may also be required prior to surgery when the underlying disease prevents effective chest excursions. Mechanical ventilators are easily applied to cats (Fig. 41-8), but careful manual ventilation is also acceptable. Care must be taken not to apply too much pressure during ventilation as this can cause lung damage.

Thoracotomy can lead to significant fluid and heat loss, and this can be especially relevant in cats due to their small body size, hence the need for regular monitoring of the patient's core body temperature. Warming methods, such as the use of warm fluids, bubble wrap application to extremities, warm air heating systems (e.g., Bair Hugger, 3M), low fresh gas flows, and heat/moisture exchangers (e.g., Thermovent) should all be considered and utilized whenever necessary. Keeping anesthetic and surgical times to a minimum can be very helpful in this regard and excessive wetting of the skin and hair is avoided during preoperative preparation and thoracic lavage.

One of the major limiting factors to successful surgery is small patient size, but it is aided by the use of fine instruments. Additional instruments that will be helpful for thoracic surgery are listed in Box 41-3 (and see Chapter 13). These include vascular clamps for the control of hemorrhage from large vessels, such as the pulmonary artery, as well as diathermy for hemorrhage from smaller vessels.

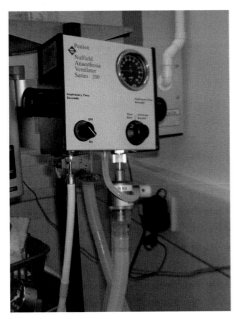

Figure 41-8 Mechanical ventilator. (© *Alison Moores; The Nuffield 200 Ventilator is produced by Penlon Ltd, Abingdon, UK.*)

Table 41-3 Intercostal approach for selected thoracic procedures[6]

Procedure or organ	Intercostal approach
Vascular anomaly (PDA, PRAA)[a]	Left 4
Pericardium	Left or right 5
Trachea/carina	5
Cranial lung lobectomy	4-5
Middle lung lobectomy	Right 5
Caudal lung lobectomy	5-6
Cranial esophagus	Left 3-4, Right 3-5
Caudal esophagus	Left or right 7-9
Thoracic duct	Left 8-10

[a]PDA, patent ductus arteriosus; PRAA, persistent right aortic arch.

Multimodal analgesia is employed, and a typical protocol would include perioperative systemic non-steroidal anti-inflammatory drugs (NSAIDs), opiates (e.g., methadone, fentanyl), and intercostal or regional sternal local anesthesia, followed by postoperative NSAIDs, opiates (e.g., methadone, buprenorphine), and interpleural local anesthesia for the duration of use of a thoracostomy tube[5] (see Chapter 2).

Lateral or intercostal thoracotomy

Intercostal thoracotomy (Box 41-4) allows access to approximately one-third of the ipsilateral hemithorax for treatment of vascular anomalies, pulmonary disease (lung lobectomy) and esophageal, tracheal or mediastinal disease. Rib resection thoracotomy has not been specifically described for cats but can be used to increase exposure via a lateral thoracotomy.

Intercostal thoracotomy can usually be performed faster in cats than dogs due to the smaller average incision length, thinner muscles, and less intraoperative bleeding associated with incision of the latissimus dorsi muscle in particular. Determining where to make the incision is dependent on the indication for surgery and the location of the lesion (Table 41-3). For those organs that traverse the length of the thoracic cavity, e.g. esophagus or trachea, radiography or CT should be used to help determine the appropriate intercostal space for maximal exposure.

To approach the thoracic cavity, the latissimus dorsi muscle can either be divided or retracted dorsally. With the latter technique the latissimus dorsi can more effectively be used to help provide an air-tight seal during closure and may result in less pain postoperatively. However, retraction of this muscle may result in a more limited thoracic exposure compared with incision, which might be a disadvantage in certain cases. Additionally, retraction is more difficult in cases where there is no surgical assistant.

Median sternotomy

Median sternotomy (Box 41-5) was first reported in cats in 1996 and described as a technically demanding procedure.[3] Median sternotomy offers excellent exposure of both hemithoraces, with access to the lungs, heart, and mediastinum. It is also the approach of choice where the location of intrathoracic disease cannot be determined,

---

Box 41-3 Useful instruments and implants for thoracic surgery in cats

Self-retaining retractors, e.g., Gelpi, Finochietto
DeBakey tissue forceps
Right-angled forceps for dissection, e.g., Mixter
Vascular clamps, e.g., Satinsky
Chest drains and adapters

Use of surgical stapling devices (see Chapter 10) is less frequent than in the dog, due in part to difficulty in placing large stapling units into the chest. Staples can be used for lobar or partial lung lobectomy, which is described in Chapter 47. Appropriate clamps should be available for placement on major blood vessels in the event of hemorrhage, which can be rapid and potentially fatal should it occur.

SURGICAL TECHNIQUES

Thoracotomy and thoracoscopy are performed to access the thoracic cavity for treatment (and/or diagnosis) of thoracic wall disease (e.g., thoracic bite wounds), pleural space disease (e.g., pyothorax, chylothorax), pulmonary disease (e.g., neoplasia, abscess), mediastinal disease (e.g., thymoma), tracheal, and esophageal disease. The incidence of thoracotomy is less in cats than dogs in referral centers,[2–4] although this may reflect fewer feline referrals rather than a lower incidence of surgical thoracic diseases in cats.

The choice of surgical approach is determined primarily by access required to the thorax. Lateral thoracotomy is sufficient if access to a limited and specific area of a hemithorax is required, but for complete thoracic exploration median sternotomy (or rarely, multiple lateral thoracotomies) is indicated. Transdiaphragmatic access to the thorax is discussed in Chapter 45.

Box 41-4 **Intercostal thoracotomy**

Following anesthesia, cats are placed in lateral recumbency. Hair is clipped from the lateral aspect of the thorax from the dorsal to ventral midline, lateral cervical region, proximal thoracic limb, and lateral aspect of the cranial abdomen. The thoracic limbs are pulled and secured cranially. A sandbag placed under the thorax increases exposure by elevating the operative hemithorax and provides improved opening of the thoracotomy incision by widening the intercostal spaces (Fig. 41-9A). It can be removed from under the cat at the end of the thoracic procedure to aid in closing the thoracotomy incision. Sandbags used as positioning aids should not interfere with the placement of air warming devices.

An incision is made over the predetermined intercostal space (see Table 41-3). The location of the initial skin incision is found by counting from the 13th rib cranially. As it is possible for cats to have more or less than the normal 13 ribs, this should be confirmed before surgery by counting ribs on the preoperative radiographs or CT. Following a skin incision from the dorsal thorax to the costochondral junction (Fig. 41-9B), a combination of sharp and blunt dissection is used to separate the subcutaneous tissue and incise the cutaneous trunci muscle. Small blood vessels are coagulated and Gelpi retractors are placed in the wound. The latissimus dorsi muscle is sharply incised or retracted dorsally as described above (Fig. 41-9C,D). Re-confirmation of the correct intercostal space can be made by counting caudally from the cranial ribs, from underneath the latissimus dorsi muscle and thoracic limb, for cranial approaches, and counting from the 13th rib for caudal approaches. Additionally, the fifth rib can be identified by the caudal insertion of the scalenus muscle or the cranial origin of the external abdominal oblique muscles. Either is usually transected to improve ventral exposure. The serratus ventralis muscle is separated in the dorsal part of the wound is separated between individual bellies, small blood vessels are coagulated and Gelpi retractors are repositioned (Fig. 41-9E). The external and internal intercostal muscles are incised midway between the ribs, with the incision continuing as far dorsal and ventral as necessary for adequate exposure (Fig. 41-9F). The dorsal incision is limited by the tubercle of the ribs and the ventral limit by the internal thoracic vasculature located ventral to the costochondral junction. Care is taken to avoid the neurovascular bundle on the caudal aspect of the rib and a smaller vessel on the cranial aspect.

It may be difficult to incise the intercostal muscles without penetrating the parietal pleura, but pleural incision must be performed with care to avoid damage to underlying structures, e.g., lung or mediastinal mass. It may be prudent to stop ventilation for a few seconds during initial pleural penetration, after which the lungs should retract from the thoracic wall and subsequent lung damage is unlikely. Moistened 10 cm × 10 cm swabs or laparotomy swabs are placed over the wound edges for protection. Thoracic exposure is obtained by replacing the Gelpi retractors between the ribs or by using small Finochietto rib retractors or abdominal retractors (Fig. 41-9G–I). The incision is lengthened dorsally and/or ventrally as necessary to increase exposure. Care is taken not to tear tissues during thoracic wall retraction.

A thoracostomy tube (see Boxes 41-6, 41-7 and 41-8) may be used if ongoing air or fluid production is anticipated and also for postoperative monitoring for complications that may result in air or fluid production. Thoracotomy closure has been described using interrupted circumcostal sutures of polydioxanone (PDS II, Ethicon) or polyglactin 910 (Vicryl, Ethicon),[4] although the author prefers the former due to its prolonged tensile strength. Sutures are preplaced with care with the blunt end of the needle passed through the intercostal space in close proximity to the rib in order to minimize nerve entrapment and damage to the intercostal vessels (Fig. 41-10A). An assistant can apply tension to the central sutures to approximate the ribs as the surgeon ties the other sutures in turn (Fig. 41-10B). Alternatively, sutures can be held with a pair of Galibans forceps during knot tying (see Chapter 13). Overlapping of adjacent ribs is avoided, although this does not seem to be a clinical problem if it occurs. The serratus ventralis and scalenus muscles are closed in one layer (Fig. 41-10C). The thoracic cavity is usually sealed at this stage, so drainage via the thoracostomy tube or thoracocentesis can be performed to allow the cat to be weaned from ventilation. There is subsequent closure of the latissimus dorsi and cutaneous trunci muscles, subcutaneous fascia (using a continuous suture pattern), and finally skin closure, followed by repeated drainage of the thoracic cavity (Fig. 41-10D,E).

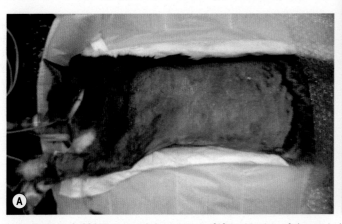

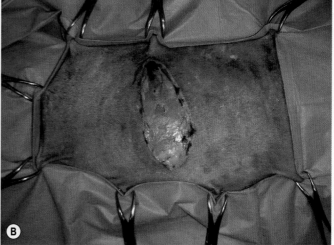

Figure 41-9 Left fifth intercostal thoracotomy. **(A)** Positioning of the cat in lateral recumbency with a sandbag under the thorax. **(B)** Initial skin incision.

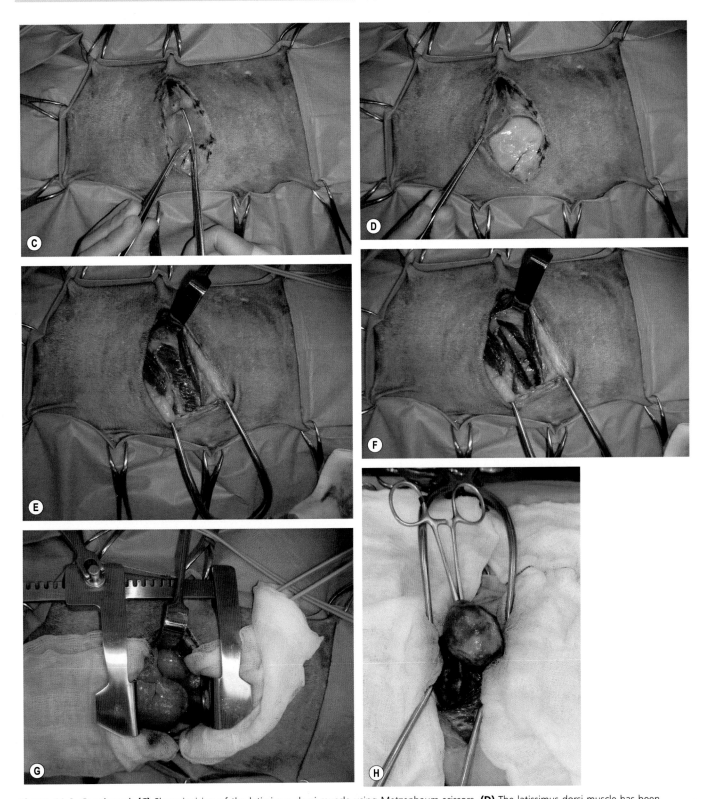

Figure 41-9, Continued **(C)** Sharp incision of the latissimus dorsi muscle using Metzenbaum scissors. **(D)** The latissimus dorsi muscle has been transected along half of its length. This can be extended dorsally as necessary for exposure of the thoracic cavity. **(E)** The serratus ventralis muscle has been separated between two of its bellies and retracted to expose the external intercostal muscle. **(F)** The external and internal intercostal muscles and pleura have been incised to expose the thoracic cavity. **(G)** Swabs are placed over the wound edges before placing Finochietto rib retractors. The latissimus dorsi muscle is retracted dorsally. **(H)** Alternatively, one or two pairs of Gelpi retractors can be used for rib retraction. In this case the cat is undergoing lung lobe resection for treatment of a pulmonary carcinoma. Laparotomy swabs to protect the wound edges are bulky in cats. A clamp is positioned on the bronchus proximal to the affected lung lobe.

although this is less common with the advent of three-dimensional imaging procedures. Difficulty in accessing dorsal structures is not as pronounced as in the average sized dog. Nine cats over a four-year period at a large referral center underwent surgery for the treatment of mediastinal masses (three cats), cor triatrium dexter, a pulmonary mass, a suspected esophageal stricture, chylothorax, pleural effusion and segmental tracheal stenosis (one of each).[3] All but one cat had a complete sternotomy, defined as complete sectioning of all sternebrae including the manubrium and xiphoid, leaving the xiphoid cartilage intact. Some surgeons will also section the xiphoid cartilage. One cat had cranial median sternotomy which included sectioning the manubrium and up to four sternebrae.

Disadvantages of this procedure compared to intercostal thoracotomy include prolonged surgical time and technical difficulty.

Thoracostomy tubes

Thoracostomy tubes are used to remove fluid or air from the thoracic cavity, due to an underlying disease process or following surgery (Boxes 41-6, 41-7 and 41-8, Fig. 41-13). It is the author's opinion that thoracostomy tubes are less well tolerated in cats than dogs, and may be associated with pain and depression. There is a recent report describing the use of small-bore wire-guided chest drains applied using a Seldinger technique.[7] This offers a viable and safe alternative to the commonly used trocar tubes and is even able to drain purulent material if used in conjunction with thoracic lavage.

Following completion of a thoracic surgical procedure, there will be residual air within the thoracic cavity and there may be the risk of ongoing air or fluid production due to the underlying disease. For those cases where there is not expected to be ongoing losses e.g., correction of a vascular anomaly or repair of a diaphragmatic defect, thoracocentesis may be sufficient to remove residual air from the thorax after a thoracic seal is achieved by wound closure. Where ongoing losses are expected, or monitoring for such potential complications required, a thoracostomy tube is inserted prior to thoracic closure (see Boxes 41-6, 41-7 and 41-8).

Tubes placed in dogs and cats after lateral thoracotomy were maintained for longer in animals with pre-existing pleural, mediastinal or pulmonary disease than those with vascular anomalies in one study.[4] Tubes were maintained in the nine cats surviving surgery for a median of 12 hours (range 20 minutes to three days;[4] unpublished data).

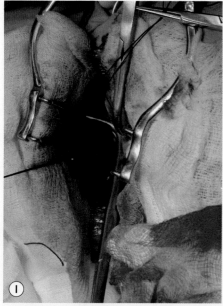

Figure 41-9, Continued **(I)** Abdominal retractors can be used during intercostal thoracotomy. Silk ligatures are being placed for removal of a lung lobe. *(A–H © Alison Moores; © Davina Anderson.)*

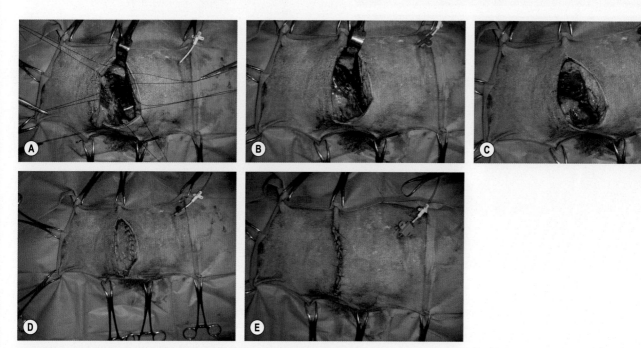

Figure 41-10 Closure of a left fifth intercostal thoracotomy. **(A)** Sutures have been preplaced circumcostally taking care to avoid intercostal vessels. **(B)** Circumcostal sutures are tied taking care not to overlap the ribs. **(C)** Closure of the serratus ventralis and scalenus muscles. **(D)** Closure of the latissimus dorsi muscle. **(E)** Closure of the skin. Note the progressive securing of a small-bore catheter which has been performed by an assistant during thoracotomy closure. *(© Alison Moores.)*

Box 41-5 **Median sternotomy**

Following anesthesia cats are placed in dorsal recumbency. Hair is clipped from the ventral and lateral aspects of the thorax as well as the ventral cervical region, proximal thoracic limbs, and cranial abdomen. Sufficient hair is removed from the lateral thorax to allow placement of thoracostomy tube(s). Routine skin preparation is performed. The cat is maintained in dorsal recumbency with the thoracic limbs pulled cranially. Sandbags used as positioning aids should not interfere with air warming devices where used.

Median sternotomy in the cat involves a midline ventral thoracic incision through the skin and subcutaneous tissue, from cranial to the manubrium to caudal to the xiphoid for complete median sternotomy. Unipolar electrocautery can be used to divide the pectoral muscles on the midline to expose the sternebrae,[3] although a suitable alternative would be sharp incision followed by use of monopolar or bipolar electrocautery to control hemorrhage. The use of electrocautery to make a groove in the midline of the sternebrae prior to sternebrae separation using an oscillating saw has been described (Fig. 41-11A).[3] The author prefers use of a scalpel blade to mark the sternebrae incision as it offers better control of the saw on the narrow bones. Alternatives to an oscillating saw include a sternal saw or use of a hammer and osteotome, or liston bone cutters. Use of a hammer and osteotome is often avoided in dogs due to the large volume of hemorrhage from the bones, but this is less of a problem in cats. Sternebrae division in cats must be performed with a high degree of precision. The bones are very narrow, such that deviation of the saw or osteotome from the midline is likely to lead to fracture through the lateral aspect of the sternebrae. Whilst this does not tend to cause problems with healing in the author's experience, it is best avoided. Similarly, excessive retraction of a partial sternotomy incision is likely to cause sternebral fracture; if increased exposure is required it would be prudent to convert to a complete median sternotomy rather than

risk fracture. Care is taken on entering the thoracic cavity, especially where there is a ventral mass such as a thymoma, to avoid hemorrhage or tissue damage.

Exposure of the thoracic cavity can be achieved using small Finochietto rib retractors, although Gelpi or handheld retractors can be used more easily than in dogs (Fig. 41-11B,C and Fig. 41-12). The wound edge is protected with moistened swabs. In small cats, a 10 cm × 10 cm swab is opened out and layered under the retractors. In larger cats laparotomy swabs can be used without hindering exposure.

Closure

A thoracostomy tube is placed as some ongoing air or fluid production is anticipated (see Boxes 41-6, 41-7 and 41-8). Closure of sternotomy wounds is described using preplaced 3.5M sutures of polypropylene (Prolene, Ethicon) in a figure-of-eight pattern,[3] although this author has also used polydioxanone (PDS II, Ethicon) or equivalent sutures. Studies of wire closure of sternotomy in dogs show figure-of-eight patterns cause the least displacement of sternebrae at high loads;[6] no such studies exist in the cat.

Reapposition of the pectoral muscles must be accurately performed to provide air-tight closure of the wound and to cover the large knots associated with using large gauge sutures for sternebral closure. Suture options include polydioxanone (PDS II, Ethicon) or polyglactin 910 (Vicryl, Ethicon), although the author prefers the former as it has prolonged tensile strength. Following pectoral muscle apposition and creation of an air-tight seal, thoracic cavity drainage can be achieved by thoracocentesis or via thoracostomy tube drainage where present. Evacuation of the thoracic cavity is required to allow spontaneous breathing and weaning from the ventilator if used. Closure of the subcutis and skin is routine.

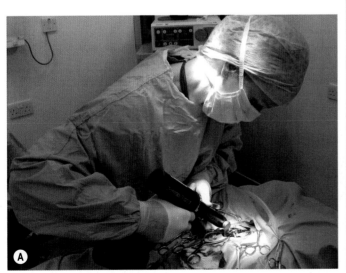
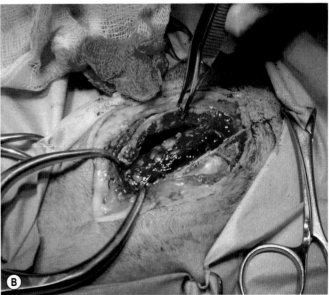

Figure 41-11 Median sternotomy for resection of thymoma. **(A)** Use of an oscillating saw for sternal osteotomy. **(B)** Cut edge of the sternebrae after median sternotomy. Note the position of the Gelpi retractors retracting the pectoral muscles.

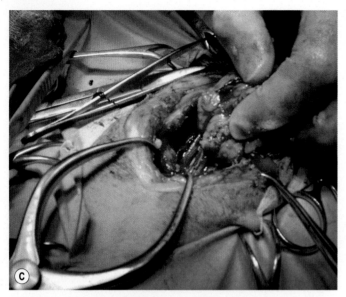

Figure 41-11, Continued (C) Gelpi retractors have been repositioned for retraction of the sternebrae. *(A–C, © Davina Anderson.)*

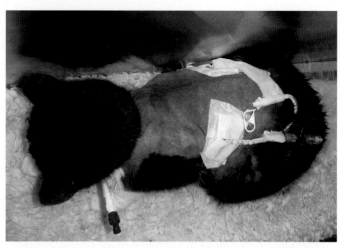

Figure 41-13 A cat with bilateral large-bore thoracostomy tubes for the treatment of pyothorax. The tubes are held closed with a plastic gate clamp and an adapter, three-way tap and bungs secure the end of the tube; the three-way tap and bung are changed daily. There is also an esophageal feeding tube. When left unsupervised the cat must wear an Elizabethan collar. *(© Alison Moores.)*

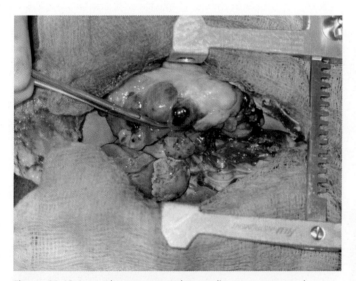

Figure 41-12 In another cat, a complete median sternotomy and retraction with Finochietto retractors provides wide exposure of the thoracic cavity. *(© Alison Moores.)*

Box 41-6 **Thoracostomy tube placement during thoracic surgery**

The tube is usually inserted via a skin incision over the dorsal third of the tenth to eleventh intercostal space, under the latissimus dorsi muscle and into the thoracic cavity at the seventh to eighth intercostal space. Tube placement is often more ventral if placed during sternotomy for practical reasons. The tube is inserted cranial to the rib to avoid damaging neurovascular structures on the caudal aspect of the rib. The tube is advanced to the second intercostal space under direct visualization from the thoracotomy incision and secured to the skin by a friction (finger trap) suture. An adapter, three-way tap, bungs, and small gate clamp are applied to the tube. The tube is left open until an air-tight seal is obtained on the thoracotomy/sternotomy incision to avoid tension pneumothorax formation.

Box 41-7 **Placement of a large-bore trocar thoracostomy tube**

Tube placement generally requires heavy sedation or anesthesia except in moribund cats. The cat is placed in lateral recumbency and the lateral thorax is clipped and aseptically prepared. The tube is placed using aseptic technique.

A skin incision is made over the ninth to tenth intercostal space. The trocar is passed through the skin incision and pushed through the underlying subcutaneous fascia and latissimus dorsi muscle. The tube is then tunneled cranially by one or two intercostal spaces, stopping on the cranial aspect of the rib to avoid the neurovascular bundle on the caudal aspect of the rib.

The tube is then held perpendicular to the skin and gripped firmly with one hand adjacent to the thoracic wall to avoid complete penetration of the thorax whilst pushing firmly on the end of the tube to penetrate the intercostal muscles and pleura. This may be difficult in the cat due to thoracic wall compliance. The tube is advanced over the trocar, which is then removed. The tube is directed cranially to approximately the second intercostal space. Placement is checked by aspiration of air or fluid and the tube is secured to skin with a friction suture.

A radiograph is taken to confirm position. The tube is adjusted or replaced as necessary, only if this can be done without breaking aseptic technique. If aseptic technique has not been maintained during radiography the tube cannot be advanced into the chest and if the tube were not in an appropriate position a new tube would then have to be placed.

The tube entry site is covered with a dressing and the tube protected with a bandage or netting vest (see Chapter 4). The cat is monitored at all times when the drain is in place. The use of an Elizabethan collar should always be considered to prevent the cat damaging or removing the tube.

Traditionally, tubes were maintained until air and/or fluid production was <2 mL/kg/day. Whilst a recent paper suggests that tubes can be removed when fluid production is higher than this, only ten cats (of which only two were postsurgical patients) were included in the study population.[8] No tube complications were noted in the nine postsurgical cats described by the author, whilst the aforementioned study reported premature removal (three of 26) and discharge around the tube (one of 26).[8]

Small-bore wire-guided chest drain placement

Placement of small-bore wire-guided drains (see Box 41-8) is easier to perform than wide-bore tubes and can easily be performed even by newly qualified veterinarians.[7] There are few complications with insertion and tubes are well tolerated. They can be placed as an alternative to needle thoracocentesis in those cats that object to thoracocentesis or if pleural fluid is difficult to drain with a needle. Sedation

---

Box 41-8 Placement of a small-bore (14G, 20 cm) wire-guided chest drain

The cat is placed in lateral or sternal recumbency and the lateral thorax is clipped and aseptically prepared. The tube is placed using aseptic technique

An optional skin incision is made over the ninth intercostal space. The introducer catheter is inserted through the thoracic wall directly into the pleural space or after tunneling subcutaneously by one or two intercostal spaces in a cranial direction (Fig. 41-14A). Entry along the caudal aspect of the rib is avoided to prevent damage to the intercostal neurovascular bundle. The introducer is advanced over the stylet, which is then removed (Fig. 41-14B). The J-guidewire is threaded through the introducer by 10 cm in a cranioventral direction (Fig. 41-14C) and the introducer catheter is removed over the wire (Fig. 41-14D). The chest tube is advanced over the guidewire into the cranial pleural space and the wire is removed (Fig. 41-14E-G). Placement is checked by aspiration

of air or fluid. The catheter is secured to the skin through the catheter suture holes using nylon (Fig. 41-10E). Excess tubing is secured with a friction suture if necessary.

The tube entry site is covered with a dressing and the tube protected with a bandage or netting vest (see Chapter 4). A radiograph is taken to confirm position. It is adjusted or replaced as necessary only if this can be done without breaking aseptic technique. If aseptic technique has not been maintained during radiography the tube cannot be advanced into the chest and if the tube were not in an appropriate position a new tube would have to be placed.

The cat is monitored at all times when the drain is in place. The use of an Elizabethan collar should always be considered to prevent the cat damaging or removing the tube.

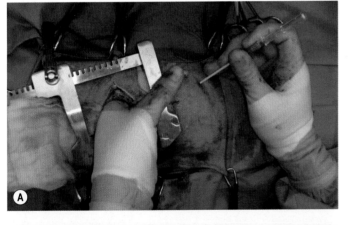
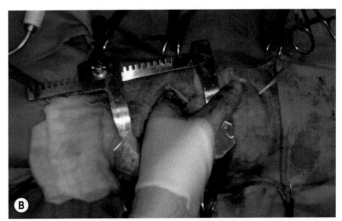
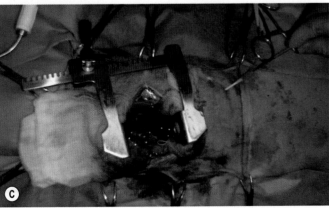
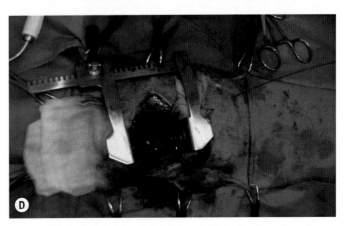

Figure 41-14 Placement of a small-bore wire-guided chest drain during thoracotomy. **(A)** An introducer catheter is inserted into the thoracic cavity. **(B)** The introducer is advanced over the stylet. The stylet is removed. **(C)** A guidewire is placed through the catheter and advanced into the thoracic cavity. **(D)** The catheter is removed leaving the wire in the thoracic cavity.

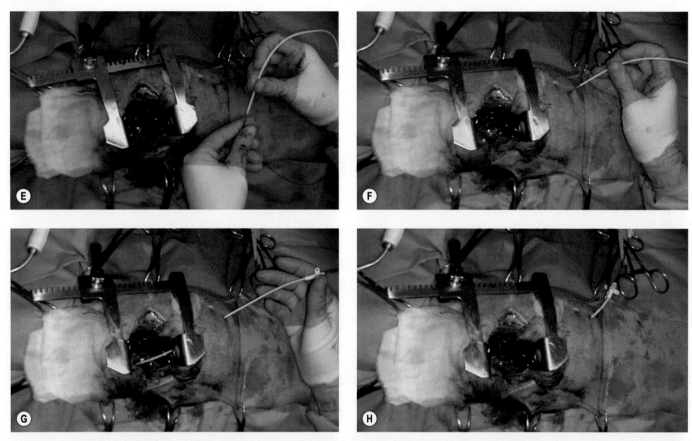

Figure 41-14, Continued (E–G) The small-bore tube is advanced over the wire into the cranial thoracic cavity. **(H)** The wire is removed and the tube can be secured to the thoracic wall. (© *Alison Moores.*)

with ketamine/midazolam or ketamine/butorphanol is usually sufficient.[7]

POSTOPERATIVE CARE

Ongoing oxygenation may be necessary in the postoperative period and can be provided using the same methods previously described (Fig. 41-15). Suction of the airway may be necessary to remove fluid (e.g., blood, pus), depending upon the surgical procedure performed (Fig. 41-16).

Cats may have thoracostomy tubes placed as part of the thoracic surgery; tube maintenance and care will play an important and significant part of the postoperative care. Postoperative nursing care including thoracostomy tube care is described in Chapter 4.

Thoracic surgery is painful and provision should be made for continuation of analgesia postoperatively. In addition to systemic analgesia, regional anesthesia can be provided with local anesthetic injections (Chapter 2). Intrapleural analgesia that produces ipsilateral somatic blocks of multiple thoracic dermatomes provides analgesia for up to 12 hours. Epidural analgesia can also be used to provide analgesia for thoracic surgery.[9] Infusion of analgesia into the thoracic cavity can be performed if there is a thoracostomy tube in place. Multimodal systemic pain relief is continued unless specifically contra-indicated (see Chapter 2). When performing thoracic wall surgery in people, it has been suggested that there is less postoperative pain after performing a muscle sparing approach by retracting the latissimus dorsi muscle

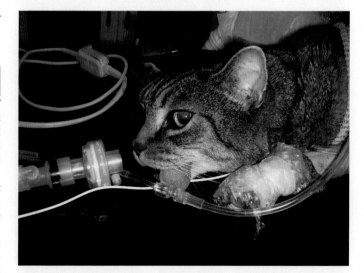

Figure 41-15 Flow-by oxygen is provided during recovery from anesthesia. (© *Alison Moores.*)

dorsally instead of incising it; this has not been investigated in animals. Closure of the thoracotomy should be performed by encircling the ribs, with the blunt end of the needle passed through the intercostal space, in close proximity to the rib in order to minimize nerve entrapment. It is important not to over-tighten the sutures to avoid subluxation of the ribs with subsequent pain.[10]

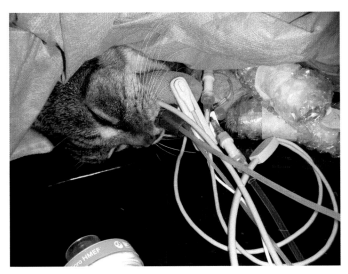

Figure 41-16 Suction of the airways may be necessary if there is fluid within the trachea, e.g., blood and pus. *(© Alison Moores.)*

Animals with indwelling thoracostomy tubes are monitored continuously, an Elizabethan collar is utilized and the drain is kept covered with dressings to prevent patient interference and inadvertent removal. The tube is kept covered with a sterile dressing and a bandage to minimize environmental contamination. Personnel handling the tube must wash their hands appropriately, wear gloves, and use a new syringe each time the tube is drained to avoid contamination. Three-way taps and clamps on the end of tubing are changed daily.

COMPLICATIONS AND PROGNOSIS

Survival to discharge of 85% was reported in 41 cats undergoing thoracic surgery, although the thoracic approaches were not reported and most cats were treated for diaphragmatic rupture, which is often classified as abdominal surgery rather than thoracic surgery.[2]

Intercostal thoracotomy

Of thirteen cats treated via an intercostal thoracotomy, nine survived to discharge (62%) and four were euthanized during surgery due to the underlying diseases.[4] Survival to discharge was significantly lower in cats than in dogs, older animals, and cats and dogs with neoplastic disease rather than non-neoplastic disease. There was no difference in the overall incidence of short-term complications between species, although complications attributed to the intercostal thoracotomy did not occur in cats (Moores, unpublished data) compared to complications such as seroma and excessive wound inflammation in 28/70 dogs.

Median sternotomy

In a short case-series there were no complications associated with median sternotomy thoracotomy,[3] although the severity of the underlying disease processes led to intraoperative euthanasia in three cats and early postoperative death of one cat. These authors also suggest that, with the use of regional local and parenteral analgesia, the procedure is not associated with excessive postoperative pain as has previously been suggested.

REFERENCES

1. Kaestner S. Anesthesia. In: Montavon PM, Voss K, Langley-Hobbs SJ, editors. Feline orthopedic surgery and musculoskeletal disease. Elsevier Edinburgh; 2009a. p. 177–98.
2. Bellenger CR, Hunt GB, Goldsmid SE, Pearson MR. Outcomes of thoracic surgery in dogs and cats. Aust Vet J 1996;74(1):25–30.
3. Burton CA, White RN. Review of the technique and complications of median sternotomy in the dog and cat. J Small Anim Pract 1996;37(11):516–22.
4. Moores AL, Halfacree ZJ, Baines SJ, Lipscomb VJ. Indications, outcomes and complications following lateral thoracotomy in dogs and cats. J Small Anim Pract 2007;48(12):695–8.
5. Kaestner S. Analgesia. In: Montavon PM, Voss K, Langley-Hobbs SJ, editors. Feline orthopedic surgery and musculoskeletal disease. Elsevier Edinburgh; 2009b. p. 199–205.
6. Davis KM, Roe SC, Mathews KG, Mente PL. Median sternotomy closure in dogs: a mechanical comparison of technique stability. Vet Surg 2006;35(3):271–7.
7. Valtolina C, Adamantos S. Evaluation of small-bore wire-guided chest drains for management of pleural space disease. J Small Anim Pract 2009;50(6): 290–7.
8. Marques AI, Tattersall J, Shaw DJ, Welsh E. Retrospective analysis of the relationship between time of thoracostomy drain removal and discharge time. J Small Anim Pract 2009;50(4):162–6.
9. Pavlidou K, Papazoglou L, Savvas I, Kazakos G. Analgesia for small animal thoracic surgery. Compend Contin Educ Vet 2009;9:432–6.
10. Rooney MB, Mehl M, Monnet E. Intercostal thoracotomy closure: transcostal sutures as a less painful alternative to circumcostal suture placement. Vet Surg 2004;33: 209–13.

Chapter |42|

Thoracoscopy

S.A. van Nimwegen, J. Kirpensteijn

There are limited descriptions of the use of thoracoscopy in cats for exploration, aspiration, and biopsy of intrathoracic tissues.[1-3] Cats are included in general texts based mainly on canine and human literature,[4-6] but specific procedural information is very sparse. Until recently however, the same was true for feline laparoscopic procedures (see Chapter 24), and there is no convincing reason not to assume that similar advantages of minimally invasive thoracic procedures apply to cats as they do to humans (including neonates of < 1 kg body weight[7]) and dogs. This chapter covers the principles of thoracoscopy in cats and describes selected surgical procedures.

BACKGROUND

Minimally invasive access to the thoracic cavity for thoracoscopic exploration and observation of intrathoracic tissues, biopsy of abnormal structures, or intrathoracic surgical procedures, also referred to as video-assisted thoracic surgery (VATS), has several advantages over conventional open thoracic procedures. Thoracotomy is associated with considerable intra- and postoperative pain, discomfort, and convalescence period, which are clearly reduced in humans when using a thoracoscopic approach[8,9] and there is also evidence to suggest the same applies to dogs.[10] Other advantages are the magnified and detailed view of intrathoracic tissues and the increased access to deep regions, which actually allows a more extensive and complete exposure of the thoracic cavity compared to open approaches. The number of applications of thoracoscopic surgery in dogs is rapidly increasing, and procedures such as the creation of a pericardial window or partial pericardectomy,[11,12] or thoracic duct ligation[13,14] are becoming the standard of care nowadays in several specialized institutions. In contrast, data on thoracoscopic surgery in cats is lacking. The number of possible thoracoscopic procedures in both dogs and cats is merely related to the surgeon's experience and skills and the willingness and creativity to convert these into an expanding range of VATS procedures. Companion animal minimally invasive surgery lags behind its human counterpart, which is primarily related to the associated costs of investment in equipment and surgical training. Nevertheless, considering the recent but revolutionary history of minimally invasive surgery in humans, both canine and feline minimally invasive surgery is likely to be increasingly applied in the near future. Moreover, the majority of advantages of minimally invasive surgery that have been described for humans are increasingly reported in veterinary patients. As with laparoscopy (see Chapter 24), the smaller average body size of cats compared to dogs requires dedicated equipment and skills, which may more often result in veterinary surgeons initially investing in minimally invasive surgery for canines rather than felines. This applies in particular to thoracoscopy, because the thorax does not expand as much as the abdominal wall does upon insufflation for laparoscopy, making the average feline thorax considerably smaller than an average canine thorax. The basic surgical principles of laparoscopic surgery also apply to thoracoscopic surgery (see Chapter 24).

ANESTHESIA

Anesthesia for thoracoscopy is essentially the same as for thoracotomy procedures, implying general anesthesia and mechanical intermittent positive pressure ventilation (IPPV). Extensive monitoring of physiologic parameters during thoracoscopy should be mandatory. In contrast to laparoscopy, insufflation of the thoracic cavity is usually not needed and not recommended because it carries the risk of significant hemodynamic compromise. Left hemithorax CO_2-insufflation using 2–5 mmHg intrathoracic pressures resulted in significant hemodynamic compromise in dogs[15,16] and is therefore advised to be used with great caution and with as low as possible pressure for as short as possible intervals.

In cats, such measurements have not been performed and intrathoracic insufflation should probably be discouraged. If established pneumothorax (after trocar placement) and altered ventilation settings (e.g., increasing ventilation rate and decreasing tidal volume) do not provide sufficient space for thoracoscopy, selective single-lung ventilation may improve the working space in one hemithorax, with less severe hemodynamic changes compared to intrathoracic insufflation.[17] One-lung ventilation is commonly applied in human thoracoscopic surgery and is considered a safe technique in dogs.[18] Again, such techniques have not been investigated in cats and caution is indicated. Single-lung ventilation can be established through selective endobronchial intubation or selective endobronchial blockade. Double lumen endobronchial tubes are too big for use in cats. Because of the relatively short distance between the branches of lobar bronchi in cats,[19] any cuff or balloon placed in a main stem bronchus may occlude branching bronchi, preventing ventilation of the cranial lung region using an endobronchial tube, especially on the right side.[20] Endobronchial blockade combined with ventilation through an endotracheal tube is commonly used in human pediatric thoracoscopy and may provide a more reliable solution to one-lung ventilation in cats.[21] However, selective endobronchial intubation or blockade is difficult to perform in cats, usually requiring endoscopic guidance using a flexible pediatric endoscope, and is not without risks. Fortunately, diagnostic thoracoscopy and most thoracoscopic procedures can be performed without single-lung ventilation.[4,7,11,13,22] At the authors' institution, thoracoscopic procedures in cats (and dogs) are performed commonly without single-lung ventilation. When required, surgical space can be increased by decreasing tidal volume in combination with an increase in ventilation rate, manual retraction of lung lobes away from the location of interest, and occasionally alternating brief periods of apnea in combination with periods of increased ventilation. Close cooperation and communication between the anesthetic and surgery teams is of major importance for thoracoscopic procedures.

EQUIPMENT, ENTRY TECHNIQUE AND CLOSURE

The equipment for thoracoscopic surgery is essentially the same as for laparoscopic surgery and is described in Chapter 24. It is even more essential in feline thoracoscopy than laparoscopy to use pediatric equipment. Trocars for thoracoscopy do not need valves or rubber washers because air should be able to enter and exit during ventilatory movements of the lungs. Dedicated thoracoscopic trocars (rigid or flexible) may be used, with blunt obturators. The same set of laparoscopic instruments can, however, also be used for thoracoscopy. The authors prefer to use threaded cannulas (most commonly the threaded laparoscopic cannulas) because of their controlled insertion, blunt tip, and firm grip in the thoracic wall (see Chapter 24). The part containing the internal valve and washer can be disconnected and removed, which also reduces cannula weight. Threaded cannulas are also very useful for initial entry into the thorax. The standard thoracoscopic entry point in lateral recumbency is in the 6th–8th intercostal space (ICS), midway between the costochondral junction and the epaxial muscles.[23] For a specific lesion, however, an entry point is selected which is a short distance away from it, to allow triangulation of the instruments and camera to the location of interest. For specific procedures, portal locations may differ depending on the size of the cat, to enable a triangulated approach. Several techniques can be used to establish pneumothorax and insert the primary trocar (Box 42-1).

Five millimeter or larger diameter instruments may be used through larger cannulas or directly through small intercostal incisions. In the case of a tumor resection or large biopsy, the use of a dedicated extraction bag or finger of a surgical glove for the removal of tissue samples suspected to be malignant may prevent port site metastasis. In many procedures, a thoracic drain is placed before closure. A drain is placed in a routine manner, tunneling through 3–4 cm subcutaneous tissue before penetrating the thoracic wall under thoracoscopic guidance. Portals are closed in two or three layers, depending on their size.

Box 42-1 **Establishing thoracoscopic entry portals**

Lateral recumbancy

Blunt mini-dissection approach for primary intercostal trocar placement: A small skin incision is made (slightly larger than the trocar diameter), the thoracic wall muscles are bluntly dissected and the parietal pleura is perforated with dissection forceps (mosquito, baby mixters, or Kelly forceps). By opening the pleura, air automatically flows into the thoracic cavity and the lungs fall away from the thoracic wall (pneumothorax). At this stage, a blunt trocar or threaded cannula can be inserted. Subsequent trocars are placed under thoracoscopic guidance. It is important to avoid the intercostal arteries running along the caudal border of each rib.

Direct primary intercostal trocar insertion: A technique that is often used for primary trocar insertion is blunt perforation of the thoracic wall through an initial small skin incision using a threaded cannula with a 0° rigid scope inserted to visualize perforation of the thoracic wall and pleura. After perforation of the pleura, air enters through the cannula into the thorax.

Dorsal recumbency

Direct primary paraxiphoid trocar insertion: Paraxiphoid trocar placement is the standard entry point in dorsal recumbency. A small skin incision is made to the right or left of the xiphoid process just caudal to the costal arch (e.g., for thoracoscopic pericardectomy, see Fig. 42-6). The threaded cannula is inserted with the endoscope mounted for visual control and gently 'screwed' through the abdominal wall and diaphragm (Fig. 42-1), slightly ventrally into the ipsilateral hemithorax. Both the left and right hemithorax can be explored using a paraxiphoid camera portal after creating a window in an avascular part of the mediastinum. In cats the mediastinum is often very thin and not filled with fat, making selective perforation relatively easy.

INDICATIONS

Thoracoscopy can be performed as a diagnostic technique or surgical approach. It is indicated in any case in which it can obviate the need for a thoracotomy or enhance a diagnostic or therapeutic procedure, provided that the surgeon has an adequate level of VATS skills. In the case of thoracic duct ligation combined with subtotal pericardectomy for idiopathic chylothorax, for instance, a thoracoscopic approach may even prevent a second thoracotomy.[24] Furthermore, VATS includes both complete thoracoscopic and thoracoscopic-assisted procedures. Thoracoscopy is contraindicated in patients with severe cardiorespiratory problems that cannot compensate for the respiratory changes inflicted by pneumothorax, such as severe cardiomyopathy or generalized lung disease requiring full utilization of tidal volume.

THORACOSCOPIC PROCEDURES

Exploration and biopsy of intrathoracic tissues

Thoracoscopic exploration can be performed for visualization and biopsy of tissues, such as lymph nodes, mediastinum, lungs,[10] pericardium, and mass lesions[9] (Fig. 42-2); for identification of underlying causes of pleural effusion[8] or spontaneous pneumothorax; and to evaluate or diagnose abnormalities found with diagnostic imaging

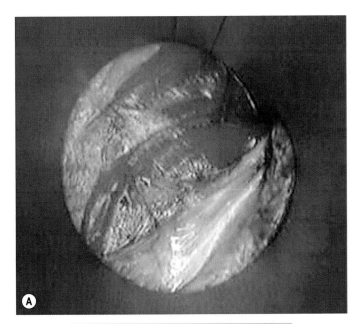

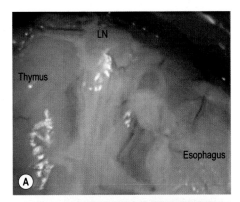

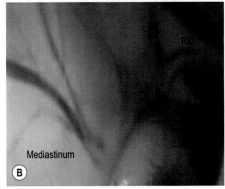

Figure 42-2 Images of thoracoscopic exploration of the left hemithorax of a cat with a persistent right aortic arch (PRAA). **(A)** Cranial view of the mediastinum with thymus, enlarged mediastinal lymph node (LN), and dilated esophagus. **(B)** Dorsal view of the aberrant mediastinum, caused by a dilated esophagus due to PRAA.

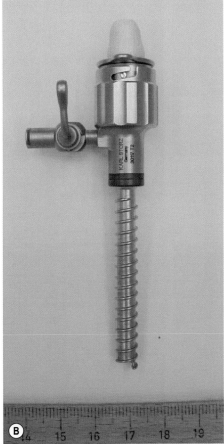

Figure 42-1 **(A)** Endoscopic image during blunt perforation of muscle and fascial layers using a threaded cannula. **(B)** Pediatric threaded cannula (3.9 mm inner diameter, centimeter scale included).

techniques, such as CT, ultrasound, or MRI (Fig. 42-3). Furthermore, thoracoscopic-assisted procedures can prevent more invasive surgery, such as thoracoscopic exploration in cases of thoracic trauma, avoiding the need for additional thoracotomies or contralateral thoracotomy (Fig. 42-4). For exploration of both thoracic compartments, a paraxiphoid camera portal with the patient in dorsal recumbency is most convenient. For exploration of one specific hemithorax, access to thoracic structures is enhanced with the patient in lateral recumbency. Biopsies of mass lesions, lymph nodes, and other non-respiratory tissues can be performed using biopsy cup forceps (Fig. 42-5; see also Chapter 24).

Biopsy of lung tissue can be performed using a pre-tied loop or extracorporeal tied ligature. The edge of a lung lobe to be biopsied is grasped with the endoscopic grasper through the pre-tied loop. The ligature is tied, ensuring that enough tissue is distal to the ligature to be able to cut a representative biopsy using scissors while enough tissue remains holding the ligature. Larger biopsies or partial lung lobectomy can be performed in a thoracoscopic-assisted approach, by exteriorizing the lung lobe through an enlarged portal and performing the partial lobectomy outside the thoracic cavity using sutures or stapler, without retracting the ribs. Endoscopic GIA staplers or linear stapler/cutters measure at least 10–12 mm in diameter and the smallest staple cartridge length is 30 mm, which requires at least 45–50 mm of space to be opened inside the thoracic cavity. Therefore, endoscopic linear staplers are too big to be used in thoracoscopic procedures in cats, but may be used in a thoracoscopic-assisted approach with enlargement of one portal to a keyhole thoracotomy to insert and open the stapler with minimal rib retraction. A lateral approach with the patient in lateral recumbency is required for partial or complete lung lobectomy. For cases involving the caudal lung lobe, the dorsal pulmonary ligament is transected using scissors and/or electrosurgery instruments.

Partial lobectomies in cats may also be performed using vessel sealer/divider devices, such as Ligasure, because these instruments can securely seal bronchi of at least 2 mm in diameter[25] and have been used successfully for pulmonary wedge resections in humans[26] and

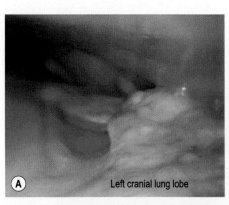
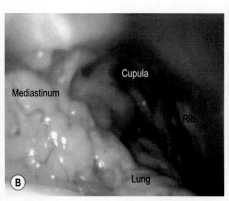
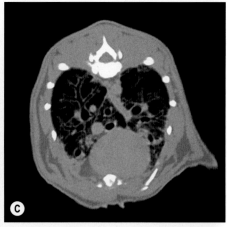

Figure 42-3 Exploratory thoracoscopy through a paraxiphoid camera port in a cat with widespread metastatic melanoma lesions in the pleura of the lungs and mediastinum. Images show the lungs and mediastinum of the left hemithorax. CT images showed marked bronchial changes and thickened pleurae and mediastinum, but not the typical signs of pulmonary metastasis.

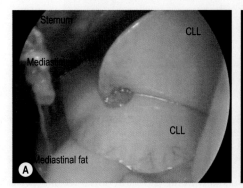
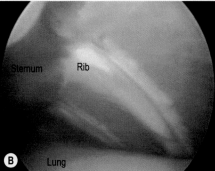
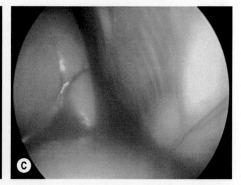

Figure 42-4 Thoracoscopic-assisted exploration of the thoracic cavity in a cat with multiple bite wounds and extensive perforative trauma of the caudal thorax and abdomen (in an open transdiaphragmatic approach to the thorax, cat in dorsal recumbency). Although extensive caudal thoracic wall trauma was present, intrathoracic trauma was limited to a single small distal lesion in the caudal part of the left cranial lung lobe (CLL), a torn mediastinum, subpleural hemorrhage (at the sternum), and self-limiting hemothorax.

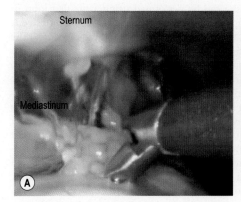
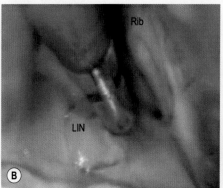
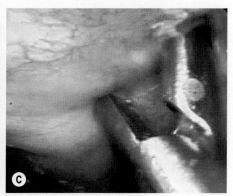

Figure 42-5 Cup forceps biopsy of a mediastinal mass. **(A)** a cranial sternal lymph node near the left cupula (middle), and a diffusely thickened parietal pleura **(B)**. Notice the thin (normal part of) mediastinum (left); cat in dorsal recumbency **(C)**.

dogs.[27] Main stem bronchi are considered too big for reliable sealing using a vessel sealer and are usually sutured intracorporally in human infants and neonates and small animals.[23,28,29] Complete lung lobectomies are considered to be difficult advanced VATS procedures,[30] and a thoracoscopic-assisted approach is generally advised in cats. When biopsying lungs for suspected malignancies, the hilar and sternal lymph nodes should also be inspected and biopsied as required.

Partial pericardectomy

The creation of a pericardial window may be indicated in cats with cardiac tamponade as a result of pericardial effusion. Partial, subphrenic (subtotal) pericardectomy may be indicated in cases of constrictive pericarditis or pericardial fibrosis (such as fibrosing pleuritis from prolonged existence of pleural effusion, infectious pericarditis, or neoplasia). Partial pericardectomy (Box 42-2) may be combined with thoracic duct ligation for treatment of idiopathic chylothorax in cats with subsequent fibrosing pleuritis.[24,31]

Thoracic duct ligation

Thoracic duct ligation (TDL) (Box 42-3) is performed as part of a treatment strategy in cats with chronic idiopathic chylothorax (see Chapter 44). TDL combined with subtotal pericardectomy may improve outcome in cases with pericardial fibrosis.[24,31] Apart from being minimally invasive, a VATS approach improves visualization of the thoracic duct.[6] In combination with pericardectomy, the VATS procedure may even prevent the need for two thoracotomies because a single open intercostal approach commonly does not allow adequate exposure of both the thoracic duct and pericardium for surgery.

Prior to surgery, it is helpful to visualize the thoracic duct using contrast CT or X-ray lymphangiography. Contrast fluid may be injected into a mesenteric lymph vessel,[6] which may, however, be difficult to cannulate in cats.[31] Other options are injection into a mesenteric lymph node or a popliteal lymph node.[34,35] Percutaneous ultrasound-guided mesenteric lymph node contrast injection was successful in dogs.[36] Lymphangiography can be repeated after surgery to investigate complete closure of the thoracic duct. During surgery, identification of thoracic duct branches can be greatly improved using a contrast fluid such as methylene blue injected in a mesenteric lymph vessel or lymph node.[31,37] In dogs, popliteal lymph node injection with methylene blue was less successful compared to injection into a mesenteric lymph node.[37] Such studies have not been performed in cats. However, identification of the thoracic duct may still be impaired because of chronic changes of the pleura and en-bloc ligation of all structures dorsal to the aorta and ventral to the sympathetic trunk may be necessary.

Additional procedures, such as thoracic omentalization, have not been proven to be of significant advantage.[38,39] Pleurodesis may be used in refractory cases of pleural effusion in humans. However, insufficient clinical data exists to support this treatment strategy in cats (and dogs).[31,40] The effectiveness of pleurodesis procedures is likely species-specific, considering the much more favorable results in humans compared to companion animals.[40–43] In dogs with idiopathic chylothorax, ablation of the cisterna chyli in addition to TDL may improve outcome.[44,45] The safety and efficacy of this treatment has not been investigated in cats.

Other procedures

Other VATS procedures that may be performed in cats in selected cases by experienced surgeons include the treatment of a persistent right aortic arch, occlusion of a patent ductus arteriosus, excision of pulmonary or other intrathoracic or mediastinal mass lesions, and treatment of diaphragmatic herniation.

COMPLICATIONS

Complications of VATS may be associated with pneumothorax, surgical technique, and the use of gas insufflation. Complications of increased intrathoracic pressures were discussed earlier in the chapter, but it is important to note that the effects of insufflating the thoracic cavity are much more severe compared to insufflation of the abdomen for laparoscopy. Initial (blind) access to the thoracic cavity carries a risk of complications such as damage to blood vessels and intrathoracic organs. It is therefore not recommended to use blind insertion

<table>
<tr><td>

Box 42-2 Partial pericardectomy

A left-paraxiphoid entry with the cat in dorsal recumbency is preferred for creation of a pericardial window or subtotal pericardectomy. After establishment of pneumothorax and entry with the endoscope (see Box 42-1), a left-sided ventral intercostal portal is made under thoracoscopic guidance in the 5th–9th intercostal space (the best location is determined from inside the thorax). The ventral mediastinum is incised using scissors, electrosurgery, or vessel sealer/divider (Ligasure), exposing the heart and right thoracic cavity. A third instrument portal can be made either in a left or right intercostal position (Fig. 42-6). The thorax is inspected and the phrenic nerves located. If the pericardium was not punctured under ultrasound guidance before surgery, it is punctured under thoracoscopic guidance using a Veress needle or making a small incision. After emptying, the ventral pericardium can be more easily grabbed using grasping forceps and pulled away from the heart and then cut using scissors or a vessel sealer/divider. After establishing an initial opening in the pericardium, a vessel sealer /divider or bipolar forceps and scissors are used to create a pericardial window of at least 3 cm diameter. Great care must be taken to stay away from the phrenic nerves. If a subtotal pericardectomy is performed, the pericardial excision is made more cranially, dorsally, and caudally, close to the phrenic nerves. Repositioning the endoscope in the right hemithorax is necessary for performing the excision on the right side.[32,33] The excised tissue is removed through one of the portals, which can be enlarged if necessary. A routine thoracic exploration is performed before placing a thoracic drain and closing the portals.

</td></tr>
</table>

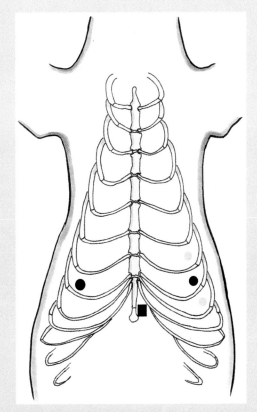

Figure 42-6 Portal positions for thoracoscopic pericardectomy in dorsal recumbency with paraxiphoid entry. ■, Camera; ●, instruments. Possible variations in positions are depicted in gray.

Box 42-3 **Thoracic duct ligation**

TDL is performed through a left lateral approach with the cat in right lateral or sternal recumbency. The authors prefer the latter. The camera portal is midway between the 9th and 10th intercostal space and two instrument portals are made in the dorsal third of the 8th or 9th and 10th or 11th intercostal spaces[7,32] (Fig. 42-7). Dissection starts by opening the mediastinum ventrolateral to the aorta. Blunt dissection is performed dorsally across the aortic surface, ventral to the thoracic duct and its branches until the right hemithoracic space is entered. Contrast studies may help visualize the duct. Dissection is performed dorsal to the thoracic duct, just ventral to the sympathetic trunk. The thoracic duct, or the dissected tissue containing it, can then be ligated or clipped. All possible thoracic duct branches should be clipped, using a 5 mm endoscopic clip applicator. However, even 5 mm clips may be too large to be effective in cats.[33] Coagulation of the tissue using bipolar forceps or a vessel sealer-divider may also be performed but may be less reliable because of the thin lymph vessel wall and poor visualization of the duct. When applied, great care must be taken to ensure proper coagulation and to prevent iatrogenic laceration of the thin wall of the thoracic duct because of tissue sticking to the device after coagulation is performed. Thoracic drainage is continued postoperatively until fluid production is significantly decreased.

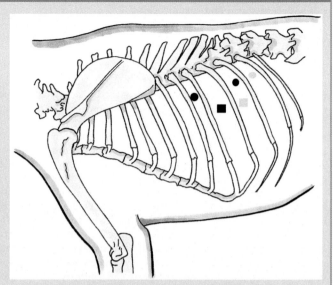

Figure 42-7 Portal positions for a VATS approach to the feline thoracic duct with the patient in right lateral or sternal recumbency. ■, Camera; ● instruments. Possible variations in positions are depicted in gray.

of sharp objects for initial entry (i.e., Veress needle and sharp trocar). Biopsy sites and trocar sites should be inspected for hemorrhage. Bipolar instruments are advised to prevent and control hemorrhage. Vascular clips are used in delicate areas (close to important nerves and major vessels to the heart and lungs). The use of monopolar devices is not recommended because of the increased chance of unintended distal or collateral effects, especially in the thoracic cavity with its thin structures and important nerves and vessels running through it. Experience and dedicated surgical technique, teamwork between surgeons and anesthetists, proper anesthetic monitoring, and the ability to readily convert to an open approach if needed will together minimize the chance for complications. Peri- and postoperative care is not essentially different from thoracotomy patients and is primarily dependent on the patient's health status and procedure performed. Postoperative thoracic drainage is indicated with most thoracic surgical procedures. The main differences between thoracoscopy and thoracotomy are reduced pain and morbidity, faster overall recovery, and shorter intensive care unit and hospital stays.

REFERENCES

1. Kovak JR, Ludwig LL, Bergman PJ, et al. Use of thoracoscopy to determine the etiology of pleural effusion in dogs and cats: 18 cases (1998–2001). J Am Vet Med Assoc 2002;221:990–4.

2. Meeking SA, Prittie J, Barton L. Myasthenia gravis associated with thymic neoplasia in a cat. J Vet Em Crit Care 2008;18:177–83.

3. Cohn LA, Norris CR, Hawkins EC, et al. Identification and characterization of an idiopathic pulmonary fibrosis-like condition in cats. J Vet Intern Med 2004;18:632–41.

4. Schmiedt C. Small animal exploratory thoracoscopy. Vet Clin North Am Small Anim Pract 2009;39:953–64.

5. Monnet E. Interventional thoracoscopy in small animals. Vet Clin North Am Small Anim Pract 2009;39:965–75.

6. McCarthy TC. Diagnostic thoracoscopy. Clin Tech Small Anim Pract 1999;14:213–19.

7. Burke RP, Jacobs JP, Cheng W, et al. Video-assisted thoracoscopic surgery for patent ductus arteriosus in low birth weight neonates and infants. Pediatrics 1999;104:227–30.

8. Paul S, Altorki NK, Sheng S, et al. Thoracoscopic lobectomy is associated with lower morbidity than open lobectomy: a propensity-matched analysis from the STS database. J Thorac Cardiovasc Surg 2010;139:366–78.

9. Meyer DM, Herbert MA, Sobhani NC, et al. Comparative clinical outcomes of thymectomy for myasthenia gravis performed by extended transsternal and minimally invasive approaches. Ann Thorac Surg 2009;87:385–90; discussion 90–1.

10. Walsh PJ, Remedios AM, Ferguson JF, et al. Thoracoscopic versus open partial pericardectomy in dogs: comparison of postoperative pain and morbidity. Vet Surg 1999;28:472–9.

11. Dupré GP, Corlouer JP, Bouvy B. Thoracoscopic pericardectomy performed without pulmonary exclusion in 9 dogs. Vet Surg 2001;30:21–7.

12. Jackson J, Richter KP, Launer DP. Thoracoscopic partial pericardiectomy in 13 dogs. J Vet Intern Med 1999;13:529–33.

13. Radlinsky MG, Mason DE, Biller DS, Olsen D. Thoracoscopic visualization and ligation of the thoracic duct in dogs. Vet Surg 2002;31:138–46.

14. Allman DA, Radlinsky MG, Ralph AG, Rawlings CA. Thoracoscopic thoracic duct ligation and thoracoscopic pericardectomy for treatment of chylothorax in dogs. Vet Surg 2010;39:21–7.

15. Daly CM, Swalec-Tobias K, Tobias AH, Ehrhart N. Cardiopulmonary effects of intrathoracic insufflation in dogs. J Am Anim Hosp Assoc 2002;38:515–20.

16. Polis I, Gasthuys F, Gielen I, et al. The effects of intrathoracic pressure during

continuous two-lung ventilation for thoracoscopy on the cardiorespiratory parameters in sevoflurane anaesthetized dogs. J Vet Med A Physiol Pathol Clin Med 2002;49:113–20.

17. Brock H, Rieger R, Gabriel C, et al. Haemodynamic changes during thoracoscopic surgery: the effects of one-lung ventilation compared with carbon dioxide insufflation. Anaesthesia 2000;55:10–16.

18. Kudnig ST, Monnet E, Riquelme M, et al. Effect of one-lung ventilation on oxygen delivery in anesthetized dogs with an open thoracic cavity. Am J Vet Res 2003;64:443–8.

19. Caccamo R, Twedt DC, Buracco P, McKiernan BC. Endoscopic bronchial anatomy in the cat. J Feline Med Surg 2007;9:140–9.

20. Bailey JE, Pablo LS. Anesthetic and physiologic considerations for veterinary endosurgery. In: Freeman LJ, editor. Veterinary endosurgery. St. Louis: Mosby; 1999. p. 24–43.

21. Hammer GB, Fitzmaurice BG, Brodsky JB. Methods for single-lung ventilation in pediatric patients. Anesth Analg 1999;89:1426–9.

22. Radlinsky MG. Complications and need for conversion from thoracoscopy to thoracotomy in small animals. Vet Clin North Am Small Anim Pract 2009;39: 977–84.

23. Potter L, Hendrickson DA. Therapeutic video-assisted thoracic surgery. In: Freeman LJ, editor. Veterinary endosurgery. St. Louis: Mosby; 1999. p. 169–87.

24. Fossum TW, Mertens MM, Miller MW, et al. Thoracic duct ligation and pericardectomy for treatment of idiopathic chylothorax. J Vet Intern Med 2004;18:307–10.

25. Santini M, Vicidomini G, Baldi A, et al. Use of an electrothermal bipolar tissue sealing system in lung surgery. Eur J Cardiothorac Surg 2006;29:226–30.

26. Kovács O, Szántó Z, Krasznai G, Herr G. Comparing bipolar electrothermal device and endostapler in endoscopic lung wedge resection. Interact Cardiovasc Thorac Surg 2009;9:11–14.

27. Sakuragi T, Okazaki Y, Mitsuoka M, et al. The utility of a reusable bipolar sealing instrument, BiClamp((R)), for pulmonary resection. Eur J Cardiothorac Surg 2008;34:505–9.

28. Rothenberg SS. First decade's experience with thoracoscopic lobectomy in infants and children. J Pediatr Surg 2008;43: 40–4.

29. Albanese CT, Sydorak RM, Tsao K, Lee H. Thoracoscopic lobectomy for prenatally diagnosed lung lesions. J Pediatr Surg 2003;38:553–5.

30. Lansdowne JL, Monnet E, Twedt DC, Dernell WS. Thoracoscopic lung lobectomy for treatment of lung tumors in dogs. Vet Surg 2005;34:530–5.

31. Fossum TW. Chylothorax in cats: is there a role for surgery? J Feline Med Surg 2001;3:73–9.

32. Radlinsky M. Rigid endoscopy: thoracoscopy. In: Lhermette P, Sobel D, editors. BSAVA manual of canine and feline endoscopy and endosurgery. Gloucester: BSAVA; 2008. p. 175–87.

33. McCarthy TC, Monnet E. Diagnostic and operative thoracoscopy. In: McCarthy TC, editor. Veterinary endoscopy for the small animal practitioner. St. Louis: Saunders; 2005. p. 229–78.

34. Naganobu K, Ohigashi Y, Akiyoshi T, et al. Lymphography of the thoracic duct by percutaneous injection of iohexol into the popliteal lymph node of dogs: experimental study and clinical application. Vet Surg 2006;35: 377–81.

35. Millward IR, Kirberger RM, Thompson PN. Comparative popliteal and mesenteric computed tomography lymphangiography of the canine thoracic duct. Vet Radiol Ultrasound 2011;52: 295–301.

36. Johnson EG, Wisner ER, Kyles A, et al. Computed tomographic lymphography of the thoracic duct by mesenteric lymph node injection. Vet Surg 2009;38: 361–7.

37. Enwiller TM, Radlinsky MG, Mason DE, Roush JK. Popliteal and mesenteric lymph node injection with methylene blue for coloration of the thoracic duct in dogs. Vet Surg 2003;32:359–64.

38. Bussadori R, Provera A, Martano M, et al. Pleural omentalisation with en bloc ligation of the thoracic duct and pericardiectomy for idiopathic chylothorax in nine dogs and four cats. Vet J 2011;188:234–6.

39. Stewart K, Padgett S. Chylothorax treated via thoracic duct ligation and omentalization. J Am Anim Hosp Assoc 2010;46:312–17.

40. Fossum TW, Forrester SD, Swenson CL, et al. Chylothorax in cats: 37 cases (1969–1989). J Am Vet Med Assoc 1991;198:672–8.

41. Colt HG, Russack V, Chiu Y, et al. A comparison of thoracoscopic talc insufflation, slurry, and mechanical abrasion pleurodesis. Chest 1997;111: 442–8.

42. Jerram RM, Fossum TW, Berridge BR, et al. The efficacy of mechanical abrasion and talc slurry as methods of pleurodesis in normal dogs. Vet Surg 1999;28: 322–32.

43. Westaby S. Principles and practice of thoracic drainage. Oxford Textbook of Surgery, chapter 41.11. 2nd ed. Oxford University Press; 2002.

44. Hayashi K, Sicard G, Gellasch K, et al. Cisterna chyli ablation with thoracic duct ligation for chylothorax: results in eight dogs. Vet Surg 2005;34: 519–23.

45. McAnulty JF. Prospective comparison of cisterna chyli ablation to pericardectomy for treatment of spontaneously occurring idiopathic chylothorax in the dog. Vet Surg 2011;40:926–34.

Chapter 43

Thoracic wall

G. Gradner

Cats can incur serious traumatic thoracic wall conditions after road traffic accidents, falls, and dog bites. Congenital conditions are encountered, such as pectus excavatum, and dependent on the severity, these may benefit from surgical correction. Neoplastic diseases in the cat, such as fibrosarcoma and osteosarcoma may also involve the thoracic wall and this chapter aims to cover the surgical management of these varying conditions.

SURGICAL ANATOMY

Bony skeleton

The bony structure of the feline thorax consists of 13 thoracic vertebrae, 13 pairs of ribs, and nine sternebrae. The first nine ribs articulate with the sternum and are called sternal ribs; the last four are called asternal ribs. Each rib articulates with the corresponding vertebra at the synovial costovertebral joints. The distal part of the rib continues as the costal cartilage to connect with the sternum. The costal cartilages of the 10th, 11th and 12th ribs unite to form the costal arch. The cartilages of the last pair of ribs end freely; these ribs are often termed 'floating ribs'. The sternum consists of eight sternebrae beginning cranially with the manubrium and ending caudally with the xiphoid cartilage of the xiphoid process. The intercostal space is filled with the internal and external intercostal muscles[1] (Fig. 43-1).

Musculature

The latissimus dorsi is a triangular muscle that originates at the spinous processes of the last thoracic and first lumbar vertebrae, extending in a cranioventral direction to insert on the humerus. When the muscle contracts the thoracic limb is retracted caudally, but excision or incision of the muscle does not seem to cause lameness. This muscle is important for reconstructive surgery of the thoracic wall. The serratus ventralis muscle extends from the caudal margin of the first eight ribs to the medial surface of the scapula. The serratus dorsalis muscle is divided into two parts. The serratus dorsalis cranialis arises via a broad aponeurosis from the superficial leaf of the thoracolumbar fascia and inserts with serrations on the cranial borders and the lateral

surfaces of ribs 2 to 10. The serratus dorsalis caudalis arises by a broad aponeurosis from the thoracolumbar fascia and extends cranioventrally to the caudal border of the 11th, 12th, 13th, and occasionally, the 10th rib. The scalenus muscle originates at the 4th and 5th cervical vertebra to insert at the 5th rib and forms a surgical landmark for thoracotomy (see Fig. 43-1). The superficial pectoral muscles originate at the cranial end of the sternum and insert at the greater tubercle of the humerus. The pectoralis profundus is a broad muscle extending between the sternum and the minor tubercle of the humerus.

The external abdominal oblique muscle covers the ventral part of the lateral thoracic wall and the lateral abdominal wall. The costal part arises from the 4th to the 12th rib; the lumbar part originates from the last rib and the thoracolumbar fascia to extend caudally. The transverse thoracic muscle lies on the inner surface of the sternum and sternal costal cartilages. When a lateral thoracotomy is performed, this muscle is a landmark for the internal thoracic artery. Sectioning of this artery should be avoided.

Vasculature

The internal thoracic artery originates from the left and right subclavian artery and passes under the transverse thoracic muscle to run caudally to form the cranial epigastric artery. The intercostal arteries and veins originate from the aorta and azygos vein; they then course ventrally along the caudal border of the rib to anastomose with the internal thoracic artery and vein. The intercostal nerves arise from the ventral branches of the thoracic nerves that run with the intercostal arteries and veins. Collateral branches of the main intercostal vessels and nerves can be found on the cranial border of the rib.[2]

GENERAL CONSIDERATIONS

Clinical signs and history

Cats with thoracic wall problems generally present in two main ways. They may present with obvious visible thoracic deformity (e.g., pectus excavatum or neoplastic masses) or abnormal thoracic movements (e.g., flail chest), usually with minimal or no signs of impedance to

DOI: 10.1016/B978-0-7020-4336-9.00043-3

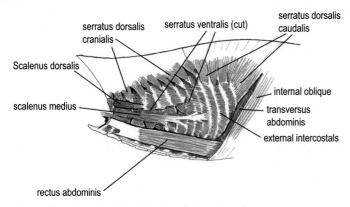

serratus dorsalis cranialis

serratus ventralis (cut)

serratus dorsalis caudalis

Scalenus dorsalis

scalenus medius

internal oblique

transversus abdominis

external intercostals

rectus abdominis

Figure 43-1 Musculature of the lateral thoracic wall.

the internal thoracic organs. Alternatively, animals are presented because of the secondary consequences of the thoracic wall conditions or trauma with resultant thoracic organ dysfunction causing clinical signs such as dyspnea, tachypnea or hypoxia.

Preoperative evaluation and stabilization of trauma patients

Cats requiring extensive surgery to the thoracic wall should always have a complete clinical examination (including a full neurologic and orthopedic examination), biochemical and hematologic analysis of blood, electrolyte levels measured, and urine analysis in order to fully evaluate the extent of the injuries and identify co-morbidities.

Thoracic trauma patients should be evaluated for breathing difficulties and treated for shock. A significant pneumothorax or a pleural effusion that is causing respiratory compromise should be drained (see Chapter 41, Box 41-2) prior to taking radiographs. An intravenous catheter should be placed for administration of fluids. Administering fluids at shock rates must be balanced against the potential to cause further respiratory compromise if fluid overload occurs with the potential for pulmonary edema. Pulmonary contusions have been reported in up to 50% of animals with thoracic trauma and are a potential indication for limited fluid volume resuscitation (see Chapter 1). Acute traumatic and neoplastic thoracic wall conditions are usually painful; analgesic drugs should be administered.

Diagnostic imaging

In trauma patients, a total body radiograph can be obtained to gain a preliminary overview of the injuries. Different studies show widely varying rates of thoracic injuries in the feline trauma patient of 11–90%.[3] Stress, multiple injuries, and the critical nature of the patient often only allow single view radiographs to be taken initially. The safest view to do first is the dorsoventral view as this avoids the patient having to lie on its side and the potential for compromise to lung expansion that this would cause. The orthogonal view can be done at a later stage when the animal is stable and sedated or anesthetized. To evaluate for metastases or primary neoplasia, a right and left-sided laterolateral view and a dorsoventral view are recommended.

Computed tomography (CT) is useful for evaluating intrathoracic disease processes and for preoperative planning for reconstructive surgery involving the thoracic wall. Tumor margins can be highlighted with contrast media and pre- or postoperative radiation therapies can be planned. Magnetic resonance imaging (MRI) is useful for investigating soft tissues and is used in human medicine for preoperative

planning and margin evaluation of intrathoracic and thoracic wall tumors. Movement of the chest during this test may cause the pictures to blur. By inducing a transient apnea the anesthetist can prevent this artifact. Ultrasound may be useful to evaluate the characteristics of a thoracic wall mass and to take ultrasound-guided biopsies. Tru-Cut biopsies, punch biopsies and trephine biopsies of the bone often require sedation or general anesthesia; if necessary, these can be performed under CT guidance.[4]

Anesthesia and analgesia

Facilities for intubation and an anesthetist familiar with intermittent positive pressure ventilation of patients should be available (see Chapter 2). Most anesthetics reduce the respiration capacity and this should be taken into consideration for patients with pneumothorax, pulmonary edema, pulmonary contusion, pleural effusion, and pneumonia, with appropriate management before anesthesia.

Thoracic surgery is painful and therefore analgesia, preferably used in a multimodal approach, should be provided pre-, intra- and postoperatively not only to reduce pain but also to minimize the overall dose requirement for anesthetics intraoperatively and to obtain optimal ventilation of the lung. Pain can be minimized by an atraumatic surgical approach, retraction rather than incision of the latissimus dorsi muscle and careful placement of the sutures used to secure the ribs or sternebrae in apposition. Multimodal analgesic techniques such as local, epidural or interpleural nerve blocks or infusions should also be considered in the preoperative plan (see Chapters 2 and 41).

SURGICAL DISEASES

Surgical diseases of the thoracic wall include congenital conditions such as pectus excavatum, traumatic lesions such as flail chest, penetrating bite wounds, and neoplasia. Many injuries or diseases will require surgical intervention and a concurrent thoracotomy may be inevitable. For further information on thoracotomy see Chapter 41.

Pectus excavatum

Pectus excavatum (PE) is a dorsoventral narrowing and inward concave deformation of the caudal sternum and associated costal cartilages. It usually extends caudally from around the 5th/6th rib and is most severe at the level of the 10th thoracic vertebra. Depending on the severity of the malformation it can lead to both displacement of the heart and lung compression.

The clinical signs of pectus excavatum can range from mild or absent, to severe. Those associated with more severe defects are growth retardation, exercise intolerance, tachypnea, cyanosis, weight loss, and vomiting. Restricted ventilation, paradoxical movement of the deformity during inspiration, and chronic alveolar collapse can contribute to exercise intolerance and hypoxemia by impairing gas exchange. Compression of the heart and kinking of great vessels can lead to heart murmurs or cardiac arrhythmias, but concurrent congenital defects are also possible and should be ruled out before surgery.

The etiology is poorly understood. Shortening of the central tendon of the diaphragm, abnormal intrauterine pressure, thickening of the substernal ligament or of the musculature of the cranial portion of the diaphragm, failure of osteogenesis or chondrogenesis, arrested sternal development, and rachitic influences have all been implicated. Multiple animals in some litters have been affected, so breeding from affected or related animals is not recommended.[5]

Frontosagittal index (FSI) is the ratio of the thoracic width at T10 as measured on a DV/VD radiograph and the distance from the center of the ventral surface of T10 or vertebrae overlying the deformity and the nearest point on the sternum as measured on a lateral radiograph.

Vertebral index (VI) is defined as the ratio of the distance from the center of the dorsal surface of the vertebral body overlying the deformity to the nearest point of the sternum and the DV diameter of the centrum of the same vertebra.

Minimum thoracic height is defined as the distance between the ventral surface of the vertebral body and dorsal surface of the sternum at the site of maximal deviation.[6]

Table 43-1 Indices used to characterize pectus excavatum in cats

	Frontosagittal index	**Vertebral index**
Normal	0.7–1.3	12.6–18.8
Mild PE	2.0	>9.0
Moderate PE	2.0–3.0	6.0–9.0
Severe PE	>3.0	<6.0

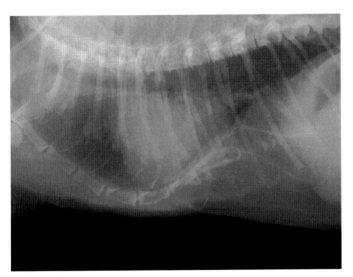

Figure 43-2 Pectus excavatum in a three-year-old cat. Note the narrow distance between the xiphoid and the caudal thoracic vertebrae leading to compression of the thoracic organs. Concurrent congenital defects are possible and have to be ruled out before surgery.

The diagnosis of pectus excavatum can be established by palpation of the thorax and by thoracic radiographs. The deformity can be assessed objectively by measuring the frontosagittal and vertebral indices on thoracic radiographs and by assessment of the minimum thoracic height. Several thoracic measurements need to be taken which are then used to calculate the frontosagittal index and the vertebral index and the minimal thoracic height (Box 43-1, Fig. 43-2). These values characterize the severity of pectus excavatum in cats (Table 43-1). The deviation of the sternum can cause rotation and displacement of the heart as well as compression of blood vessels and lung lobes. Cats with high values are more likely to have impaired ventilation or ECG changes.

The need for surgical intervention (see Box 43-2), or the ability to treat the condition conservatively is dependent on the severity and presence of clinical signs. Surgical treatment of a moderate pectus excavatum depends on the clinical findings; a severe pectus excavatum is likely to require surgical treatment if the condition of the patient allows it. Mild pectus excavatum is often an incidental finding with no clinical relevance.

The prognosis depends on the severity of concomitant lung injuries: it worsens with cardiac dysrhythmias, the need for mechanical ventilation, and concurrent injuries.

Flail chest

Dog bite injuries are the most common causes of flail chest in cats, followed by blunt trauma. A flail chest results from a segmental fracture and/or dislocation of two or more adjacent ribs. The section of unstable ribs moves paradoxically during respiration. During inspiration the flail segment collapses inward; during expiration it moves outward. Air is shunted from the lung under the flail segment to the opposite hemithorax (Fig. 43-3).

The diagnosis is made by visualization of the unstable flail segment. The concurrent lung trauma and pain will often cause dyspnea and tachypnea. Lung contusions result in decreased bronchovesicular sounds; decreased or hyper-resonant lung sounds are found with pneumothorax. In some cases subcutaneous emphysema is found. Thoracic radiography and CT will show the rib fractures.

Stabilization of the patient is the main priority, and this involves securing a patent airway, assessing for adequate ventilation, and establishing oxygenation. If pulse oximetry shows an oxygen saturation of less than 92% at a FiO2 of 21%, supplemental oxygen is needed by face mask, oxygen cage, or a nasopharyngeal or nasotracheal oxygen tube could be inserted. Endotracheal intubation may be necessary if the saturation cannot be kept above 92%.[7] Electrocardiography (ECG) may identify cardiac dysrhythmias although they may not be present until 12 to 48 hours after injury. Pain management should be initiated at this time. If possible, the patient should be placed in lateral recumbency; to inhibit paradoxical movement the flail segment should be down. Reduced volume resuscitation (see Chapter 1) is implemented to avoid pulmonary edema.[8]

The prognosis for a cat with flail chest depends on the severity of concomitant lung injuries. In mild cases the prognosis is favorable, whereas in severe cases with established clinical signs it is guarded. Prognosis worsens with cardiac dysrhythmias, the need for mechanical ventilation, and concurrent injuries. In a clinical study, the outcomes of 24 cases of flail chests were compared (21 dogs and three cats): nine flail chests were surgically stabilized and 15 were not stabilized. There was no significant difference in hospitalization time or outcome.[9]

Crushing injuries and bite wounds

Types of crushing injuries include perforating and non-perforating bite wounds and other incidents where a compressive injury occurs to the thorax, e.g., an object falling on to the cat. Dog bite wounds involving the chest wall are the most common crush injury to the feline thoracic wall. Most cats sustain severe damage to the chest wall,

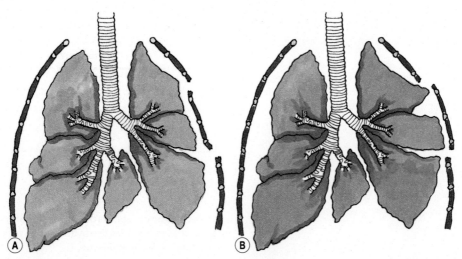

Figure 43-3 Schematic drawings showing the air movement with flail chest. **(A)** During inspiration the negative pressure causes movement of the flail segment into the thorax. **(B)** During expiration air from the unaffected hemithorax pushes the flail segment outward.

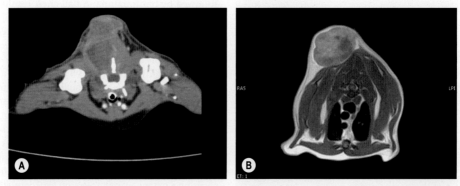

Figure 43-4 Advanced imaging is helpful in presurgical planning and to estimate the extent and depth of the tumor. **(A)** Contrast enhanced computed tomographic image of a fibrosarcoma in the cat. **(B)** A magnetic resonance imaging scan of a cat with a thoracic wall fibrosarcoma. *(B, Courtesy of the University of Cambridge.)*

with devitalized muscle tissue, fractured ribs and sternebrae, pneumothorax, and internal organ damage. The degree of skin damage may be misleading; major internal organ injury may be present despite the patient only presenting with minor skin wounds or skin bruising. After a crush injury, devitalized tissues and serum accumulation provide a good medium for growing inoculated bacteria. Puncture bite wounds by cats do not cause crushing injuries but they enclose bacteria in the tissue where abscesses can form. These may extend into the thorax causing pyothorax (see Chapter 44).

A thorough clinical examination that also rules out further injury sites is recommended. Twenty five percent of bite wounds involve multiple parts of the body.[10] Radiography, CT, and ultrasound are currently the most useful diagnostic imaging modalities. In cases of thoracic wall injury, it is advisable to check for rib fractures, lung contusions, spinal injuries, pneumothorax, and hemothorax. Open and closed pneumothoraces should be differentiated.

In a study of 185 dogs and 11 cats that underwent thoracotomy (of which 35% of dogs and 36% of cats sustained a dog bite injury) there was a mortality rate of 7% with exploratory thoracotomy and 8% mortality without surgery in those patients treated for bite wounds. This has to be interpreted with caution because animals undergoing thoracotomy presented with more severe injuries necessitating surgical intervention.

Neoplasia

Cats with thoracic wall tumors are usually presented with a recently recognized acute or chronic visible swelling at the affected site. Three-view radiographs can lead to a presumptive diagnosis of thoracic wall tumor, especially in cases with a soft tissue mass, osteolysis or osteo-proliferation, and can be useful for exclusion of metastasis. Additional diagnostics valuable for presurgical planning include contrast CT, MRI or scintigraphy.[11] These advanced imaging modalities can be used to evaluate the invasiveness of the tumor (Fig. 43-4) and to assess for metastasis.

It is difficult to distinguish inflammatory or reactive bone proliferation from neoplasia solely on cytologic examination from fine needle aspirates.[12] The definitive diagnosis can usually be obtained with histopathologic examination of biopsies using a Jamshidi biopsy needle. With soft tissue neoplasia, Tru-Cut or wedge biopsies are often required for diagnosis. In cases with anemia, e.g., due to presurgical radiation therapy, a blood transfusion might be necessary before surgery (see Chapter 5). Inappetence or increased nutritional demands may have to be addressed before surgery (see Chapter 4). In cases with adhesion formation between thoracic structures, such as lung or pericardium, the attached organ should be removed en bloc with the underlying neoplasm.

Osteosarcoma

Primary bone tumors of the thoracic wall are uncommon in cats (4.9 per 100 000 cases).[13] No breed or gender predisposition was found with osteosarcomas in cats. The average age was 10.1 years, ranging from one to 17 years.[14]

Osteosarcomas in cats behave differently to those in dogs: the metastatic rate was found to be only 10%, therefore local destruction seems to be more of a concern than metastasis with feline osteosarcomas.[15] When metastasis occurs, it is usually to the lungs. The skull is most commonly affected; however, osteosarcomas have also been diagnosed infrequently in the ribs and sternebrae of the cat.[14] In one report of 78 cats with osteosarcomas, 54% were located axially and only one osteosarcoma was located on a rib.[14]

The median survival time of seven cats with axial osteosarcomas treated surgically was 13 months versus 22.2 months for cats with appendicular osteosarcomas treated with amputation, which may indicate a worse prognosis for thoracic wall osteosarcomas, likely to be due to the inability to achieve wide resections of the lesion.[14]

Chondrosarcoma

The characteristics and biologic behavior of chondrosarcoma in cats are not well defined. An incidence rate of 2% of chondrosarcoma in vaccine-associated sarcomas was found in an immunohistochemical study. Twenty of 67 cats (30% of the cases) with chondrosarcoma showed involvement of subcutaneous sites and of these 10% were in the thoracic region.[16] In two of these cats (3%), the tumor affected the sternum and/or ribs.

The median survival time for cats with chondrosarcoma is difficult to predict as it has rarely been reported.[17] Where amputation or radical surgery is possible, recurrence and metastasis are low.

Feline osteochondromatosis

Osteochondromatosis in cats accounts for approximately 20% of primary bone tumors. Most cats are young (two to four years old) when the exostosis is discovered. Sites of skeletal involvement are the rib cage, scapulae, vertebral column, skull, pelvis, and limbs (Fig. 43-5).

Feline osteochondromatosis lesions show progressive enlargement and continuous growth throughout the cat's life. Viral particles causing feline leukemia or transmissible feline sarcoma have consistently been found in the neoplastic cartilage; detection of such viral particles is a prerequisite for diagnosing this disease. The tendency for malignant transformation into an osteosarcoma or a chondrosarcoma is an indication for removal of the feline osteochondroma.[18]

Fibrosarcoma (FSA)

Fibrosarcomas are one of the most common feline subcutaneous neoplasms. They are locally aggressive tumors with a moderate metastatic rate of up to 22.5% and a local recurrence rate as high as 67%.[19] Complete excision has been shown to improve survival rate and decrease the likelihood of tumor recurrence. Preoperative radiation could also be considered (see Chapter 15). Vaccine-associated sarcomas can involve the thoracic wall and this condition is covered in detail in Chapter 22.

The only factor found to influence the length of disease-free intervals of cats with thoracic wall fibrosarcoma was whether margins of tissue obtained at the time of surgery contained tumor cells. Surgery alone is seldom curative and radiation therapy is mandatory for disease control.[20] Recurrence rates range from 31% to 55%.[21]

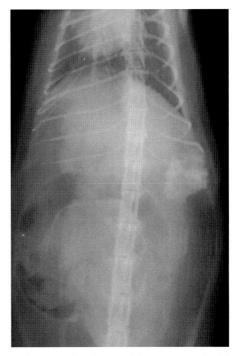

Figure 43-5 Feline osteochondromatosis in an 11-month-old cat. This dorsoventral radiograph shows right-sided involvement of the 12th and 13th rib. Differentials were osteosarcoma and chondrosarcoma, which were excluded by the results of Jamshidi needle biopsy.

Mast cell tumor

Mast cell tumors are the second most common feline cutaneous tumor; they account for approximately 20% of feline cutaneous tumors in the US.[15] There are two cutaneous forms of mast cell tumors in cats: the mastocytic form, which is the most common one, and the histiocytic (atypical) form. The latter occurs in cats under the age of four and it generally regresses spontaneously.

The prognosis for a mast cell tumor depends on the histologic grade. Multiple lesions of the pleomorphic phenotype with high KIT immunoreactivity score, which is a mast cell growth factor receptor, and high mitotic and Ki67 indices correlate with an unfavorable outcome. Therefore, immunohistochemical staining is an important step for gaining a prognosis.[15] Twenty per cent of mast cell tumors show malignant behavior. Local recurrence rates of 0–24% after surgical excision have been reported.[22] A more aggressive approach for histologically anaplastic mastocytic tumors may be necessary. The histiocytic form may regress spontaneously.

SURGERY FOR THORACIC WALL CONDITIONS

Surgery of the thoracic wall always requires special instrumentation because a 'simple' wound exploration might result in an open thoracic wall. Instruments that may be useful to include in a kit are listed in Table 43-2. When performing thoracic wall surgery in cats, it is often more practical to suture the drape onto the skin in order to avoid interference with the towel clamps. A thoracotomy may be necessary (see Chapter 41) and anesthetists need to be prepared to perform intermittent positive pressure ventilation (IPPV) (see Chapter 2).

Table 43-2 An instrument kit for thoracic wall surgery

Soft tissue instruments	Quantity
Bard Parker handle No 3	1
Bowl for warmed flushing solution	1
Swabs with radiodense marker	10
Backhaus towel clamps	10
Mayo scissors	1
Wire cutting scissors	1
Metzenbaum scissors	1
Mayo-Hegar needle holder	1
Adson Brown forceps	2
DeBakey forceps	1
Halstead mosquito forceps straight	5
Halstead mosquito forceps bent	5
Special thoracic instruments	
Gelpi retractor	1
Small Finochietto retractor	1
Beckmann retractor	1
Warm Ringer's solution	1
Poole suction tip and suction	1
Polydioxanone	
Polyglecaprone 25, Polyglactin 910, Polyglycol acid	
Thoracic drain	1
Monopolar or bipolar cautery	1
Cotton swabs, sterile	1
Periosteal elevator	1
Bone cutting forceps (Liston)	1

Pectus excavatum

Surgical intervention may be necessary for pectus excavatum when the defect is considerable and associated with clinical signs. The condition is treated by external splinting or bone resection, dependent on the age of the cat. In animals younger than 4 months of age, where the sternum is compliant and non-ossified, the treatment of choice is an external splint with percutaneously placed circumsternal sutures (Box 43-2). The goal of this treatment is to pull the sternum outward and maintain this position while the sternum matures and becomes non-compliant in the corrected position.

In a case report of a Siamese kitten of five months of age, the flattened shape deformity was corrected by a 1.5 mm Kirschner pin inserted with a handheld Jacobs chuck longitudinally through the manubrium in a cranial to caudal direction. From the manubrium the pin was inserted into the second, third, and fourth sternebrae to align and reduce the deformity. The abrupt depression deformity was corrected with an external splint through the 4th, 5th, and 6th interster-nebral cartilages.[24]

For animals older than four months, and thus with less mobile sternebrae, a variety of different techniques have been reported. In one report a total resection of the sternum and the associated cartilages

Box 43-2 External splinting with percutaneous circumsternal sutures

This technique is used in kittens less than four months old. The kitten is placed in dorsal recumbency and a U-shaped splint is modeled out of a thermoplastic casting material at a slightly greater width than the sternum. Four to six pairs of holes are made in the splint. While the splint is left to harden, sutures are placed around the sternum, preferably incorporating the costal cartilage (45° angle) to reduce the risk of suture pulling through the soft sternal bone (Fig. 43-6). The splint is padded and the sutures are passed through the predrilled holes. Large 2/0 monofilament absorbable (e.g., polydioxanone) or non-absorbable (e.g., polypropylene) suture material is recommended. The sutures are pre-placed and the most caudal sutures are tied first. The splint is left in place for 10–21 days. Intraoperative complications of this technique are penetration of heart, lung or internal thoracic vessels; postoperative complications include suture abscesses, mild superficial dermatitis, and skin abrasions. Because of rapid growth the splint size may need to be adjusted.[6]

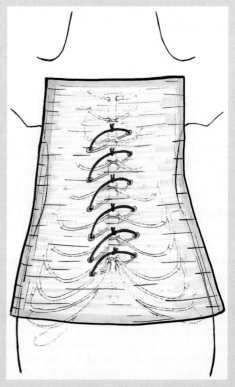

Figure 43-6 Diagram illustrating external splint on the ventral thorax with percutaneous circumsternal sutures placed at a 45° angle between the ribs.

was performed. After a midline skin incision the superficial and deep pectoralis muscles and the rectus abdominis muscles were elevated and the sternum, with the adjacent ribs, was removed using a rongeur, taking care not to lacerate the internal thoracic artery. The remaining ribs and intercostal muscles were apposed with a large monofilament suture in an interrupted or horizontal mattress suture pattern. Placement of a thoracostomy tube, closure of the thoracic wall, and a light support wrap completed the surgical procedure.[20] A total or partial sternectomy is feasible in small animals. A wedge ostectomy of the sternum combined with an external splint has also been described. With cats older than four months it may be advisable to use a more stable internal splint.[23]

The use of internal splinting to realign a non-compliant sternum in a cat with pectus excavatum was described in a five-month-old domestic short-hair kitten. At the maximal point of deformity a small section of the 5th to 8th ribs was removed without destroying the periosteum on the costectomy site. At the chondral junction between the 4th and the 5th sternebra, a wedge-shaped piece of cartilage was removed, with the base of the wedge positioned ventrally. A 2 mm veterinary cuttable plate, contoured at the rostral end to accommodate the normal dorsal deviation of the cranial portion of the sternum covered the length of the entire sternum and was fixed with 2/0 polydioxanone suture material around the sternebrae, ribs, and through plate holes. Three months later the plate was removed.[17]

Postoperative care

Depending on the treatment chosen, the kitten must be monitored closely for breathing difficulties during the first 24 hours and oxygen must be provided as needed. Bandages placed too tightly or placed under anesthesia can progress to be life-threateningly restrictive and should therefore be applied with great care. Feeding per os or via a feeding tube is introduced as soon as the animal is fully awake.

Flail chest

Several techniques for stabilization of a flail chest (Box 43-3) have been introduced, but attention has been focused on the underlying pulmonary injuries as a cause of respiratory dysfunction. Stabilization of the flail segment is often not required and is not commonly performed but is still recommended if either a thoracotomy is needed to address associated injuries, if rib fractures may cause further injury, or if conservative medical management is ineffective.

Postoperative management

Continued conservative treatment consists of oxygen supplementation, rest, hydration, and nutrition. Pain management is mandatory; prophylactic antibiotics are only necessary if there are signs of bronchopneumonia or concurrent injuries such as bite wounds. Recumbent cats should be turned every four to six hours. A thoracotomy tube to eliminate pneumothorax may be necessary.

Monitoring consists of measuring the oxygen saturation every two to four hours initially. Arterial blood gas analysis should be performed every 12 to 24 hours, dependent on the patient's recovery. ECG monitoring, blood pressure, and urinary output are evaluated. External splints are left for two to four weeks after callus formation is detected or the flail segment is stabilized. Bandaging the thorax is contraindicated and may further compromise ventilation. Diuretics are not recommended for treating pulmonary contusions unless fluid overload and pulmonary edema are present. Corticosteroids are contraindicated because they predispose to pneumonia.

Bite wounds

In cases of bite wounds, exploratory surgery is always indicated.[25-27] Intrathoracic injuries caused by penetrating or crushing teeth are often not visible, making surgical exploration necessary. The elastic skin can follow the movement of the jaws, often leaving just small teeth marks while the muscles and organs underneath may be severely damaged. This is called the iceberg-effect, because on the surface of water only the smallest part of the iceberg is seen. No standard protocol is available for the treatment of bite wounds in dogs and cats. Thoracotomy is recommended in more severe cases where penetrating wounds are apparent or internal organs have been damaged.[28] With an open pneumothorax the wound should be covered with a sterile occlusive

Box 43-3 Surgical stabilization of a flail chest

For external stabilization of a flail chest strong plastic material, e.g., from a buster collar, a wire coat hanger, or aluminium rods is molded to conform to the thoracic wall and 2/0 to 0 suture material (e.g., nylon) is passed using a large curved needle around the affected ribs and then through the plastic splint in predrilled holes or around the wire of the hanger. The circumcostal sutures are passed at two sites, one ventrally and one dorsally, to avoid a pivot point of the flail segment. Some padding is applied between the skin and the splint. The splint should be extended cranially and caudally over the unaffected ribs to help stabilize the flail segment (Fig. 43-7). Internal stabilization, consisting of interfragmentary wire and suture approximation, may be required for large thoracic defects, multiple unstable rib fractures, or for an open pneumothorax.

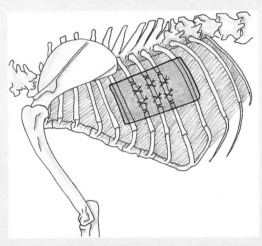

Figure 43-7 External splinting of a flail chest. To develop a flail chest at least two neighbouring ribs must be broken both proximally and distally. These floating ribs can be stabilized against the thoracic wall with an external plastic splint or with part of a metal coat hanger.

bandage and air should be removed from the interpleural space via thoracocentesis. The use of a sterile swab secured on the thorax with cling film has proven to be useful. The animal has to be closely monitored to avoid a tension pneumothorax. In cats with severe lung contusions and atelectasis, surgery should be postponed until sufficient recovery has occurred from these injuries and the anesthetic risk has been minimized. In the presence of lung contusions, fluid should be administered cautiously (see Chapter 2). Analgesia, oxygen, and antibiotics should be administered.

After stabilization, judicious surgical debridement to remove any devitalized fat and muscle as well as copious lavage is recommended.[29-32] Before lavage, tissue samples from the wound bed are taken for culture and sensitivity testing. In the presence of an open pneumothorax, high pressure flushing should be avoided in order to avoid introducing infected material into the chest.

When treating a bite wound with possible tearing of the intercostal musculature, the surgeon and the anesthetist have to be prepared for a thoracotomy and the possibility of lung lacerations, bronchial, and/or tracheal injuries.[28] All devitalized tissue must be removed and local muscle flaps, such as the latissimus dorsi muscle, may be needed to close thoracic wall defects. Broken ribs are generally not repaired and are normally left in situ. However, in cases with lacerated lung lobes a total or partial lung lobectomy may be necessary and the adjacent fractured rib can be removed to avoid further injury. A chest drain should be placed after debridement when entering the chest or when severe pneumothorax is present.

Postoperative management

Antibiotic treatment in bite wound victims is highly controversial both in the veterinary and human medical literature. The efficacy of prophylactic antibiotics in significantly reducing the incidence of post-bite wound infections is unproven; this may be due to the fact that no single antimicrobial agent has been demonstrated to be effective against most of the potential pathogens. In a study the most common aerobes identified were: *Pasteurella* spp., *Streptococcus* spp., *Staphylococcus* spp.[33] The most common anaerobes identified were: *Fusobacterium* spp. and *Bacteroides* spp.[34] Ampicillin and either fluorquinolone or aminoglycoside antibiotics are recommended. In cases of confirmed wound infection, re-culturing is advisable to monitor efficacy of treatment.[35]

With severe soft tissue trauma, the risk of systemic inflammatory response syndrome (SIRS) and sepsis increases. Patients in this 'at risk' group should be in an intensive care unit with optimal systemic and nutritional support.

Bone neoplasia

Reconstruction of the thoracic wall (Box 43-4) is often necessary after en bloc resection of masses. Surprisingly large portions of thoracic wall can be removed as long as an airtight seal can be obtained after excision. Removal of up to six ribs (including the first) has been reported in dogs without increased risk of ventilatory complications.[36] When fewer than five ribs are removed, prosthetic mesh and either autogenous muscle or omental pedicle flap can be used alone or in combination.[37] Additional rigid support to prevent paradoxical movement may be necessary if more than five ribs are removed; however, reconstruction without the use of foreign material is preferred in oncologic surgery.

Seroma formation has been reported in up to 50% of the patients and a closed suction drain should be placed.[38] Drains should always

exit close to the wound margins because of the risk of tumors seeding into the surrounding tissue.

THORACIC WALL RECONSTRUCTION

The most common indication for thoracic wall reconstruction is after en bloc resection of a thoracic wall neoplasm. Other possible indications are severe thoracic wall trauma, chronic infections of the thoracic wall, and severe congenital defects involving the thoracic wall. Reconstruction requires an airtight seal to prevent pneumothorax and rigid repair to prevent excessive paradoxical movement.

Autogenous techniques

Latissimus dorsi muscle

The latissimus dorsi muscle can be used as a muscle flap or myocutaneous flap and it is the most commonly used autogenous technique for closure and reconstruction of chest wall defects (Box 43-5). This

---

Box 43-4 **Thoracic wall resection for neoplasia**

With a sterile surgical marker pen, the extent of surgical resection required should be marked 2–4 cm radially from the outlined edge of the gross tumor. Instruments should not breach these margins. The deep margin must extend at least one (preferably two) intact fascial plane(s) below the tumor. In cases with a mass involving the lateral thoracic wall, a full depth body wall resection may be required to achieve clean margins. Because of retraction of the loose skin in cats, tacking sutures to connect the deep margin to the skin are recommended to maintain orientation.

The skin covering the tumor is incised and retracted and muscles not invaded by the neoplasm are spared for closure. The thorax is entered through an unaffected intercostal space and the tumor extension can be estimated intraoperatively by palpation and also by thoracoscopic techniques. Surgical treatment involves complete resection of the affected ribs with proximal and distal disarticulation and removal of adjacent ribs to obtain a 2–3 cm margin. The use of rib cutters 2–3 cm from the tumor margins has also been described. Disarticulation may be better for osteosarcomas because of the risk of intramedullary extension of the tumor. The adjacent arteries and veins are cauterized or ligated. Adhesions between the thoracic wall and underlying organs may require lung lobectomy or pericardectomy.

Box 43-5 **Latissimus dorsi muscle flap**

The flap is created by identifying the origins and insertions of the latissimus dorsi muscle (Fig. 43-8). This triangular muscle has its base along the lumbodorsal fascia associated with the spinous processes of the lumbar and last seven or eight thoracic vertebrae and its insertion on the teres tuberosity of the humerus. The dorsal border runs from the acromion to the head of the 13th rib and the ventral border is either the ventral border of the muscle or the incised edge of the latissimus dorsi that has been removed.[36] Some intercostal branches supply the muscle and may have to be cauterized for transposition of the flap.

Preoperative measurements have to be taken before creation of the flap: the length of the flap decreases the more the flap is rotated. At the height of the acromion, but caudal to the border of the triceps muscle a slight depression can be felt; this is where the thoracodorsal artery arises. For the dorsal flap border an oblique line is drawn from the acromion to the head of the 13th rib. The ventral border is defined by the skin fold, which extends to the lower third of the humerus and runs parallel to the dorsal line. The caudal margin of the flap is the 13th rib. This muscle can be exposed through the primary surgical approach or incisions are made parallel to the muscle fibers. The intercostal arteries supplying the dorsal part of the muscle have to be cauterized or ligated when the flap is raised after freeing the dorsal, caudal, and ventral borders.

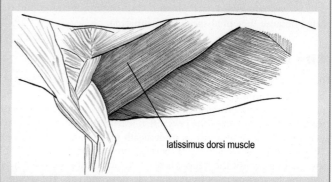

latissimus dorsi muscle

Figure 43-8 Superficial musculature of the cat showing the latissimus dorsi muscle.

flap is based on the thoracodorsal artery arising at the caudal depression of the shoulder (see Chapter 19).

Diaphragmatic advancement

Advancement of the diaphragm is a very useful technique for closure of caudal thoracic defects involving the 9th to the 13th ribs. Normal function can be restored by advancement of the diaphragm and fixing it to the remaining rib or muscular fascia.[18] If more than four ribs have to be removed, expansion of the caudal lung lobe may be compromised and therefore its removal should be considered[39] (Fig. 43-9).

Deep pectoral muscle flap

This muscle flap can be used for reconstruction of the cranial and ventral thoracic wall and is based on the lateral thoracic and external thoracic artery (Box 43-6).

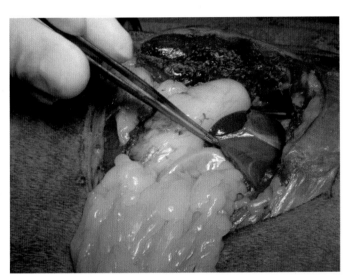

Figure 43-9 Reconstruction of the right caudal thoracic wall after removal of a tumor involving the last four ribs. The diaphragm is moved cranially and secured with encircling sutures on the 9th rib and with simple continuous sutures to the internal and external intercostal muscles. It can be advanced as far cranially as the 8th rib; if more cranial advancement is required then lobectomy of the caudal lung lobe may be necessary.

Box 43-6 Deep pectoral muscle flap

This muscle has its origin at the sternebrae and has its insertion on the lesser tubercle of the humerus with an aponeurosis to the greater tubercle. The lateral thoracic artery and external thoracic artery enter the muscle cranially; a segmental blood supply from the internal thoracic artery enters the muscle along the sternum. This flap can either be divided along the long sternal origin of the muscle or on the insertion on the humerus with division of the lateral and external thoracic arteries.[40] This flap is limited cranially by the superficial pectoral muscle. By cutting the muscle from the greater and lesser tubercle of the humerus it can be rotated cranially and dorsally. Based on the segmental branches of the internal thoracic artery, defects across the midline on the contralateral side can be covered. The deep pectoral muscle is incised along the sternum but the cranial portion of the sternal attachment and as many branches of the internal thoracic artery as possible should be preserved.

Omentum

An omental flap can be used in combination with muscular flaps (Fig. 43-10) or to cover synthetic mesh that has been used over thoracic wall defects, The omentum provides lymphatic drainage, blood supply, minimizes mesh-induced pleuritis, and provides an airtight seal. Creation of an omental flap is described in Chapter 19.

Autologous or synthetic reconstruction

Polypropylene mesh

A polypropylene mesh is most commonly used for reconstruction of large defects in small animal surgery (see Chapter 10). The mesh is cut slightly larger than necessary as the edge is folded to achieve a double thickness margin of approximately 1 cm around the entire periphery of the prosthesis[41] (Fig. 43-11). The cut edge should be external to the body cavity to prevent contact of the sharp edges with the lung or other organs. Alternatively, the mesh may be folded in half

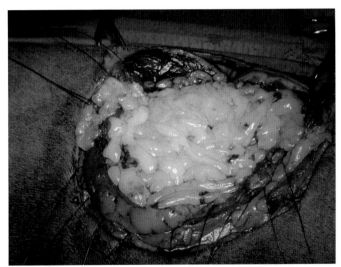

Figure 43-10 Thoracic reconstruction. Reinforcement of the caudal thoracic wall wound with a double layer of omentum before it is closed with muscular flaps. The omentum is fixed with pre-placed simple interrupted sutures.

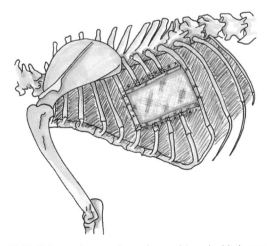

Figure 43-11 Polypropylene mesh can be used in a double layer or the edge can be folded over by one centimeter to improve the suture holding properties and to have rounded smoother margins towards the inner organs.

to uniformly double the thickness present at the defect. The mesh is sutured under slight tension and a monofilament suture such as polypropylene, polydioxanone, or polyethylene is used. Simple interrupted or mattress sutures are applied. Soft tissue coverage is achieved by undermining and transposing the local musculature, subcutaneous tissue, and skin. Seroma formation can be prevented with active drains and may be less common with concurrent usage of the omentum. Omentum can be elongated and used as a double sheet to cover the mesh (see above and Chapter 19). Polypropylene mesh is infiltrated uniformly with fibrous tissue to a 3–4 mm thickness at six weeks post implantation. The monofilament properties of the polypropylene prevent bacteria from being trapped by the fibers of the mesh.[42]

Small intestinal submucosa (SIS)

Small intestinal submucosa is used for reconstruction of abdominal wall deficits, enhancement of tendons and reconstruction of inner organs.[43] In human medicine, it is also used for chest wall reconstruction. There are no reports of its use for thoracic wall reconstruction in cats but it has potential for use in this situation.

POSTOPERATIVE CARE

Pneumothorax, hemothorax, pulmonary edema, hypoventilation, hypothermia, circulatory shock, acid-base disorders, and oliguria may arise after thoracic wall surgery. Placement of a thoracostomy tube before closure is always indicated when the thorax is entered. The thoracostomy tube should remain open until the thoracic wall is closed to prevent tension pneumothorax. After surgery, the pleural space is evacuated hourly to test for the presence of air or blood with a maximum negative pressure of 2–3 mL in the syringe.

Complications increase the longer a thoracic drain is left in,[44] so it should be removed once it has ceased to be useful. To treat persistent pneumothorax, continuous rather than intermittent suction may be required. To treat hemothorax, several options exist depending on the severity of hemorrhage including fluid replacement, administration of whole blood, autotransfusion of blood, and reoperating to address the source of hemorrhage.

Hypoventilation leads to respiratory acidosis. Causes include anesthetic drugs, pneumo- or hemothorax, tight thoracic bandages, and pain. Hypoventilation is confirmed when the $PaCO_2$ is greater than 50 mmHg. Supplemental oxygen is sometimes indicated after thoracic surgery. Ventilatory support is rarely necessary after surgery; maintenance of 5 cm H_2O positive end-expiratory pressure therapy during thoracotomy decreases the degree of hypoxemia secondary to alveolar collapse during surgery.

A bandage placed under anesthesia or sedation is contraindicated and can lead to severe respiratory distress when the thorax expands in the recovery period. A light bandage can be applied when the animal is fully awake, to protect the wound and the drain.[37]

COMPLICATIONS

Most common complications are seroma formation, recurrence of the resected neoplasia, emphysema, pleural effusion, peripheral edema, pulmonary edema, and infection. In cats with neoplasia, pedicle flaps are preferred for thoracic wall reconstruction over foreign material (mesh) especially when the possibility exists that the tumor is not completely resected.

After autogenous reconstruction of chest wall defects, partial or complete muscle flap failure can occur and this can be a cause of seroma. Therefore, the cause of the seroma should be investigated if it does not resolve spontaneously.

REFERENCES

1. Hunt GB. Thoracic wall anatomy and surgical approaches. In: Bockman DJ, Hold DE, editors. BSAVA manual of canine and feline head, neck and thoracic surgery. 1st ed. Gloucester: British Veterinary Association; 2005. p. 135–48.
2. Hermanson JW, Evans HE. The muscular system. In: Evans HE, editor. Miller's anatomy of the dog. 3rd ed. Philadelphia: Sauders Company; 1993. p. 303.
3. Zulauf D, Kaser Hotz B, Hässig M, et al. Radiographic examination and outcome in consecutive feline trauma patients. Vet Comp Orthopaed Traumatol 2008;1: 36–40.
4. Davis KM, Hardie EM, Lascelles BDLX, Hansen B. Feline Fibrosarcoma: perioperative management. Comp Contin Ed Vet 2007;12:712–37.
5. Orton CE. Thoracic wall. In: Slatter D, editor. Textbook of small animal surgery. 3rd ed. Philadelphia: Saunders; 2002. p. 381.
6. Sturgess CP, Waters L, Gruffydd-Jones TJ, et al. An investigation into the association between whole blood and tissue taurine

7. levels in flat chests and pectus excavatum in neonatal Burmese kittens. Vet Record 1997;141:566–70.
7. Abato E, Byers CG. Flail chest. Standards of care 2009;9:1–7.
8. Hahn KA, Endicott MM, King GK, Harris-King FD. Evaluation of radiotherapy alone or in combination with doxorubicin chemotherapy for the treatment of cats with incompletely excised soft tissue sarcomas: 71 cases (1998-1999). J Am Vet Med Assoc 2007;231:742–5.
9. Olson D, Renberg W, Hauptman JG, et al. Clinical Management of Flail Chest in Dogs and Cats: A retrospective study of 24 cases (1989-1999). J Am Anim Hosp Assoc 2002;38:315–20.
10. Kolata RJ, Kraut NH, Johnston DE. Patterns of trauma in urban dogs and cats: A study of 1000 cases. J Am Vet Med Assoc 1974;164:499–502.
11. Rosetti E, Bertolini G, Zotti A. Multilobular tumour of bone of the thoracic wall in a cat. J Feline Med Surg 2007;9:254–7.

12. Stockhaus C, Teske E. Klinische Erfahrung mit der zytologischen Diagnostik beim Hund. Schweizer Archive für Tierheilkunde 2002;143:233–40.
13. Dernell WS. Tumours of the skeletal system. In: Dobson JM, Lascell BDX, editors. BSAVA manual of canine and feline oncology. 2nd ed. Gloucester: BSAVA; 2003. p. 179–96.
14. Kessler M, Tassani-Prell M, von Bomhard D, Matis U. Das Osteosarkom der Katze: epidemiologische, klinische und röntgenologische Befunde bei 78 Tieren (1990–1995) Tierärztl Prax 1997;25: 275–283.
15. Sabattini S, Bettini G. Prognostic value of histologic and immunohistochemical features in feline cutaneous mast cell tumors. Vet Pathol 2010;47(4): 643–53.
16. Nieto A, Sanchez MA, Martinez E, Rollan E. Immunohistochemical expression of p53, fibroblast growth factor-b, and transforming growth factor-α in feline vaccine associated sarcomas. Vet Pathol 2003;40:651–8.

17. Risselada M, de Rooster H, Liuti T, et al. Use of internal splinting to realign a noncompliant sternum in a cat with pectus excavatum. J Am Vet Med Assoc 2006;228:1047–52.

18. Gradner G, Weissenböck H, Kneissl S, et al. Use of latissimus dorsi and abdominal external oblique muscle for reconstruction of a thoracic wall defect in a cat with feline osteochondromatosis. J Feline Med Surg 2008;10:88–94.

19. Cronin K, Page RL, Spodnick G, et al. Radiation therapy and surgery for fibrosarcoma in 33 cats. Vet Radiol Ultrasound 1998;39:51–6.

20. Hershey AE, Sorenmo KU, Hendrick MJ, et al. Prognosis for presumed feline vaccine associated sarcoma after excision: 61 cases (1986–1996). J Am Vet Med Assoc 2000;216(1):58–61.

21. Cohen M, Wright JC, Brawner WR, et al. Use of surgery and electron beam irradiation, with or without chemotherapy, for treatment of vaccine-associated sarcomas in cats: 78 cases (1996–2000). J Am Vet Med Assoc 2001;219(11):1582–9.

22. Thamm DH, Vail DM. Mast cell tumors. In: Withrow S, Vail DM, editors. Small animal clinical oncology. 4th ed. Philadelphia: WB Saunders; 2007. p. 402–21.

23. Shires PK, Waldron DR, Payne J. Pectus excavatum by percutaneous suturing and temporary external coaptation in a kitten. J Am Vet Med Assoc 1988;194:1065–7.

24. Crigel MH, Moissonnier P. Pectus excavatum surgically repaired using sternum alignment and splint techniques in a young cat. J Small Anim Pract 2005;46:352–6.

25. Holt DE, Griffin GM. Dog bite wounds: bacteriology and treatment outcome in 37 cases. J Am Anim Hosp Assoc 2001;37:453–60.

26. Scheepens ETF, Peeters ME, Eplattenier HFL, Kirpensteijn J. Thoracic bite trauma in dogs: A comparison of clinical and radiological parameters with surgical results. J Small Anim Pract 2006;47:721–6.

27. Shamir MH, Leisner S, Klement E, et al. Dog bite wounds in dogs and cats: a retrospective study in 196 cases. J Vet Med Assoc 2002;49:107–12.

28. Zook EG, Miller M, Van Beek AL, Wavek P. Successful treatment protocol for canine fang injuries. J Trauma 1980;20:243–7.

29. Davidson EB. Managing bite wounds in dogs and cats – part I. Comp Contin Ed Vet 1998;20:811–20.

30. Davidson EB. Managing bite wounds in dogs and cats – part II. Comp Contin Ed Vet 1998;20:974–90.

31. Shahar R, Shamir M, Johnston DE. A technique for management of bite wounds of the thoracic wall in small dogs. Vet Surg 1997;26:45–50.

32. Scheepens ETF, Peeters ME, L'Eplattenier HF, Kirpensteijn J. Thoracic bite trauma in dogs: a comparison of clinical and radiological parameters with surgical results. J Small Anim Pract 2006;47:712–26.

33. Cowell K, Penwick C. Dog bite wounds: A study of 93 cases. Comp Contin Ed Vet 1989;11:313–20.

34. Talan DA, Citron DM, Abrahamian FM, et al. Bacteriologic analysis of infected dog and cat bites. N Eng J Med 1999;340:85–92.

35. Goldstein EJ, Richwald GA. Human and animal bite wounds. Am Fam Phys 1995;36:101–9.

36. Liptak JM, Dernell WS, Rizzo SA, et al. Reconstruction of chest wall defects after rib tumor resection: A comparison of autogenous, prosthetic, and composite techniques in 44 dogs. Vet Surg 2008;37:479–87.

37. Orton EC. Body cavities and hernias, thoracic wall. In: Slatter D, editor. Texbook of small animal surgery. 3rd ed. Philadelphia: Saunders; 2003. p. 373–87.

38. Bowman KLT, Birchard SJ, Bright RM. Complications associated with the implantation of polypropylene mesh in dogs and cats: a retrospective study of 21 cases (1984–1996). J Am Anim Hosp Assoc 1998;34:225–33.

39. Aronson M. Diaphragmatic advancement for defects of the caudal thoracic wall in the dog. Vet Surg 1984;13:26–8.

40. Baines S. Pedicle muscle flaps. In: Williams J, Moores A, editors. BSAVA manual of canine and feline wound management and reconstruction. 2nd ed. Gloucester: BSAVA; 2010. p. 159–200.

41. Bright RM. Reconstruction of thoracic wall defects using Marlex mesh. J Am Anim Hosp Assoc 1981;17:415–20.

42. Usher FC, Gannon JP. Marlex mesh, a new plastic mesh for replacing tissue defects. Am Med Assoc Arch Surg 1959;78:131–7.

43. Badylak SF. Small intestinal submucosa: A biomaterial conducive to smart tissue remodelling. In: Bell E, editor. Tissue engineering: Current prospectives. Cambridge, AM: Burkhause; 1993. p. 179–89.

44. Tattersall JA, Welsh E. Factors influencing the short-term outcome following thoracic surgery in 98 dogs. J Small Anim Pract 2006;47(12):715–20.

Chapter |44|

Pleura

A.L. Moores

Pleural diseases are a significant cause of respiratory distress in cats and while life-threatening if severe, they can often be managed successfully. Thirty years ago, all cats with pleural fluid due to thymic lymphosarcoma or pulmonary carcinoma were immediately euthanized according to one study.[1] Now, advancements in diagnostic procedures, critical care management, surgical techniques, and adjunctive therapies mean that most pleural diseases have a better outcome.

SURGICAL ANATOMY AND PATHOPHYSIOLOGY

The pleura is a serous membrane that lines the mediastinum, pericardium, diaphragm and thoracic wall (parietal pleural), and the lungs (visceral or pulmonary pleura) (Fig. 44-1). A fold of pleura encloses the caudal vena cava. The left and right pleural cavities are potential spaces in normal cats, containing a small volume of serous fluid for lubrication. The mediastinal pleura is often incomplete, allowing communication between the pleural cavities. The blood supply to the parietal pleura is from the arteries of the thoracic wall, i.e., the intercostal, diaphragmatic, and pericardial arteries. The pulmonary and bronchial circulation supplies the visceral pleura. The pulmonary ligaments are fairly avascular.

Lymphatic drainage from the thoracic wall and pleura is to the cranial sternal and cranial mediastinal lymph nodes.

The cisterna chyli in cats is bipartite, arising ventral to the last thoracic to third lumbar vertebrae, lying both dorsal and ventral to the aorta and in close association with the crura of the diaphragm. The thoracic duct, which actually comprises multiple collateral ducts, arises from the cisterna chyli and passes through the aortic hiatus on the left dorsal aspect of the aorta, before entering the left jugular vein.

Pleural effusion may occur when there is an increase in systemic or pleural capillary hydrostatic pressure (e.g., congestive heart failure), a decrease in plasma oncotic pressure (e.g., hypoalbuminemia), increased capillary permeability (e.g., inflammation), or lymphatic obstruction. More simply, the rate of fluid production into the pleural space is greater than the rate of fluid drainage from it. Hemorrhagic effusions may occur due to bleeding from vessel erosion (e.g., neoplasia, infection), trauma or coagulopathy.

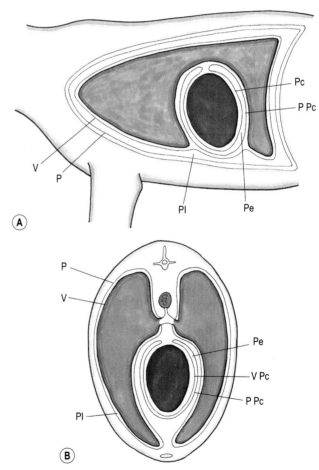

Figure 44-1 Pleural anatomy. P, parietal pleura; Pl, pleural cavity; P Pc, parietal pericardium; Pe, pericardial cavity; V , visceral pleura; V Pc, visceral pericardium.

© 2014 Elsevier Ltd
DOI: 10.1016/B978-0-7020-4336-9.00044-5

GENERAL CONSIDERATIONS AND DIAGNOSTIC PROCEDURES

Clinical signs and physical examination

While pleural disease in cats will have the same clinical effects as in dogs, the symptoms are often less apparent due to the differences in physical activity, and as such, owners will usually not notice the early changes in behavior and respiration that may be detected in dogs. Signs are often not detected until the disease is in the advanced stages and causing respiratory distress, open mouth breathing, and cyanosis. Indeed, one study reported that breathing abnormalities were not noted by 40% of owners with dyspneic cats.[2]

The clinical signs of pleural disease most often reflect the presence of fluid, air or soft tissue in the pleural space, with the most common signs relating to incomplete lung expansion. The respiratory pattern is usually short and shallow, in contrast to that seen with many other diseases of the respiratory tract. However, as with other respiratory conditions, cats with pleural disease may choose to limit their movement and often adopt a position that aids more effective breathing (usually a sternal position), with or without elbow abduction. Paradoxical abdominal effort can occur with severe disease. Depending on the degree of respiratory compromise, cats may also have other clinical signs including reduced appetite, anorexia and weight loss, lethargy, and depression.

In one study of 73 cats with pleural fluid, the main presenting complaints were dyspnea/tachypnea (69%), lethargy/weakness (36%), inappetence/weight loss (27%), dysphagia/regurgitation (12%), and cough (12%). Physical examination findings included dyspnea (59%), muffled cardiac and breath sounds (41%), tachypnea (38%), poor body condition (33%), hypothermia (21%), pyrexia (18%), reduced thoracic compressibility (14%), and tachycardia (8%).[3]

In light of the fragile nature of many of these patients, the first part of the examination of a dyspneic cat should just involve careful observation of the respiratory pattern and an assessment of the cat's general condition, taking care to minimize stress and handling. If necessary, oxygen support should be provided before any physical examination is undertaken. Careful auscultation should then be performed to elucidate whether or not there is a reduction/absence of normal lung sounds and if so, in which areas of the thorax such deficits are present. Gentle percussion over all the lung fields can also be extremely useful, with dull, hyporesonant or absent sounds being suggestive of pleural fluid or a large mass lesion, in which case these abnormalities are likely to be in the dependent part of the thorax. Hyper-resonance is indicative of a pneumothorax and this is most likely to be heard in the dorsal part of the thorax (see Chapter 41, Table 41-2).

Emergency management

The reason it is so important to avoid stress during the initial handling of the cat is because it can increase respiratory effort and, in severely ill cats, this can even lead to respiratory arrest. If used, supplementation of oxygen can be provided via facemask, flow-by technique (administering the oxygen close to but not covering the face) or by placing the cat in an oxygen cage. An oxygen cage allows for careful observation without direct handling but does not easily allow diagnostic and therapeutic techniques to be performed. Thoracocentesis (ideally ultrasound-guided) should be performed early on in markedly dyspneic cats before any procedure other than oxygenation, including the placement of an intravenous catheter, as the stress of handling for catheter placement may be sufficient to cause respiratory arrest. Thoracocentesis is often the most important therapeutic intervention in pleural diseases causing air or fluid production, with the advantage that this technique is also diagnostic for many conditions.

Diagnostic imaging

Radiography is often not performed until after thoracocentesis. Movement artifacts are a significant problem and may limit the film's diagnostic quality. Other imaging modalities, e.g., ultrasonography, may be preferred or used concurrently. Radiography can identify pleural fluid and air, with the dorsoventral view the most useful for detection of small volumes of air or fluid (Figs 44-2 and 44-3). Ventrodorsal radiography is avoided as it can lead to marked respiratory

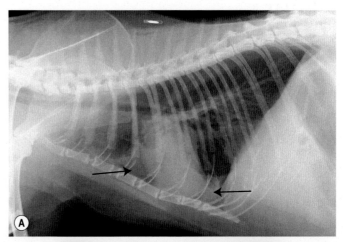

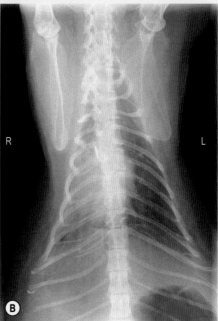

Figure 44-2 (A) Lateral and **(B)** dorsoventral (DV) radiographs of the thorax. A small volume pleural effusion is evident in the lateral radiograph (arrows). In the DV radiograph, a mediastinal shift of the cardiac silhouette is present. The right lung lobes are collapsed causing an even increase in soft tissue opacity throughout the right hemithorax. The most likely cause is a right lateral recumbent position for some length of time before the DV radiograph was taken. A small amount of pleural effusion cannot be excluded on this radiograph.

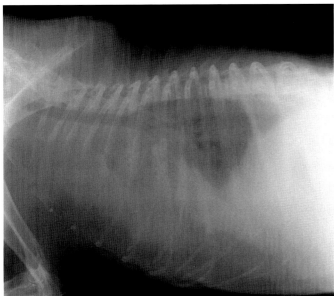

Figure 44-3 Lateral radiograph of the thorax showing a large volume pleural effusion.

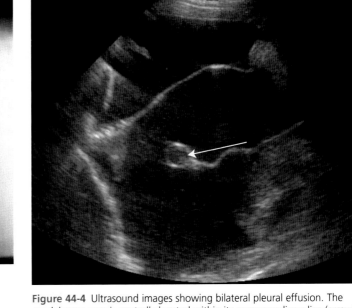

Figure 44-4 Ultrasound images showing bilateral pleural effusion. The caudal vena cava is centrally located within its corresponding plica (arrow).

distress by causing collapse of the dorsal part of the lungs. Underlying causes of large volume pleural fluid cannot often be identified radiographically prior to thoracocentesis as fluid obscures soft tissue structures. Radiography is, however, useful for evaluating underlying diseases after fluid has been removed and can also be used to assess the completeness of thoracocentesis. Due to superimposition of mediastinal structures, especially in the cranial mediastinum, small mediastinal masses may be difficult to detect radiographically although there may be widening of the mediastinum. Large masses can usually be easily identified.

Ultrasound is the diagnostic imaging modality of choice to identify the presence of pleural fluid and has the advantage that it can be performed with the cat in almost any body position to minimize further respiratory difficulties (Fig. 44-4). Ultrasound also facilitates guided thoracocentesis of small volumes of fluid and identification of possible underlying causes, e.g., abscess. Ultrasound is an excellent way to assess mediastinal masses and is a simple method to aid procurement of cells or tissue by aspiration or needle core biopsy techniques. It can also be a useful way to assess the progression of treatment, as a cadaver study of estimation of fluid volume showed a good correlation with absolute volume,[4] making it an effective method for comparing sequential fluid volumes. Ultrasound is less useful in the presence of air as the ultrasound waves are reflected at the soft tissue–air interface.

Advanced imaging techniques can offer the most information on pleural disease. Computed tomography scans are generally significantly faster to perform than MRI and movement of the thorax is a particular problem with MRI, resulting in distracting artefacts (see Chapter 8). There will inevitably be some movement blur during computed tomography (CT), as there is for radiography and MRI, but this can be minimized by hyperventilation prior to scanning during the expiratory pause. CT allows effective visualization of the entire thoracic cavity for assessment of the volume of fluid/air, possible underlying causes, and other concurrent mediastinal diseases (see Chapter 8). The CT findings in normal cats and those with pleural, pulmonary, and mediastinal diseases have been described.[5,6]

Laboratory analysis and etiology

Serum biochemistry, hematology and FIV/FeLV testing should be performed to rule out concurrent disease. Heartworm antibody testing is performed in areas where the disease is endemic.

Pus, blood, and chyle generally have a characteristic gross appearance, but laboratory testing is always necessary to confirm the diagnosis. Pleural fluid analysis should include cell count, cytology, aerobic and anaerobic bacteriological and fungal culture. Transudates and exudates can be accurately differentiated, with pleural fluid lactate dehydrogenase concentration and pleural fluid/serum total protein ratio being reported as the most the reliable parameters (sensitivity of 100% and 91% and specificity of 100%, respectively). However, additional parameters such as the pleural fluid/serum cholesterol ratio and serum/effusion cholesterol gradient can also help in classifying the effusion if necessary.[7]

Tables 44-1 and 44-2 show the incidence and underlying causes of pleural fluid submitted to a laboratory for analysis.[3] No underlying cause was identified in 23% of cats. As expected, FIP affected predominantly young cats and neoplastic conditions, other than thymic lymphoma, older cats.

Simultaneous pleural and peritoneal effusion is most common in dogs and cats with neoplastic and cardiovascular diseases and non-neoplastic liver disease. It develops most rapidly in those with infectious causes of pleuritis and/or peritonitis and pancreatitis, although the description in the literature does not differentiate dogs and cats.[8] The prognosis of double effusions is grave as it is usually an indication of severe disease.

Thoracoscopy

Thoracoscopy (see Chapter 42) has been described in the cat as a less invasive technique than thoracotomy to examine the thoracic cavity and obtain tissue for histologic evaluation.[9] However, this can be challenging in the face of a pleural effusion and full thoracic drainage is required before thoracoscopy is performed, to enable maximum visualization of the pleural cavity.

Table 44-1 Types of pleural effusion and potential underlying causes of each type of effusion[3]

Effusion	Incidence (%)	Examples of underlying causes
Chylous	31	Idiopathic Cardiac disease Mediastinal mass Dirofilariasis Pericardial effusion Lung lobe torsion Congenital thoracic duct anomaly Pulmonary disease Trauma
Neoplastic	21	Mesothelioma Metastatic malignant melanoma Disseminated histiocytic sarcoma
Septic exudate – Pyothorax	15	Puncture wound Lung lobe abscess Intrabronchial plant material Foreign body granuloma Perforating esophageal disease Iatrogenic
Modified transudate	13	Heart failure Lung lobe torsion Neoplasia Diaphragmatic rupture Pancreatitis
Non-septic purulent exudate	11	Feline infectious peritonitis
Blood PCV/TP > 50% peripheral blood	10	Trauma Coagulopathy Blood vessel erosion by neoplasia or inflammation Dirofilariasis Pulmonary fat embolization
Transudate		Pulmonary tumor Acquired heart disease Congenital PPDH Thymic lymphosarcoma Diaphragmatic rupture Perinephric pseudocyst
Miscellaneous		Urine Bile Eosinophilic, e.g., aleurostrongylosis

Table 44-2 Underlying causes of pleural effusion based on pleural fluid analysis ($n = 82$ cats)[3]

Underlying disease	Incidence (%)
Pyothorax	18
Mediastinal lymphoma	17
Feline infectious peritonitis	10
Trauma	10
Pulmonary neoplasia	6
Hypertrophic cardiomyopathy	6
Unspecified mediastinal mass	5
Pulmonary thromboemboli	1
Pericardioperitoneal hernia	1
Heartworm disease	1
Restrictive cardiomyopathy	1
Unknown	23

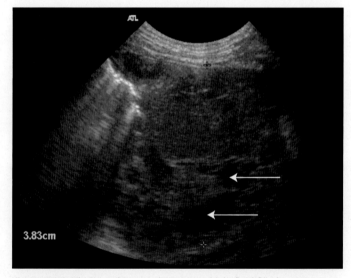

Figure 44-5 Ultrasound image showing multiple fluid-filled cavities (arrows) consistent with pulmonary abscessation.

SURGICAL DISEASES

Pyothorax

Pyothorax is an inflammatory disease of the pleural space caused by inoculation of the pleural space with microorganisms. Cats with pyothorax may be younger than the general hospital population and more likely to come from multi-cat households and there is no sex predisposition. The causative organism is usually a bacterium and it was originally thought these came from the oral cavity following a cat bite, or the environment by direct penetration of the thoracic wall. However, in one large study only 14% of cats had a history of a bite or other trauma[10] and the inciting cause often remains undetected. It has been recently suggested that the most common cause (56%) is parapneumonic spread of infection after colonization and invasion of lung tissue by oropharyngeal flora.[2] Postmortem studies of cats with pyothorax showed underlying causes in less than half of cases and these included: lung lobe abscesses (Fig. 44-5), puncture wounds, intrabronchial plant material, and foreign body granuloma.[10] Iatrogenic infection occurred in 14% of cats with chylothorax treated by thoracocentesis or surgery.[11]

A positive bacterial culture was obtained in 96% of cats clinically suspected to have pyothorax, of which 89% were obligate anaerobes.[12]

Table 44-3 Bacterial isolates from cases of feline pyothorax[10,12]

Bacteria	Incidence (%)
Aerobic	
Pasteurella	13–39
Unidentified non-enteric bacteria	5
Actinomyces spp.	4–15
Other	5
Anaerobic	
Clostridium	0–48
Bacteroides spp.	19–20
Peptostreptococcus anaerobius	17
Fusobacterium spp.	14–21
Porphyromonas spp.	10
Prevotella spp.	8
Other	16
Negative culture	4

Table 44-4 Typical clinical signs and physical examination findings in cats with pyothorax[2,10,15]

Clinical signs	Incidence (%)
Decreased appetite/anorexia	21–83
Lethargy	36–80
Dyspnea	59–79
Hypersalivation	18
Weight loss	14–36
Cough	26
Vomiting	15
Pain	13
Ocular/nasal discharge	9
Physical examination findings	
Increased respiratory effort	81–94
Abnormal lung sounds	97
Abnormal mucous membrane color	97
Poor pulse quality	68
Mental dullness	96
Dehydration	7–93
Poor body condition	37–67
Tachycardia	21–64
Pyrexia	29–50
Hypothermia	15
Muffled heart sounds	14–37

Forty-four per cent of these cats had a mixture of facultative bacteria and obligate anaerobes and an average of 2.1 obligate anaerobic and 1.2 aerobic bacterial species were isolated per cat. Table 44-3 shows the bacterial isolates from feline cases of pyothorax from two studies. Of the facultative bacteria isolated, most were non-enteric (especially *Pasteurella*), in contrast to dogs in which the Enterobacteriaceae (especially *E. coli*) were more common.[12] At the time of the study, the *Pasteurella* species were sensitive to those antibiotics they were tested against. Eight percent of cats with pyothorax had *Actinomyces* species isolated, which is usually considered to be associated with grass awns in dogs, but there appears to be less of an association in cats. Almost a quarter of cats are reported to have unusual causative organisms isolated including *Candida albicans, Salmonella, Cryptococcus, Rhodococcus, Blastomyces,* and *Mycoplasma* species.[2,13,14]

Typical clinical signs and physical examination findings are shown in Table 44-4. In one study 30% of cats had a current or recent history of upper respiratory tract infection.[2] Dehydration in most cats and poor body condition in up to two-thirds suggest the disease is not immediately apparent to owners.[10] Average time from onset of clinical signs to referral was up to 40 days.[2,15] Changes on serum biochemistry and hematology included hyponatremia, hypochloremia, hypocalcemia, hypoalbuminemia, high aspartate aminotransferase activity, high total bilirubin concentration, elevated mean white blood cell and neutrophil counts, presence of band neutrophils, and anemia.[2,10,15,16] Hypersalivation and a lower heart rate were significantly related to mortality, as was cholesterol and lower white blood cell count.[10] Just over half of cats that had enough information for assessment were diagnosed with sepsis or systemic inflammatory response syndrome.[10]

Radiography was used for the diagnosis of pleural fluid in all cases;[2,10] 76–89% had bilateral effusion, and 40% in one study also had evidence of concurrent pneumonia.[2]

Abnormalities of color, texture, and odor will be noted on gross fluid samples but the definitive diagnosis of an exudate requires pleural fluid analysis including cell counts and cytologic identification of degenerate neutrophils with or without the presence of intracellular bacteria. Cats are more likely than dogs to have bacteria identified on pleural fluid cytology (91% compared with 68% dogs with positive bacterial culture).[2,12] Failure to demonstrate bacteria cytologically may be related to recent antibiotic administration or inappropriate techniques. Fluid samples should be submitted for aerobic and anaerobic bacteriologic and fungal culture and antimicrobial sensitivity testing to identify causative organisms and provide the appropriate treatment.

Feline pyothorax is usually treated medically as a first-line approach. Intravenous fluid therapy is instituted to correct dehydration and electrolyte abnormalities, and thoracocentesis is performed to relieve dyspnea and obtain a fluid sample prior to antibiotic administration. Results of bacterial studies recommend that initial antibiotics be directed against both anaerobic bacteria (e.g., ampicillin, amoxicillin-clavulanic acid, clindamycin or metronidazole) and facultative bacteria (e.g., ceftizoxime).[10] These drugs have good pleural penetration and low toxicity. Although amikacin and gentamicin have good activity against *E. coli* and other Enterobacteriaceae, their poor pleural penetration and the low incidence of Enterobacteriaceae in feline pyothorax limits their usefulness as a first-line antibiotic, although retrospective case series show that veterinarians have been prescribing them clinically.[10] Obligate anaerobic bacteria are inherently resistant to aminoglycosides and quinolones and there may be inhibition of trimethoprim-sulfonamide by inhibitors within the exudate.[12] The most commonly used antibiotics in a published retrospective study pending culture results were ampicillin (83%), gentamicin (62%), metronidazole (42%), the cephalosporins (23%), enrofloxaxin

(19%), and clindamycin (17%).[10] Most cats were treated with multiple classes of drugs but further information on specific combinations was not reported.[10] Antibiotic use is prolonged, with a mean duration of 30–50 days.[2,15]

Thoracostomy tube use has been related to increased survival.[10] Bilateral tube use has been recommended for bilateral effusion.[2] The use of routine lavage in feline pyothorax is controversial; however, the cats in the more recent studies underwent therapeutic lavage with isotonic saline or compound sodium lactate, with the occasional addition of an antibiotic solution.[2,15] The authors argued that lavage may decrease the time that tubes need to be maintained, thus reducing tube-associated pain, risk of nosocomial infection and hospitalization times. Cats have been successfully treated with small-bore wire-guided chest tubes placed by a Seldinger technique, which can usually be placed with the cat sedated rather than anesthetized.[17] Lavage was performed two to six times daily and none of the tubes became occluded, suggesting that they can be successfully used and potentially reduce the morbidity associated with the large-bore tubes.

Indications for surgery include failure of medical therapy or identification of an obvious surgical cause such as an abscess on diagnostic imaging (see Fig. 44-5). It appears that the requirement for surgery following medical management is low; of 35 cats that underwent thoracic lavage and survived the placement of drains in one study, only one cat required thoracotomy.[2,15]

In the largest case series of pyothorax in cats, 26% of cases were euthanized without treatment, due to either financial constraints or a poor perceived prognosis, and a further 11% died within 24 hours of presentation.[10] Overall, 66% of cats that were treated survived, with 78% survival of those still alive 24 hours after admission. Of those cats available for follow up, only one (5%) had disease recurrence. Better survival rates were reported in studies where thoracostomy tubes were placed in all patients and thoracic lavage was performed (77–93%).[2,15]

The surgical approach in cases of feline pyothorax would usually be guided by diagnostic imaging results. If a specific lesion is identified (e.g., lung lobe abscess) then a lateral thoracotomy is indicated. For non-specific causes or multiple lesions then a median sternotomy is selected to access the entire chest for thorough exploration.

Chylothorax

Chylothorax is the pathological accumulation of chyle in the pleural space. Experimentally, chylothorax has been induced in cats following ligation of the cranial vena cava although it is interesting to note that resolution of the chylothorax was noted in some cases, presumably due to the development of collateral lymphatic circulation in the thorax and abdomen.[18] However, in the clinical situation the majority of cases of chylothorax are idiopathic in nature. It is obviously important to rule out the presence of underlying diseases that can cause leakage of chyle from the thoracic duct, either due to increased pressure in the thoracic duct or interference with chyle flow through the duct (Fig. 44-6). Right-sided heart failure does not commonly cause chylothorax in cats. Chylothorax is occasionally caused by traumatic disruption of the thoracic duct following trauma or as a surgical complication e.g., transection of the left brachiocephalic vein.[11,19,20] Reported causes of chylothorax in the cat are listed in Box 44-1.

Pure bred cats are reported to be more commonly affected with chylothorax.[11] The mean age of presentation is reported to be six years (range six months to 14 years) with older cats being more likely to develop chylothorax, which may be related to its association with neoplasia. There is no reported sex predisposition.[11] The presenting complaint and physical examination findings include dyspnea (84%) and coughing (30%).[11]

Chylous fluid is typically white but is often pink due to the presence of erythrocytes. However, it is vital to confirm whether or not any suspected chylous fluid is truly chyle by performing a biochemical

Figure 44-6 Schematic showing the pathophysiology of chylothorax

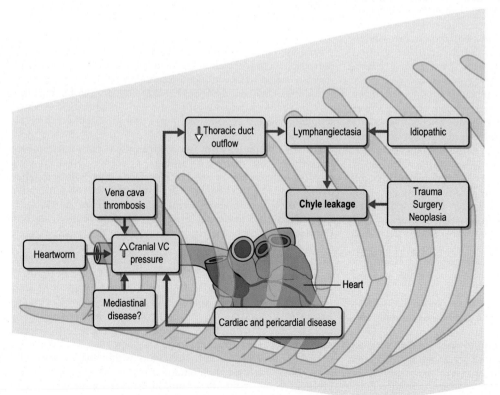

Heart disease
   a. Cardiomyopathy (hypertrophic, restrictive and unclassified) either idiopathic or secondary to thyrotoxicosis
   b. Congenital cardiac disease (such as tetralogy of Fallot, tricuspid or mitral valve dysplasia) resulting in congestive heart failure
Dirofilariasis (in endemic areas)
Pericardial disease (causing pericardial effusion or restrictive pericarditis)
Venous obstruction
   Thrombosis of the cranial vena cava (e.g., as a complication of a jugular catheter)
   Cryptococcal mediastinal granuloma (precaval syndrome)
Cranial mediastinal mass
   Mediastinal lymphosarcoma
   Thymoma
   Lymphangiosarcoma
Lung lobe torsion
Pulmonary neoplasia
Trauma
Congenital thoracic duct anomalies e.g., lack of continuity of the thoracic duct

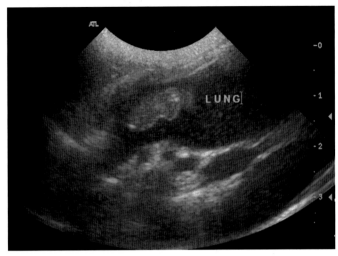

Figure 44-7 Ultrasound image of a consolidated lung lobe surrounded by hyperechoic pleural effusion. Failure of the lung to re-expand after fluid drainage may suggest constrictive pleuritis.

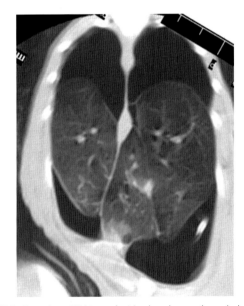

Figure 44-8 Conscious CT image (cat in dorsal recumbancy) showing cortication of the lung lobes and thickening of the pleura, consistent with constrictive pleuritis.

analysis on the effusion. True chyle has a cholesterol to triglyceride ratio of <1 with significantly greater triglyceride in pleural fluid than serum. Cytology classically reveals predominantly a mixture of small and large lymphocytes, with increasing numbers of neutrophils, macrophages and mesothelial cells seen in chronic cases. Cytology and bacteriologic culture must be performed to rule out concurrent pyothorax, especially in cats that have had repeated thoracocentesis. Once the effusion has been confirmed to be truly chylous in nature, investigation of any potential underlying causes should focus on careful imaging evaluation of the thorax and particularly the heart.

Most cases resulting from trauma or surgical complications will usually resolve with intermittent thoracocentesis.[11] Medical or surgical management of specific underlying causes may also lead to resolution of the effusion. However, cats managed with long-term periodic thoracocentesis may develop complications including iatrogenic pyothorax or fibrosing pleuritis.

Medical management of idiopathic chylothorax can be attempted by intermittent thoracocentesis to manage any respiratory distress, a low fat diet, and an oral benzopyrone, i.e., rutin. This approach occasionally leads to complete or partial resolution of the effusion but the success rates are low. As a result of the limited efficacy of this treatment surgery is usually recommended for cats with idiopathic chylothorax failing to show significant improvement after 14 days of medical therapy. Surgical management of cats with chylothorax is discussed below.

Constrictive (or restrictive) pleuritis was associated with chylothorax in ten of 15 of cats in one study.[21] In another study the chronic presence of chylous fluid led to moderate to severe fibrosing pleuritis in five of ten cats,[22] which may result in an inability of atelectic lung lobes to re-expand after removal of fluid. Constrictive pleuritis has also been associated with other pleural effusions, e.g., FIP.[23] Ongoing respiratory distress may be evident and the condition carries a guarded prognosis. Diagnostic imaging shows atelectic lung lobes with rounded edges (Figs 44-7 and 44-8).[21] Decortication has been described to remove fibrous tissue from lung parenchyma and allow pulmonary expansion, but this procedure has also been associated with

pneumothorax and pulmonary edema[24] so cannot be routinely recommended. Some cats may have ongoing non-chylous fluid production after thoracic duct ligation. Pericardectomy is recommended if it has not already been performed.[22]

Mediastinal masses

Mediastinal masses are uncommon in the cat.[25] However, they are an important cause of disease, with signs that can be attributed to the pleural cavity as they can cause dyspnea, coughing (either due to direct compression of lungs or the presence of pleural fluid), lethargy, and weight loss. More specific physical examination findings may include reduced compressibility of the cranial thorax and caval syndrome due to the fact that both thymoma and thymic lymphoma can be very large (>10 cm) at the time of diagnosis.[25] The presence of a secondary pleural effusion can make the diagnosis, especially by radiography, difficult, thereby increasing the challenge to the clinician.

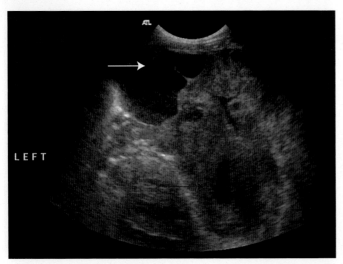

Figure 44-9 Ultrasound image showing anechoic pleural effusion (arrow) and a large heterogeneous cranial mediastinal mass (red arrow).

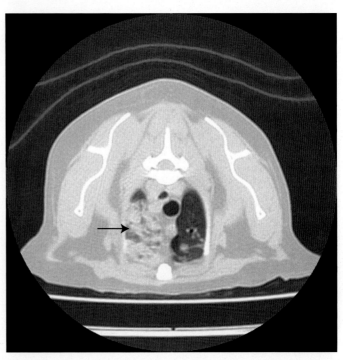

Figure 44-10 Computed tomography image showing a cavitary mass (arrow) in the right cranial hemithorax.

Table 44-5 Causes of thymic pathology in 30 cats[25]

Cause	Incidence (%)
Thymoma	63
Thymic hyperplasia	17
Thymic branchial cyst formation or cystic change	7
Congenital thymic hypoplasia	3
Thymic hemorrhage	3
Thymic amyloidosis	3

Differential diagnoses of mediastinal masses in cats include: thymic lymphoma, thymoma (which may be solid or cystic), thymic hyperplasia, other cystic lesions (from the thymic branchial or pharyngeal arches including thyroglossal duct cysts, parathyroid gland, thymus and idiopathic cysts), and thymolipoma. The causes of thymic pathology reported in 30 cats are listed in Table 44-5.

The diagnosis of a mediastinal mass relies predominantly on imaging. Radiology is usually sufficient but more information about local invasion and metastatic disease can be obtained using ultrasound and computed tomography (Figs 44-9 and 44-10). However, cytologic or histopathologic assessment is required for a definitive diagnosis.

Thymic lymphoma is more common than thymoma in cats, a reverse of the trend seen in dogs.[25] It generally presents in young cats and in one study four out of eight cats tested were positive for FeLV infection. It frequently spreads locally (lung, pericardium, and body wall) and metastasizes. Thymic lymphoma is not a surgical disease but is generally considered to respond well to chemotherapy or radiotherapy.

Thymoma is a tumor of thymic epithelial cells with benign lymphoid proliferation. The predominance of epithelial or lymphoid cells may vary between thymomas and can sometimes make differentiation from lymphoma difficult, especially on cytology. Cystic lesions may be present and in one report cholesterol-rich fluid was isolated.[26]

Squamous cell carcinoma has been reported arising from thymomas.[27] Thymoma generally affects older cats than those with lymphoma and is not usually associated with FeLV infection. Thymomas are usually biologically benign and tend to be non-invasive and non-metastatic, with a low mitotic rate. Staging in people and dogs is based on invasiveness rather than histopathologic features but this has not yet been related to prognosis in cats.[28] In one study, of 11 tumors in nine cats (two were recurrences), four were encapsulated/non-adherent and seven adherent to the pericardium and pleura.[28] Of the latter, four were poorly encapsulated. Radiation therapy has been described and while complete responses were rare, median survival approached two years, so it may have a role to play in the therapy of invasive thymoma.[29] Chemotherapy is reported to be unrewarding.[28] Surgical management of thymomas is described and discussed below.

Thymic masses may result in paraneoplastic syndromes (Table 44-6) that may resolve after mass resection.[30]

The prognosis for lymphangiomas, multilocular thymic cysts, and cystic thymomas managed surgically can be excellent.[35]

Pneumothorax

Traumatic pneumothorax may occur due to discontinuity of the thoracic wall or intrathoracic structures following trauma (Box 44-2). Spontaneous pneumothorax (the accumulation of pleural air in the absence of trauma) is less common in cats than dogs.[36]

The clinical presentation is similar to that for pleural effusion. However, development of tension pneumothorax, in which a massive accumulation of air in the pleural space due to skin or soft tissue acting as a one-way valve for the entry of air, may rapidly lead to circulatory and respiratory arrest. Radiography can be used to diagnose pneumothorax (see Chapter 8), but computed tomography is often required to identify and localize potential underlying causes.

There are several reports of iatrogenic pneumothorax, including creation of a bronchopleural fistula after thoracocentesis,[37] bronchial

Table 44-6 Paraneoplastic syndromes associated with thymic tumors

Paraneoplastic syndromes and conditions related to thyroid disease	Pathophysiology	Clinical signs
Skin diseases including: Basement membrane immune complex deposition; superficial necrolytic dermatitis; pemphigus foliaceus; exfoliative dermatitis[25]	Histopathologic evidence of a cell-poor hydropic interface dermatitis of the surface and follicular epithelium	Non-pruritic scaling dermatits
Myasthenia gravis[31]	Autoantibodies to the acetylcholine receptor	Dysphagia/regurgitation (megaesophagus) Reduced ocular reflexes Neck ventroflexion, weakness
Polymyositis including myocarditis[31,32]		Muscle weakness, difficulty swallowing
Hypercalcemia[33]	Production of parathyroid hormone-like substances	Polyuria/polydypsia, clinical signs of urolithiasis or urinary tract infection,
Granulocytopenia[34]	Immune-mediated destruction of peripheral granulocytes	

Box 44-2 Causes of traumatic and spontaneous pneumothorax

Traumatic pneumothorax

Open – disruption of the neck or thoracic wall:
   Bite wounds (see Chapter 43), gunshot wounds, shearing injuries, laceration from rib fractures
   Iatrogenic – thoracotomy dehiscence
Closed – leakage from internal structures:
   Trachea, e.g., foreign body
   Esophagus, e.g., foreign body (see Chapter 27)
   Alveoli and small airways, e.g., blunt trauma
   Cystic thymoma
   Iatrogenic, e.g., lung disease following thoracocentesis or drain placement, thoracic disc fenestration, venepuncture
   Anesthesia, e.g., iatrogenic endotracheal tube-related injury (see Chapter 46) or positive-pressure ventilation

Spontaneous pneumothorax

Primary pneumothorax: pulmonary bullae
Secondary pneumothorax (sequel to underlying lung disease):
   Parasitic infection – *Dirofilaria immitis, Aelurostrongylus abstrusus*
   Feline asthma (small airway disease)
   Eosinophilic small airway inflammation

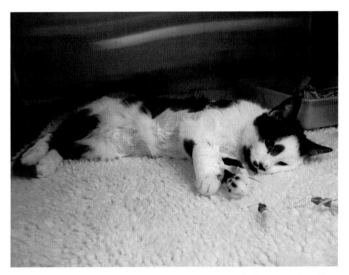

Figure 44-11 A six month old male kitten presented after a road traffic accident with dyspnea and tachypnea due to a traumatic hemothorax.

rupture during handling of a kitten for venepuncture,[38] and during anesthesia (possible causes including tracheal disruption, barotrauma or a closed pop-off valve while using high oxygen flows).[39,40]

Traumatic pneumothorax and pneumothorax due to an underlying disease, e.g., small airway disease or parasitic disease, are managed initially by thoracocentesis, with thoracostomy tube placement used in persistent cases. Resolution typically occurs following healing of the damaged tissue. In one report two cats with small airway disease were treated by thoracocentesis followed by medical management of the underlying disease. The authors suggested the use of more aggressive medical management should the pneumothorax recur but caution that surgical resection may not prevent leakage from another diseased portion of lung in the future.[41] A recent report of 35 cats with spontaneous pneumothorax showed that in cats with an established

etiology, pneumothorax occurred due to underlying lung disease, such as inflammatory airway disease, neoplasia, heartworm infection, pulmonary abscess and lungworm infection. Many cats were managed successfully with specific therapy for their primary lung disease, and needle thoracocentesis in some cases, without the need for surgery. Cats therefore seem to have a better prognosis with medical therapy than dogs.[42] Pulmonary bulla formation was described in conjunction with bronchopulmonary dysplasia, which may represent an underlying cause.[36] Areas of emphysema can be removed by partial lung lobectomy; however, as there is no evidence that emphysematous lesions will cause recurrence of pneumothorax the author would leave extensive lesions in situ if surgical resection is not feasible at the time of surgery.

Hemothorax

Hemothorax is diagnosed if the packed cell volume of pleural fluid is greater than half that of peripheral blood. Reported causes include trauma (Fig. 44-11), cardiopulmonary resuscitation, clotting disorders, blood vessel wall invasion (inflammation, neoplasia), *Dirofilaria immitis* infestation and pulmonary fat embolization.[3,43] Fluid resuscitation and use of blood products may be necessary following major hemorrhage, and surgical intervention may be required to identify and control the source of hemorrhage.

Neoplastic effusion

Neoplastic effusion is a rare cause of pleural effusion in the cat. However, possible underlying neoplasms include mesothelioma, pulmonary carcinoma, metastatic malignant melanoma and disseminated histiocytic sarcoma. Diagnosis is by identifying neoplastic cells on cytology although it can be difficult to differentiate reactive and neoplastic mesothelial cells. Histopathology and, if necessary or possible, immunohistochemistry on samples collected by ultrasound-guided biopsy, thoracoscopy or thoracotomy should provide a definitive diagnosis. Gross inspection of the pleural and pericardial surfaces usually demonstrates nodular lesions but because the disease may be microscopic it is recommended that biopsies should be taken from all cats with pleural effusion undergoing thoracoscopy or thoracotomy. Thoracic omentalization has been described in a cat with refractory neoplastic pleural effusion that required frequent thoracocentesis.[44] Intracavitary carboplatin, as has been reported to be successful in the dog, has been used to treat presumed mesothelioma although the survival time was only 120 days in the single case reported.[45]

PREPARATION FOR SURGERY

Preparation of a cat for thoracotomy and the thoractomy procedure are described in detail in Chapter 41. Anesthesia considerations for a cat undergoing thoracic surgery are covered in Chapter 2. The lymphangiography procedures that are often recommended prior to and post thoracic duct ligation are described below.

Lymphangiography

Mesenteric

Mesenteric lymphangiography is performed pre ligation of the thoracic duct to aid its identification and post ligation to assess the success of the procedure.[46] Oil or cream is administered per os within the 12 hours prior to surgery to enhance identification of the lymphatic vessels. The cat is positioned in right lateral recumbency to perform a left paracostal incision. A mesenteric lymphatic vessel is catheterized distal to a mesenteric lymph node. A water-soluble iodinated contrast agent is then injected and fluoroscopy or radiography is performed. Methylene blue can also be given via the lymphatic vessel to help identify the thoracic duct and toxicosis has not been reported.

Mesenteric lymphangiography can be difficult to perform due to the small size of lymphatic vessels and care must be taken to minimize leakage of contrast from the catheter site during post-duct ligation lymphangiography. Furthermore, it may be difficult to demonstrate that all lymphatic vessels have been ligated.

Popliteal

An alternative is percutaneous CT lymphography with ultrasound-guided administration of iohexol into the popliteal lymph node, followed by immediate helical CT acquisition, which allows reliable delineation of the thoracic duct after CT scanning.[47] For popliteal lymphangiography, 1.5 mL of iohexol (300 mg/mL) is injected into the popliteal lymph node.

SURGICAL TECHNIQUES

There are a limited number of surgical techniques that are performed for pleural disease and these will be described below. In Chapter 41, the techniques of thoracocentesis, thoracic drain placement, and thoracotomy are described. To date, a surgical procedure to treat chylothorax successfully in all cats remains elusive. Options include thoracic duct ligation (see Box 44-4), pericardectomy (see Chapter 48), and omentalization (see Box 44-2 and Chapter 19).

Thoracic duct ligation

Lymphangiography performed prior to thoracic duct ligation is generally recommended and has been reported to demonstrate lymphangiectasia in most cats, although some have normal lymphangiograms.[11,46]

Thoracic duct ligation alone, performed via a left 8th to 10th intercostal thoracotomy, has a reported success rate of up to 53%, with the effusion typically resolving within a week.[11,46,48] The addition of pericardectomy was proposed as some animals also have marked thickening of the pericardium that may impede chyle drainage into the venous circulation. Pericardectomy can be achieved via a second thoracotomy at the left 5th intercostal space or, alternatively, median sternotomy may be performed to facilitate concurrent thoracic duct ligation and pericardectomy (see Chapter 48). Resolution of chylothorax was seen in eight of ten cats undergoing thoracic duct ligation and pericardectomy, although in some of these patients the procedures were performed during two separate surgeries (Box 44-3).[47]

It should be noted that identification of the thoracic duct branches is extremely challenging in cats and in the aforementioned study the authors suggested their high success rate could be attributed to surgeon experience and the use of magnification techniques.[47] There is no reported correlation between chronicity of chylothorax and success of surgery or for the extent of fibrosing pleuritis in those cats where it is present.[47] For those cases where thoracic duct ligation has failed, repeat thoracotomy to attempt further ligation may be of benefit. Although it has not been assessed in many cats, pleural omentalization does not seem to improve success rates and is not necessarily recommended at initial surgery,[49,50] the reason being that the omental lymphatic vessels ultimately drain into the chysterna chyli and thoracic duct so this procedure may have little impact on the volume of fluid produced. Despite the lack of evidence for efficacy, omentalization has often been performed concurrently if a second surgery is required and there is one report of resolution of chylothorax when omentalization was the sole procedure performed.[51] Omentalization may not, however, prevent the development of fibrosing or constrictive pleuritis. Pleuroperitoneal shunting and pleurodesis have been described with little success.[11] A pleural port has been described allowing drainage using a 7-French fenestrated tube in the pleural cavity via a subcutaneous hub surgically placed over the dorsolateral abdominal epaxial musculature. A Huber needle is inserted into the hub for intermittent thoracic drainage (Box 44-4).[52]

Box 44-3 Aims of surgical treatment of chylothorax

Thoracic duct: ligation: promotes the formation of new lymphaticovenous anastomoses 5-14 days after surgery.
Pericardectomy: improves passage of chyle across the lymphaticovenous junction
Omentalization: absorption of chyle from the pleural space

Box 44-4 **Management of chylothorax**[22,53]

Thoracic duct ligation

Following mesenteric / popliteal lymphangiography the cat is positioned in right lateral recumbency and a left 8th to 10th intercostal thoracotomy performed. The more caudal the incision the more likely it is that all branches of the thoracic duct will be ligated but the incision should not be further caudal than the 10th intercostal space or it may impede upon the diaphragm. It is important to note that this surgery is undertaken on the contralateral side to dogs due to differences in thoracic duct anatomy. Following the thoracotomy an en bloc ligation is performed on all structures dorsal to the aorta and ventral to the thoracic vertebrae using non-absorbable suture (e.g., polypropylene) or, alternatively, hemostatic clips are placed on individual thoracic duct branches. Post-ligation lymphangiography is then performed.

Pericardectomy

This can be performed either via the same incision or a separate 5th intercostal thoracotomy on the left side (for detailed description of pericardectomy see Chapter 48).

Omentalization

This would usually be performed through the same intercostal incision as the thoracic duct ligation and then a further diaphragmatic incision is made to retrieve the omentum from the greater curvature of the stomach (see Chapter 19). Note that there is no evidence supporting the routine use of omentalization for the treatment of chylothorax.

Box 44.5 **Thymoma resection**

Thymomas are typically removed via a median sternotomy (see Chapter 41). Care must be taken performing the sternotomy, including the placement of retractors and opening of the thoracic cavity, in case there is sternal involvement of the mass. Careful initial visual inspection of the pericardium, blood vessels (particularly the cranial vena cava and internal thoracic arteries) and pleura is essential to establish whether or not there is invasion into these tissues before dissection is started. Then, where possible, the mass is removed by a combination of sharp and blunt dissection, taking care not to damage the other thoracic structures. Bipolar or monopolar cautery and suction is essential for this procedure as hemorrhage may be profuse. Pericardectomy (see Chapter 48) can also be performed if there is pericardial invasion. If there invasion of the venous system, e.g., the vena cavae, venotomy can be performed to remove a tumor thrombus.

As these masses are generally slow growing, it is acceptable to perform cytoreductive surgery rather than surgery with curative intent, to minimize complications in removing very invasive masses, as complete excision is rarely achievable.

Thymectomy

Thymomas are generally removed via median sternotomy although it is important to note that intercostal thoracotomy is possible in selected cases (Box 44.5, Figs 44-12 and 44-13).[28] While asymptomatic mediastinal cysts do not need surgical resection, in people surgical resection is often performed to differentiate cysts from neoplastic disease, which is difficult without histopathology. In a report describing eight of nine cats diagnosed with a mediastinal cyst as an

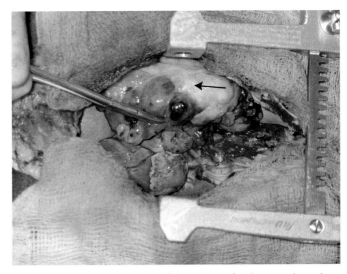

Figure 44-12 Median sternotomy for resection of a thymoma (arrow).

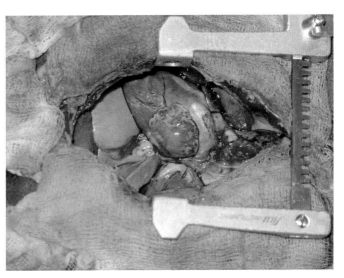

Figure 44-13 The cat in Figure 44-12 after successful resection of a thymoma. Subtotal pericardectomy has been performed due to adhesions of the thymoma to the pericardium.

incidental finding, there was no evidence of respiratory disease and all cats remained asymptomatic up to three years later.[54] However, cysts that are causing clinical signs should be removed.

Eight of nine cats with thymomas survived surgery and lived for a mean of five years with one- and three-year survival rates of 89% and 74%, respectively. In a second study, ten of 12 cats survived surgery with a median survival of 21 months.[55] Debulking or cytoreductive surgery should be performed if the thymoma cannot be removed due to invasiveness but complications associated with this include significant hemorrhage. Post-thymectomy myasthenia gravis has been reported.[55,56]

POSTOPERATIVE CARE

After thoracotomy, thoracocentesis, and thoracic drain placement, it is essential to provide cats with a multi-disciplinary approach to postoperative care and the reader is directed to Chapters 2 to 4 for details of this very important subject.

COMPLICATIONS AND PROGNOSIS

There are two specific feline studies that discuss outcomes of pyothorax.[2,10] Cats that survive the initial hospitalization period and have thoracostomy tubes inserted to aid management of pyothorax appear to have a good outcome, with 66–95% of cases treated successfully. Recurrence rates also appear to be low in this species.

The prognosis for simultaneous pleural and peritoneal effusions is poor due to their association with neoplastic and advanced stage cardiovascular and liver disease.

Studies have suggested that there is a better outcome in cats when chylothorax is treated with thoracic duct ligation in combination with pericardectomy compared with thoracic duct ligation alone, although further work is required in this area to fully establish the most effective treatment of this condition in cats. Fibrosing pleuritis has been associated with chylothorax in up to 67% of cats in one study[21] and carries a guarded prognosis. Cats with chylothorax managed with long-term periodic thoracocentesis may develop complications including iatrogenic pyothorax or fibrosing pleuritis.

The prognosis of traumatic pneumothorax in the cat is dependent on the severity and concurrent injuries; however, most will resolve with conservative thoracocentesis. The prognosis for spontaneous pneumothorax in the cat also appears good when they are treated conservatively.

REFERENCES

1. Gruffydd-Jones TJ, Flecknell PA. The prognosis and treatment related to the gross appearance and laboratory characteristics of pathological thoracic fluids in the cat. J Small Anim Pract 1978;19:315–28.

2. Barrs VR, Allan GS, Martin P, et al. Feline pyothorax: a retrospective study of 27 cases in Australia. J Feline Med Surg 2005;7:211–22.

3. Davies C, Forrester SD. Pleural effusion in cats: 82 cases (1987 to 1995). J Small Anim Pract 1996;37:217–24.

4. Shimali J, Cripps PJ, Newitt AL. Sonographic pleural fluid volume estimation in cats. J Feline Med Surg 2010;12:113–16.

5. Samii VF, Biller DS, Koblik PD. Normal cross-sectional anatomy of the feline thorax and abdomen: comparison of computed tomography and cadaver anatomy. Vet Radiol Ultrasound 1998;39:504–11.

6. Henninger W. Use of computed tomography in the diseased feline thorax. J Small Anim Pract 2003;44:56–64.

7. Zoia A, Slater LA, Heller J, et al. A new approach to pleural effusion in cats: markers for distinguishing transudates from exudates. J Feline Med Surg 2009;11:847–55.

8. Steyn PF, Wittum TE. Radiographic, epidemiologic, and clinical aspects of simultaneous pleural and peritoneal effusions in dogs and cats: 48 cases (1982–1991). J Am Vet Med Assoc 1993;202:307–12.

9. Kovak JR, Ludwig LL, Bergman PJ, et al. Use of thoracoscopy to determine the etiology of pleural effusion in dogs and cats: 18 cases (1998–2001). J Am Vet Med Assoc 2002;221:990–4.

10. Waddell LS, Brady CA, Drobatz KJ. Risk factors, prognostic indicators, and outcome of pyothorax in cats: 80 cases (1986–1999). J Am Vet Med Assoc 2002;221:819–24.

11. Fossum TW, Forrester SD, Swenson CL, et al. Chylothorax in cats: 37 cases (1969–1989). J Am Vet Med Assoc 1991;198(4):672–8.

12. Walker AL, Jang SS, Hirsh DC. Bacteria associated with pyothorax of dogs and cats: 98 cases (1989–1998). J Am Vet Med Assoc 2000;216:359–63.

13. McCaw D, Franklin R, Fales W, et al. Pyothorax caused by Candida albicans in a cat. J Am Vet Med Assoc 1984;185(3):311–12.

14. Sherding RG. Diseases of the pleural cavity. In: Sherding RG, editor. The Cat: Diseases and clinical management, Vol. 1. 2nd ed. New York: Churchill Livingstone; 1994. p. 1063–71.

15. Demetriou JL, Foale RD, Ladlow J, et al. Canine and feline pyothorax: a retrospective study of 50 cases in the UK and Ireland. J Small Anim Pract 2002;43:388–94.

16. Ottenjann M, Weingart C, Arndt G, Kohn B. Characterization of the anemia of inflammatory disease in cats with abscesses, pyothorax, or fat necrosis. J Vet Intern Med 2006;20:1143–50.

17. Valtolina C, Adamantos S. Evaluation of small-bore wire-guided chest drains for management of pleural space disease. J Small Anim Pract 2009;50:290–7.

18. Blalock A, Cunningham RS, Robinson CS. Experimental production of chylothorax by occlusion of the superior vena cava. Ann Surg 1936;104:359–64. 212:652–7.

19. Meincke JE, Hobbie WV Jr, Barto LR. Traumatic chylothorax with associated diaphragmatic hernias in the cat. J Am Vet Med Assoc 1969;155:15–20.

20. Greenberg MJ, Weisse CW. Spontaneous resolution of iatrogenic chylothorax in a cat. J Am Vet Med Assoc 2005;226:1667–70, 1659.

21. Suess Jr, RP, Flanders JA, Beck KA, Earnest-Koons K. Constrictive pleuritis in cats with chylothorax: 10 cases (1983–1991). J Am Anim Hosp Assoc 1994;30:70–7.

22. Fossum TW, Mertens MM, Miller MW, et al. Thoracic duct ligation and pericardectomy for treatment of idiopathic chylothorax. J Vet Intern Med 2004;18:307–10.

23. Stevenson RG, Tilt SE, Purdy JG. Case report. Feline infectious peritonitis and pleurisy. Can Vet J 1971;12:97–9.

24. Fossum TW, Evering WN, Miller MW, et al. Severe bilateral fibrosing pleuritis associated with chronic chylothorax in five cats and two dogs. J Am Vet Med Assoc 1992;201:317–24.

25. Day MJ. Review of thymic pathology in 30 cats and 36 dogs. J Small Anim Pract 1997;38(9):393–403.

26. Galloway PE, Barr FJ, Holt PE, et al. Cystic thymoma in a cat with cholesterol-rich fluid and an unusual ultrasonographic appearance. J Small Anim Pract 1997;38:220–4.

27. Carpenter JL, Valentine BA. Squamous cell carcinoma arising in two feline thymomas. Vet Pathol 1992;29:541–3.

28. Zitz JC, Birchard SJ, Couto GC, et al. Results of excision of thymoma in cats and dogs: 20 cases (1984–2005). J Am Vet Med Assoc 2008;232(8):1186–92.

29. Smith AN, Wright JC, Brawner WR Jr, et al. Radiation therapy in the treatment of canine and feline thymomas: a retrospective study (1985–1999). J Am Anim Hosp Assoc 2001;37:489–96.

30. Forster-Van Hijfte MA, Curtis CF, White RN. Resolution of exfoliative dermatitis and Malassezia pachydermatis overgrowth in a cat after surgical thymoma resection. J Small Anim Pract 1997;38:451–4.

31. Scott-Moncrieff JC, Cook JR Jr, Lantz GC. Acquired myasthenia gravis in a cat with thymoma. J Am Vet Med Assoc 1990;196(8):1291–3.

32. Carpenter JL, Holzworth J. Thymoma in 11 cats. J Am Vet Med Assoc 1982;181(3):248–51.

33. Savary KC, Price GS, Vaden SL. Hypercalcemia in cats: a retrospective study of 71 cases (1991–1997). J Vet Intern Med 2000;14:184–9.

34. Fidel JL, Pargass IS, Dark MJ, Holmes SP. Granulocytopenia associated with thymoma in a domestic shorthaired cat. J Am Anim Hosp Assoc 2008;44:210–17.

35. Malik R, Gabor L, Hunt GB, et al. Benign cranial mediastinal lesions in three cats. Aust Vet J 1997;75:183–7.

36. Milne ME, McCowan C, Landon BP. Spontaneous feline pneumothorax caused by ruptured pulmonary bullae associated with possible bronchopulmonary dysplasia. J Am Anim Hosp Assoc 2010;46:138–42.

37. Fife WD, Côté E. What is your diagnosis? Pleural effusion, pneumothorax, lung collapse and bronchopleural fistula in a cat. J Am Vet Med Assoc 2000;216:1215–16.

38. Godfrey DR. Bronchial rupture and fatal tension pneumothorax following routine venipuncture in a kitten. J Am Anim Hosp Assoc 1997;33:260–3.

39. Brown DC, Holt D. Subcutaneous emphysema, pneumothorax, pneumomediastinum, and pneumopericardium associated with positive-pressure ventilation in a cat. J Am Vet Med Assoc 1995;206:997–9.

40. Evans AT. Anesthesia case of the month. Pneumothorax, pneumomediastinum and subcutaneous emphysema in a cat due to barotrauma after equipment failure during anesthesia. J Am Vet Med Assoc 1998;212:30–2.

41. White HL, Rozanski EA, Tidwell AS, et al. Spontaneous pneumothorax in two cats with small airway disease. J Am Vet Med Assoc 2003;222:1547, 1573–5.

42. Mooney ET, Rozanski EA, King RG, Sharp CR. Spontaneous pneumothorax in 35 cats (2001–2010). J Feline Med Surg 2012;14:384–91.

43. Sierra E, Rodríguez F, Herráez P, et al. Post-traumatic fat embolism causing haemothorax in a cat. Vet Rec 2007;161(5):170–2.

44. Talavera J, Agut A, Fernández Del Palacio J, et al. Thoracic omentalization for long-term management of neoplastic pleural effusion in a cat. J Am Vet Med Assoc 2009;234:1299–302.

45. Sparkes A, Murphy S, McConnell F, et al. Palliative intracavitary carboplatin therapy in a cat with suspected pleural mesothelioma. J Feline Med Surg 2005;7:313–16.

46. Kerpsack SJ, McLoughlin MA, Birchard SJ, et al. Evaluation of mesenteric lymphangiography and thoracic duct ligation in cats with chylothorax: 19 cases (1987–1992). J Am Vet Med Assoc 1994;205:711–15.

47. Lee N, Won S, Choi M, et al. Thoracic duct lymphography in cats by popliteal lymph node iohexol injection. Vet Radiol Ultrasound 2011. [Epub ahead of print]

48. Fossum TW, Jacobs RM, Birchard SJ. Evaluation of cholesterol and triglyceride concentrations in differentiating chylous and nonchylous pleural effusions in dogs and cats. J Am Vet Med Assoc 1986;188:49–51.

49. Bussadori R, Provera A, Martano M, et al. Pleural omentalisation with en bloc ligation of the thoracic duct and pericardiectomy for idiopathic chylothorax in nine dogs and four cats. Vet J 2011;188:234–6.

50. Stewart K, Padgett S. Chylothorax treated via thoracic duct ligation and omentalization. J Am Anim Hosp Assoc 2010;46:312–17.

51. Lafond E, Weirich WE, Salisbury SK. Omentalization of the thorax for treatment of idiopathic chylothorax with constrictive pleuritis in a cat. J Am Anim Hosp Assoc 2002;38:74–8.

52. Brooks AC, Hardie RJ. Use of the Pleural Port device for management of pleural effusion in six dogs and four cats. Vet Surg 2011;40:935–41.

53. Fossum TW, Birchard SJ, Arnold PA. Mesenteric lymphography and ligation of the thoracic duct in a cat with chylothorax. J Am Vet Med Assoc 1985;187(10):1036–7.

54. Zekas LJ, Adams MW. Cranial mediastinal cysts in 9 cats. Veterinary Radiology & Ultrasound 2002;43(5):413–18.

55. Gores BR, Berg J, Carpenter JL, et al. Surgical treatment of thymoma in cats: 12 cases (1987–1992). J Am Vet Med Assoc 1994;204:1782–5.

56. Singh A, Boston SE, Poma R. Thymoma-associated exfoliative dermatitis with post-thymectomy myasthenia gravis in a cat. Can Vet J 2010;51(7):757–60.

Chapter 45

Diaphragm

D.A. Yool

Traumatic diaphragmatic ruptures are common in cats and are life-threatening injuries that generally require prompt surgical attention. Other forms of congenital and acquired diaphragmatic defects also occur although to a much lesser degree. This chapter reviews the diagnosis and surgical management of diaphragmatic defects in the cat.

SURGICAL ANATOMY

The diaphragm is a musculotendinous sheet with a strong central tendon anchored to the costal arch and vertebrae by the sternal, costal, and lumbar muscles (Fig. 45-1).[1,2] The paired lumbar muscles form the diaphragmatic crura that originate from the ventral aspect of the third and fourth lumbar vertebrae and run forward to form the central portion of the dorsal diaphragm.[3] The paired costal and unpaired sternal muscles anchor the central tendon to the costal arch and xiphisternum.[1,2]

There are three apertures in the diaphragm.[1,3] The caval foramen allows passage of the caudal vena cava. It is the most ventral aperture and is located in the central tendon to the right of midline.[3] The esophageal hiatus is located on the midline dorsal to the caval foramen. The esophagus and paired vagal nerves pass through it.[3] The aortic hiatus is the most dorsal aperture. It is located between the left and right diaphragmatic crura and is bordered dorsally by the lumbar vertebrae. The aorta, the azygous and hemiazygous veins, and the lumbar cistern of the thoracic duct pass through this.[3] The splanchnic nerves and sympathetic chain also cross the diaphragm between the lateral part of each crus and the 13th rib.[3]

The phrenicoabdominal arteries (branches of the abdominal aorta) give rise to the phrenic arteries that divide across the base of the crura, run ventrally down the central tendon and supply the costal and sternal diaphragmatic muscles.[4] These vessels anastomose with the intercostal arteries of the costal arch.[4] The left and right phrenic nerves supply motor innervation to the diaphragm.[2]

DIAGNOSIS AND GENERAL CONSIDERATIONS

There are several forms of diaphragmatic defect. Pleuroperitoneal defects are common and usually acquired following trauma. They allow communication of the pleural and peritoneal cavities (Fig. 45-2). Peritoneopericardial hernias (PPDHs) are uncommon congenital defects caused by failure of formation of the diaphragm and pericardium.[5] They allow the pericardial and peritoneal spaces to communicate but the pleural cavities remain intact (Fig. 45-2). Sliding hiatal hernias occasionally develop, enabling cranial displacement of the terminal esophagus and gastric fundus through the esophageal hiatus into the mediastinum (Fig. 45-3). The severity of signs associated with these defects varies between individuals but surgery is generally indicated.

Clinical signs

Cats with diaphragmatic ruptures often present with concurrent injuries and these may be of more consequence at initial presentation than the diaphragm injury. Clinical signs are usually related to respiratory compromise with tachypnea and/or dyspnea. In chronic cases the signs may be more attributable to compression of the gastrointestinal tract in the thoracic cavity.

Diagnostic imaging

A diagnosis of diaphragmatic disease is usually made from plain radiography or abdominal ultrasound but contrast radiography or CT is sometimes necessary. Loss of the diaphragmatic contour is found consistently in most cases but is not specific and can be associated with other pleural diseases such as pleural effusion. The presence of portions of the gastrointestinal tract within the thoracic cavity, recognized by luminal gas, ingesta or barium, is characteristic of the condition. Parenchymatous organs may also be delineated running forward from the abdomen into the thorax.[6,7] The cardiac silhouette and lungs

DOI: 10.1016/B978-0-7020-4336-9.00045-7

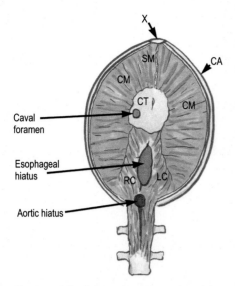

Figure 45-1 Diagram of diaphragmatic anatomy viewed from the abdominal (concave) surface with the animal positioned in dorsal recumbency (mimicking the presentation at surgery). CA, costal arch; CM, costal muscles (left and right); CT, central tendon; LC, left crus; RC, right crus; SM, sternal muscle (unpaired); V, 4th lumbar vertebra; X, xiphisternum.

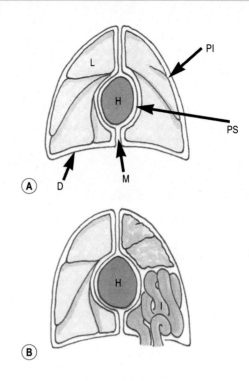

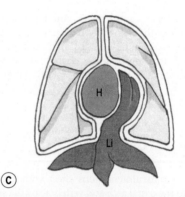

Figure 45-2 Schematics of pleuroperitoneal and peritoneopericardial hernias (PPDHs). **(A)** Intact diaphragm and thoracic wall from dorsoventral projection. **(B)** Pleuroperitoneal hernia with intestinal herniation into the thorax. **(C)** PPDH with liver herniated into the pericardial sac causing cardiac displacement; note that the pleural cavities are intact. D, diaphragm; H, heart; I, intestine; L, lung; Li, liver; M, mediastinum; Pl, pleural cavity; PS, pericardial sac.

are often displaced cranially or dorsally.[7,8] Pleural effusions can mask many of the characteristic radiographic features and repeating radiographic studies following thoracocentesis can help to resolve key features enabling a diagnosis to be confirmed.[6]

SURGICAL DISEASES

Congenital pleuroperitoneal hernias

Congenital pleuroperitoneal hernias are thought to account for less than 10% of pleuroperitoneal defects in cats.[9,10] There are only a handful of confirmed cases that have been classified as congenital because of the presence of a hernial sac[11-15] or because of the early onset of signs.[16] Congenital defects can affect most areas of the diaphragm with involvement of the central tendon,[13,14] the sternal muscle,[12] most of the left side of the diaphragm including the left crus[16] and the right crus[11,15] being reported. Liver and falciform fat are most commonly herniated, although two cases have contained the majority of the abdominal viscera.[14,16] Some cats have presented with signs of dyspnea at an early age.[11,16] Others have been diagnosed with congenital hernias as incidental findings during the investigation of unrelated diseases[12,13,15] or during abdominal surgery[14] and the oldest reported age at diagnosis was 11 years.[13]

In humans, congenital pleuroperitoneal hernias are thought to have a genetic basis.[17] An autosomal recessive pattern of inheritance has also been proposed in dogs,[18,19] although teratogens can induce diaphragmatic hernia formation in animal models.[20] The etiopathogenesis of congenital pleuroperitoneal hernias in the cat is unknown but it is prudent to advise against breeding from affected animals.

The investigation and management of congenital pleuroperitoneal hernias is identical to that of acquired pleuroperitoneal ruptures.

Acquired pleuroperitoneal ruptures

The majority of pleuroperitoneal defects (over 85%) are acquired traumatic ruptures.[3,9] These are usually caused by blunt abdominal trauma and are associated with immediate herniation of abdominal organs because of the sudden increase in intra-abdominal pressure.[21,22] Vehicular trauma is the commonest cause, but falls and dog attacks are also reported.[23-25] Occasionally, diaphragmatic ruptures are caused by penetrating diaphragmatic injuries.[23,24] In these cases, organs may not herniate immediately and the ruptures may only become clinically apparent some time after the initial injury. There is a single case report of an acquired pleuroperitoneal rupture associated with the collagen defect, cutaneous asthenia, in a cat.[26]

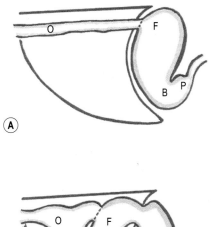

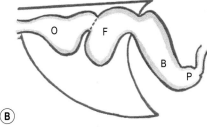

Figure 45-3 Schematics of sliding hiatal hernia (lateral projection). **(A)** before herniation. **(B)** during herniation. The gastroesophageal junction and proximal fundus slide in and out of the mediastinum through the esophageal hiatus. Dotted line: gastroesophageal junction; B, gastric body; F, gastric fundus; O, esophagus; P, pylorus.

Most traumatic diaphragmatic ruptures are single tears through the sternal and costal muscles.[3,27,28] Four percent of cases have multiple ruptures.[3] Some ruptures involve the central tendon but the crura are very strong and rarely rupture.[3,29] The most common rupture is a unilateral costal muscle tear in the ventral diaphragm below the level of the esophageal hiatus.[3,27,28] Sixty percent of tears are circumferential with muscle tearing parallel to the rib or avulsing from it completely.[28] Radial tears and combined radial and circumferential tears also occur.[28]

The liver is the most commonly herniated organ.[3,10,28,30] The small intestine, stomach, spleen, omentum, and pancreas also frequently become herniated.[3,10,30] Rarely, kidney, colon or cecum are involved.[10,30–34] Right-sided hernias tend to contain liver, small intestines, and pancreas and left-sided hernias tend to contain stomach, spleen, and small intestine.[28]

Pleuroperitoneal defects usually lead to respiratory compromise due to compression of lung by herniated organs and poor diaphragmatic function.[21,22,24,27,29] Pleural effusions may develop from transudation following venous congestion of herniated liver lobes and the effusion can contribute to the dyspnea.[3,27,29] Ventilation-perfusion mismatches occur in the collapsed areas of lung[22,29] and concurrent pulmonary contusion, pneumothorax, fractured ribs or flail chest may also contribute to respiratory compromise.[27,29,35]

In addition to dyspnea, injury of herniated organs may lead to clinical signs. Displaced, twisted liver lobes become congested, ischemic, and friable[3,22] and displaced portions of the gastrointestinal tract may become obstructed or devitalized.[29] Displacement or compression of the hepatobiliary tree has been associated with obstructive jaundice.[36] Herniation of part or all of the stomach may lead to gastric dilatation and volvulus (GDV).[37] This may cause obstructive shock, gastric necrosis, and severe respiratory compromise due to compression of lung by the dilated stomach.[30] Rarely, perforation and rupture of organs lead to hemothorax, chylothorax or urothorax.[28,31,32,38]

Uterine herniation and bile leakage are reported in the dog but have not been reported in the cat to date.[30,33,34,39–41]

Forty-seven percent of cats diagnosed with diaphragmatic rupture have a history of witnessed trauma and most of the remainder have clinical findings suggestive of recent trauma.[24] The diagnosis is usually reached within seven days of the original trauma. Almost one-quarter of patients have concurrent injuries including fractured ribs, fractured limbs or other external abdominal wall ruptures.[24] In patients diagnosed within a few days of trauma, the commonest presenting signs are tachypnea and dyspnea.[10,21,24,27,28,30] However, approximately 10% of patients have signs of gastrointestinal dysfunction such as vomiting and, in some of these cases, these are the only clinical signs of disease.[24,28] Some patients do not develop signs immediately following trauma or have non-specific signs that delay investigation such as anorexia or lethargy.[28] Patients in which the diagnosis is made several weeks following trauma are more likely to present with signs of gastrointestinal dysfunction (50% of cases) and dyspnea is less prevalent (38% of cases).[42] Additional common clinical findings include muffled lung and heart sounds and hyporesonant thoracic percussion. Often, borborygmi can be heard in the thoracic cavity indicating herniation of portions of the gastrointestinal tract.[10] Abdominal palpation may reveal a comparatively empty abdomen or apparent loss of key organs, such as the spleen, that have been displaced. Occasionally, pleuroperitoneal ruptures are identified as incidental findings with no overt clinical signs.[42]

The diagnosis of pleuroperitoneal rupture is usually confirmed using plain radiography or abdominal ultrasound but contrast radiography or CT is sometimes necessary.[6,7,15,43,44] There are several key diagnostic radiographic features (Fig. 45-4). Loss of the diaphragmatic contour is found consistently in most cases but is not specific and can be associated with other pleural diseases such as pleural effusion.[6,7] The presence of portions of the gastrointestinal tract within the thoracic cavity, recognized by luminal gas, ingesta or barium, is characteristic of the condition.[6,7] Parenchymatous organs may also be delineated running forward from the abdomen into the thorax.[6,7] The cardiac silhouette and lungs are often displaced cranially or dorsally.[7,8] Pleural effusions can mask many of the characteristic radiographic features and repeating radiographic studies following thoracocentesis can help to resolve key features, enabling a diagnosis to be confirmed.[6]

Indicators of diaphragmatic rupture may also be seen on abdominal radiographs. Cranial displacement of the gastric axis is associated with liver herniation (see Fig. 45-6A).[7] Gastrointestinal contrast studies delineate fluid-filled intestinal loops within the thorax although these are usually not required to confirm a diagnosis (Fig. 45-5).[6,7] Positive contrast peritoneography is a more definitive test of diaphragmatic integrity (Box 45-1).[6,15]

The diaphragm is difficult to visualize with ultrasound unless abdominal or pleural fluid is present but transhepatic and intercostal ultrasound can be used to identify herniated organs within the thorax.[44] It is important to distinguish herniated liver lobe from consolidated lung and from mirror artifact.[44,45]

Most cases with congenital or acquired pleuroperitoneal defects are managed surgically following a short period of stabilization.

Congenital peritoneopericardial hernia

PPDH is considered to be a congenital condition in the cat although rare examples of traumatic PPDH are described in humans.[46–48] During normal development, the pericardial cavity separates from the common pleuroperitoneal cavity before the pleural and peritoneal cavities separate. If these two processes fail during development,[5] the pericardium and ventral diaphragm fuse to form a stoma in the central diaphragm immediately dorsal to the xiphisternum. In some cases,

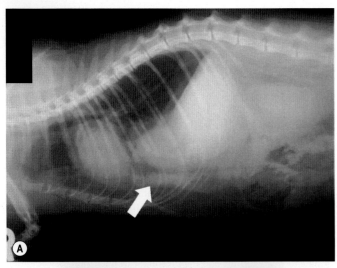

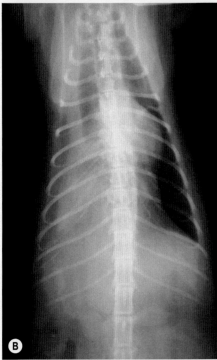

Figure 45-4 Thoracic radiographs of cat with a pleuroperitoneal rupture. **(A)** Lateral view: the ventral diaphragmatic contour is obliterated. A parenchymatous organ (spleen) is seen traversing the diaphragmatic line into the thorax (arrow). **(B)** Dorsoventral view: the left diaphragmatic contour is obliterated, there is left-sided pleural effusion and the heart is displaced towards the right. *(With kind permission of the Image Archives of R(D)SVS, University of Edinburgh.)*

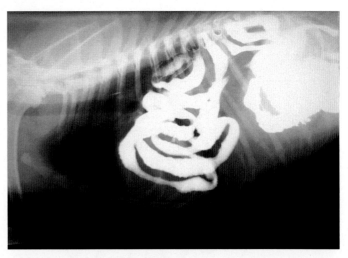

Figure 45-5 Thoracic radiograph of a cat with a pleuroperitoneal rupture following an upper gastrointestinal contrast study: contrast delineates the lumen of intestinal loops within the thorax.

Box 45-1 **Positive contrast peritoneopraphy**

The patient is sedated or anesthetized and the umbilical region is clipped and aseptically prepared to allow contrast to be injected into the abdomen by paracentesis. A site is selected for needle insertion 1 cm to the right of midline in front of the umbilicus. Palpate the abdomen to locate underlying viscera such as the spleen or bladder before injection. Introduce a short 23G needle through the abdominal wall attached to a syringe containing a suitable volume of low-osmolar, non-ionic contrast agent (e.g., 2 mL/kg iohexol at 300 mg/mL [Omnipaque, Nycomed Amersham]). Warming the contrast agent to body temperature will reduce discomfort associated with injection. Before injection, aspirate to ensure that abdominal viscera have not been penetrated. A small amount of blood may be aspirated into the hub of the syringe. If larger volumes of blood, urine or intestinal contents are aspirated, withdraw the needle. Inject contrast into the peritoneal cavity. If resistance is met during injection, withdraw the needle and start again. Leave the patient for two to five minutes before radiographing the thorax and abdomen to give time for contrast to distribute. Gentle balloting of the abdomen may facilitate contrast distribution. If contrast passes in front of the diaphragm into the thorax, this is diagnostic for the presence of a diaphragmatic defect. However, false negative results may occur if omentum or other viscera block the diaphragmatic defect. Contrast can also be injected into the retroperitoneal space in fat animals, in which case it will not redistribute far from the site of injection.[6]

---

the caudal sternebrae and cranial linea alba may also be malformed producing concurrent ventral body wall hernias, sternal defects or pectus excavatum.[46,48,49]

PPDH may remain clinically silent for some time before causing clinical signs and the median age at diagnosis is over four years.[46] Respiratory and gastrointestinal dysfunction are reported with equal frequency.[46,47] Rarely, cardiac tamponade develops due to the presence of large volumes of herniated organs or the development of intrapericardial cysts from incarcerated hepatobiliary tissue, omentum or falciform fat.[50–52] Forty percent of cases have no clinical signs, with PPDH diagnosed as an incidental finding.[46,47,49]

PPDH shares many of the clinical features of pleuroperitoneal hernias including muffling and displacement of the cardiac apex beat, dyspnea, and thoracic borborygmi.[46,47,49] Concurrent cranial ventral abdominal wall hernias (located cranial to the umbilicus) or sternal defects are occasionally palpable and increase suspicion of PPDH.[47,49] Rarely, signs of cardiac tamponade occur (open-mouth breathing, lethargy, weak femoral pulses, distended jugular veins, tachycardia).[50–52]

The key radiographic differences that distinguish PPDH from pleuroperitoneal defects are that the herniated organs are centered around the heart causing mediastinal widening and that the diaphragmatic contour is preserved on ventrodorsal views bilaterally although the cupula of the diaphragm is effaced (Fig. 45-6).[6] PPDH may be

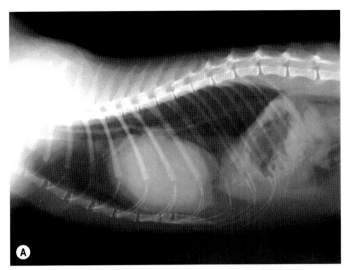

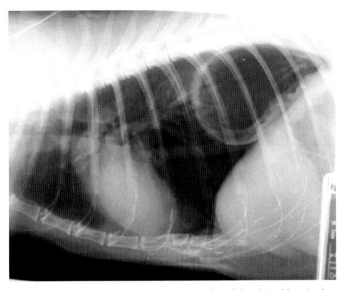

Figure 45-7 Thoracic radiograph of a cat with a sliding hiatal hernia that presented for dyspnea with herniation of the fundus into the mediastinal space. Diagnosis was delayed for some time in this case due to the lack of gastrointestinal signs and the dynamic nature of the hernia preventing earlier radiographic diagnosis.

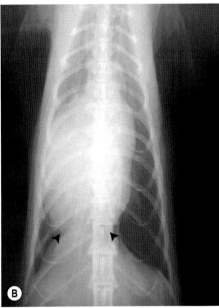

Figure 45-6 Thoracic radiographs of a cat with a PPDH. **(A)** Lateral view: the cardiac silhouette appears enlarged giving the impression of cardiomegaly. The cupula of the diaphragm is effaced by soft tissue and there is increased contact between the diaphragm and pericardium. Forward displacement of the gastric axis due to liver herniation can also be seen (apparent microhepatica). **(B)** Dorsoventral view: the cupula of the diaphragm is effaced by soft tissue (arrowheads) but the diaphragmatic line is otherwise intact, distinguishing PPDH from pleuroperitoneal hernia (compare to Figure 45-4B). *(With kind permission of the Image Archives of R(D)SVS, University of Edinburgh.)*

Hiatal hernia

Hernias affecting the esophageal hiatus of the cat are rare. The most frequently reported is the sliding hiatal hernia that allows dynamic displacement of the terminal abdominal esophagus, gastric cardia, and proximal fundus through the esophageal hiatus into the mediastinum.[53] Sliding hiatal hernias may be congenital or traumatic.[54] Traumatic hernias occur due to blunt abdominal trauma or due to increased inspiratory effort.[53,54,55] Occasionally, pleuroperitoneal hernias and ruptures may also extend into the esophageal hiatus.[12]

Sliding hiatal hernias lead to dysfunction of the lower esophageal sphincter and reflux of gastric contents into the distal esophagus causing reflux esophagitis, megaesophagus, and aspiration pneumonia.[53] A putative link between a recent history of general anesthesia and the onset of signs has highlighted the possibility that some asymptomatic congenital hernias may become symptomatic only after anesthesia-induced reflux of material into the esophagus.[54] Regurgitation is the major presenting sign in most cases (89%).[54] Dyspnea is reported in only 7% of cases.[54] Occasionally, hiatal hernias are diagnosed as incidental findings during investigation of other diseases.[54]

Confirming the diagnosis of sliding hiatal hernia can be difficult as the hernia is dynamic and may contain no abdominal organs at the time of investigation. Plain radiography may demonstrate a soft tissue density or a hollow viscus in the caudal dorsal thorax causing mediastinal widening (Fig. 45-7).[54] Non-specific findings include megaesophagus and aspiration pneumonia.[54] Contrast radiography increases the specificity of these studies as rugal folds may be delineated in the herniated gastric fundus within the thorax.[54] Fluoroscopic studies may demonstrate dynamic herniation of the fundus during swallowing and endoscopy may demonstrate distal esophagitis suggestive of a reflux disorder.[54] Occasionally, displacement of the fundus through the esophageal cardia can be identified using endoscopy to confirm the diagnosis.[54]

Asymptomatic cases probably do not warrant specific therapy. Medical therapy to manage reflux esophagitis (antacid therapy and the use of prokinetic agents including cisapride and metoclopramide) in combination with weight loss has been described but may be

mistaken for generalized cardiomegaly or pericardial effusion radiographically but cardiac ultrasound can distinguish between these conditions.

PPDH has been successfully managed both conservatively and surgically.[46] The decision of whether or not to operate can be difficult as some patients present with non-specific signs that may be caused by other diseases or have the hernia identified as an incidental finding. Conservative management can be considered in asymptomatic patients but surveillance for deterioration is required.[46] Surgical repair of the hernia is recommended in animals that have symptoms associated with organ herniation.[46]

insufficient to control signs.[53,54,] Surgery (combined herniorrhaphy, esophagopexy, and gastropexy) has the highest success rate in the long-term management of the condition.[53,56]

PREOPERATIVE CONSIDERATIONS

Timing of surgery

The timing of surgery is dependent on the severity of clinical signs and degree of organ compromise. PPDHs and hiatal hernias may not cause life-threatening signs and are often repaired as elective procedures.[46,54] Pleuroperitoneal defects are more likely to cause dyspnea and require urgent correction but most cases will still benefit from a period of stabilization prior to surgery. One of the major advances in the management of pleuroperitoneal ruptures was the realization that survival rates improved following 12 to 24 hours of stabilization.[30] Survival rates have remained high recently despite earlier surgical intervention. This may reflect earlier recognition of the condition and advances in the management of shock and anesthesia.[23] It is still recommended that patients receive at least a short period of preoperative stabilization unless there are specific indications to proceed immediately to surgery. The key components of preoperative stabilization are fluid resuscitation, pain relief, cage rest and oxygen supplementation. Thoracocentesis may help relieve dyspnea preoperatively in patients with large pleural effusions or pneumothorax.

Indications to proceed rapidly to surgery without further stabilization include patient deterioration despite supportive care, the presence of the stomach within the thoracic cavity (which may develop into GDV), and evidence of organ rupture or uncontrolled hemorrhage.[27]

Anesthesia

Anesthesia for patients with diaphragmatic defects (see Chapter 2) carries additional risks compared to other abdominal surgeries. Pneumothorax develops intraoperatively when pleuroperitoneal defects are repaired and may also develop during PPDH and hiatal hernia repairs. Positioning in dorsal recumbency for surgery causes further compression of the lungs and displacement of the heart, exacerbating cardiovascular and respiratory compromise.[30] The time between induction of anesthesia and reduction of the hernia should be as short as possible.[28] If tolerated, pre-clip and pre-oxygenate the patient before inducing anesthesia. Use intravenous agents to achieve rapid induction of anesthesia and endotracheal intubation. Be prepared to start intermittent positive pressure ventilation as soon as the patient is intubated.[27,30] Elevate the thorax in relation to the abdomen to limit lung compression by herniated organs before the hernia is reduced.[30]

SURGICAL TECHNIQUES

Surgical approach

The standard approach for the repair of all diaphragmatic defects is a ventral midline abdominal celiotomy.[10,47] This approach enables the entire diaphragm and abdominal contents to be thoroughly assessed. It can also be extended by median sternotomy to manage thoracic adhesions, for example, in patients with chronic pleuroperitoneal defects (Fig. 45-8).[3,42] The prepared surgical field should include the ventral thorax to enable the incision to be extended cranially if required.[42] Elevate the thorax in relation to the abdomen to aid

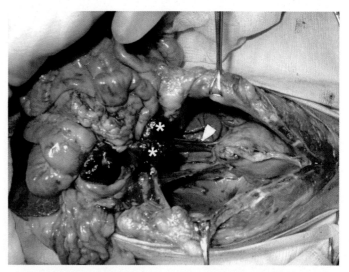

Figure 45-8 Intraoperative view of a cat with a chronic pleuroperitoneal rupture of 12 months' duration with herniation of the small intestine and omentum. The hernia could not be reduced from an abdominal approach so the incision was extended by median sternotomy. The combined approach to the abdominal and thoracic cavities is shown (head to right). Following reduction of the hernia, two liver lobes appear fibrotic and distorted (asterisks). Repair of this defect was complicated as it extended into the caval foramen (arrowhead shows caudal vena cava). *(Image courtesy of E.M. Welsh with permission.)*

reduction of hernia contents and remove the falciform ligament and fat to improve visualization.[9,30]

Some authors have recommended an intercostal thoracotomy approach as this enables the diaphragm to be repaired from the convex surface and thoracic adhesions can be disrupted.[57] However, the side of the hernia must be accurately identified preoperatively and there is no facility for evaluating the contralateral hemi-diaphragm for additional injuries or for fully evaluating abdominal organs for injury following reduction of the hernia.[3] The transthoracic approach across the 9th intercostal spaces has also been described as it gives better access to the diaphragm but this approach offers little advantage and several disadvantages compared to ventral midline celiotomy.[3] Neither thoracic approach is recommended routinely.

Pleuroperitoneal repair

Primary repair of the muscular tear or avulsion will be sufficient to treat most affected cats (Box 45-2). Some large diaphragmatic defects cannot be reconstructed easily. Large costal defects can be repaired by moving the point of reattachment of the diaphragm forwards as far as the 9th rib, obliterating the costodiaphragmatic recess. Synthetic meshes (e.g., polypropylene) have been used to successfully repair large diaphragmatic defects in dogs and could also be used in cats.[61] A double layer of porcine small intestinal submucosa has been used to repair a congenital diaphragmatic defect in a kitten.[43] The collagen sheet forms a biological scaffold that is replaced by host tissues within a few weeks.[62] This will not restrict subsequent growth of the diaphragm as the patient grows and will not cause long-term foreign body reaction, both problems encountered with synthetic meshes in humans that may have relevance in cats.[43,63] However, the collagen sheets are weaker than synthetic meshes initially and the feline case report, although documenting successful resolution of signs, described partial breakdown of the repair.[43] Muscle flaps generated from the transverse abdominis muscle have also been used to repair diaphragmatic defects.[64,65] The flap is made by incising the peritoneum and

Box 45-2 **Primary diaphragmatic (pleuroperitoneal) repair**

The cat is positioned in dorsal recumbency and clipped and prepared for aseptic surgery. A wide clip extending from caudal to the pubis to the cranial aspect of the thorax is recommended in case the incision needs to be extended into the thorax.

A ventral midline abdominal celiotomy is performed. The falciform ligament and fat are removed to improve visualization. During surgery, most diaphragmatic defects are easily identified but the liver and stomach should be retracted to enable the caval foramen, central tendon, and the dorsal diaphragm lateral to the crura to be checked for defects. Once the defect is identified, the hernia is reduced by applying gentle traction to herniated omentum, small intestine, stomach or spleen, and finally the displaced liver lobes are repositioned. Traction should not be applied directly to the liver lobes as they may be congested and friable so a finger or instrument may be used to hook under the liver lobe within the thorax and gently lift and push it back into the abdomen.[30] If the hernia/rupture cannot be reduced, it may be necessary to enlarge the defect by incising the hernial ring.[30] The incision is made from the edge of the defect running ventrally towards the costal arch or sternum as this area is most accessible for repair. Rarely, adhesions form between the herniated organs and the diaphragm or thoracic organs.[28,30] Diaphragmatic adhesions can be managed by gentle dissection but intrathoracic adhesions may require extension of the incision by median sternotomy and lung lobectomy or other intrathoracic procedures.[42]

It is critical to ensure that all sutures engage healthy tissue during herniorrhaphy and that the repair is not under tension. If the edges of the hernial ring appear unhealthy or devitalized, they are sharply excised until a bleeding surface is achieved. Most defects can be closed easily by direct apposition of the edges using simple appositional interrupted or continuous suture patterns but care is taken not to restrict the caval foramen if the hernia extends into this area (Fig. 45-8).[9] Simple continuous patterns are easier to place and enable tension to be evenly distributed along the suture line. Synthetic monofilament absorbable suture material that retains strength adequately to allow repair of tendon and muscle (e.g., polydioxanone II) is recommended. Start suturing at the dorsal (least accessible) portion of the defect and continue ventrally into the more accessible area (Fig. 45-9A).[3] Sometimes, the costal muscles avulse

from the costal arch leaving no lateral muscle remnant to suture to. To repair these defects the avulsed muscle is anchored to the ribs at the point of detachment using circumcostal sutures (Fig. 45-9B).[58]

After repair of the diaphragmatic defect, residual air in the thorax can be removed intraoperatively by needle thoracocentesis through either the diaphragm or an intercostal space (Fig. 45-10).[3,23,59] Thoracostomy tubes may also be placed but must enter the chest through an intercostal space and not through the defect in the diaphragm. Forced expansion of lungs to expel air from the thorax before tying the final suture must be avoided as it is associated with a high fatal complication rate through the development of re-expansion pulmonary edema.[28,30,60]

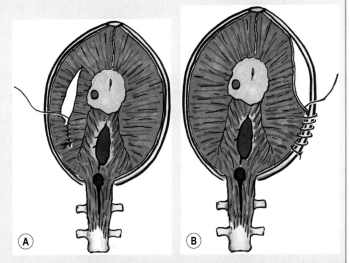

Figure 45-9 Diagrams of suture placement during hernia repair. **(A)** Mid costal, sternal, and central tendon ruptures are repaired by apposing the edges of the defects. Note that the suture line is started dorsally in the least accessible portion of the diaphragm. **(B)** Avulsion of the diaphragm from the costal arch is repaired by anchoring the diaphragm to the costal arch using circumcostal sutures.

transverse abdominis muscle to create a muscle pedicle with its base along the costal arch.[65] The flap is elevated into the diaphragmatic defect with the peritoneal surface facing the thorax. It has the advantages of not causing foreign body reactions and adapting to the growth of the patient.

Displacement of part or all of the stomach during diaphragmatic rupture can lead to GDV in the cat.[37] Affected patients require immediate surgery but preoperative orogastric intubation may help to stabilize the patient. If this is not possible, gastrocentesis may be performed through an intercostal space.[30] Gastropexy to prevent recurrence of GDV has been performed in some cases following gastric repositioning but, to date, recurrent GDV has not been reported in the cat following diaphragmatic rupture repair so it is uncertain whether or not this additional procedure is warranted.[37]

PPDH repair

PPDH repair follows the same principles as pleuroperitoneal herniorrhaphy (Box 45-2) and is usually straightforward.[47,49] Although adhesions between the herniated organs and pericardium are occasionally

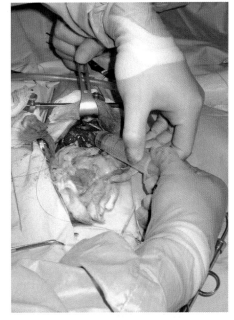

Figure 45-10 Intraoperative view of needle thoracocentesis through the diaphragm to establish negative pressure in the thorax after hernia repair.

Section | 6 | Thorax

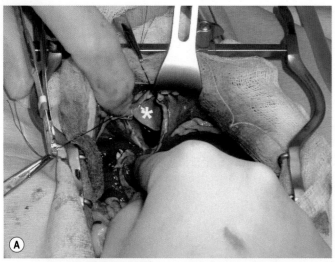
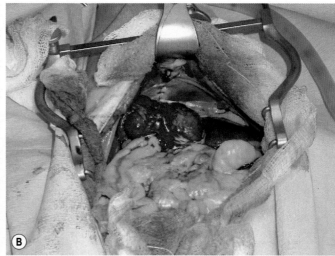

Figure 45-11 Intraoperative views during PPDH repair. A ventral midline celiotomy incision has been made and the falciform fat has been excised to improve exposure. **(A)** The heart (asterisk) can be seen through the PPDH following reduction of herniated liver lobes. **(B)** The defect is closed by apposing the edges using a continuous suture pattern starting dorsally.

Box 45-3 Sliding hiatal hernia repair

The cat is positioned in dorsal recumbency and clipped and prepared for aseptic surgery. A wide clip extending from caudal to the pubis to the cranial aspect of the thorax is recommended in case the incision needs to be extended into the thorax. A ventral midline abdominal celiotomy is performed. The falciform ligament and fat are removed to improve visualization. Following reduction of the hernia, the peritoneum is bluntly dissected as it reflects from the gastric cardia onto the diaphragm at the esophageal hiatus. This will expose the underlying fascia and ventral branch of the vagal nerve (Fig. 45-12A). The dissection is confined to the ventral half of the circumference of the esophageal hiatus to avoid damaging the dorsal vagal branch and continued for a short distance between the esophageal wall and pleura to mobilize the terminal esophagus and enable it to be drawn back into the abdomen (Fig. 45-12B). Pneumothorax may develop during this dissection if the mediastinal pleura is penetrated. A lubricated stomach tube (e.g., 26 French) is passed along the esophagus and into the stomach to act as a guide during partial closure of the esophageal hiatus. Caudal traction is applied to pull the terminal portion of the esophagus into the abdomen. Starting ventrally, the esophageal hiatus is partially closed using a series of simple interrupted polypropylene sutures and bites of the ventral esophageal muscle are incorporated in the last two sutures to anchor the esophagus in its new position. The stomach tube prevents excessive closure of the hiatus to avoid impairing esophageal emptying. Finally, a left-sided gastropexy (incisional or tube) is performed between the gastric fundus and left body wall to maintain slight caudal traction on the esophageal cardia (Fig. 45-12C).

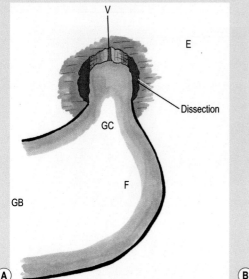
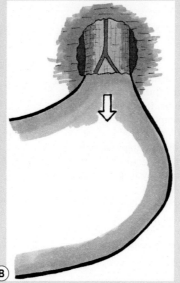
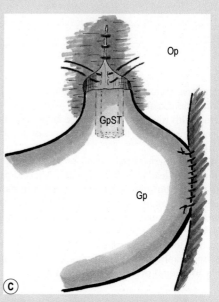

Figure 45-12 Diagram of sliding hiatal hernia repair. **(A)** Bluntly dissect around the ventral two-thirds of the esophageal wall as it passes through the esophageal hiatus. **(B)** Apply caudal traction (arrow) to pull the terminal esophagus into the abdominal cavity. **(C)** Partly close the esophageal hiatus, incorporating the muscular wall of the esophagus in the last two sutures to anchor it in position and perform a left-sided gastropexy to prevent excessive reduction in the size of the hiatus (dotted line indicates presence of stomach tube). E, terminal esophagus; F, gastric fundus; GB, gastric body; GC, gastric cardia; Gp, gastropexy; V, ventral branch of the vagus.

encountered and must be dissected,[46,47] adhesions to the epicardium have not been reported. Following reduction of the defect, the hernia is repaired by direct apposition of the edges of the hernial ring (Fig. 45-11). The pericardium does not need to be dissected from the diaphragm at the edge of the ring and should be left undisturbed to reduce the risk of pleural complications.[51] Air is evacuated from the pericardium by pericardiocentesis through the diaphragm before abdominal closure. If there are concurrent sternal or abdominal wall defects, these are repaired at the same time. Sternal defects can be apposed using cerclage wire in a similar fashion to closure of median sternotomy incisions.

Sliding hiatal hernia repair

Sliding hiatal hernia repair has two components, partial closure of the hernia ring and left-sided gastropexy (Box 45-3).[54,56]

POSTOPERATIVE CARE

Animals may still become dyspneic following diaphragmatic surgery because of residual pneumothorax, concurrent thoracic injuries, re-expansion pulmonary edema, pleural effusion, or recurrence of the hernia. Cats should be monitored carefully for dyspnea for at least 24 hours following surgery and should be investigated if signs occur. Patients should be exercise restricted for ten days following surgery and receive analgesia as required.

COMPLICATIONS AND PROGNOSIS

PPDH is associated with a 14% postoperative mortality rate.[46] The prognosis for cats with traumatic pleuroperitoneal ruptures is good, with up to 92% of cases surviving at least until discharge.[59] The prognosis for chronic pleuroperitoneal rupture repair is sometimes cited to be worse but a comparatively recent report suggests that the survival rate is similar (86%).[42]

Most complications that are fatal occur within 24 hours of surgery and the complications are fatal due to the respiratory compromise that they cause.[10,28,42,59] Re-expansion pulmonary edema is a major cause of dyspnea and develops within 24 hours of surgery. This syndrome is seen following forced re-expansion of collapsed lungs and is usually fatal.[60] However, the risk of developing this syndrome is greatly reduced by ensuring that the lungs are never forcibly over-inflated during hernia repair.[30] Other causes of dyspnea postoperatively include pneumothorax, pleural effusion, and pulmonary contusion.

Some patients have contraction of the abdominal wall due to the reduced volume of abdominal contents associated with chronic herniation of abdominal organs into the thorax. This may complicate hernia repair as the abdominal wall may be difficult to close following return of herniated organs to the abdomen.[3] Excessive intra-abdominal pressure can restrict diaphragmatic movement postoperatively and lead to vascular injury to abdominal organs that may prove life threatening. Splenectomy or partial hepatectomy may be necessary to facilitate closure.[27] Other uncommon complications include megaesophagus, regurgitation, and reherniation.[3,24,57,66]

REFERENCES

1. Sieck GC, Roy RR, Powell P, et al. Muscle fiber type distribution and architecture of the cat diaphragm. J Appl Physiol 1983;55:1386–92.
2. Hermanson JW, Evans HE. The muscular system. In: Evans HE, editor. Miller's anatomy of the dog. 3rd ed. Philadelphia: W. B. Saunders; 1993. p. 258–384.
3. Wilson III GP 3rd, Hayes HM Jr. Diaphragmatic hernia in the dog and cat: a 25-year overview. Semin Vet Med Surg (Small Anim) 1986;1:318–26.
4. Evans HE. The heart and arteries. In: Evans HE, editor. Miller's anatomy of the dog. 3rd ed. Philadelphia: W. B. Saunders; 1993. p. 586–681.
5. Noden MD, de Lahunta A. Respiratory system and partitioning of body cavities. In: Stamathis G, editor. The embryology of domestic animals – developmental mechanisms and malformations. Baltimore: Williams & Wilkins; 1985. p. 279–91.
6. Williams J, Leveille R, Myer CW. Imaging modalities used to confirm diaphragmatic hernia in small animals. Comp Cont Ed Pract Vet 1998;20(11):1199–209.
7. Sullivan M, Lee R. Radiological features of 80 cases of diaphragmatic rupture. J Small Anim Pract 1989;30(12):561–6.
8. Marolf A, Kraft S, Lowry J, et al. Radiographic diagnosis–right kidney herniation in a cat. Vet Radiol Ultrasound 2002;43(3):237–40.
9. al-Nakeeb SM. Canine and feline traumatic diaphragmatic hernias. J Am Vet Med Assoc 1971;159:1422–7.
10. Wilson GP 3rd, Newton CD, Burt JK. A review of 116 diaphragmatic hernias in dogs and cats. J Am Vet Med Assoc 1971;159:1142–5.
11. Mann FA, Aronson E. Surgical correction of a true congenital pleuroperitoneal diaphragmatic hernia in a cat. J Am Anim Hosp Assoc 1991;27:501–7.
12. Cariou MP, Shihab N, Kenny P, Baines SJ. Surgical management of an incidentally diagnosed true pleuroperitoneal hernia in a cat. J Feline Med Surg 2009;11:873–7.
13. Voges AK, Bertrand S, Hill RC, et al. True diaphragmatic hernia in a cat. Vet Radiol Ultrasound 1997;38:116–19.
14. Briscoe G. Hernia through the central tendon of the diaphragm (cat). J Anat 1928;62(Pt 2):224–6.
15. Parry A. Positive contrast peritoneography in the diagnosis of a pleuroperitoneal diaphragmatic hernia in a cat. J Feline Med Surg 2010;12:141–3.
16. Keep JM. Congenital diaphragmatic hernia in a cat. Aust Vet J 1950;26(8):193–6.
17. Pober BR, Russell MK, Ackerman KG. Congenital diaphragmatic hernia overview. GeneReviews (Internet) 2006 2010 Mar 16 (cited 2010 20 August); Available from: http://www.ncbi.nlm.nih.gov/books/NBK1359/
18. Feldman DB, Bree MM, Cohen BJ. Congenital diaphragmatic hernia in neonatal dogs. J Am Vet Med Assoc 1968;153:942–4.
19. Valentine BA, Cooper BJ, Dietze AE, Noden DM. Canine congenital diaphragmatic hernia. J Vet Intern Med 1988;2:109–12.
20. Clugston RD, Greer JJ. Diaphragm development and congenital diaphragmatic hernia. Semin Pediatr Surg 2007;16:94–100.
21. Ragni RA, Hotston Moore A. Diaphragmatic rupture in dogs and cats – part 1: diagnosis. UK Vet 2007;12(2):22–9.
22. Worth AJ, Machon RG. Traumatic diaphragmatic herniation: pathophysiology and management. Comp Cont Educ Pract Vet 2005;27:178–91.
23. Gibson TW, Brisson BA, Sears W. Perioperative survival rates after surgery for diaphragmatic hernia in dogs and cats:

92 cases (1990–2002). J Am Vet Med Assoc 2005;227:105–9.

24. Schmiedt CW, Tobias KM, Stevenson MA. Traumatic diaphragmatic hernia in cats: 34 cases (1991–2001). J Am Vet Med Assoc 2003;222(9):1237–40.

25. Vnuk D, Pirkić B, Maticić D, et al. Feline high-rise syndrome: 119 cases (1998–2001). J Feline Med Surg 2004;6(5):305–12.

26. Benitah N, Matousek JL, Barnes RF, et al. Diaphragmatic and perineal hernias associated with cutaneous asthenia in a cat. J Am Vet Med Assoc 2004;224(5):706–9, 698.

27. Burton C, White R. Surgical approach to a ruptured diaphragm in the cat. In Pract 1997;19:298–305.

28. Garson HL, Dodman NH, Baker GJ. Diaphragmatic hernia. Analysis of fifty-six cases in dogs and cats. J Small Anim Pract 1980;21:469–81.

29. Hunt GB, Johnson KA. Diaphragmatic, pericardial, and hiatal hernia. In: Slatter DH, editor. Textbook of small animal surgery. 3rd ed. Philadelphia: Saunders; 2003. p. 471–87.

30. Sullivan M, Reid J. Management of 60 cases of diaphragmatic rupture. J Small Anim Pract 1990;31:425–30.

31. Katic N, Bartolomaeus E, Böhler A, Dupré G. Traumatic diaphragmatic rupture in a cat with partial kidney displacement into the thorax. J Small Anim Pract 2007;48(12):705–8.

32. Störk CK, Hamaide AJ, Schwedes C, et al. Hemiurothorax following diaphragmatic hernia and kidney prolapse in a cat. J Feline Med Surg 2003;5(2):91–6.

33 Bellenger CR, Milstein M, McDonell W. Herniation of gravid uterus into the thorax of a dog. Mod Vet Pract 1975;56(8):553–5.

34. Sullivan JL, Puckett JR, Sevedge JP. Ruptured diaphragm with herniation of the gravid uterus and abdominal viscera. J Am Vet Med Assoc 1969;155(6):941–2.

35. Kraje BJ, Kraje AC, Rohrbach BW, et al. Intrathoracic and concurrent orthopedic injury associated with traumatic rib fracture in cats: 75 cases (1980–1998). J Am Vet Med Assoc 2000;216(1):51–4.

36. Cornell KK, Jakovljevic S, Waters DJ, et al. Extrahepatic biliary obstruction secondary to diaphragmatic hernia in two cats. J Am Anim Hosp Assoc 1993;29(6):502–7.

37. Formaggini L, Schmidt K, De Lorenzi D. Gastric dilatation-volvulus associated with diaphragmatic hernia in three cats: clinical presentation, surgical treatment and presumptive aetiology. J Feline Med Surg 2008;10(2):198–201.

38. Meincke JE, Hobbie WV Jr, Barto LR. Traumatic chylothorax with associated diaphragmatic hernias in the cat. J Am Vet Med Assoc 1969;155(1):15–20.

39. Lin JL, Lee CS, Chen PW, et al. Complications during labour in a chihuahua due to diaphragmatic hernia. Vet Rec 2007;161(3):103–4.

40. Bellenger CR, Trim C, Summer-Smith G. Bile pleuritis in a dog. J Small Anim Pract 1975;16(9):575–7.

41. Donald CE, Lee R, Sullivan M. Diaphragmatic rupture and biliary tract damage. J Small Anim Pract 1985;26:61–6.

42. Minihan AC, Berg J, Evans KL. Chronic diaphragmatic hernia in 34 dogs and 16 cats. J Am Anim Hosp Assoc 2004;40(1):51–63.

43. Andreoni AA, Voss K. Reconstruction of a large diaphragmatic defect in a kitten using small intestinal submucosa (SIS). J Feline Med Surg 2009;11(12):1019–22.

44. Spattini G, Rossi F, Vignoli M, Lamb CR. Use of ultrasound to diagnose diaphragmatic rupture in dogs and cats. Vet Radiol Ultrasound 2003;44(2):226–30.

45. Reichle JK, Wisner ER. Non-cardiac thoracic ultrasound in 75 feline and canine patients. Vet Radiol Ultrasound 2000;41(2):154–62.

46. Reimer SB, Kyles AE, Filipowicz DE, Gregory CR. Long-term outcome of cats treated conservatively or surgically for peritoneopericardial diaphragmatic hernia: 66 cases (1987–2002). J Am Vet Med Assoc 2004;224:728–32.

47. Neiger R. Peritoneopericardial diaphragmatic hernia in cats. Comp Cont Ed Pract Vet 1996;18(5):461–79.

48. Reina A, Vidaña E, Soriano P, et al. Traumatic intrapericardial diaphragmatic hernia: case report and literature review. Injury 2001;32(2):153–6.

49. Wallace J, Mullen HS, Lesser MB. A technique for surgical correction of peritoneal pericardial diaphragmatic hernia in dogs and cats. J Am Anim Hosp Assoc 1992;28:503–10.

50. Liptak JM, Bissett SA, Allan GS, et al. Hepatic cysts incarcerated in a peritoneopericardial diaphragmatic hernia. J Feline Med Surg 2002;4(2):123–5.

51. Scruggs SM, Bright JM. Chronic cardiac tamponade in a cat caused by an intrapericardial biliary cyst. J Feline Med Surg 2010;12(4):338–40.

52. Less RD, Bright JM, Orton EC. Intrapericardial cyst causing cardiac tamponade in a cat. J Am Anim Hosp Assoc 2000;36(2):115–19.

53. Sivacolundhu RK, Read RA, Marchevsky AM. Hiatal hernia controversies – a review of pathophysiology and treatment options. Aust Vet J 2002;80(1–2):48–53.

54. Lorinson D, Bright RM. Long-term outcome of medical and surgical treatment of hiatal hernias in dogs and cats: 27 cases (1978–1996). J Am Vet Med Assoc 1998;213:381–4.

55. Arndt JW, Marks SL, Kneller SK. What is your diagnosis? Hiatal hernia due to laryngeal squamous cell carcinoma. J Am Vet Med Assoc 2006;228(5):693–4.

56. Prymak C, Saunders HM, Washabau RJ. Hiatal hernia repair by restoration and stabilization of normal anatomy. An evaluation in four dogs and one cat. Vet Surg 1989;18(5):386–91.

57. Stokhof AA. Diagnosis and treatment of acquired diaphragmatic hernia by thoracotomy in 49 dogs and 72 cats. Vet Q 1986;8(3):177–83.

58. Fossum TW. Surgery of the lower respiratory system: pleural cavity and diaphragm. In: Fossum TW, editor. Small animal surgery. St Louis: Mosby Elsevier; 2007. p. 896–929.

59. Bellenger CR, Hunt GB, Goldsmid SE, Pearson MR. Outcomes of thoracic surgery in dogs and cats. Aust Vet J 1996;74(1):25–30.

60. Stampley AR, Waldron DR. Reexpansion pulmonary edema after surgery to repair a diaphragmatic hernia in a cat. J Am Vet Med Assoc 1993;203(12):1699–701.

61. Bowman KL, Birchard SJ, Bright RM. Complications associated with the implantation of polypropylene mesh in dogs and cats: a retrospective study of 21 cases (1984–1996). J Am Anim Hosp Assoc 1998;34(3):225–33.

62. Brown CN, Finch JG. Which mesh for hernia repair? Ann R Coll Surg Engl 2010;92(4):272–8.

63. Smith MJ, Paran TS, Quinn F, Corbally MT. The SIS extracellular matrix scaffold-preliminary results of use in congenital diaphragmatic hernia (CDH) repair. Pediatr Surg Int 2004;20(11–12):859–62.

64. Furneaux RW, Hudson MD. Autogenous muscle flap repair of a diaphragmatic hernia. Feline Pract 1976;6(1):20–4.

65. Helphrey ML. Abdominal flap graft for repair of chronic diaphragmatic hernia in the dog. J Am Vet Med Assoc 1982;181(8):791–3.

66. Joseph R, Kuzi S, Lavy E, Aroch I. Transient megaoesophagus and oesophagitis following diaphragmatic rupture repair in a cat. J Feline Med Surg 2008;10(3):284–90.

Chapter |46|

Trachea and bronchus

E. Hardie

Tracheal problems in cats can be life threatening. Surgical intervention may be required for removal of foreign bodies or focal masses. Tracheal avulsion has a good success rate after surgical repair with the right preparation of the patient, the surgical team, and anesthetist. The small size of the cat's trachea and the propensity to produce thick secretions contribute to blockage of the lumen, tracheotomy tubes, and tracheostomy incisions. A tracheotomy should not be done in cats unless there are facilities to provide continuous monitoring postoperatively, and even then the morbidity is high. This chapter will review the anatomy, clinical signs, and imaging of the different tracheal disorders in cats, and give details on how to perform surgery for these conditions.

SURGICAL ANATOMY

The trachea extends from the cricoid cartilage to the carina. The normal cat trachea ranges from 7–10 mm in diameter[1] and has 38–43 tracheal cartilages.[2] These cartilage rings are composed of hyaline cartilage and are incomplete for a short distance dorsally. The dorsal space is filled with loose connective tissue covered by the trachealis muscle, which attaches to the external surface of the tracheal rings.[3] Adjacent cartilage rings are joined by fibroelastic annular ligaments, which fuse with the perichondrium. The inner surface of the trachea is covered with respiratory epithelium supported by the submucosa. The tissue at the dorsal aspect of the trachea (muscle, connective tissue, submucosa, and mucosa) is commonly referred to as the dorsal tracheal membrane (Fig. 46-1).

The blood supply to the trachea is segmental, coming from the cranial thyroid, caudal thyroid, and the bronchoesophageal arteries. The vascular pedicles are on the lateral aspects of the trachea. Venous drainage occurs through the thyroid, internal jugular, and bronchoesophageal veins. Sympathetic innervation is from the sympathetic trunk, while parasympathetic innervation is from the recurrent laryngeal nerve.[4]

The cervical trachea lies dorsal and medial to the sternohyoideus and sternothyroideus muscles. It is ventral to the longus colli and longus capitus muscles. The carotid sheaths are dorsal to the trachea in the cranial half of the neck and lateral to the trachea in the caudal half of the neck. The esophagus is dorsal in the cranial neck and is on

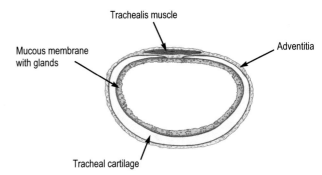

Figure 46-1 Cross-section of the feline trachea. The muscle attaches on the outside of the cartilage ring and the ring only has a very narrow defect dorsally.

the left dorsolateral or left lateral aspect in the caudal neck. The recurrent laryngeal nerves are on the dorsolateral aspects of the trachea. The thyroid and parathyroid glands are on the lateral aspects of the trachea in the cranial neck (Fig. 46-2).

As the trachea passes through the thoracic inlet and into the mediastinum, it passes dorsal to the jugular veins, which join to become the cranial vena cava. Within the thorax,[5] the aortic arch, left subclavian artery and brachiocephalic trunk lie on the left aspect of the trachea. The right subclavian artery and right vagus nerve are directly lateral to the trachea. The azygos vein crosses the right side of the trachea cranial to the carina. The esophagus moves from the left aspect of the trachea to dorsal as it approaches the carina. The trachea bifurcates into the main stem bronchi between the pulmonary arteries and veins. The main stem bronchi in the cat are short, quickly branching into lower level bronchi.

GENERAL CONSIDERATIONS AND DIAGNOSTIC PROCEDURES

The major surgical conditions of the feline trachea are tracheal disruption due to trauma or intubation, tracheal collapse, and tracheal obstruction due to foreign bodies, masses or stenosis.

© 2014 Elsevier Ltd
DOI: 10.1016/B978-0-7020-4336-9.00046-9

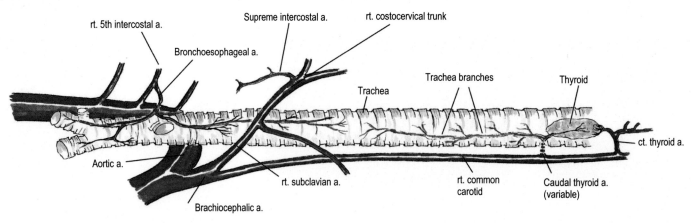

Figure 46-2 The blood supply to the feline trachea.

Clinical signs

Clinical signs of tracheal disease are those of respiratory distress: increased respiratory rate, increased respiratory effort, cyanosis, and/or open-mouth breathing. If the integrity of the trachea is compromised, subcutaneous emphysema may be observed. Other clinical signs include inspiratory stridor, coughing or gagging, exercise intolerance, self-limitation of vigorous movement, and a distinct preference for a sternal position. Patients with chronic disease may experience anorexia and weight loss.

Emergency management

Emergency stabilization of the patient involves administering oxygen by facemask or placing the cat in an oxygen-rich environment, and administering sedation (e.g., acepromazine, butorphanol), if indicated. An indwelling intravenous catheter is placed so that the cat can be quickly anesthetized if there is a need to control respiration. Corticosteroids are administered if airway swelling is suspected. In severe cases, intubation may be needed. Tracheostomy should be avoided unless absolutely necessary, due to the cat's propensity to produce large quantities of mucus that easily plug the narrow tracheostomy tubes that fit in the feline trachea.

Diagnostic imaging

Radiographs of the neck and thorax often yield a diagnosis and should be performed before other diagnostic tests. If the equipment to take a standing lateral radiograph is present, the cat can be maintained in a sternal position while the radiographs are obtained. All radiographs for tracheal measurements should be taken with the cat in a sternal position. For additional lateral views then the cat is repositioned for a minimal amount of time to enable each radiograph to be taken. In between radiographs, the cat is placed once again in sternal recumbency and a facemask or flow-by technique is used to administer oxygen.

Radiographic signs are dependent on the lesion. If obstruction is present, the foreign body or mass may be observed in the lumen of the trachea (Fig. 46-3). Stenosis or extratracheal compressive masses will cause a narrowing of the tracheal lumen. Tracheal collapse may be difficult to recognize without fluoroscopy, but narrowing of the cervical trachea along the affected segment should be observed on radiographs taken during inspiration (Fig. 46-4). The diameter of the cervical trachea of normal cats is 18–20% of the diameter of the thoracic inlet on lateral radiographs, depending on breed.[6] Acute rupture will result in air outside the tracheal lumen. Depending on the

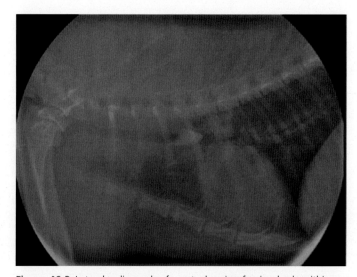

Figure 46-3 Lateral radiograph of a cat, showing foreign body within the lumen of the trachea. *(Image © Michael Tivers, reprinted with kind permission.)*

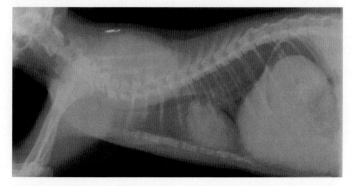

Figure 46-4 Lateral radiograph of a cat, showing tracheal narrowing at the thoracic inlet.

location of the rupture, subcutaneous emphysema, air trapping in muscle and fascial planes, pneumomediastinum or pneumothorax may be observed (Fig. 46-5).

The level of tracheal obstruction will influence the pulmonary radiographic changes. Extrathoracic tracheal obstruction may result in poorly inflated lung fields, a high and domed diaphragm, or

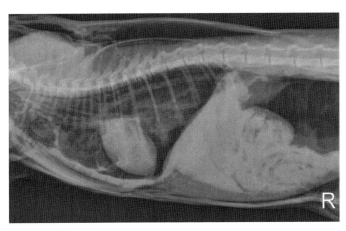

Figure 46-5 Lateral radiograph of a cat, showing subcutaneous emphysema and pneumomediastinum due to iatrogenic tracheal rupture.

Box 46-1 **Tracheal masses in the cat**

Neoplastic[13–29]

Lymphoma/lymphosarcoma (11 cats)
Adenocarcinoma (seven cats)
Squamous cell carcinoma (three cats)
Carcinoma (two cats)
Seromucinous carcinoma (one cat)
Neuroendocrine carcinoma (one cat)
Histiocytic sarcoma (one cat)
Adenoma (one cat)

Non-neoplastic[19,30–34]

Myiasis due to *Cuterebra* larvae (four cats)
Lymphocytic/plasmacytic inflammation (two cats)
Granuloma due to mycobacterial infection (one cat)
Zygomycosis (one cat)
Polyp (one cat)

pulmonary edema. Intrathoracic tracheal obstruction may result in hyperlucent lung fields, prominent pulmonary vasculature and a flattened diaphragm due to over-expansion of the lungs and air trapping.

Tracheal endoscopy may be needed to fully characterize a lesion, but requires general anesthesia. If compromise of the integrity of the trachea is suspected, great care must be taken not to worsen the condition during intubation. Ideally, the cat is pre-oxygenated by facemask or flow-by, anesthesia is induced and maintained using injectable anesthetic agents, and oxygen is administered using a facemask or an endotracheal tube placed cranial to the lesion. If needed, a small endotracheal tube or a small-bore catheter may be passed distal to the lesion before and after scoping, if adequate oxygenation cannot be maintained by other means. If neoplasia is suspected, cytology and biopsy samples are obtained as needed to identify and stage the tumor. The surgeon should be prepared to correct the lesion immediately following the scoping procedure.

SURGICAL DISEASES

Foreign bodies

Tracheal foreign bodies reported in cats include grass awns, tree needles, a twig, bark, wood mulch, gravel, small stones, teeth, bones, a bullet, and a safety pin.[7] Young cats may be predisposed to this condition in that six of 12 cats in the largest published case series were 18 months or younger.[7] The duration of observed clinical signs ranges from one to 21 days. Unless they are very small, e.g., tree needles,[8] foreign bodies tend to lodge at or immediately cranial to the tracheal bifurcation, rather than in the bronchi, presumably due to the small diameter of the feline trachea and bronchi. Plain radiographs are usually sufficient for diagnosis. Many objects are radio-opaque and those that are not will be highlighted as a soft tissue density surrounded by tracheal air. Methods used to retrieve foreign bodies include removal using endoscopic guidance,[9] removal using fluoroscopic guidance,[7] and surgical removal.[10] Non-surgical removal is preferred because of the need for a thoracotomy to approach the carina.

Endoscopic removal involves visualization of the foreign body using a rigid or flexible endoscope. The foreign body is grasped with forceps or enclosed in a snare. Small objects may be grasped with forceps passed through the biopsy channel of the scope, but larger forceps must be carefully passed alongside the scope. Balloons have been passed beyond the foreign body under endoscopic or fluoroscopic guidance, inflated, and then pulled towards the larynx.[11,12] A case series described successful removal of tracheal foreign bodies from ten cats using grasping forceps with a length of 58.7 cm from the tip to the handle.[7] The forceps were placed, then the object was grasped and withdrawn, under fluoroscopic guidance. Two of these cases involved repeated unsuccessful attempts to remove the foreign body under endoscopic guidance, followed by successful use of the fluoroscopically guided forceps. The particular forceps used was of a custom design, but long-handled grasping forceps are common in minimally invasive surgery packs.

Once the object has been removed, tracheoscopy/bronchoscopy should be performed to ensure that the inhaled object(s) was completely removed and that there was no iatrogenic damage of the trachea. If the foreign body cannot be removed or if smaller foreign objects are observed in the bronchi, beyond the reach of any endoscopic forceps, the object(s) may be removed using tracheotomy.

Tracheal masses

Tracheal masses are less common than laryngeal masses in the cat, but do occur. Neoplasia is most common (Box 46-1).

From the literature, the age at time of diagnosis of neoplastic masses ranged from two to 18 years, with all cats, except one with squamous cell carcinoma, being over six years of age, with a median age of 9.5 years.[14,29] Affected breeds included domestic short-haired (DSH), domestic long-haired (DLH), Siamese, Himalayan, and Persian cats.

Non-neoplastic masses are less common than neoplastic conditions (Box 46-1). Cats with myiasis were one to two years of age, while the other non-neoplastic masses were found in older cats. The masses were observed as focal soft tissue opacities within the trachea, focal annular thickening of the trachea or focal narrowing of the trachea on radiographs. Tracheoscopy allowed direct observation of masses (Fig. 46-6), removal of one of four *Cuterebra* larvae, and tissue removal for diagnostic purposes and/or debulking of the obstruction. Histology provided definitive diagnosis, but cytology was less reliable, most notably when lymphocytic/plasmacytic inflammation was found. Subsequent histologic examination found neoplasia in some of these instances.

Treatment of tumors differed according to tumor type. Treatment of lymphoma/lymphosarcoma with surgical resection/anastomosis, radiation therapy, and/or chemotherapy resulted in disease-free intervals of up to 19 months.[13,15,24,25] Resection/anastomosis resulting in complete removal of adenocarcinomas has resulted in long-term

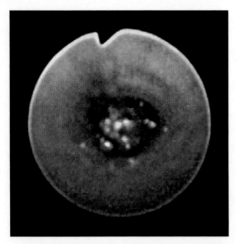

Figure 46-6 Intraluminal tracheal mass viewed through an endoscope.

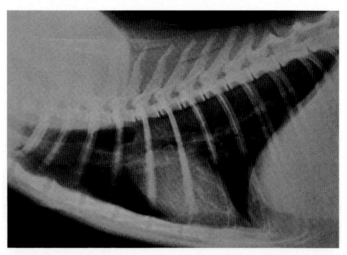

Figure 46-7 Lateral radiograph of a cat, showing the pseudoairway associated with tracheal avulsion. *(Image © Robert White, reprinted with kind permission.)*

survival, while partial removal has resulted in disease-free intervals up to one year.[13,18,19,22,25] Tracheal stenting relieved respiratory distress due to tracheal stenosis, but progression of carcinoma within the lung resulted in recurrent respiratory distress in six weeks.[27] Definitive treatment of tracheal seromucinous, squamous cell or neuroendocrine carcinoma has not been described. Surgical removal of a *Cuterebra* larva through a tracheotomy incision resolved disease in three cats, but one cat developed tracheal collapse in the region of the tracheotomy six years later.[27,30,31] The cat with mycobacterial infection died of other causes six months after excisional biopsy of the tracheal lesion and a course of appropriate antibiotic therapy.[33] Excisional biopsy of the tracheal polyp using the endoscopic biopsy forceps resulted in resolution of clinical signs for four months, after which the cat was lost to follow up.[32]

Tracheal avulsion

Tracheal avulsion is a traumatic lesion, thought to be caused by sudden hyperextension of the neck while the carina remains in a fixed position.[35-40] Separation of the tracheal wall usually occurs just cranial to the carina. Depending on the degree of disruption, signs of respiratory distress will be present immediately or will be delayed. In cats with delayed clinical signs, the tissues surrounding the intrathoracic trachea maintain the airway, creating a pseudotrachea, and signs become apparent only when further motion results in sudden disruption of the remaining tissues or stenosis develops at the ends of the pseudotrachea, causing severe air trapping in the lung. Tracheal avulsion typically occurs in young adult cats with a history of known or presumed trauma, with times to presentation being one to 28 days after the traumatic episode. The onset of respiratory distress is often sudden and severe.

If the animal is examined at the time of the injury and signs of respiratory distress are not present, radiographic findings associated with tracheal avulsion may easily be missed. These signs include separation of tracheal rings, focal tracheal narrowing, and the presence of air outside the trachea. Radiographic findings in cats exhibiting respiratory distress include obviously separated tracheal rings with an associated gas-filled diverticulum or dilated pseudotrachea (Fig. 46-7), stenosis of the tracheal lumen at the junctions of normal and avulsed tracheal tissue, pneumomediastinum, and over-inflation/hyperlucency of the lung fields associated with air trapping.

Resolution of clinical signs with conservative therapy has been reported in one cat, but most cats with this condition need resection of the affected segment because the degree of stenosis at the ends of

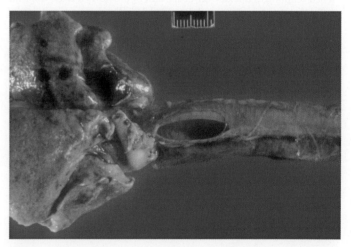

Figure 46-8 Dorsal view of a cadaveric cat trachea, showing the dorsal linear tear created by over-expansion of an endotracheal tube cuff.

the affected tracheal segment worsens with time. Long-term resolution of clinical signs was documented in 18 of 20 cats treated with immediate repair or resection/anastomosis of the affected tracheal segment and followed for five months to seven years after surgery.[37-40] Two cats did not survive the surgical procedure.

Iatrogenic tracheal rupture

Iatrogenic injury to the dorsal tracheal membrane may occur in cats undergoing endotracheal tube intubation.[1,40-44] The majority of reported injuries are associated with dental procedures and appear to be secondary to endotracheal tube cuff over-inflation. Most ruptures occur at the thoracic inlet, the site at which the endotracheal tube cuff is routinely placed. Both high pressure, low volume cuffs and low pressure, high volume cuffs have been associated with injury. The average volume of air required for endotracheal cuff inflation resulting in an air-tight seal in the normal cat trachea is 1.6 mL. Studies in cat cadavers determined that inflation volumes over 6 mL resulted in tracheal rupture.[1] The ruptures were linear tears at the junction of the dorsal tracheal membrane and the tracheal cartilage (Fig. 46-8). The mediastinum remained intact when rupture occurred.

The predominant clinical signs in cats with tracheal rupture were subcutaneous emphysema (37/38 reported cases), dyspnea (11/38 cases), anorexia (8/38 cases), coughing (6/38 cases), lethargy (5/38 cases), and respiratory stridor (4/38 cases).[1,41-44] Clinical signs were noted four hours to 14 days after the anesthetic episode. Subcutaneous emphysema and pneumomediastinum were present in 28/29 cases in which thoracic radiographs were obtained (see Fig. 46-5). The tear in the dorsal membrane was observed in 9/11 cases in which tracheoscopy was used and was confirmed on necropsy in one case.

Of the 38 reported cases, one died while being radiographed. Conservative treatment, consisting of oxygen supplementation, sedation, cage rest, and antibiotic therapy when indicated, was successful in 22 cases. Time to resolution of clinical signs ranged from 24 hours to five weeks. Fifteen cats with severe respiratory distress unresponsive to conservative therapy underwent surgical treatment. Of these cases, five of 15 died as a result of intraoperative or postoperative complications and ten recovered (although one cat required temporary postoperative ventilator support).

Tracheal collapse

Tracheal collapse has been reported in nine cats.[27,45-48] Clinical signs reported in these cats included intermittent dyspnea, which worsened with exertion, episodes of severe respiratory distress requiring oxygen therapy, coughing, cyanosis, and syncope. Cats with upper airway obstruction had stertor, stridor, or a loud purring noise during inspiration. On physical examination, the affected trachea was easily compressed and palpation elicited a cough. Narrowing of the affected tracheal segment was observed on lateral radiographs obtained during inspiration. On bronchoscopy or fluoroscopy, dynamic narrowing of the affected trachea occurred on inspiration.

Five cats with cranial upper airway obstruction (congenital cranial cervical tracheal stenosis, laryngeal mass, nasal lymphoma, nasal adenocarcinoma, histiocytic sarcoma) had secondary collapse of the cervical trachea just cranial to the thoracic inlet.[45,46] The tracheal collapse resolved with removal of the obstruction (chemotherapy of the nasal lymphoma and removal of the laryngeal mass) in two cats. Two cats with dynamic tracheal collapse secondary to previous intubation or tracheal surgery were successfully treated with tracheal stenting.[27] One case of cervical tracheal collapse secondary to suspected trauma was successfully treated in a four-year-old Siamese cat using a spiral ring prosthesis.[48] One case of primary cervical tracheal collapse in a seven-year-old DSH was successfully treated with prosthetic tracheal rings.[47]

Bronchoesophageal fistula

Bronchoesophageal fistula is a rarely reported cause of chronic cough and vomiting in young cats.[49] A congenital cause was suspected in the two reported cases because they were young cats with no history of an esophageal foreign body. On radiographs, a large soft tissue mass in the left caudal hemi-thorax was observed. At surgery, the mass was found to be an abscess communicating with the lumen of the esophagus. Lobectomy of the affected lung lobe, with repair of the esophageal defect, successfully resolved disease.

PREPARATION FOR SURGERY

Anesthetic considerations

The anesthesia and surgery teams must communicate and cooperate fully to maintain respiratory function while surgery is being

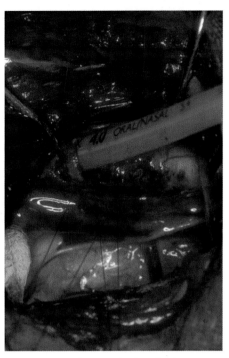

Figure 46-9 Intraoperative photograph of tracheal resection-anastomosis, showing placement of the endotracheal tube in distal segment and use of simple interrupted sutures for alignment and traction.

performed. Because each anesthetic recovery is risky in patients with respiratory compromise, invasive diagnostic procedures and surgical treatment are ideally planned for one anesthetic episode. If tracheal wall compromise is suspected, preparations should be made for treatment of sudden development of pneumothorax during the anesthetic episode.[50]

The cat is pre-oxygenated prior to induction of anesthesia. Anesthesia is best induced and maintained using injectable anesthetics, in which case the endotracheal tube is used solely to support respiratory function. The endotracheal tube is usually placed cranial to the lesion to avoid injury. Endoscopic guidance has been used for precise distal placement of an endotracheal tube in a case involving a carinal tear.[44] Tracheal surgery is considered to be contaminated and prophylactic antibiotics should be administered prior to the start of surgery.

During the surgical procedure, the anesthetist and the surgeon work together to maintain the airway, using sterile endotracheal tubes (or smaller tubes and catheters) passed into the distal airway, as needed. Unless the surgery is at the carina, the orally placed endotracheal tube can be passed distal to the surgery site once the obstruction is removed or the defect is located. If a tear is present at the carina, it may be necessary to alternate oxygenation using a sterile small tube passed through the surgery site (Fig. 46-9) and periods of apnea, during which the surgeon works. Once tracheal surgery is complete, the endotracheal tube is placed cranial to the lesion, to avoid compromise of the surgery site during extubation.

SURGICAL TECHNIQUES

Approaches to the trachea

As the approach to the trachea is lesion dependent, the surgeon should make every effort to clearly identify the location of the lesion

The cat is positioned in dorsal recumbency with the head extended and the forelimbs pulled caudally and tied back. A sandbag placed under the neck may be used to elevate the trachea. A ventral midline cervical incision is made extending from the larynx to the manubrium. The sternohyoideus and sternothyroideus muscles are separated or cut in a lengthwise direction (the muscles spiral more in the cat than in the dog, often preventing complete exposure using only blunt dissection). Carefully placed small Weitlaner retractors are used to hold the muscles laterally. The trachea is directly below the muscles. Dissection of the lateral aspects of the trachea should be limited and performed with care, to avoid damage to the recurrent laryngeal nerves and the tracheal blood supply. Traction sutures placed around the ventral aspect of the tracheal rings can be used to gently roll the dorsal aspect of the trachea into the view of the surgeon. If exposure to the trachea in the thoracic inlet is needed, the incision is extended over the thoracic midline and the first three sternebrae are split. Care must be taken to clearly identify and protect the jugular veins as they pass ventral to the trachea and join to form the cranial vena cava.

Box 46-3 **Approach to the thoracic trachea**

While ventral midline approaches to the thoracic trachea have been described, the preferred approach is a standard or modified right lateral 3rd–4th intercostal space thoracotomy (see Chapter 41). Once the thorax is open, the right cranial lung is packed caudally using wet gauze sponges. The trachea, esophagus, cranial vena cava, vagus nerve, recurrent laryngeal nerves, and azygos vein are identified as they are encountered. The vessels and nerves are retracted as needed, using soft loop retractors. The azygos vein may be ligated and cut, if necessary. Traction sutures placed around tracheal rings are used to manipulate the trachea so that the surgeon can gain access to all aspects of the trachea.

Appropriate nerve blocks, infusion of peri-incisional tissues with bupivacaine, and/or placement and use of a wound infusion catheter[51] to administer bupivicaine help reduce pain and anxiety during the postoperative period. A thoracic drainage tube (see Chapter 41) is placed prior to closure of the body wall incisions if the chest cavity was exposed. This tube is maintained for 12–24 hours to assure that no further air leakage occurs.

Box 46-4 **Tracheal resection and reconstruction**

A surgical approach is made to the trachea depending on the site of the lesion to be removed. An uncuffed endotracheal tube is placed through the larynx and the tip of the tube is located cranial to the proposed cranial extent of the site of resection. Intermittent positive pressure ventilation through this tube is used to maintain oxygenation. The tracheal section to be excised is identified. Once the caudal site of resection is identified, the surgeon should have available a sterile cuffed endotracheal tube of the appropriate size. The trachea is severed and the endotracheal tube is placed into the caudal segment. The cuff is inflated and oxygenation is maintained using this tube (see Fig. 46-9). If the incision is close to the carina, a tube small enough to be wedged into a mainstem bronchus may be needed to maintain oxygenation. Alternatively, the surgeon can intermittently occlude the tracheal opening while oxygen is delivered through a needle placed directly through the bronchial wall.

The site of the cranial resection is identified and severed. Three or four simple interrupted sutures of 4/0 monofilament absorbable suture material are pre-placed around the tracheal rings of each segment (Fig. 46-9). These sutures are used to manipulate and align the tracheal segments. They allow the trachea to be 'rolled' to allow exposure of the left side, which is opposite the surgeon. Additional simple interrupted sutures are placed around or through the rings and are used to suture the defect in the dorsal tracheal membrane. Depending on the location of the anastomosis, the orally placed endotracheal tube can be advanced past the defect and the distal tube withdrawn early in the process, or the distal tube/needle can be used until the last portion of the defect is closed. Once the defect is closed, the endotracheal tube is withdrawn cranial to the suture line and the suture line is checked for any air leaks by placing saline on the area and observing for air bubbles during positive pressure ventilation.

prior to surgery (Boxes 46-2 and 46-3). Surgical instruments for performing tracheal surgery in cats need to be delicate. Many surgeons use a microsurgical pack supplemented with a few general surgery instruments. The use of magnification is recommended. Use of traction sutures for retraction helps to keep the small surgical field free of instruments and fingers.

Tracheotomy or bronchotomy

Incisions into the trachea are made between adjacent tracheal rings. A carinal tracheotomy can be used to access the lumen of the main stem bronchi. Traction sutures may be placed around the rings to hold the incision open, while sutures placed around both rings on either side of the opening allow the surgeon to rapidly close the incision during ventilation, which may make passing a tube into the distal segment(s) unnecessary. Ideally, the incision should not extend more than two-thirds around the ventral aspect of the trachea. If needed, sterile endoscopic or minimally invasive surgery instruments can be used to retrieve foreign bodies or to perform excisional biopsies through a limited tracheal approach. If a 360° circumferential incision or laceration is present, the operation becomes similar to a tracheal resection-anastomosis. The incision is closed using simple interrupted 4/0 absorbable monofilament sutures placed through or around the adjacent tracheal rings.

If traumatic laceration or rupture has created a lengthwise defect in the trachea, repair depends on whether the dorsal tracheal membrane or the tracheal rings are affected. The dorsal tracheal membrane is sutured using simple interrupted sutures or a continuous suture, using 4/0 or 5/0 monofilament absorbable suture material. If a lengthwise cut through the tracheal rings is present, simple interrupted sutures of 4/0 monofilament suture are placed around or through the rings on either side of the cut. If a long defect is present, the surgeon should consider placing prosthetic tracheal rings to support the trachea during healing. Care must be taken to ensure that no suture entering the tracheal lumen punctures or entraps an endotracheal tube cuff, if present.

Tracheal resection and reconstruction

Tracheal resection (Box 46-4) is performed for tracheal masses or stenosis. The amount of trachea that can safely be removed has not been identified in the cat, but successful removal of four rings has been reported.[24] The author has removed five rings of the cervical trachea in a cat with a tracheal granuloma, without the need to place the neck in ventroflexion during healing. In cases of tracheal avulsion, the unaffected rings at either end of the avulsion will be separated by the pseudotrachea.

Box 46-5 **Temporary tracheostomy**

To perform temporary tracheostomy, a ventral cervical midline approach is used. The skin is incised from the level of the cricoid cartilage 2–3 cm caudally. The sternohyoideus muscles are separated to expose the trachea. A ventral incision is made between tracheal rings anywhere from tracheal ring 2–5. Long suture loops are placed around the rings on either side of the incision. The incision is pulled open using the loops and a pediatric tracheostomy tube is placed. The muscles and skin are partially closed around the opening. Disinfectant ointment is placed on the tissues around the opening. The opening is covered with a sterile gauze swab that has been split to fit around the tube. Umbilical tapes are tied to wings of the tube and then tied around the neck. The suture loops are maintained so that the tracheal opening can easily be accessed in the event of tube dislodgement.

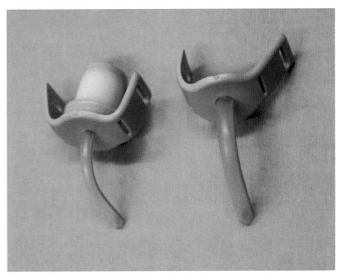

Figure 46-10 Tracheostomy tubes suitable for cats do not have inner cannulas. A 3 mm tracheostomy tube (left) with connector for an endotracheal tube; 4 mm tracheosotomy tube (right) with no connector.

Tracheostomy

Temporary tracheostomy

Temporary tracheostomy (Box 46-5) is performed to provide an airway for a cat with a life-threatening upper airway obstruction. In a study of 23 cats treated with temporary tracheostomy, 13 had laryngeal masses, five had trauma to the upper airway and five had upper airway swelling.[52] Major complications (complete tube occlusion with mucus or tube dislodgement) occurred in ten cats, while minor complications (partial tube obstruction, hyperthermia, pneumomediastinum, subcutaneous emphysema, edema at the tracheostomy site, Horner syndrome, iatrogenic laryngeal paralysis, cough, vomiting associated with suction, stay suture dislodgement) occurred in 17 cats. The tubes remained in place for one to 11 days, with a median of three days. These results suggest that while temporary tracheostomy can be life-saving, major complications should be anticipated and the cat should be closely monitored. Interestingly, in a study of 35 cats with laryngeal disease performed at another institution, none of the cats were managed with temporary tracheostomy, suggesting that alternative methods of managing upper airway obstruction are often effective.[53]

Tubes of the appropriate size for cats do not have an inner cannula (Fig. 46-10) and must be cleaned and suctioned on a regular schedule. Nebulization helps prevent thick mucous plugs. Given the high rate of complications, 24 hour surveillance is critical to the successful use of temporary tracheostomy in cats. Placing a spare tracheostomy tube, injectable anesthetic drugs, cotton tip applicators, and a suction tip next to the cage saves time in the event of tube occlusion or dislodgement.

Permanent tracheostomy

Permanent tracheostomy is used when upper airway obstruction cannot be resolved (Box 46-6). However, it is a fairly risky procedure. Overall, 46% of cats in two studies of permanent tracheostomy died of stomal or airway obstruction shortly after the procedure was performed.[52,54] The procedure was most successful in cats without airway inflammation, particularly if the primary disease could be resolved.

In a study of 21 cats, permanent tracheostomy was performed as a treatment for neoplasia (eight cats), inflammation of the larynx (five cats), laryngeal paralysis/collapse (four cats), trauma (three cats) and laryngeal mass of unknown cause (one cat).[54] Fourteen cats had dyspnea shortly after surgery (mainly due to mucous plugs), and six cats died while still in the hospital. From the fifteen cats that were discharged, five cats died within two months due to obstruction of

Box 46-6 **Permanent tracheostomy**

Prior to performing the procedure, the cat is placed in a normal standing position and the neck is carefully palpated to assess if loose skin surrounding the planned stoma will occlude the opening. If so, the surgeon must plan to excise the excess skin. Once anesthetized, the cat is placed in dorsal recumbency and a ventral midline skin incision is made over the cranial trachea. The sternohyoideus muscles are separated and sutured together dorsal to the trachea, using horizontal mattress sutures. A rectangular cut is made in the ventral one-third of the trachea for a length of 3–4 rings. The outer tracheal tissues are dissected from the mucosa, if possible, resulting in a ventral rectangle covered only by mucosa. The mucosa is incised along the ventral midline, folded over the edges of the cut tracheal rings, and sutured to the adjacent skin using simple interrupted sutures of 4/0 monofilament non-absorbable suture material. The cranial and caudal tissues are closed routinely from side to side. The cut edge of the skin at the cranial and caudal aspects of the stoma is sutured to the cut edge of the stoma. Excess skin is excised as needed.

the stoma and seven cats were euthanized three to 420 days (median 35 days) after surgery, mainly due to progression of neoplasia. Cats with inflammatory laryngeal disease were seven times more likely to die after the procedure than cats with other diseases, presumably because mucus production was more pronounced in these cats. Two cats with resolved upper airway obstruction were alive three months and five years after surgery.

In a separate study, of seven cats with permanent tracheostomy performed as treatment for neoplasia or granulomatous laryngeal disease, all cats were discharged from the hospital.[52] Two cats died due to obstruction of the stoma two and 42 days after discharge, one cat died of unknown causes 182 days after discharge, three cats were euthanized at seven to 281 days due to progression of disease and one cat with granulomatous disease was alive 4.5 years after discharge.

To prevent occlusion of the stoma with mucous plugs, routine humidification is needed for at least eight weeks after the procedure is performed. If secretions are thick and crusty, nebulization may be needed as often as every two to four hours. A clean suction catheter

Extraluminal

A routine approach to the cervical trachea is used. The recurrent laryngeal nerves are identified and protected. If a spiral prosthesis is chosen, a small dissection is made on one side of the trachea at the cranial aspect of the length to be supported. The prosthesis is introduced into the defect and 'spiralled' caudally, using minimal dissection as needed to advance through the peritracheal tissues. Every attempt is made to preserve the tracheal vessels. If prosthetic tracheal rings are chosen, a small lateral peritracheal dissection is made at each site of ring placement and a curved hemostat is passed dorsally around the trachea, grasping the end of the C-shaped ring. The ring is positioned with the opening on the ventral aspect of the trachea. Rings are placed approximately 5–8 mm apart. In each instance, the prosthesis is secured to the trachea using simple interrupted non-absorbable 4/0 sutures placed on the ventral, lateral, and dorsal aspects of the trachea. Each suture is placed around a tracheal ring or through the dorsal tracheal membrane, as indicated. The ends of the suture may be left long until the end of the procedure and used as traction sutures to assist in tracheal manipulation. Care must be taken to use an endotracheal tube without a cuff or to move the cuff out of the way while suturing. Closure is routine.

Intraluminal

Prior to placement, the cat is placed under anesthesia and the endotracheal tube is positioned just caudal to the larynx. Using a radio-opaque marker of known length to determine magnification, the maximal diameter of the trachea is measured while positive pressure ventilation (20 cm of H_2O) is maintained. The measurement is corrected for magnification and a self-expanding nitinol stent (see Chapter 10) that is 10–15% wider than the maximal diameter, and is at least 2 cm longer than the narrowed tracheal segment, is chosen. A bronchoscopic adapter is attached to the endotracheal tube and the stent delivery system is placed through the endotracheal tube and into the trachea under fluoroscopic guidance. The stent is positioned across the narrowed region and care is taken to make sure that the stent is distal to the endotracheal tube (preventing deployment of the stent within the tube). There may be advantages to stenting the whole trachea, rather than just the narrowed area, to avoid the risk of recurrent collapse beyond the limits of the stent. The stent is deployed slowly by withdrawing the outer sheath of the delivery system under fluoroscopic guidance. The stent can be re-constrained and repositioned up until 70% has been deployed. Once the stent is fully deployed, the delivery system is slowly withdrawn. Both lateral (Fig. 46-11) and ventrodorsal radiographs are taken to record the site of stent placement.

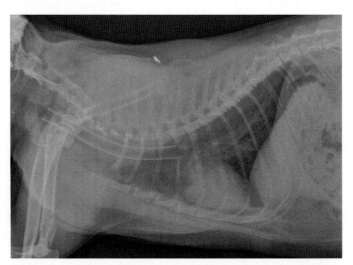

Figure 46-11 Lateral radiograph of a cat, showing a tracheal stent in place.

POSTOPERATIVE CARE

Cats undergoing tracheal surgery are at risk for acute respiratory compromise, even after surgery. The patient should be recovered in an oxygen cage to reduce the work of breathing. Once respiratory rate and effort are within normal limits in the oxygen cage, the cat is transitioned to room air in the oxygen cage. If respiratory rate and effort remain normal, the cat is moved to a regular cage with continuing 24 hour surveillance. Respiratory rate and effort are recorded on a regular basis, as they may alert the surgeon to developing complications. Because minimal airway swelling or mucus production can result in acute obstruction, a plan must be devised ahead of time to handle this complication. Anesthetic drugs, endotracheal or tracheostomy tubes, suction catheters and any other needed equipment should be stored within easy reach of the cage. Corticosteroids may be administered to control airway swelling. Antibiotics are given if ongoing infection is anticipated. Antitussives may be used to control coughing. Analgesics will allow the cat to breathe more comfortably, encouraging deep breaths.

Careful training of the owner is critical to the success of the surgery. The owner should be trained to recognize and report subtle signs of respiratory distress. There must be a workable plan for exercise restriction. Owners bringing home cats with healing tracheostomies must be prepared for 24 hour surveillance for signs of respiratory distress, as well as humidification and nebulization chores. They must be properly instructed on airway suctioning and stomal cleaning. Even after the tracheostomies have healed, the cats are at risk of obstruction due to stenosis of the opening and ongoing formation of mucous plugs.

should always be at hand. In the hospital, suctioning should be used only when necessary and suction pressure should be below 120 mmHg. At home, owners should be taught how to use a catheter and syringe to suction the trachea in the event of an emergency. Stomal cleaning should be limited to gentle removal of occluding crusts using saline-moistened cotton tip applicators or gauze.

Tracheal Stenting

Both extraluminal and intraluminal stents (see Chapter 10) have been used in cats (Box 46-7). Extraluminal stents have been used to treat collapse of the cervical trachea to the level of the thoracic inlet.[47,48] Intraluminal stents have been used to treat tracheal collapse secondary to endotracheal tube or surgical injury, as well as tracheal obstruction secondary to neoplasia (see Box 46-7).[27]

COMPLICATIONS AND PROGNOSIS

Complications associated with tracheostomy are detailed above. Potential complications associated with other tracheal surgeries include inability to oxygenate the patient during surgery, airway obstruction associated with swelling or mucus production, dehiscence (leading to pneumomediastinum or pneumothorax), tracheal stenosis, tracheal collapse, tracheal necrosis, and laryngeal paralysis.

Reported complications in the immediate postoperative period are postoperative swelling, excessive mucus production, pneumothorax and pulmonary edema.[1,31,40,50] Two cases of iatrogenic laryngeal paralysis have been reported, one associated with prosthetic tracheal ring placement[47] and the other with tracheal resection-anastomosis.[37] One of these cats had no obvious clinical signs and one developed exercise-related respiratory distress and stridor two months after surgery, which responded to conservative therapy. Tracheal collapse has been reported six years after tracheotomy for *Cuterebra* larva removal.[27] Recurrence or progression of neoplastic disease,

particularly after partial resection, has been reported.[13,18,22,25] There are no reports of postsurgical tracheal necrosis or symptomatic postsurgical tracheal stenosis in the cat.

Potential complications of intraluminal tracheal stenting include migration, stent collapse or breakage, collapse in an unstented region, coughing, formation of excess granulation within the trachea, pneumomediastinum, pneumonia, acute death, and progression of neoplastic disease. Coughing and progression of neoplastic disease have been reported in cats.[27] Restenting in cases where collapse has occurred in an unstented region is not generally recommended.

REFERENCES

1. Hardie EM, Spodnick GJ, Gilson SD, et al. Tracheal rupture in cats: 16 cases (1983–1998). J Am Vet Med Assoc 1999;214:508–12.

2. Light GS. Respiratory System. In: Hudson LC, Hamilton WP, editors. Atlas of feline anatomy for veterinarians. Philadelphia: W.B. Saunders; 1993.

3. Nickel R, Schummer A, Seiferle A, et al. The Viscera of the Domestic Mammals. 1st English Edition ed. New York: Verlag Paul Parey-Springer-Velag; 1973.

4. Roach W, Krahwinkel D. Obstructive lesions and traumatic injuries of the canine and feline tracheas. Compend Contin Educ Vet 2009;31:86–93.

5. Samii VF, Biller DS, Koblik PD. Normal cross-sectional anatomy of the feline thorax and abdomen: comparison of computed tomography and cadaver anatomy. Vet Radiol Ultrasound 1998;39:504–11.

6. Hammond G, Geary M, Coleman E, Gunn-Moore D. Radiographic measurements of the trachea in domestic shorthair and Persian cats. J Feline Med Surg. 2011;13:881–4.

7. Tivers MS, Moore AH. Tracheal foreign bodies in the cat and the use of fluoroscopy for removal: 12 cases. J Small Anim Pract 2006;47:155–9.

8. Dimski DS. Tracheal obstruction caused by tree needles in a cat. J Am Vet Assoc 1991;199:477–8.

9. Jones BD, Roudebush P. The use of fiberoptic endoscopy in the diagnosis and treatment of tracheobronchial foreign bodies. J Am Anim Hosp Assoc 1984;20: 497–504.

10. Eyster GE, Evans AT, O'Handley P, Steffes J. Surgical removal of a foreign body from the tracheal bifurcation of a cat. J Am Anim Hosp Assoc 1976;12:481–3.

11. Pratschke KM, Hughes JM, Guerin SR, Bellenger CR. Foley catheter technique for removal of a tracheal foreign body in a cat. Vet Rec 1999;144:181–2.

12. Goodnight ME, Scansen BA, Kidder AC, et al. Use of a unique method for removal of a foreign body from the trachea of a cat. J Am Vet Med Assoc 2010;237: 689–94.

13. Beaumont PR. Intratracheal neoplasia in two cats. J Small Anim Pract 1982;23: 29–35.

14. Brown MR, Rogers KS. Primary tracheal tumors in dogs and cats. Compendium on Continuing Education for the Practicing Veterinarian 2003;25: 854–9.

15. Brown MR, Rogers KS, Mansell KJ, Barton C. Primary intratracheal lymphosarcoma in four cats. J Am Anim Hosp Assoc 2003;39:468–72.

16. Cain GR, Manley P. Tracheal adenocarcinoma in a cat. J Am Vet Med Assoc 1983;182:614–16.

17. Carlisle CH, Biery DN, Thrall DE. Tracheal and laryngeal tumors in the dog and cat: literature review and 13 additional patients. Vet Radiol 1991;32:229–35.

18. Evers P, Sukhiani HR, Sumner-Smith G, Binnington A. Tracheal adenocarcinoma in two domestic shorthaired cats. J Small Anim Pract 1994;35:217–20.

19. Jakubiak MJ, Siedlecki CT, Zenger E, et al. Laryngeal, laryngotracheal, and tracheal masses in cats: 27 cases (1998–2003). J Am Anim Hosp Assoc 2005;41: 310–16.

20. Kim DY, Kim JR, Taylor HW, Lee YS. Primary extranodal lymphosarcoma of the trachea in a cat. J Vet Med Sci 1996;58:703–6.

21. Lobetti RG, Williams MC. Anaplastic tracheal squamous cell carcinoma in a cat. J S Afr Vet Assoc 1992;63:132–3.

22. Neer TM, Zeman D. Tracheal adenocarcinoma in a cat and review of the literature. J Am Anim Hosp Assoc 1987;23:377–80.

23. Rossi G, Magi GE, Tarantino C, et al. Tracheobronchial neuroendocrine carcinoma in a cat. J Comp Pathol 2007;137:165–8.

24. Schneider PR, Smith CW, Feller DL. Histiocytic lymphosarcoma of the trachea in a cat. J Am Anim Hosp Assoc 1979;14:485–7.

25. Zimmermann U, Muller F, Pfleghaar S. Tracheal neoplasms of differing origin in two cats. / Zwei Fälle von histogenetisch unterschiedlichen Trachealtumoren bei Katzen. Kleintierpraxis 1992;37:409–12.

26. Glock R. Primary pulmonary adenomas of the feline. Iowa State University Veterinarian 1961;23:155–6.

27. Culp WT, Weisse C, Cole SG, Solomon JA. Intraluminal tracheal stenting for treatment of tracheal narrowing in three cats. Vet Surg 2007;36: 107–13.

28. Bell R, Philbey AW, Martineau H, et al. Dynamic tracheal collapse associated with disseminated histiocytic sarcoma in a cat. J Small Anim Pract 2006;47:461–4.

29. Veith LA. Squamous cell carcinoma of the trachea in a cat. Feline Pract 1974;4: 30–2.

30. Bordelon JT, Newcomb BT, Rochat MC. Surgical removal of a Cuterebra larva from the cervical trachea of a cat. J Am Anim Hosp Assoc 2009;45:52–4.

31. Dvorak LD, Bay JD, Crouch DT, Corwin RM. Successful treatment of intratracheal cuterebrosis in two cats. J Am Anim Hosp Assoc 2000;36:304–8.

32. Sheaffer KA, Dillon AR. Obstructive tracheal mass due to an inflammatory polyp in a cat. J Am Anim Hosp Assoc 1996;32:431–4.

33. De Lorenzi D, Solano-Gallego L. Tracheal granuloma because of infection with a novel mycobacterial species in an old FIV-positive cat. J Small Anim Pract 2009;50:143–6.

34. Snyder KD, Spaulding K, Edwards J. Imaging diagnosis – tracheobronchial zygomycosis in a cat. Vet Radiol Ultrasound 2010;51:617–20.

35. Burton C. Surgical diseases of the trachea in the dog and cat. In Pract 2003;25:514–27.

36. White RN, Oakley MR. Left principal bronchus rupture in a cat. J Small Anim Pract 2001;42:495–8.

37. White RN, Burton CA. Surgical management of intrathoracic tracheal avulsion in cats: long-term results in 9 consecutive cases. Vet Surg 2000;29: 430–1.

38. Griffiths LG, Sullivan M, Lerche P. Intrathoracic tracheal avulsion and pseudodiverticulum following pneumomediastinum in a cat. Vet Rec 1998;142:693–6.

39. White RN, Milner HR. Intrathoracic tracheal avulsion in three cats. J Small Anim Pract 1995;36:343–7.

40. Lawrence DT, Lang J, Culvenor J, et al. Intrathoracic tracheal rupture. J Feline Med Surg 1999;1:43–51.

41. Bhandal J, Kuzma A. Tracheal rupture in a cat: diagnosis by computed tomography. Can Vet J 2008;49:595–7.

42. Mitchell SL, McCarthy R, Rudloff E, Pernell RT. Tracheal rupture associated with intubation in cats: 20 cases (1996–1998). J Am Vet Med Assoc 2000;216:1592–5.

43. McMillan FD. Iatrogenic tracheal stenosis in a cat. J Am Anim Hosp Assoc 1985;21:747–50.

44. Kästner SB, Grundmann S, Bettschart-Wolfensberger R. Unstable endobronchial intubation in a cat undergoing tracheal laceration repair. Vet Anaesth Analg 2004;31:227–30.

45. Fujita M, Miura H, Yasuda D, et al. Tracheal narrowing secondary to airway obstruction in two cats. J Small Anim Pract 2004;45:29–31.

46. Hendricks JC, O'Brien JA. Tracheal collapse in two cats. J Am Vet Med Assoc 1985;187:418–19.

47. Mims HL, Hancock RB, Leib MS, Waldron DR. Primary tracheal collapse in a cat. J Am Anim Hosp Assoc 2008;44:149–53.

48. Foley RH, Krarup A. Prosthetic repair of tracheal collapse in a dyspneic cat. Feline Pract 1991;19:16–21.

49. Muir P, Bjorling DE. Successful surgical treatment of a broncho-oesophageal fistula in a cat. Vet Record 1994;134:475–6.

50. Zambelli AB. Pneumomediastinum, pneumothorax and pneumoretroperitoneum following endoscopic retrieval of a tracheal foreign body from a cat. J S Afr Vet Assoc 2006;77: 45–50.

51. Davis KM, Hardie EM, Lascelles BD, Hansen B. Feline fibrosarcoma: perioperative management. Compend Contin Educ Vet 2007;29:716–20, 722–729 passim.

52. Guenther-Yenke CL, Rozanski EA. Tracheostomy in cats: 23 cases (1998–2006). J Feline Med Surg 2007;9: 451–7.

53. Taylor SS, Harvey AM, Barr FJ, et al. Laryngeal disease in cats: a retrospective study of 35 cases. J Feline Med Surg 2009;11:954–62.

54. Stepnik MW, Mehl ML, Hardie EM, et al. Outcome of permanent tracheostomy for treatment of upper airway obstruction in cats: 21 cases (1990–2007). J Am Vet Med Assoc 2009;234:638–43.

Chapter 47

Lung

A.L. Moores

Diffuse lung disease in cats is rarely treated surgically. However, cats with certain discrete or lobular lung diseases may respond well to surgical management. Recent advances in diagnostic imaging have led to the improvement of diagnosis and localization of lung disease, and access to the thoracic cavity is easily achieved by intercostal thoracotomy for individual lung lobectomy or pneumonectomy where appropriate. Median sternotomy may be required for bilateral lung surgery or for exploratory thoracotomy, but it is more technically challenging than the intercostal approach. Thoracoscopy can also be used in cats to assess the lungs and obtain tissue samples for laboratory interpretation.

SURGICAL ANATOMY

The lungs expand to fill most of the thoracic cavity. The smaller left lung is divided into cranial and caudal lobes by interlobular fissures, with the left cranial lobe having a further partial division into cranial and caudal parts. The right lung is divided into cranial, middle, caudal, and accessory lobes (Fig. 47-1) and the hilus of the accessory lung lobe passes dorsal to the caudal vena cava to sit medial to the plica vena cava. Laterally the lungs are bordered by the thoracic wall and caudally by the diaphragm, separated by the pleura and the pleural space. Cranially the lungs are adjacent to the thymus when it is prominent in the younger cat.

Blood supply

The functional blood supply to the lungs for gas exchange is via the pulmonary arteries, which arise from the right ventricular outflow tract. The blood then returns to the left atrium via the pulmonary veins. The pulmonary arteries lie dorsal and lateral to the bronchi while the veins are ventral and medial. The terminal alveoli have a dense capillary bed to facilitate gas exchange. The nutritional blood supply to the lungs is provided by the bronchial vessels, which arise from the thoracic aorta.

Innervation

The innervation of the lungs is autonomic. Bronchiolar constriction occurs with parasympathetic stimulation of bronchiolar smooth muscle via the vagus nerves. There is also a parasympathetic supply to the bronchioles and alveoli. Sympathetic stimulation via the vagus and stellate cardiac nerves (the right and left pulmonary plexuses) leads to bronchiolar dilatation. The pulmonary plexuses also carry sensory fibers from the lung parenchyma and vasculature.

Regional lymph nodes

Lymphatic drainage from the lungs is to the left, right, and medial tracheobronchial lymph nodes lying to the left, right, and caudal to the tracheal bifurcation, respectively. Subsequent drainage is to the cranial mediastinal lymph nodes ventral or medial to the trachea at the level of the first two ribs.

GENERAL CONSIDERATIONS AND DIAGNOSTIC PROCEDURES

Clinical signs

Cats with pulmonary disease do not commonly present with obvious signs of respiratory distress unless the condition is at an advanced stage. Early clinical signs may be vague and non-specific and not pathognomonic for a particular disease. Clinical signs specifically relating to the respiratory tract include dyspnea, wheezing, tachypnea, coughing, epistaxis, and hemoptysis.

Diagnostic imaging

A full radiographic assessment of the lungs should ideally include left and right lateral projections. However, if the patient is unstable it is important that emergency procedures (e.g., thoracocentesis) are

© 2014 Elsevier Ltd
DOI: 10.1016/B978-0-7020-4336-9.00047-0

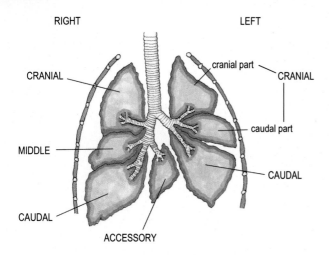

RIGHT   LEFT

CRANIAL

cranial part — CRANIAL

caudal part

MIDDLE

CAUDAL

CAUDAL

ACCESSORY

Figure 47-1 Schematic diagram illustrating the anatomy of the feline lung.

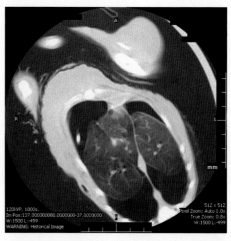

Figure 47-2 Conscious computed tomographic image (cat in dorsal recumbency) showing cortication of the lung lobes and thickening of the pleura. *(© Alison Moores.)*

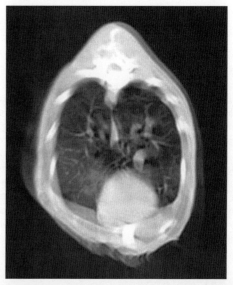

Figure 47-3 Transverse CT image of a conscious cat positioned in a custom-made Perspex box. Blurring of the images is caused by movement of the cat during the scanning procedure. *(© Alison Moores.)*

performed prior to radiography as the stress of handling and positioning for radiography could precipitate respiratory arrest. Inflated views taken under anesthesia are always preferable if possible as this provides additional information, such as a higher likelihood of identifying the presence of small primary or metastatic nodules. However, sedation and/or anesthesia are only advisable in patients who are clinically stable. If the patient is dyspneic a single dorsoventral radiograph may be the only possible view obtainable in the initial stages of assessment. However, it is always important to note that one limitation of radiography is that it is not always possible to correctly identify the anatomical location of disease or the primary disease focus (e.g., bronchial, interstitial, alveolar).[1]

Advanced imaging techniques such as ultrasound, computed tomography (CT), and scintigraphy may identify abnormalities not visible on radiography (e.g., lung metastases) and may also further facilitate surgical planning e.g., by identifying affected lung lobes to guide surgical approach.[2]

Some abnormalities may be seen with ultrasound, such as consolidation, atelectasis, and pulmonary masses.[2] However, the technical difficulties of ultrasound of the lungs caused by the inability of ultrasound waves to pass through air limit its usefulness to lesions located in an entire lung lobe or at the periphery of lung lobes adjacent to the thoracic wall.[3,4]

CT is the preferred imaging modality for pulmonary disease and the CT findings in normal cats and those with pleural, pulmonary, and mediastinal diseases have been well described (Box 47-1).[2,5,6] CT can be successfully performed without chemical restraint in cats by using a positioning device,[7] but it is more usual to perform CT under sedation or general anesthesia. There will inevitably be some movement blur during CT as there is for radiography and MRI, but this can be minimized by hyperventilation prior to scanning and then undertaking the scan during the expiratory pause (Figs 47-2 and 47-3).[6] Aspiration of any pleural fluid or air that may be present prior to CT will improve pulmonary parenchymal visualization by allowing increased lung inflation,[8] while the administration of intravenous contrast agents can also improve the detection of pulmonary lesions.[7,8] CT provided additional correct diagnoses in 28% of cats undergoing conscious CT compared to conscious radiography, as well as further additional information in 74% of cats. Overall, 40% of cats undergoing both techniques had a significant different disease or prognosis following CT imaging (Box 47-2).

Box 47-1 Advantages of computed tomography over thoracic radiography[2,5,7]

Not affected by pleural effusion

Eliminates superimposition of lung

Can differentiate pleural, pulmonary, mediastinal, and thoracic wall opacities

Can differentiate lung patterns, e.g., mass lesion, consolidation, bronchopneumonia, atelectasis

Can differentiate diseases, e.g., consolidation, lung lobe torsion, infarction, bronchiectasis

Samples can be obtained by aspiration or needle core biopsy under CT guidance

Allows more accurate surgical planning

Most accurate imaging technique for the recognition of lymph node and pulmonary metastatic disease

Can identify fluid within mass lesions, e.g., abscess, necrotic neoplasia

Box 47-2 **Differential diagnoses for common radiographic and computed tomographic patterns of lung disease**[2,9–15]

Solid radio-opaque pulmonary mass

Primary neoplasia

Metastatic neoplasia

Abscess/foreign body

Granuloma including fungal granuloma (e.g., aspergillosis)

Cyst

Infarction

Localized hemorrhage/hematoma

Localized pneumonia

Diaphragmatic hernia with incarceration of abdominal contents
e.g., liver

Ectopic hepatic parenchyma

Cavitary masses

Granuloma

Abscess/foreign body

Cavitary infarcts

Primary neoplasia

Metastatic neoplasia

Parasitic disease, e.g., *Paragonimus* spp.[a]

Multiple pulmonary masses

Primary pulmonary neoplasia

Primary neoplasia with pulmonary metastasis

Multiple different primary neoplasms

Metastatic neoplasia from a non-pulmonary location

Disseminated pulmonary patterns

Primary neoplasia

Metastatic neoplasia

Pneumonia

Hemorrhage

Edema

Granuloma

Fibrosis

Pulmonary consolidation

Pneumonia

Infarction

Contusion

Primary neoplasia

Lung lobe torsion

[a]Note: infection is rare outside endemic areas in Asia and Africa.

Biopsy and laboratory analysis

Fluid obtained by bronchoalveolar lavage (BAL) should always be examined cytologically for evidence of neoplastic or inflammatory cells and for evidence of active infection but samples are more likely to be diagnostic for neoplastic disease when there are large lesions involving central rather than peripheral lung.[16] The limitations of BAL include failure to sample a representative area of disease, low cellularity, the difficulty sometimes encountered differentiating neoplasia from epithelial hyperplasia, the presence of marked inflammation

obscuring and hindering identification of other cells, and the inability to analyze cells in relation to airway architecture.[1] In addition, many different underlying diseases, including neoplasia and septic or nonseptic inflammation can all lead to neutrophilic inflammation being present, thereby sometimes making it difficult to make a definitive diagnosis by cytology alone.[1] Hemosiderosis on tracheal wash samples is common but a non-specific finding.[17] Any fluid obtained by either BAL or tracheal wash techniques should always be submitted for culture, although there may not be a correlation between culture results from BAL and lung tissue obtained by biopsy if aspiration of oral and pharyngeal bacteria into the lower airways has occurred during the sampling procedure, so every care should be taken to avoid this if possible.[1]

Where radiography and cytology from BAL fail to establish a diagnosis, obtaining a biopsy for histologic analysis may be useful. Transthoracic fine needle aspiration can be performed blindly after a lesion has been identified on diagnostic imaging or, more preferably, using ultrasound, fluoroscopic or CT guidance.[4,18,19] Ultrasound-guided aspiration can either be performed conscious or with sedation,[4] but undertaking a biopsy procedure necessitates deep sedation or anesthesia. Aspirates can certainly help differentiate neoplastic from nonneoplastic disease and therefore guide clinical decision making, but biopsy is often required to determine exact tumor types.[4] A solid tissue sample is also more likely to be diagnostic for diseases affecting pulmonary architecture, e.g., fibrosis, emphysema, bronchiectasis.[20] Contraindications for obtaining biopsies include coagulopathies, pulmonary bullae, severely compromised pulmonary function, and pulmonary hypertension.[4] Potential complications encountered after a biopsy procedure include pneumothorax or pulmonary hemorrhage,[4,19] and it is important to counsel owners in this regard before such a procedure is performed.

In most instances, obtaining a tissue sample for histology requires open thoracotomy (see Chapter 41), but where available, thoracoscopy in the cat is considered a less invasive technique than thoracotomy for examining the thoracic cavity and obtaining tissue for histologic evaluation[21] and should always be considered (see Chapter 42).

SURGICAL DISEASES

Primary pulmonary neoplasia

Primary pulmonary neoplasia is rare in cats, with a reported annual incidence in one study of 2.2 per 100 000 cats,[22] while a further study reported an incidence of pulmonary neoplasia of 0.38% of cats examined at necropsy.[23] Affected cats are generally middle to old-aged and tumor development is independent of feline immunodeficiency virus or feline leukemia virus infection.[24] No predisposing causes of feline pulmonary neoplasia have been identified.[24] Most tumors encountered are malignant and of epithelial origin (98–100%), of which adenocarcinomas are the most common (85–100%).[10,12,25] Adenocarcinomas are not easily differentiated by topographic nomenclature (bronchial versus bronchiolar versus bronchioloalveolar) due to the extent of disease at diagnosis, and some are classified as adenosquamous carcinomas if there is significant squamous differentiation.[26] It is therefore more common to describe them as differentiated or undifferentiated, which is more useful clinically as it relates to prognosis.[10] Undifferentiated adenocarcinomas appear to occur most commonly (43–69%) and are more invasive and metastatic than the less frequently reported differentiated adenocarcinomas.[10,25,26] Other epithelial malignancies such as anaplastic carcinoma and squamous cell carcinoma appear to be less common, while sarcomas and benign

Box 47-3 **Pulmonary tumors reported in the cat**[13,25–27,30–36,38,75]

Malignant

Epithelial

Adenocarcinoma[a], comprising:

  Differentiated adenocarcinomas: bronchogenic, bronchial, and bronchial gland adenocarcinoma; bronchioalveolar carcinoma; squamous/adenosquamous carcinoma
  Undifferentiated adenocarcinoma[b]

Alveolar-cell carcinoma (anaplastic small-cell and large-cell types, and adenomatosis type)

Squamous cell carcinoma

Anaplastic carcinoma

Carcinosarcoma

Non-epithelial

Sarcoma, e.g., pulmonary intravascular hemangiosarcoma, fibrosarcoma; spindle cell sarcoma with elements of cartilage and bone

Lymphomatoid granulomatosis

Malignant fibrous histiocytoma

Benign

Adenoma

Chondromatous hamartoma

---

[a]Most common. Due to advanced disease at the time of diagnosis, adenocarcinomas are not easily differentiated by topographical nomenclature.

[b]Higher incidence than in dogs.

Table 47-1 Reported clinical signs of 86 cats with pulmonary neoplasia[25,28]

Related to the respiratory tract	
Dyspnea	40%
Wheezing	40%
Tachypnea	30%
Coughing	27%
Hemoptysis	1%
Non-specific clinical signs	
Weight loss	47%
Lethargy	40%
Decreased appetite	30%
Ataxia	21%
Vomiting, regurgitation	19%
Lameness	12–25%
Diarrhea	9%
Polyuria/polydipsia	3%

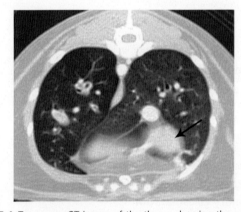

Figure 47-4 Transverse CT image of the thorax showing the presence of a mass in the accessory lung lobe just ventral to the caudal vena cava (arrow). Differential diagnoses include primary neoplasm and abscess. (© Alison Moores.)

tumors are rarely reported.[10,27,28] Other reported pulmonary tumors in cats are listed in Box 47-3. Additionally, there has been a report of a mediastinal mass in a cat, which was consistent with bronchogenic adenocarcinoma. The author suggested that it originated from an accessory embryonic lung.[29]

The reported clinical signs of cats with pulmonary neoplasia are summarized in Table 47-1. Interestingly, respiratory signs are reported to only occur in 33–62% of cats,[10,12,25,27,28] and in some cats lameness was the only presenting complaint. Lameness may occur from metastatic spread to the digits, appendicular bones or skeletal muscles or, more rarely, hypertrophic osteopathy.[34,39,47] Invasion of the esophagus may cause gastrointestinal signs such as vomiting or regurgitation.[24,27]

Significant changes on serum biochemistry and hematology are unusual.[25] Paraneoplastic conditions are occasionally recognized, including hypercalcemia, thrombocytopenia and leukocytosis, and are most likely due to humoral factors produced by the tumor.[41–43] Such paraneoplastic syndromes may resolve after tumor excision,[41] but specific further medical management is still required in some cases.

Imaging

When diagnosing pulmonary neoplasia via radiography, a variety and sometimes a combination of patterns may be present including a solid circumscribed mass, lobar consolidation, a nodular interstitial pattern, or a diffuse alveolar/reticulonodular pattern (Figs 47-4 and 47-5).[12] Solitary masses tend to be well circumscribed whereas multiple masses are usually more poorly circumscribed.[12] Mass lesions may also be

cavitated (0–22%) or calcified (6–12%) (Fig. 47-6).[12,27] When comparing three large studies of feline primary pulmonary tumors, the radiographic presentations are found to vary (Table 47-2)[12,25,27] with no recognized association between the radiographic findings and the tumor type.[12,25] In a further study in which 79 of 86 cats with pulmonary neoplasia had radiographs taken, 53 cats had single or multiple masses and the remaining cats had a pleural effusion. The 86 cats subsequently had a postmortem or surgery and 40 cats were found to have a single well-circumscribed mass, 37 had lobar consolidation (Fig. 47-7), and nine had multiple masses.[25] Further postmortem studies have shown that multiple lung lobes are often affected in cats with a diffuse radiographic pattern and radiography may fail to identify single or multiple masses subsequently found on direct visualization of the lungs.[12,27]

When evaluating the most common location for primary pulmonary neoplasia, one study showed an approximately even distribution

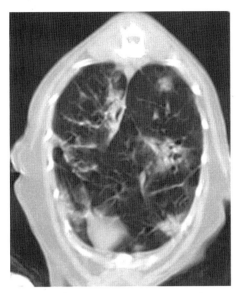

Figure 47-5 Transverse CT image showing a mixed infiltrate. (© Alison Moores.)

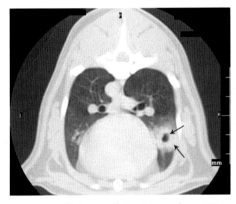

Figure 47-6 Transverse CT image of the thorax of a cat. Rounded area of dense alveolar infiltration with centrally located gas-filled cavity. Differential diagnoses include primary neoplasm with cavitation and abscess. (© Alison Moores.)

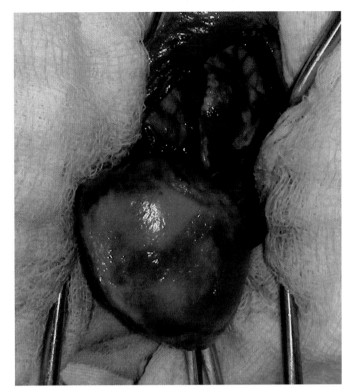

Figure 47-7 A consolidated lung lobe seen via an intercostal thoracotomy. Histopathology of the lobe demonstrated a moderately differentiated adenocarcinoma. (© Alison Moores.)

Table 47-2 Radiographic presentation of cats with primary pulmonary neoplasia[12,27,28]

Radiographic description	Incidence
Solid, circumscribed mass	39%
Lobar consolidation	23%
Diffuse alveolar or reticulo-nodular pattern	33%
Multiple diffuse nodules/nodular interstitial pattern[a]	45%
Multiple small circumscribed nodules	15%
Normal	8%
Pleural effusion	49%

[a]± solitary mass – 44.
Multiple radiographic findings were present in some cats.[28]

of pulmonary tumors between left unilateral, right unilateral and bilateral disease, but another study reported a low incidence of bilateral disease.[12,27] However, it does appear that the caudal lung lobes are more commonly affected than the cranial lobes.[10,12,27] Squamous cell carcinomas and bronchioloalveolar carcinomas are reported to primarily affect the middle and peripheral parts of the lungs whereas focal adenocarcinomas may occur throughout any region of the lung lobe.[12] Reported incidences of pleural effusion and lymphadenomegaly also vary, with 9–65% cats reported as having a concurrent pleural effusion.[10,12,25,27] Rarely, non-neoplastic disease such as ectopic hepatic parenchyma mimics lung neoplasia on radiography.[9] Further complication can arise from the fact that pulmonary neoplasia may look similar radiographically and histopathologically to fibrotic interstitial lung disease and both diseases may exist concurrently.[44] Radiography may fail to detect neoplasia, either because it is not recognized or the radiographic changes are misinterpreted, and therefore it is not possible to ascertain estimates for false positive or false negative diagnoses based on radiographic studies alone.[12]

Ultrasonography can detect pulmonary masses that contact the thoracic wall, but the interposition of air in normal lung tissue will preclude visualization of many mass lesions. Ultrasonography can be useful for assessing regional lymph nodes but CT allows more accurate localization of masses and detection of smaller macroscopic disease than radiography.[2]

Cytology

Cytology is a useful diagnostic tool for pulmonary neoplasia[10,25] and samples can be obtained by transthoracic or transbronchial aspiration or by bronchial brushing. A correct diagnosis was obtained in 80–86% of the cats in which samples were obtained by blind or guided fine needle aspiration through the thoracic wall and assessed cytologically.[10,25] However, as needle tract implantation of neoplastic cells on the thoracic wall after ultrasound-guided fine needle aspiration of a pulmonary adenocarcinoma has been reported,[45] care should be taken to consider this possibility whenever fine needle aspirates are planned.

Cytology can also be useful in the assessment of pleural fluid or BAL fluid for malignant cells, but as their presence is variable the absence of neoplastic cells does not rule out disease.[1,25,27] Furthermore, as sarcomas do not typically exfoliate well, the diagnostic value of pleural fluid or a BAL for sarcomas may be less than that for carcinomas.[1] False positive diagnosis of neoplasia on BAL cytology has been reported only rarely in cats with inflammatory disease, but care should always be taken with interpretation in the presence of marked inflammation.[1] Immunohistochemistry of biopsy samples can be used to characterize the cell of origin.[1,24] Inflammation and hemosiderosis is common in BAL samples from cats with confirmed or suspected pulmonary neoplasia (100 and 79%, respectively).[17]

Aerobic and anaerobic bacterial culture and fungal culture should always be performed to rule out pulmonary abscess as a differential diagnosis or to recognize concurrent infection associated with a neoplasm.[17,46]

Metastasis

Metastases are found in up to 76% of cats with primary pulmonary neoplasia at the time of diagnosis.[10,12,25] Tumors will most commonly metastasize to other pulmonary tissue and the regional lymph nodes; hilar lymphadenopathy has been reported to be seen radiographically in 5–29% cats at the time of diagnosis of pulmonary neoplasia.[10,12,25,27] However, metastatic lesions may not be detected on thoracic radiography,[24,27] and furthermore it is important to note that lymphadenomegaly is not always due to metastatic disease even if a primary tumor is identified.[10] In a study of 86 cats, metastatic lesions were identified in 76% of the patients, with metastasis to the bronchial lymph nodes occuring in 45% of the cats, to the pleural cavity in 30%, and to extrathoracic sites in 16%.[25] However, as described previously, the accuracy of radiography for the diagnosis of pleural metastasis and lymph node involvement in one study was 70% and 62%, respectively,[12] and CT is generally considered to be more sensitive than radiography for detecting pulmonary metastatic disease.[2]

Digital bone, muscle, and skin are reported sites of metastasis for bronchogenic adenocarcinomas and these metastatic lesions account for nearly 90% of all feline digital carcinomas.[24,40] In one study describing digital metastasis, the cats presented with lameness rather than with clinical evidence of respiratory disease. A third of the cats had multiple digital involvement either on the same or multiple feet, with 75% affecting the weight bearing digits.[40] Unlike humans, metastatic carcinomas in cats can cross phalangeal joints.[24,40] However, although rare, lameness can sometimes be due to hypertrophic osteopathy secondary to pulmonary neoplasia and, in such cases, the lameness and radiographic changes identified within the bone may resolve with excision of the primary mass.[34]

Tumor embolization of the brachial and femoral arteries, resulting in lameness or ischemic neuromyopathy, has been described.[47,48] There are also occasional reports of tumor metastasis to the posterior segment of the eye, often in conjunction with digital metastases, with histopathology suggesting angioinvasive properties of the tumor.[29,49] Posterior segment analysis should therefore be an important part of the physical examination. Numerous other sites of metastasis of pulmonary neoplasia have been reported including intrathoracic structures (diaphragm, parietal pleura, mediastinum, heart, and esophagus), abdominal organs (liver, spleen, kidney, intestines, bladder, pancreas, adrenal gland), the brain, and salivary glands.[9,10,12,27,28,39,40,42,49,50]

Treatment options

The majority of cats presented with pulmonary neoplasia (75%) had inoperable disease due to extensive primary disease or metastatic spread.[28] In a retrospective study of 86 cats with primary pulmonary neoplasia, two died and 63 (76%) were euthanized shortly after initial examination.[25] However, a single pulmonary neoplasm in the absence of metastatic disease can be treated by lung lobectomy, usually via an intercostal thoracotomy (Fig. 47-7). It is important to note that if adhesions are present then removal of multiple lobes may be necessary to ensure a compartmental resection is achieved. The median survival time in a series of 21 cats with pulmonary carcinomas, mostly with a single solitary lesion, was 115 days, with death or euthanasia related to metastatic disease.[10] Cats with moderately differentiated tumors had an increased probability of survival compared with those with poorly differentiated tumors (median 698 vs 75 days, respectively), whereas clinical findings and the specific tumor histologic type did not influence survival.[10,25] Although not examined statistically, cats without tracheobronchial lymphadenomegaly appeared to have a longer survival time than those without lymph node enlargement (median 412 vs 73 days).[10] The prognosis for cats with more diffuse lesions or lung consolidation is not known but in one study half of the cats examined at necropsy showed local invasion of parietal pleura, mediastinum, esophagus, pericardium, and the diaphragm.[27] Adhesions to local structures, including the thoracic vertebral bodies, diaphragm, and other lung lobes may also occur[43,51] and this possibility must always be considered when planning the surgical resection of a mass.

Cats with metastatic digital carcinoma, all treated by digit amputation, had a median survival time from presentation of only 67 days, even though some tumors were histopathologically well differentiated. Although histopathologic analysis of the resected digits is a method for obtaining a diagnosis for the pulmonary tumor, surgery is unlikely to be curative and so may not be indicated.[40] The short survival and absence of respiratory clinical signs suggest that thoracotomy will not improve survival.[40]

It has been suggested that adjunctive chemotherapy is required to reduce local recurrence and metastasis of pulmonary neoplasia,[52] but no effective protocols have been established[53] and there are currently only limited reports of its success, i.e., one cat with adenocarcinoma treated by pneumonectomy and mitoxantrone survived for 34 months.[54] In a study of 18 feline pulmonary carcinomas and adenosquamous carcinomas evaluated immunohistochemically, all tumors expressed one or more proteins associated with multidrug resistance to chemotherapy agents, including doxorubicin, vincristine, and cisplatin, which may result in a poor response to treatment.[52] COX-2 inhibitors are also unlikely to be beneficial due to the absence of COX-2 expression seen in eight pulmonary adenocarcinomas assessed by immunohistochemistry.[55] Radiation therapy is not an option as normal lung tissue would undergo significant pathology from radiation exposure.[56]

Pulmonary metastatic neoplasia

The lungs are the most common site for metastatic disease.[16] It is also important to recognize the fact that metastatic disease may sometimes represent the first evidence of primary neoplastic disease.[16] The typical radiographic or CT findings of pulmonary metastatic disease in cats have been well reported. A study of 25 cats showed most had interstitial nodules (eight well defined, ten ill defined); seven cats had diffuse pulmonary patterns, of which some had concurrent alveolar consolidation, ill-defined interstitial nodules, and/or pleural effusion (Figs 47-8 to 47-11).[57] Diffuse or ill-defined disease is more common than well-circumscribed nodules, especially for metastatic mammary

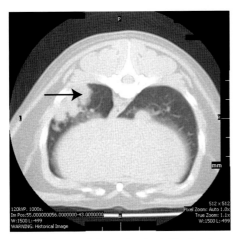

Figure 47-8 Rounded area of dense alveolar infiltration (arrow). Changes may be consistent with primary or secondary neoplasia as well as inflammatory disease. *(© Alison Moores.)*

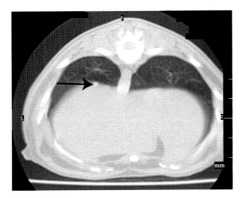

Figure 47-9 Metastatic nodule (arrow) in the left caudal lung lobe shown on a transverse CT image. Partial volume artifact is causing partial superimpositioning of the diaphragm and this nodule. *(© Alison Moores.)*

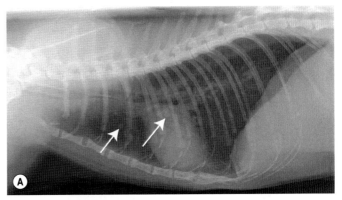

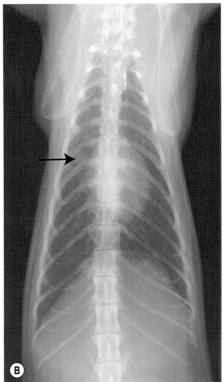

Figure 47-10 Left lateral **(A)** and dorsoventral **(B)** radiographs showing multiple well defined soft tissue nodules (arrows) throughout the lung parenchyma. These changes are consistent with metastatic disease. *(© Alison Moores.)*

neoplasia and other tumors of epithelial origin, probably due to metastasis via the lymphatic system.[57] Most pulmonary lesions (92%) are generalized[57] but metastatic nodules tend to be in the middle or peripheral portions of lung and typically consist of several large masses and a number of smaller masses, which are generally smaller and well circumscribed compared with primary masses.[13] Cavitation is rarely described, which is in contrast to that described in primary neoplasms.[13]

Primary and metastatic mass lesions are not reliably visualized radiographically until they are 0.6–1 cm in diameter, when they represent advanced disease.[16] It has been suggested that lesions of 0.3–0.5 cm are the absolute lower limit for radiographic identification[58] because it can be difficult to differentiate metastatic disease from other pulmonary diseases resulting in a similar radiographic pattern (e.g., pneumonia, hemorrhage, or edema).[57] Unrelated neoplastic or non-neoplastic pulmonary masses may occur in animals with concurrent neoplastic disease at another location,[59] underlining the fact that pulmonary masses may not necessarily represent metastatic disease. Therefore, in order to ensure an accurate diagnosis is always reached, consideration should be given to undertaking ultrasound-guided fine needle aspiration of consolidated areas of lung or nodular lesions.[57] If cytology proves to be inadequate, it may in some circumstances be appropriate to undertake thoracoscopy or

thoracotomy to allow biopsy samples to be collected. Metastatectomy may be appropriate for single or small pulmonary metastatic masses secondary to primary tumors with a low metastatic rate, slow progression of disease, and long median survival, but such cases need to be assessed and staged carefully.

Lung lobe torsion

Lung lobe torsion is rare in cats but when it occurs, as is the case in dogs, the right cranial and right middle lobes are reported to be the most commonly affected lobes.[60-62] Torsion can occur spontaneously,[60,63] but most reported cases have an underlying respiratory disease identified or suggested, e.g., feline asthma,[64] or it may be associated with pleural effusion, including chylothorax. The torsion is considered to be the primary disease if the effusion resolves after lung

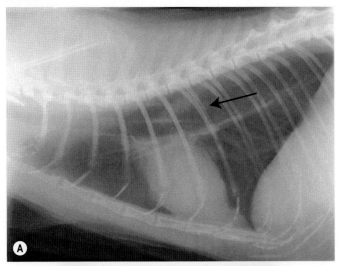

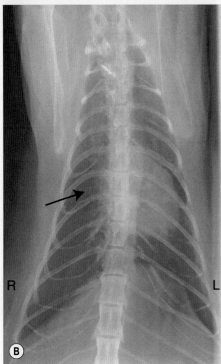

Figure 47-11 (A) Lateral and **(B)** dorsoventral radiographs of the thorax showing a nodule of soft tissue opacity (arrows) in the seventh right intercostal space, just lateral to the cardiac silhouette (dorsoventral view) and between the carina and the aorta (lateral view). (© *Alison Moores.*)

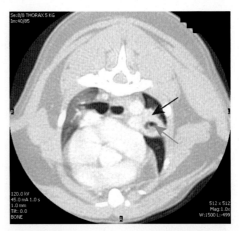

Figure 47-12 Transverse CT image of the thorax of a cat. Rounded area of dense alveolar infiltration (red arrow) with centrally located gas-filled cavity (orange arrow) represented a lung abscess. (© *Alison Moores.*)

lobectomy, whereas it is considered a sequela if the identified effusion does not resolve. Both scenarios have been reported in cats.[61,65]

The clinical signs of lobar torsion include respiratory difficulty, lethargy and epistaxis.[60] Diagnostic techniques useful in such cases include radiography, ultrasonography, CT, and bronchoscopy[8,60,62,63] and it is recommended that a combination of these is used when the diagnosis is difficult to make, especially on radiography. Typical radiographic findings include pleural effusion, dorsal displacement of the trachea, twisting of the carina, an inability to visualize the affected bronchus, increased lung lobe opacity, and a vesicular lung pattern (gas bubbles).[60] A recent report describes the diagnosis by virtual bronchoscopy using CT.[8] Treatment is lung lobectomy via an

intercostal thoracotomy and it is important to note that the lung should be removed without derotating it to limit release of inflammatory mediators into the systemic circulation.[61] Although there are only a few case reports in the literature, the prognosis is considered to be good, assuming there is no underlying effusion.

Pulmonary embolism

Pulmonary thromboembolism is a medical condition, but it may occur as a complication in cats with surgical disease. Fat embolization of the lung can occur as a rare complication of orthopedic surgery and may be fatal.[66]

Pulmonary thromboembolism is the term applied when there is obstruction to flow within the pulmonary vasculature by a thrombus or embolus. Possible underlying causes include cardiac disease and neoplasia.[67] Thrombi typically form in the right side of the heart or systemic veins and may occur in conjunction with systemic arterial thromboembolism.[67] Affected cats often have marked respiratory distress, that is non-responsive to oxygen and progresses to respiratory failure.[68] The radiographic changes described in these cases include pulmonary vessel abnormalities, peripheral lung lucency, atelectesis, and pleural effusion.[67] CT has been described to identify the thrombus and characterize blood flow.[69] However the condition is diagnosed, the prognosis is poor with reported fatality rates of 72–100%.[67]

Pulmonary abscesses, granulomas and foreign bodies

Pulmonary abscesses are uncommon in cats but potential underlying causes include trauma, foreign material, neoplasia, parasitic infection, infective emboli, or pneumonitis.[8,70,71] Abscesses secondary to foreign body (grass awn) inhalation most frequently affect the right and left caudal and accessory lung lobes (Figs 47-12 and 74-13).[71] Primary abscesses without a causal foreign body are typically treated by lung lobectomy, as left untreated they may rupture leading to pyothorax.

Although a rare condition, many cats affected by pulmonary aspergillosis have concurrent viral, endoparasitic, or endocrine diseases, which may make them susceptible to infection.[11] Clinical signs include lethargy, depression, and gastrointestinal signs but pleural effusions are an uncommon finding.[11] Due to the poor response rates most cases of pulmonary aspergillosis are diagnosed on postmortem

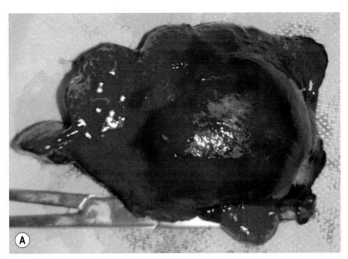

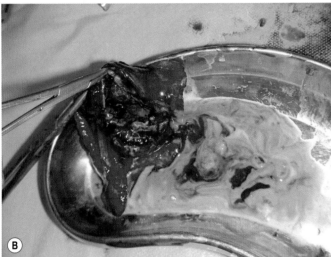

Figure 47-13 Lung lobe of a cat. **(A)** A large swelling contained **(B)** purulent material and a grass awn. *(© Alison Moores.)*

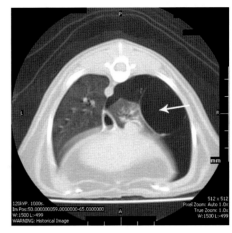

Figure 47-14 Transverse CT image of the thorax showing lobar emphysema of the right caudal lung lobe (arrow). *(© Alison Moores.)*

examination, but in one case report an extensive pulmonary abscess caused by *Aspergillus fumigatus* was successfully treated by left-sided pneumonectomy and itraconazole; however, there was no evidence of disseminated disease.[11] Other reported fungal granulomas in cat lungs include *Paecilomyces lilacinus* and *Cladophialophora bantiana*, which were successfully treated by lung lobectomy and adjuvant itraconazole.[72,73]

Pneumonia

Lung lobectomy is rarely necessary for the treatment of pneumonia in cats as most respond to medical therapy.[74] However, surgery may be necessary to remove a nidus of infection in focal pneumonia or to allow collection of lung tissue for culture and histopathology to aid in choosing appropriate therapy for diffuse pneumonia.[74]

Lung laceration

Lung laceration can occur as a complication of needle thoracocentesis or thoracostomy tube placement. It can be minimized by using small-bore wire-guided chest drains rather than trocar style drains.[37] Laceration may also be caused by trauma, e.g., blunt thoracic trauma, penetrating thoracic injury, bite wounds, or rib fractures with medial

displacement of fracture ends. It may result in pneumothorax and hemorrhage. Mild cases can be managed with intermittent thoracocentesis and supportive treatment, such as fluid therapy and oxygen supplementation. Surgery is indicated if the pneumothorax does not resolve or if there is extensive hemorrhage. Severe cases may lead to tension pneumothorax and in such cases rapid surgical intervention, often with lung lobectomy, may be necessary.

Pulmonary bulla and pneumothorax of pulmonary origin

Based on information in dogs with primary spontaneous pneumothorax, it was thought that medical treatment of this condition would be associated with a high rate of recurrence. A recent study reports that cats who present with spontaneous pneumothorax typically had inflammatory airway disease, neoplasia, heartworm infection, pulmonary abscess, or lungworm infection.[76] It was shown that cats could be treated successfully with non-surgical therapies and appeared to have a better prognosis than previously extrapolated from canine studies.[76] Pulmonary bullae formation is rare in cats. It has been described in conjunction with bronchopulmonary dysplasia, which may represent the underlying cause.[77] Persistent pneumothorax in cats with pulmonary bullae unresponsive to medical therapy could be treated by lobectomy of affected lobe(s), usually via a median sternotomy unless there is a specific indication for intercostal thoracotomy (Fig. 47-14). Areas of emphysema can be removed by partial lung lobectomy but as there is no evidence that emphysematous lesions will cause recurrence of pneumothorax the author would leave extensive lesions in situ if surgical resection is not feasible.

PREOPERATIVE CONSIDERATIONS

Cats with lung disease should be carefully assessed prior to anesthesia. Thoracocentesis should be performed prior to sedation or anesthesia in all cats with known or presumed pleural space disease to remove any pleural effusion or air that may compromise respiration while under anesthesia. A period of oxygenation in a calm environment prior to induction is beneficial and recommended (Fig. 47-15). Selection of an appropriate pre-anesthetic medication and induction agent will depend on the ANA score of the cat and the underlying disease,[78]

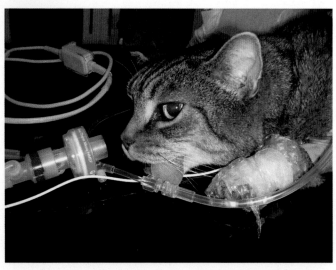

Figure 47-15 Oxygen is provided both prior to and on recovery from anesthesia. *(© Alison Moores.)*

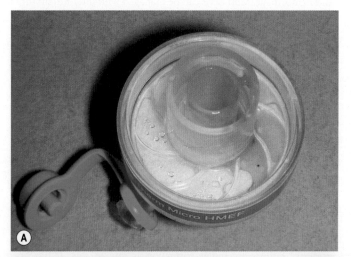

(A)

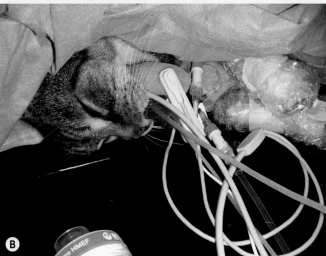

(B)

Figure 47-16 (A) A Thermovent filled with purulent material that had also caused partial obstruction of the endotracheal tube causing hypoxemia. **(B)** The airway is suctioned. *(© Alison Moores.)*

but mask induction is generally not recommended for cats with respiratory disease. Multimodal analgesia is preferred and for thoracotomy would typically include the use of systemic opiates and regional local anesthetic techniques. Intermittent positive pressure ventilation (IPPV), either via a mechanical ventilator or manually via the anesthetic breathing bag, is required whenever the thoracic cavity is opened. IPPV may also be beneficial before surgery in cats with pleural disease. Positive end-expiratory pressure ventilation may improve oxygenation in cats with hypoxemia due to poor ventilation. Obstruction of the endotracheal tube leading to hypoxemia can occur with secretions from the respiratory tract, such as pus from a pulmonary abscess. If such obstruction occurs, the endotracheal tube should be replaced and the airway suctioned (Fig. 47-16).[71] For further information on anesthesia of cats undergoing thoracic surgery see Chapter 2 and Chapter 4.

SURGICAL MANAGEMENT AND TECHNIQUES

A cat with lung disease may benefit from biopsy of the affected lung tissue to assist in obtaining a definitive diagnosis. However, biopsy is not always necessary and, where possible, definitive diagnoses should be reached in a minimally invasive manner. If the decision is made that a cat is a candidate for more extensive surgery then the choice of which surgery to perform is dependent on the extent of the disease and the choices of technique available, which include partial and complete lung lobectomy or pneumonectomy.

Lung biopsy and aspiration

Biopsy of lung tissue (Box 47-4) can be performed via intercostal thoracotomy, median sternotomy, keyhole thoracotomy, or thoracoscopy (see Chapter 42).

Box 47-4 Lung biopsy

Fine needle aspirate

Aspiration can be performed under ultrasound guidance or at surgery. Technique for aspiration is similar to other tissues, with introduction of a small gauge needle into the lung followed by gentle aspiration. The lung should be examined for air leakage during surgery or it can be assessed via ultrasonography.

Biopsy

A keyhole intercostal thoracotomy incision is useful for generalized interstitial disease. The site of intercostal thoracotomy is chosen dependent on the lung lobe affected (see Chapter 41). The lung lobe to be biopsied is gently exteriorized, a TA stapler placed and fired to apply a double or triple row of staggered staples, depending upon the size of stapler chosen. Ligatures can also be placed to obtain a biopsy in the same manner as for partial lung lobectomy if staples are not available (see Box 47-5).

Samples collected should be submitted for fungal, aerobic and anaerobic bacterial culture, and sensitivity testing and histopathology as appropriate.

Box 47-5 **Lung lobectomy**

The thoracotomy incision is made at the appropriate intercostal space according to the lung lobe affected (see Chapter 41). The diseased lung lobe(s) are examined to confirm which lobe(s) are affected.

Adjacent lung lobes may need to be retracted to allow access to the affected lobe, which can simply be achieved using a moistened swab. Care should be taken to avoid reduced ventilation and hypoxemia and the retracted lung lobe may have to be returned to its normal position should this occur. The pulmonary ligament between the caudal edge of the hilus and the mediastinal pleura must be transected for caudal lung lobectomy to be performed, which can be difficult for large lung lesions (Fig. 47-18A). The disease process and the size and location of the lesion within the lobe will dictate whether it is easier to perform lung lobectomy with the lung lobe remaining in the thoracic cavity or after exteriorization through the thoracotomy (Fig. 47-18B). Care should be taken during manipulation not to rupture the lung, damage surrounding structures, compromise venous return to the heart, or apply undue pressure to the heart.

Stapled lung lobectomy

Stapling is generally performed using a vascular thoracoabdominal stapler (TA 30 V), which places a triple staggered row of 3.5 mm titanium staples. The stapler is placed transversely across the lobar bronchus and pulmonary artery/vein supplying the affected lung lobe without the need for them to be dissected from each other (Fig. 47-18C). In some situations, for example where disease affects the hilus of the lung, a combination of ligatures and sutures may be the easiest way to achieve lung lobectomy. It is acceptable for some lung tissue to be included in the stapler and this may be necessary in some cases where there is not a clear separation of lung lobes by the interlobular fissures. Care is taken to ensure that no additional tissue, such as mediastinum or adjacent pulmonary blood vessels, has become incorporated into the stapler before the stapler is closed and fired. A large clamp is placed across the lung lobe distal to the staple to prevent spillage of blood or abnormal tissue or cells from the resected lobe and it is particularly important to avoid contamination of the thoracic cavity with blood or exudate from a pulmonary tumor. The lung lobe is transected using a scalpel blade (or scissors) distal to the stapler using the stapler itself as a guide (Fig. 47-18D). The stapler is removed and the bronchus and blood vessels examined for complete firing of the staple line (Fig. 47-18E). Failure of some or all or the staples to fire can result in brisk arterial or venous hemorrhage, so appropriate vascular clamps should be readily available to clamp bleeding vessels prior to ligating them. However, it is not necessary to oversew the staple line.

Sutured lung lobectomy

Blood vessels and bronchi can be ligated individually with suture material or en bloc.[81] It is easier to obtain a wider margin of normal tissue at the hilus of the lung lobe with ligation than stapling, especially if the bronchi and blood vessels have been dissected from each other. This is important where disease involves the bronchus or hilus of the lung rather than the middle or periphery of the lung. The bronchi can be carefully dissected from the blood vessels using blunt dissection (Fig. 47-19A) but care must be taken to avoid sharp dissection or penetration of blood vessels during blunt dissection. Such dissection may be difficult or impossible if there is severe inflammatory or neoplastic disease around the hilus as there may be adhesions to local structures and an increased local blood supply. Following dissection of the bronchi and vessels, a double ligature of a monofilament absorbable or non-absorbable suture with high tensile strength, for example 1.5–2M polydioxanone or polypropylene, is placed proximally around both the artery and vein (Fig. 47-19B). Care must be taken to avoid the right or left pulmonary trunks and the vessels supplying other lobes. A third suture is placed at least 5 mm distally, although occasionally the presence of a large lung mass dictates that this distance must be less, and the vessels are transected between the proximal and distal sutures. Appropriate vascular clamps (see Chapter 13) should be readily available to clamp bleeding vessels should there be a technical error with suture placement, before reapplication of sutures proximal to the clamp is attempted. The bronchus is similarly ligated and transected if there is no cartilage present. If the bronchus is transected in the cartilaginous portion it can either be simply ligated or it may be oversewn using a similar suture material. En bloc resection is performed in a similar manner but the artery, vein, and bronchus are ligated together, usually with a larger gauge (2–3M) suture material as described above. It should be noted that there may be communication between the pulmonary parenchymal tissues at adjacent lung lobes, due to incomplete interlobular fissures. These can be ligated before transection.

Samples should be submitted for fungal, aerobic, and anaerobic bacterial culture and sensitivity testing and histopathology as appropriate.

Closure

Prior to thoracic closure following partial or complete lung lobectomy or pneumonectomy, the sutures or staples are checked for security and then the hilus should be flooded with warm sterile saline to look for air leaks (Fig. 47-20). Additional sutures or staples are then placed as necessary before a chest drain is placed, the saline suctioned, a swab count performed, and the thoracotomy incision closed (see Chapter 41).

Lung lobectomy

Lung lobectomy is indicated for single lesions such as foreign bodies not removable via bronchoscopy, pulmonary abscesses, single pulmonary neoplasms, or metastases. Lung lobectomy (Box 47-5) is usually performed via a thoracotomy (see Chapter 41) although thorascopic-assisted lung lobectomy (see Chapter 42) is also possible.

Lobectomy of a single lung lobe or multiple lobes within a hemithorax is most easily performed by intercostal thoracotomy, at the fifth intercostal space for cranial and middle lobes and the sixth space for caudal and accessory lobes (Fig. 47-17; see Chapter 41). Complete examination of the whole hemithorax is limited via an intercostal approach, as although most of the ipsilateral lung lobes can be examined, access to the mediastinum is limited and there is almost no visualization of the contralateral hemithorax. Median sternotomy for lung lobectomy is required when all the lung lobes must be individually examined to look for underlying pathology or if lobes from both hemithoraces need resection. Access to the hilus is more difficult via median sternotomy but it is easier to reduce adhesions and assess invasion of local structures. Closure of the hilar blood vessels and

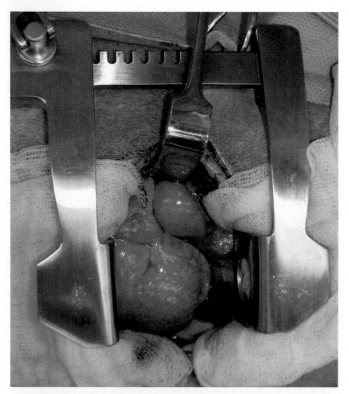

Figure 47-17 Left sixth intercostal thoracotomy for lung lobectomy. Small Finochietto rib retractors and a handheld retractor aid visualization but complete examination of the left hemithorax is not possible. There is easy access to the hilus for lung lobectomy. *(© Alison Moores.)*

bronchi for complete lung lobectomy can be achieved by ligation or the use of surgical staples.[79,80] While the use of stapling is considered to be a faster method of ligation than individually ligating bronchi and blood vessels, it may not be any faster than en bloc ligation. The author prefers ligation in small cats where placement of the stapler is limited by access into the thoracic cavity, as in these instances there may actually be little difference in the time taken to ligate using sutures and application of a stapler. Staplers are also more expensive than sutures.

It is important to assess at surgery whether disease affects part or all of the lung, and specifically whether it involves the hilus, as this can affect the ability to remove a lobe using staples and may influence outcome of the underlying disease, e.g., neoplasia. Disease of the mid or peripheral parts of lung may be amenable to partial lung lobectomy (Box 47-6), which can also be performed via thoracoscopy (see Chapter 42).

Pneumonectomy

Pneumonectomy (Box 47-7) is the resection of all lung tissue from one hemithorax.[79] It has been described in cats with chronic pyothorax,[79] pulmonary neoplasia,[54,81] and pneumonia.[74] Right-sided pneumonectomy, which removes more than 50% of lung volume, has been successfully reported in the cat, despite initial reservations that this would not be tolerated in small animals.[79,81] Care must be taken when considering pneumonectomy to ensure that the remaining lung lobes are healthy enough to support respiratory functions.

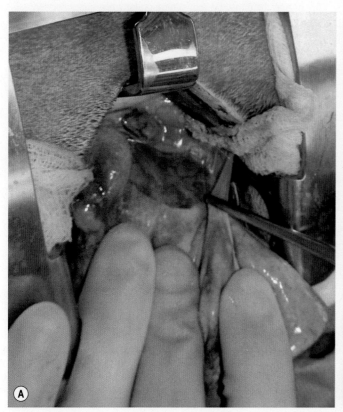

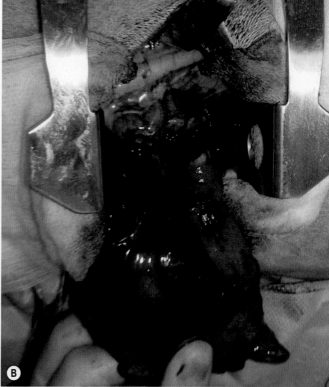

Figure 47-18 (A) The pulmonary ligament is shown between the caudal edge of the hilus and the mediastinal pleura. It must be transected to allow caudal lung lobectomy. **(B)** Exteriorization of a lung lobe prior to lung lobectomy.

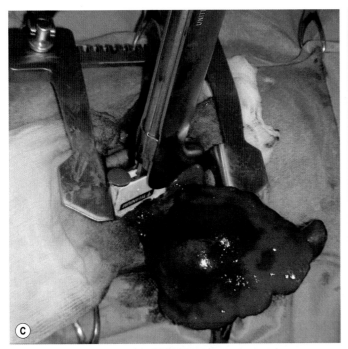

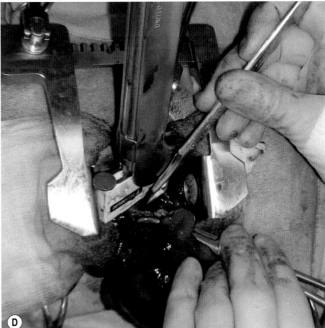

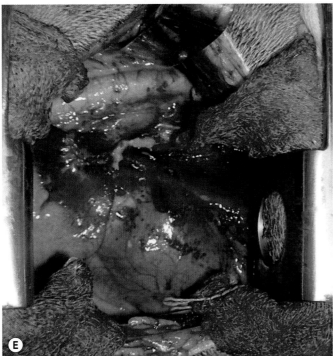

Figure 47-18, Continued (C) A vascular thoracoabdominal stapler is placed transversely across the lobar bronchus and pulmonary artery and vein supplying the affected lung lobe. **(D)** A large clamp is placed across the lung lobe distal to the stapler to prevent spillage of blood or abnormal tissue or cells from the resected lobe. The lung lobe is transected using a scalpel blade distal to the stapler using the stapler itself as a guide. **(E)** The stapler is removed and the bronchus and blood vessels examined for complete firing of the staple line. *(© Alison Moores.)*

POSTOPERATIVE CARE AND COMPLICATIONS

The postoperative care of patients undergoing pulmonary surgery is an extremely important part of management. Particularly in cats, due to their small size, heat loss resulting in a drop in core body temperature after open thoracotomy is common, so every effort should be made to prevent this during and after surgery. Close monitoring in a suitable intensive care facility is required so that any changes in parameters are noted quickly. For further more detailed information on the postoperative monitoring of these patients the reader is referred to Chapters 3, 4, and 41.

Complications associated with lung lobectomy include pneumothorax, hemorrhage (from hilar blood vessels or disruption of pleural adhesions) and damage to local structures (e.g., diaphragm, adjacent pulmonary vessels, heart).[74,79,80] Disruption of a staple line can result in pneumothorax and hemothorax and may be due to placing too much tissue within the staple thus preventing normal firing, failure of the staples to fire, or residual disease at the staple line.[80]

Reported complications after thoracoscopic lung biopsy in dogs and cats include hypoxemia, pneumothorax, pulmonary hemorrhage, and wound healing complications.[1]

Damage to the bronchus or pulmonary vessels during high partial lung lobectomy may necessitate complete lung lobectomy.

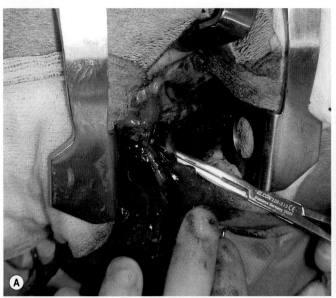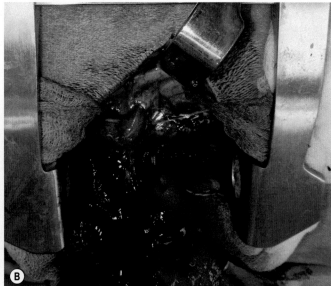

Figure 47-19 Lung lobectomy using ligatures. **(A)** Dissection around a pulmonary blood vessel. **(B)** Ligatures have been placed on the pulmonary vessels prior to transection. (© *Alison Moores.*)

Box 47-6 **Partial lung lobectomy**

Partial lung lobectomy may be performed for disease within the distal two-thirds of a lung lobe. It is an alternative to complete lung lobectomy and is useful to preserve lung tissue where there is disease distally in multiple lung lobes e.g., bullae, metastatic tumors. It is technically easier to perform partial lung lobectomy with staples than by suturing. A thoracoabdominal stapler is placed across the lung lobe proximal to the lesion. The TA 30 vascular staple may not be suitable due to the short length of the staple lines. Staples with heights of 3.5 mm or 4.8 mm are selected depending upon the thickness of the lung parenchyma; 3.5 mm staples are most commonly used. Care is taken to ensure that no additional tissue, such as mediastinum or adjacent lung, has become incorporated into the stapler before it is closed and fired. A large clamp is placed across the lung lobe distal to the stapler to prevent spillage of blood or abnormal tissue or cells from the resected lobe and it is particularly important to avoid contamination of the thoracic cavity with blood or exudate from a pulmonary tumor. The lung lobe is transected using a scalpel blade (or scissors) distal to the stapler, using the stapler itself as a guide. The stapler is removed and the lung examined for complete firing of the staple line. Failure of some of all or the staples to fire can result in arterial or venous hemorrhage or air leakage, so appropriate vascular clamps should be readily available to clamp bleeding vessels prior to ligating them or reapplying a stapler. It is not necessary to oversew the staple line. Small areas of hemorrhage or air leakage can be controlled using ligatures or small staples.

Partial lung lobectomy using sutures can be performed by placing a continuous overlapping suture pattern of 1.5M polydioxanone or polypropylene or other suitable suture 0.5 cm proximal to the proposed transection site of lung. The suture should be tight enough to achieve hemostasis and pneumostasis. Crushing forceps are applied distal to the suture line and the lung is transected between the clamp and the suture. A simple continuous suture of the same material is placed along the free lung edge distal to the overlapping sutures.

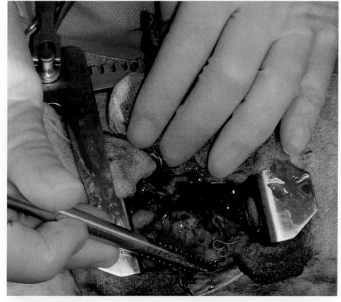

Figure 47-20 Following lung lobectomy, the hilus is flooded with warm sterile saline to look for air leaks. (© *Alison Moores.*)

Box 47-7 **Pneumonectomy**

The approach to pneumonectomy is performed as described for lung lobectomy (see Box 47-5), but all affected lung lobes of one hemithorax are resected. Lung lobes can be removed individually or en mass more proximally, with ligation and transection of the right or left main stem bronchus and lobar pulmonary artery/vein. Alternatively, staples may be used. If it is difficult to access the lung hilus due to the extent of lung disease, it may be preferable to clamp the hilus and transect the lung lobes distally before ligating the bronchi and blood vessels. Care should be taken that the clamp does not become dislodged before the blood vessels have been ligated. A 5 mm cuff of artery and vein should be left distal to the ligatures to minimize the risk of the suture falling off. The end of the bronchus is usually oversewn. The type of staple or suture material and size to use is described in Box 47-5.

PROGNOSIS

The prognosis following lung lobectomy depends upon the underlying cause. Most cats tolerate thoracotomy and lung lobectomy well unless there is severe underlying disease. Indeed, respiratory function in cats is often improved if the diseased lung has been acting as a shunt and inhibiting complete oxygen saturation. Compensatory mechanisms in remaining lung occur after lung lobectomy to increase residual lung volume and total lung capacity.[79,81] In studies of normal dogs, where less than 50% of lung is removed, compensation occurs by recruitment of existing mechanisms, such as remodeling the alveolar-capillary network.[81] Where more than 50% of lung tissue is removed, there is also regenerative growth of remaining lung tissue.[81]

REFERENCES

1. Norris CR, Griffey SM, Samii VF, et al. Thoracic radiography, BAL cytopathology, and pulmonary parenchymal histopathology: a comparison of diagnostic results in 11 cats. J Am Anim Hosp Assoc 2002;38(4):337–45.

2. Schwarz LA, Tidwell AS. Alternative imaging of the lung. Clin Tech Small Anim Pract 1999;14:187–206.

3. Reichle JK, Wisner ER. Non-cardiac thoracic ultrasound in 75 feline and canine patients. Vet Radiol Ultrasound 2000;41(2):154–62.

4. Wood EF, O'Brien RT, Young KM. Ultrasound-guided fine-needle aspiration of focal parenchymal lesions of the lung in dogs and cats. J Vet Intern Med 1998;12:338–42.

5. Samii VF, Biller DS, Koblik PD. Normal cross-sectional anatomy of the feline thorax and abdomen: comparison of CT and cadaver anatomy. Vet Radiol Ultrasound 1998;39:504–11.

6. Henninger W. Use of CT in the diseased feline thorax. J Small Anim Pract 2003;44:56–64.

7. Oliveira CR, Mitchell MA, O'Brien RT. Thoracic computed tomography in feline patients without use of chemical restraint. Vet Radiol Ultrasound 2011;52(4):368–76.

8. Schultz RM, Zwingenberger A. Radiographic, computed tomographic, and ultrasonographic findings with migrating intrathoracic grass awns in dogs and cats. Vet Radiol Ultrasound 2008;49(3):249–55.

9. Dhaliwal RS, Lacey JK. Ectopic hepatic parenchyma attached to the diaphragm: simulating a pulmonary mass in a cat. J Am Anim Hosp Assoc 2009;45(1):39–42.

10. Hahn KA, McEntee MF. Prognosis factors for survival in cats after removal of a primary lung tumor: 21 cases (1979–1994). Vet Surg 1998;27:307–11.

11. Hazell KL, Swift IM, Sullivan N. Successful treatment of pulmonary aspergillosis in a cat. Aust Vet J 2011;89:101–4.

12. Koblik, PD. Radiographic appearance of primary lung tumors in cats. Veterinary Radiology 1986;27:66–73.

13. Miles KG. A review of primary lung tumors in the dog and cat. Vet Radiol Ultrasound 1988;29:122–8.

14. White JD, Tisdall PL, Norris JM, Malik R. Diaphragmatic hernia in a cat mimicking a pulmonary mass. J Feline Med Surg 2003;5(3):197–201.

15. Rossi F, Vignoli M, Sarli G, et al. Unusual radiographic appearance of lung carcinoma in a cat. J Small Anim Pract 2003;44:273–6.

16. Madewell BR, Theilen GH. Tumors of the respiratory tract and thorax. In: Madewell BR, Theilen GH, editors. Veterinary cancer medicine. 2nd ed. Philadelphia: Lea & Febiger; 1987. p. 535–65.

17. DeHeer HL, McManus P. Frequency and severity of tracheal wash hemosiderosis and association with underlying disease in 96 cats: 2002–2003. Vet Clin Pathol 2005;34:17–22.

18. McMillan MC, Kleine LJ, Carpenter JL. Fluoroscopically guided percutaneous fine-needle aspiration biopsy of thoracic lesions in dogs and cats. Vet Radiol 1988;29:194–7.

19. Zekas LJ, Crawford JT, O'Brien RT. Computed tomography-guided fine-needle aspirate and tissue-core biopsy of intrathoracic lesions in thirty dogs and cats. Vet Radiol Ultrasound 2005;46:200–4.

20. Norris CR, Samii VF. Clinical, radiographic and pathologic features of bronchiectasis in cats: 12 cases (1987–1999). J Am Vet Med Assoc 2000;216:530–4.

21. Kovak JR, Ludwig LL, Bergman PJ, et al. Use of thoracoscopy to determine the etiology of pleural effusion in dogs and cats: 18 cases (1998–2001). J Am Vet Med Assoc 2002;221:990–4.

22. Dorn CR, Taylor DO, Schneider R, et al. Survey of Animal Neoplasms in Alameda and Contra Costa Counties, California. II. Cancer morbidity in dogs and cats from Alameda County. J Nat Cancer Inst 1968;40:307–18.

23. Moulton JE. Tumors of the respiratory system. In: Moulton JE, editor. Tumors in domestic animals. 2nd ed. Berkeley: University of California press; 1978. p. 216–30.

24. Petterino C, Guazzi P, Ferro S, Castagnaro M. Bronchogenic adenocarcinoma in a cat: an unusual case of metastasis to the skin. Vet Clin Pathol 2005;34:401–4.

25. Hahn KA, McEntee MF. Primary lung tumors in cats: 86 cases (1979–1994). J Am Vet Med Assoc 1997;211:1257–60.

26. Moulton JE, von Tscharner C, Schneider R. Classification of lung carcinomas in the dog and cat. Vet Pathol 1981;18:513–28.

27. Barr F, Gruffydd-Jones T, Brown P, et al. Primary lung tumors in cats. J Small Anim Pract 1987;28:1115–25.

28. Mehlhaff CJ, Mooney S. Primary pulmonary neoplasia in the dog and cat. Vet Clin North Am Small Anim Pract 1985;15:1061–7.

29. Gionfriddo JR, Fix AS, Niyo Y, et al. Ocular manifestations of a metastatic pulmonary adenocarcinoma in a cat. J Am Vet Med Assoc 1990;197(3):372–4.

30. Dhaliwal RS, Kufuor-Mensah E. Metastatic squamous cell carcinoma in a cat. J Feline Med Surg 2007;9:61–6.

31. Drolet R, Phaneuf JB. Pulmonary chondromatous hamartoma in a young cat. Vet Rec 1983;113:541–2.

32. Ghisleni G, Grieco V, Mazzotti M, et al. Pulmonary carcinosarcoma in a cat. J Vet Diagn Invest 2003;15(2):170–3.

33. Goodwin J-K, Lawrence DT, Bellah JR, et al. A large solitary pulmonary fibrosarcoma in a cat. J Am Anim Hosp Assoc 1991;27:327–30.

34. Grierson JM, Burton CA, Brearley MJ. Hypertrophic osteopathy secondary to pulmonary sarcoma in a cat. Vet Comp Oncol 2003;1:227–31.

35. Pool RR, Mantos JJ, Bodle JE, et al. Primary lung carcinoma with skeletal metastases in the cat. Feline Pract 1974;4:36–41.

36. Scott-Moncrieff JC, Elliott GS, Radovsky A, Blevins WE. Pulmonary squamous cell carcinoma with multiple digital metastases in a cat. J Sm Anim Pract 1989;30:696–9.

37. Valtolina C, Adamantos S. Evaluation of small-bore wire-guided chest drains for management of pleural space disease. J Sm Anim Pract 2009;50:290–7.

38. Yamagami T, Nomura K, Fujita M, et al. Pulmonary intravascular hemangiosarcoma in a cat. J Vet Med Sci 2006;68:731–3.

39. Moore AS, Middleton DJ. Pulmonary adenocarcinoma in three cats with

non-respiratory signs only. J Sm Anim Pract 1982;23:501–9, 14.

40. Gottfried SD, Popovitch CA, Goldschmidt MH, Schelling C. Metastatic digital carcinoma in the cat: a retrospective study of 36 cats (1992–1998). J Am Anim Hosp Assoc 2000;36:501–9.

41. Schoen K, Block G, Newell SM, Coronado GS. Hypercalcemia of malignancy in a cat with bronchogenic adenocarcinoma. J Am Anim Hosp Assoc 2010;46:265–7.

42. Anderson TE, Legendre AM, McEntee MM. Probable hypercalcemia of malignancy in a cat with bronchogenic adenocarcinoma. J Am Anim Hosp Assoc 2000;36:52–5.

43. Dole RS, MacPhail CM, Lappin MR. Paraneoplastic leukocytosis with mature neutrophilia in a cat with pulmonary squamous cell carcinoma. J Feline Med Surg 2004;6:391–5.

44. Cohn LA, Norris CR, Hawkins EC, et al. Identification and characterization of an idiopathic pulmonary fibrosis-like condition in cats. J Vet Intern Med 2004;18:632–41.

45. Vignoli M, Rossi F, Chierici C, et al. Needle tract implantation after fine needle aspiration biopsy (FNAB) of transitional cell carcinoma of the urinary bladder and adenocarcinoma of the lung. Schweiz Arch Tierheilkd 2007;149: 314–18.

46. Forman MA, Johnson LR, Jang S, Foley JE. Lower respiratory tract infection due to Capnocytophaga cynodegmi in a cat with pulmonary carcinoma. J Feline Med Surg 2005;7:227–31.

47. Ibarrola P, German AJ, Stell AJ, et al. Appendicular arterial tumor embolization in two cats with pulmonary carcinoma. J Am Vet Med Assoc 2004;225:1065–9, 1048–9.

48. Sykes JE. Ischemic neuromyopathy due to peripheral arterial embolization of an adenocarcinoma in a cat. J Feline Med Surg 2003;5:353–6.

49. Cassotis NJ, Dubielzig RR, Gilger BC, Davidson MG. Angioinvasive pulmonary carcinoma with posterior segment metastasis in four cats. Vet Ophthalmol 1999;2:125–31.

50. Hamilton HB, Severin GA, Nold J. Pulmonary squamous cell carcinoma with intraocular metastasis in a cat. J Am Vet Med Assoc 1984;185:307–9.

51. Byers CG, Tumulty JW, Stefanacci JD. What Is Your Diagnosis? Journal of the American Veterinary Medical Association 2006;228:1341–2.

52. Hifumi T, Miyoshi N, Kawaguchi H, et al. Immunohistochemical detection of proteins associated with multidrug resistance to anti-cancer drugs in canine and feline primary pulmonary carcinoma. J Vet Med Sci 2010;72:665–8.

53. Richard WN, Guillermo CC. Lung tumors. In: Nelson RW, Couto CG, editors. Small animal internal medicine. 3rd ed. Missouri: Mosby; 2005. p. 317–19.

54. Clements DN, Hogan AM, Cave TA. Treatment of a well differentiated pulmonary adenocarcinoma in a cat by pneumonectomy and adjuvant mitoxantrone chemotherapy. J Feline Med Surg 2004;6:199–205.

55. Beam SL, Rassnick KM, Moore AS, McDonough SP. An immunohistochemical study of cyclooxygenase-2 expression in various feline neoplasms. Vet Pathol 2003;40:496–500.

56. Withrow SJ. Lung cancer. In: Withrow SJ, MacEwan EG, editors. Small animal clinical oncology. 2nd ed. Philadelphia: WB Saunders CO; 2001. p. 361–70.

57. Forrest LJ, Graybush CA. Radiographic patterns of pulmonary metastasis in 25 cats. Vet Radiol Ultrasound 1998;39: 4–8.

58. Suter PF, Carrig CB, O'Brien TR, Koller D. Radiographic recognition of primary and metastatic pulmonary neoplasms of dogs and cats. J Am Vet Radio 1974;15: 3–25.

59. Nafe LA, Hayes AA, Patnaik AK. Mammary tumors and unassociated pulmonary masses in two cats. J Am Vet Med Assoc 1979;175:1194–5.

60. d'Anjou MA, Tidwell AS, Hecht S. Radiographic diagnosis of lung lobe torsion. Vet Radiol Ultrasound 2005;46: 478–84.

61. Mclane MJ, Buote NJ. Lung lobe torsion associated with chylothorax in a cat. J Feline Med Surg 2011;13:135–8.

62. Brown NO, Zontine WJ. Lung lobe torsion in the cat. Vet Radiol Ultrasound 1976;17:219–23.

63. Millard RP, Myers JR, Novo RE. Spontaneous lung lobe torsion in a cat. J Vet Intern Med 2008;22:671–3.

64. Dye TL, Teague HD, Poundstone ML. Lung lobe torsion in a cat with chronic feline asthma. J Am Anim Hosp Assoc 1998;34:493–5.

65. Kerpsack SK, McLoughlin MA, Graves TK, et al. Chylothorax associated with lung lobe torsion and a peritoneopericardial diaphragmatic hernia in a cat. J Am Anim Hosp Assoc 1994;30:351–4.

66. Schwarz T, Crawford PE, Owen MR, et al. Fatal pulmonary fat embolism during humeral fracture repair in a cat. J Small Anim Pract 2001;42:195–8.

67. Norris CR, Griffey SM, Samii VF. Pulmonary thromboembolism in cats: 29 cases (1987–1997). J Am Vet Med Assoc 1999;215:1650–4.

68. Schermerhorn T, Pembleton-Corbett JR, Kornreich B. Pulmonary thromboembolism in cats. J Vet Intern Med 2004;18:533–5.

69. Hylands R. Pulmonary thromboembolism. Can Vet J 2006;47:385–6, 388.

70. Crisp MS, Birchard SJ, Lawrence AE, Fingeroth J. Pulmonary abscess caused by a Mycoplasma sp in a cat. J Am Vet Med Assoc 1987;191:340–2.

71. Wegner K, Pablo L. Anesthesia case of the month. Pulmonary abscess formation. J Am Vet Med Assoc 2006;228:850–3.

72. Evans N, Gunew M, Marshall R, et al. Focal pulmonary granuloma caused by Cladophialophora bantiana in a domestic short haired cat. Med Mycol 2011;49: 194–7.

73. Pawloski DR, Brunker JD, Singh K, Sutton DA. Pulmonary Paecilomyces lilacinus Infection in a Cat. J Am Anim Hosp Assoc 2010;46(3):197–202.

74. Murphy ST, Mathews KG, Ellison GW, Bellah JR. Pulmonary lobectomy in the management of pneumonia in five cats. J Small Anim Pract 1997;38(4):159–62.

75. Valentine BA, Blue JT, Zimmer JF, et al. Pulmonary lymphomatoid granulomatosis in a cat. J Vet Diagn Invest 2000;12:465–7.

76. Mooney ET, Rozanski EA, King RG, Sharp CR. Spontaneous pneumothorax in 35 cats (2001–2010). J Feline Med Surg 2012;14(6):384–91.

77. Milne ME, McCowan C, Landon BP. Spontaneous feline pneumothorax caused by ruptured pulmonary bullae associated with possible bronchopulmonary dysplasia. J Am Anim Hosp Assoc 2010;46(2):138–42.

78. Kaestner S. Anesthesia. In: Montavon PM, Voss K, Langley-Hobbs SJ, editors. Feline orthopedic surgery and musculoskeletal disease. Edinburgh: Elsevier; 2009. p. 177–98.

79. Crawford AH, Halfacree ZJ, Lee KC, Brockman DJ. Clinical outcome following pneumonectomy for management of chronic pyothorax in four cats. J Feline Med Surg 2011;13:762–7.

80. LaRue SM, Withrow SJ, Wykes PM. Lung resection using surgical staples in dogs and cats. Vet Surg 1987;16: 238–40.

81. Liptak JM, Monnet E, Dernell WS, et al. Pneumonectomy: four case studies and a comparative review. J Small Anim Pract 2004;45:441–7.

Chapter |48|

Heart

R. Burrow

Heart disease is common in cats but there are few feline cardiac conditions that are treated surgically. Of these, patent ductus arteriosus (PDA) and symptomatic, medically unresponsive bradycardias are the most frequent indications for performing cardiac surgery. Both conditions are rare in cats.

The commonest cardiac surgical procedure performed in cats is subtotal pericardectomy; the commonest indication for performing this procedure is chylothorax, which has a number of potential underlying causes, only one of which is cardiac disease.

The basic requirements for anesthesia and postoperative care for cats undergoing cardiac surgeries, and many of the potential postoperative complications are as for patients undergoing sternotomy or thoracotomy for other reasons. Specific postoperative requirements will depend on the underlying disease and the patient's clinical status. In this chapter the most commonly performed surgical cardiac procedures are discussed.

SURGICAL ANATOMY

There is little variability in normal thoracic conformation and heart shape between cat breeds. The normal feline heart is slender in appearance on a lateral thoracic radiograph and it appears more horizontal in its orientation within the thorax than in the dog; with increasing age this can become more marked.[1] The heart lies within the mediastinum in the mid thorax, approximately between the 3rd and 6th intercostal spaces.

The right atrium and ventricle form the craniodorsal part of the heart. The right atrium receives blood from the cranial and caudal vena cavae, and from the coronary vessels via the coronary sinus. The right atrial appendage arises from the cranial aspect of the right atrium and extends ventrally. The right ventricle is arciform in cross section; it lies cranial and ventral to the left ventricle. Blood is ejected from the right ventricle through the pulmonic valve into the pulmonary trunk. The initial part of the pulmonary trunk is within the pericardium, the ventral, lateral and caudal surfaces are covered by serous pericardium, and this portion of the pulmonary trunk is usually masked by fat. The pulmonary trunk contacts the aorta along its entire medial surface. The pulmonary trunk divides into the right and left

pulmonary arteries. The fibrous pericardium attaches to the distal fourth of the pulmonary trunk and the terminal portion of the pulmonary trunk can be examined without opening the pericardium.

The left atrium and ventricle form the caudodorsal part of the heart. The left atrium forms the left dorsocaudal part of the base of the heart. The left atrial appendage is a cranial extension of the left atrium. It is located caudal to the pulmonary trunk and lies along the right atrial appendage, caudal to and separated from it by the pulmonary trunk. Blood enters the left atrium from the pulmonary veins, which open into its dorsal aspect; the individual pulmonary veins may fuse but usually remain separate and enter the left atrium separately. The left ventricle is cone shaped and its apex forms the apex of the heart. Blood is ejected from the left ventricle through the aortic valve into the aorta, near the center of the heart base. The initial part of the aorta, the ascending portion, is mainly located within the pericardium. It continues for a short distance cranially before passing dorsocaudally and to the left by forming a U-bend, the aortic arch. Two great vessels leave the aortic arch to supply the head, neck, and thoracic limbs: the brachiocephalic trunk and the left subclavian artery. The ligamentum arteriosum, the connective tissue remnant of the fetal ductus arteriosus, arises near the bifurcation of the pulmonary trunk and passes to the aorta. The aorta then continues caudally as the descending aorta.

The right and left vagus nerves pass caudally in the dorsal mediastinal pleura. The left vagus nerve passes over the ligamentum arteriosum, and is a landmark used during the surgical treatment of PDA. The left recurrent laryngeal nerve leaves the left vagus nerve just cranial to the ductus and it passes around the caudal aspect of the ductus.

The pericardium forms a double layered sac that surrounds the heart, the initial portion of the ascending aorta, pulmonary trunk, termination of the vena cavae, and the pulmonary veins. It attaches near/at the base of the heart to the aortic arch, pulmonary trunk, left atrium at the level of the pulmonary veins and dorsal to the interatrial groove on the right side. The outer fibrous layer is termed the parietal pericardium, the inner serous membrane the visceral pericardium, which is adherent to the epicardium. At its apex the pericardium is continued as a flattened band, the caudoventral mediastinal reflection, which attaches to the ventral part of the muscular insertion of the diaphragm. The right and left phrenic nerves run across the dorsal third of the pericardium and must be identified and preserved during pericardectomy. Paired pericardiophrenic blood vessels from the

DOI: 10.1016/B978-0-7020-4336-9.00048-2

internal thoracic arteries run with the phrenic nerves. Pericardial blood vessels, also arising from the internal thoracic arteries, run within the pericardium passing in a caudoventral direction. With pericardial disease or pericardial and/or pleural effusion the pericardium can become thickened and these vessels will become more prominent.

GENERAL CONSIDERATIONS

Specific investigations will depend on the patient's history, clinical signs, findings on clinical examination, and differential diagnoses but will usually include a minimum of hematology, serum biochemistry, and thoracic radiography. Specific blood tests to assess for infections such as feline coronavirus, leukemia, and immunodeficiency viruses may be indicated. For investigation of suspected cardiac disease electrocardiography (ECG), echocardiography and, uncommonly, angiography are indicated. Pleural and/or pericardial effusions should be sampled for biochemistry, cytology, and bacterial and/or fungal culture as appropriate. Blood coagulation screen should be performed if a hemorrhagic effusion is identified. Advanced imaging of the thorax using computed tomography may be appropriate in cases (e.g., chylothorax or other pleural effusions) where intrathoracic neoplasia is a differential diagnosis.

SURGICAL DISEASES

Patent ductus arteriosus

The ductus arteriosus carries blood from the pulmonary artery to the aorta in the fetus. Within hours of the birth the ductus normally closes in response to an increase in the oxygen tension of the blood; failure of closure allows continual shunting of blood between the left and right sides of the heart. After birth, the blood pressure in the pulmonary artery reduces and the systemic blood pressure increases. Typically this pressure differential is such that blood shunts continuously through the cardiac cycle, from the higher pressure aorta to the lower pressure pulmonary artery (i.e., left to right shunting) if the ductus remains patent. The secondary changes that occur with increased blood flowing in the pulmonary artery are pulmonary over-circulation, left atrial dilatation, left ventricular dilatation with eccentric hypertrophy, dilatation of the aortic arch to the level of the origin of the PDA, and dilatation of the pulmonary trunk. As a consequence of the left to right shunting and left-sided volume overload, left-sided congestive heart failure (CHF) commonly develops. The size of the shunt will determine volume of blood shunting, which in turn determines the onset and severity of secondary consequences. As a sequel to the increased blood flow in the pulmonary vessels, resistance to blood flow and pulmonary hypertension can develop. If the pulmonary arterial pressure is greater than the aortic pressure for some or all of the cardiac cycle, blood flow through the PDA will reverse. Blood will then flow from the pulmonary artery into the aorta (i.e., right to left shunting). Right to left shunting can also occur from birth, and usually occurs when the ductus is large and tubular without narrowing at the pulmonary ostium, and this may reflect retention of fetal pulmonary vasculature. Right to left shunting, termed Eisenmenger's physiology, is rarely reported in cats,[2,3] although it is suggested that it is more likely to develop over time in cats than dogs.[4] Surgical treatment of the PDA is contraindicated in patients with right to left shunting.

PDA is a rarely diagnosed congenital heart disease in the cat, with few cases of this condition reported in the English language veterinary literature so it is difficult to make conclusions about the presentation, investigative findings, and the outcome with medical or surgical treatment. This contrasts with dogs, where PDA is one of the more commonly diagnosed congenital heart diseases[5,6] and it is well documented.

Most dogs are diagnosed as puppies, whilst the condition is asymptomatic, by auscultation of a pathognomic continuous murmur. It is suggested that the situation may be similar in cats, and certainly the majority of cats reported with PDAs are less than one year of age. However, in an abstract reporting 21 cases of PDAs in cats approximately two-thirds had a continuous murmur but the remainder were described to have systolic murmurs and approximately only one-third of the cats in the study were asymptomatic at presentation. Their presenting complaints included abnormal respiration, exercise intolerance/lethargy, stunted growth, and poor weight gain.[7]

The murmur is well described in dogs; it may be accompanied by a thrill felt at the heart base, and by hyperkinetic pulses. The point of maximal intensity of the murmur lies over the main pulmonary artery at the dorsocranial heart base and may radiate cranially to the thoracic inlet and to the right heart base. It is suggested that in cats the continuous murmur of a PDA may be best heard slightly more ventrally than this typical location in dogs. Femoral pulses may be more difficult to assess in cats;[8] hyperkinetic pulses may be noted.

Diagnosis

Thoracic radiographic changes are variable and will depend on the size of the PDA and any consequential left-sided heart failure. Cardiomegaly, shifting of the cardiac apex to the left, a ductus aneurysmal bump, and pulmonary over-circulation are all common radiographic findings. If the patient presents in left-sided heart failure, pulmonary venous congestion and pulmonary edema will be present.

Diagnosis is usually confirmed with echocardiography using a right parasternal short axis or left parasternal cranial window (Fig. 48-1). Initially, there may be no changes in chamber size or myocardial contractility but eventually the consequences of left to right shunting may result in dilatation of the left atrium, aorta, and main pulmonary artery and dilatation and hypertrophy of the left ventricle, all recognizable on echocardiography (Fig. 48-2). Left ventricular systolic function may become impaired. If a left-to-right shunting PDA is identified, Doppler studies can be performed and will show characteristic high velocity turbulent flow from the aorta, through the ductus and into the main pulmonary artery (Fig. 48-3). This PDA peak velocity will

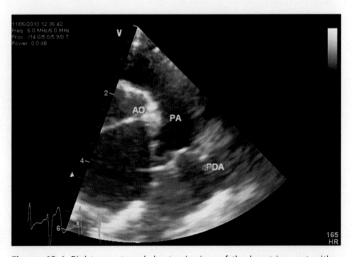

Figure 48-1 Right parasternal short axis view of the heart in a cat with a patent ductus arteriosus (PDA). This image was taken at the level of the pulmonary artery and shows the PDA. *(Courtesy Dr Jo Dukes-McEwan.)*

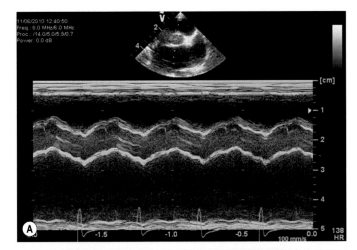

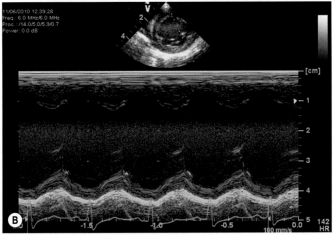

Figure 48-2 A cat with a left-to-right shunting patent ductus arteriosus (PDA). **(A)** Aortic M-mode image showing marked left atrial dilatation relative to the size of the aorta. **(B)** M-mode image of the left ventricle showing left ventricular dilatation, relative wall thinning and impaired systolic function. *(Courtesy Dr Jo Dukes-McEwan.)*

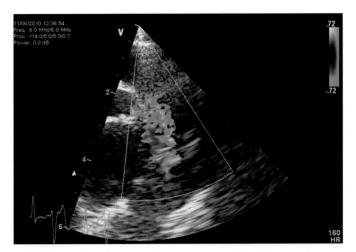

Figure 48-3 Right parasternal short axis view of the heart in a cat with a patent ductus arteriosus (PDA). This image was taken at the level of the pulmonary artery with color flow Doppler showing turbulent flow across the PDA. *(Courtesy Dr Jo Dukes-McEwan.)*

decrease if pulmonary pressures increase, prior to exceeding systemic pressures. However, note that this decrease may be reactive pulmonary hypertension as a consequence of the pulmonary over-circulation and closure of the PDA may resolve the mild pulmonary hypertension when assessed after surgery. Mild increase of velocity in the left ventricular outflow tract and mild aortic and pulmonic insufficiency may also be recognized. Mitral regurgitation is secondary to the left-sided dilation and may be significant.

Thorough echocardiography should be performed in cats because concurrent, but unspecified, congenital heart defects may be present; these were found in 29% of cats in one study.[7]

If the diagnosis of suspected PDA cannot be confirmed by echocardiography, or the presence of other congenital heart anomalies is suspected, cardiac catheterization and angiocardiography may be helpful, but this investigative procedure is rarely required to confirm diagnosis of PDA.

ECG is non-specific; it usually shows tall R waves and wide P waves due to atrial enlargement. Arrhythmias such as atrial fibrillation, supraventricular or ventricular arrhythmias, and ventricular premature complexes may be present.

Treatment

Patients with CHF and pulmonary edema at the time of diagnosis should be treated for several days with furosemide and angiotensin-converting enzyme (ACE) inhibitors before proceeding to anesthesia and surgery. In patients that are older at the time of diagnosis, with a small PDA, conservative management may be appropriate, although generally surgery is still recommended.

Pericardial disease

Congenital pericardial diseases are infrequently diagnosed and most have an excellent prognosis with surgical treatment. The most common condition in dogs and cats is peritoneopericardial diaphragmatic hernia (PPDH);[9] it is more common in cats (see Chapter 45).

Intrapericardial cysts

Intrapericardial 'cysts' are rarely reported.[10-14] These are usually not true cysts but encapsulated adipose tissue or organizing cystic hematomas. The cyst may be attached to the apex of the pericardium by a pedicle. They may arise if a PPDH containing herniated omentum or falciform fat closes before birth, trapping the fat within the pericardial sac. Cystic changes of herniated and incarcerated liver tissue may also occur in association with PPDH in cats. Intrapericardial cysts cause clinical signs either directly associated with their presence, or due to an associated effusion causing cardiac tamponade. Diagnosis can usually be made by radiography (Fig. 48-4) and/or ultrasound examination of the cranial abdomen and heart. Treatment is by subtotal pericardectomy (see Box 48-4), removal of the cyst (and pedicle if present), and repair of the PPDH (Chapter 45, 45.4.3) if present.

Congenital pericardial defects are very rare. Clinical signs may develop if the size of the defect is such that a portion of the heart can herniate through the defect, as cardiac function will then be compromised. This condition is treated by subtotal pericardectomy.

Pericardial effusion

The commonest acquired pericardial disease in both cats and dogs is pericardial effusion (PE), but the incidence, presentation and underlying causes have differences between these species. Clinically significant PE is very uncommon in cats, and this species rarely presents with cardiac tamponade. In both species PEs remain asymptomatic if the

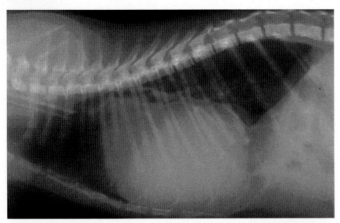

Figure 48-4 Lateral thoracic radiograph of a young, anesthetised cat with a peritoneopericardial diaphragmatic hernia (PPDH). The cardiac silhouette is markedly enlarged and silhouettes with the diaphragm. The distal intrathoracic trachea is displaced dorsally over the cranial border of the cardiac silhouette.

Box 48-1 Possible causes of pericardial effusion in cats

Congestive heart failure (various cardiac pathologies including hypertrophic cardiomyopathy, dilated cardiomyopathy, pulmonic stenosis)

Feline infectious peritonitis

Peritoneopericardial diaphragmatic hernia

Cardiac neoplasia (e.g., lymphoma, hemangiosarcoma, rhabdomyosarcoma)

Heart base tumors

Pericardial tumor (e.g., mesothelioma)

Systemic inflammation and infection

Uremia

Coagulopathies (e.g., warfarin toxicity, disseminated intravascular coagulation)

Trauma

Intrapericardial cyst

Bacterial pericarditis

Figure 48-5 (A) Dorsoventral and **(B)** lateral thoracic radiographs of a cat with a pericardial effusion. There is a small volume of pleural fluid. The underlying heart disease in this cat was severe hypertrophic cardiomyopathy. *(Courtesy Dr Jo Dukes-McEwan.)*

---

effusion is small and the pericardium remains slightly compliant, or if a larger effusion accumulates slowly allowing the pericardial sac to accommodate to some extent. Cardiac tamponade results when the amount of fluid (or cyst/mass) reaches a volume such that it exerts a pressure equal to or greater than normal cardiac diastolic pressures. The heart is compressed externally and cannot fill effectively during diastole. Right ventricular filling is reduced first, and may progress to compromise left ventricular filling and cardiac output. Systemic venous pressure and capillary hydrostatic pressure increase whilst cardiac output is reduced. Cats with cardiac tamponade usually develop pleural effusion and present with tachypnea and increased respiratory effort.

PE in cats is most commonly part of a more generalized disease (Box 48-1). Myocardial disease is the commonest underlying cause.[15] Small volume clinically insignificant PEs have been reported in approximately | 45% of cats with CHF,[16,17] while PEs are rarely reported

in dogs with CHF. The other most frequent underlying cause of PE in cats is feline infectious peritonitis. The commonest causes of PE in dogs are idiopathic hemorrhagic pericardial effusion (IPHE), which is unreported in the cat, and cardiac-related neoplasia. In dogs, hemangiosarcoma, usually of the right side of the heart, is the most common neoplastic cause of PE, aortic body tumors also occur with some frequency, mesotheliomas occur less commonly, and other tumors are also reported. These tumors are rarely diagnosed as a cause of PE in cats; lymphoma is the most common underlying tumor associated with the effusion.

The classic radiographic appearance of PE is general cardiomegaly (globoid heart) and sharp borders to the cardiac silhouette (Fig. 48-5). If the PE has accumulated rapidly without time for adaptation, cardiac tamponade may occur without the classic radiographic signs being present. Pleural effusion is usually present in cats with significant PE and may partly obscure the cardiac silhouette.

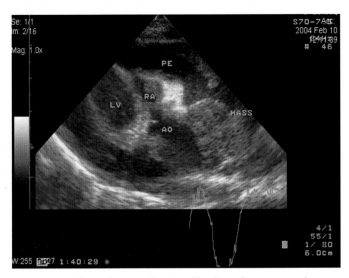

Figure 48-6 Echocardiogram of a cat with a heart base mass and an associated pericardial effusion (PE). *(Courtesy Dr Jo Dukes-McEwan.)*

A definitive diagnosis of PE is made by echocardiography, which allows cardiac disease or mass lesions to be excluded. The pericardial fluid is seen as an anechoic/slightly anechoic circular region surrounding the heart, within the thin hyperechoic line representing the pericardium. Although an uncommon cause of PE in cats, mass lesions affecting the heart may be seen on ultrasound examination. A thorough examination of the heart should be performed prior to pericardiocentesis because masses are most likely to be identified whilst surrounded by fluid (Fig. 48-6).

ECG findings in the dog can include reduced amplitude QRS complexes, electrical alternans and ST segment depression, but low voltage QRS complexes are normal in cats.

Cardiac tamponade should be treated immediately by pericardiocentesis (Box 48-2). Any pleural effusion should also be drained. Cats with significant PE may benefit from subtotal pericardectomy (see Box 48-4).

Chylothorax and fibrosing pericarditis

Fibrosing pleuritis (see Chapter 44) can develop secondary to any prolonged hemorrhagic, exudative, or chylous effusion. In these circumstances the pericardium is subject to the same environment and is also likely to become thickened and less compliant and there may be a consequential increase in venous pressures. Even a modest increase could cause the formation of extra lymphatics in the cranial thorax; these lymphatics may then leak. Thus a thickened, noncompliant pericardium may contribute to the development of chylothorax, and conversely chylothorax may cause pericardial thickening or fibrosing pericarditis. The actual role that the pericardium has in the development of and progression of chylothorax is unknown but pericardectomy, in combination with thoracic duct ligation with or without thoracic omentalization, has been shown in several small case series to achieve a successful resolution of the disease in approximately 75–80% cats.[18,19] Subtotal pericardectomy (see Box 48-4) has been successful in some cats as the sole treatment of chylothorax. It has also been suggested that it may be used to treat and/or prevent the serosanguinous effusions that occasionally occur in some patients after thoracic duct ligation.[18] Further studies are required to investigate these apparent benefits of pericardectomy.

Constrictive pericardial disease

Rarely, the visceral and/or parietal pericardial thickening can restrict ventricular filling in the absence of a PE, resulting in constrictive pericarditis. In some cases a small PE may be present, which would be insufficient to cause cardiac tamponade if the pericardial changes were absent, a situation that is called constrictive-effusive pericarditis. This condition is rarely diagnosed in cats, but it has been reported in a cat with dilated cardiomyopathy.[20] It is uncommon in dogs; underlying causes have included IPHE, intrapericardial foreign body, chronic septic pericarditis, and traumatic pericardial hemorrhage. Diagnosis can be difficult, and is easier if a small volume of PE is present. Thoracic radiographs may show mild to moderate cardiomegaly, pleural effusion, and distension of the caudal vena cava. Echocardiography may demonstrate suggestive changes such as flattening of the left ventricular free wall in diastole and abnormal septal motion. Invasive hemodynamic studies to measure central venous pressure changes may be needed to confirm the diagnosis.

Treatment is subtotal pericardectomy (see Box 48-4). The surgery is easier, complications fewer, and the outcome good if only the parietal pericardium is involved. If the visceral pericardium (epicardium) is also involved, and is fused to the parietal layer, subtotal pericardectomy is a more difficult and traumatic procedure. Stripping of this layer can result in severe hemorrhage from the myocardium, tachyarrhythmias, and pulmonary thromboembolism postoperatively.

561

Symptomatic bradycardia of cardiac origin

Symptomatic bradyarrhymia is one of the indications for pacemaker implantation in cats. Affected cats may have signs of hypoperfusion, and/or CHF, and/or syncope or seizure-like episodes due to atrioventricular (AV) block and normokalemic atrial standstill. Bradyarrhythmias are often asymptomatic in cats, and hence do not require treatment, as cats can have stable and relatively fast escape rhythms (90–120 beats per minute),[21] unlike dogs.

In dogs, electrodes are usually placed via a transvenous route, whilst in cats, generally, epicardial electrodes are placed using a surgical approach. This is because in cats the transvenous route is technically more difficult, and complications such as thromboembolism and obstruction to venous return causing chylothorax occur more commonly.[22]

A thorough history, clinical examination, and patient assessment are necessary to ensure that any non-cardiac disease is identified and eliminated as a cause of the bradycardia.

An ECG is necessary to diagnose the bradycardia. There is an absence of P waves and a slow supraventricular or ventricular escape rhythm with persistent atrial standstill. High grade second degree AV block is characterized by frequent 'dropped' QRS complexes, and usually does not respond to atropine. Third degree AV block has a complete dissociation of P waves and QRS complexes, there is a slow ventricular escape rhythm, and the arrhythmia is non-responsive to atropine.

PREOPERATIVE PREPARATION

It is essential to prepare thoroughly for cardiac and pericardial surgery. The correct instrumentation should be available for the surgeon (see Chapter 13). The anesthesia technique selected, the ability to be able to continually monitor anesthesia and respond to changes, the need for intermittent positive pressure ventilation (IPPV), and the ability to be able to provide appropriate levels of postoperative care are integral to the success of any thoracic surgery (see Chapters 2 and 3).

Surgical approaches to the heart.

The heart and associated structures can be approached from intercostal thoracotomies (see Chapter 41, Box 41-4) and median sternotomy (see Chapter 41, Box 41-5). The approach will depend on the procedure that is to be performed. Access to the apex of the heart for pacemaker lead implantation can also be achieved through a cranial midline celiotomy combined with caudal median sternotomy or a transdiaphragmatic incision.

Intercostal thoracotomies performed through the left 4th, 5th or 6th intercostal spaces have all been reported to achieve good access for surgical ligation of PDAs in cats.[2,23,24] In dogs a 4th intercostal space is the recommended approach; in cats the 4th or 5th space is generally recommended[25] due to the slightly more caudal location of the heart in this species.

Approach to the pericardium

Pericardectomy can be performed via several approaches. The final decision will depend on the indication for surgery and surgeon preference. If the primary reason for performing thoracic surgery is pericardectomy, a 5th left or right intercostal thoracotomy is recommended; excellent access is also obtained by median sternotomy. If a lateralized heart base mass is confirmed in a patient with a PE, the thoracotomy should be performed on the side of the mass. If a heart base mass is suspected, or has been identified involving both sides of the heart base, a median sternotomy may be the preferred approach.[26] A median sternotomy gives good access to both the left and right sides of the heart and allows easier identification of both phrenic nerves at surgery. Thus, pericardectomy may be technically easier via median sternotomy. A median sternotomy also reduces the requirement for manipulation of the heart during surgery, and thus reduces the likelihood of associated intraoperative arrhythmias and it allows exploration of both the right and left sides of the heart base if required.

When pericardectomy is performed as an adjunct to thoracic duct ligation (TDL) for the treatment of chylothorax it is usually possible to perform pericardectomy from an 8th, 9th or 10th left intercostal thoractomy (i.e., the same approach through which TDL is performed). If the access achieved from the caudal thoracotomies used for TDL is inadequate for pericardectomy a separate 5th left intercostal thoracotomy incision can be made.

Pericardectomy can also be performed thoracoscopically (see Chapter 42, Box 42-2).

Access to the apex of the heart for epicardial pacemaker implantation has been achieved via a 5th or 6th left or right lateral thoracotomy, midline cranial celiotomy and caudal sternotomy, and a cranial midline celiotomy and transdiaphragmatic approach.[27–30] The latter gives adequate access to the apex of the heart and is a less traumatic procedure for the patient, avoiding some of the additional postoperative management considerations and potential complications associated with thoracotomy and sternotomy.

SURGICAL MANAGEMENT AND TECHNIQUES

Ligation of a patent ductus arteriosus

It is widely accepted that prompt surgical treatment (Box 48-3) should be performed in young patients diagnosed with PDA to avoid the development of CHF or pulmonary hypertension. There are two described methods of open PDA ligation: the conventional approach and the Jackson–Henderson approach (Box 48-3).

The use of a vascular clip to occlude a ductus has been reported in a cat where safe dissection around the far wall of the ductus was considered impossible[3] and more recently for PDA occlusion in dogs.[32,33] It appears to be a suitable alternative to suture ligation and avoids 'blind' dissection around the far side of the ductus.

The use of vascular occluding devices is extensively reported for treatment of PDAs in dogs and has a similar rate of complications and outcome whilst avoiding an invasive surgical procedure. The femoral artery is generally used for catheter introduction to place the occluding device. This vessel is very small in cats, restricting the size of introducer or delivery catheter that can be placed and several authors have suggested that feline PDAs are only amenable to surgical ligation.[34,35] Transvenous embolization with detachable coils has been reported for successful occlusion of PDAs in two cats using the femoral vein to gain vascular access, and this technique may prove to be a good alternative to surgical closure of PDAs in cats.[36]

Subtotal pericardectomy

Subtotal pericardectomy is performed for PEs, restrictive pericarditis, symptomatic pericardial cysts, congenital or acquired pericardial defects, with herniation of the heart, and chylothorax. Generally, subtotal pericardectomy (Box 48-4) is performed via a right or left 5th intercostal thoracotomy although a median sternotomy can also be used.

Box 48-3 **Ligation of patent ductus arteriosus**

A 4th or 5th left intercostal thoracotomy is made (see Box 41-4). The left cranial lung lobe is reflected caudally using a saline soaked swab. The ductus is identified between the aorta positioned dorsally and the pulmonary artery ventrally. If not immediately evident, the ductus should be easily identified by palpation, as obvious fremitus will be present. The vagus nerve is identified as it runs over the ductus, and several stay sutures are placed in the mediastinal pleura above or below the vagus nerve. The mediastinal tissue is carefully incised and the vagus nerve is retracted dorsally or ventrally, respectively. The caudal aspect of the ductus is dissected using roght-angled forceps (Mixter forceps), passed parallel to the transverse plane. Dissection may be entirely external to the pericardium, or extended so that the pericardium is opened, depending on the individual ductus anatomy. The cranial aspect of the ductus is dissected with the tips of the forceps angles approximately 45° caudally. Dissection is continued caudally around the medial ductal wall; this must be performed with extreme care and patience to avoid damage to the vessels. A double strand or loop of 3M or 4M silk is soaked in saline and knotted near one end. Once dissection around the medial aspect of the ductus is complete and the tips of the forceps can be seen at the caudal border of the ductus, the knotted suture material is placed between the tips of the forceps and is very carefully passed around the ductus by slowly withdrawing the forceps. The knot is then cut and removed.

Ligation

The suture on the aortic side is tied first. As the PDA is ligated, in response to the pressure changes there may be a vagally mediated bradycardia (Branham's sign) so an anticholinergic agent such as atropine should be available for administration in this event. It is recommended that the ligature is tied slowly over several minutes to avoid this reflex. The suture on the pulmonic side is then tied and it is confirmed by auscultation using an esophageal stethoscope that the murmur has resolved. There should now be no fremitus on digital palpation. Stay sutures and the swab retracting the left cranial lung lobe are removed and the thorax is lavaged with warm sterile saline. A thoracostomy tube is placed (see Box 41-6) and closure of the thorax is routine.

The Jackson–Henderson approach[31]

The Jackson–Henderson approach is an alternate technique of PDA ligation that avoids dissection of the medial aspect of the PDA. The ductus is dissected on the cranial and caudal aspect as described above. The mediastinal pleura is incised between the origin of the left subclavian artery to the origin of the first intercostal artery dorsal to the aorta and the connective tissues on the medial aspect of the aorta at this level are bluntly dissected. A pair of right-angled forceps is passed immediately cranial to the ductus and around the medial aspect of the aorta so their tips can be seen dorsal to the aorta at the site where the mediastinum has been dissected. A knotted loop of 3M or 4M silk is placed in the tips of the forceps and the forceps are gently removed so that the suture material passes from dorsal to ventral around the medial aspect of the aorta immediately cranial to the ductus. This dissection around the medial aspect of the aorta is repeated immediately caudal to the ductus, the free end of the suture material passed into the tips of the forceps, and as they are withdrawn the suture material is taken around the caudal aspect of the ductus. Ligation then proceeds as described above.

Total pericardectomy

Although total pericardectomy (Box 48-5) may be appropriate in the management of some neoplastic or infectious pericardial diseases, it is very rarely indicated. It is a more challenging surgery with a greater risk of serious complications than subtotal pericardectomy.

Box 48-4 **Subtotal pericardectomy**

For subtotal pericardectomy the cat is positioned in lateral recumbency and a right or left 5th intercostal thoracotomy performed (see Box 41-4). A T-shaped incision is made in the pericardium: the base of the T extends from the apex of the heart, and the arms of the T extend around the circumference of the heart just ventral to the phrenic nerves. Stay sutures can be placed in the pericardium just ventral to the phrenic nerve to aid dissection and manipulation. If the pericardium is thickened the pericardial vessels can be hypertrophied and hemorrhage from these vessels can be marked so use of electrocautery applied to individual vessels, or in a cutting/coagulating mode, or use of a vessel sealing device prior to cutting the pericardium is recommended (see Chapter 13). The heart can gently be retracted by an assistant to aid access to the contralateral side of the heart if performing pericardectomy via intercostal thoracotomy. The contralateral phrenic nerve must be identified and preserved. This manipulation can cause arrhythmias and temporary reduction in venous return and cardiac output. The caudoventral mediastinal reflection is ligated, or alternatively a vessel sealing device can be applied to this structure to achieve hemostasis and this tissue is then divided.

After subtotal pericardectomy the excised pericardium is submitted for histopathologic analysis, and bacterial and/or fungal culture if considered appropriate. The pleural cavity is lavaged with sterile saline and the remaining pericardium is checked to ensure there is no ongoing hemorrhage. A thoracostomy tube is placed (see Chapter 41) and closure of the thorax is routine. The thoracostomy tube is drained on closure of the thorax, and again once the patient is positioned in sternal recumbency in recovery.

Epicardial pacemaker implantation

Anesthesia can worsen bradycardias and it is thus recommended that patients undergoing pacemaker implantation have temporary pacing under anesthesia until the permanent pacemaker has been implanted. Transthoracic pacing patches attached to an external pacer are useful in small patients, although their use results in patient movement, but neuromuscular blockade reduces this.

The author recommends a cranial midline celiotomy and transdiaphragmatic approach (Box 48-6). This gives good access whilst avoiding the invasiveness and potential complications of sternotomy or intercostal thoracotomy. If access is inadequate, the celiotomy incision can be extended to a caudal sternotomy.

Alternate approaches for epicardial pacemaker implantation include modifying the transdiaphragmatic approach by extending the cranial celiotomy by the addition of a caudal sternotomy or placement via a 5th or 6th left or right thoracotomy. A standard intercostal approach is made and the epicardial lead is secured as described for a midline celiotomy/transdiaphragmatic approach. The lead is exited through a stab incision made in the intercostal muscles at an intercostal site one to two intercostal spaces caudal or cranial to the site of surgical entry into the thorax. Several sites of generator placement have been described including a subcutaneous site overlying the craniolateral abdomen, the caudal thorax, and with and without suture anchorage to local structures such as an adjacent rib. A second incision may be necessary to implant the generator when using an intercostal approach for pacemaker placement. An alternate site for generator placement and anchorage, if the latissimus dorsi was retracted dorsally rather than incised during thoracotomy, is under this muscle adjacent to the thoracotomy site (but not overlying it). The generator can then be sutured to the external thoracic muscles.

Box 48-5 **Total pericardectomy**

This surgery for total pericardectomy is performed with the cat in dorsal recumbency via median sternotomy (see Box 41-5). The phrenic nerves are identified as they cross the pericardium. They are preserved by very careful dissection to free them from the pericardium; fine ophthalmic surgical scissors may be helpful to perform this delicate dissection. The apex of the heart is gently shifted to the right side of the thorax to aid access to the left heart base using the surgeon's or surgical assistant's fingers, or a malleable retractor wrapped in a saline-moistened surgical sponge, and likewise the apex is gently shifted to the left to improve access to the right side. The apex of the heart is gently moved in a cranial direction to access the caudal heart base. The anesthetist should be warned prior to these manipulations as they can result in a reduction in cardiac output or arrhythmias. Dissection should be temporarily halted to allow recovery (and adjustment of retraction if necessary) in the event of reduced cardiac output and/or arrhythmias. Saline-moistened umbilical tape is placed around the phrenic nerves once they have been freed from the pericardium, so they can gently be retracted away from the heart. The pericardium is incised/entered towards the apex of the heart and any PE is removed by suction. The pericardium is then incised towards the heart base. Once nearing the base of the heart, stay sutures are placed in the pericardium on either side of the incision to allow retraction and aid exposure so that the great vessels can clearly be identified and avoided. The pericardium is then dissected circumferentially around the heart base, close to the great vessels[26] leaving a small remaining 'rim' of pericardium (approximately 5 mm). Great care must be taken to avoid the heart base and great vessels being injured by sharp dissection, or by thermal trauma if using electrocautery or a vessel sealing device to achieve hemostasis of the pericardial vessels.

After total pericardectomy the excised pericardium is submitted for histopathologic analysis, and bacterial and/or fungal culture if considered appropriate. The pleural cavity is lavaged with sterile saline and the remaining rim of pericardium is checked to ensure there is no ongoing hemorrhage. A thoracostomy tube is placed (see Chapter 41) and closure of the thorax is routine. The thoracostomy tube is drained on closure of the thorax, and again once the patient is positioned in sternal recumbency in recovery, and thereafter as necessary.

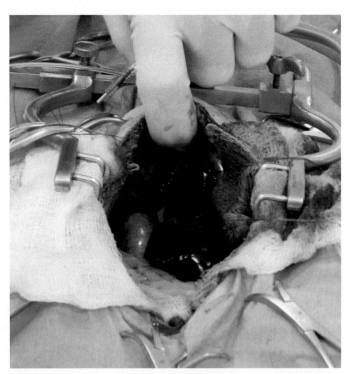

Figure 48-7 Intraoperative view during the approach for epicardial electrode placement by a caudal celiotomy and transdiaphragmatic approach. The liver and gall bladder are seen immediately caudal to the diaphragm which has been incised and is being retracted by stay sutures to aid exposure.

Box 48-6 **Epicardial pacemaker implantation through a cranial celiotomy and transdiaphragmatic approach**

An incision is made from the xiphoid and extending caudally up to the umbilicus. Self-retaining retractors are placed to facilitate access. Neuromuscular blockade may also facilitate surgery. The diaphragm is incised at its midline attachment to the sternum or just to the left of the midline. This incision is extended towards the central tendon. Stay sutures are placed in the diaphragm on either side of the incision to allow retraction and aid exposure (Fig. 48-7). The apex of the heart is readily identified, the pericardium is grasped at its apex using forceps and a 1–2 cm incision is made to allow access to the apex of the heart. Stay sutures can be placed in the pericardium on either side of the incision to aid manipulation. An epicardial pacemaker lead is placed in an avascular area at the apex of the left ventricle using either a non-sutured screw-in corkscrew electrode (according to manufacturer directions) or a sutured electrode (Fig. 48-8). If using a sutured technique, the electrode is anchored to the heart with three or four sutures (depending on the actual electrode being used) of 2M polypropylene; pre-placing the sutures before tying is helpful. If the

incision in the pericardium is small and herniation of the heart through this defect is impossible it can be left unsutured, otherwise it is repaired using 1.5M monofilament absorbable material placed in a simple continuous pattern. The end of the lead is exited from the thorax through a small stab incision through the diaphragm lateral to the incision made to enter the thorax, leaving a loop of epicardial lead within the pleural cavity to allow for cardiac and respiratory movements, activity, etc., in the conscious patient and thus avoid tension on the lead. The pulse generator is connected to the lead and covered in a saline-soaked swab, or surrounded by abdominal tissues (e.g., omentum) to activate the system (which is unipolar, requiring contact with the body).

Any external pacing is stopped and it is confirmed that the implanted system is achieving pacing as planned, and threshold tests and impedance can be interrogated with an appropriate programmer. The lead can be anchored with a suture to the diaphragm at its entry to the peritoneal cavity but if doing this care must be taken not to

Box 48-6 **Continued**

damage the insulation layer of the lead. The diaphragmatic incision is closed routinely and the pleural cavity is evacuated via needle or cannula drainage across the diaphragm.

Alternatively, a thoracostomy tube can be placed. Some reports describe leaving the pulse generator free within the abdomen, but generally it is recommended that the generator is anchored in a 'pocket' within the abdominal wall. A pocket just large enough to accommodate the transducer is made in the left cranioventral abdominal wall between the transversus abdominis and internal abdominal oblique muscles (Fig. 48-9). A loop of lead is left within the abdomen to avoid tension on the fixation, as above. Any excess lead is loosely coiled around the generator. Usually the generator has a small hole at an edge to allow it to be sutured and anchored to the local tissues. The incision in the internal abdominal oblique is closed using 2M or 3 M polydioxanone placed in a simple continuous pattern. Abdominal closure is routine. A postoperative radiograph of the lateral and/or dorsoventral thorax/abdomen is taken prior to recovery from anesthesia to confirm the electrode, lead, and pacemaker locations and to confirm that the lead is not kinked (Fig. 48-10).

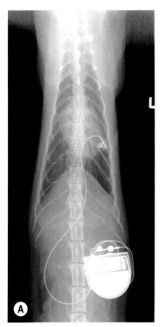
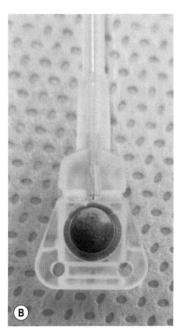
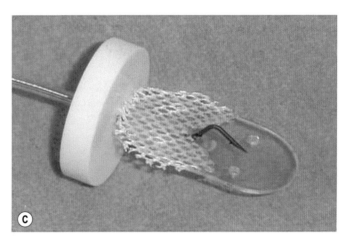

Figure 48-8 Electrodes that can be used for pacemakers in cats. **(A)** A non-sutured screw-in electrode has been used in this cat, that is 'self' anchored to the left ventricular wall at the apex. This postoperative radiograph also shows the transducer placed within the abdomen. Excess lead has been coiled around the transducer. The lead and transducer are then tucked into a pocket made between the internal abdominal oblique and transverse abdominal muscles of the left body wall. **(B)** Epicardial electrode. This type of electrode is placed onto the left ventricle at its apex and is anchored to the heart by sutures placed between holes in the end of the electrode and the left ventricular muscle. An additional suture is placed around the base of the electrode through the left ventricular muscle, providing additional anchorage. **(C)** Epicardial electrode. This type has a barbed point that is embedded into the left ventricular muscle at the apex; the electrode is then secured to the left ventricle by placing sutures through the holes in the end of the electrode to the ventricular muscle. The circular white disk at the base of the electrode is removed prior to implantation.

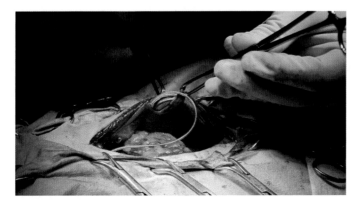

Figure 48-9 A pocket is made in the left cranioventral abdominal wall between the tranversus abdominis and internal abdominal oblique muscles for implantation of the pacemaker.

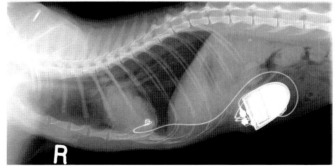

Figure 48-10 A postoperative radiograph is taken to confirm correct electrode, lead, and pacemaker locations and to confirm that the lead is not kinked.

POSTOPERATIVE CARE

General postoperative considerations after heart surgery include monitoring respiration (rate, effort), heart (arrhthymias, murmurs, rate), analgesic requirements, and management of the thoracostomy tube. Postoperative nursing after thoracic surgery and postoperative monitoring are covered in Chapters 3 and 4.

Thoracostomy tube

The thoracostomy tube is drained immediately on closure of the thorax and again once the patient is positioned in sternal recumbency in recovery. The thoracostomy tube is maintained whilst there is a significant volume of fluid being aspirated. For information about when to remove the tube see Chapter 41. Minimal fluid and air production is expected following uneventful PDA ligation and the thoracostomy tube can usually be removed in recovery or within several hours of completion of surgery. Intravenous fluid therapy with crystalloids is continued cautiously (2–4 mL/kg/hour) after heart surgery to avoid volume overload until patients are eating in recovery.

COMPLICATIONS AND PROGNOSIS

Complications after heart and pericardial surgery can range from minor and treatable to serious or even fatal, the most common including hemorrhage, pain, arrythmias, and cardiac arrest.

Patent ductus arteriosus

There is little data available in cats, but the anticipated potential complications are those reported in dogs. The most serious, potentially fatal intraoperative complication is rupture of the PDA, aorta or pulmonary artery during dissection around the ductus. Small tears to these vessels may be managed by the immediate application of digital pressure, but continued dissection may result in further hemorrhage as the tear in the damaged vessel may enlarge. A decision must be made whether to continue with surgery, or abandon the procedure on this occasion but second surgeries can be difficult due to scarring and fibrosis at the surgical site. If hemorrhage is marked, a vascular occlusion clamp (Satinsky) is applied to the aorta cranial to the ductus and caudal to the brachycephalic and left subclavian arteries. This allows blood flow to continue to the head and heart. Another vascular clamp is placed across the aorta caudal to the ductus to prevent retrograde aortic hemorrhage. Hemorrhage from the ductus will now be from the pulmonary artery, which is a lower pressure system so hemorrhage should not be as severe. Various techniques are suggested for resolving intraoperative hemorrhage including vascular repair using 1M polypropylene if the tear can be identified, ductal closure using polytetrafluoroethylene felt pledget buttressed mattress sutures, or ductal division between clamps and oversewing of the ductal edges.

In dogs, surgical mortality of less than 2% is achievable by experienced surgeons.[37–39] There is inadequate information available in cats to report an expected surgical outcome although the mortality rates are higher than in dogs for the few feline cases reported to date.

Outcome in dogs is excellent, but residual shunting has been reported in over 20% of cases.[40] Ductal division and oversewing of ductal ends prevents residual flow but is not recommended because it is more difficult than ligation and the risk of fatal intraoperative hemorrhage is not justified against the potential benefits gained.

Other rare postoperative complications in dogs include rupture of an aortic aneurysmal dilation with fatal hemorrhage, recanalization of the ductus with recurrent blood flow through the shunt, and bacterial colonization of the ductus, none of which have been reported in cats.

Pericardectomy

Failure to seal/ligate pericardial blood vessels cut during pericardectomy will result in postoperative hemorrhage, and occasionally a further surgery may be necessary to address this hemorrhage.

Epicardial pacemaker

Complications associated specifically with epicardial pacemaker implantation include displacement of the pacemaker electrode with accompanying loss of pacing, infection, seroma, and migration of the generator.

REFERENCES

1. Moon ML, Keene BW, Lessard P, et al. Age related changes in the feline cardiac silhouette. Vet Radiol Ultrasound 1993;34:315–20.

2. Jeraj K, Ogburn P, Lord PF, Wilson JW. Patent ductus arteriosus and pulmonary hypertension in a cat. J Am Vet Med Assoc 1978;172:1432–6.

3. Connolly DJ, Lamb CR, Boswood A. Right-to-left shunting patent ductus arteriosus with pulmonary hypertension in a cat. J Small Anim Pract 2003;44:184–8.

4. Martin M, Dukes-McEwan J. Congenital heart disease. In: Luis Fuentes EV, Johnson LR, Dennis S, editors. BSAVA Manual of canine and feline cardiorespiratory medicine. 2nd ed. Gloucester: BSAVA; 2010. p. 239.

5. Patterson DF. Canine congenital heart disease: epidemiology and etiological hypotheses. J Small Anim Pract 1971;12:263–87.

6. Buchanan JW. Causes and prevalence of cardiovascular disease. In: Kirk RW, Bonagura JD, editors. Kirk's current veterinary therapy. Philadelphia: WB Saunders; 1992. p. 647.

7. Hitchcock LS, Lehmkuhl LB, Bonagura JD, et al. Patent ductus arteriosus in cats: 21 cases. J Vet Int Med 2000;14:338(abstract).

8. Ware WA. The cardiovascular examination. In: Cardiovascular disease in small animal medicine (2007). London: Manson Publishing Ltd; 2007. p. 30.

9. Miller MW, Sisson D. Pericardial disorders. In: Ettinger SJ, Feldman EC, editors. Textbook of veterinary internal medicine. 5th ed. Philadelphia: WB Saunders; 2000. p. 923–36.

10. Marion J, Schwartz A, Ettinger S, et al. Pericardial effusion in a young dog. J Am Vet Med Assoc 1970;157:1055–63.

11. Sisson D, Thomas WP, Reed J, et al. Intrapericardial cysts in the dog. J Vet Int Med 1993;7:364–9.

12. Simpson DJ, Hunt GB, Church DB, et al. Benign masses in the pericardium of 2 dogs. Aust Vet J 1999;77:225–59.

13. Less RD, Bright JM, Orton EC. Intrapericardial cyst causing cardiac tamponade in a cat. J Am Anim Hosp Assoc 2000;36:115–19.

14. Loureiro J, Burrow R, Dukes-McEwan J. Canine intrapericardial cyst – complicated

surgical correction of an unusual cause of right heart failure. J Small Anim Pract 2009;50:492–7.

15. Davidson BJ, Paling AC, Lahmers SL, Nelson OL. Disease association and clinical assessment of the feline pericardial effusion. J Am Anim Hosp Assoc 2008;44:5–9.

16. Lui SK. Acquired cardiac lesions leading to congestive heart failure in the cat. Am J Vet Res 1970;31:2071–88.

17. Liu SK, Tashjian RJ, Patnaik AK. Congestive heart failure in the cat. J Am Vet Med Assoc 1970;156:1319–30.

18. Fossum TW, Mertens MM, Miller MW, et al. Thoracic duct ligation and pericardectomy for treatment of idiopathic chylothorax. J Vet Int Med 2004;18:307–10.

19. Bussadori R, Provera A, Martano M, et al. Pleural omentalisation with en bloc ligation of the thoracic duct and pericardiectomy for idiopathic chylothorax in nine dogs and four cats. Vet J 2011;188:234–6.

20. Bunch SE, Bolton GR, Hornbuckle EW. Pericardial effusion with restrictive pericarditis associated with congestive cardiomyopathy in a cat. J Am Anim Hosp Assoc 1981;17:739.

21. Ware WA. Management of arrhythmias. In: Cardiovascular disease in small animal medicine. London: Manson Publishing Ltd; 2007. p. 211.

22. Dennis S. Antiarrhythmic therapies. In: Luis Fuentes EV, Johnson LR, Dennis S, editors. BSAVA Manual of canine and feline cardiorespiratory medicine. 2nd ed. Gloucester: BSAVA; 2010. p. 183.

23. Cohen JS, Tilley LP, Liu S, et al. Patent ductus arteriosus in five cats. J Am Anim Hosp Assoc 1975;11:95–101.

24. Jones CL, Buchanan JW. Patent ductus arteriosus: anatomy and surgery in a cat. J Am Vet Med Assoc 1981;179:364–9.

25. Orton CE. Cardiac surgery. In: Slatter D, editor. Textbook of small animal surgery, vol. 1. 3rd ed. Philadelphia: WB Saunders; 2003. p. 958.

26. Fossum TW. Surgery of the cardiovascular system. In: Small animal surgery. 3rd ed. Missouri: Mosby Elsevier; 2007. p. 805.

27. Bonagura JD, Helphrey ML, Muir WW. Complications associated with permanent pacemaker implantation in the dog. J Am Vet Med Assoc 1983;182:149–55.

28. Fingeroth JM, Birchard SJ. Transdiaphragmatic approach for permanent cardiac pacemaker implantation in dogs. Vet Surg 1986;15:329–33.

29. Fox PR, Matthiesen DT, Purse D, Brown NO. Ventral abdominal, transdiaphragmatic approach for implantation of cardiac pacemakers in the dog. J Am Vet Med Assoc 1986;189:1303–8.

30. Fox PR, Moise NS, Woodfield JA, Darke PG. Techniques and complications of pacemaker implantation in four cats. J Am Vet Med Assoc 1991;12:1742–53.

31. Jackson WF, Henderson RA. Ligature placement in closure of patent ductus arteriosus. J Am Anim Hosp Assoc 1979;15:55–8.

32. Boothe HW. Use of ligating clips for patent ductus arteriosus surgery in small animals. Vet Rep 1989;2:6–9.

33. Borenstein N, Behr L, Chetboul V, et al. Minimally invasive patent ductus arteriosus occlusion in 5 dogs. Vet Surg 2004;33:309–13.

34. Stafford-Johnson M. Decision making in suspected congenital heart disease in cats and dogs. In Pract 2006;28:538–43.

35. MacDonald KA. Congenital heart disease of puppies and kittens. Vet Clin Small Anim 2006;36:503–31.

36. Schneider M, Hildebrandt N. Transvenous embolization of the patent ductus arteriosus with detachable coils in 2 cats. J Vet Int Med 2003;17:349–53.

37. Eyster GE, Eyster JT, Cords GB, Johnston J. Patent ductus arteriosus in the dog: characteristics of occurrence and results of surgery in one hundred consecutive cases. J Am Vet Med Assoc 1986;168:435–8.

38. Buchanan JW. Patent ductus arteriosus. Semin Vet Med Surg Small Anim 1994;9:168–76.

39. Hunt GB, Simpson DJ, Beck JA, et al. Intra-operative haemorrhage during patent ductus arteriosus ligation in dogs. Vet Surg 2001;30:58–63.

40. Stanley BJ, Luis-Fuentes V, Darke PG. Comparison of the incidence of residual shunting between two surgical techniques used for ligation of patent ductus arteriosus in the dog. Vet Surg 2003;32:231–7.

Section | 7 |

S.J. Langley-Hobbs, J.F. Ladlow, J.L. Demetriou

The head and neck

The final part of the book covers surgery of the head and neck in the cat. In the first chapter, conditions affecting all the parts of the head that have not been covered in previous chapters are described, for example salivary gland disease. In subsequent chapters, conditions of the throat area, including the pharynx and larynx are described. Some diseases will affect more than one organ or region; polyps are a notable disease in cats that can affect the middle ear but also have clinical signs that are attributable to a nasopharyngeal location.

Aural anatomy is consistent across most cat breeds so ear disease attributable solely to conformational defects is not common. However, ear disease is still a significant problem in the cat and surgery in the form of partial or complete aural resection can be curative for some conditions, most notably tumors. Surgery for nasal disease is most commonly performed for nasal planum tumors or chronic nasal disease associated with foreign bodies.

Thyroid disease in cats is common and surgery is one treatment option to consider alongside medical management and radioactive iodine therapy. In the chapter on the thyroid and parathyroid gland, decision making with regard to the best treatment for the individual cat is covered.

The feline head is a site that is commonly affected by neoplasia and therefore surgical management of neoplasia, including maxillectomy and mandibulectomy and the resection of brain tumors, is discussed. Although these may be advanced surgical procedures that would be best performed at a specialist center, an understanding of what is entailed is important to be able to discuss the most appropriate treatment options with owners of affected cats.

In the penultimate chapter of the book, management of eyelid and orbital disease is covered. There are already entire textbooks dedicated to ocular disease in the cat and it was not the aim of this textbook to fully cover surgical management of all eye disease in this chapter. Instead, some conditions that might be treated by a more general surgeon, as opposed to an ophthalmologist, are described, such as eyelid surgery and enucleation.

The final chapter provides in-depth descriptions of brain surgery, including pituitary gland resection for pituitary dependent hyperadrenocorticism in the cat, a procedure that is currently being performed at specialist centers to successfully treat this condition.

Chapter |49|

Head

S.J. Langley-Hobbs

A variety of conditions affect the feline head, some of which are common. If disease is located in an area that is readily visible to the owner (e.g., neoplasms or inflammatory conditions of the skin) then early recognition and prompt treatment is possible. However, other conditions that are located in regions that are not easily visible (e.g., inside the mouth) are often only detected at a later stage when the cat becomes clinically affected: late diagnosis and the invasive nature of some conditions of the head can influence the prognosis. In this chapter some general information will be given about head examination, imaging, and some of the common diseases, with more specific sections on the tongue, tonsils, salivary glands, chin, cheeks, and lips. The reader is referred to other chapters in this part (Chapters 50 to 58) for detailed information on other organs or parts of the head.

SURGICAL ANATOMY

Lips, cheeks and mouth

The lips in the cat are small and relatively immobile compared to the dog. They form a large rima oris, with the upper and lower lips meeting at the commissure caudally. The lips consist of skin, muscle, and mucosa and contain numerous small scattered salivary glands. The cheeks form the buccal vestibule, which receives salivary secretions from the parotid, molar, and zygomatic salivary glands. The hard palate separates the oral and nasal cavities and is formed from the incisive, maxillary, and palatine bones. The oral aspect of the hard palate is covered by thick mucosa with transverse folds (rugae) that are continuous with the gingiva rostrally, laterally, and the soft palate caudally. The floor of the oral cavity is supported by paired mylohyoideus muscles passing between the mandibular bodies. The ventral oral mucosa has two protuberances to either side of the lingual frenulum known as sublingual caruncles, marking the opening of the mandibular and sublingual salivary ducts.[1]

The tissues of the lips and cheek are supplied by the facial artery and infraorbital artery. The facial nerve provides motor innervation to these structures and the trigeminal nerve sensory innervation.

Tongue

The tongue is an integral and functional part of the oral cavity. It is composed primarily of skeletal muscle. The body of the tongue is joined to the floor of the oral cavity by an oral fold called the frenulum. The cat has multiple caudal-facing filiform papillae on the dorsal surface of the tongue that assist with the prehension of food and water and they are also used for grooming.

The intrinsic muscles of the tongue consist of longitudinal, transverse, and perpendicular fibres. The extrinsic muscles have an osseous origin and radiate into the tongue, and they include the styloglossal, hypoglossal, and genioglossal muscles.[2] The mylohyoid muscle suspends the tongue between the mandibular bodies and is important for the induction of deglutition.

The vascular supply to the tongue is primarily from the paired lingual artery, supplemented by the paired sublingual artery, and both of these arteries arise from the linguofacial trunk. The innervation of the tongue is from the lingual branch of the mandibular nerve, the chorda tympanii of the intermediofacial nerve, the glossopharyngeal nerve, and the vagal nerve.[2] These nerves are individually responsible for sensations such as pain, heat, and taste. The hypoglossal nerve is responsible for motor function, and damage to this nerve will result in paralysis of the tongue.[2]

Tonsils

The two palatine tonsils are located in the lateral pharyngeal walls and they consist of multiple subepithelial lymph nodules. They have efferent lymphatics only and their function is to provide an immunologic barrier to protect the respiratory and alimentary systems. They are located in a fossa, the medial wall of which is formed by a falciform fold from the soft palate, the tonsilar fold.[2]

Salivary glands

Cats have five major salivary glands (parotid, mandibular, sublingual, molar, and zygomatic) (Fig. 49-1); the molar gland is absent in the dog and humans. The mandibular and sublingual glands empty by

© 2014 Elsevier Ltd
DOI: 10.1016/B978-0-7020-4336-9.00049-4

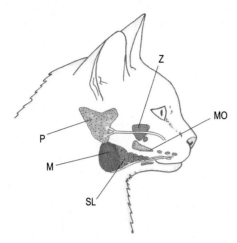

Figure 49-1 Diagram showing the salivary glands of the cat. M, mandibular; Mo, molar; P, parotid; SL, sublingual; Z, zygomatic.

separate duct systems, which may exit to a common papilla (sublingual caruncle) just lateral to the frenulum of the tongue.

The parotid gland is the largest salivary gland. It lies ventral to the ear canal and it slightly overlaps the masseter muscle. The posterior facial vein enters its ventral border. The parotid duct leaves cranioventrally, passes over the masseter muscle, and enters the mouth in a small papilla opposite the most prominent cusp of the last premolar tooth. Some accessory parotid gland tissue can be seen at the cranial end of the duct just in front of the zygomatic gland.[1]

The mandibular gland lies caudal to the masseter muscle and ventral to the parotid. The posterior facial vein crosses over the mandibular gland. The mandibular duct leaves the gland medially and runs craniomedially in close association with the sublingual gland. It passes between the extrinsic muscles of the tongue and then continues craniad against the oral mucosa, running parallel to the mandible to open at the apex of the sublingual papilla, accompanied by the sublingual duct.[1]

The sublingual gland is closely associated with the mandibular gland caudally. It extends cranially with the sublingual duct, running in close association with the mandibular duct.[1]

The molar gland lies between the mucosa of the lips and the orbicularis oris muscle. It is a triangular-shaped gland, wider caudally. It extends to a level between the first premolar and the canine. Molar ducts open directly through the mucosa into the oral cavity, with the mandibular duct lying close or adjacent to it. Other separate openings may be present.

The zygomatic gland is usually ovoid or pyramidal in shape and it lies between the zygomatic arch in the lower part of the orbit in contact with the ventral orbit. The ventral aspect of the gland rests against the mucosa of the mouth caudal to the molar teeth. The major duct leaves the ventral part of the gland and enters the oral cavity through the mucosa about 3 mm caudal to the molar tooth. Minor ducts may also be present.

GENERAL CONSIDERATIONS

Cats that have undergone trauma rather than those presenting for chronic or non-traumatic disease may have other life-threatening injuries that require immediate attention and it is therefore important that the reader is familiar with the preoperative assessment of these cases (see Chapter 1). For example, a cat with an avulsed chin may also have concurrent mandibular or maxillary fractures or brain injury. Once the

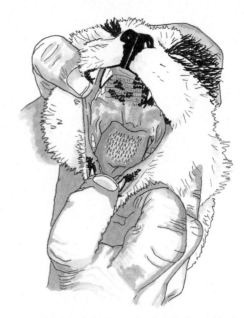

Figure 49-2 Examination of the cat's mouth is facilitated by holding the head steady with one hand and using the first finger of the other hand to open the lower jaw.

animal is stable, further examination of the head injuries can be undertaken. For uncooperative cats this may need to be performed under sedation or general anesthesia.

Clinical examination and signs

Clinical signs of oral injury or disease include hypersalivation, loss of appetite or fastidiousness, and difficulty in swallowing or prehending food. Affected animals may be in poor condition due to a reduced intake of food. Halitosis with or without hemorrhage from the mouth may also be reported.

A thorough examination of the head should involve a visual inspection looking for asymmetry, swellings, ulceration, and trauma. The mandibular salivary glands and the submandibular lymph nodes should be palpated just caudal to the skull. Injury to the chin and lips will usually be obvious to the observer, except perhaps in long-haired cats. The inside of the mouth can be inspected in amenable animals by placing the first finger on the lower incisors and pulling the chin distally, keeping the thumb and middle finger of the other hand on the lips just caudal to the canine teeth (Fig. 49-2). The hard palate should be inspected for signs of trauma or bruising. The dental arcades should be evaluated for tartar and broken or missing teeth. Trauma or disease of the rostral tongue should be easy to identify, but conditions affecting the caudal portion can be missed. To aid visualization of the caudal part of the mouth it is useful to place a finger on the tongue to depress it. Normally, the tonsils in a cat are not visible; however, with certain diseases the tonsils may protrude from the crypt and show a change in size and appearance. Salivary gland conditions can result in ranulas (Fig. 49-3). A finger can be used to press dorsally in the intermandibular space causing displacement of the tongue so that the subglossal area can be inspected. A common location of squamous cell carcinomas is in the sublingual area near to the frenulum of the tongue.

In older animals or those with suspected concurrent disease or trauma, further investigations may be indicated, such as biochemical and hematologic analysis of blood to help identify any abnormalities that may require further management.

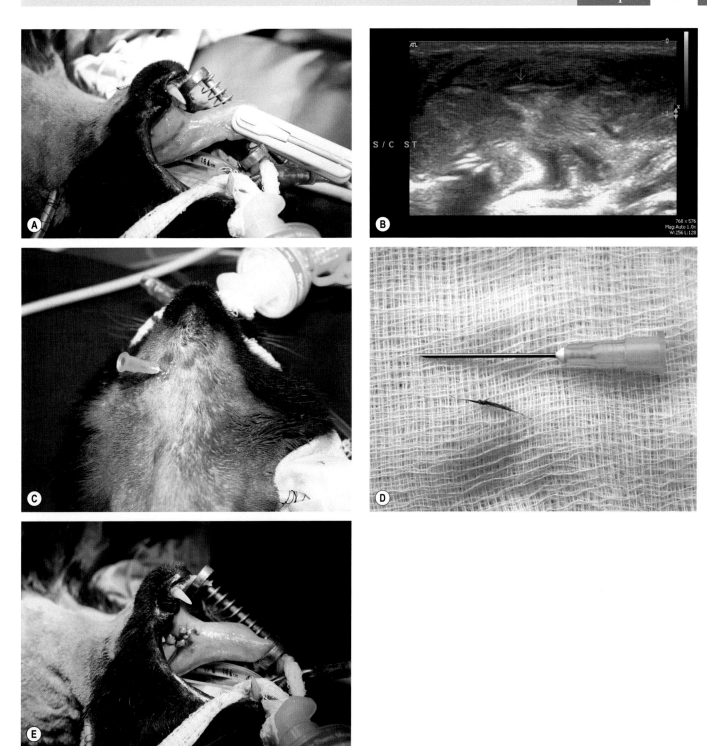

Figure 49-3 An 18-year-old cat presented with a three week history of progressive increase in difficulty eating and a mild pyrexia. There was a firm intermandibular swelling and purulent material was aspirated from this mass. **(A)** On oral examination there was sublingual swelling and a ranula. **(B)** Ultrasound evaluation revealed a structure suspected to be a foreign body (arrow). **(C)** A needle was placed preoperatively with the tip adjacent to the suspected foreign body to aid surgical exploration. **(D)** A grass seed was removed at surgery. **(E)** The ranula was marsupialized in an attempt to decrease its size. An esophagostomy tube was placed for postoperative feeding until the cat was able to prehend orally again.

Feline orofacial pain syndrome

A condition known as feline orofacial pain syndrome (FOPS) has been described in one study.[3] This is a pain disorder of cats relating to behavioral signs of oral discomfort and tongue mutilation. The condition primarily affects Burmese cats and is characterized by an episodic, typically unilateral discomfort with pain-free intervals. The discomfort is apparently triggered, in many cases, by mouth movements. The majority of cases in this study had a history of mild oral lesions and a small number of cases experienced their first sign of discomfort during eruption of their permanent teeth. The degree of pain these cats express seems to be unrelated to the severity of oral lesions and is therefore thought to be a neuropathic or anxiety-related condition.

Diagnostic imaging

In cases of suspected neoplasia, a baseline check for metastases should be performed and include three-view thoracic radiographs (see Chapter 9). Survey radiographs of the affected area of the head can provide useful information about whether underlying bone is involved and radiographs will be necessary in trauma cases to assess for the presence of fractures. Intraoral and oblique radiographs can be particularly useful as they avoid superimposition of bony structures.

More advanced imaging such as computed tomography or magnetic resonance imaging may be indicated in certain situations such as cases with neoplasia, prior to surgical planning or radiation therapy. Ultrasonography can be useful for investigation of soft tissue inflammation of the tongue and detection of foreign bodies (Fig. 49-3B) and it has been used in one study to help delineate soft tissue margins of lingual squamous cell carcinoma.[4]

Biopsy

It can be difficult to determine whether a lesion is neoplastic or inflammatory from the visual or radiographic appearance alone and this is particularly the case for oral lesions in the cat where inflammatory lesions (e.g., hyperplastic gingival, eosinophilic granuloma complex) are common and can be aggressive. The primary lesion may be initially evaluated by fine needle aspiration to provide a rapid preliminary cytological assessment. Regional lymph nodes, whether enlarged or not, need to be assessed via fine needle aspiration and cytologic examination.

If sedation is required to obtain the aspirate, it is also recommended to consider taking a biopsy. A biopsy is crucial for obtaining a sample for histopathologic examination to enable an accurate diagnosis and plan appropriate treatment; biopsy of masses should be undertaken prior to attempting surgical resection. It is important to obtain a deep sample as oral lesions are frequently infected, necrotic, or inflamed. Large samples that include healthy tissue at the edge and also include deeper areas of the lesion will increase the diagnostic yield. Lesions such as feline oral squamous cell carcinoma should never be biopsied through the skin but rather through an intraoral incision. An intraoral biopsy prevents seeding of the tumor into the surrounding normal external tissues. These tissues may be required for local reconstruction after oral tumor excision and, thus, need to be preserved without tumor contamination. For more details on different biopsy procedures see Chapter 14.

SURGICAL DISEASES OF THE HEAD

Many conditions around the head will not be confined to a single organ or area. Neoplasia, for example, may primarily appear to affect the chin or lips but closer inspection and further imaging may reveal invasion into the bone of the mandible or maxilla. For further information on diseases of the different parts of the head the reader is referred to Chapters 50 to 58.

Neoplasia of the head

Oral neoplasia overall is common in cats, accounting for 3–12% of all feline neoplasms.[4] Differential diagnoses in cats with oral masses include dental disease, malignant tumors, benign abnormalities (e.g.,

ranulas), and infections.[5–8] Neoplasias affecting the mandible and maxilla are discussed in detail in Chapter 55.

In feline cases of oral pharyngeal neoplasia the tongue is the most frequent tumor site, followed by the gingiva.[6] In a survey of 340 cats with cutaneous neoplasia, the head was the most common site for basal cell tumors, mast cell tumors, and squamous cell carcinomas.[9] The general characteristics of skin tumors are discussed in detail in Chapter 20.

Squamous cell carcinoma

Oral squamous cell carcinoma is a malignant tumor that may occur anywhere within the oral cavity. It is locally invasive, infrequently metastasizes to ipsilateral regional lymph nodes, and rarely spreads to distant sites. Given the local invasiveness the prognosis for this fast-growing, invasive tumor in cats is grave, so it is vital to identify and treat the condition early. The average reported duration of survival after diagnosis of this tumor has been reported as two months.[8] There is no sex or breed predisposition, although entire male cats were more commonly affected in one study.[8] The gingiva, tongue, and sublingual region are the most commonly reported sites of squamous cell carcinoma.[6,8]

Mucosal ulceration, necrosis, and severe suppurative inflammation are commonly associated with oral squamous cell carcinoma. There may also be mucosal swelling in the absence of ulceration, or animals may be presented solely for chin enlargement. Gingival squamous cell carcinoma often invades the underlying mandible or maxilla, leading to severe and extensive tumor involvement of the bone in that area and marked osteolysis on radiographs. In addition to osteolysis, there is commonly periosteal new bone formation and osseous metaplasia of tumor stroma detected on radiography and computed tomography (CT) evaluation.[8]

Although several environmental risk factors have been recognized, the cause of feline oral squamous cell carcinoma remains poorly defined. Various potential contributing factors have been suggested (Box 49-1).[7]

To date, no therapies or combinations of therapy have shown great success in treating this tumor. Local and regional disease control is the treatment goal. Surgery such as mandibulectomy (see Chapter 55), radiation therapy (see Chapter 15), or radiation therapy combined with chemotherapy (see Chapter 16) are the principal treatment modalities used. The one-year survival rate is generally less than 10%, with a median survival time of approximately three months for most therapies. The overall poor survival times in cats with oral squamous cell carcinoma may reflect the tumor's location and aggressive behavior, as sublingual and maxillary tumors are rarely resectable, and also the fact that this tumor is often diagnosed late in the course of the disease. Assessing an individual patient's tumor stage and location is critical in advising an owner regarding possible treatment options and likely outcome. Early diagnosis followed by aggressive local treatment and appropriate supportive care is the best way to improve survival times. Recurrence despite aggressive surgical resection is common, thus multimodality therapy appears to be indicated.

Box 49-1 Potential contributing causes to feline squamous cell carcinoma[7]

Passive smoking
Flea control collars
Flea shampoos (decreased risk)
Diet

Fibrosarcoma

Feline fibrosarcoma is one of the most common subcutaneous neoplasms in cats and the second most common feline oral neoplasm in one survey of 371 cases.[5] It is a locally aggressive tumor with a moderate metastatic rate and high recurrence rates.[10] Oral fibrosarcoma affects cats of a wide age range, but with a median age of 10 years.[5] The tumor is usually located in the gingiva or palate, arising from the submucosal stroma. It is locally infiltrative and causes local destruction of bone and muscle.[5] Aggressive surgical excision is the treatment of choice, but unfortunately recurrence rate is high due to poor local disease control.

Inflammatory disorders of the head

Proliferative inflammatory eosinophilic granulomatosis is a common disease of the head in cats and it may be localized to the skin, the mucocutaneous junctions or the oral cavity. The disease has three different manifestations: indolent ulcer, eosinophilic plaque, and eosinophilic granuloma. The last mentioned form can affect the cheek, the tongue, and the palate. Pain does not appear to be a common feature, but the nodular form in the oral cavity may make deglutition difficult.

The eosinophilic granuloma complex was reported in 17 related Norwegian forest cats and the high prevalence of the disease in this population is suggestive of a genetic background.[11] There may also be a viral etiology. The lesions of acute feline calicivirus infection can appear similar; they are of a transient vesiculo-ulcerative nature and involve, to varying degrees, the palate, tongue, gingiva, lips, nasal philtrum, and oral fauces. Chronic ulceroproliferative faucitis is a specific but uncommon sequela to persistent feline calicivirus oral carriage.[12]

These lesions can be treated by medical management, surgical resection alone or in combination with therapeutics.

Abscessation

Abscesses around the head are common sequelae to cat fight or bite injuries. The normal flora of the cat's mouth includes strains of hemolytic staphylococci, β-hemolytic streptococci, *Pasteurella multocida*, *Escherichia coli*, and fusiforms[13] so abscesses are often associated with these bacteria. Affected animals may present with depression, difficulty eating, pyrexia, and obvious swelling. In early cases, careful inspection may be required to find a puncture hole or small scab. Treatment is usually successful by provision for ventral drainage and parenteral antibiotics. In more severe cases, in animals that are also systemically unwell (e.g., with pyrexia, dehydration, etc.), more intensive treatment would be recommended with intravenous fluids, drainage, and flushing the abscess cavity in combination with systemic intravenous antibiosis. Skin necrosis may occur secondarily to a large abscess that has formed rapidly causing local ischemia of the skin: the dead skin will slough or can be debrided as part of the management (Fig. 49-4). These lesions are also very painful so analgesics should be administered. Unless contraindicated, non-steroidal anti-inflammatory drugs are recommended in these cases. Alternatively, opioids can be administered to hospitalized patients.

SURGICAL DISEASES OF THE TONGUE

The feline tongue is particularly prone to trauma and foreign bodies due to its barbed nature. Neoplasms are occasionally diagnosed but animals are often only presented at an advanced stage as these are most commonly sublingual so are easily missed in the early stage of the disease. It is important to fully evaluate the tongue, examining both the caudal aspect and sublingual area, to avoid missing foreign bodies or masses.

Tongue trauma

The tongue is prone to injury in the cat either as a result of self-inflicted injury as the cat bites its own tongue during a traumatic incident (Fig. 49-5) or from a foreign body such as a fishing hook or needle and thread. Small lesions can be left to heal by second intention. More severe lacerations should be repaired using simple interrupted sutures of absorbable suture material such as 2M poliglecaprone or polyglyconate. If a proportion of the tongue is lost due to necrosis or trauma then intravenous fluids and provision for feeding

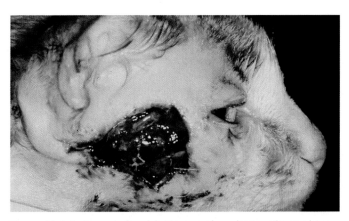

Figure 49-4 A stray cat after debridement of an abscess. The overlying skin was necrotic and required resection. A large deficit was present on the cheek of the cat, that healed by second intention with appropriate wound management. *(Courtesy of Tanya Mills.)*

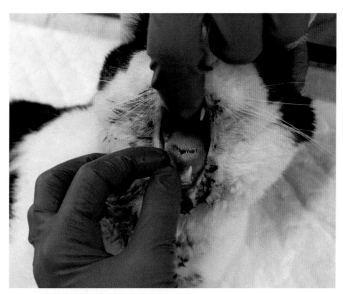

Figure 49-5 A five-year-old male domestic short-haired cat that presented after a suspected road traffic accident. There was a full thickness central wound on the tongue suspected to be secondary to the cat biting through the tongue. The lateral margins of the tongue were intact and no specific treatment was required aside from placement of a feeding tube to bypass the mouth while the laceration healed.

via a tube may be required in some cases until the cat is able to prehend food on its own. In dogs, resection of up to 50% of the tongue can be performed without major complications; however, conclusive evidence regarding the success of glossectomy in cats is unavailable. Cats are generally less tolerant than dogs of procedures that affect their ability to eat (e.g., mandibulectomies and maxillectomies) so therefore their postoperative recovery from large glossectomies (up to 50%) is less predictable. In addition to difficulties in eating, the ability to groom, which is an important aspect of their behavior, will also be severely compromised.

Foreign bodies

Gastrointestinal foreign bodies are relatively common in cats. Fastidious grooming habits and the anatomy of the tongue with its backward facing barbs makes expulsion of sticky foreign material difficult in the cat. Thread and sewing needles are common gastrointestinal foreign bodies and the thread is most commonly anchored at either the tongue or the pylorus – a thorough examination of the mouth, including the sublingual area, is necessary for the thread or a needle.[14] In a review of 24 cats with gastrointestinal linear foreign bodies, 13 had the linear foreign bodies wrapped around either the base of the tongue or in the sublingual area at presentation, but in six of these cats this was missed at first inspection.[15] Cutting and the release of the foreign body may be successful in some cats and can avoid the need for intestinal surgery if clinical signs do not warrant immediate surgical intervention.[15] When considering conservative management it is important to hospitalize the cat and monitor it clinically, radiographically, and hematalogically for any changes that may indicate the need for subsequent surgical intervention[15] (see Chapter 29).

Neoplasia of the tongue

Reported lingual neoplasms in the cat include squamous cell carcinoma,[5,7] fibrosarcoma and lymphoma,[16] which represent the majority (approximately 24%) of all oral tumors in this species. The most common site of oral squamous cell carcinoma (SCC) is in the sublingual area in the ventral portion of the tongue near the frenulum (Fig. 49-6). Mucosal ulceration, necrosis, and severe suppurative inflammation are common findings with SCC. In one study, cats with lingual SCC were younger (mean, 11.9 years) compared to cats with gingival SCC (mean, 13.6 years).[8] Ultrasonography may be used to help

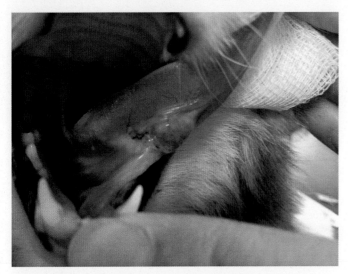

Figure 49-6 Lingual squamous cell carcinoma in a cat.

delineate soft tissue margins of lingual SCC. Treatment can be attempted by wide surgical excision, which may necessitate concurrent mandibulectomy, followed with radiation and chemotherapy, but prognosis is guarded (one year survival of <25%) as it is not often possible to achieve local control.[17]

Inflammatory disease of the tongue

Eosinophilic granulomas can affect the tongue. These lesions can be treated by medical management, surgical resection alone, or in combination with therapeutics. Laser-assisted surgery had been reported for one cat with a lesion involving the caudal tongue and pharynx.[18] After surgery the cat recovered rapidly on steroids, and its condition and quality of life improved greatly. Conventional surgery was not felt to be appropriate in this case because of the vascular nature of the tongue and pharynx.

Thyroglossal duct cyst

The thyroglossal duct is a tract that connects the foramen cecum at the base of the tongue to the thyroid gland as the gland undergoes embryologic descent to the trachea. Thyroglossal cysts have been reported in two cats with cervical masses[19,20] and they will be discussed further in Chapter 53.

SURGICAL DISEASES OF THE SALIVARY GLANDS

Salivary gland neoplasia, sialoadenitis, and mucoceles have all been reported in cats.

Neoplasia of the salivary glands and duct

The predominant presenting sign for animals with salivary gland neoplasia is that of a mass being noted by the owner. Other common complaints included halitosis, dysphagia, and exophthalmia.[21] Adenocarcinoma is the most commonly reported tumor affecting the salivary gland in cats,[5,21] with the mandibular and parotid glands most frequently affected[22,23] (Fig. 49-7). Metastasis is rare, but has been reported locally and distally to draining lymph nodes, liver, and lung, as well as the spleen.[24-26] Thirty cats with histopathologically confirmed salivary gland neoplasia were retrospectively reviewed in a multi-institutional study.[21] Siamese cats were over-represented, indicating a possible breed predisposition.[21] The median survival time for the thirty cats in this study was 516 days.[21] Other salivary gland tumors are rarely reported in cats (Box 49-2).

Adenocarcinoma has also been reported affecting the salivary duct in five cats.[30] The cats ranged in age from seven–13 years, and two of the cats were Siamese. The minor salivary gland was involved in four of the five cats. Two cats had local metastasis at the time of diagnosis.

Necrotizing sialoadenitis

Necrotizing sialometaplasia is an ischemic disease of the salivary glands. Unilateral swelling of mandibular salivary glands in two cats, aged nine and seven years, was diagnosed as necrotizing sialometaplasia.[34] Salivary gland infarction has been reported in eleven cats, representing 13% of salivary gland disease cases in a review of 85 cats.[23] Unilateral mandibular salivary glands were affected in all 13 cases and males and females were equally represented.

Histologic features are used to differentiate the disease from other salivary gland lesions, particularly neoplasia, and they include lobular

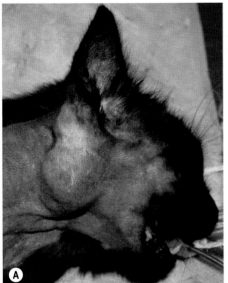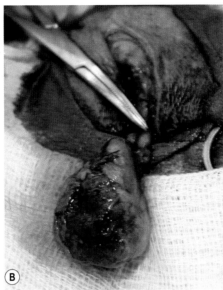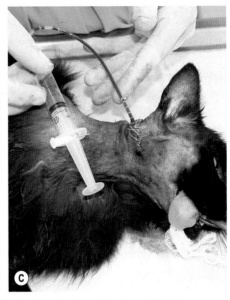

Figure 49-7 Salivary adenocarcinoma affecting the right mandibular salivary gland in a nine-year-old male domestic short-haired cat. **(A)** A large mass is visible on the caudolateral aspect of the jaw of the cat just ventral to the ear. **(B)** The salivary gland has been dissected and is shown just prior to duct ligation to include some of the monostomatic parts of the sublingual glands that are closely associated. **(C)** A closed suction drain has been placed at the end of surgery. *(Courtesy of Jon Hall.)*

Box 49-2 Salivary gland tumors in the cat

Adenocarcinomas[21]
Sebaceous carcinoma[27]
Basal cell adenocarcinomas[28]
Epithelial-myoepithelial carcinoma[29]
Salivary duct adenocarcinomas[30]
Malignant mixed tumor/carcinosarcoma[31,32]
Oncocytoma[33]

---

necrosis of salivary tissue, squamous metaplasia conforming to duct and/or acinar outlines, preservation of salivary lobular morphology, and variable inflammation and granulation tissue.[34] The treatment is surgical excision (see below). In dogs, the disease is extremely painful but recovery from surgery in the two cats reported in one study was uneventful.[34] Although the precise etiology remains unclear, a vascular lesion seems likely. The prognosis following surgical excision appears favorable.

Salivary mucocele

Salivary mucoceles are formed by the extravasation and accumulation of saliva in tissues adjacent to a salivary gland. The accumulated saliva incites an inflammatory response, leading to a walled-off accumulation of mucoid fluid. Trauma can cause salivary mucoceles; however, most cases are presumed to be idiopathic.

Salivary mucoceles are uncommon in cats although case reports exist.[35–41] All the salivary glands, except the molar gland, can be affected and in one series of seven cats with this condition the sublingual gland was involved in five cases and the mucocele formed a ranula in all of the cases.[42]

The mass is usually detected by careful physical examination.[42] A unilateral fluctuant non-painful mass, close to the salivary glands, in the sublingual or cervical area or on the buccal mucosal surface is found on visual and physical examination.[42] The cat may present with dysphagia, exophthalmia, and dyspnea depending on which gland is involved. Intermittent vomiting, ptyalism, and lethargy have also been reported.[42] If a ranula is large enough, respiratory stridor or respiratory distress may be present. Clinical signs largely depend on the location and size of the mucocele. Differential diagnoses include an abscess, neoplasia, a foreign body, and a granuloma.[42]

The diagnosis of salivary mucoceles involves aspiration of a thick, stringy, golden (or often dark pink due to the presence of erythrocytes) fluid with low cellularity from the mass. Staining of the aspirated fluid with periodic acid Schiff stain will confirm the presence of saliva. Sialography may be useful for identifying specific gland involvement when it is not readily apparent. Other diagnostic imaging tests (radiography, ultrasonography, computed tomography) may help rule out other disease processes, such as a foreign object or involvement or invasion of multiple tissues, but are unlikely to definitively identify a salivary mucocele.

Treatment options include draining the mucocele, marsupialization, and removing the involved gland. Drainage alone is likely to result in recurrence unless the source of mucus is addressed. Marsupialization, which involves excising an elliptical section of mucosa over the mucocele, draining the saliva, and apposing the mucosal surface to underlying connective tissue, does not address the underlying problem. Because of potential complications such as frequent recurrence and the fact that future surgical intervention would be difficult, marsupialization is not the preferred procedure unless the primary problem can be identified and treated concurrently (see Fig. 49-3). Thus, surgically excising the affected gland is the recommended treatment in all cases (see below). In one series of seven cats with salivary mucoceles, with a follow up ranging from two months to 13 years, no signs of recurrence were seen in any of the cats after salivary gland resection.[42]

Three dogs and one cat were diagnosed at the University of Pennsylvania Veterinary Hospital as having parotid salivary duct rupture and fistula as a result of previous surgery. Sialography was used to confirm the diagnosis. Two animals were treated by ligation, and two by anastomosis of the parotid duct. All four animals returned to normal after treatment.[43]

SURGICAL DISEASES OF THE LIPS AND CHEEK

Cleft lips

Cleft lips or harelips (cheiloschisis) can be unilateral or bilateral and are considered rare in the cat.[44] They are congenital defects either seen in isolation or in conjunction with cleft palate (see Chapter 56) and normally affecting the upper lip.[44] There are reports of a heritable tendency in Siamese but teratogenic drugs such as griseofulvin are also implicated in the pathogenesis of this condition.[45,46] Surgery can be attempted in cases that have associated clinical signs such as recurrent infections, nasal discharge, oronasal fistulae.

Neoplasia

Neoplastic lesions of the lips and cheek in the cat include squamous cell sarcoma (Fig. 49-8), fibrosarcoma, neurofibroma, melanoma, mast cell tumor, basal cell carcinoma, hemangiosarcoma, labial granuloma, eosinophilic granuloma, labial ulcer, or rodent ulcer.[5,47,48]

Some lesions of the lip may be amenable to resection and reconstruction with local skin flaps or geometric closure techniques.[49] The angularis oris axial pattern dermal flap has been used for reconstruction of a large ventral chin and rostral lip wound in the cat.[50]

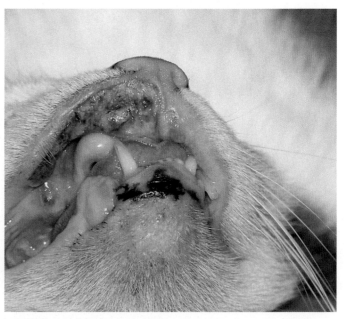

Figure 49-8 Squamous cell carcinoma of the lip in an eight-year-old female tortoiseshell (calico) and white cat.

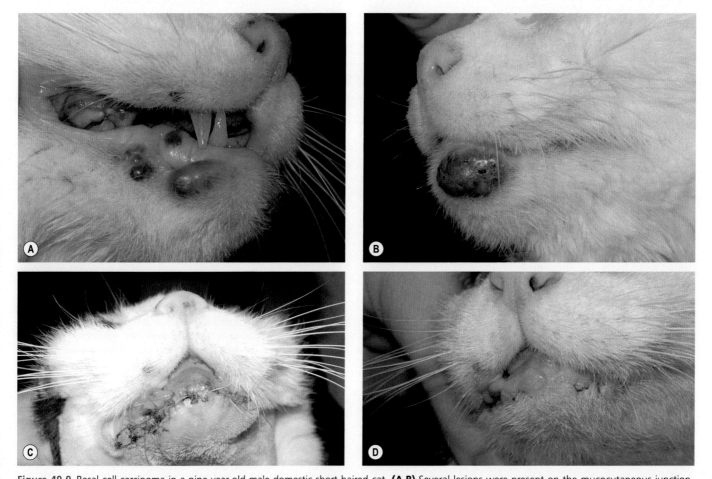

Figure 49-9 Basal cell carcinoma in a nine-year-old male domestic short-haired cat. (A,B) Several lesions were present on the mucocutaneous junction of the lip and chin. (C) The masses were excised by performing an elliptical excision with minimal margins of normal tissue. (D) The cat three weeks postoperative; the excision site healed without complication.

SURGICAL DISEASES OF THE CHIN

Conditions affecting the skin of the chin may have spread from the adjacent mandible, or the primary lesion in the chin may invade the bone. For chin lesions localized to the skin (Fig. 49-9) the reader is referred to Chapter 20 and for lesions with mandibular involvement see Chapter 55.

Chin avulsion

Mandibular fractures[51] may be accompanied by skinning of the lower jaw[44] whereby the whole submental area becomes separated from the horizontal rami of the mandible (Fig. 49-10). The chin usually separates at the junction between the gum and the teeth so there is usually insufficient tissue remaining on the mandible to ensure a secure repair and sutures must be anchored to teeth or bone (see below).

Neoplasia

SCC is the most common tumor found affecting the chin of the cat. This tumor is usually locally aggressive and invades adjacent bone, so radical excision will involve mandibulectomy (Chapter 55). Inflammatory or infectious lesions may be difficult to distinguish from neoplastic lesions so prior investigations including local and thoracic radiography and biopsy of the mass and local lymph node aspiration are recommended to enable diagnosis prior to the decision to perform radical surgery.

Other tumors affecting the feline chin, including fibrosarcoma and osteosarcoma, are discussed in Chapter 56, and skin tumors in Chapter 20.

SURGICAL DISEASES OF THE TONSIL

Neoplasia of the tonsil

SCC was the commonest tonsilar tumor in a review of oral neoplasia in cats[5] (Fig. 49-11). Affected cats had mucosal ulceration, necrosis and severe suppurative inflammation.[5] Tonsillar SCCs have a high rate of metastasis to regional lymph nodes and distal organs and therefore a very poor prognosis after local excision. Four cats with tonsillar SCC and one cat with SCC affecting the cheek were given a combination of radiation and carboplatin chemotherapy. They had a mean survival of 724 days and the median had not been reached because of continued survival of four cats.[52]

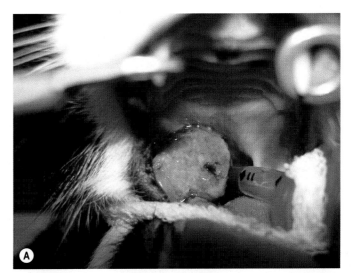

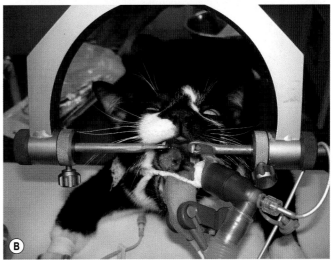

Figure 49-11 A three-year-old male neutered domestic short-haired cat with a tonsillar lesion extending to the base of the tongue. The histopathologic diagnosis was of a marked pyogranulomatous reaction of the right tonsil. **(A)** The large tonsillar mass was causing increased respiratory noise and halitosis. **(B)** The mass was excised by a combination of sharp and blunt dissection and with the use of diathermy. Positioning the cat for intraoral surgery was facilitated by use of a custom-made device through which the canine teeth were placed.

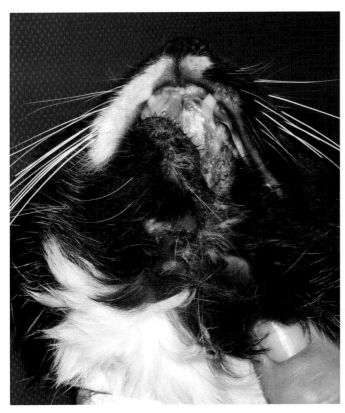

Figure 49-10 Chin degloving injury in a two-year-old male entire cat.

Lymphoma can affect the feline tonsils[5] and is usually accompanied by lymphadenopathy. Cervical lymphadenopathy, ipsi- or contralateral, is a common presenting sign, even with very small primary cancers. Fine needle aspirates of these lymph nodes or excisional biopsy of the tonsil will confirm the diagnosis. In spite of being apparently confined to the tonsil, this disease is considered systemic at diagnosis in more than 90% of patients.

Simple tonsillectomy is almost never curative but, when performed, it probably should be done bilaterally because of the high percentage of bilateral disease. Cervical lymphadenectomy, especially for large and fixed nodes, is rarely curative and should be considered diagnostic only.

Other tumors, especially malignant melanoma, may also metastasize to the tonsil.

PREPARATION FOR SURGERY

Several factors must be considered prior to oral surgery in the cat. The patient should have had thorough investigations including lymph node and mass aspirates, radiography, and coagulation profiles where deemed appropriate. Blood typing or cross-matching should be considered in cats where blood loss is anticipated (see Chapter 5).

Cats with oral masses can have complicated endotracheal intubation. Equipment to perform an emergency tracheostomy (see Chapter 46), endotracheal tubes of multiple sizes, and suction should be available at the time of induction and recovery from surgery.

An appropriately sized mouth gag is useful for intraoral surgery to maintain an open mouth and thereby facilitate access to the intraoral structures (see Fig. 49-12). There is a risk of aspiration of blood and fluids during surgery so the pharyngeal area should be packed with a swab or bandage.

Povidone iodine solution or 0.2% chlorhexidene solution is used for aseptic preparation of the oral cavity. Eye lubrication should be used and care taken to prevent antiseptic solutions entering the eye.

If it is anticipated that the cat may have difficulty or reluctance to prehend food postoperatively then the cat should be prepared for a feeding tube to be placed, with an adequate area of hair clipped and the equipment prepared and assembled for tube placement (see Chapter 12).

SURGICAL TECHNIQUES

Glossectomy

Removal of part of the tongue or partial glossectomy is performed to treat small neoplasms or traumatic lesions affecting the tip or side (Box 49-3). It is not known exactly how much of the tongue can be removed in the cat while preserving function, though in the dog up to 50% can be effectively removed. It must be noted, however, that postoperative recovery may become more complicated with increasing volumes of resection. The tongue is very vascular so precautions must be taken to prevent aspiration of blood. The cat may also be reluctant to eat postoperatively so placement of a feeding tube should be considered (see Chapter 12). Grooming will also be interfered with and provision should be made to attend to this.

Salivary gland resection

Salivary glands are resected if they are neoplastic, affected by necrotizing sialoadenitis, or for definitive treatment of salivary mucoceles. Surgical treatment consists of removing the entire mandibular–sublingual salivary chain on the affected side with marsupialization if a ranula is present. In dogs, the mandibular and sublingual glands are intimately associated so both glands are removed together if disease affects one of the two glands. In cats, the two glands are separate so it may not be necessary to remove both glands; however, there is insufficient literature published on this to determine whether resection of only the affected gland will be effective treatment. In a case series of seven cats with salivary mucoceles, five were treated surgically. Three had the entire mandibular-sublingual chain removed, and the sublingual chain alone was removed in one cat. In all cats marsupialization, lancing, or resection of the mucocele was performed concurrent to surgical resection of the glands.[42] The glands can be removed with the cat positioned in dorsal or dorsolateral recumbency and both techniques are described (Box 49-4).

Resection of the parotid and molar salivary glands is performed less frequently but descriptions of the surgical techniques are provided in Boxes 49-5 and 49-6.[6] There is one report in the literature of a feline zygomatic salivary cyst that was removed through a lateral orbitotomy and partial zygomatic arch resection (Box 49-7).

Box 49-3 Glossectomy

The cat is positioned in sternal recumbency with the mouth held open with a mouth gag.

Transverse glossectomy

Stay sutures are placed both in the rostral aspect of the tongue, that will be removed, and in the caudal part, that are to remain (Fig. 49-12). Horizontal mattress sutures are placed about 5 mm caudal to the incision line and about 3 mm apart using 3/0 polydioxanone. The tongue is then incised cranial to this line of sutures. Mucosal surfaces are then apposed with simple interrupted sutures.

Wedge glossectomy

A small margin of normal tissue should be removed from around the tumor. Simple interrupted sutures are pre-placed prior to tumor excision (Fig. 49-13). The pre-placed sutures are tightened and additional sutures placed to appose the mucosal edges on the dorsal and ventral tongue surfaces.

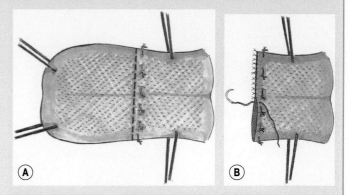

(A) **(B)**

Figure 49-12 Transverse glossectomy in the cat. **(A)** Stay sutures facilitate manipulation of the tongue. **(B)** Pre-placed sutures reduce hemorrhage prior to placing additional sutures after resection of part of the tongue.

Box 49-3 **Continued**

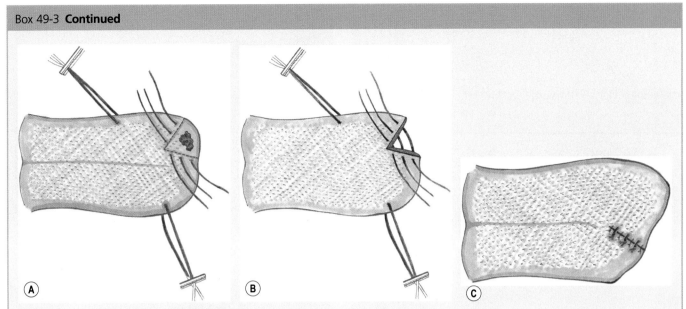

Figure 49-13 Partial wedge glossectomy. **(A)** Stay sutures are placed to help stabilize the tongue prior to resection of the mass. Pre-placed sutures are placed across where the mass will be removed. **(B)** The pre-placed sutures are shown after mass resection. **(C)** The sutures are then tightened and additional simple interrupted sutures placed to appose the ventral and dorsal mucosal surfaces.

Box 49-4 **Mandibular and sublingual sialadenectomy**

Dorsal recumbency[53]

The cat is positioned in dorsal recumbency. The incision starts just caudal to the mandibular symphysis on the affected side and extends caudally parallel to the mandibular ramus to a point caudal to the ear canal (Fig. 49-14A). The platysma muscle is incised to facilitate identification of the external jugular bifurcation. The mandibular lymph nodes must be identified: they lie more ventral to the salivary gland at this location (Fig. 49-14B). The mandibular gland sits just caudal to the ramus of the mandible at or cranial to this birfurcation of the external jugular vein and dorsal to the lymph nodes. Blunt dissection is performed to expose the mandibular salivary gland. The thin salivary gland capsule is incised and bluntly dissected off the gland to allow ligation of the great auricular artery and vein that lie medially (Fig. 49-14C). The gland complex is then retracted caudally to allow blunt dissection of the sublingual gland under (dorsal to) the digastricus muscle (Fig. 49-14D). A hemostat is placed from rostral to caudal under the digastricus muscle. The salivary gland complex and ducts are gently pulled under the external jugular birfurcation and digastricus muscle (Fig. 49-14E).

The mylohyoideus muscle needs to be incised for best exposure of the rostral glandular tissue and lingual nerve. The duct is ligated with 1M, 1.5M or 2M polypropylene and transected as far rostrally as possible in an attempt to remove all salivary tissue and particularly if a ranula is present. If during dissection the duct tears rostral to the planned ligation site then further dissection is not necessary to perform ligation. The aim is to remove all the salivary gland tissue or the mandibular gland and sublingual gland complex.

The digastric, mylohyoideus, and platysma muscles and the salivary gland capsule and subcutaneous tissues are reapposed with an absorbable monofilament suture such as 1.5M poliglecaprone.[53]

Dorsolateral recumbency[54]

The cat is positioned in dorsolateral recumbency with a small sandbag under the neck. A small incision is made directly over the salivary gland. The platysma muscle is divided and the gland located dorsal to the lymph nodes. The thin capsule is incised and the glandular tissue grasped with an Allis tissue forceps or thumb forceps and retracted to facilitate dissection. The branches of the great auricular artery and vein that enter the gland on the dorsomedial aspect are ligated. Dissection is continued rostrally along the duct and sublingual glands under the mandibular ramus.

The mylohyoideus muscle needs to be incised for best exposure of the rostral glandular tissue and lingual nerve. The duct is ligated with 1M, 1.5M or 2M polypropylene and transected as far rostrally as possible in an attempt to remove all salivary tissue and particularly if a ranula is present. If during dissection the duct tears rostral to the planned ligation site then further dissection is not necessary to perform ligation. The aim is to remove all the salivary gland tissue or the mandibular gland and sublingual gland complex.

The digastric, mylohyoideus, and platysma muscles and the salivary gland capsule and subcutaneous tissues are reapposed with an absorbable monofilament suture such as 1.5M poliglecaprone.[53]

Marsupialization

This should be performed in conjunction with salivary gland resection. The ranula is incised at the most dependent or swollen aspect, taking care not to cause iatrogenic damage to any vital structures. Then simple interrupted sutures or a simple continuous pattern using small gauge absorbable suture (1.5–2M poliglecaprone) can be used for suturing the stoma (see Fig. 49-3).

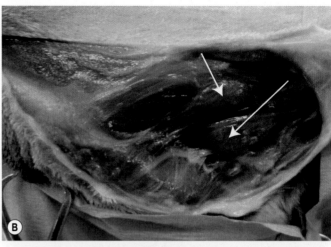

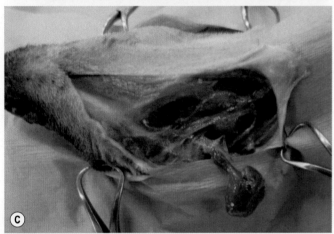

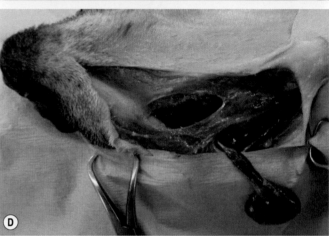

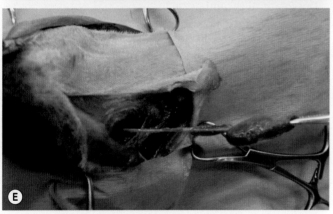

Figure 49-14 Salivary gland resection demonstrated on a cat cadaver. **(A)** The cat is positioned in dorsal recumbency and the skin incision extends parallel to the mandible from caudal to the symphysis to caudal to the level of the ear canal. **(B)** The mandibular lymph nodes (arrows) are visible in this cat just between and axial to the external jugular birfurcation. **(C)** The mandibular salivary gland was located by blunt dissection just dorsal to the mandibular lymph node. **(D)** The gland is carefully dissected out and the sublingual gland complex and duct are clearly visible. **(E)** The glands and ducts are brought under the external jugular vein to aid further rostral dissection.

Removal of the zygomatic salivary gland via a ventral transconjunctival approach is possible in dogs,

Facial reconstructive surgery

Reconstruction of facial defects can be very challenging, even in the hands of an experienced surgeon. Most defects can be repaired using local available tissues. Lip defects can be reconstructed using geometric closure techniques and advancement of local tissues. Forehead defects can be reconstructed using skin grafts, caudal auricular flaps, or rotational or transposition flaps. Care must be taken to minimize tension on eyelids and maintain the integrity of the facial nerve. Cheek defects can be reconstructed using local advancement, superficial

temporal, omocervical, and caudal auricular flaps.[49] Descriptions of skin flaps used for facial reconstruction are provided in Chapter 19.

Chin avulsion repair

Surgical repair of chin avulsion can be prone to failure if the avulsive and contractive forces that are tending to pull the chin off the mandible are not taken into consideration. The gum is not a strong enough tissue to provide sufficient holding power for sutures as the sutures have a tendency to cheese-wire through. To avoid this from happening the sutures need to be anchored around structures like the canine teeth or small holes in the mandible if the canine teeth are missing (Box 49-8).

Box 49-5 Parotid gland sialadenectomy[55]

The cat is positioned in lateral recumbency and the skin incised over the vertical ear canal to a point just dorsal to the mandibular ramus. The thin platysma muscle is incised to expose the parotid salivary gland and the parotidoauricularis muscle. The muscle is incised and retracted ventrally. The caudal auricular vein is ligated and divided. The gland is dissected away from the underlying tissue starting at the dorsal caudal aspect of the gland. Care must be taken at the base of the ear canal due to the close proximity of the facial nerve. At the craniodorsal aspect of the V-shaped gland the superficial temporal vein is identified and ligated. Once the gland has been dissected out the parotid duct is ligated and divided. The parotidoauricularlis muscle is reapposed with cruciate or horizontal mattress sutures followed by reapposition of the platysma muscle, subcutaneous tissue, and skin.

Adhesions to adjacent structures can make dissection challenging. Facial nerve paralysis and hemorrhage from the external carotid vessels are possible complications of parotid gland resection.

Box 49-6 Molar gland sialadenectomy

The cat is positioned in lateral or dorsal recumbency with a mouth gag in place. A longitudinal intraoral incision is made from caudal to the angle of the mouth (angularis oris) to a point immediately cranial to the masseter muscle. It is important not to lacerate the deep facial vein, which courses along the cranial aspect of the masseter muscle. The molar gland is visible immediately below the mucosal surface. The gland is dissected free by using a combination of sharp and blunt dissection, and the associated vessels and duct are ligated. The mucosa is closed routinely with absorbable sutures.

Box 49-7 Zygomatic gland sialadenectomy[37]

The cat is positioned in lateral recumbency. A lateral orbitotomy with partial zygomatic arch resection is performed. A skin incision is made along the dorsal border of the zygomatic arch immediately ventral to the globe. The periosteum of the zygomatic arch is incised and the orbital fascia is reflected dorsally, and the masseter aponeurosis ventrally. The dorsal half of the zygomatic arch is removed for a distance of 2 cm using an air-powered high speed burr or rongeurs.

The zygomatic salivary gland is located deep to the orbital fat. The gland is reflected dorsally and dissected free, removing as much of the duct as possible.

The wound is closed with simple interrupted sutures of absorbable suture material such as polyglactin 910 or poliglecaprone in the periosteum, masseter aponeurosis, and orbital fascia. The skin is closed routinely.

Box 49-8 Chin avulsion repair (Fig. 49-15)

The lower lip is reflected and the surface is debrided. Non-absorbable sutures of 3M prolene or polydioxanone are passed through the skin around the canine tooth and sutured firmly around the canine tooth. This is repeated on the opposite side. If the canine teeth are broken then the lip should be secured to the mandible through predrilled holes.

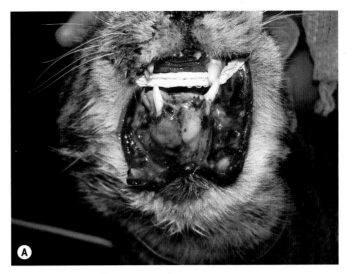

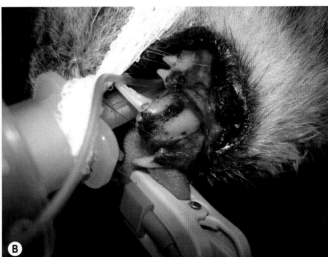

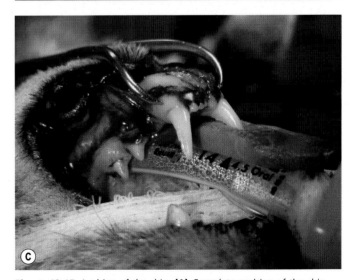

Figure 49-15 Avulsion of the chin. **(A)** Complete avulsion of the chin in a 18-month-old tabby cat involved in a road traffic accident. The mandible is exposed and the wound is markedly contaminated and the chin significantly distracted. **(B)** After initial clipping of hair and cleaning of the wound a symphyseal separation is clearly visible. **(C)** The symphysis is reduced with pointed reduction forceps prior to stabilization with a cerclage wire.[51]

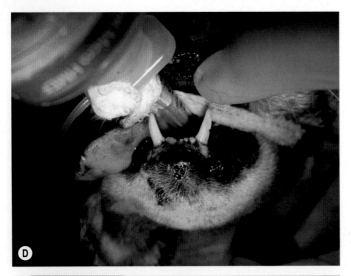

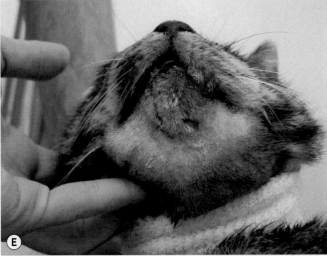

Figure 49-15, Continued **(D)** The avulsed skin is secured back in an anatomical position by placement of non-absorbable sutures around the lower canine teeth. **(E)** Two days postoperative. There is significant swelling and edema of the chin but the skin apposition has been maintained and the skin appears warm and viable.

Box 49-9 Tonsillectomy

The cat is positioned in sternal recumbency with a mouth gag in place. The tonsil is grasped with Allis tissue forceps or curved mosquito forceps and pulled out of its crypt. The base of the tonsil is transected with a scalpel blade, sharp scissors, electrosurgery, or laser. Hemostasis is achieved with digital pressure, electrosurgery, or laser. Large tumors may require ligation at the base with 1.5 or 2M absorbable suture material. After removal of the tonsil the crypt can be closed with a simple interrupted or continuous suture pattern.[56]

Tonsillectomy

Tonsillectomy (Box 49-9) is rarely indicated in the cat but in the rare instances of suspected neoplasia of the gland it may be performed for tonsil resection and to collect tissue for histopathologic analysis (see Fig. 49-11).

POSTOPERATIVE CARE

Supportive care is critical during treatment of cats with oral disease. These cats are often in pain. The use of analgesics should be considered in all patients and particularly those with large tumors, tumors that have ulcerated, painful metastatic lesions, or after trauma.

Adequate nutrition is also critical in supportive care. Cats may be in a poor nutritional state because of their difficulty or inability to eat. The pre-emptive placement of an esophageal feeding tube or gastrostomy tube may be necessary (see Chapter 12). If oral feeding is possible then soft food that can be lapped should be offered.

An Elizabethan collar is often required after surgery has been performed on or around the head to prevent self-trauma of the surgical site. Effective nursing care of cats after head surgery is an important component of the recovery (see Chapter 4).

COMPLICATIONS AND PROGNOSIS

Incisional breakdown soon after surgery is not uncommon, particularly after resection of oral masses. It is not always essential to resuture these lesions as many will subsequently heal by second intention. The oral cavity has a good blood supply so infection of the superficial tissues is not common. Infection in the mandible can be problematic and difficult to resolve. Delayed hemorrhage can occur following oral mass resection, so careful postoperative monitoring is imperative and the judicious use of sedatives for the first 12 hours following surgery can help prevent this.

Anorexia following any oral surgery appears to be more common in the cat compared with the dog, therefore the use of assisted feeding, via pre-placed feeding tubes is often required. Esophagostomy tubes are relatively easily placed and maintained (see Chapter 12).

Recurrence of masses is a distinct probability for many neoplastic oral lesions as it is often not feasible to remove these lesions with large margins. Fibrosarcoma and SCCs are tumors that are particularly liable to recur at the site of previous resection. The use of adjunctive therapies (e.g., radiotherapy) should be considered for these neoplasms (see Chapter 15). The prognosis for the cat is dependent on the type of tumor or disease, the size of the lesion, and whether it is in a position that will allow resection with adequate margins of normal tissue to increase the chance of a complete excision. Details on the prognosis of different diseases are discussed above in the relevant sections.

Salivary gland surgery

Damage to salivary ducts or glands can result in mucoceles or ranulas. These may be temporary complications, particularly after radical tumor excision; once the postsurgical inflammation has subsided these will usually resolve spontaneously. If this is not the case, then removal of the offending salivary gland may be necessary. Adhesions of salivary glands to adjacent structures can make dissection challenging. Nerves and blood vessels are often intimately associated with the glands and their ducts, and damage to these structures is possible during dissection. Temporary or permanent nerve deficits can be the result. Hemorrhage is also a distinct possibility if there are adhesions to underlying or overlying blood vessels.

REFERENCES

1. Crouch JE. Text atlas of cat anatomy. Philadelphia: Lea & Febiger; 1969. p. 131–40.

2. Konig HE, Liebich HG. Veterinary anatomy of domestic mammals. 3rd ed. Stuttgart: Schattauer; 2007. p. 661–76.

3. Rusbridge C, Heath S, Gunn-Moore DA, et al. Feline orofacial pain syndrome (FOPS): a retrospective study of 113 cases. J Feline Med Surg 2010;12(6):498–508. Epub 2010 May 6.

4. Solano M, Penninck DG. Ultrasonography of the canine, feline and equine tongue: normal findings and case history reports. Vet Radiol Ultrasound 1996;37:206–13.

5. Stebbins KE, Morse CC, Goldschmidt MH. Feline oral neoplasia: a ten-year survey. Vet Pathol 1989;26:121–8.

6. Vos JH, van der Gaag I. Canine and feline oral-pharyngeal tumours. J Vet Med Ser A 1987;34:420–7.

7. Brodey RS. Alimentary tract neoplasms in the cat: a clinicopathologic survey of 46 cases. Am J Vet Res 1966;27:74–80.

8. Martin CK, Tannehill-Gregg SH, Wolfe TD, Rosol TJ. Bone-invasive oral squamous cell carcinoma in cats: pathology and expression of parathyroid hormone-related protein. Vet Pathol 2011;48;302–12.

9. Miller MA, Nelson SL, Turk JR, et al. Cutaneous neoplasia in 340 cats. Veterinary Pathology 1991;28:389–95.

10. Davis KM, Hardie EM, Lascelles BD, Hansen B. Feline fibrosarcoma: perioperative management. Compend Contin Educ Vet 2007;29:712–29.

11. Leistra WH, van Oost BA, Willemse T. Non-pruritic granuloma in Norwegian forest cats. Vet Rec 2005;156:575–7.

12. Reubel GH, Hoffmann DE, Pedersen NC. Acute and chronic faucitis of domestic cats. A feline calicivirus-induced disease. Vet Clin North Am Small Anim Pract 1992;22:1347–60.

13. Smith JE. Symposium on diseases in cats – III. Some pathogenic bacteria in cats with special reference to their public health significance. J Smal Anim Pract 1964;5:517–24.

14. Felts JF, Fox PR, Burk RL. Thread and sewing needles as gastrointestinal foreign bodies in the cat: a review of 64 cases. J Am Vet Med Assoc 1984;184:56–9.

15. Basher AW, Fowler JD. Conservative versus surgical management of gastrointestinal linear foreign bodies in the cat. Vet Surg 1987;16:135–8.

16. Bound NJ, Priestnall SL, Cariou MP. Lingual and renal lymphoma in a cat. J Feline Med Surg 2011;13:272–5.

17. Withrow SJ Vail DM. Cancer of the gastrointestinal tract. In: Withrow SJ, Vail DM, editors. Small animal clinical oncology. 4th ed. Elsevier; 2007. p. 455–510.

18. Kovács K, Jakab C, Szász AM. Laser-assisted removal of a feline eosinophilic granuloma from the back of the tongue. Acta Vet Hung 2009;57:417–26.

19. Giles JT 3rd, Rochat MC, Snider TA. Surgical management of a thyroglossal duct cyst in a cat. J Am Vet Med Assoc 2007;230:686–9.

20. Kallet AJ, Richter KP, Feldman EC, Brum DE. Primary hyperparathyroidism in cats: seven cases (1984–1989). J Am Vet Med Assoc 1991;199:1767–71.

21. Hammer A, Getzy D, Ogilvie G, et al. Salivary gland neoplasia in the dog and cat: survival times and prognostic factors. J Am Anim Hosp Assoc 2001;37:478–82.

22. Carberry CA, Flanders JA, Harvey HJ, Ryan AM. Salivary gland tumors in dogs and cats: a literature and case review. J Am Anim Hosp Assoc 1998;24:561–7.

23. Spangler WL, Culbertson MR. Salivary gland disease in dogs and cats: 245 cases (1985–1988). J Am Vet Med Assoc 1991;198:465–9.

24. Volmer C, Benal Y, Caplier L, et al. Atypical vimentin expression in a feline salivary gland adenocarcinoma with widespread metastases. J Vet Med Sci 2009;71:1681–4.

25. Mazzullo G, Sfacteria A, Ianelli N, et al. Carcinoma of the submandibular salivary glands with multiple metastases in a cat. Vet Clin Pathol 2005;34:61–4.

26. Burek KA, Munn RJ, Madewell BR. Metastatic adenocarcinoma of a minor salivary gland in a cat. Zentralbl Veterinarmed A 1994;41:485–90.

27. Sozmen M, Brown PJ, Eveson JW. Sebaceous carcinoma of the salivary gland in a cat. J Vet Med A Physiol Pathol Clin Med 2002;49:425–7.

28. Sozmen M, Brown PJ, Eveson JW. Salivary gland basal cell adenocarcinoma: a report of cases in a cat and two dogs. J Vet Med A Physiol Pathol Clin Med 2003;50:399–401.

29. Sozmen M, Brown PJ, Eveson J, Scott HW. Epithelial-myoepithelial carcinoma of the salivary gland in two cats. Eur J Vet Pathol 1998;4:93–6.

30. Sozmen M, Brown PJ, Eveson JW. Salivary duct carcinoma in five cats. J Comp Pathol 1999;121:311–19.

31. Kim H, Nakaichi M, Itamoto K, Taura Y. Malignant mixed tumor in the salivary gland of a cat. J Vet Sci 2008;9:331–3.

32. Carpenter JL, Bernstein M. Malignant mixed (pleomorphic) mandibular salivary gland tumors in a cat. J Am An Hosp Assoc 1991;27:581–3.

33. Brocks BA, Peeters ME, Kimpfler S. Oncocytoma in the mandibular salivary gland of a cat. J Feline Med Surg 2008;10:188–91.

34. Brown PJ, Bradshaw JM, Sozmen M, Campbell RH. Feline necrotising sialometaplasia: a report of two cases. J Feline Med Surg 2004;6:279–81.

35. Harrison JD, Garrett JR. An ultrastructural and histochemical study of a naturally occurring salivary mucocele in a cat. J Comp Pathol 1975;85:411–16.

36. Rahal SC, Nunes AL, Teixeira CR, Cruz ML. Salivary mucocele in a wild cat. Can Vet J 2003;44:933–4.

37. Speakman AJ, Baines SJ, Williams JM, Kelly DF. Zygomatic salivary cyst with mucocele formation in a cat. J Small Anim Pract 1997;38:468–70.

38. Feinman JM. Pharyngeal mucocele and respiratory distress in a cat. J Am Vet Med Assoc 1990;197:1179–80.

39. Wallace LJ, Guffy MM, Gray AP, Clifford JH. Anterior cervical sialocele (salivary cyst) in a domestic cat. J Am Anim Hosp Assoc 1972;8:74–8.

40. Hawe RS. Parotid salivary sialocele in a cat. Feline Pract 1998;26:6–8.

41. Rahal SC, Mamprim MJ, Caporali EH, et al. Temporomandibular joint ankylosis and salivary mucocele in a cat: case report. Arq Bras Med Vet Zootec 2007;59:140–4.

42. Kiefer KM, Davis GJ. Salivary mucoceles in cats: A retrospective study of seven cases 2007: http://veterinarymedicine.dvm360.com/vetmed/Medicine/ArticleStandard/Article/detail/456165.

43. Harvey C. Parotid salivary gland duct rupture and fistula in the dog and cat. J Small Anim Pract 1977;18:163–8.

44. Prescott CW. Some oral lesions in the cat. Aust Vet J 1971;47(2):41–5.

45. Loevy HT. Cytogenic analysis of Siamese cats with cleft palate. J Dent Res 1974;53:453–6.

46. Scott FW, LaHunta A, Schultz RD, et al. Teratogenesis in cats associated with griseofulvin therapy. Teratology 1974;11:79.

47. Miller MA, Ramos JA, Kreeger JM. Cutaneous vascular neoplasia in fifteen cats: clinical, morphologic, and immunohistochemical studies. Vet Pathol 1992;29:329–36.

48. Levene A. Upper digestive tract neoplasia in the cat (A comparative study). J Laryngol Otol 1984;98:1221–4.

49. Degner DA. Facial reconstructive surgery. Clin Tech Small Anim Pract 2007;22(2):82–8.

50. Bradford M, Degner DA, Bhandal J. Use of the angularis oris cutaneous flap for repair of a rostral mandibular skin defect in a cat. Vet Comp Orthop Traumatol 2011;24:303–6.

51. Voss K, Langley-Hobbs SJ, Grundmann S, Montavon PM. Mandible and maxilla. In: Montavon PM, Voss K, Langley-Hobbs SJ, editors. Feline orthopedic surgery and musculoskeletal disease. Edinburgh: Elsevier; 2009. p. 311–28.

52. Fidel J, Lyons J, Tripp C, et al. Treatment of oral squamous cell carcinoma with accelerated radiation therapy and concomitant carboplatin in cats. J Vet Intern Med 2011;25:504–10.

53. Ritter MJ, Stanley BS. Salivary glands. In: Tobias KM, Johnston SA, editors. Veterinary surgery small animal. Missouri: Elsevier; 2012. p. 1439–47.

54. Dunning D. Tongue, lips, cheeks, pharynx, and salivary glands. In: Slatter D, editor. Textbook of small animal surgery. 3rd ed. Saunders; 2002. p. 553–61.

55. Smith MM, Waldron DR. Approach to the parotid salivary gland. In: Atlas of approaches for general surgery of the dog and cat. Philadelphia: WB Saunders; 1993. p. 88.

56. Anderson GM. Soft tissues of the oral cavity. In: Tobias KM, Johnston SA, editors. Veterinary surgery small animal. Missouri: Elsevier; 2012. p. 1425–37.

Chapter 50

Ear

S.J. Baines

Aural conditions in cats are common. Many of these have underlying causes that will respond effectively to medical management, but in some cases surgery is indicated either as the primary treatment option or due to failure to respond to other treatment regimens. The approach to aural disease, the surgical diseases that affect the feline ear, and the surgical management of these diseases will be discussed in the following chapter.

SURGICAL ANATOMY

The ear is a sensory organ that receives and transforms the vibrations perceived as sound into neural impulses conveyed to the brain. The ear is composed of the pinna, external ear canal (comprising vertical and horizontal ear canals), the middle ear, and the inner ear (Fig. 50-1).

Pinna

The pinna is a broad skin-covered extension of the external ear canal cartilages that helps to collect and localize the origin of sound waves. It is also important in non-verbal communication between cats and other animals, including humans. Ear position, in association with other changes in facial expression, can convey feelings such as fear, anger, happiness, and curiosity.

The size and shape of the pinna varies according to breed, although less so in the cat than the dog. Most cats, except Scottish Folds, have erect pinnae unless they are diseased. The pinna is triangular in appearance with the base of the triangle attached to the head. It has a relatively hairless and more glabrous rostralateral concave surface and a haired caudomedial surface. The auricular cartilage of the pinna is elastic with small perforations through which blood vessels pass. Rupture of these blood vessels may lead to an aural hematoma.

External ear canal

The external ear canal opening is formed by the auricular and scutiform cartilages. The large auricular cartilage is cone shaped from its origin at the annular cartilage to the external auditory meatus, and it

then flares to form the pinna. The helix is the edge of the pinna and the scapha is the center. The antihelix is a ridge with a prominent tubercle on the medial aspect of the auricular cartilage at the opening of the vertical canal. The tragus is the lateral rim of the opening to the external ear canal. The antitragus is caudal to the tragus and separated from it by the inter-tragic notch. The tragohelicine fissure lies between the tragus and helix. The funnel-shaped cavum conchae

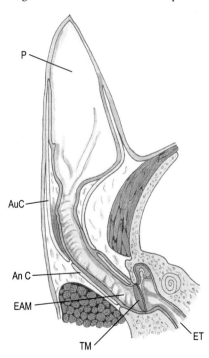

An C = annular cartilage, AuC = auricular cartilage,
P = pinna, TM = tympanic membrane

EAM = external acoustic meatus
ET - opening to eustachian tube

Figure 50-1 Diagram illustrating the anatomy of the feline ear. *(Reprinted from Slatter DH (2003) Textbook of Small Animal Surgery 3e, with permission from Elsevier.)*

© 2014 Elsevier Ltd
DOI: 10.1016/B978-0-7020-4336-9.00050-0

forms the vertical canal and, along with the tragus, antitragus, and antihelix, the external auditory meatus. As the auricular cartilage approaches the horizontal canal it is replaced by the annular cartilage. The annular cartilage ends just before the tympanic membrane and the osseous external auditory meatus, which is an extension of the temporal bone containing the cochlea and peripheral vestibular apparatus. This canal ends at the tympanic bulla and the external acoustic meatus.

There are numerous muscles of the external ear canal and groups of muscles act to move the ear in particular directions. These groups are rostro-auricular, caudo-auricular and ventro-auricular. The innervation of the external ear is provided by cervical and cranial nerves. Sensory input is via the branches of the 2nd cervical nerve dorsally (greater occipital nerve) and ventrally (transverse cervical and greater auricular nerves) and the facial nerve and mandibular branch of the trigeminal nerve.

Blood supply to the labyrinth is provided by the vertebral artery via its basilar branches and blood supply to the rest of the ear is from the external carotid artery and its branches (caudal, intermediate, lateral, medial, and deep auricular arteries) and the superficial temporal artery via the rostral auricular artery. Blood is drained by satellite veins.

The skin of the ear canal contains sebaceous glands, which produce an oily substance, and ceruminous glands (modified apocrine glands), which secrete a milky white fluid that turns brown on exposure to air. The combined product of these glands is cerumen. Cerumen, along with trapped debris, is carried away from the tympanic membrane by migration of the epithelial cells lining the canal. The functions of cerumen are: to protect the ear canals and tympanic membrane by entrapping microorganisms and their products and mechanically removing them; to keep the ear canals moist, allowing normal desquamation of the epithelium; to contribute to the barrier function of the epidermis; and to have an antibacterial action mediated via sebaceous gland-derived fatty acids.

Middle ear

The tympanic membrane is part of the mechanism of hearing. Vibrations detected by the tympanic membrane are transmitted via the ossicles (malleus, incus, and stapes) to the vestibular (oval) window. The tympanic membrane slants downward and inward obliquely, so that it forms an angle of 30–45° with the floor of the horizontal canal. This may be a mechanism to allow a larger tympanic membrane to fit in a given size of ear canal, thus decreasing the acoustic pressure in the ear canal needed to produce perceptible vibrations in the cochlea. However, this anatomic arrangement means that debris tends to accumulate at the junction of the ventral horizontal ear canal and the tympanic membrane.

The tympanic membrane is a concave, semi-transparent epithelial structure. The *umbo* is the most depressed part and is formed where the tip of the manubrium of the malleus pulls the tympanic membrane medially. The tympanic membrane is divided into two parts. The *pars flaccida* is the smaller, dorsal opaque portion that is pink, loosely attached, and contains small blood vessels. The *pars tensa* is the large gray, semi-transparent ventral portion. In cats, it may be difficult to appreciate the pars flaccida as it is much smaller. Epithelial migration begins with the germinal epithelium at the umbo, and therefore this area should not be damaged during myringotomy.

The tympanic membrane has four layers. The outermost layer is a continuation of the lining of the external ear canal. Medial to this is the fibrous stratum that consists of two layers of collagen fibers. The inner layer is composed of modified respiratory epithelium, which lacks goblet cells and cilia normally found in respiratory epithelium. The tympanic membrane is thin in the center and thicker at the periphery, where the fibrous layers thicken to form the tympanic

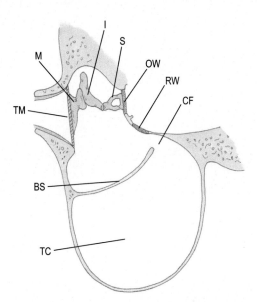

TC = tympanic cavity, BS = bony septum, TM = tympanic membrane, M = malleus, I = incus, S = stapes, OW = oval window, RW = round window, CF = communicating fissure.

Figure 50-2 Diagram illustrating the feline tympanic bulla. *(Reprinted from Slatter DH (2003) Textbook of Small Animal Surgery 3e, with permission from Elsevier.)*

annulus. If the tympanic membrane is perforated, it will heal by proliferation of the fibrous layer, which results in a thickened, opaque membrane in contrast to the normal translucent structure.

The normal barrier function of the tympanic membrane is impaired with acute inflammation and this may lead to transtympanic migration of bacteria with resulting otitis media, and absorption of topical medication with resulting ototoxicity. With chronic inflammation, the tympanic membrane becomes thickened and this is less of a concern.

The middle ear is an air-filled cavity lined by a pseudostratified ciliated columnar epithelium containing goblet cells, which is continuous with the pharynx via the Eustachian tube. It is separated from the external ear canal by the tympanic membrane. There are mucus-producing glands in the tympanic cavity, but not in the external ear canal and thus if mucus is present in the horizontal ear canal, it must have originated in the tympanic cavity, which indicates a defect in the tympanic membrane. The tympanic cavity is not sterile and bacteria found in the tympanic cavity are similar to those found in the nasopharynx and not the external ear canal.

The middle ear cavity contains three parts: the dorsal epitympanic recess (or attic), the tympanic cavity proper, and the tympanic bulla (Fig. 50-2).

The *epitympanic recess* is located dorsally and is the smallest chamber. It contains two of the three ossicles, the malleus and incus, and the facial nerve canal. The ossicles have synovial articulations with each other, with fibrous ligaments for support.

The *tympanic cavity proper* (mesotympanum) is adjacent to the tympanic membrane and contains the stapes and part of the malleus. The stapes is attached to the vestibular (oval) window, which communicates directly with the inner ear. The manubrium of the malleus attaches to the fibrous layer of the pars tensa, and may be seen through the normal tympanic membrane as the stria mallearis. The manubrium of the malleus is much straighter in the cat compared to the C-shape in the dog.

The *tympanic bulla* (hypotympanum) is the largest of the three compartments of the tympanic cavity, and is located in the ventromedial part of the tympanic cavity. In cats, a bony shelf separates the tympanic cavity proper from the tympanic bulla almost completely, with a small defect in the shelf located just lateral and caudal to the round window in the medial caudal part of the tympanic cavity proper. This makes access to the tympanic bulla from the tympanic cavity proper via a myringotomy difficult.

The bony eminence (*promontory*) is on the medial wall of the tympanic cavity proper, directly opposite the mid-dorsal region of the tympanic membrane. It may occasionally be visible through the tympanic membrane. The oval (vestibular) window is dorsal to the cochlear promontory and is covered by the stapes. Medial to the promontory is the round (cochlea) window of the inner ear. The cervical sympathetic nerves run through the tympanic cavity proper, coursing submucosally across the promontory, and thus they are susceptible to damage when performing a myringotomy or middle ear lavage.

The medial wall of the tympanic cavity proper also contains the Eustachian tube opening rostrally. The Eustachian tube is lined by ciliated pseudostratified columnar epithelium that includes goblet cells. The Eustachian tube is normally collapsed, but will inflate when the pressure in the tympanic cavity and medial aspect of the tympanic membrane is equalized with the pressure on the lateral surface of the tympanic membrane. The tensor veli palatini muscle supports the lateral wall of the auditory tube and contraction of this muscle and the levator veli palatini keeps the pharyngeal opening of the Eustachian tube open.

Inner ear

The *inner ear* is composed of the cochlea, vestibule, and semicircular canals which are housed in a membranous labyrinth, surrounded by a bony labyrinth in the petrous temporal bone, located deep to the tympanic bulla dorsomedially.

Vibrations from the tympanic membrane are transmitted from the malleus to the incus and then stapes. The stapes then transmits this vibration to the inner ear via the vestibular (oval) window and movement of the fluid in the inner ear (perilymph) converts mechanical energy (vibrations) to electrochemical energy (nerve impulses), which is then transmitted to the auditory cortex in the temporal lobe of the cerebral cortex. The cochlear (round) window is located at the caudal end of the promontory. It is covered by a mucous membrane and communicates with the inner ear. The round window functions as a pressure relief valve, bulging into the tympanic cavity as the pressure rises in the inner ear.

The *vestibular* system mediates the control of posture and movements of the body and eyes relative to the external environment. Sensory information from vestibular, somatosensory, and visual receptors and motor information from the cerebellum and cerebral cortex are integrated and processed centrally allowing appropriate co-ordination of the relevant muscle movements. The vestibular system is divided into a peripheral component located in the inner ear and a central component, located in the central nervous system (CNS). Three major CNS areas receive projections from the peripheral sensory receptors of the vestibular system: the cerebral cortex, the spinal cord, and the cerebellum.

GENERAL CONSIDERATIONS

History

A detailed and logical history is of paramount importance and, in common with other problems that are considered more purely 'dermatological', will guide the selection of additional diagnostic tests and may go a long way to providing a diagnosis.

Important findings to determine include details of the onset, duration, and progression of the clinical signs and a consideration of

whether the disease is unilateral or bilateral. Unilateral disease is more consistent with foreign bodies, ear tumors, and polyps, whereas generalized dermatopathies are more likely to be bilateral. Seasonal disease suggests allergic reactions, which is an important cause of ear disease in cats. The age of the patient may also guide the diagnosis, as young animals are more likely to have mites, young adult animals are more prone to allergies, and older animals more prone to tumors and immune-mediated disease. The owner's approach to parasite control should be ascertained as fleas and mites commonly affect the head and neck.

Other health matters are also important. Recently rescued cats may have unknown underlying medical disorders, free-roaming cats are at increased risk of contagious diseases, and viral status may be important as chronic otitis media is often linked to chronic upper respiratory tract virus infection and retrovirus infection.

The owner's normal treatment regime, response to prior treatment, and compliance with treatment should be determined.

The owner may report head shaking, ear twitching, fits of ear scratching, particularly after manipulation of the ear, change in eating habits, change in behavior, and vocalization. Clinical signs may be unilateral or bilateral, persistent or intermittent, and acute or chronic. Pain when eating may indicate otitis media that has extended to involve the tissues around the tympanic cavity and temporomandibular joint. A history of upper respiratory tract disease, e.g., sneezing, ocular discharge, and nasal discharge may be present in cats with ascending otitis media.

Clinical signs

Clinical signs of external ear canal disease include otorrhea, head shaking, and scratching at the ear. External ear canal or middle ear disease may cause pain on opening the mouth and facial nerve paralysis.

Clinical signs of middle ear disease include shaking the head and pawing at the ear. An intermittent and temporary tilt of the head, caused by irritation, pain, and discomfort rather than neurologic dysfunction, may be seen.

Involvement of the facial nerve will result in paralysis of the lip or ear, widened palpebral fissure, reduced palpebral reflexes, and drooling. Involvement of the cervical sympathetic trunk will result in Horner syndrome (miosis, ptosis, enophthalmos, and protrusion of the nictitans gland) and involvement of the parasympathetic fibers in the facial nerve may result in keratoconjunctivitis sicca. An ophthalmologic examination may show signs of CNS disease in cats with central vestibular syndrome.

Clinical signs of vestibular disease include a head tilt towards the affected side or wide excursions of the head if the disease is bilateral, asymmetric ataxia, typically with leaning, stumbling, falling or rolling to the affected side, or symmetric ataxia if both sides are equally affected, and spontaneous horizontal or rotatory nystagmus, with the fast phase away from the affected side. Nausea and vomiting may be seen due to vestibular input to the vomiting center in the brainstem. Peripheral vestibular disease should be differentiated from central vestibular disease (Table 50-1). Rarely, extension of inner ear disease into the CNS may cause brainstem dysfunction. Neurologic signs indicating middle ear involvement may be seen in 25% of cats with external ear canal tumors.

Involvement of the inner ear may cause deafness (sensorineural deafness), as may obstruction of the external ear canal, rupture of the tympanic membrane, disruption of the ossicles, and middle ear disease (conductive deafness). Conductive deafness is usually not complete and there may be differences between the ears in a hearing impaired animal.

Involvement of the nasopharynx is uncommon, but signs such as gagging, upper respiratory tract dyspnea, and stertor may be seen, with

Table 50-1 Neurologic findings in vestibular system dysfunction

Clinical signs	Peripheral vestibular disease	Central vestibular disease
Head tilt	Towards the lesion	Towards the lesion (or away from the lesion with paradoxical disease)
Spontaneous nystagmus	Horizontal or rotatory with the fast phase away from the side of the lesion, rarely positional	Horizontal, rotatory, vertical and/or positional, with the fast phase toward or away from the lesion; the direction may change with head position
Paresis/proprioceptive deficits	None	Common ipsilateral to the lesion
Mentation	Normal to disorientated	Depressed, stuporous, obtunded or comatose
Cranial nerve deficits	Ipsilateral CN VII deficit	Unilateral or bilateral CN V, VII, IX, X and XII deficits
Horner syndrome	Common ipsilateral	Uncommon
Head tremors	None	Seen with concurrent cerebellar dysfunction
Circling	Infrequent, may occur toward side of lesion	Usually toward the side of the lesion

---

Box 50-1 Points to consider in a cat with suspected ear disease

1. Does the patient definitely have ear disease?
2. Is the ear disease limited to the external ear canal, the middle ear or the inner ear or some combination of these?
3. Is the ear drum intact?
4. What is the primary cause or causes of the ear disease and are there any predisposing factors or perpetuating factors?
5. What treatment is most appropriate?
6. How often should re-examination be performed to monitor the success of treatment?

---

thick discharge draining from the Eustachian tube or the presence of a nasopharyngeal polyp.

Marked pain on palpation of the base of the ear canal and on traction of the pinna may be seen in animals with otitis media.

DIAGNOSTIC PROCEDURES

Examination of the patient, using various means, is indicated to answer the questions listed in Box 50-1.

Physical examination

Examination of the ear should be performed in any cat with skin disease and conversely, a dermatologic examination should be performed in any cat with ear disease, as most dermatopathies will also affect the ear. A general examination of the patient is needed to determine if the ear disease is the only abnormality, or if there are concurrent medical or dermatologic problems. Otitis may occur as a paraneoplastic syndrome, e.g., in cats with mast cell disease.

Examination of the pinna for primary lesions, such as macules, papules, plaques, pustules, and alopecia, as well as secondary lesions such as scale and crusts should be performed to help identify the nature of the pinnal disease.

The external ear canals are palpated for thickening, calcification, exudate, and pain or discomfort. The external auditory meatus is examined for the presence of exudate, masses, and foreign material. Pain on palpation of the ear canal and fluid within the canal increase the suspicion of otitis media associated with chronic otitis externa.

The oropharynx should be examined because of the close association of pharyngeal disease and middle ear disease, particularly from nasopharyngeal polyps and palatine defects. Pain on palpation of the tympanic bulla or on opening the mouth may be seen with middle ear disease.

A neurologic examination should be performed to examine for the presence of abnormalities that might indicate middle ear or inner ear disease, such as vestibular signs (ataxia, nystagmus, head tilt, and circling or falling to the affected side), facial paresis, Horner syndrome, and keratoconjunctivitis sicca. An ophthalmologic examination may reveal evidence of inflammatory CNS disease.

Otoscopy

Otoscopy should be performed on every animal with otitis externa. Many cats may require sedation or anesthesia for a complete examination. If a ruptured tympanic membrane is suspected, ideally the examination should be performed under general anesthesia so that a cuffed endotracheal tube may be placed to prevent aspiration of fluid and discharge from the Eustachian tube into the pharynx.

Both ears should be examined, even in animals with unilateral signs, as bilateral disease of different severities may be present. The less affected ear should be examined first and a new otoscope cone should be used for each ear. If a large amount of discharge is present, the ears may need to be flushed before examination can be conducted. In animals with marked erythema, proliferation, stenosis or ulceration, administration of topical or systemic corticosteroids for seven–14 days may be needed to decrease the inflammation and pain and open up the external ear canals so that a full examination may be performed. The use of a video-otoscope (Fig. 50-3A), rather than a hand-held otoscope (Fig. 50-3B) has a number of advantages to consider (Box 50-2).

To examine the ear, the tip of the otoscope cone should be introduced into the ear canal pointing ventrally, with concurrent upward and outward traction on the pinna. There is a ridge of cartilage on the dorsal surface of the ear canal where the vertical canal meets the horizontal canal, and the otoscope must be passed below this ridge, while pulling on the pinna.

The lining of the normal ear canal is pink and glistening with few hairs and the dermal blood vessels should be apparent. One of the first signs of inflammation in the ear canal is inability to see these vessels as a result of thickening of the epidermis or dermal edema. In the presence of inflammation, the epidermis becomes reddened. Excessive waxy secretions and ceruminous gland hyperplasia may be seen which creates a cobblestone appearance to the lining, which may

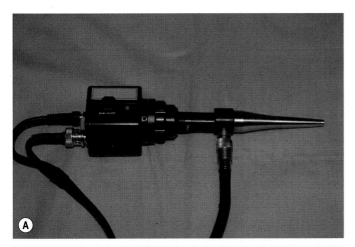

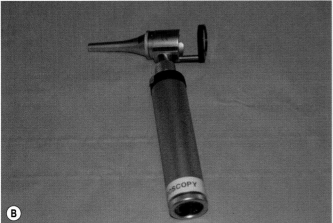

Figure 50-3 Equipment used for evaluation of the external ear canal and tympanic membrane. **(A)** Video-otoscope. **(B)** Handheld otoscope.

Box 50-2 **Advantage of using a video-otoscope compared with otoscopic examination**

Higher degree of magnification
Broader field of vision
Brighter illumination
Reduction in shadowing as the light is at the tip of the cone
Electronic image capture
Ability to perform ear flushing and biopsies under direct visualization

---

progress to polyp formation. Defective epithelial migration, as a result of damage to the tympanic membrane or inflammation of the ear canal, leads to the accumulation of cerumen, which may therefore indicate previous or current ear canal disease. Recurrence of cerumen after removal indicates continued external ear canal disease. Cerumen in cats tends to be moist and is seldom dry and flaky as it can be in dogs.

The presence, location, and degree of inflammation, stenosis, ulceration, and proliferative changes should be noted. The size of the vertical and horizontal canals and the type, location, and quantity of debris or exudate should also be noted. The consistency, color and amount of any exudate should be determined. Samples should be collected for cytology and culture and sensitivity testing.

Ulceration of the ear canal is often associated with a Gram negative infection, e.g., *Pseudomonas*, but may also be caused by inappropriate cleaning with cotton-tipped applicators. Foreign bodies such as plant awns, impacted wax, and concreted otic preparations may be present. Plant awns should be removed with forceps and impacted wax and otic preparation should be softened with ceruminolytic agents and removed by flushing or with endoscopic forceps. Masses in the external ear canal should be biopsied with forceps.

The tympanic membrane is assessed for presence, integrity, color, and texture. If the tympanic membrane cannot be assessed due to debris in the external ear canal, this should be cleaned thoroughly to allow inspection of the tympanic membrane. If the tympanic membrane cannot be assessed due to stenosis of the canal, then a number of tests may be used to assess its presence and integrity. A small diameter (3.5 or 5 French) red rubber catheter may be inserted into the ear canal until it stops and then gently removed and advanced to get a feel for the rigidity of the 'stop'. The 'stop' will be 'spongy' if the ear drum is intact and more rigid if it is not intact, and the catheter is therefore contacting the medial wall of the tympanic bulla.

Alternatively, positive contrast ear canalography (see below) or tympanometry may be used. A warmed, colored solution (e.g., fluorescein or povidone-iodine) may be infused via the ear canal in the conscious patient; the appearance of this fluid at the external nares or the patient snorting it through the oropharynx indicates that the tympanic membrane is not intact and the fluid has passed via the Eustachian tube into the pharynx. However, this carries the risk of introducing potentially ototoxic substances into the middle ear. A simpler method in the anesthetized patient is to lavage the external ear canal with warm saline and, if bubbles of air rise through the fluid when the animal breathes, then the tympanic membrane is not intact.

Otitis media may be present when the tympanum is discolored gray or brown. An intact tympanum does not rule out otitis media, although with otitis media the tympanic membrane does not usually have a normal opacity and color, and a ruptured tympanic membrane is not an absolute indicator of otitis media in the absence of other abnormal findings. Bulging of the membrane towards the observer may indicate fluid accumulation in the middle ear and retraction of the tympanic membrane suggests a partially filled middle ear with obstruction of the Eustachian tube.

It is not possible to differentiate a thickened tympanic membrane caused by chronic inflammation from a thickened tympanic membrane caused by previous or current otitis media without advanced imaging, a myringotomy, or surgical exploration via bulla osteotomy. Animals with otitis media and an open ear drum often have a copious malodorous liquid discharge on otoscopy, with magnetic discharge along the floor of the horizontal canal.

Clinical pathology

Both cytology and culture have a role to play in the diagnosis of ear disease and these tests are complementary to each other. Many infections are polymicrobial with mixed infections of bacteria (cocci and rods) and yeast. Cytology may reveal *Malassezia*, which would not be reported if only bacterial culture was performed. Conversely, culture may show bacteria that were not identified on cytology as mucus may protect them from cytology stains. Bacteria may be obtained from many samples, but the presence of a host inflammatory response on cytology suggests that organisms cultured are pathogens rather than contaminants.

Cytology

Cytologic examination of otic exudate is a simple, practical, and cheap diagnostic test that provides rapid results to help identify the primary cause and perpetuating factors in animals with ear disease. Cytologic examination of exudate should be repeated while treating the disease and it should not be assumed that the changes present at previous examinations are representative of the current status of the ear canal.

The main use of cytology is to identify and characterize microbial overgrowth or infection, which then guides therapeutic decisions and allows response to therapy to be monitored. Bacterial overgrowth is uncommon in cats compared to dogs and therefore culture is indicated when bacteria are seen. Cytology may identify the primary cause of otitis in some cases, although this is less important than other dermatologic testing.

Samples should be taken from both ears and should be taken before use of any cleaning agent or therapy. A cytology sample may be obtained by using a cotton-tipped applicator inserted gently into the external ear canal. Samples obtained from the deeper horizontal canal are more clinically relevant than samples obtained from the vertical canal, although this is best performed with the animal under anesthesia. In cats with otitis media, samples obtained from the tympanic cavity are more representative. The swab is then rolled onto a clean glass microscope slide, evenly distributing a thin layer of material. Cerumen has a high lipid content and briefly heating the slide will fix the material to the slide and avoid loss of the sample in the stain solvent. A simple, rapid in-house stain using a modified Wright's stain (e.g. DiffQuick) is adequate. A Gram stain is more time consuming and may not be necessary as most cocci found in the ear are Gram positive and most rods are Gram negative. If parasites are suspected, mounting the otic exudate in a few drops of mineral oil on a slide followed by a coverslip is suitable and this should be performed in all cats with otitis externa. Examination for *Demodex* should similarly be performed in adult cats with pruritic otitis externa as this condition is uncommon but certainly underdiagnosed.[1]

It is tempting to make conclusions about the etiology of the ear disease (e.g., parasites, bacteria or yeast) based on the color, texture, and smell of the discharge, but these observations are not reliable and the diagnosis should rest on more objective tests.

The normal cerumen is waxy and yellow and, due to the high lipid content, does not take up stain and therefore a cytology slide from a normal ear should be almost colorless. Normal cornified squamous epithelial cells and desquamated keratinocytes may be seen. Small numbers of resident bacteria may be identified in 71% of cats,[2] usually Gram positive cocci: coagulase negative *Staphylococcus* spp., coagulase positive *Staphylococcus* spp., and *Streptococcus* spp. Rods are rarely found in the normal ear canal, with the exception of *Corynebacterium*.[2,3] Bacteria found in the presence of leukocytes should be considered an abnormal finding. *Malassezia* is a normal resident of the feline ear canal, being found in 23% to 83% of normal cats,[2,4] but it is also an opportunistic pathogen and is found in 64% of cats with otitis externa.[5] Abnormal findings include increased numbers of *Malassezia* organisms (greater than 12 organisms per high dry [×40 objective] field).[6] Less than two organisms is considered normal and two to 11 is considered a gray zone. This cut off has a specificity of 100% and sensitivity of 63% for Malassezia infection in cats.

Bacteria identified on cytology may be normal flora, bacterial overgrowth in the debris and on the epithelial surface, or true infection. Semiquantitative cytologic criteria may help to identify the clinical importance of bacteria. Four or fewer bacteria per high dry field may be considered normal, five to 14 is of unknown importance, and 15 or more is abnormal.[6] This cut off has 100% specificity and 63% sensitivity in cats. The presence of a large number of leukocytes, which are not usually found in normal cerumen, particularly if they contain phagocytosed bacteria, also provides evidence in support of true infection, although leukocytes may be seen in other forms of ear disease, e.g., immune-mediated dermatopathies.

Cytology may also identify parasites such as *Otodectes cynotis*, which is responsible for up to 50% of all cases of otitis externa in cats, as well as other mites such as *Demodex*, *Notoedres cati*, and *Neotrombicula autumnalis*.

Cytology may also be used in the evaluation of masses involving the external ear canal.[7] In one study of 27 masses from 25 cats, fine needle aspirate cytology showed a good level of agreement with the final histologic diagnosis and was able to differentiate all inflammatory polyps from other tumors. However, cytology was less useful in differentiating between benign and malignant neoplasia, being correct in 22 out of 27 masses (81.5%).[7]

Culture

Culture is needed to identify the species of bacteria and the antimicrobial sensitivity of the isolates. However, culture should be used in conjunction with cytology to avoid making therapeutic decisions based on isolation of bacteria of no clinical relevance. Culture and sensitivity testing may not be a cost-effective and relevant test, because clinical response to topical therapy may not correlate with in vitro sensitivity as topical agents reach very high concentrations in the ear canal.

In cats with otitis media, the most common bacterial pathogen is *Staphylococcus intermedius*, although other organisms including streptococci spp, *Pseudomonas*, *Proteus*, *Bordetella*, *Bacteroides*, *Fusobacterium*, and *Mycoplasma* have been reported.[8] Bacterial resistance is not usually a problem in feline otitis media compared with the situation in dogs. Bacteria of the same species isolated from the middle ear and the horizontal ear canal may display different antibiotic sensitivity patterns in up to 80% of cases.[9]

Dermatophyte culture is recommended in cats with otitis externa, particularly if they are young, free-roaming or have been recently acquired from a rescue shelter.

Serology

Serology for antigens or antibodies may be of use for some infectious diseases, e.g., *Toxoplasma* and *Neospora*. These tests may also be performed on the cerebral spinal fluid (CSF). CSF analysis may help to confirm central vestibular syndrome, but is generally not disease-specific. This should be performed after advanced imaging of the brain by computed tomography (CT) or preferably magnetic resonance imaging (MRI). The risk of CNS trauma and cerebellar herniation should be considered against the likely diagnostic benefit of this test.

Biopsy

Skin biopsy of the ear is an underused diagnostic test. It is recommended when an immune-mediated, proliferative or neoplastic disease is suspected.

Diagnostic imaging

Diagnostic imaging is often useful in the diagnosis of ear disease, mainly to investigate those parts of the ear that cannot be visualized directly on examination. Diagnostic imaging of the thorax and (other potential sites of metastasis) should be performed if neoplasia is suspected. Diagnostic imaging should be performed before otoscopy and certainly before administration of any medication or lavage fluid into the ear canal as these may mimic findings of otitis externa or media and lead to a false positive diagnosis.

The selection of the most appropriate diagnostic imaging technique depends on the particular question being asked and the differential diagnoses being considered.[10] For instance, in an animal with otitis externa with suspected otitis media, radiography or CT is appropriate, with CT having a role to play even if radiographs do not reveal any abnormality. In a cat with a suspected nasopharyngeal polyp, a CT has greater sensitivity for detection of a mass in the middle ear and nasopharynx, although these areas can still be imaged with radiographs. An MRI scan has the greatest sensitivity, particularly for acute otitis media, but assessment of the bony structures of the middle ear is difficult with MRI. In a cat with signs of vestibular disease, an MRI provides the most useful information for evaluation of inner ear structures, but a CT may be useful to assess the middle ear if otitis interna arose from otitis media.

Radiography

Radiography is the mainstay of diagnostic imaging for the ear in most private practices. It is cheap and relatively easy to perform and produces a global view of the region being examined. However, great care must be taken to use good technique and positioning to get radiographic images of diagnostic quality. This usually means general anesthesia for positioning. The greatest disadvantage is superimposition of overlying structures, which is a particular problem when imaging the head.

Projections include lateral, dorsoventral or ventrodorsal, latero 20° ventral-laterodorsal oblique, rostro 10° ventral-caudodorsal closed-mouth oblique[11] and rostro 30° ventral–caudodorsal open-mouth oblique.[12] The ventrodorsal view is better for evaluating a patient with otitis externa, although positioning is easier for the dorsoventral view. Of the two rostroventral-caudodorsal oblique projections, the 10° closed-mouth oblique is more accurate and easier to perform, although there is no difference in the accuracy of these views for the detection of fluid in the middle ear.[13]

Radiographs are useful for evaluating the osseous tympanic cavity and evaluating the external ear canals for chronic changes, such as stenosis and mineralization. In otitis externa, radiographic findings include stenosis or mineralization of the wall of the ear canal and soft tissue opacity within the canal, representing a mass or debris.

The tympanic bulla is a thin-walled gas-filled structure with well-defined, smooth borders. Sclerosis of the wall of the tympanic bulla may be seen in older animals or following resolution of middle ear disease. The external acoustic meatus is rounded with distinct smooth margins.

In otitis media, soft tissue opacity in the tympanic cavity (representing fluid or a soft tissue mass), sclerosis of the wall of the bulla or petrous temporal bone, bony proliferation of the bulla or petrous temporal bone, lysis of the bony wall of the tympanic bulla, and signs of concurrent otitis externa may be seen. Lysis of the adjacent calvarium may be seen with aggressive tumors. Radiographs are remarkably insensitive for the diagnosis of middle ear disease in the absence of osseous changes.

Contrast radiography may be of use on occasion. Positive contrast canalography, after instillation of a water contrast iodinated solution into the external ear canal, may be used to assess the integrity of the tympanic membrane and to assess the integrity of the external ear canal, e.g., in patients with suspected ear canal avulsion or stenosis, and the success of any repair.[14–16] Water soluble iodine-containing contrast medium (1–2 mL) is instilled into the ear canal with the patient either in lateral recumbency, or, preferably in ventral recumbency so that a dorsoventral projection may be used to compare both external ear canals at the same time. In normal canine ears, positive contrast canalography was more sensitive than otoscopy in identifying iatrogenic tympanic membrane perforation.[16] Positive contrast

sinography may also be used in patients with chronic draining tracts after total ear canal ablation or accidental trauma to the ear canal (See Fig. 50-9B).

Inner ear disease rarely produces signs visible radiographically.

Ultrasound

Ultrasonography is not commonly used, but has several potential advantages, as it is relatively quick, non-invasive and may be used in conscious patients.[17] In a normal animal, air in the external ear canal and middle ear prevents transmission of ultrasound waves, but if the external ear canal is filled with fluid, e.g., saline, or if the middle ear contains soft tissue or fluid as a result of disease, then these structures may be examined. In one study ultrasonography was more accurate than radiography in the detection of fluid in the middle ear in feline cadavers, although both modalities were inferior to CT.[18]

Computed tomography

CT is more sensitive than radiography for examination of the ear, particularly the middle ear, and for assessment of other structures such as the draining lymph nodes. CT can also differentiate between soft tissue and fluid within the middle ear and intravenous contrast will allow the vascularity of a lesion to be identified. The principles of interpretation and diagnostic imaging findings with the various disease processes are similar to radiography, but findings are more readily identified on transverse CT images as there is no superimposition of structures compared to radiographs. CT may therefore be of use for detection of soft tissue changes, delineation of tumors and detection of subtle bony lysis and proliferation.

Caution should be exercised when evaluating the thickness of the tympanic bulla wall in animals with fluid in the middle ear, as the thickness of the wall of a fluid-filled bulla appears greater than that of an air-filled bulla, due to a volume averaging artifact.[19]

CT evaluation of the peripheral vestibular system is useful if radiographs have not provided a diagnosis, if a mass lesion such as a polyp or tumor is considered likely, or if the patient is a potential surgical candidate. However, CT is less useful for the evaluation of the central vestibular system.

CT has been found to be a more sensitive but less specific modality for the diagnosis of middle ear disease, although neither modality was able to detect early lesions associated with otitis media/interna when there was no osseous involvement.[20] Another study showed that CT and radiographs have a similar sensitivity for detection of otitis media.[21] Sensitivity is increased if a smaller slice thickness is chosen.[10] Otitis interna is difficult to diagnose with CT except where there is marked destruction of the inner ear.

Magnetic resonance imaging

MRI produces images with better soft tissue contrast than radiography or CT and is indicated if peripheral or CNS disorders are suspected, such as tumors, inflammatory lesions, or abscesses associated with ear disease.[22] However, osseous lesions of the middle ear are difficult to assess with MRI and MRI requires general anesthesia. MRI is superior to radiography in the detection of middle ear disease in cats.[23]

MRI provides superior soft tissue resolution that aids the diagnosis of neoplastic and inflammatory diseases of the central vestibular system.

MRI findings of middle ear disease include medium signal intensity material in the tympanic bulla (TB) on T1W (isointense to brain tissue) and hyperintense on T2W and enhancement of inner margin of TB post-contrast. Soft tissue will enhance with gadolinium whereas fluid will not.

MRI findings of otitis interna are lack of signal intensity of the labyrinthine fluid on T2W sequences[24] and meningeal enhancement on post-contrast T1W sequences.[25]

Sampling the middle ear and myringotomy

Samples of fluid from the middle ear are required to make a diagnosis of otitis media. A myringotomy may be needed if the material in the middle ear is too thick to aspirate (see Box 50-7).

Additional tests

Hearing test

This is the simplest method of evaluating the hearing ability, although it does not detect a unilateral hearing disability. The patient is placed in a familiar environment and a sound is produced out of sight. The sound should be within the normal range of hearing for the species and should be considered loud by the observer. A response is considered positive if the animal appears startled and looks around to find the source of the sound, whereas a response is considered negative if the animal is not disturbed and its behavior is not changed.

Tympanometry

Tympanometry is the continuous recording of middle ear impedance as the air pressure in the ear is systematically increased or decreased. It is a sensitive, rapid, and simple measure of the integrity of the tympanic membrane and the function of the middle ear. It involves closure of the external ear canal with a rubber plug which contains three channels: one for introducing the sound stimulus, one for receiving the sound stimulus, and one to allow pressure variation. At the moment, this is more of a research tool than a useful clinical tool.

Brainstem-evoked auditory responses (BEAR)

This is used to assess the integrity and function of the peripheral and central auditory pathways and for indirect assessment of the closely associated vestibular pathways. This test is a recording of sound-evoked electrical activity in the auditory pathway between the cochlea and the auditory cortex. Sedation or anesthesia is required for this test to be conducted. Small (27G) needle electrodes are placed subcutaneously in the skin of the head and connected to an amplifier. The brain activity is measured after delivery of clicks at 10–20Hz through earphones in the external ear canal.[26–28]

SURGICAL DISEASES OF THE PINNA

Trauma

Wounds to the pinna are relatively common after cat fights, but they have also been reported in cats with frostbite. These wounds are classified according to the depth of the wound. The wounds may involve: skin on one side of the pinna; skin on one side of the pinna and cartilage; and full thickness defects involving skin on both sides of the pinna and cartilage.

Small linear lacerations involving one skin surface only may be left to heal by second intention after appropriate local wound management as the cartilage will splint the wound and prevent deformity of the pinna. Larger lacerations that result in two-sided or three-sided flaps should be closed primarily if possible, as second intention

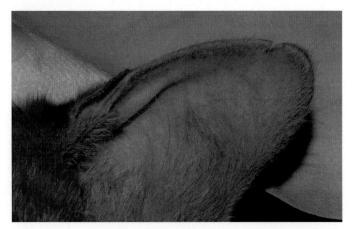

Figure 50-4 Old laceration wound to the margin of the pinna left to heal by second intention.

healing may result in malalignment or pinnal deformity as a result of wound contraction.

Wounds that involve the cartilage take longer to heal by second intention as the cartilage support is lost and healing is delayed until there is fibrous union of the cartilage. This may result in pinnal deformity. Surgical closure provides a more rapid and cosmetic result. Sutures should be placed to appose the edges of the cartilage and the skin edges, either with separate sutures in each tissue plane, or with vertical mattress sutures with deep bites in the cartilage and superficial bites in the skin.

Wounds that involve both skin surfaces and the cartilage will have a better cosmetic outcome if sutured, although these wounds may be left to heal by second intention (Fig. 50-4). Lacerations on the ear margin may widen with time as a result of contracture if allowed to heal by second intention, but if closed, wounds in this location may result in 'cupping' or folding of the ear margin as a result of contraction. Small wounds on the margin of the pinna may be treated with partial amputation of the pinna (subtotal pinnectomy) to avoid these cosmetic changes.

Traumatic wounds resulting in large wounds with substantial loss of tissue may be reconstructed with a distant direct flap from the adjacent skin, although the erect nature of the feline pinna makes apposition of the pinna to the skin more challenging than the same technique in a dog with a pendulous pinna.

Aural hematoma

Aural hematoma (Fig. 50-5) is a common disorder of the pinna, resulting either from trauma, which may be self-trauma due to head shaking or scratching, or external trauma, e.g., from a cat-fight wound, or from immune-mediated disease.[29] In cats, otitis externa associated with ear mites is often noted and is usually unilateral. Hemorrhage results in sanguinous fluid accumulating between the cartilage and skin on the concave inner surface of the pinna, although analysis of this fluid suggests an exudate rather than frank blood.[29] Further head shaking or self-trauma results in continuing bleeding and formation of a hematoma. Left untreated, the hematoma matures, leaving a sanguinous seroma, and then granulation tissue forms on the wall of the cavity. Contraction and fibrosis then result in pinnal deformity ('cauliflower ear') and thickening.

Therapeutic options for aural hematoma comprise: identification and, if possible, treatment of the underlying cause; prevention of further self-trauma, by using an Elizabethan collar and specific therapy

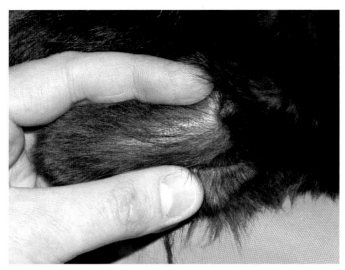

Figure 50-5 Aural hematoma on the concave (inner) aspect of the pinna results in convex appearance due to accumulation of sanguinous fluid.

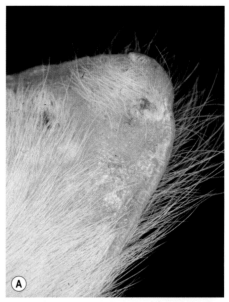

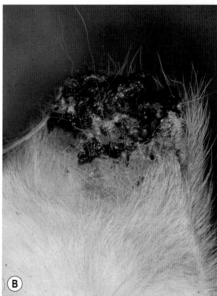

Figure 50-6 Pinnal squamous cell carcinoma. Typical crusting, erosive, and ulcerated lesions of SCC in a cat showing **(A)** early and **(B)** late lesions in the same cat.

for any underlying cause; drainage of the hematoma cavity; and apposition of the skin and cartilage to allow healing to progress without significant deformity.

Drainage of the hematoma may be achieved in several ways. Needle aspiration of the hematoma is the simplest method, but may not be effective if the hematoma is chronic and may need to be repeated if the hematoma recurs before the cavity has been obliterated. Corticosteroids may be used to reduce local inflammation, reduce head shaking and self-trauma, and suppress an autoimmune reaction if one is present.[29,30] Although these are probably best given systemically, as administration into the hematoma cavity has the potential to maintain the separation between the cartilage and skin and prolong healing.

There are a variety of surgical options reported for aural hematoma management[31-36] (see Box 50-13).

Pinnal neoplasia

Tumors arising from the ear are uncommon in cats, and usually affect the pinna and external ear canal. Benign tumors are less common than malignant tumors, although the most frequent proliferative lesion is the inflammatory polyp. Benign tumors are less likely to be ulcerated, tend to have a narrow base of attachment, are more likely to be lobulated and typically do not invade the ear cartilage.[37]

Clinical signs depend on the location and size of the tumor, degree of ulceration and local invasion, and the presence or absence of distant metastases. As with all tumors and suspected tumors, cytologic or histologic diagnosis of the primary tumor and assessment of regional lymph node involvement and depending on tumor type, distant metastasis, is indicated.

Many tumors of the pinna are actinically induced and therefore reducing exposure to UV light by keeping the cat indoors, by UV shields on windows and by applying infant-safe sunscreen to the pinnae and nose may prevent tumor formation.

Squamous cell carcinoma (SCC)

SCC is the most common tumor of the feline pinna (Fig. 50-6). SCC usually affects light-colored cats exposed to UVB.[38] These tumors are often actinically induced as a result of DNA damage following exposure to solar radiation. Tumors are more frequent in regions with the highest solar radiation. In such regions, the incidence of cutaneous SCC has been reported to be 27 cases per 100 000 cats.[39] Thin-haired and light-colored cats are at risk, with white cats being 13 times more likely to develop this tumor.[39] Lesions are most common where the hair is thin and exposure to the sun is greatest, i.e., pinna, especially the concave aspect and base, eyelids and nasal planum. SCCs are discussed further in Chapter 20.

Mutations in the *p53* gene have been found in the majority of cats with premalignant actinic lesions and SCC of the pinna.[40,41] No causative association between pinnal SCC and feline leukemia virus (FeLV) or feline immunodeficiency virus (FIV) has been found,[42] but papillomavirus group antigens have been found in multicentric SCC in situ lesions (Bowens disease).[43,44]

For peripheral lesions that are large enough, fine needle aspirate cytology may yield a tentative diagnosis although the associated inflammation may hinder this. For small, superficial lesions, excisional biopsy is the most appropriate diagnostic step and histologic examination should provide a definitive diagnosis with information about vascular invasion and completeness of margins. Histologic examination of pre-malignant lesions may yield a diagnosis of actinic keratosis.

Evaluation for other primary lesions, particularly on the nasal planum and eyelids, assessment of the regional lymph nodes and, in the more invasive tumors, thoracic radiographs or CT are indicated to stage the disease. Approximately 15% of cats will have multicentric actinic lesions.[45]

Treatment options for SCC include wide surgical excision, often comprising pinnectomy (Fig. 50-7), cryosurgery, laser ablation, radiotherapy, strontium plesiotherapy, photodynamic therapy (Fig. 50-8),

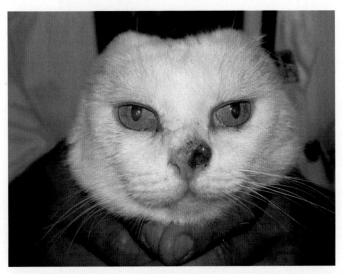

Figure 50-7 An adult cat with nasal squamous cell carcinoma that had bilateral pinnectomy for pinnal squamous cell carcinoma some years previously.

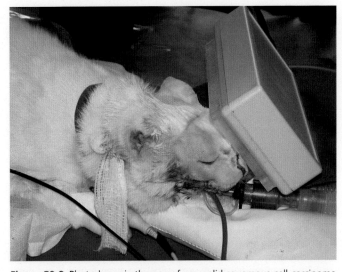

Figure 50-8 Photodynamic therapy of an eyelid squamous cell carcinoma lesion in an adult cat with recent nasal planum excision for SCC and a previous right pinnectomy for SCC.

and chemotherapy.[38] Surgical excision is curative for peripheral lesions and allows the histologic assessment of margins. Pinnectomy is simple to perform, cosmetically acceptable and the best option for long-term local control (Box 50-12). In one study, 18 cats treated with surgical excision had no local recurrence and a median disease-free interval of 681 days and median survival time of 799 days.[38]

Cryosurgery is less satisfactory but may be considered if pinnectomy is not anatomically possible or if owners would not accept the cosmetic appearance. It has the disadvantages that only small (<5 mm), superficial lesions may be treated and no surgical margins can be assessed. In one study, 12 cats with pinnal and eyelid lesions were treated successfully with a complete response after one treatment cycle, although cats with nasal planum lesions did not respond as well, with 20% being treatment failures.[46]

Photodynamic therapy may be used for superficial lesions, although tumor responses are variable and the disease-free interval is lower than with other therapies, but the cosmetic effect may be better.[47–49] The photosensitizing agent may be administered systemically (e.g., aluminium phthalocyanine tetrasulphonate) or topically (e.g., 5-amino levulinic acid). The initial response has been reported to be good (up to 100%), but the duration has been short, ranging from two to 18 months.[47–49] In one study, all aural lesions showed a complete response, possibly because light is more able to penetrate the thin tissue of the pinna.[48]

Local hyperthermia has been used, with an overall response rate of 68%.[50] Megavoltage radiotherapy is not associated with a good response rate or survival time and may cause side effects to the pinna and external ear canal, such as ulceration and fibrosis. Strontium plesiotherapy is effective for superficial lesions and is relatively inexpensive.

Intralesional chemotherapy using cisplatin, carboplatin and 5-fluorouracil have been used for nasal planum lesions and allow the local administration of drugs that would be fatal if given systemically.[51,52] Systemic chemotherapy with bleomycin and 13-cis retinoic acid may provide a small improvement in disease-free interval and survival time in cats with more aggressive or advanced disease.[53,54] Apparent clinical resolution of actinic keratosis and SCC has been reported in one cat following topical therapy with 5% imiquimod cream.[55]

Further sun exposure should be avoided and all cutaneous sites predisposed to the development of this tumor should be monitored for the development of new lesions.

Other tumors that affect the pinna include basal cell tumor, hemangioma, hemangiosarcoma, soft tissue sarcoma, rhabdomyoma, mast cell tumor, melanoma, and papilloma/fibropapilloma. For more details on these tumors please see Chapter 20.

Dermatopathy

Dermatoses that affect the pinna may be described according to the nature of the lesions, e.g., crusting/scaling, alopecia, ulceration or plaques/nodules, and according to the etiology, e.g., infectious, parasitic, immune-mediated, and neoplastic. These are listed in Table 50-2.

Although some dermatoses may only affect the pinna, most pinna dermatoses are part of a more generalized disorder, which may be limited to the skin or be systemic. A complete physical and dermatologic examination is therefore indicated. Although many of these disorders are the domain of the dermatologist, the surgeon should be aware of these conditions as they may require biopsy or surgical excision and they may be dermatologic indicators of local or systemic ill-health that may require surgical management, e.g., aural hematoma in otitis externa, alopecia in hyperthyroidism, exfoliative dermatitis in thymoma.

Table 50-2 Differential diagnoses for pinnal dermatoses

Etiology	Nature of lesion			
	Crusts/scales	**Alopecia**	**Ulceration**	**Plaques/nodules**
Infectious	Dermatophytosis *Malassezia* *Leishmania* Feline cowpox virus	Dermatophytosis *Leishmania*	*Leishmania*	Dermatophytosis Deep mycosis *Leishmania*
Parasitic	*Notoedres cati* (scabies) *Demodex* Trombiculosis Lice Flea-bite dermatitis	*Demodex*		Ticks
Allergic	Mosquito-bite hypersensitivity	Eosinophilic granuloma Miliary dermatitis Food allergy Atopy	Mosquito-bite hypersensitivity	
Hormonal		Hyperthyroidism Hyperadrenocorticism and pinna folding		
Immune-mediated	Pemphigus DLE/SLE Vasculitis Thrombovascular/cold agglutinin disease Adverse drug reactions Auricular chondritis		Pemphigus DLE/SLE Vasculitis Thrombovascular/cold agglutinin disease Adverse drug reactions Auricular chondritis	
Environmental	Actinic keratosis Frostbite			Foreign body
Hereditary	Primary seborrhea	Pattern baldness Congenital hypotrichosis		
Neoplastic	Epidermotropic T-cell lymphoma	Epidermotropic T-cell lymphoma	Squamous cell carcinoma Epidermotropic T-cell lymphoma	Squamous cell carcinoma Basal cell tumor Hemangioma Hemangiosarcoma Mast cell tumor Melanoma Epidermotropic T-cell lymphoma
Miscellaneous	Trauma	Feline pinnal alopecia Topical corticosteroid use		Aural hematoma

SURGICAL DISEASES OF THE EAR CANAL

Otitis externa

Otitis externa is the most common disease of the external ear canal, with a prevalence of 2–6% in cats.[56] It is defined as inflammation of the external ear canal with a multifactorial etiology. It is a syndrome rather than a diagnosis and it should not be assumed that it is infectious in nature. In cats, otitis is the third most common dermatologic problem after abscesses and flea infestations.[57] In some cats, extension of the infection from the external ear canal and middle ear into the surrounding soft tissues results in the development of a para-aural abscess and discharging sinus.[58] Abscesses are almost exclusively unilateral.

The factors involved in the development of otitis externa may be divided into:[56,59] (1) primary causes, which directly initiate the inflammation of the ear canal; (2) predisposing causes, which increase the

risk of developing otitis externa and work together with the primary or perpetuating causes to result in clinical disease, but rarely cause disease on their own; and (3) perpetuating causes, which contribute to the persistence of the disease once established and prevent its resolution (Box 50-3). As with many dermatologic conditions, otitis may be categorized into those diseases that are treatable and curable and those that may be controlled and managed.

Compared to the dog, otitis externa is much less common in the cat, which may reflect the fact that cats are much less likely to be affected by a chronic skin disease that acts as a primary cause. It tends to affect younger cats (one to two years old), ectoparasites are more common (responsible for approximately 50% of cases of otitis externa), and the role of bacterial pathogens, in particular *Pseudomonas*, is less important.

The successful management of otitis externa depends on identification and treatment of both the primary cause and predisposing factors, while considering whether the presence of perpetuating factors will thwart the therapeutic plan. Failure to identify and address the primary

Box 50-3 Causes of otitis externa

Primary causes

Parasites
- *Otodectes cynotis*
- *Demodex cati*
- *Sarcoptes scabiei*
- *Notoedres cati*
- *Cheyletiella*
- *Trombicula*
- Ticks

Foreign bodies

Hypersensitivity and allergic diseases
- Atopy
- Food allergy
- Contact allergy

Keratinization disorders
- Facial dermatosis of Persian cats

Autoimmune diseases
- Pemphigus foliaceous
- Pemphigus erythematosus
- Drug reactions

Infectious agents (primary otitis media)
- *Mycoplasma*
- *Bordetella*

Predisposing causes

Congenital anatomic and conformational factors

Acquired conformational factors
- Mass in the external ear canal
- Trauma to the external ear canal and pinna
- Stenosis of the ear canal
- Hair in the ear canal

Excessive moisture in the ear canal

Iatrogenic factors
- Mechanical cleaning
- Removal of hair
- Irritating topical treatment
- Systemic antimicrobial therapy selecting for resistant strains of bacteria

Immunosuppression
- FeLV
- FIV

Systemic disease
- Metabolic disease
- Endocrinopathy

Perpetuating causes

Bacteria
- *Staphylococcus intermedius*
- *Pseudomonas* spp.
- *Streptococcus* spp.
- *Proteus* spp.
- *Pasteurella multocida*
- *E. coli*
- *Klebsiella*
- *Corynebacterium* spp.
- *Enterococcus* spp.

Yeasts
- *Malassezia pachydermatis*
- *Candida* spp.

Chronic hyperplasia of the external ear canal

Ulceration of the ear canal

Stenosis of the ear canal

Otitis media

Chronic upper respiratory tract infection

---

and/or predisposing factors is the most common cause of chronic recurrent otitis externa. Chronic inflammation of the ear canal leads to the development of perpetuating factors (hyperplasia of the integument, fibrosis of the ear canal, erosion and ulceration of the integument, and otitis media), which may be the major reason for treatment failure, regardless of the primary cause. However, identification of the primary cause may not be possible until secondary infections and predisposing factors are identified, treated, and eliminated if possible. In particular, bacterial and fungal pathogens involved in the process are rarely the sole primary cause and therefore simply addressing these pathogens alone may lead to treatment failure.

If treatment is not effective, recurrent infections with increasing likelihood of resistant organisms and secondary changes in the ear canal, which will then act as perpetuating causes, are likely. This may lead to a chronic end-stage ear, for which medical therapy will no longer provide a solution and a surgical salvage procedure is required.

Primary otitis externa is not common in cats and generally it occurs because there has been a change in the microenvironment of the external ear canal to favor bacterial growth, especially when the pathogens are either small (*Proteus mirabilis*, *Pseudomonas aeruginosa* or *Pasteurella multocida*) or large (*E. coli*) rods.

Initial therapy for pathogens is topical antimicrobial therapy when bacteria are implicated, with systemic use in animals with severe or resistant infection, and topical antifungal agents (e.g., clotrimazole or miconazole) when there is fungal infection, with systemic therapy (fluconazole 50 mg PO q12–24h) or itraconazole (5 mg/kg PO q12h) for resistant infections. Secondary therapeutics include specific therapy for ectoparasites and flushing of wax, debris, and discharge from the ear canals. Short-term therapy with topical or systemic corticosteroids may be required in animals with stenosis of the ear canals resulting from chronic inflammation.

Flushing the ear canal under general anesthesia is necessary for the resolution of many cases of otitis, particularly in chronic cases and where topical therapy has not been effective (see below).

Obstructive otitis

The most common causes are polyps, tumors, stenosis secondary to inflammation, ear deformity as a result of untreated aural hematoma, and concretions of debris in the ear canal. The clinical signs are chronic, recurrent otitis externa/media, head shaking, and a malodorous suppurative discharge. This condition is usually unilateral, although that caused by polyps may be bilateral. Mast cell tumors, particularly in Siamese cats, may cause obstructive ear canal lesions. This is commonly a chronic condition and therefore otitis media may be present and need specific therapy. Patients have commonly been treated with a variety of antibiotics, and culture and sensitivity testing to ensure the use of an appropriate agent at the time of definitive therapy to deal with the obstructive lesion is recommended. If the obstruction is caused by a mass, then surgical removal of the mass by traction (if a polyp) or removal of a part of, or the whole of the external ear canal is required. If the obstruction is due to stenosis caused by pinnal or ear canal deformity or chronic hyperplastic changes, then this may be improved with a short course of prednisolone (1–2 mg/kg PO q24h for 14 days, then tapering over 14 days). This treatment may need to be repeated periodically to maintain patency in animals with chronic disease. For cats that fail to respond to therapy with corticosteroids, then surgical resolution of the obstruction is indicated.

Proliferative necrotizing otitis

This is a rare syndrome that manifests with sharply marginated erythematous crusted plaques with erosions and/or ulcers beneath them. The lesions are present on the inner aspect of the pinnae, the external ear canal, and sometimes the pre-auricular region of the face. Histologic changes are striking, with parakeratosis, follicular acanthosis, dyskeratotic epidermal cells, and folliculitis. The etiology is unknown, but drug reactions have been proposed. Infection, presumed to be secondary, is often present, but responds poorly to antimicrobial therapy. The disease may regress slowly in some animals by the time they are 12 to 24 months of age and in others there is a response to topical tacrolimus with or without prednisolone.[60] It is seen primarily in young kittens from two to six months of age, but there are reports of older animals (three to five years old) being affected.[60]

Ceruminous cystomatosis or benign proliferative ceruminous cysts

This is a disorder of unknown cause that manifests by multiple, small (<2 mm) often coalescing papules, vesicles, nodules or plaques that are pigmented dark blue, brown or black in the external ear canal or concave surface of the pinna. A yellow-brown fluid may be obtained on aspiration or puncture. Many cats are unaffected by this disorder, although in some cats the lesions may predispose to the development of otitis externa as the lesions alter the conformation of the ear canal. In other cats it is noted after otitis externa. Biopsy may be needed to rule out neoplasia. In symptomatic cats treatment consists of surgical removal of the cysts, lancing them with a blade or use of topical chemical cautery with silver nitrate or trichloroacetic acid.

Neoplasia

Tumors of the external ear canal are uncommon, representing approximately 1–2% of all tumors in cats.[37,61] External ear canal tumors are more aggressive in cats compared to dogs, with more than 85% of feline tumors being malignant.[37] Tumors arise mainly from the epithelium and adnexal structures of the auditory meatus and both vertical and horizontal canals are equally affected. Benign tumors include ceruminous gland adenoma and sebaceous adenoma. The most common malignant tumor is the ceruminous gland adenocarcinoma, but SCC, sebaceous gland adenocarcinoma and carcinomas of unknown origin have also been described.

Tumors of the ear canal are often locally invasive, but slow to metastasize, although some tumors present with a much more malignant phenotype, with early spread to the lymph nodes and lungs. The degree of local invasion is a prognostic indicator in these tumors.[37]

Clinical signs are typically aural discharge, which may be dark or bloody and foul-smelling, and the presence of a mass that can be identified clinically in approximately half the cats.[37] Malodor, pruritus, and signs of pain may be seen less commonly with malignant tumors and are rare with benign tumors. Secondary infection, as a result of impairment of the normal epithelial barrier function, is frequent. The first diagnostic step is otoscopic examination, although as these tumors are usually painful a detailed otoscopic examination is difficult without chemical restraint.

Cytologic examination of a fine needle aspirate is a useful screening test and will provide a diagnosis of ceruminous gland adenocarcinoma in 86% of cases and a diagnosis of a benign tumor in 80% of cases.[7] However, histologic examination of tissue remains the gold standard for diagnosis.

Clinical staging for malignant ear canal tumors comprises baseline hematologic and biochemical screens, evaluation and aspiration of the draining lymph nodes, and thoracic diagnostic imaging using radiographs or CT. Radiographs or CT may demonstrate stenosis of the ear canal, mineralization of the soft tissues, destruction of the bony wall of the tympanic bulla or calvarium, and fluid or soft tissue within the tympanic bulla. MRI may be indicated in cats with neurologic signs that cannot be explained by middle ear disease alone. Five of 56 cats with various carcinomas of the ear canal had evidence of lymph node metastasis, but none had evidence of pulmonary metastasis ante mortem, although metastases were found in one cat post mortem.[37]

Surgery is the main mode of therapy for external ear canal tumors. However, the invasive nature of these tumors means that complete excision may not be possible. Conservative surgical techniques such as lateral wall resection (LWR) or vertical canal ablation (VCA) tend to result in incomplete excision and early recurrence. A more aggressive surgical approach, such as total ear canal ablation and lateral bulla osteotomy (TECA/LBO) is more likely to result in complete excision.[62] Adjuvant radiotherapy may be of use if clean surgical margins are not achieved and chemotherapy may be of use for tumors with a high metastatic potential.[63] The presence of neurologic signs at the time of diagnosis, a diagnosis of SCC, or a carcinoma of unknown origin and histological evidence of invasion into blood vessels or lymphatics are associated with a poor prognosis.[37]

Ceruminous gland adenocarcinoma

This is the most common tumor of the external ear canal in cats.[62,64] Ceruminous glands are modified apocrine sweat glands that underlie the superficial epithelium and their secretory products, along with that of the sebaceous glands and desquamated epithelium, make up earwax. Malignant ceruminous gland tumors occur more frequently than their benign counterpart in cats in contrast to dogs.[64]

Ceruminous gland adenocarcinomas often destroy the adjacent soft tissues and may metastasize, but this tumor type has the longest median survival time of the malignant tumors if treated aggressively.[37] Following TECA/LBO the median disease-free interval was 42 months, with a one-year survival rate of 75% and a 25% local recurrence rate, whereas with LWR these figures were ten months, 33% and 67%, respectively.[62] Adjuvant therapy may be needed in patients with advanced disease. In one study of six cats with macroscopic and microscopic disease treated with 48 Gy of megavoltage radiation, a few cats achieved a complete response, but most eventually developed local recurrence or metastases.[63]

Squamous cell carcinoma

SCC of the external ear canal is a very aggressive tumor. The tumors are locally invasive, ulcerated, and painful. In this location, SCC is more likely to invade into the ear canal and adjacent structures and cause facial nerve paralysis, Horner syndrome, and deafness.

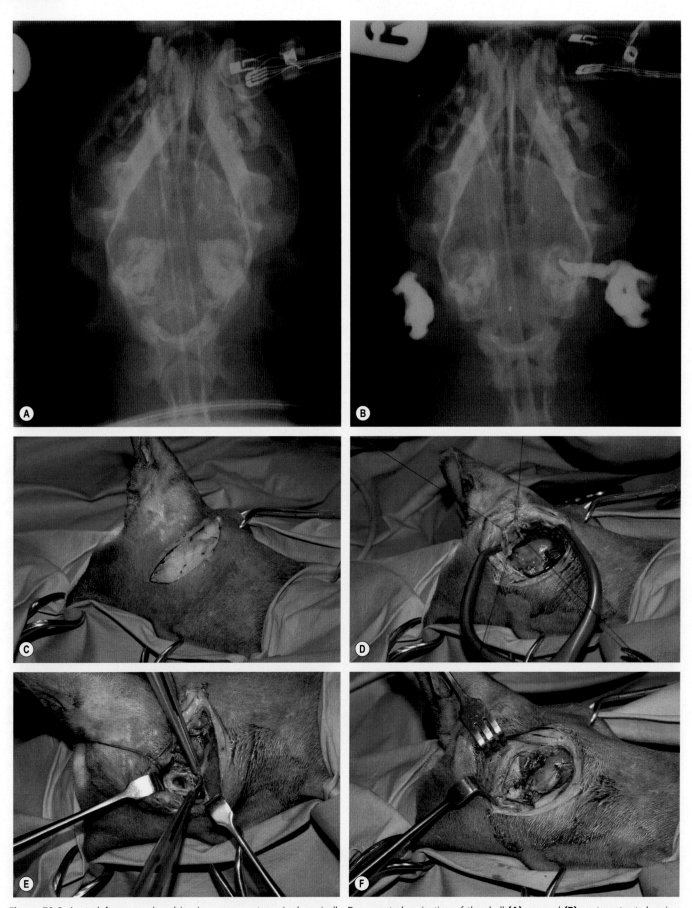

Figure 50-9 Acute left ear canal avulsion in a young cat repaired surgically. Dorsoventral projection of the skull **(A)** pre-and **(B)** post-contrast showing loss of gas shadow within the right external ear canal and lack of positive contrast filling the external ear canal. **(C)** A curvilinear incision is made caudal and ventral to the pinna. **(D)** The distal external ear canal is identified and stay sutures placed. **(E)** The proximal external ear canal is identified. **(F)** The external ear canal is repaired with interrupted sutures.

Eventually, invasion into the brain or brainstem may occur. These tumors are difficult to excise completely and they do not respond well to adjuvant chemotherapy or radiotherapy. Meningeal carcinomatosis and associated neurologic signs have been reported secondary to this tumor.[65]

Trauma

Trauma to the external ear canal may be caused by road traffic accidents and fight wounds. This may be serious enough to cause separation of the auricular and annular cartilages[15,66] or avulsion of the annular cartilage from the osseous external auditory meatus.[67] Acutely, signs of trauma predominate, but chronically the ear canal may become stenosed or closed, with the development of a draining sinus.

In acute cases the ends of the ear canal may be identified and sutured in apposition (Fig. 50-9). In more chronic cases this may not be possible and a salvage surgical procedure, such as suturing the end of the horizontal canal to the skin surface while leaving the vertical ear canal in situ, a VCA or a total ear canal ablation may be required.[15,66,68]

Congenital disorders

Congenital absence of portions of the external ear canal is rarely encountered. Recurrent ear pain and draining tracts may be the result. Similar surgical techniques as for trauma to the external ear canal, including primary anastomosis of the ear canal, may be used.[69]

SURGICAL DISEASES OF THE MIDDLE EAR

Otitis media

Otitis media is inflammation of the middle ear. It is a relatively common disease process that often goes unrecognized. Otitis media is generally assumed to be less common in cats compared with dogs, although it is not clear whether this is a true species difference, or because it less recognized in cats. Otitis media may be difficult to diagnose as it is often masked by concurrent otitis externa. Because of this difficulty, in most cats with otitis media the disease is chronic. Otitis media may actually be easier to diagnose in cats compared to dogs as their ear canal is relatively short.

In some animals the disorder is asymptomatic and an incidental finding,[70] although the lack of clinical signs may reflect the inability of the owner to recognize a problem or the clinician to identify any abnormality on examination. Fluid may be found in the middle ear of cats with no clinical signs of ear disease. This fluid may be associated with the presence of palatine defects[71,72] or sinonasal disease, such as nasopharyngeal lymphoma and sinusitis,[73] and it is suspected that Eustachian tube dysfunction is present in these cats. In one study, the prevalence of non-neoplastic middle ear disease in 66 cats was 6%[74] and in another study of 3442 cats was 1.7%, with 44% affected bilaterally and 56% unilaterally. Only 10% of affected cats had clinical signs related to middle ear disease, namely peripheral vestibular disease and Horner syndrome.[70]

Otitis media may be primary or secondary and can also be iatrogenic. In the cat, primary otitis media occurs as a result of infection ascending via the Eustachian tube to the middle ear, following upper respiratory tract infection or as a result of Eustachian tube dysfunction as a result of nasopharyngeal disease or anatomic abnormalities in this area.[75] This is supported by the fact that the pathogens involved are consistent with respiratory tract pathogens. Organisms cultured

Box 50-4 Treatment plan for otitis media

1. Gain access to the middle ear, directly if the tympanic membrane is not intact, or via myringotomy (see Box 50-7) if it is still intact
2. Collect samples for cytology and bacterial culture
3. Flush the tympanic bulla, until the fluid removed is clear
4. Infuse topical medications into the bulla
5. Reduce inflammation with systemic corticosteroids
6. Administer systemic and topical antimicrobials
7. Consider the use of systemic antifungal agents if *Malassezia* suspected or confirmed
8. Administer additional analgesia as required
9. Recheck frequently, e.g., every one to two weeks initially, and re-treat two to three times
10. Treat for a sufficient length of time, e.g., four to eight weeks
11. Consider surgery in severe, chronic or refractory cases

from the middle ear in cats with otitis media include streptococci and staphylococci and organisms that are more difficult to culture, such as *Mycoplasma* and *Bordetella*,[76] although culture is by no means positive in all cases.

Cats may develop secondary otitis media as a result of damage to the tympanic membrane from ear mites, a foreign body or by extension of a polyp through the tympanic membrane. Acute otitis media may be encountered after iatrogenic damage to the tympanic membrane during cleaning or investigation of otitis externa.

Infective otitis media is treated with systemic antibiotics for three to six weeks in the first instance. Ideally, the choice of antibiotic should be based on culture and sensitivity testing of material obtained by otoscopy (if the tympanic membrane is ruptured) or myringotomy (if the tympanic membrane is intact). If concurrent otitis externa is present, this should be treated.

Conservative management of otitis media may not be successful in the long term and a bulla osteotomy may be required to achieve surgical drainage and to remove any abnormal tissue, e.g., thickened epithelium or polyps. An LBO is indicated if there is concurrent external ear canal disease that is to be managed with a total ear canal ablation, whereas a ventral bulla osteotomy (VBO) is indicated if external ear canal disease is absent or may be managed non-surgically.

Treatment of otitis media

A framework of steps for the treatment of otitis media is listed in Box 50-4.[77]

Administration of topical agents directly into the middle ear should be done with caution after due consideration of the likely benefit of therapy (i.e., successful resolution of the condition that has not responded to more conservative measures) versus the potential adverse effects (i.e., ototoxicity). Topical agents normally recommended are fluoroquinolones (e.g., enrofloxacin) and ticarcillin or ceftazidime. Neurologic complications after flushing of the middle ear may be seen, but are usually transient and resolve within 24 hours. However, hospitalization for at least 24 hours may be prudent so that the clinician can assess the effect of the treatment and so that the cat may be fully recovered before discharge to the owner.

Middle ear polyps

This condition is dealt with in Chapter 51.

Neoplasia

Tumors affecting the middle ear are rare in cats and there is little information on their true incidence and etiology. The few cases reported include carcinoma, SCC, adenocarcinoma, lymphoma, and fibrosarcoma.[45,76,78-86] Of these, SCC, which is also the most common oropharyngeal neoplasm, is the most common tumor. Middle ear tumors are locally invasive, but metastasis is rare and tends to be to the lymph nodes.

Cats usually present with clinical signs of otitis media that is refractory to medical therapy. Clinical signs may progress to otitis interna or otitis externa, facial nerve paralysis, laryngeal paralysis, Horner's syndrome, keratoconjunctivitis sicca, and exposure keratitis, and may rarely extend into the pharynx. Clinical signs may not differentiate between an inflammatory polyp and true neoplasia, as the neurologic signs of secondary infection of a polyp may be severe.[87]

Diagnosis via otoscopy may be possible if the tympanic membrane is irregular, bulging or ruptured. However, diagnostic imaging, either CT, MRI or radiography, is normally required to demonstrate a mass in the tympanic bulla, although this will not indicate the tumor type. Fine needle aspiration via the external ear canal may be possible and may yield a diagnosis, particularly with lymphoma. Histologic examination of tissue samples taken percutaneously may be possible if there is extensive invasion of tissues outside of the middle ear.

Surgery may be performed for local control, either via a LBO or VBO, depending on the involvement of the external ear canal, although complete surgical excision is not commonly possible.[37,76,88] Adjuvant radiotherapy may be indicated for long-term local control. Tumors are often not diagnosed until advanced disease is present, e.g., marked ataxia and inappetence, and the prognosis is guarded to poor.

Cholesteatoma

Cholesteatomas have not been described clinically in cats, although they may be induced experimentally by ligation of the external auditory canal.[89]

SURGICAL DISEASES OF THE INNER EAR

Surgery is rarely indicated for disease of the inner ear, but conditions affecting this area may occur as an extension of middle ear disease or as complications of aural surgery, such as bulla osteotomy, ototoxic agents, and ear flushing.

Deafness

Congenital deafness has been reported in white cats.[90] Acquired deafness may be sensorineural or conductive. Causes of acquired deafness include drug toxicity, noise trauma, infection, aging, middle ear effusion, excess cerumen production, and physical trauma.[91,92] Deafness may be acquired following ear cleaning under general anesthesia and concurrent vestibular dysfunction was noted in some animals, with resolution of these signs in all cases.[93] Deafness or impaired hearing will be seen postoperatively after total ear canal ablation.

Vestibular syndrome

Common clinical signs of vestibular disease are head tilt, nystagmus, and ataxia, which may be present as single entities or a combination. Neurologic examination of the patient will allow differentiation of peripheral versus central vestibular disease (see Table 50-1), which

---

- Cats with vestibular signs need a careful physical and neurologic examination to determine whether peripheral or central vestibular disease is present (see Table 50-1)
- If clinical signs of otitis externa or otitis media are present, then it is likely that the vestibular signs are associated with the otitis media
- Otitis media can occur without signs of otitis externa, making the diagnosis of otitis media difficult. Neurologic examination and diagnostic imaging may be required to make a diagnosis of otitis media

Table 50-3 Diseases causing central vestibular signs

Type of disease	Disease
Degenerative	Cerebellar cortical abiotrophy
	Lysosomal storage diseases
Anomalous	Hydrocephalus
Nutritional	Thiamine deficiency
Neoplasia	Meningioma
	Lymphoma
	Oligodendroglioma
	Medulloblastoma
Toxic	Metronidazole
	Lead
Trauma	
Vascular	Feline ischemic encephalopathy

will then guide the diagnostic approach. Important points related to vestibular disease in cats are listed in Box 50-5.

Peripheral vestibular dysfunction results from diseases of the inner and middle ear affecting the receptors in the labyrinth and the vestibular portion of cranial nerve VIII. Central vestibular dysfunction results from disease affecting the brainstem and cerebellum. Central vestibular diseases are listed in Table 50-3 and are not considered further here, but should be considered as differential diagnoses for cats presenting with vestibular disease.

The three major differential diagnoses for cats with peripheral vestibular disease are otitis interna/media, nasopharyngeal polyps (see Chapter 51), and idiopathic feline vestibular disease.[94,95] The damaged vestibular system can compensate over time; however, residual neurologic deficits such as a head tilt are relatively common and recurrence of clinical signs may be seen at times of stress, recurrent disease or after anesthesia.[96-98] Supportive care for cats with vestibular disease is important to manage the clinical signs such as inappetence, vomiting, salivation, and nausea that accompany vestibular dysfunction.[99-101]

Inflammation/infection

Most animals with otitis interna have otitis media, and extension of otitis media is the most common cause of otitis interna.[102] Bacterial otitis interna or labyrinthitis may cause peripheral vestibular dysfunction. Organisms commonly isolated include *Staphylococcus, Streptococcus, Pasteurella, Proteus, E. coli, Enterococcus, Pseudomonas,* and obligate anaerobes. Treatment comprises long-term (six to eight weeks) antibiotic therapy. Refractory cases may need surgical drainage of the tympanic bulla.[102,103] Progression to brainstem dysfunction, with the development of central vestibular signs, altered mentation, abnormal posture and gait, cranial nerve deficits, and seizures, may be seen in severe cases. Diagnosis is by MRI and CSF analysis and the prognosis is good to excellent with surgical management and appropriate antibiotic therapy, despite the severe and apparently life-threatening presentation.[104]

Cryptococcosis usually causes central vestibular signs, but cats with peripheral vestibular disorders have been described. All animals responded well to surgical drainage and medical therapy with ketoconazole, fluconazole or itraconazole.[105] Resolution of the neurologic signs may take two to six weeks and often some neurologic deficits, e.g., a head tilt, remain.

Neoplasia

Tumors affecting the peripheral vestibular system are dealt with above in the section on the middle ear, as these regions are commonly affected together, particularly by carcinomas.[79,81,83,86] Surgery for biopsy or therapy may be considered as for middle ear neoplasia, but cure of the disease and resolution of the neurologic signs are unlikely. Craniectomy and VBO has been described for the management of middle ear tumors with medial extension in two cats with prolonged postoperative survival.[106]

Ototoxicity

Peripheral vestibular disease may be induced by ototoxic agents, i.e., those agents that may damage the cochlear or vestibular apparatus when administered orally, parenterally or topically. The round window membrane is more permeable to drugs in the presence of otitis media.[107] Ototoxicity results from damage to the hair cells in the cochlea or in the vestibular apparatus and results in hearing deficits, vestibular signs or both, which may be very obvious or more subtle. In cats, vestibular signs tend to predominate, whereas in dogs deafness is more usual.

A large number of agents have been described as ototoxic or potentially ototoxic, but much of the information is of poor quality as it is anecdotal, based on extrapolation from other species, or found as a result of using drugs in far higher concentrations than used clinically.[108-110] In addition, many reports describe ototoxicity experimentally in normal animals, whereas in animals with otitis, the susceptibility to ototoxic agents may be different. For further information on flushing solutions and therapeutic agents see below.

External trauma

Peripheral vestibular signs may follow head trauma, particularly where there is fracture of the petrosal temporal bone or tympanic bulla, or gunshot injury.[111] This may be accompanied by facial nerve paresis or paralysis. Treatment is supportive, along with management of other injuries sustained as a result of the trauma.

Iatrogenic trauma

Peripheral vestibular disease may be seen after bulla osteotomy, particularly where vigorous curettage of the petrous temporal bone has been performed.

Idiopathic feline vestibular syndrome (IFVS)

This is a disorder of peracute peripheral vestibular dysfunction, usually found in young to middle-aged cats, especially in the summer months. No cause is known, although comparisons have been drawn with Meniere disease in man, where abnormal endolymphatic flow or electrolyte abnormalities in the perilymph have been suggested.[94] Bilateral disease is uncommon (less than 10%) and concurrent facial nerve paralysis or Horner syndrome is not expected.

IFVS may be preceded by upper respiratory tract disease and clinical signs of excessive vocalization, which may be related to general disorientation, have been reported.[94,112] A diagnosis is made by excluding other causes of vestibular disease. Treatment consists of supportive nursing care for the disorientation and anorexia. The prognosis for recovery is good, although this may take two to four weeks and approximately 25% of cats will have residual neurologic deficits such as a head tilt. In addition, recurrence of clinical signs may occur.[94]

Anomalous vestibular disorders

Congenital vestibular disorders have been reported in Siamese and Burmese kittens.[23,102] Signs of peripheral vestibular dysfunction and concurrent deafness are seen at three to four weeks of age, with clinical improvement in three to four months. The cause is unknown.

FLUSHING THE EAR CANAL AND MYRINGOTOMY

Flushing the ear canal under general anesthesia is necessary for the resolution of many cases of otitis, particularly in chronic cases and where topical therapy has not been effective. In animals with marked stenosis of the ear canal caused by inflammation, flushing may need to be delayed until the ear canal is patent following the use of topical or systemic corticosteroids. Indications for otic flushing are listed in Box 50-6. Flushing of the ear canal should be followed by a regime of owner-administered ear cleaning once or twice daily and this should be demonstrated to the client prior to flushing, when the ear may be less painful. Ear flushing is described in Box 50-7.

Myringotomy involves making a hole in the tympanic membrane with a needle or myringotomy knife and sampling the contents of the middle ear and may be used as a diagnostic test in middle ear disease. In animals with otitis media and a persistent pressure change in the tympanic cavity, myringotomy will equalize the pressure and reduce pain and is therefore therapeutic.

Aural solutions and therapeutics

Careful consideration should be given to the contents of any topical preparation used in the external ear canal, particularly if there is a

---

Box 50-6 Indications for otic flushing

- Failure of owner-administered topical therapy to resolve the problem in a reasonable period of time, usually within four weeks
- Presence of aural discharge that may harbor microorganisms and prevent topical agents reaching adequate concentrations
- Suspicion of otitis media, foreign body or neoplasia
- If a full and detailed examination of the ear canal and tympanic membrane and/or myringotomy is required
- If foreign bodies are present

Box 50-7 Ear flushing and myringotomy

The cat is generally placed in lateral recumbency with the caudal head and neck elevated to allow fluid exiting the bulla via the Eustachian tubes to flow rostrally out of the nares. Care should be taken to keep the flushing solution and associated debris and potential pathogens out of the patient's eyes.

Ear flushing

The ear canal should be alternately flushed and then suctioned to remove the instilled fluid to improve visibility. A syringe and a red rubber or polypropylene catheter (3.5–5 French) may be used for this purpose. Alternatively, a catheter may be attached to a bag of warmed saline and continuous lavage provided with intermittent suction. Samples should always be collected for cytology and culture and the need for a myringotomy should be considered.

Once samples have been taken for clinical pathology, a ceruminolytic agent may be applied to break down waxy and adherent materials and hasten the cleaning process. However, most ceruminolytic agents are potentially ototoxic, so caution should be exercised, particularly if the tympanic membrane is not intact. The ear should be lavaged thoroughly with saline afterwards, particularly if the tympanic membrane is perforated.

Myringotomy

A 20G or 22G spinal needle of appropriate length (at least 1.5 inches) may be used. This is introduced into the pars tensa of the tympanic membrane at either the 5 o'clock or 7 o'clock position (i.e., caudoventrally) to keep away from the germinal epithelium and blood vessels overlying the manubrium of the malleus. Fluid is either aspirated directly, or 1 mL of saline is instilled and then aspirated with a syringe. Samples should be obtained for cytology and culture and sensitivity, and this may be followed by therapeutic lavage.

---

clinical suspicion or knowledge that the tympanic membrane is not intact.[109] Many ear-cleaning solutions contain a mixture of ototoxic substances and, of these, chlorhexidine is probably the most toxic, particularly in cats. Similarly, most otic preparations for the treatment of otitis externa contain potentially ototoxic agents. Other potentially ototoxic agents in cats include aminoglycosides, furosemide, bumetanide, and fipronil. In humans, ethacrynic acid and antibiotics such as erythromycin, minocycline, chloramphenicol, vancomycin, and topical polymyxin B have been reported to cause vestibular signs, but this has not been reported in cats. Treatment comprises stopping the potentially ototoxic medication and provision of supportive care. The prognosis for recovery is good in most cases.

The following drugs may be considered safe, or perhaps more correctly, less ototoxic: fluoroquinolones, aqueous penicillin G, some semisynthetic penicillins (carbenacillin and ticarcillin) and some cephalosporins (ceftazidime and cefmenoxime), clotrimazole, miconazole, nystatin and tolnaftate, the aqueous forms of dexamethasone and fluocinolone, and some flushing agents (squalene and Tris-EDTA).[77,113] The only safe solution for lavage of the middle ear, or of the external ear canal if the tympanic membrane is ruptured is a sterile isotonic crystalloid, such as saline. Antiseptics and known ototoxic agents should be avoided.

Complications

Complications from ear flushing are more common in cats than dogs, although it is important to consider that some of these may also result from the presence of uncontrolled otitis externa/media. Complications include pain and neurologic signs (facial nerve paresis, Horner

syndrome, vestibular, deafness). Most complications are transient, but permanent neurologic complications may occur and flushing the ear canal should never be considered as a routine or prophylactic procedure. Complications are avoided by using good chemical restraint (general anesthesia), gentle atraumatic technique, avoiding ototoxic agents, and either avoiding ceruminolytic agents or ensuring that these agents are thoroughly flushed out with saline after their administration.

Fluid in the middle ear will dampen hearing and fluid introduced during lavage of the middle ear may take seven to ten days to be absorbed, with resultant impaired hearing during this time. The normal tympanic membrane heals in three to five weeks.

PREPARATION FOR SURGERY

Preparation of the external surfaces of the ear may be readily achieved, but the external ear canal cannot be cleaned as effectively and it should be considered that surgery in this location constitutes clean-contaminated or contaminated surgery. In animals with established infectious otitis, then surgery may be classified as dirty, although in these patients, an effort to control the local infection may be made before beginning surgery. Thus perioperative antimicrobial prophylaxis may be indicated, although some consideration should be given to delaying antibiotic administration until samples have been obtained for culture.

A pharyngeal pack should be placed whenever intervention (surgery or otoscopy) is performed in a patient that might have a defect in the tympanic membrane, as fluid may exit the tympanic bulla via the auditory tube. The eyes should be protected with a topical agent to protect them against damage from the skin preparation agent.

SURGICAL TECHNIQUES

Lateral wall resection

A LWR is the removal of the lateral wall of the vertical part of the external ear canal, with subsequent apposition of the skin surface to the integument of the remaining vertical canal (Fig. 50-10 and Box 50-8). It is indicated in the management of otitis externa where an improvement in the local microenvironment following the procedure will allow for either resolution of the condition or improved access for treatment, for removal of small masses from the lateral wall of the vertical canal and, uncommonly, to gain surgical access to the horizontal part of the ear canal. It is important to realize that for most animals with otitis externa, this procedure is not curative, and the animal will need continued therapy. For cats with chronic otitis externa affecting the remaining external ear canal or otitis media, this procedure is likely to be unsuccessful. This procedure is uncommonly performed in cats.

Vertical canal ablation

A VCA is the removal of the entire vertical part of the external ear canal with subsequent apposition of the ends of the horizontal part of the ear canal to the skin (Box 50-9). It is indicated for otitis externa that affects only the vertical ear canal, trauma, and small masses of the vertical canal. The advantages of this technique are that, compared to a total ear canal ablation, it is technically simpler, with fewer complications, and preserves hearing. The main disadvantage is that otitis externa rarely solely involve the vertical canal, and usually persistent otitis externa in the remaining part of the ear canal renders this surgical technique a failure. This surgery is very uncommonly performed in cats.

A variation of this procedure, the 'pull-through' technique, involves making an incision around the external auditory meatus and dissecting the vertical canal free of its attachments, before pulling it through a defect in the skin made at the junction of the horizontal and vertical canals and then creating a new opening as for the standard technique.[114,115]

Total ear canal ablation and lateral bulla osteotomy

Total ear canal ablation (Fig. 50-12) is the excision of both the vertical and horizontal parts of the external ear canal to the level of the osseous external acoustic meatus (Box 50-10). A LBO is always performed concurrently to investigate the contents of the tympanic bulla and manage concurrent middle ear disease.

In the cat, the main indication for TECA/LBO is neoplasia of the external ear canal, although other indications include chronic otitis externa, trauma, and congenital malformations.[37,62,64,88,104,116–119]

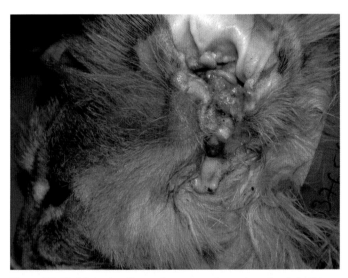

Figure 50-10 A lateral wall resection was performed previously in this adult domestic short-haired cat. There is evidence of continuing otitis externa.

A variation of this procedure, a subtotal ear canal ablation, has been recommended for animals with minimal pathologic changes in the distal ear canal.[120] The technique involves resection of the proximal (ventral) half of the vertical ear canal and the entire horizontal canal. The remaining distal (dorsal) vertical canal is then closed to create a small, blind-ending auricular cavity with preservation of the entire circumference of the annular cartilage. Potential advantages include less dissection and maintenance of a normal ear carriage and potential disadvantages include necessity for continued medical therapy if not all the diseased tissue is removed.

Box 50-8 Lateral wall resection

The cat is positioned in lateral recumbency. Two vertically directed incisions are made in the skin, one from the tragohelicine fissure and one from the intertragic notch, approximately 1.5 times the length of the vertical canal. The soft tissue is then cleared from the lateral wall of the vertical canal and similar incisions are made in the vertical canal, removing approximately 50% of the circumference of the ear canal. The resulting cartilage flap is reflected distally and the proximal two-thirds is amputated, leaving a small portion ventral to the opening of the horizontal canal as a drainage board. The surrounding skin is then apposed to the integument of the external ear canal with simple interrupted sutures of a monofilament non-absorbable suture material (e.g.,1.5 M Nylon).

Box 50-9 Vertical canal ablation

The cat is positioned in lateral recumbency with the affected ear uppermost (Fig. 50-11A). A circular incision is made around the external auditory meatus, and the incision is then extended ventrally over the vertical part of the external ear canal (Fig. 50-11B). The tissue of the parotid salivary gland is bluntly dissected to expose the vertical ear canal. Dissection of the vertical part of the external ear canal then proceeds with a mixture of sharp and blunt dissection, making an effort to stay as close to the cartilage of the ear canal as possible (Fig. 50-11C). When the vertical canal is fully exposed circumferentially the dorsal two-thirds of the vertical canal is amputated. Incisions are made in the remaining vertical canal rostrally and caudally to the level of the junction of the vertical canal and horizontal canal, and the resulting flaps are sutured to the surrounding skin as dorsal and ventral drainage boards.

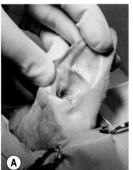 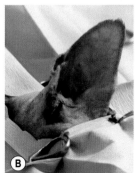 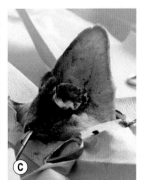 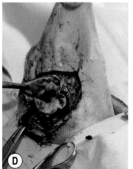 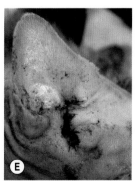

Figure 50-11 Vertical canal ablation in an elderly cat with a ceruminous gland adenoma affecting the vertical ear canal. **(A)** The ear is manually extended to tense the skin prior to making the first incision. **(B)** A T-shaped skin incision is made around the external ear canal opening and extending down distal to the ear canal. **(C)** The incision is extended around the external ear canal opening. **(D)** The vertical ear canal is dissected out by a combination of sharp and blunt dissection, keeping close to the cartilage. **(E)** At the end of surgery after resection of the vertical ear canal, dorsal and ventral flaps are sutured to the surrounding skin, and the original skin incision is closed. *(Courtesy of Jon Hall.)*

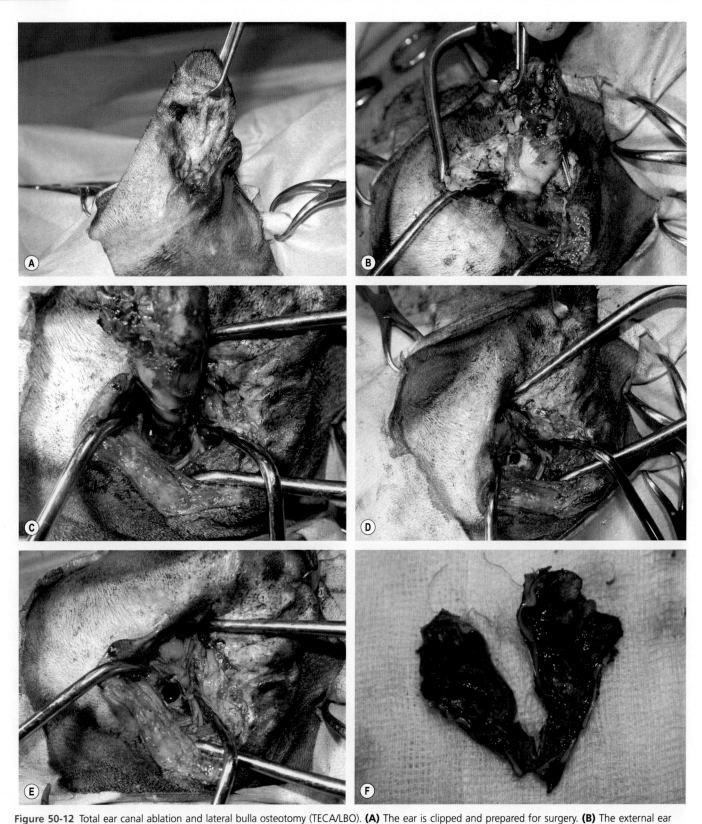

Figure 50-12 Total ear canal ablation and lateral bulla osteotomy (TECA/LBO). **(A)** The ear is clipped and prepared for surgery. **(B)** The external ear canal is dissected out. **(C)** The junction of the external ear canal and osseous external acoustic meatus and facial nerve are identified. **(D)** The external ear canal is amputated from the osseous external acoustic meatus. **(E)** A lateral bulla osteotomy is performed. **(F)** The excised external ear canal is shown after bisection; there are chronic proliferative changes in the integument and intraluminal discharge and debris.

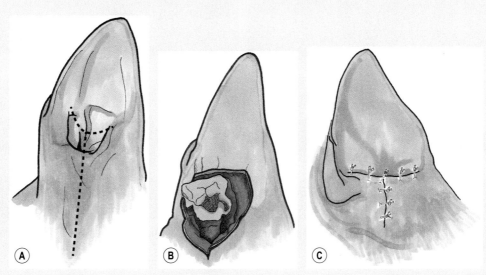

Box 50-10 Total ear canal ablation and lateral bulla osteotomy (TECA/LBO)

The cat is placed in lateral recumbency with the affected ear uppermost. The neck is extended over a small sandbag or towel. An incision is made around the opening of the external ear canal, which may be extended ventrally with a linear incision over the vertical ear canal (Fig. 50-13A). The tissue of the parotid salivary gland is bluntly dissected to expose the vertical ear canal. Dissection of the external ear canal then proceeds with a mixture of sharp and blunt dissection, making an effort to stay as close to the cartilage of the ear canal as possible (Fig. 50-13B). This process proceeds deeper until the external acoustic meatus is encountered. Care is taken to avoid the facial nerve, which exits the skull via the stylomastoid foramen caudal to the ear canal and courses rostrally around the ventral aspect of the ear canal. The external ear canal is excised with a scalpel blade while protecting the facial nerve. Remnants of epithelium attached to the opening of the external acoustic meatus are removed.

The opening to the bulla is enlarged with rongeurs by removing bone ventral to the external acoustic meatus. The bony shelf between the small dorsolateral compartment and the larger ventromedial compartment is opened with rongeurs. A curette is used to remove the epithelial lining and debris from the tympanic bulla and lavage and suction is used to remove debris and discharge. Samples should be submitted for culture. The dorsal (epitympanic recess and auditory ossicles) and dorsomedial (promontory and inner ear structures) regions are avoided to reduce the incidence of iatrogenic vestibular defects.[118] A wound drain is not routinely used.

The deeper tissues are closed with small gauge synthetic monofilament suture material in a simple interrupted or purse-string suture, taking care to avoid the facial nerve. Final incisional closure is routine (Fig. 50-13C).

Figure 50-13 Total ear canal ablation and lateral bulla osteotomy (TECA/LBO). **(A)** A T-shaped skin incision extends around the opening of the external ear canal and extends distally over the vertical ear. **(B)** The incision is continued around the opening of the external ear canal and the dissection is continued close to the ear canal down to the external acoustic meatus and a lateral bulla osteotomy is performed. **(C)** Final appearance after skin closure.

Another variation of this procedure uses a ventrally based single pedicle advancement flap to maintain normal ear carriage after total ear canal ablation.[121] The complication rate of this procedure was not different from the standard procedure.

Ventral bulla osteotomy

VBO (Figs 50-14 and 50-15) is indicated for diagnostic and therapeutic purposes in cats with middle ear disease (Box 50-11). This includes mass lesions of the middle ear, primarily middle ear polyps, but including other tumors, and otitis media, where medical therapy alone or with myringotomy and lavage are not sufficient and where there is no concurrent otitis externa, for which a total ear canal ablation and LBO would be indicated.

Pinnectomy

A partial or total pinna removal or pinnectomy (Box 50-12) is performed for resection of traumatic lesions or neoplasia. The most common indication is pinnal SCC (see Fig. 50-7).

Aural hematoma drainage

A surgical drain[31,32] or teat cannula[33] may be implanted to provide longer term continuous drainage (Box 50-13), but this may be ineffective if there is a substantial quantity of fibrin in the hematoma cavity. Incisional drainage is usually needed for a chronic hematoma.

Postoperative application of a sterile dressing and a bandage provides optimal aseptic care, may contribute to maintaining apposition between the skin and cartilage, and helps to retain an implanted drain, but bandaging the ear and head in cats can be difficult to maintain and achieve without complications.

POSTOPERATIVE CARE

Surgery of the external ear canal and middle ear has the potential to be painful and a robust and effective analgesia plan should be made, with repeated assessment of the patient and adjustment of this plan

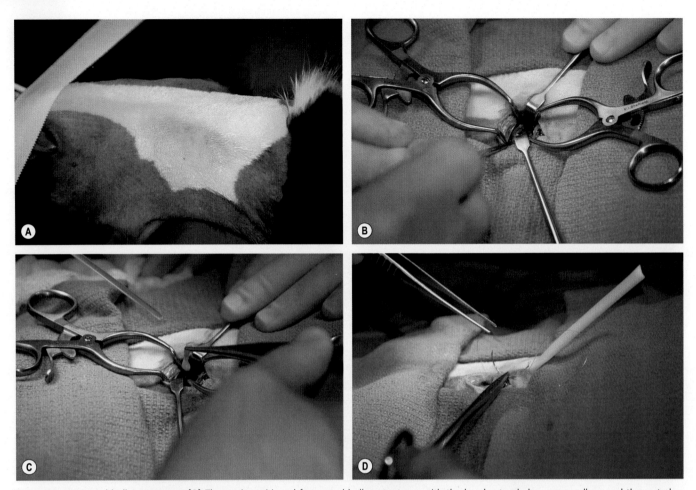

Figure 50-14 Ventral bulla osteotomy. **(A)** The cat is positioned for ventral bulla osteotomy with the head extended over a sandbag and the rostral aspect taped down. **(B)** Multiple retractors are used to assist in exposing the ventral aspect of the tympanic bulla. **(C)** Removal of thick fluid from the bulla after osteotomy. **(D)** Placement of a Penrose drain prior to closure.

as needed. A pre-emptive multimodal analgesic plan should be employed, with opiates and non-steroidal anti-inflammatory drugs (NSAIDs) given preoperatively (unless there is a contraindication to NSAID use), with additional opiates given during the anesthetic as required (e.g., fentanyl infusion). Postoperatively, opiates, either as bolus doses or as a continuous rate infusion, should be continued along with NSAIDs. Local anesthesia may be used singly, e.g., as a splash block, or as multiple doses, e.g., with a wound diffusion catheter. Lidocaine or ketamine may be added as a continuous rate infusion if additional analgesia is required.

The use of antibiotics postoperatively depends on the assessment of standard criteria, such as the US National Research Council classification of the wound, the duration of the anesthesia and surgery, and the patient's general health status. Bandaging the ears is difficult to achieve satisfactorily and the use of a bandage which passes round the neck has the potential to obstruct venous and lymphatic flow or cause asphyxia, and these are not recommended. A patient with an open wound or a surgical drain needs particular care of the wound using standard aseptic technique.

Patients with pre-existing or iatrogenic postoperative facial nerve paresis or paralysis need to have an artificial tear replacement used to prevent the eye from drying due to the loss of the blink response and the loss of the parasympathetic supply to the lacrimal gland. Patients with vestibular syndrome are often disorientated and require additional nursing care, particularly with respect to eating and drinking.

COMPLICATIONS AND PROGNOSIS

Most complications associated with surgical procedures of the ear result from total ear canal ablation and LBO. The complication rate in cats is similar to that in dogs, although there may be a greater incidence of neurologic complications, particularly Horner syndrome and permanent facial nerve paralysis, in cats compared to dogs.[88,119]

Hemorrhage

Intraoperative hemorrhage may be clinically significant, particularly if it arises from trauma to the retroglenoid vein or branches of the carotid artery, but in most cases it is not. However, bleeding impairs the surgeon's view of the intraoperative site and this may increase the risk of iatrogenic damage to structures in the surgical field. Concerns about the significance of hemorrhage may result in the surgeon rushing or abbreviating the procedure, which may increase the risk of

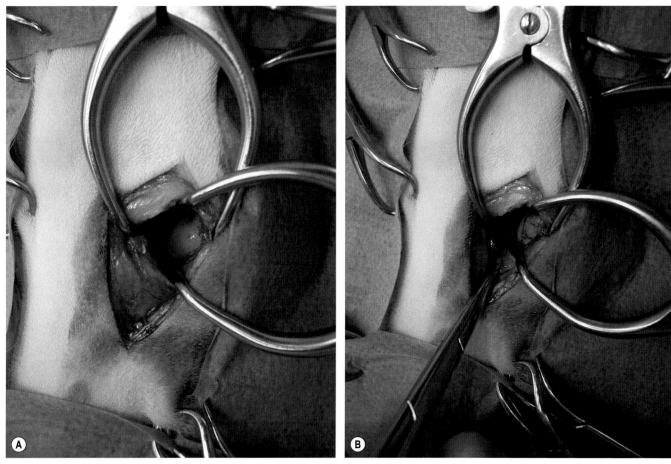

Figure 50-15 Ventral bulla osteotomy in a domestic short-hair cat with a middle ear polyp and secondary otitis media. **(A)** The ventral aspect of the tympanic bulla had been exposed by soft tissue dissection using a standard ventral approach. **(B)** A square section of the ventral bulla has been cut using an osteotome and mallet.

complications relating to incomplete removal of the integument from the tympanic cavity.

Acute wound complications

Acute wound complications include incisional hematoma, incisional dehiscence, extended wound drainage, wound infection, and acute cellulitis and abscessation. Wound contamination is difficult to avoid and some degree of minor wound swelling, exudation or dehiscence is not uncommon, but rarely requires any further attention.

Local wound care, establishing drainage and antibiotic therapy, followed by second intention healing will normally result in resolution of these problems.

Necrosis of the pinna is very uncommon and is normally caused by disruption of the proximal edge of the caudal pinnal margin.[118]

Fistulous tract

A chronic draining tract or fistula may develop postoperatively. Prior to fistula development signs of fluid accumulation and pain in the middle ear may be subtle, including pain on opening of the mouth (yawning or eating) and scratching or shaking of the head. Clinical examination often reveals marked pain on palpation of the previous surgical site and bulla. The most common reason for the fistula is incomplete removal of the secretory epithelium from the tympanic cavity, although osteomyelitis of the auditory ossicles, inadequate drainage of the middle ear through the Eustachian tube and damage to the parotid salivary gland have also been implicated. Antibiotic therapy alone is usually not successful in resolving this problem and surgical exploration of the tract and re-exploration of the middle ear via a lateral approach is likely to be needed.

Nerve damage

Iatrogenic facial nerve damage is a relatively common complication after total ear canal ablation and bulla osteotomy and is transient in the majority of cases if the nerve has not been severed. Regular inspection of the eye and application of a tear replacement is required until the palpebral response returns. Horner's syndrome (Fig. 50-19) is much more common in the cat than in the dog, and is generally transient,[117] lasting three to four weeks. Vestibular syndrome is very uncommon and normally results from excessive and inappropriate curettage of the dorsomedial region of the tympanic cavity (Fig. 50-20). The clinical signs are usually temporary. Hypoglossal nerve deficits are very uncommon and may be associated with a VBO or extensive ventral dissection during a LBO. Pre-existing signs of vestibular syndrome, particularly a head tilt, may persist after resolution of the cause of the problem.

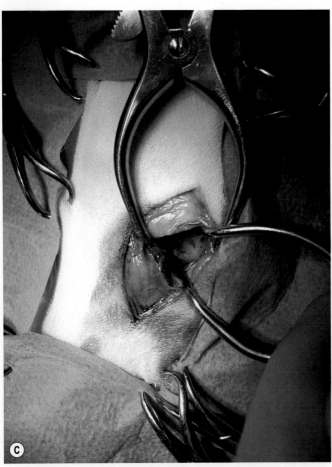
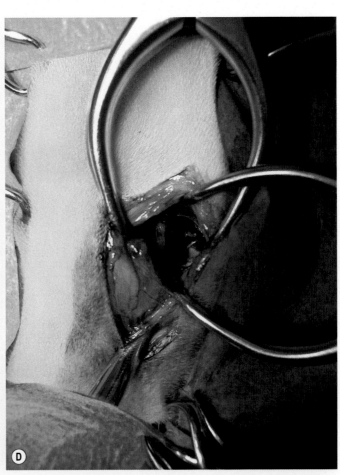

Figure 50-15, Continued (C) Removal of this bone gives good exposure to the bulla cavity, which is full of purulent fluid. Samples are collected for analysis, after which the fluid is aspirated and the bulla flushed. **(D)** The tympanic bulla is shown after removal of purulent fluid and a small polyp; both bulla cavities were opened and flushed. Great care is taken not to damage nerves on the dorsomedial wall during surgery. *(Courtesy of Laura Owen.)*

Box 50-11 Ventral bulla osteotomy

VBO is performed with the cat in dorsal recumbency, with the head and neck extended over a sandbag (Fig. 50-14A). The maxilla may be taped to the surgical table to stabilize the skull. With the cat anesthetized, the ventral aspect of the tympanic bulla is relatively easy to palpate. Other palpable landmarks include body and ramus of the mandible, the digastricus muscle, which is a relatively large curved tubular muscle that inserts on the caudoventral mandible, and the wing of the atlas.

A skin incision is made in a paramedian location, just medial to the digastricus muscle, approximately mid-way between the ventral aspect of the body of the mandible and the midline (Fig. 50-16A). This incision is centered between the angular process of the mandible and the wing of the atlas. Blunt dissection is continued through the subcutaneous tissue and platysma and sphincter colli muscles. Blunt dissection is then continued between the digastricus muscle laterally and the styloglossus and hyoglossus muscles are identified medially. The lingual artery and hypoglossal nerve are identified on the lateral border of the hyoglossus muscle and are retracted medially with this muscle. The linguofacial vein may be identified on the medial border of the digastricus muscle further caudally and should be avoided.

Exposure of the tympanic bulla (Fig. 50-16B) is achieved with hand-held (e.g., Senn) or self-retaining (e.g., Gelpi or Weitlaner) retractors. The soft tissue is elevated from the ventral aspect of the bulla with a periosteal elevator and an opening is made into the

tympanic bulla with a drill bit or Steinmann pin and hand chuck. The bone of the tympanic bulla may be chronically thickened or weakened by the presence of middle ear disease and care should be taken when performing the osteotomy. The hole is then enlarged with rongeurs. Samples of fluid or tissue are taken for culture and histology. This approach will provide access to the large ventromedial compartment of the bulla (see Fig. 50-2), which contains the round window. Care is taken to avoid damage to the cervical sympathetic nerves that lie on the surface of the promontory on the dorsomedial wall in this compartment. The ventral portion of the transverse septum is then opened as for entry into the bulla and the hole enlarged with rongeurs to gain access to the smaller dorsolateral compartment, which is where most polyps originate. This bone is thin and fragile and should be removed with care. Making this hole as laterally as possible will reduce the risk of damage to the bone promontory (Fig. 50-16C).

The origin of the polyp is removed by traction and any thickened lining of the bulla is removed by curettage. Care is taken to avoid curettage of the caudomedial and dorsal parts of the tympanic bulla to prevent damage to the round and oval windows and the ossicles. The tympanic bulla is lavaged with saline and a passive or active drain may be placed prior to closure if the bulla contains infected material that cannot be completely removed at surgery. The wound is closed by approximating the tissues in the same layers as encountered on the approach.

Box 50-11 **Continued**

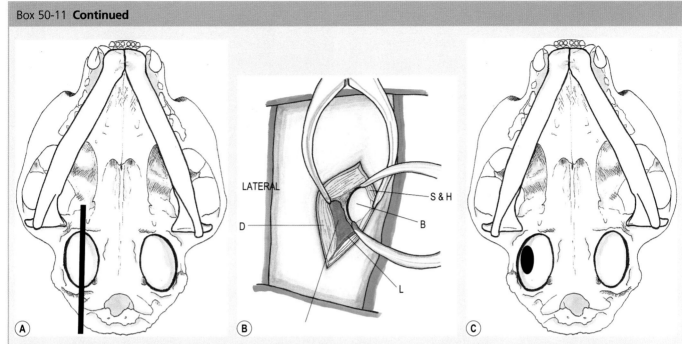

Figure 50-16 **(A)** The skin incision is made mid-way between the midline of the cat and the caudal ramus, centered over the tympanic bulla. **(B)** The bulla is exposed. **(C)** The ventral bulla osteotomy in the tympanic bulla is made on the lateral aspect of the bulla, in order to avoid damage to the promontory. B, bulla; D, digastricus muscle; L, linguofacial artery; MSG, mandibular salivary gland; S&H styloglossal and hypoglossal muscles.

Box 50-12 **Pinnectomy**

The pinna is transected at least 1 cm from the margins of the lesion (Fig. 50-17A). Scissors can be used to perform the amputation. The skin edges are then apposed with non-absorbable simple interrupted or continuous sutures, aiming to pull the thicker skin from the convex surface over the edge of the cartilage and apposing with it the thinner skin on the concave pinna (Fig. 50-17B).

The resected pinna is submitted for histopathologic analysis

Deafness or impaired hearing will be seen postoperatively after total ear canal ablation, although many patients with obstruction to the external ear canal, a disrupted tympanic membrane, or middle ear disease will have impaired hearing prior to surgery and a change may not be appreciated postoperatively.[118]

Change in cosmetic appearance

Removal of the external ear canal and loss of the external auditory meatus will result in a minor change in the animal's cosmetic

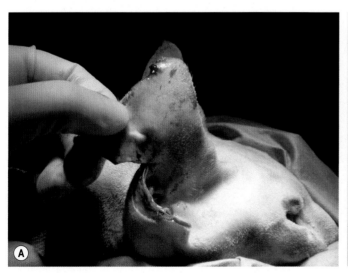
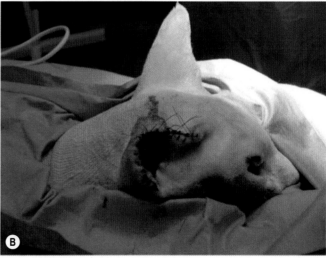

Figure 50-17 Pinnectomy in an 11-year-old female neutered Burmese cat for squamous cell carcinoma. **(A)** The pinna is resected close to the base using scissors, taking slightly more cartilage than skin to facilitate closure. **(B)** The skin is apposed using simple interrupted sutures. *(Courtesy of Jane Ladlow.)*

611

Box 50-13 Aural hematoma drainage

An incision is made in the skin of the concave aspect of the pinna into the hematoma and the contents (seroma fluid and fibrin and granulation tissue) are evacuated. Through-and-through mattress sutures are then placed parallel to the blood vessels in the pinna to avoid vascular compromise from the sutures, taking care to avoid the vessels with the suture needle (Fig. 50-18). Alternatively, after the skin is incised, the edges of the skin may be sutured to the wound bed with a simple continuous suture.[34] An alternative to a single large incision is the use of multiple smaller incisions, e.g., created with a 4–6 mm dermal biopsy punch[35] or a carbon dioxide laser,[36] although this method provides less access to drain any solid contents from the hematoma cavity.

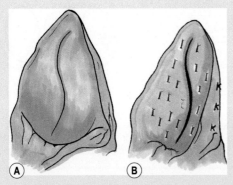

Figure 50-18 (A) Aural hematoma bulging on the concave inner pinna. **(B)** An S-shaped or sinusoidal incision is made along the length of the hematoma to drain the contents. The cavity is then closed down with multiple through-and-through mattress sutures placed parallel to blood vessels to avoid vascular compromise.

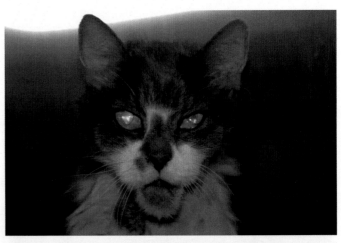

Figure 50-19 Marked Horner syndrome after ventral bulla osteotomy.

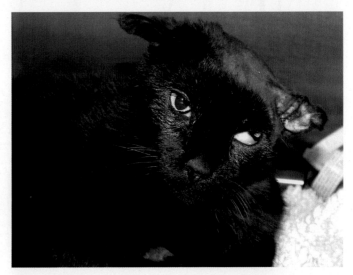

Figure 50-20 Horner syndrome and vestibular syndrome in a cat following total ear canal ablation and lateral bulla osteotomy.

Box 50-14 Reasons for failure of aural surgery in cats

Poor surgical technique, e.g., failure to drain the horizontal canal properly
Poor patient selection, i.e., chronic irreversible changes in the remaining ear canal
Failure to control the underlying ear disease
Unremitting otitis media

appearance. Of more importance is the alteration in ear carriage, with ventral deviation of the pinna, particularly if a large area of skin surrounding the external auditory meatus is removed. This cosmetic change may be avoided by using a ventrally-based advancement flap to provide more local skin for closure of the defect.[121]

Failure of surgery

It is important to realize that LWR or VCA does not provide a solution to all cases of chronic ear disease. The reasons for failure of LWR or VCA are listed in Box 50-14.

REFERENCES

1. Kontos V, Sotiraki S, Himonas C. Two rare disorders in the cat: demodectic otitis externa and sarcoptic mange. Feline Pract 1998;26(6):18–20.

2. Tater KC, Scott DW, Miller WH Jr, Erb HN. The cytology of the external ear canal in the normal dog and cat. J Vet Med A Physiol Pathol Clin Med 2003;50(7):370–4.

3. Uchida Y, Nakade T, Kitazawa K. Clinico-microbiological study of the normal and otitic external ear canals in dogs and cats. Nihon Juigaku Zasshi 1990;52(2):415–17.

4. Baxter M. The association of *Pityrosporum pachydermatis* with the normal external ear canal of dogs and cats. J Small Anim Pract 1976;17(4):231–4.

5. Nardoni S, Mancianti F, Rum A, Corazza M. Isolation of *Malassezia* species from healthy cats and cats with otitis. J Feline Med Surg 2005;7(3):141–5.

6. Ginel PJ, Lucena R, Rodriguez JC, Ortega J. A semiquantitative cytological evaluation of normal and pathological samples from the external ear canal of dogs and cats. Vet Dermat 2002;13(3):151–6.

7. De Lorenzi D, Bonfanti U, Masserdotti C, Tranquillo M. Fine-needle biopsy of external ear canal masses in the cat: cytologic results and histologic correlations in 27 cases. Vet Clin Pathol 2005;34(2):100–5.

8. Foster AP, DeBoer DJ. The role of Pseudomonas in canine ear disease. Compend Cont Educ Pract Vet 1998;20(8):909–19.

9. Cole LK, Kwochka KW, Kowalski JJ, Hillier A. Microbial flora and antimicrobial susceptibility patterns of isolated pathogens from the horizontal ear canal and middle ear in dogs with otitis media. J Am Vet Med Assoc 1998;212(4):534–8.

10. Garosi LS, Dennis R, Schwarz T. Review of diagnostic imaging of ear diseases in the dog and cat. Vet Radiol Ultrasound 2003;44(2):137–46.

11. Hofer P, Meisen N, Bartholdi S, Kaser-Hotz B. A new radiographic view of the feline tympanic bullae. Vet Radiol Ultrasound 1995;36(1):14–15.

12. Bischoff MG, Kneller SK. Diagnostic imaging of the canine and feline ear. Vet Clin North Am Small Anim Pract 2004;34(2):437–58.

13. Hammond GJ, Sullivan M, Weinrauch S, King AM. A comparison of the rostrocaudal open mouth and rostro 10 degrees ventro-caudodorsal oblique radiographic views for imaging fluid in the feline tympanic bulla. Vet Radiol Ultrasound 2005;46(3):205–9.

14. Eom KD, Lee HC, Yoon JH. Canalographic evaluation of the external ear canal in dogs. Vet Radiol Ultrasound 2000;41(3):231–4.

15. Tivers MS, Brockman DJ. Separation of the auricular and annular ear cartilages: surgical repair technique and clinical use in dogs and cats. Vet Surg 2009;38(3):349–54.

16. Trower ND, Gregory SP, Renfrew H, Lamb CR. Evaluation of the canine tympanic membrane by positive contrast ear canalography. Vet Rec 1998;142(4):78–81.

17. Benigni L, Lamb C. Diagnostic imaging of ear disease in the dog and cat. In Pract 2006;28(3):122–30.

18. King AM, Weinrauch SA, Doust R, et al. Comparison of ultrasonography, radiography and a single computed tomography slice for fluid identification within the feline tympanic bulla. Vet J 2007;173(3):638–44.

19. Barthez PY, Koblik PD, Hornof WJ, et al. Apparent wall thickening in fluid filled versus air filled tympanic bulla in computed tomography. Vet Radiol Ultrasound 1996;37(2):95–8.

20. Remedios AM, Fowler JD, Pharr JW. A comparison of radiographic versus surgical diagnosis of otitis-media. J Am Anim Hosp Assoc 1991;27(2):183–8.

21. Love NE, Kramer RW, Spodnick GJ, Thrall DE. Radiographic and computed tomographic evaluation of otitis media in the dog. Vet Radiol Ultrasound 1995;36(5):375–9.

22. Klopp LS, Hathcock JT, Sorjonen DC. Magnetic resonance imaging features of brain stem abscessation in two cats. Vet Radiol Ultrasound 2000;41(4):300–7.

23. Allgoewer I, Lucas S, Schmitz SA. Magnetic resonance imaging of the normal and diseased feline middle ear. Vet Radiol Ultrasound 2000;41(5):413–18.

24. Garosi LS, Dennis R, Penderis J, et al. Results of magnetic resonance imaging in dogs with vestibular disorders: 85 cases (1996–1999). Journal of the American Veterinary Medical Association 2001;218(3):385–91.

25. Mellema LM, Samii VF, Vernau KM, LeCouteur RA. Meningeal enhancement on magnetic resonance imaging in 15 dogs and 3 cats. Veterinary Radiology & Ultrasound 2002;43(1):10–15.

26. Farley GR, Starr A. Middle and long latency auditory evoked potentials in cat. I. Component definition and dependence on behavioral factors. Hear Res 1983;10(2):117–38.

27. Starr A, Farley GR. Middle and long latency auditory evoked potentials in cat. II. Component distributions and dependence on stimulus factors. Hear Res 1983;10(2):139–52.

28. Strain GM, Tedford BL, Littlefield-Chabaud MA, Treviño LT. Air- and bone-conduction brainstem auditory evoked potentials and flash visual evoked potentials in cats. Am J Vet Res 1998;59(2):135–7.

29. Kuwahara J. Canine and feline aural hematoma: clinical, experimental, and clinicopathologic observations. Am J Vet Res 1986;47(10):2300–8.

30. Kuwahara J. Canine and feline aural hematoma: results of treatment with corticosteroids. J Am Anim Hosp Assoc 1986;22(5):641–7.

31. Swaim SF, Bradley DM. Evaluation of closed-suction drainage for treating auricular hematomas. J Am Anim Hosp Assoc 1996;32(1):36–43.

32. Joyce JA. Treatment of canine aural hematoma using an indwelling drain and corticosteroids. J Small Anim Pract 1994;35(7):341–4.

33. Wilson JW. Treatment of auricular hematoma, using a teat tube. J Am Vet Med Assoc 1983;182(10):1081–3.

34. Weber HO. A technique for surgical treatment of aural hematoma in dogs and cats. Vet Med Small Anim Clin 1979;74(9):1271.

35. Neunzig RJ. A modified surgical procedure for treating canine and feline aural hematoma. Vet Med Small Anim Clin 1983;78(6):927–9.

36. Dye TL, Teague HD, Ostwald DA. Evaluation of a technique using the carbon dioxide laser for the treatment of aural hematomas. J Am Anim Hosp Assoc 2002;38(4):385–90.

37. London CA, Dubilzeig RR, Vail DM, et al. Evaluation of dogs and cats with tumors of the ear canal: 145 cases (1978–1992). J Am Vet Med Assoc 1996;208(9):1413–18.

38. Lana SE, Ogilvie GK, Withrow SJ, et al. Feline cutaneous squamous cell carcinoma of the nasal planum and the pinnae: 61 cases. J Am Anim Hosp Assoc 1997;33(4):329–32.

39. Dorn CR, Taylor DON. Sunlight exposure and risk of developing cutaneous and oral squamous cell carcinomas in white cats. J Natl Cancer Inst 1971;46(5):1073–8.

40. Nasir L, Krasner H, Argyle DJ, Williams A. Immunocytochemical analysis of the tumour suppressor protein (p53) in feline neoplasia. Cancer Letters 2000;155(1):1–7.

41. Teifke JP, Lohr CV. Immunohistochemical detection of P53 overexpression in paraffin wax-embedded squamous cell carcinomas of cattle, horses, cats and dogs. J Comp Pathol 1996;114(2):205–10.

42. Hutson CA, Rideout BA, Pedersen NC. Neoplasia associated with feline immunodeficiency virus infection in cats of southern California. Journal of the American Veterinary Medical Association 1991;199(10):1357–62.

43. O'Neill SH, Newkirk KM, Anis EA. Detection of human papillomavirus DNA in feline premalignant and invasive squamous cell carcinoma. Vet Dermatol 2011;22(1):68–74.

44. Schwittlick U, Bock P, Lapp S, et al. Feline papillomavirus infection in a cat with Bowen-like disease and cutaneous squamous cell carcinoma. Schweiz Arch Tierheilkd 2011;153(12):573–7.

45. Fan TM, de Lorimier LP. Inflammatory polyps and aural neoplasia. Vet Clin North Am Small Anim Pract 2004;34(2):489–509.

46. Clarke RE. Cryosurgical treatment of feline cutaneous squamous cell carcinoma. Aust Vet Pract 1991;21(3):148–53.

47. Hahn KA, Panjehpour M, Legendre AM. Photodynamic therapy response in cats with cutaneous squamous cell carcinoma as a function of fluence. Vet Dermatol 1998;9(1):3–7.

48. Peaston AE, Leach MW, Higgins RJ. Photodynamic therapy for nasal and aural squamous cell carcinoma in cats. J Am Vet Med Assoc 1993;202(8):1261–5.

49. Stell AJ, Dobson JM, Langmack K. Photodynamic therapy of feline superficial squamous cell carcinoma

using topical 5-aminolaevulinic acid. J Small Anim Pract 2001;42(4):164–9.

50. Grier RL, Brewer WG, Theilen GH. Hyperthermic treatment of superficial tumors in cats and dogs. J Am Vet Med Assoc 1980;177(3):227–33.

51. Orenberg EK, Luck EE, Brown DM, Kitchell BE. Implant delivery system: intralesional delivery of chemotherapeutic agents for treatment of spontaneous skin tumors in veterinary patients. Clin Dermatol 1991;9(4): 561–8.

52. Theon AP, VanVechten MK, Madewell BR. Intratumoral administration of carboplatin for treatment of squamous cell carcinomas of the nasal plane in cats. AmJ Vet Res 1996;57(2):205–10.

53. Buhles WC, Theilen GH. Preliminary evaluation of bleomycin in feline and canine squamous cell carcinoma. Am J Vet Res 1973;34(2):289–91.

54. Evans AG, Madewell BR, Stannard AA. A trial of 13-cis-retinoic acid for treatment of squamous cell carcinoma and preneoplastic lesions of the head in cats. Am J Vet Res 1985;46(12):2553–7.

55. Peters-Kennedy J, Scott DW, Miller WH. Apparent clinical resolution of pinnal actinic keratoses and squamous cell carcinoma in a cat using topical imiquimod 5% cream. J Feline Med Surg 2008;10(6):593–9.

56. August JR. Otitis externa. A disease of multifactorial etiology. Vet Clin North Am Small Anim Pract 1988;18(4): 731–42.

57. Hill PB, Lo A, Eden CA, et al. Survey of the prevalence, diagnosis and treatment of dermatological conditions in small animals in general practice. Vet Rec 2006;158(16):533–9.

58. Lane JG, Watkins PE. Para-aural abscess in the dog and cat. J Small Anim Pract 1986;27(8):521–31.

59. Murphy KM. A review of techniques for the investigation of otitis externa and otitis media. Clin Tech Small Anim Pract 2001;16(4):236–41.

60. Mauldin EA, Ness TA, Goldschmidt MH. Proliferative and necrotizing otitis externa in four cats. Vet Dermatol 2007;18(5):370–7.

61. Legendre AM, Krahwinkel DJ. Feline ear tumors. J Am Anim Hosp Assoc 1981;17(6):1035–7.

62. Marino DJ, MacDonald JM, Matthiesen DT, Patnaik AK. Results of Surgery in Cats with Ceruminous Gland Adenocarcinoma. J Am Anim Hosp Assoc 1994;30(1):54–8.

63. Théon AP, Barthez PY, Madewell BR, Griffey SM. Radiation therapy of ceruminous gland carcinomas in dogs and cats. J Am Vet Med Assoc 1994;205(4):566–9.

64. Moisan PG, Watson GL. Ceruminous gland tumors in dogs and cats: a review

of 124 cases. J Am Anim Hosp Assoc 1996;32(5):448–52.

65. Salvadori C, Cantile C, Arispici M. Meningeal carcinomatosis in two cats. J Comp Pathol 2004;131(2–3):246–51.

66. Clarke SP. Surgical management of acute ear canal separation in a cat. J Feline Med Surg 2004;6(4):283–6.

67. Smeak DD. Traumatic separation of the annular cartilage from the external auditory meatus in a cat. J Am Vet Med Assoc 1997;211(4):448–50.

68. Boothe HW, Hobson HP, McDonald DE. Treatment of traumatic separation of the auricular and annular cartilages without ablation: results in five dogs. Vet Surg 1996;25(5):376–9.

69. Coomer AR, Bacon N. Primary anastomosis of segmental external auditory canal atresia in a cat. J Feline Med Surg 2009;11(10):864–8.

70. Schlicksup MD, Van Winkle TJ, Holt DE. Prevalence of clinical abnormalities in cats found to have nonneoplastic middle ear disease at necropsy: 59 cases (1991–2007). J Am Vet Med Assoc 2009;235(7):841–3.

71. Gregory SP. Middle ear disease associated with congenital palatine defects in seven dogs and one cat. J Small Anim Pract 2000;41(9):398–401.

72. Woodbridge NT, Baines EA, Baines SJ. Otitis media in five cats associated with soft palate abnormalities. Vet Rec 2012;171:124–5.

73. Detweiler DA, Johnson LR, Kass PH, Wisner ER. Computed tomographic evidence of bulla effusion in cats with sinonasal disease: 2001–2004. J Vet Intern Med 2006;20(5):1080–4.

74. Lawson D. Otitis media in the cat. Vet Rec 1957;69:643–7.

75. Tos M, Wiederhold M, Larsen P. Experimental long-term tubal occlusion in cats. A quantitative histopathological study. Acta Otolaryngol 1984;97(5–6): 580–92.

76. Trevor PB, Martin RA. Tympanic bulla osteotomy for treatment of middle-ear disease in cats: 19 cases (1984–1991). J Am Vet Med Assoc 1993;202(1):123–8.

77. Gotthelf LN. Diagnosis and treatment of otitis media in dogs and cats. Vet Clin North Am Small Anim Pract 2004;34(2):469–87.

78. de Lorimier LP, Alexander SD, Fan TM. T-cell lymphoma of the tympanic bulla in a feline leukemia virus-negative cat. Can Vet J 2003;44(12):987–9.

79. Fiorito DA. Oral and peripheral vestibular signs in a cat with squamous-cell carcinoma. J Am Vet Med Assoc 1986;188(1):71–2.

80. Hayden DW. Squamous cell carcinoma in a cat with intraocular and orbital metastases. Vet Pathol 1976;13:332–6.

81. Indrieri RJ, Taylor RF. Vestibular dysfunction caused by squamous cell

carcinoma involving the middle ear and inner ear in two cats. J Am Vet Med Assoc 1984;184(4):471–3.

82. Lane IF, Hall DG. Adenocarcinoma of the middle ear with osteolysis of the tympanic bulla in a cat. J Am Vet Med Assoc 1992;201(3):463–5.

83. Pentlarge VW. Peripheral vestibular disease in a cat with middle and inner ear squamous cell carcinoma. Comp Cont Educ Pract Vet 1984;6(8):731–3.

84. Rendano VT, Delahunta A, King JM. Extracranial neoplasia with facial nerve paralysis in two cats. J Am Anim Hosp Assoc 1980;16(6):921–5.

85. Stone EA, Goldschmidt MH, Littman MP. Squamous cell carcinoma of the middle ear in a cat. J Small Anim Pract 1983;24(10):647–51.

86. Busch DS, Noxon JO, Miller LD. Laryngeal paralysis and peripheral vestibular disease in a cat. J Am Anim Hosp Assoc 1992;28(1):82–6.

87. Cook LB, Bergman RL, Bahr A, Boothe HW. Inflammatory polyp in the middle ear with secondary suppurative meningoencephalitis in a cat. Vet Radiol Ultrasound 2003;44(6):648–51.

88. Williams JM, White RAS. Total ear canal ablation combined with lateral bulla osteotomy in the cat. J Small Anim Pract 1992;33(5):225–7.

89. McGinn MD, Chole RA, Henry KR. Cholesteatoma induction. Consequences of external auditory canal ligation in gerbils, cats, hamsters, guinea pigs, mice and rats. Acta Otolaryngol 1984;97(3–4):297–304.

90. Bergsma DR, Brown DS. White fur, blue eyes and deafness in the domestic cat. J Hered 1971;62:171–85.

91. Strain GM. Aetiology, prevalence and diagnosis of deafness in dogs and cats. Br Vet J 1996;152:17–36.

92. Strain GM. Congenital deafness and its recognition. Vet Clin North Am 1999;29:895–907.

93. Stevens-Sparks CK, Strain GM. Post-anesthesia deafness in dogs and cats following dental and ear cleaning procedures. Vet Anaesth Analg 2010;37(4):347–51.

94. Burke EE, Moise NS, de Lahunta A, Erb HN. Review of idiopathic feline vestibular syndrome in 75 cats. J Am Vet Med Assoc 1985;187(9):941–3.

95. Negrin A, Cherubini GB, Lamb C, et al. Clinical signs, magnetic resonance imaging findings and outcome in 77 cats with vestibular disease: a retrospective study. J Feline Med Surg 2010;12: 291–9.

96. Bagley RS. Recognition and localization of intracranial disease. Vet Clin North Am Small Anim Pract 1996;26(4): 667–709.

97. Chrisman CL. Vestibular Diseases. Vet Clin North Am 1980;10(1):103–29.

98. Thomas WB. Vestibular dysfunction. Vet Clin North Am Small Anim Pract 2000;30(1):227–49.

99. Tighilet B, Lacour M. Pharmacological activity of the Ginkgo biloba extract (EGb 761) on equilibrium function recovery in the unilateral vestibular neurectomized cat. J Vestib Res 1995;5(3):187–200.

100. Tighilet B, Leonard J, Lacour M. Betahistine dihydrochloride treatment facilitates vestibular compensation in the cat. J Vestib Res 1995;5(1):53–66.

101. Tighilet B, Mourre C, Trottier S, Lacour M. Histaminergic ligands improve vestibular compensation in the cat: behavioural, neurochemical and molecular evidence. Eur J Pharmacol 2007;568(1–3):149–63.

102. Vernau KM, LeCouteur RA. Feline vestibular disorders. Part II: diagnostic approach and differential diagnosis. J Feline Med Surg 1999;1(2):81–8.

103. LeCouteur RA, Vernau KM. Feline vestibular disorders. Part I: anatomy and clinical signs. J Feline Med Surg 1999;1(2):71–80.

104. van der Gaag I. The pathology of the external ear canal in dogs and cats. Vet Q 1986;8(4):307–17.

105. Beatty JA, Barrs VR, Swinney GR, et al. Peripheral vestibular disease associated with cryptococcosis in three cats. J Feline Med Surg 2000;2:29–34.

106. Lucroy MD, Vernau KM, Samii VF, LeCouteur RA. Middle ear tumours with brainstem extension treated by ventral bulla osteotomy and craniectomy in two cats. Vet Comp Oncol 2004;2(4):234–42.

107. Merchant SR. Ototoxicity. Vet Clin North Am Small Anim Pract 1994;24(5):971–80.

108. Callaghan D, Culley CD. Ototoxicity in the dog and cat. Vet Rec 1985;117(11):291.

109. Lane JG. Ototoxicity in the dog and cat. Vet Rec 1985;117(4):94.

110. Willoughby K. Chlorhexidine and ototoxicity in cats. Vet Rec 1989;124(20):547.

111. Podell M, Kerpsack SJ, Fenner WR. What is your diagnosis? Prog Vet Neurol 1992;3:21–3.

112. LeCouteur RA. Feline vestibular diseases – new developments. J Feline Med Surg 2003;5(2):101–8.

113. Martín Barrasa JL, Lupiola Gómez P, González Lama Z, Tejedor Junco MT. Antibacterial susceptibility patterns of Pseudomonas strains isolated from chronic canine otitis externa. J Vet Med B Infect Dis Vet Public Health 2000;47(3):191–6.

114. Tirgari M. Long-term evaluation of the pull-through technique for vertical canal ablation for the treatment of otitis externa in dogs and cats. J Small Anim Pract 1988;29(3):165–75.

115. Tirgari M, Pinniger RS. Pull-through technique for vertical canal ablation for the treatment of otitis externa in dogs and cats. J Small Anim Pract 1986;27(3):123–31.

116. Day DG, Couto CG, Weisbrode SE, Smeak DD. Basal cell carcinoma in two cats. J Am Anim Hosp Assoc 1994;30(3):265–9.

117. Smeak DD, Dehoff WD. Total ear canal ablation: clinical results in the dog and cat. Vet Surg 1986;15(2):161–70.

118. Smeak DD, Kerpsack SJ. Total ear canal ablation and lateral bulla osteotomy for management of end-stage otitis. Semin Vet Med Surg Small Anim 1993;8(1):30–41.

119. Bacon NJ, Gilbert RL, Bostock DE, White RA. Total ear canal ablation in the cat: indications, morbidity and long-term survival. J Small Anim Pract 2003;44(10):430–4.

120. Mathews KG, Hardie EM, Murphy KM. Subtotal ear canal ablation in 18 dogs and one cat with minimal distal ear canal pathology. J Am Anim Hosp Assoc 2006;42(5):371–80.

121. McNabb AH, Flanders JA. Cosmetic results of a ventrally based advancement flap for closure of total ear canal ablations in 6 cats: 2002–2003. Vet Surg 2004;33(5):435–9.

Chapter |51|

Pharynx

S.J. Baines

The pharynx is a small anatomic region that is often forgotten or overlooked compared to the adjacent nasal passages, oropharynx, and oral cavity. However, a variety of clinical conditions relating to the nasopharynx have been described, comprising infectious (viral, bacterial, and fungal), inflammatory and neoplastic etiologies, along with anatomic abnormalities and foreign bodies.[1] In cats with nasopharyngeal mass lesions, the most common inflammatory causes are polyps and cryptococcosis, and the most common neoplastic cause is lymphoma.[2] Surgical intervention for disorders of the nasopharynx is not commonly performed, with the exception of nasopharyngeal polyps, stenosis and, occasionally, foreign bodies.

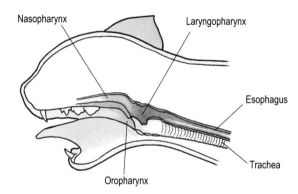

Figure 51-1 Diagram showing the regions of the pharynx in the cat.

SURGICAL ANATOMY

The pharynx is the crossroads where the ventrally located oral cavity can pass food to the dorsally located esophagus while the dorsally located nasal cavity can conduct air to the ventrally located larynx and trachea. The greatest risk of this design of the upper aerodigestive tract is flooding of the respiratory tract with ingested food and fluid, and the pharynx has a number of mechanisms to avoid this. The pharynx is equipped with valves to direct the flow of food, it is distensible so it can receive large boluses of food, and it is muscular so that it can move the boluses on quickly.

The pharynx comprises the caudal aspects of the oral and nasal cavities at the confluence of the digestive and respiratory tracts. The pharynx is a short fibromuscular tube divided into three compartments: the oropharynx, the nasopharynx and the laryngopharynx (Fig. 51-1).

The walls and roof of the pharynx are lined by an elastic mucous membrane, beneath which sit three sets of horseshoe-shaped constrictors, with the muscles on each side meeting the contralateral muscle at a median raphe. These muscles arise from the hard palate, hyoid, and larynx and are known as the rostral, middle, and caudal constrictors. The caudal constrictor muscle is subdivided into the cricopharyngeal and thyropharyngeal muscles. The pharynx is surrounded by loose connective tissue, which allows it to dilate when needed. Vessels, including the common, internal and external carotid arteries, and

nerves, including the glossopharyngeal, vagus, hypoglossal, and cervical sympathetic nerves, run in this tissue. Adjacent structures include the retropharyngeal and mandibular lymph nodes, the mandibular, sublingual and molar salivary glands, and the hyoid apparatus.

Surgical diseases of the oral cavity are described in Chapter 49, the ear in Chapter 50, the larynx in Chapter 52, and the nasal cavity is described in Chapter 54. This chapter will deal primarily with the nasopharynx, as many oropharyngeal disorders also affect the oral cavity. However, the pharynx is a common space and diseases of the nasopharynx may affect all parts of the pharynx. Extension of nasal cavity disease into the nasopharynx and vice versa is relatively common and the chapters dealing with these diseases should be read in conjunction.

Nasopharynx

The nasopharynx is the caudal portion of the nasal cavity that connects the nasal cavity to the larynx. It extends from the choanae rostrally to the intrapharyngeal opening caudally. The choanae are fixed apertures in the roof of the rostral aspect of the nasopharynx, either side of the vomer bone. The intrapharyngeal opening is the opening of the nasopharynx over the caudal free border of the soft palate. Only its floor is mobile and the rest of the nasopharynx moves little and remains patent. The pharyngeal tonsil is located in the nasopharynx

© 2014 Elsevier Ltd
DOI: 10.1016/B978-0-7020-4336-9.00051-2

and the auditory or Eustachian tubes open on the lateral wall of the nasopharynx, via a 4 mm long slit, dorsal to the middle of the soft palate, immediately rostral to a small mucosal cushion. The intrapharyngeal opening is closed during swallowing to isolate the nasopharynx and nasal cavity from the oropharynx and laryngopharynx and prevent reflux of food and fluid into the nasal cavity.

Oropharynx

The oropharynx is the caudal portion of the oral cavity, whose borders are the soft palate dorsally, the root of the tongue ventrally, and the tonsillar fossae laterally. The palatine tonsils are located in the oropharynx, along with lymphoid tissue in the lateral walls of the oropharynx and the base of the tongue (lingual tonsils). In the cat, the palatine tonsil is very small and not covered by a mucosal fold. The efferent lymphatics of the palatine tonsil drain into the retropharyngeal lymph node. The muscular wall of the pharynx and the base of the tongue act together during deglutition to move the food bolus into the laryngopharynx.

Laryngopharynx

The laryngopharynx is a short passage dorsal to the larynx that connects the caudal aspect of the nasopharynx to the proximal esophagus. The pharyngeal muscles (constrictors, shorteners, and dilators) control the size and shape of the nasopharynx and laryngopharynx and co-ordinate swallowing.

GENERAL CONSIDERATIONS

History

The owner should be asked questions about the animal's general physical condition, appetite, ability to eat and drink, and activity level. Presence of more specific signs such as abnormal respiratory noises, coughing, gagging, retching, regurgitation, vomiting, and dyspnea should be ascertained.

Clinical signs

The clinical signs of nasopharyngeal disease are stertor, open-mouth breathing (Fig. 51-2), repeated attempts at swallowing, nasal discharge, and reverse sneezing. The clinical signs of oropharyngeal or laryngopharyngeal disease are pain, anorexia, dysphagia, and stridor.

Coughing, vomiting, and regurgitation may also be present and it may be difficult to localize the disease to one portion of the pharynx or differentiate pharyngeal from esophageal, laryngeal or tracheal disease. The presence of anorexia, drooling saliva, and weak swallowing efforts, which may not be associated with eating or drinking, typifies acute pharyngeal disease. In chronic pharyngeal disease, gagging and regurgitation or vomiting predominate and halitosis may be noted with neoplasia or foreign bodies.

Cats with nasal disease more commonly have a history of nasal discharge and sneezing, whereas cats with nasopharyngeal disease more commonly have stertorous respiration, change in phonation, and weight loss,[3] although nasal discharge and sneezing may still be present.

Dyspnea

Difficulty breathing is usually due to obstruction of the nasopharynx or oropharynx. Small obstructive lesions of the laryngopharynx will

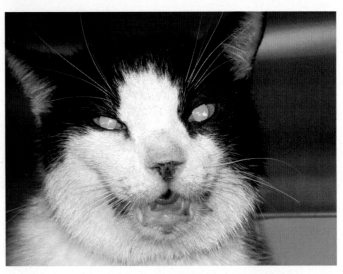

Figure 51-2 A middle-aged cat was presented with open-mouth breathing associated with an obstructive pharyngeal mass.

impair the passage of food into the digestive tract, but larger lesions may also obstruct the nasopharynx.

Obstruction of the nasal passages and nasopharynx may show a similar stridorous respiration and it may be difficult to differentiate these clinically in the absence of other clinical signs such as sneezing and nasal discharge, which suggest nasal cavity disease. Disorders of the caudal nasopharynx may encroach on the caudal turbinates and cause sneezing. Dyspnea caused by nasopharyngeal disease should not be life threatening since the animal can breathe via the oropharynx. However, some animals will avoid mouth breathing, which will exacerbate the clinical signs. Obstruction of the caudal nasopharynx results in a stertorous respiration.

Cats may not show obvious clinical signs even with severe nasopharyngeal obstruction. They are often reluctant to show open-mouth breathing, but are able to ventilate with the mouth almost closed and the lips parted. Closure of the mouth and examination of the animal's breathing pattern and tolerance of this maneuver may help diagnose nasopharyngeal disease, but is not without risk in animals with marked obstruction. Measurement of airflow at the external nares with a glass slide or cotton wool offers a less invasive means of achieving this.

Dyspnea caused by obstruction of the oropharynx is more readily diagnosed, as a mass or edema is usually apparent on clinical and/or oral examination, along with 'gargling' type respiratory sounds.

Dysphagia

Difficulty swallowing or dysphagia is usually due to obstruction of the oropharynx or laryngopharynx, although large lesions in the nasopharynx will encroach on the oropharynx and also cause dysphagia. Dysphagia resulting from an abnormality in the pharyngeal phase of swallowing is usually manifested by gagging, choking, and repeated swallowing of the same bolus of food. Cats may also show repeated attempts at swallowing or gulping when not eating. Coughing may be present if food is aspirated into the larynx. If swallowing is painful, the animal may attempt to eat, but then stop and turn away from the food, often exhibiting drooling of saliva. If the cat gives up eating very quickly, the dysphagia may simply be assessed as inappetence, although drooling saliva suggests pharyngeal disease as the cause. The cat may also paw at its nose and mouth, particularly with acute disease. Dyspnea and dysphagia may also result in aerophagia.

Reverse sneezing

Reverse sneezing may accompany inflammation of the nasopharyngeal mucosa and is caused by asynchronous closing of the intrapharyngeal opening independent of swallowing. This results in acute onset of marked dyspnea with repeated short snoring sounds and extension of the neck caused by forced inhalation via the nose against a closed nasopharynx. The clinical signs are usually less marked in the cat than in the dog. Diagnosis is by recognition of this pattern of behavior as animals do not often display these signs when presented for examination. Symptomatic treatment comprises stimulation of the swallowing reflex by massaging the throat or occluding the nares, so that the intrapharyngeal opening may re-open. Treatment of the underlying nasopharyngeal irritation or inflammation may resolve the problem.

Other signs

The regional lymph nodes (mandibular and retropharyngeal) may be enlarged with pharyngeal disease. Clinical signs of external ear canal disease, including aural discharge and a mass may be present; these have been identified with both nasopharyngeal polyps and lymphoma.[3]

Clinical signs of otitis media, peripheral vestibular disease, and Horner syndrome may be seen if the lesion also involves the tympanic bulla or if the lesion obstructs the auditory tube. Facial nerve dysfunction may be seen if a more extensive lesion has broken out through the tympanic bulla. Invasive lesions of the nasopharynx (neoplasia, cryptococcosis) may cause central neurologic signs if they erode into the calvarium. A neurologic examination should be performed if clinical signs suggest extension into the calvarium, particularly ophthalmoplegia and vestibular signs. A fundic examination should be performed if cryptococcosis is suspected.

Physical examination

Evaluation of the pharynx begins with watching the animal's behavior at rest, listening for abnormal respiratory noises, such as stertor or stridor, and then while eating or drinking. This is followed by examination of the external nares and the oral cavity in the conscious animal. Since pharyngeal disease and ear disease may be associated, the external ear canals should be examined at this stage.

In a compliant animal, the soft palate may be palpated and pushed dorsally to identify nasopharyngeal mass lesions, although only a brief examination will be possible. For a right-handed operator, the cat's head is supported in the left hand, with the index finger and fourth finger on either side of the temporomandibular junction, with the palm supporting the head. The mouth is then opened using pressure from the middle finger on the mandible and then the right index finger is introduced into the mouth to palpate the soft palate.[3] The effect of opening the mouth on the nature of any respiratory noises is assessed.

Anesthesia

Physical examination of the conscious animal is followed by examination of the pharynx under a light plane of anesthetic (Fig. 51-3). Anesthesia should be induced with an intravenous agent so that rapid induction and rapid intubation and control of the airway can be achieved in patients with an obstructive lesion. Use of an intravenous agent also allows anesthesia to be maintained without the presence of an endotracheal tube if a more detailed examination of the pharynx is required without an endotracheal tube in place. The endotracheal tube cuff should be inflated, and the caudal pharynx should be packed

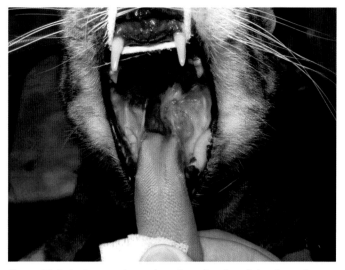

Figure 51-3 A pharyngeal mass is evaluated under a light plane of anesthesia prior to endotracheal intubation.

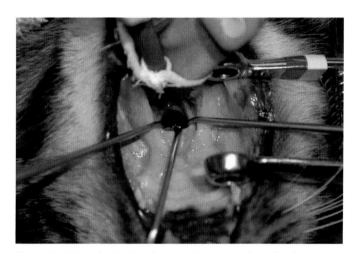

Figure 51-4 Spay hooks have been used to retract the soft palate rostrally in this anesthetized cat with a nasopharyngeal polyp.

with gauze if this does not impair the examination, to prevent aspiration of blood or other fluids. The pharynx is a very sensitive area and manipulations may cause the animal to wake up. To avoid having a very deep plane of anesthesia, a local anesthetic technique, such as topical administration of lidocaine trickled from the external nares or direct administration to the pharyngeal mucosa may be used. This may also avoid excessive vagal stimulation from intrapharyngeal manipulation, which may cause a clinically significant bradycardia.

Endoscopy

The oral cavity, soft palate, base of the tongue, palatine tonsils, and laryngopharynx may be examined directly with a laryngoscope. During initial examination, the soft palate may be elevated dorsally with a retractor or tongue depressor to visualize the laryngopharynx and dorsal nasopharynx. The soft palate may be elevated dorsally against the dorsal wall of the nasopharynx to evaluate for large obstructive lesions.

Once the animal is anesthetized, it may be placed in dorsal recumbency and a more detailed examination of the pharynx can be performed. Palpation of the soft palate, followed by rostral retraction with an instrument, e.g., a spay hook, is performed (Fig. 51-4). In cats, the cranial nasopharynx and choanae may be exposed in this manner. In one series of 53 cats with nasopharyngeal disease, 23 cats (43.4%) had soft palate palpation performed and in 82% of these a palpable mass was identified.[3] Palpation is of limited value for masses located dorsal to the hard palate, but diagnostic imaging or endoscopy (see Chapter 9) will identify these.[3]

Visualization of the nasopharynx is achieved by retrograde rhinoscopy (see Chapter 9) with an endoscope passed into the oral cavity and retroflexed 180°. A limited examination of the nasopharynx may be achieved with a dental mirror and a light source and the soft palate may be retracted with a tissue hook or stay suture to increase visibility. On endoscopy, mass lesions may be visualized, although in some cases visualization is obscured by pus, blood or mucus. Flushing of the site with saline, either via the endoscope or via the external nares, may clear the field and improve visualization. In one study of endoscopic examination of the choanae in 27 cats with signs of upper respiratory tract disease, gross abnormalities were identified in 85% of the cats, with a mass (44%), rhinitis (25%), foreign bodies (7%), follicles (3.5%), and deformed choanae (3.5%) being noted.[4]

A technique to perform nasopharyngoscopy via gastrotomy has been described that allows the use of a larger endoscope which does not have to be retroflexed, but since this involves an additional surgical approach it is not recommended unless there is no alternative method of examination.[5] However, this method does allow larger diameter instruments to be used and has been successful in removing a large (3.5 cm long) polyp.[5]

The caudal nasal cavity and rostral nasopharynx may be examined with a rigid (2–4 mm) arthroscope or flexible endoscope passed via the external nares. If anterior rhinoscopy is also required, it is performed after retrograde pharyngoscopy to avoid causing hemorrhage that might obscure the view.[4]

Diagnostic imaging

Radiographs should include the nasal and oral cavity rostrally and the proximal trachea caudally, and should be taken at inspiration to increase the volume of gas in the pharynx. The high inherent contrast of this area allows delineation of the nasopharynx, oropharynx and laryngopharynx, and soft palate. Examination of the nasopharynx is impaired by superimposition of the bones of the skull and the presence of the endotracheal tube and other anesthetic monitoring devices. If evaluation of the external ear canal and tympanic bullae is required, additional projections are needed. Masses, radiopaque foreign bodies (Fig. 51-5), and secretions may be identified with radiography, but apart from these lesions, radiography may offer little more information than a thorough endoscopic examination. In animals where swallowing is impaired, or in whom the clinical signs are suggestive of this, radiographs of the thorax should be taken to rule out aspiration pneumonia and megaesophagus.

Contrast radiographs following administration of contrast medium via the ventral nasal meatus may aid in the diagnosis of nasopharyngeal disease, e.g., stenosis.[6] Fluoroscopy is of theoretical use in the evaluation of animals with dysphagia, but these examinations are very difficult to perform in cats. Ultrasonography may be of use for soft tissue or fluid-filled masses encroaching on the pharynx, or assessment of the retropharyngeal lymph node, and may guide sampling of these areas.

Computed tomography (CT), with and without contrast, is the most useful modality for evaluating the nasopharynx (Fig. 51-6) and allows investigation of the status of the regional lymph nodes. Both bone and soft tissue windows should be evaluated and it is important to differentiate between a soft tissue mass and mucus in the pharynx.[3] The nasal passages, external ear canals, and tympanic bullae should be assessed at the same time. Fluid within the tympanic bullae may

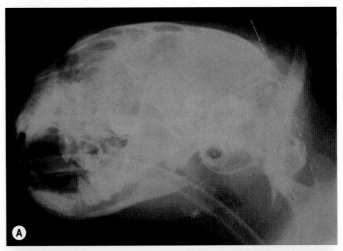

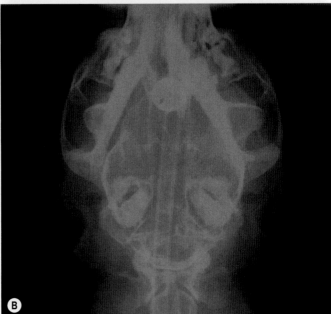

Figure 51-5 A cat with a history of nasal discharge. (A) Lateral and (B) dorsoventral radiographs of the skull show a radiopaque metallic foreign body in nasopharyngeal meatus that was found to be a bell. The foreign body was removed by flushing from the external nares.

be seen in animals with nasopharyngeal masses, most likely due to obstruction of the pharyngeal opening of the auditory tube.[7,8] Magnetic resonance imaging (MRI) examination may allow a better appreciation of the relationship of a soft tissue mass to the surrounding soft tissues of the nasopharynx[6] (Fig. 51-7) and is the imaging modality of choice if intracranial extension of a mass is suspected.[7]

Biopsy

Diagnosis may require biopsy of a lesion, particularly masses that do not have the gross appearance of a nasopharyngeal polyp. Fine needle aspirates or Tru-Cut biopsies may be taken under direct visualization, taking care to avoid the large blood vessels that lie lateral to the pharynx. Anterograde flushing of the nasopharynx from the external nares may also allow pieces of tissue or foreign bodies to be recovered, as well as producing temporary alleviation of clinical signs in animals

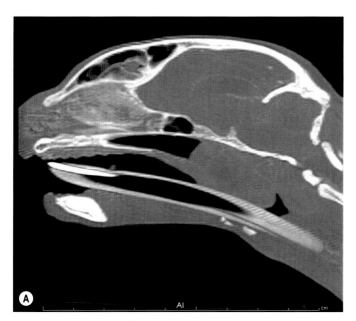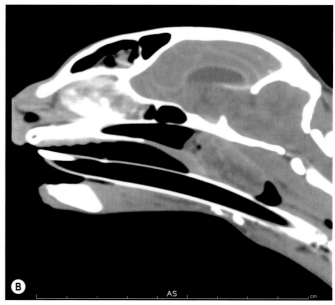

Figure 51-6 A cat with a history of inspiratory stertor. CT image of the head reconstructed in the sagittal plane post-contrast administration showing a large heterogeneously enhancing nasopharyngeal mass. **(A)** Bone window (width 2000, level 350). **(B)** Soft tissue window (width 400, level 40).

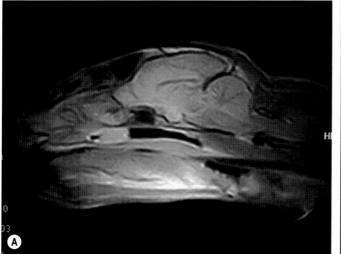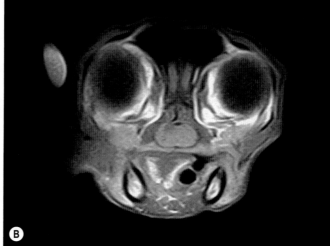

Figure 51-7 (A) Sagittal and **(B)** transverse MRI images show a rostral nasopharyngeal mass that obstructs the majority of the nasopharynx.

where obstruction is due to a friable mass or thick fluid. In animals presenting with clinical signs consistent with nasal or nasopharyngeal disease, direct visualization of the nasopharynx and biopsy of any lesions is a simple, inexpensive technique with a high diagnostic yield and is preferred to biopsies achieved via rhinoscopy.[3] In one study of 38 cats with endoscopically detected nasopharyngeal masses, a histologic sample of diagnostic quality was obtained in 34 of them (89%).[9] Forty per cent of these cats also had a co-existent nasal mass.

In another study of 27 cats with signs of upper respiratory tract disease, histologic or cytologic samples were retrieved in 18 animals.[4] Diagnoses included neoplasia (nine cats), rhinitis/hyperplasia (seven cats), polyp (one cat) and cryptococcosis (one cat). In cats with a mass lesion at the choanae, the diagnosis was neoplasia in 58%, polyp in 18%, rhinitis in 18%, and unknown in 9%. Thick tenacious mucus may also appear as a mass lesion.[8] In 30 cats with nasopharyngeal masses, squash preparation cytology showed a good agreement (90%) with histology, although the agreement was poorest for lymphoid lesions.[9] The histologic diagnoses were benign inflammatory/ hyperplastic lesions (11 cats), lymphoma (12 cats), carcinoma (five cats), and sarcoma (two cats).

SURGICAL DISEASES

Nasopharyngeal polyps are the most commonly described entity, but this disorder may not be the most common disease. In a review of 53 cats with nasopharyngeal disease, the most common diagnosis was lymphoma in 49% of cats, with nasopharyngeal polyps being reported in 28%. The remaining 23% of cats had other tumors including squamous cell carcinoma, adenocarcinoma, spindle cell carcinoma, rhabdomyosarcoma, and lymphoplasmacytic rhinitis/pharyngitis.[3]

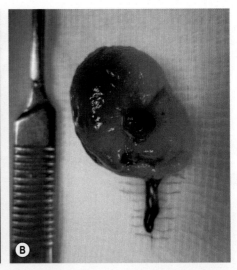

Figure 51-8 A cat with a history of inspiratory stertor. **(A)** A spay hook has been used to retract the soft palate rostrally and visualize a large nasopharyngeal polyp. **(B)** The polyp was removed by gentle traction and the typical stalk can be seen.

The mean age at presentation aids in prioritizing the differential diagnosis list—cats with nasopharyngeal polyps have a mean age of three years (range four months to seven years) and those with lymphoma are 10.7 years (range five–19 years).

Polyps

Nasopharyngeal polyp is the name given to a benign proliferation arising from the respiratory epithelium that may be found in the nasopharynx. The most common type of polyp originates in the middle ear or auditory tube and extends via the auditory tube into the nasopharynx (Fig. 51-8). In this location the polyp may grow to a large size (>3 cm). A middle ear polyp is the name given to a polyp that originates in the middle ear and/or Eustachian tube and grows through the tympanic membrane into the external ear canal, although the term nasopharyngeal polyp is often used to refer to both these entities. The middle ear mucosa may be diffusely inflamed with a polypoid lining. These may occasionally be bilateral, either at the same time or sequentially.[10,11] In some cats, polyp tissue may be present in both locations.[10,12] Inflammatory polyps of the nasal turbinates (IPNT) that may extend into the nasopharynx have also been described as a distinct entity.[13-15] These have been reported to be more common in Italy[14] than other European countries.

The cause of the polyps is unknown, although it has been proposed that they originate from a congenital defect (e.g., remnants of the branchial arches[16]) or middle ear disease,[17] or as a result of chronic inflammation, infectious or otherwise, which may either initiate or potentiate the growth of the polyp. Soft palate hypoplasia was reported in one cat with a nasopharyngeal polyp.[18] The polyps are associated with inflammation and are often secondary to bacterial infection, although it is not clear whether the polyp causes the inflammation or the inflammation causes the proliferation of the mucosa. Feline calicivirus, which is an infectious agent known to colonize cats, has been isolated from the nasopharynx of cats with polyps and from an inflammatory polyp in one cat.[19] However, other studies have not consistently amplified RNA or DNA of infectious agents, including feline herpesvirus-1 (FHV-1), feline calicivirus (FCV), *Mycoplasma* species, *Bartonella* species, and *Chlamydophila felis* from polyp tissue and there was no difference in the amplification rates in normal and affected cats.[11,20] In addition, a previous history of recent upper respiratory tract infection is not commonly reported in cats with polyps.[11]

Most affected cats are young adults, although polyps have been reported in older cats up to 15 years old. Clinical signs are referable to an obstructive lesion at the level of the nasopharynx or disease of the middle ear or external ear canal. Inspiratory dyspnea and stertor are the primary signs, but dysphagia, gagging or reluctance to eat may also be seen. Occasionally, polyps may cause life-threatening upper airway obstruction, either with normal activity[21] or on recovery from anesthesia if a polyp is not suspected and diagnosed.[19,20] Acquired megaesophagus has also been reported,[10,22] which resolves on removal of the polyp. In one cat this was associated with a large (7 cm long) nasopharyngeal polyp that extended into the cranial esophagus.[22] Pulmonary hypertension, presumed to be due to chronic upper airway obstruction, is reported in one cat.[10] Clinical signs of nasal cavity disease, i.e., sneezing and nasal discharge, are generally uncommon, unless secondary infection extends from the nasopharynx to the nasal cavity. However, similar polyps may also be found in the nasal cavities, and clinical signs of nasal cavity disease such as sneezing, epistaxis, and stertor may be seen with polyps in this location.[13,14]

A middle ear polyp is the most common mass identified in the external ear canal in the cat. In most cats, the polyp does not extend beyond the horizontal canal, but in some cats it may be visible in the external ear canal. Middle ear polyps may cause signs of otitis externa (e.g., head shaking, scratching at the ear, and aural discharge) or otitis media/interna (e.g., Horner syndrome [Fig. 51-9], head tilt, ataxia, and nystagmus).

Examination of the oral cavity may reveal ventral depression of the soft palate and resistance to gentle dorsal pressure on the soft palate. Less than half of affected cats have a visible mass on physical examination.[23] Rostral retraction of the soft palate may improve visualization of smaller or more rostral lesions. Large lesions may obstruct the larynx and may cause difficulty on endotracheal intubation. Radiography or CT examination will reveal a soft tissue mass in the nasopharynx, which may depress the soft palate ventrally. More than 80% of cats have evidence of middle ear disease on diagnostic imaging (Figs 51-10 and 51-11).[24]

Grossly, nasopharyngeal polyps appear as a mass of red or pink friable tissue and are rounded, often with a long pedicle. They are composed of loosely arranged well-vascularized fibrous connective tissue with scattered lymphocytes, plasma cells, and neutrophils, covered by a layer of stratified squamous or ciliated columnar epithelium, which may be ulcerated. Inflammatory cells, primarily

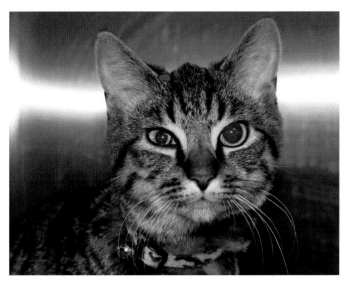

Figure 51-9 A cat with a nasopharyngeal polyp and associated middle ear disease with right-sided Horner syndrome, showing miosis, ptosis, and enophthalmus.

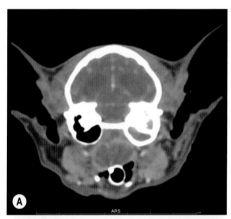

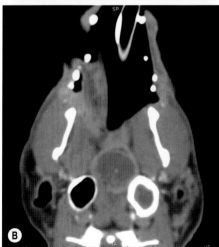

Figure 51-10 A cat with a history of inspiratory stertor and otitis media/interna due to a nasopharyngeal polyp. **(A)** Transverse plane and **(B)** dorsal plane reconstruction CT images of the head show sclerosis and thickening of the left tympanic bulla, filling of the bulla with hyperattenuating material, and a large hyperattenuating nasopharyngeal mass with a rim of contrast enhancement.

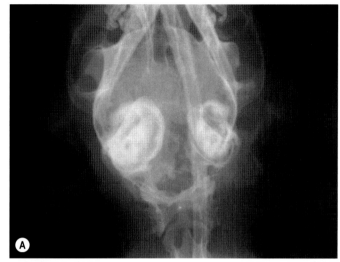

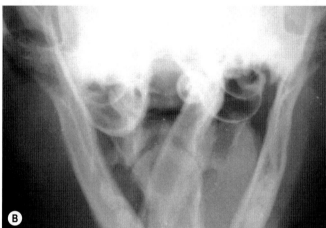

Figure 51-11 A cat with clinical signs of otitis media and otitis interna, associated with the presence of a nasopharyngeal polyp. **(A)** Ventrodorsal and **(B)** open-mouth rostrocaudal radiographic projections show thickening of the wall of the right tympanic bulla and increased opacity within the bulla associated with otitis media.

lymphocytes, plasma cells and macrophages, are present within the stroma.

Nasal polyps arising from the nasal passages are solid and white to pink on gross examination.[13] Histologically, nasal polyps arising from the nasal turbinates consist of fibrous connective tissue and woven bone and erythrocyte-filled spaces, covered by ciliated columnar epithelium. These lesions have more in common with nasal hamartomas seen in humans[13] and have also been described as hemangiomas, fibrous dysplasia, ossifying fibroma, and aneurysmal bone cysts.[13,14]

Recommended therapy for nasopharyngeal polyps is traction/avulsion,[17,23] ventral bulla osteotomy,[23,25] or lateral bulla osteotomy with total ear canal ablation[12,23] depending on the location, with or without post-treatment corticosteroids. Corticosteroid therapy has been recommended for either polyps with middle ear involvement[23] or for all polyps.[26] In one study, the recurrence rate after traction/avulsion alone was 64% and after traction/avulsion and postoperative corticosteroids at anti-inflammatory doses (1–2 mg/kg/day for two weeks, tapered over two weeks) the recurrence rate in cats with no aural involvement was 0%.[23] Recurrence was higher with aural polyps (50%) compared to nasopharyngeal polyps (11%). Overall, traction/avulsion may result in a 33–55% recurrence rate[11,23,27] and this method of treatment should be generally limited to those cats without an aural component, where recurrence may be as low as 0%. A ventral bulla osteotomy (VBO) in patients with middle ear disease reduces the recurrence rate to 0–8%.[26,28,29] It has therefore been suggested that traction/avulsion followed by corticosteroid therapy is a suitable first-line treatment for polyps, even if middle ear changes are present. Surgery, usually a VBO, may then be used if the condition fails to resolve or recurs, if the clinical signs are severe on first presentation, or if there is no nasopharyngeal component to apply traction to.[23,30] Recurrence may recur months to years after removal.[30]

Pharyngeal neoplasia

Most tumors of the nasopharynx are malignant. Lymphoma is the most common nasopharyngeal tumor in the cat,[3,31] followed by squamous cell carcinoma and soft tissue sarcomas. The most common oropharyngeal tumor type is squamous cell carcinoma.[32] Melanoma

occasionally occurs in the pharynx, but advanced disease is usually present at presentation.

These tumors usually arise in the rostral nasopharynx and the nasal cavity is usually spared. The clinical signs are stertor and dyspnea without nasal discharge, although some animals will develop large obstructive lesions in the nasal cavity with no nasal discharge or sneezing. If hemorrhage occurs secondary to the tumor, this may be seen as epistaxis, but the blood may pass caudally and be swallowed and then recognized as melena. Approximately 50% of cats with sinonasal masses will show extension into the nasopharynx on CT examination.[33]

Diagnosis may be by direct inspection or radiography or CT examination (Fig. 51-12). There are no gross or diagnostic imaging findings that allow differentiation of the histologic type and definitive diagnosis requires a cytologic or histologic diagnosis. The prognosis for nasopharyngeal lymphoma is fair with chemotherapy, but it is

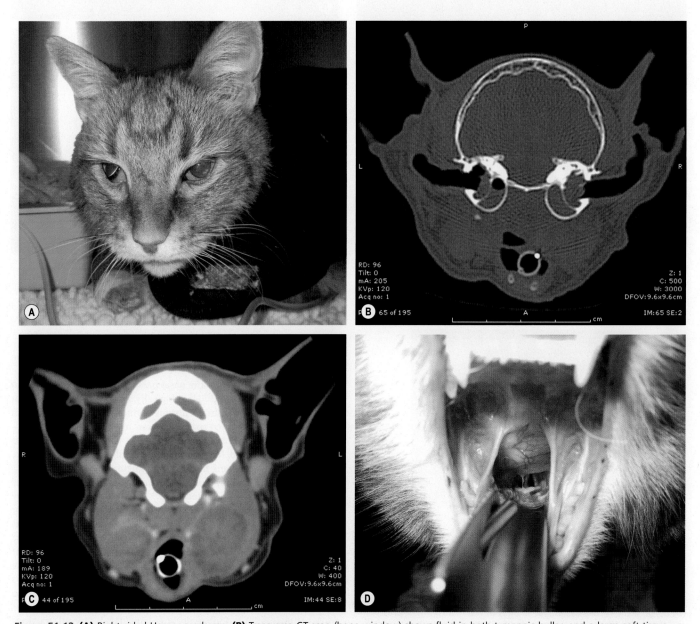

Figure 51-12 (A) Right-sided Horner syndrome. **(B)** Transverse CT scan (bone window) shows fluid in both tympanic bullae and a large soft tissue pharyngeal mass. **(C)** Transverse CT scan (soft tissue window) post-contrast shows enlargement of the mandibular lymph nodes bilaterally. **(D)** On oral examination under anesthesia there is ventral displacement of the soft palate by the mass.

difficult to provide more than a palliative reduction in tumor volume with surgery for animals with carcinoma.

Lymphoma

Lymphoma may affect the nasal cavity and may extend into the nasopharynx.[34] In one study of cats with lymphoma of the nasal passages and nasopharynx, the nasal passages were the most common site (82%), with fewer cats having isolated nasopharyngeal lymphoma (10%) or involvement of both sites (12%). Immunoblastic lymphoma is the most common histologic diagnosis and the majority are B-cell lymphoma.[34] Cytology may yield a diagnosis in a high proportion of cases, but some samples are misclassified as inflammatory lesions and normal lymphoid tissue.[34] Panhyperproteinemia, usually due to dehydration, and hypocholesterolemia, associated with reduced appetite, are seen in a proportion of cats.

Cats may have a long remission time after radiotherapy or chemotherapy.[7,35,36] Control of local disease is important with regards to survival times, although up to 30% of cats with nasal lymphoma will develop lymphoma at other sites, notably the kidney, brain, and lymph nodes.[36] Central nervous system (CNS) involvement may also arise by direct extension.[7] CNS signs include oculomotor nerve deficits. A multicenter study of 118 cats which were treated with either radiotherapy alone, chemotherapy and radiotherapy, or chemotherapy alone found no significant difference in survival times between the three treatment groups, with mean survival times of 473 days for radiotherapy and chemotherapy, 1431 days for radiotherapy alone, and 320 days for chemotherapy alone.[35] The inclusion of radiotherapy in the treatment protocol did, however, significantly improve the overall survival.

Sarcoma

Although squamous cell carcinoma affecting the head and neck is more commonly seen in the oral cavity affecting the tongue, maxilla, mandible, and buccal mucosa, it is occasionally found affecting the mucosa of the soft palate and pharynx.[37] Sarcomas are uncommon, but soft tissue sarcoma, osteosarcoma, and chondrosarcoma may be encountered. Little is known about the most appropriate therapy and the prognosis.

Craniopharyngioma

Craniopharyngioma (Rathke's pouch tumor) is derived from nests of epithelium of the primordial craniopharyngeal canal (Rathke's pouch). Rathke's pouch is a diverticulum arising from the embryonic buccal cavity, from which the anterior pituitary gland develops. Craniopharyngiomas are composed of well-differentiated epithelial elements, including cysts and ameloblasts, and bone. The tumor is usually noted first intracranially, above the sella turcica, and the pharyngeal component is secondary. Reports of this tumor in cats are rare.[38] Clinical signs include initial dyspnea and nasal discharge, followed by cranial nerve signs, resulting in an abnormal appearance to the pupil, blindness, and vestibular signs. There are no reports of successful treatment.

Foreign bodies

Occasionally, foreign bodies may be encountered in the nasopharynx. The usual route of entry is from the caudal pharynx rostrally into the nasopharynx, after ingestion, regurgitation or vomiting, although direct entry from the nasal passages may occur. The most commonly reported foreign body is a blade of grass that moves rostrally and becomes trapped in the nasopharynx.[39,40] Other items that are chewed

may become lodged in the nasopharynx, particularly if the animal coughs while ingesting them. Other items reported are avian bones,[41] fish bones,[42] trichobezoars,[1] tablets,[8] and sewing needles.[1]

Consistent signs of a grass foreign body are persistent dry coughing or gagging, with harsh tracheal sounds but no pyrexia.[39] Palpation of the throat usually elicits a marked swallowing response. Foreign bodies usually cause an acute onset of clinical signs, which may worsen as secondary inflammation develops and pyrexia and halitosis ensue.[41,42] Since cats are relatively fastidious eaters, identification of an ingested foreign body should always prompt consideration of whether the cat is exhibiting pica or polyphagia.

Diagnosis may be achieved by imaging or endoscopy (Fig. 51-13). Care should be taken to differentiate osseous foreign bodies from the mineralized hyoid apparatus. The foreign bodies may be covered with mucus or exudate (Fig. 51-14) or may be partially embedded in the mucosa, which makes identifying them and removing them more difficult. Foreign bodies may also lodge in the oropharynx, particularly in the piriform recesses, including the areas just lateral to the glossoepiglottic folds, and the tonsillar crypts.

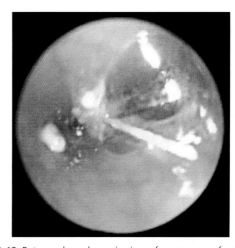

Figure 51-13 Retrograde endoscopic view of a grass awn foreign body in the nasopharynx.

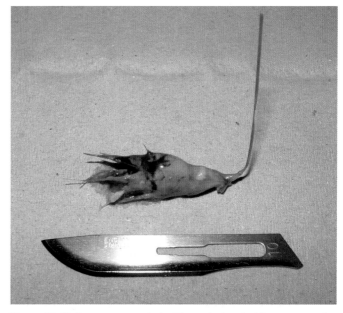

Figure 51-14 A grass awn coated with purulent material was removed from a cat with a chronic history of nasal discharge and sneezing.

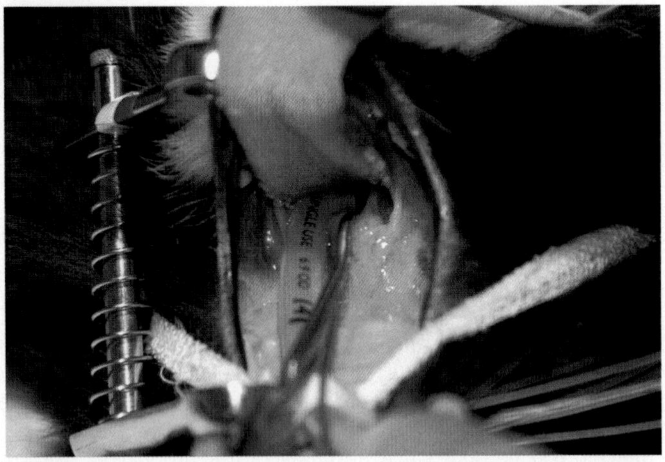

Figure 51-15 A spay hook has been used for rostral retraction of the soft palate in a cat with a nasopharyngeal foreign body.

Removal of most foreign bodies may be achieved under direct visualization following rostral retraction of the soft palate (Fig. 51-15). Small fragments of plant material may be removed endoscopically with grasping forceps or may be moved into the pharynx after flushing the nasal cavity from the external nares or by passing a small catheter or endoscope caudally from the external nares. If foreign bodies are located more rostrally, an incision in the soft palate may be required for access, but this is not commonly required. The nasal cavity and nasopharynx should be flushed with saline after removal of the foreign body.

Recovery is generally good, although one cat is reported to have developed a permanent change in voice after lodgment of an osseous foreign body in the pharynx.[41]

Trauma

Blunt trauma to the nasopharynx may be caused by a fall from a height ('high-rise syndrome'). A fissure of the hard palate with or without the soft palate may be seen. The oral mucoperiosteum may also be split or may remain intact over the split hard palate. Penetrating injuries to the pharynx, such as those caused by oropharyngeal stick injuries in dogs, are rare in cats.[43] Clinical signs may be referable to the traumatic injury itself, the presence of foreign material, or the development of an abscess and include oral pain, hypersalivation, and reluctance to close the mouth.

Occasionally, cats will develop penetrating injuries to the pharynx caused by playing with thread to which a needle is attached. Orthogonal radiographic projections should be used to localize the needle, but removal may be either straightforward or very time consuming. Care should be taken to ensure that the clinical signs match the presence of the foreign body, since this may be an old lesion.

Linear foreign bodies anchored in the oropharynx at the base of the tongue may be encountered, although the clinical signs are referable to obstruction of and leakage from the proximal intestinal tract following plication caused by peristalsis against a fixed foreign body.

Pharyngeal mucocele

Pharyngeal mucocele is uncommon in dogs and rare in cats.[44] Clinical signs of pharyngeal mucocele include dyspnea, gagging, and coughing, and a ranula and cervical swelling may also be seen. Excision of the ipsilateral mandibular and sublingual salivary glands results in resolution of the problem (see Chapter 49).

Choanal atresia

This is the most common congenital nasal abnormality in humans and is a common cause of neonatal respiratory distress. However, it is rare in the cat.[45] The cause is failure of the buccopharyngeal membrane to break down, leading to unilateral or bilateral obstruction at the level of the choanae. Although the condition in humans is often osseous, the few cases reported in animals have been soft tissue in nature.

The clinical signs are respiratory distress from birth. In bilateral atresia, the animal must breathe through its mouth and clinical signs are seen from birth, but in unilateral atresia, the airflow via the unaffected side may be sufficient and diagnosis may be delayed until a later date, or until other pharyngeal disease occurs. There will be reduced or no airflow via the nasal passages on the affected side and nasal discharge may be present.

Diagnosis is via endoscopic examination and/or failure of a catheter passed through the external nares to reach the nasopharynx. Treatment by balloon dilation and temporary stenting with a segment of feeding tube, followed by systemic corticosteroids, has been reported.[45]

Nasopharyngeal stenosis

Congenital nasopharyngeal stenosis caused by soft palate dysgenesis has been reported in a cat with clinical signs, from eight weeks of age.[46] In this animal, the caudal free border of the soft palate was attached to the caudal pharyngeal wall, with only a small oval slit allowing communication between the nasopharynx and the oropharynx. Clinical signs of inspiratory stridor were associated with marked laryngeal edema. Resolution of the edema following treatment with oral corticosteroids resulted in resolution of the clinical signs apart from a mild inspiratory stertor and no further treatment was pursued.

Acquired stenosis of the nasopharynx may occur secondary to inflammation caused by upper respiratory tract infection, nasal regurgitation of food and/or fluid, possibly under anesthesia, ingestion of caustic substances, trauma, or surgery. A thin membrane of inflammatory origin develops across the nasopharynx, partially or completing occluding it.[47] Many animals show acute onset of clinical signs following upper respiratory tract infection, persistence of clinical signs for several months with little progression and failure to respond to medical therapy for upper respiratory tract infection.[48]

Clinical signs include snuffling respiratory sounds and partial nasal obstruction, but nasal discharge is not common. Little or no airflow may be found at the level of the external nares. Stenosis of the nasopharynx may impair the normal function of the muscles and the intrapharyngeal opening may not close during deglutition, thus resulting in reflux and worsening inflammation.

Endoscopic examination of the nasopharynx and choanae will show marked narrowing of the lumen (Fig. 51-16).[48] Failure to be able to pass a catheter from the external nares via the ventral nasal meatus to the nasopharynx may confirm a physical obstruction.[47] Radiographs, CT or MRI will also provide a diagnosis (Fig. 51-17).

Histologic examination of the excised tissue reveals diffuse submucosal fibrosis with infiltration by lymphocytes, mast cells, and eosinophils, consistent with a diagnosis of chronic inflammatory rhinitis.[47]

Treatment options for nasopharyngeal stenosis are described below.

Nasopharyngitis

Inflammation of the nasopharynx may occur with nasal cavity disease or separately. Nasal cavity disease may lead to secondary nasopharyngeal disease due to the exposure of the mucosa to draining

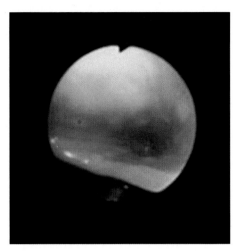

Figure 51-16 Endoscopic evaluation shows marked nasopharyngeal stenosis.

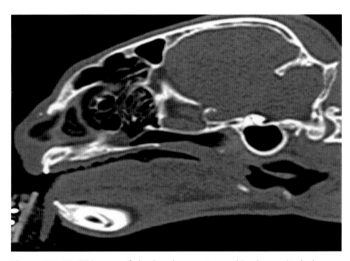

Figure 51-17 CT image of the head reconstructed in the sagittal plane showing nasopharyngeal stenosis and obliteration of the nasopharyngeal lumen. *(Courtesy of Rob White.)*

infected secretions.[49] Inflammatory conditions of the oral cavity and oropharynx are common and include gingivitis-periodontitis related to dental plaque and calculus, and gingivitis–stomatitis–pharyngitis complex.[50]

Causes of pharyngitis include trauma, foreign bodies within the pharynx or penetrating injuries, insect bites or stings, allergic reactions, reaction to ingested caustic agents, infectious agents, lymphoma, chronic stomatitis–pharyngitis complex, and eosinophilic granuloma complex.

The clinical signs are stertor, reverse sneezing, and dyspnea with the mouth closed. On inspection the mucosa may appear diffusely swollen and erythematous and may be ulcerated.

Viral nasopharyngitis

This may be caused by FHV-1 and FCV infections. These pathogens account for the vast majority of feline upper respiratory infections and affect the nasal cavity, nasopharynx, and pharynx. Pain on eating, anorexia, salivation, inflammation of the pharyngeal mucosa, and pain on palpation of the pharyngeal mucosa are the clinical signs. Although this is not a surgical disease, it is a common disease that

should be considered as a differential diagnosis for acute onset clinical signs referable to the pharynx.

Fungal nasopharyngitis

Fungal infection of the nasopharynx by *Cryptococcus*, *Aspergillus*, phaeohyphomycosis, blastomycosis, histoplasmosis, trichosporonosis, and sporotrichosis has been reported.[2]

Cryptococcus

Cryptococcus usually affects the rostral nasal cavity, but nasopharyngeal involvement comprising fungal granulomas causing respiratory obstruction may be seen.[8] Extension to cause meningitis has been reported. Two species, *C. neoformans*, which has a global distribution, and *C. gattii*, which has a more limited distribution to Australia and the Pacific north west of the US, have been isolated. Diagnosis is by cytology and/or histology and culture of lesions. Serology, using a latex agglutination test, is a sensitive and specific test for cryptococcal antigens.

Removal of as much of the lesion as possible via flushing or surgery is recommended to alleviate the airway obstruction and to reduce the bulk of the disease to be treated medically. Medical therapy with oral itraconazole (50–100 mg per cat once daily with food) or fluconazole (30–50 mg per cat q12–24h) is recommended. Itraconazole is cheaper and may be used as the first-line treatment, although it may induce a reversible hepatopathy, manifest by inappetence and vomiting, at higher doses. However, fluconazole penetrates the blood–brain barrier even in the absence of inflammation and should be used if there is CNS involvement. Medical therapy should continue until resolution of all clinical signs and until the antigen titer declines to zero, which may take three to 12 months.

Aspergillus

Aspergillus is an uncommon cause of nasal and nasopharyngeal disease in the cat. This is a more aggressive disease in the cat than in the dog, caused by fungi of the genera *Aspergillus* and *Neosartorya*.[2,51] Brachycephalic cats seem predisposed, which contrasts with the predisposition of mesaticephalic and dolichocephalic dogs to the disease.[2]

Although some cats will present with primarily nasal passage disease, there is a propensity for extension of infection beyond the nasal passages and sinuses to involve adjacent structures such as the orbit, palate, cribriform plate, and nasopharynx.[51] Up to 70% of cats with upper respiratory tract aspergillosis will present with a mass lesion in the caudal nasal passage or nasopharynx.[2,52]

Recommendations for therapy comprise surgical debridement of lesions followed by anti-fungal therapy with topical clotrimazole[52–54] or systemic drugs such as itraconazole (10 mg/kg PO q24h), fluconazole (7.5 mg/kg PO q12h), posaconazole (5 mg/kg PO q24h), voriconazole (10 mg/kg PO q24h), or caspofungin.[51,55]

Bacterial nasopharyngitis

Primary bacterial nasopharyngitis is uncommon, although secondary infection may be seen in animals with bacterial rhinitis, cleft palate, oronasal fistula, foreign body, nasopharyngeal polyp, or incompetence of the nasopharyngeal opening. Bacteria reported include *Bordetella bronchiseptica*, *Mycobacteria* spp., and *Actinomyces* spp. *Chlamydophila felis* and *Mycoplasma* spp. have also been implicated.

Feline chronic gingivitis–stomatitis–pharyngitis complex

This is an inflammatory disease of unknown etiology characterized by lymphocytic/plasmacytic infiltration of the oral and pharyngeal

627

mucosa. Lesions are inflammatory, proliferative, and ulcerative. The etiology is unknown, but a number of factors have been suggested as causative or contributory, such as bacterial, viral, and systemic disease. Dental disease, diet, oral conformation, and genetic factors (e.g., immune status) may also be contributing factors.[50]

Clinical signs are anorexia, difficulty in eating, halitosis, and ptyalism. Diffuse or focal inflammation, which may be proliferative or ulcerative, particularly along the gingival margins and at the lateral oropharynx and glossopalatine arches, may be seen on oral examination. A thorough dental examination and FeLV/FIV testing should be performed. The diagnosis is confirmed with a biopsy of the affected mucosa (e.g., with a Keyes biopsy punch).

In animals with dental disease, appropriate dental cleaning, prophylaxis and teeth extraction may result in a temporary improvement in clinical signs. Immunosuppressive therapy with corticosteroids and/or other agents such as chlorambucil or gold salts may be required. Antibiotics with an anaerobic spectrum such as metronidazole or clindamycin may be effective in the initial stages of the disease, but recurrence of clinical signs is often seen after stopping therapy.

Caustic agent ingestion

Cats are more selective than dogs and voluntary ingestion of caustic substances such as phenolic or alkaline compounds is uncommon.

Electric burn

Electrical burns affecting the oral cavity and pharynx may be caused by biting through an electric cable. Oral pain and ptyalism may be seen and many animals will have dyspnea from associated pulmonary edema.

Nasopharyngeal turbinates in brachycephalic cats

Nasal turbinates may protrude caudally from the choanae into the nasopharynx in brachycephalic (e.g., Persian and Himalayan) cats and can easily be seen on retrograde pharyngoscopy.[56] The median age at presentation was lower for cats with nasopharyngeal turbinates (three years, range two to four years) than those without (11 years, range 6.5–16 years). While it is clear that these turbinates cause some degree of airway obstruction, the significance of this clinical finding is uncertain.

SURGICAL TECHNIQUES

When performing pharyngeal surgery it is important that a cuffed endotracheal tube is used and the low pressure cuff is fully inflated to prevent aspiration of blood and secretions.

Surgical approach to the nasopharynx

Oral examination of the pharynx and rostral retraction of the palate with a hook (see Fig. 51-4) or stay suture (Fig. 51-18) give good access to the nasopharynx in the cat. If this is not sufficient, then the rostral nasopharynx may be approached via a midline incision in the soft palate.[8,19] This may be a small incision just caudal to the hard palate to gain access to the rostral nasopharynx, or may be extended caudally to the caudal free border of the soft palate. Ideally, the caudal soft palate should be left intact to facilitate closure and help support the tissue during healing. The incision may be continued rostrally with an incision in the mucoperiosteum of the hard palate, followed by

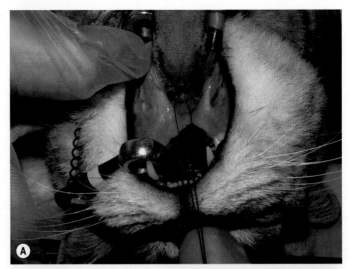

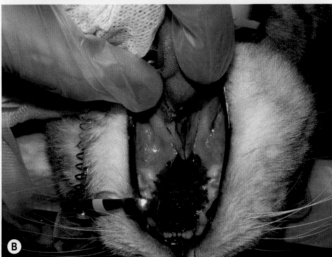

Figure 51-18 (A) A stay suture in the caudal border of the soft palate. **(B)** The stay suture is used to retract the palate rostrally.

ventral rhinotomy. The incision should be closed in three layers, namely the nasal mucosa, the muscularis, and the oral mucosa. Simple continuous sutures using small gauge synthetic monofilament absorbable suture are recommended. Healing is usually rapid.

Mandibular symphysiotomy has been described to improve access to the nasopharynx via the soft palate incision.[57] In this technique, a ventral midline incision is made through the skin from the basihyoid bone to the rostral lip, extending through the mylohyoideus with separation of the paired geniohyoideus muscles. An incision in the mucosa is made rostrally in the midline and then deviating laterally at the frenulum. The mandibular symphysis is exposed and split and gentle retraction exposes the genioglossus muscles. The genioglossus is bluntly separated from the geniohyoideus and severed close to its attachment on the mandible. The incision is deepened by blunt separation between the styloglossus and mylohyoideus. The incision in the mucosa is continued caudally, lateral to the sublingual and mandibular salivary ducts to the level of the glossopalatine arch. This procedure is reported to be well tolerated, with animals eating soft food the day after surgery and no complications have been described.[57]

A dorsal rhinotomy (see Chapter 54) with turbinectomy has been described to remove IPNT with marked nasopharyngeal extension,[13] but this is likely to be rarely needed.

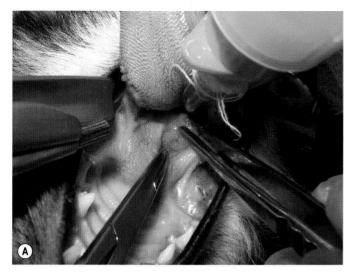

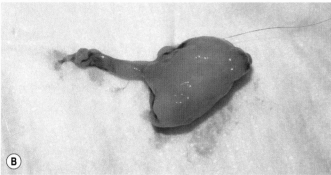

Figure 51-19 (A) The soft palate is retracted rostrally by use of a small mosquito hemostat so the polyp can be visualized. **(B)** The polyp after removal by gentle traction showing the classic tail.

Removal of polyps: traction/avulsion

If the polyp is palpable, it may be possible to displace it caudally into the oropharynx by caudodorsal pressure on the soft palate. If this is not possible, the soft palate is retracted rostrally (Fig. 51-19) and the base of the polyp examined. The polyp is grasped at its base or stalk with forceps and, after ensuring that no pharyngeal mucosa is included in the forceps, gentle continuous traction is used to remove the polyp. Hemorrhage is controlled by pressure with a gauze swab. It is important not to crush the base of the polyp with forceps, otherwise it may break at this point leaving remnants attached to the middle ear or Eustachian tube. The polyp should be examined to ensure it has a long, tapered stalk (Fig. 51-19B).

The polyp should be submitted for histologic examination to confirm the suspected diagnosis and to rule out other causes of a nasopharyngeal mass, e.g., lymphoma.

Removal of foreign bodies

Foreign bodies may be removed by rhinoscopy, either from an antero-grade or retrograde approach, with appropriate grasping instruments. Alternatively, flushing saline through the nasal passages from a rostral to caudal direction may dislodge the foreign material. In animals with secondary bacterial infection and/or copious mucoid or purulent discharge, treatment with antibiotics for a short period may resolve the infection so that the foreign material may be identified. Caudal retraction of the soft palate with instruments or a stay suture as described

for nasopharyngeal polyps may be needed. Ventral or, rarely, a dorsal rhinotomy may be needed to remove foreign material that cannot be retrieved non-surgically.

Ventral bulla osteotomy (VBO)

Vental bulla osteotomy is indicated for nasopharyngeal polyps if they recur after traction/avulsion, if the clinical signs are severe on first presentation, or if there is no nasopharyngeal component to apply traction to.[23,30] The surgical technique is described in Chapter 50 (see Box 50-11).

Nasopharyngeal stenosis

Treatment of nasopharyngeal stenosis in the cat involves surgical resection of the obstruction, forcibly opening the narrowed area by passage of a structure that enlarges the aperture or by placement of a stent to maintain a passage.

Resection of the membranous tissue can be performed via an incision in the soft palate (Fig. 51-20 and Box 51-1).[15,47] This technique was reported to be successful in four cats, with no recurrence, although dehiscence of the soft palate incision in one animal necessitated a second surgery.[47] However, other authors have described recurrence of this condition with this technique.[48,58,59] Ablation of the membrane with a holmium : YAG laser has also been reported, although this was not successful. Resection of the membranous tissue followed by reconstruction of the dorsal nasopharyngeal wall with an advancement flap from the caudal nasopharynx has been described (Box 51-1).[60] This technique was performed due to concerns about postoperative webbing and recurrence with the first technique, particularly if denuded mucosa is left in situ, as described in the cat[58] and dog.[48]

Dilation (Box 51-1) is performed with surgical instruments (artery forceps), bougies or balloon catheters.[6,15,59,61] It usually produces a prompt resolution of clinical signs, but recurrence in the short term after one procedure has been reported, which was successfully managed by repeating the procedure.[6,59,61] Recurrence of stenosis after a single procedure has prompted other authors to try an alternative procedure, but the long-term improvement seen after repeating the procedure suggests that this represents a good first option. Postoperatively, corticosteroids have been given at various doses, from 0.25 mg/kg q24 h for seven days to 2 mg/kg q24h for ten days, then tapered. Long term, clinical signs are resolved or much improved, although a variable degree of stenosis at the site may be seen on endoscopic examination. Balloon dilation was reported to be unsuccessful in one case, but this involved introduction of a 10 French Swann-Ganz catheter and 10 mm balloon via the oral cavity and only short-term corticosteroids were given, both of which may have contributed to failure.[58]

Stents may be used to maintain patency while the denuded epithelium is restored to prevent recurrence. A braided wire prosthesis (Wallstent, Schneider US Stent Division) was placed in one cat following failure of an open surgical approach and balloon dilation[58] and a balloon-expandable metallic stent (Palmaz Genesis; Cordis) was placed in three cats.[62] Granulation tissue formation, tissue ingrowth requiring placement of a covered stent and need to resect the end of the stent because of dysphagia, hairball entrapment, and discomfort during swallowing were complications reported, but were successfully managed.[58,62] Recommendations have been made that covered stents are used in animals with complete nasopharyngeal stenosis, animals with caudal stenosis have serial balloon dilation prior to stent placement, and 1 cm of unstented soft palate is left caudal to the stent.[62]

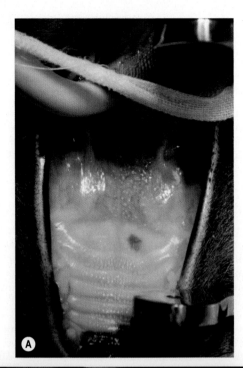

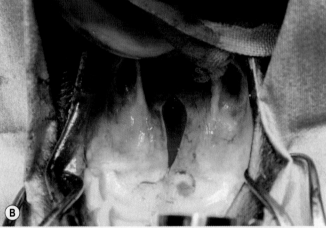

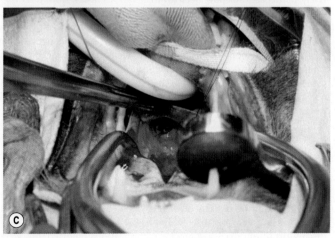

Figure 51-20 (A) Nasopharyngeal stenosis. **(B)** An incision has been made in the soft palate and the narrowed nasopharynx is visible. **(C)** The stenotic area is resected. *(Courtesy of Rob White.)*

Box 51-1 **Treatment options for nasopharyngeal stenosis**

Resection

The cat is positioned in dorsal recumbency with the mouth held in an open position by use of a mouth gag. A midline soft palate incision is made and stay sutures placed in the palate edges to retract them.[47] The obstructing membrane is excised by the use of iris scissors or small Metzenbaum scissors. The incision in the soft palate is then closed in three layers, namely the nasal mucosa, the muscularis, and the oral mucosa. Simple continuous sutures using small gauge synthetic monofilament absorbable suture are recommended.

Resection and reconstruction[60]

The cat is placed in dorsal recumbency. A midline incision is made in the soft palate to the level of the hard palate and the caudal edges retracted by the use of stay sutures. The scar tissue forming the obstructive membrane between the soft palate and dorsal nasopharynx is excised with iris scissors. Cannulation from the external nares is repeated to verify that the passages are now patent. The defect in the dorsal nasopharyngeal wall is then reconstructed with a pedicle advancement flap from the caudal nasopharynx and cranial laryngopharynx and closed in two layers (submucosa and mucosa) using small gauge synthetic monofilament absorbable suture material. The incision in the soft palate is then closed in three layers, namely the nasal mucosa, the muscularis, and the oral mucosa. Simple continuous sutures using small gauge synthetic monofilament absorbable suture are recommended.

Dilation

A 5 French balloon catheter with a 10 mm or 15 mm balloon is introduced via the external nares to pass across the stenotic region, either directly, or over a guidewire, if the balloon catheter cannot be passed alone. A smaller catheter is usually passed first and then the effect of the procedure monitored either by direct visualization via retrograde pharyngoscopy[59,60] or fluoroscopy.[6] A larger catheter can then be passed if it is felt that the opening into the caudal nares was still too small. The procedure can be repeated at a subsequent time if re-stenosis occurs.

Stenting[62]

Retroflex rhinoscopy and simultaneous fluoroscopy are used during balloon dilatation and stent placement. Stent sizes are determined on the basis of computed tomography measurements and stent availability. In one report on three cats, stents sized 8 mm × 16 mm, 9 mm × 17 mm, and 9 mm × 19 mm were used.[62] If there is a complete membrane across the nasopharynx then dilation with a balloon, as described above, is performed first. Stent location is then identified via fluoroscopy and rhinoscopy and the stent centered over the lesion; 1 cm of unstented soft palate should be left caudal to the stent to allow for normal nasopharyngeal closure during swallowing. Stents are inflated to the recommended pressures for the individual balloons (8 to 12 atmospheres or pressure).

Recommendations have been made that covered balloon-expandable metallic stents are used in animals with a closed membrane, although these are more expensive than the uncovered versions.[62] A covered stent is not considered necessary with an open nasopharyngeal stenosis.

POSTOPERATIVE CARE

Cats should be monitored in the immediate postoperative period for respiratory distress resulting from pharyngeal edema. Rarely, a tracheostomy tube (see Chapter 46) may be needed on recovery. Intravenous fluids are administered until the cat is able to drink voluntarily. Water and then food may be offered once the cat has recovered and there is no evidence of respiratory distress. Soft food should be fed for two to three weeks in cats with nasopharyngeal disease or surgical intervention of the nasopharynx. An esophagostomy tube may be placed in cats that are inappetent prior to surgery if it is suspected that they will not return to prompt feeding postoperatively. This includes cats with marked vestibular syndrome undergoing a VBO.

Corticosteroids may be given if pharyngeal edema is present or it is suspected it will develop. Antimicrobial agents may be indicated if an infectious process is present. Potentiated amoxicillin represents a good empirical choice, since the likely organisms are flora from the oral cavity and pharynx.

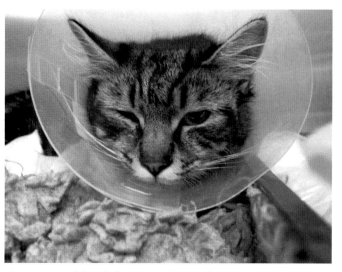

Figure 51-21 Right-sided Horner syndrome after removal of a nasopharyngeal polyp by traction. This is a common complication and resolved within two weeks of surgery.

COMPLICATIONS

Inflammation, edema and infection

Swelling from inflammation and edema may be seen after manipulation of the tissues as they are exquisitely sensitive to trauma and handling. Swelling causes increased airway resistance and increased negative pressure on inspiration, which will worsen airway obstruction and contribute to further edema and worsening airway obstruction. This complication is reduced by gentle atraumatic handling of tissues and the use of fine, sharp instruments appropriate to their purpose. Stay sutures should be used instead of retractors where possible and electrosurgery should not be used for incision or hemostasis. Anti-inflammatory doses of corticosteroids may be used if there is pre-existing edema or if it is predicted to develop postoperatively. Animals with respiratory tract disease or surgery involving the respiratory tract should be subject to continuous monitoring until the dyspnea has resolved.

Wound infection and drainage is uncommon, even though procedures of the nasopharynx and middle ear are clean-contaminated to dirty, due in part to the excellent blood supply. Dehiscence of the palate incision is a potential complication.[47]

Aspiration pneumonia is avoided by using a cuffed endotracheal tube and a pharyngeal pack if possible, ensuring adequate hemostasis, removal of all blood and fluid at the end of the procedure with suction and not feeding the animal until fully conscious with a normal swallowing reflex. Pulmonary dysfunction caused by aspiration pneumonia may be exacerbated by pulmonary edema in those patients with respiratory tract obstruction.

Hemorrhage

Bleeding is common during procedures of the pharynx due to its excellent blood supply, although it is usually mild and manageable with simple procedures, e.g., direct pressure. However, continued hemorrhage may cause aspiration of blood into the lower airway and the development of pneumonia, and blood clots may exacerbate respiratory obstruction still further. Prevention of hemorrhage involves the application of the basic principles of hemostasis, avoiding methods that cause tissue trauma. Hemorrhage may be seen after sharp surgical procedures as well as after traction/avulsion of polyps and balloon dilation of stenotic lesions. Conchal necrosis and nasal discharge are also reported after balloon dilation of nasopharyngeal stenosis.[59]

Neurologic complications

Damage to the facial and hypoglossal nerves is possible during surgery of the middle ear, although this is less likely in the cat than the dog.[25,26,63]

Horner syndrome (Fig. 51-21) is a common complication after removal of nasopharyngeal or middle ear polyps. It can occasionally occur after traction/avulsion and is common after VBO, usually due to curettage of the ventromedial compartment. In most animals, the clinical signs resolve in one to three weeks,[12] although cats in which clinical signs persist beyond six weeks are unlikely to recover fully. Even in those animals where it persists, functional impairment is uncommon.

Clinical signs of peripheral vestibular disease may be seen in up to 40% of cats, if curettage of the tympanic bulla is too vigorous and causes damage to the round or oval windows or vestibulocochlear apparatus. These signs are generally transient in cats and resolve within two weeks.[28] However, cats with preoperative vestibular syndrome may have persistence of clinical signs postoperatively, particularly the head tilt.[12]

Many cats with nasopharyngeal polyps are deaf as assessed by brainstem auditory evoked potentials. In one study, none of six cats showed an improvement in hearing ability in the postoperative period.[12] Lack of reformation of the tympanic cavity and damage to the auditory ossicles during surgery has the potential to render the patient deaf.

Bradycardia after nasopharyngeal stimulation, necessitating administration of atropine, has been reported.[6]

REFERENCES

1. Haynes KJ, Anderson SE, Laszlo MP. Nasopharyngeal trichobezoar foreign body in a cat. J Feline Med Surg 2010;12(11):878–81.

2. Barrs VR, Beatty JA, Lingard AE, et al. Feline sino-orbital aspergillosis: An emerging clinical syndrome? Aust Vet J 2007;85(3):N23.

3. Allen HS, Broussard J, Noone K. Nasopharyngeal diseases in cats: A retrospective study of 53 cases (1991–1998). J Am Anim Hosp Assoc 1999;35(6):457–61.

4. Willard MD, Radlinsky MA. Endoscopic examination of the choanae in dogs and cats: 118 cases (1988–1998). J Am Vet Med Assoc 1999;215(9):1301–5.

5. Esterline ML, Radlinsky MG, Schermerhorn T. Endoscopic removal of nasal polyps in a cat using a novel surgical approach. J Feline Med Surg 2005;7(2):121–4.

6. Boswood A, Lamb CR, Brockman DJ, et al. Balloon dilatation of nasopharyngeal stenosis in a cat. Vet Radiol Ultrasound 2003;44(1):53–5.

7. Chang Y, Thompson H, Reed N, Penderis J. Clinical and magnetic resonance imaging features of nasopharyngeal lymphoma in two cats with concurrent intracranial mass. J Small Anim Pract 2006;47(11):678–81.

8. Malik R, Martin P, Wigney DI, et al. Nasopharyngeal cryptococcosis. Aust Vet J 1999;75:483–8.

9. De Lorenzi D, Bertoncello D, Bottero E. Squash-preparation cytology from nasopharyngeal masses in the cat: cytological results and histological correlations in 30 cases. J Feline Med Surg 2008;10(1):55–60.

10. MacPhail CM, Innocenti CM, Kudnig ST, et al. Atypical manifestations of feline inflammatory polyps in three cats. J Feline Med Surg 2007;9(3):219–25.

11. Veir JK, Lappin MR, Foley JE, Getzy DM. Feline inflammatory polyps: historical, clinical, and PCR findings for feline calici virus and feline herpes virus-1 in 28 cases. J Feline Med Surg 2002;4(4):195–9.

12. Anders BB, Hoelzler MG, Scavelli TD, et al. Analysis of auditory and neurologic effects associated with ventral bulla osteotomy for removal of inflammatory polyps or nasopharyngeal masses in cats. J Am Vet Med Assoc 2008;233(4):580–5.

13. Greci V, Mortellaro CM, Olivero D, et al. Inflammatory polyps of the nasal turbinates of cats: an argument for designation as feline mesenchymal hamartoma. J Feline Med Surg 2011;13:2 13–19.

14. Galloway PE, Kyles A, Henderson JP. Nasal polyps in a cat. J Small Anim Pract 1997;38(2):78–80.

15. Henderson SM, Bradley K, Day MJ, et al. Investigation of nasal disease in the cat – a retrospective study of 77 cases. J Feline Med Surg 2004;6:245–57.

16. Baker G. Nasopharyngeal polyps in cats. Vet Rec 1982;111(2):43.

17. Pope ER. Feline inflammatory polyps. Semin Vet Med Surg (Small Anim) 1995;10(2):87–93.

18. Bedford PGC, Coulson A, Sharp NJ, Longstaffe JA. Nasopharyngeal polyps in the cat. Vet Rec 1981;109(25-2):551–3.

19. Parker NR, Binnington AG. Nasopharyngeal polyps in cats: Three case reports and a review of the literature. J Am Anim Hosp Assoc 1985;21(4): 473–8.

20. Klose TC, MacPhail CM, Schultheiss PC, et al. Prevalence of select infectious agents in inflammatory aural and nasopharyngeal polyps from client-owned cats. J Feline Med Surg 2010;12(10): 769–74.

21. Stanton ME, Wheaton LG, Render JA, Blevins WE. Pharyngeal polyps in two feline siblings. J Am Vet Med Assoc 1985;186(12):1311–13.

22. Byron JK, Shadwick SR, Bennett AR. Megaesophagus in a 6-month-old cat secondary to a nasopharyngeal polyp. J Feline Med Surg 2010;12(4):322–4.

23. Anderson DM, Robinson RK, White RAS. Management of inflammatory polyps in 37 cats. Vet Rec 2000;147(24):684–7.

24. Seitz SE, Losonsky JM, Marretta SM. Computed tomographic appearance of inflammatory polyps in three cats. Vet Radiol Ultrasound 1996;37(2):99–104.

25. Ader PL, Boothe HW. Ventral bulla osteotomy in the cat. J Am Anim Hosp Assoc 1979;15(6):757–62.

26. Kapatkin AS, Matthiesen DT, Noone KE, et al. Results of surgery and long-term follow-up in 31 cats with nasopharyngeal polyps. J Am Anim Hosp Assoc 1990;26(4):387–92.

27. Harvey CE, Goldschmidt MH. Inflammatory polypoid growths in the ear canal of cats. J Small Anim Pract 1978;669–77.

28. Faulkner JE, Budsberg SC. Results of ventral bulla osteotomy for treatment of middle-ear polyps in cats. J Am Anim Hosp Assoc 1990;26(5):496–9.

29. Trevor PB, Martin RA. Tympanic bulla osteotomy for treatment of middle ear disease in cats: 19 cases(1984–1991). J Am Vet Med Assoc 1993;202:123–8.

30. Lane JG, Orr CM, Lucke VM, Gruffydd-Jones TJ. Nasopharyngeal polyps arising in the middle ear of the cat. J Small Anim Pract 1981;22(8):511–22.

31. Hunt GB, Perkins MC, Foster SF, et al. Nasopharyngeal disorders of dogs and cats: A review and retrospective study.

Comp Cont Educ Pract Vet 2002;24(3): 184–200.

32. Cotter SM. Oral Pharyngeal Neoplasms in the Cat. J Am Anim Hosp Assoc 1981;17(6):917–20.

33. Schoenborn WC, Wisner ER, Kass PP, Dale M. Retrospective assessment of computed tomographic imaging of feline sinonasal disease in 62 cats. Vet Radiol Ultrasound 2003;44:185–95.

34. Little L, Patel R, Goldschmidt M. Nasal and nasopharyngeal lymphoma in cats: 50 cases (1989–2005). Vet Pathol 2007;44:885–92.

35. Haney SM, Beaver L, Turrel J, et al. Survival Analysis of 97 Cats with Nasal Lymphoma: A Multi-Institutional Retrospective Study (1986–2006). J Vet Intern Med 2009;23:287–94.

36. Sfiligoi G, Theon AP, Kent MS. Response of nineteen cats with nasal lymphoma to radiation therapy and chemotherapy. Vet Radiol Ultrasound 2007;48:388–93.

37. Gendler A, Lewis JR, Reetz JA, Schwarz T. Computed tomographic features of oral squamous cell carcinoma in cats: 18 cases (2002–2008). J Am Vet Med Assoc 2010;236(3):319–25.

38. Nagata T, Nakayama H, Uchida K, et al. Two cases of feline malignant craniopharyngioma. Vet Pathol 2005;42(5):663–5.

39. Riley P. Nasopharyngeal grass foreign body in eight cats. J Am Vet Med Assoc 1993;202(2):299–300.

40. Rocken H. Unusual foreign body in the laryngeal-pharyngeal cavity of a cat. Prakt Tierarzt 1987;68:55.

41. Rendano VT, Zimmer JF, Wallach MS, et al. Impaction of the pharynx, larynx, and esophagus by avian bones in the dog and cat. Vet Radiol 1988;29(5):213–16.

42. Phillipson MH, Leveque JI, Leveque NW. A case report. Foreign body in the pharynx of a cat. J Am Vet Med Assoc 1960;136:70.

43. Bright SR, Mellanby RJ, Williams JM. Oropharyngeal stick injury in a Bengal cat. J Feline Med Surg 2002;4(3):153–5.

44. Feinman JM. Pharyngeal mucocele and respiratory distress in a cat. J Am Vet Med Assoc 1990;197(9):1179–80.

45. Khoo AM, Marchevsky AM, Barrs VR, Beatty JA. Choanal atresia in a Himalayan cat - first reported case and successful treatment. J Feline Med Surg 2007;9(4): 346–9.

46. Talavera Lopez J, Josefa Fernandez Del Palacio MA, Cano FG, Del Rio AB. Nasopharyngeal stenosis secondary to soft palate dysgenesis in a cat. Vet J 2009;181(2):200–4.

47. Mitten RW. Nasopharyngeal stenosis in four cats. J Small Anim Pract 1988;29(6):341–5.

48. Coolman BR, Marretta SM, McKiernan BC, Zachary JF. Choanal atresia and secondary nasopharyngeal stenosis in a dog. J Am Anim Hosp Assoc 1998;34(6): 497–501.

49. August JR, Bahr A. Chronic upper respiratory disease: principles of diagnosis and management, In: August JR, editor. Consultations in feline internal medicine. St Louis: Elsevier; 2006. p. 347–60.

50. Diehl K, Rosychuk RAW. Feline gingivitis stomatitis pharyngitis. Vet Clin North Am Small Anim Pract 1993;23(1): 139–53.

51. Giordano C, Gianella P, Bo S, et al. Invasive mould infections of the naso-orbital region of cats: a case involving *Aspergillus fumigatus* and an aetiological review. J Feline Med Surg 2010;12:714–23.

52. Whitney BL, Broussard J, Stefanacci JD. Four cats with fungal rhinitis. J Feline Med Surg 2005;7(1):53–8.

53. Hamilton HL, Whitley RD, McLaughlin SA. Exophthalmos secondary to aspergillosis in a cat. J Am Anim Hosp Assoc 2000;36:343–7.

54. Tomsa K, Glaus TM, Zimmer C, Greene CE. Fungal rhinitis and sinusitis in three cats. J Am Vet Med Assoc 2003;222(10): 1380–4.

55. McLellan GJ, Aquino SM, Mason DR, et al. Use of posaconazole in the management of invasive orbital aspergillosis in a cat. J Am Anim Hosp Assoc 2006;42(4):302–7.

56. Ginn JA, Kumar MS, McKiernan BC, Powers BE. Nasopharyngeal turbinates in brachycephalic dogs and cats. J Am Anim Hosp Assoc 2008;44(5):243–9.

57. Curley BM, Nelson AW, Kainer RA. Mandibular symphysiotomy in the dog and cat: a surgical approach to the nasopharynx. J Am Vet Med Assoc 1972;160(7):981–7.

58. Novo RE, Kramek B. Surgical repair of nasopharyngeal stenosis in a cat using a stent. J Am Anim Hosp Assoc 1999;35(3):251–6.

59. Glaus TM, Tomsa K, Reusch CE. Balloon dilation for the treatment of chronic recurrent nasopharyngeal stenosis in a cat. J Small Anim Pract 2002;43(2):88–90.

60. Griffon DJ, Tasker S. Use of a mucosal advancement flap for the treatment of nasopharyngeal stenosis in a cat. J Small Anim Pract 2000;41(2):71–3.

61. Glaus TM, Gerber B, Tomsa K, et al. Reproducible and long-lasting success of balloon dilation of nasopharyngeal stenosis in cats. Vet Rec 2005;157(9): 257–9.

62. Berent AC, Weisse C, Todd K, et al. Use of a balloon-expandable metallic stent for treatment of nasopharyngeal stenosis in dogs and cats: six cases (2005–2007). J Am Vet Med Assoc 2008;233(9): 1432–40.

63. Little CJL, Lane JG. The Surgical Anatomy of the Feline Bulla Tympanica. J Small Anim Pract 1986;27(6):371–8.

Chapter |52|

Larynx

B. Kirby

Surgical conditions of the feline larynx are relatively uncommon. Laryngeal paralysis, laryngeal neoplasia, and laryngeal inflammatory disease are the most common feline laryngeal conditions reported in the veterinary literature. However, there are relatively few reports and these often involve single or small numbers of cats. Laryngeal trauma and laryngeal foreign body are also sporadically reported.

As in other species, the clinical signs of laryngeal disease in cats can be peracute in onset, severe, and rapidly fatal without appropriate intervention. The propensity for laryngospasm in the cat may make orotracheal intubation challenging, particularly in emergency presentations of laryngeal disease. It is critically important to be prepared for emergency temporary tracheostomy in cats with laryngeal disease. In this chapter the surgical treatment of the common laryngeal conditions in cats will be described.

SURGICAL ANATOMY

The larynx is situated between the pharynx and first tracheal cartilage ring. It serves as a conduit for passage of air between the pharynx and trachea. The larynx functions in phonation, regulation of airflow through its lumen, and protection of the lower airway during swallowing. The larynx consists of a set of complicated cartilages, ligaments, and muscles (Figs 52-1 and 52-2). The five laryngeal cartilages are the epiglottis, thyroid cartilage, cricoid cartilage, and paired arytenoid cartilages. The epiglottis is the most rostral of the laryngeal cartilages. It is triangular in shape and composed of flexible fibrocartilage. It is attached by a fold of mucous membrane to the root of the tongue.[1] The epiglottis, together with the laryngeal adductors, covers the laryngeal opening during swallowing, allowing food and fluid to pass over it and into the esophagus.[1] The thyroid cartilage is the largest of the laryngeal cartilages. It is U-shaped, continuous ventrally and forms approximately two-thirds of the circumference of the larynx. It is attached cranially to the hyoid bone and articulates dorsally with the cricoid cartilage. The cricoid cartilage is signet ring shaped, with its broader part dorsad. Its caudal border is connected to the first tracheal ring. It articulates with the arytenoid cartilages on each side in addition to its thyroid cartilage articulation. The paired arytenoid cartilages are pyramidal in shape, with the base and sides nearly equilateral triangles. The arytenoid cartilages articulate with the cricoid and thyroid cartilages.

The vocal folds, thyroarytenoid muscles, and cricoarytenoid dorsalis and lateralis muscles attach to the arytenoid cartilages. Movements produced by these muscles and the vocal folds, open and close the rima glottidis, the laryngeal airway. There are two pairs of tissue folds at the cranial end of the feline larynx; the false vocal cords that lie more cranially and laterally, while the true vocal cords lie more caudally and nearer the median plane. The laryngeal ventricles are reported to lie between the true and false vocal cords on each side.[2] However, laryngeal ventricles are also reported not to exist in feline species.[3] To the author's knowledge, eversion of laryngeal ventricles has not been described in the cat, though this is commonly observed in dogs with brachycephalic upper airway syndrome.

The false and true vocal cords are most easily visualized by ventral laryngotomy.[2] The false vocal cords, often appearing tannish in color, extend from the arytenoid cartilages to the epiglottis. The true vocal

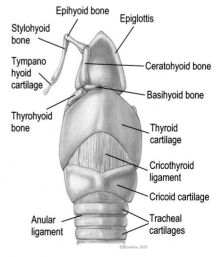

Figure 52-1 The feline larynx ventral view (arytenoid cartilages not visible) with hyoid apparatus on the right-hand side. *(Medical illustrations © Wm. P. Hamilton 2010.)*

© 2014 Elsevier Ltd
DOI: 10.1016/B978-0-7020-4336-9.00052-4

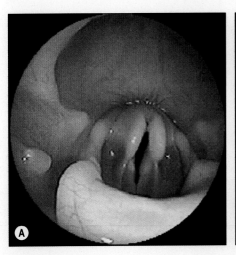

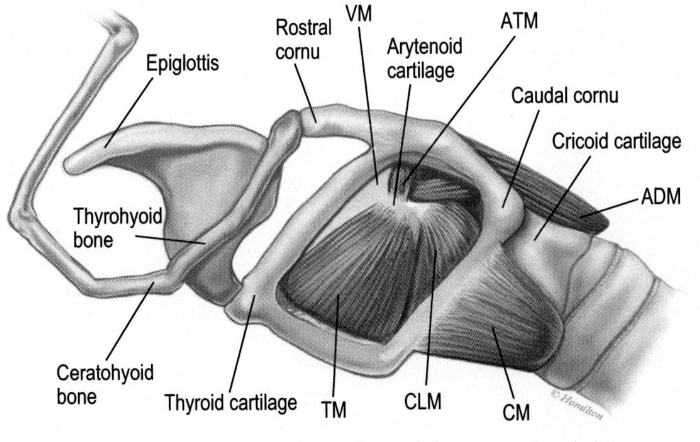

Figure 52-2 Illustration of the intrinsic musculature of the feline larynx, lateral view with window in thyroid cartilage. ATM, arytenoideus transversus muscle; ADM, arytenoideus dorsalis muscle (more commonly referred to as cricoarytenoideus dorsalis muscle); TM, thyroarytenoideus muscle; CLM, cricoarytenoideus lateralis muscle; CM, cricothyroideus muscle; VM, ventricularis muscle. *(Medical illustrations © Wm. P. Hamilton 2010.)*

cords, appearing as whitish bands, extend from the arytenoid cartilages to the thyroid cartilages. Conflicting reports of the presence of muscle in feline vocal cords exist, with one report stating that feline vocal cords do not contain muscle, in contrast to the dog and horse,[4] while another report cites extremely rapid twitching of the vocalis muscle running within the vocal folds as the mechanism of purring.[5] The feline cuneiform and corniculate processes are inconspicuous when viewed per os (Fig. 52-3A), while these structures are easily identified in dogs (Fig. 52-3B).[2] The larynx is elevated and depressed by action of the thyrohyoideus and sternothyroideus muscles, respectively. The laryngeal lumen is lined by mucous membrane.

The larynx is innervated by branches of the vagus. The vagus gives rise to the cranial laryngeal nerve which separates into an internal and external branch.[6] The cricothyroid muscle is innervated by the external branch, while the internal branch provides sensory innervation to the laryngeal muscles and mucosal surfaces.[6,7] The recurrent laryngeal nerves separate from the vagus at the thoracic inlet. The right recurrent laryngeal nerve passes around the subclavian artery before coursing cranially and traveling up the neck, while the left recurrent laryngeal nerve passes around the aortic arch on the left side before coursing cranially.[4] The recurrent laryngeal nerves terminate as caudal laryngeal nerves, innervating ipsilateral thyroarytenoideus, arytenoideus, and cricoarytenoideus muscles. The cricoarytenoideus dorsalis muscle is the only intrinsic laryngeal muscle responsible for abduction of the vocal cords, thus its critical role in respiratory dysfunction in laryngeal paralysis.

In all species studied, the left recurrent laryngeal nerve is more commonly involved than the right in laryngeal paralysis. The left recurrent laryngeal nerve has a longer course and fewer nerve fibers compared to the right,[4] which is postulated to account for its susceptibility to injury and the more common occurrence of left laryngeal hemiplegia. Interestingly, experimental left recurrent laryngeal denervation by resection of 30 mm length of the nerve in cats did not result in clinical signs of respiratory obstruction up to one month after surgery.[8] At one month, functional electrical stimulation of the laryngeal adductors restored mobility of the vocal folds and improved vocalization.[8]

GENERAL CONSIDERATIONS

Clinical examination

Clinical signs of laryngeal disease in cats are often vague and nonspecific. Most commonly reported clinical signs include tachypnea or dyspnea, inspiratory noise or stridor, dysphagia, weight loss, change in vocalization, coughing independent of eating, coughing and gagging when eating, and lethargy. Absence of purring is reported in cats with laryngeal paralysis and resumption of purring has been reported after surgery in some cats.[4] Absence of purring and a change in voice is also reported in cats with laryngeal tumors.[9] Laryngeal stridor in cats with laryngeal paralysis has been described as frequently having a distinct whistling component that can be less easy to recognize as part of the respiratory cycle.[7] Detection of this whistling sound may be facilitated by auscultation of the laryngeal region. Careful palpation of the cervical area to detect masses and compression of the cranial thorax to assess for a mediastinal mass are also important in the physical examination of cats with suspected laryngeal disease.

Diagnostic investigation in cats with clinical evidence of airway obstruction must be undertaken with care to minimize the risk of iatrogenic induction of life-threatening dyspnea. Routine analysis of blood and urine is recommended to rule out concurrent disease, particularly in geriatric cats. In addition to detailed general clinical examination, a complete neurologic examination is recommended.

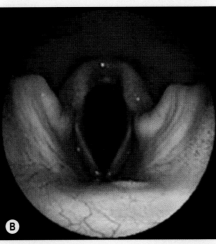

Figure 52-3 (A) Per os endoscopic view of normal feline larynx. **(B)** Per os endoscopic view of normal canine larynx. *(Photographs courtesy of Dr Nicole van Israël, ACAPULCO cardiopulmonary referrals, Masta, BE.)*

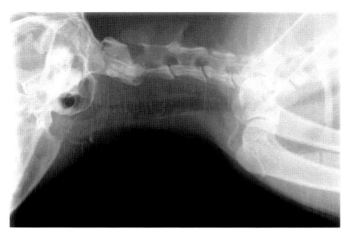

Figure 52-4 Lateral cervical radiographic view showing laryngeal soft tissue mass in a cat. Histologic examination of excisional biopsy of the mass revealed pyogranulomatous inflammation.

Diagnostic imaging

Radiography

Radiographic examination of the thorax and neck is recommended, but extreme care in restraint and positioning is required. Sedation or general anesthesia may be required in some cases to obtain diagnostic quality radiographs. Radiographic evidence of airway obstruction may be observed, including hyperinflation of the lungs, prominent caudal displacement of the larynx, and presence of air in the pharynx, larynx, esophagus, and stomach. Mass lesions in the larynx, cervical soft tissues, thoracic inlet, or thorax may be observed (Fig. 52-4).

Sonography

Sonographic examination of the larynx has been reported in 30 cats.[10] In five of these 30 cats, the larynx was normal. Vocal fold movement in the normal cats was difficult to identify. The presence and location of cysts and masses were accurately identified in nine cats and the authors considered echolaryngography likely superior to laryngoscopy for identification of cysts and soft tissue masses and cited the clinical advantage that echolaryngography could be performed in these animals without sedation or anesthesia. In eight cats with laryngeal paralysis and/or laryngeal collapse, poor movement of the vocal folds was observed, but further studies and further refinement of the technique are needed for its use in laryngeal paralysis.

Computed tomography (CT)/magnetic resonance imaging (MRI)

The use of advanced imaging techniques in the evaluation of laryngeal conditions in the dog has been reported.[11] Findings of laryngeal paralysis were identified by CT in unanesthetized dogs, including failure of arytenoid cartilage abduction and a narrow rima glottis. CT and MRI have not (to the author's knowledge) yet been evaluated in the cat, but based on the canine study these imaging modalities may have a role to play in the evaluation of laryngeal conditions in this species, although the precise nature of their role remains to be fully defined.

Laryngoscopy

Definitive diagnosis of feline laryngeal disease is most often achieved by direct laryngoscopy per os under a light plane of anesthesia. Direct laryngoscopy can be achieved with a handheld laryngoscope or an endoscope. Direct laryngoscopy allows assessment of laryngeal function as well as observation for laryngeal masses (Fig. 52-5) or other

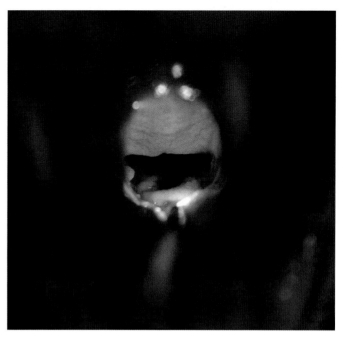

Figure 52-5 Endoscopic view of a feline laryngeal soft tissue mass. Histologic diagnosis was squamous cell carcinoma. *(Photograph courtesy of Jon Hall, Cambridge University, UK.)*

lesions, which can usually be sampled by fine needle aspiration or biopsy per os. Anesthesia is required for direct laryngoscopy. Protocols for sedation and anesthesia appear to vary widely. Similar to other species, general anesthesia may obliterate laryngeal function in normal animals. Particular care is required to distinguish sedative or anesthetic drug-induced laryngeal paralysis from the clinical disease. Additionally, it is important to recognize the potential presence of paradoxical laryngeal movement which could be mistaken for normal laryngeal abduction/adduction; this can be avoided by assessing laryngeal movement in time with each phase of the respiratory cycle. Care is also required to avoid contact with laryngeal structures during direct laryngoscopy due to the propensity for laryngospasm in cats. Complete recovery of base-line response after spraying the larynx of normal cats required 17–100 minutes for 2% lidocaine and 61–256 minutes for 10% lidocaine in one study.[12] Assessment of laryngeal function is therefore impossible following local anesthetic administration.

A prospective, randomized clinical trial of anesthetic induction agents for assessment of laryngeal function by videoendoscopy in healthy adult cats premedicated with methadone has recently been reported.[13] Induction by slow infusion of midazolam and ketamine to effect preserved arytenoid movement better in comparison to induction with propofol or alfaxolone. However, arytenoid movement was completely obliterated in three cats in the midazolam-ketamine group and three cats in the propofol group. The obliteration of laryngeal function in these normal cats highlights the difficulty of making a definitive diagnosis of laryngeal paralysis in this species. Competent laryngeal protective reflexes were maintained in normal cats anesthetized with ketamine and administered barium suspension orally.[14] Barium was aspirated into the pharynx and cranial part of the trachea in these cats, but not into the lower respiratory tract.

Administration of doxapram hydrochloride to stimulate more vigorous laryngeal motion in anesthetized patients to assist in the diagnosis of laryngeal paralysis has been described in healthy dogs[15] and recommended by one author as a useful technique in the cat.[16] Safety and efficacy of doxapram administration in cats with laryngeal paralysis has not been documented, to the author's knowledge.

In the author's experience of direct laryngoscopy in cats with laryngeal paralysis, changes observed grossly in affected cats are similar to those observed in dogs with laryngeal paralysis, although much more subtle. Edema of the laryngeal mucosa is generally apparent, but erythema and hyperemia commonly seen in affected dogs is not a prominent feature in cats. Median displacement of the arytenoid cartilages and vocal folds with resultant narrowing of the rima glottis may be appreciated in cats, although the propensity for laryngospasm and complete obliteration of the rima glottis in this species tends to mask the abnormal position in many cats. It is particularly important to avoid depressing the epiglottis with the laryngoscope blade in cats during direct laryngoscopy, as this induces laryngospasm in most cats. Cranial retraction on the tongue together with positioning the laryngoscope blade directly ventral to the epiglottis allows good visualization of laryngeal function in most cats. Paradoxical movement of the arytenoids and vocal folds as observed in dogs has not been observed by the author in cats with laryngeal paralysis.

SURGICAL DISEASES

Laryngeal paralysis

No breed or sex predilection has been reported yet for feline laryngeal paralysis. A congenital form of laryngeal paralysis has been hypothesized with the observance of laryngeal paralysis in kittens and cats less than two years or age; however, this form of the disease appears to be exceedingly rare.[17] In contrast to dogs, where laryngeal paralysis is most often considered to be idiopathic or part of a poorly characterized general neuropathy, laryngeal paralysis in cats is often non-idiopathic in origin. Feline laryngeal paralysis has been diagnosed in association with neoplastic infiltration of the vagus nerve in lymphosarcoma, in extranodal lymphosarcoma, as an iatrogenic complication of thyroidectomy and other surgical procedures of the neck, as a symptom of lead toxicosis, and as part of a progressive generalized neuromuscular disorder.[17,18] Unilateral laryngeal paralysis has also been observed in a cat with clinical signs of peripheral vestibular disease, ataxia, and dyspnea diagnosed with adenocarcinoma of the tympanic bulla and Wallerian degeneration of the right recurrent laryngeal nerve.[6] So-called idiopathic laryngeal paralysis also occurs in cats. However, the frequency of non-idiopathic etiology of feline laryngeal paralysis warrants careful and thorough clinical and diagnostic evaluation of all cats with suspected laryngeal paralysis for underlying specific etiology.

Ninety-nine cats with a diagnosis of laryngeal paralysis were identified in a search of the Veterinary Medicine Data Base from January 1986 through April 2008.[19] Fourteen of these 99 cats met the inclusion criteria for their evaluation of unilateral arytenoid lateralization for the treatment of laryngeal paralysis in cats. Proposed etiology of laryngeal paralysis in these animals included congenital (one cat), traumatic (two cats), idiopathic (seven cats), polyneuropathy/ polymyopathy (three cats), and iatrogenic (one cat). Concurrent disease, most commonly azotemia, was reported in 11/14 cats. Ten of 14 cats were diagnosed with bilateral laryngeal paralysis, three were left unilateral, and one was right unilateral. All 14 cats were treated with unilateral arytenoid lateralization. Minor variations in technique included degree of disarticulation of the larynx; suture placement (arytenoid to thyroid versus arytenoid to cricoid cartilages); and type, size, and number of strands of suture material used. Intraoperative complications were observed in three of 14 cats (21%) including fracture of the muscular process in two and laryngeal displacement in one. Postoperative complications were reported in seven of 14 cats (50%) but were treatable and/or considered minor. All 14 cats were

discharged alive and there was no reported aspiration pneumonia. The incidence of aspiration pneumonia in dogs following unilateral arytenoid lateralization is 8–18%. The authors concluded that the prognosis for resolution of respiratory compromise in cats with laryngeal paralysis treated with unilateral arytenoid lateralization appears good.

In a retrospective study of laryngeal paralysis in 16 cats,[17] bilateral laryngeal paralysis was reported in 12 cats. In the cats with unilateral laryngeal paralysis, the left side was affected. Three of the four unilaterally affected cats were managed medically, while seven of 12 bilaterally affected cats were managed surgically. Long-term outcome was considered successful in four of seven surgically managed cats. A variety of surgical techniques were used in these cats including unilateral or bilateral arytenoid lateralization, ventriculocordectomy, and partial arytenoidectomy. A retrospective study of ten cats, with arytenoid lateralization for laryngeal paralysis was reported by Hardie et al.[20] Nine of these ten cats had bilateral laryngeal paralysis. Concurrent medical problems were diagnosed in seven of these ten cats, including hyperthyroidism, renal insufficiency, congestive heart failure, hypertension, thyroid adenocarcinoma, and mycoplasma pneumonia. Of these ten cats, seven had unilateral arytenoid lateralization, one had bilateral arytenoid lateralization, and two had staged bilateral procedures. All three cats with bilateral procedures developed aspiration pneumonia and died.

Although case numbers are small in these studies, the development of aspiration pneumonia in all three cats with bilateral arytenoid lateralization but in none of the seven cats with unilateral arytenoid lateralization in Hardie's study and in none of 14 cats with unilateral arytenoid lateralization in Thunberg and Lantz's study suggests that unilateral arytenoid lateralization should be considered the current preferred technique.

Laryngeal masses

Benign and malignant laryngeal masses have been reported in cats, although laryngeal neoplasia is considered rare in both dogs and cats. In a 10-year survey of laryngeal neoplasia, 13 dogs and 11 cats were reported.[21] In contrast to canine laryngeal neoplasia, where no single tumor type predominated, lymphosarcoma of the larynx was predominant in cats in this survey.[21] However, six of nine cats with laryngeal neoplasia in a retrospective study of tracheostomy were diagnosed with squamous cell carcinoma while only one cat was diagnosed with lymphosarcoma.[22] Adenocarcinoma has also been reported in the larynx of cats.[21-26]

Inflammatory laryngeal disease (Fig. 52-6) resulting in acute upper airway obstruction has been reported in eight cats in two separate publications.[27,28] Inflammatory laryngeal disease was also reported in six of 27 cats with laryngeal, laryngotracheal, and tracheal masses,[25] in three of 13 cats with laryngeal masses,[22] and in two of seven cats with miscellaneous conditions of the larynx.[26] This relatively high incidence of inflammatory disease of the larynx in cats with laryngeal mass lesions highlights the importance of a cytologic or histologic diagnosis both for treatment and prognosis. Neoplastic and inflammatory lesions are not distinguishable on gross examination or radiographic examination. Feline inflammatory laryngeal disease is most commonly described as granulomatous or pyogranulomatous, although neutrophilic and lymphoplasmacytic inflammation has also been reported.[22,27,28] A second biopsy has been recommended for cats with a diagnosis of lymphoid hyperplasia of laryngeal, laryngotracheal, and tracheal masses, as five of 27 cats with this diagnosis on initial biopsy were subsequently diagnosed with neoplasia on a second biopsy.[25] A combination of surgical treatment (either by excision via ventral laryngotomy or, if accessible, per os) and prolonged medical therapy with corticosteroids is recommended for

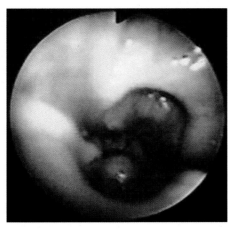

Figure 52-6 Per os endoscopic view of feline laryngeal inflammatory disease diagnosed by fine needle aspiration cytology and confirmed by histopathology at necropsy.

inflammatory laryngeal disease in cats with histologically confirmed diagnoses.[27]

PREOPERATIVE CONSIDERATIONS

Cats with respiratory compromise are predisposed to acute functional decompensation in stressful situations. Preoperative management should be aimed at minimizing stress, with anesthetic premedication and induction in a quiet environment. Preoxygenation is useful, provided the method of delivering supplemental oxygen is not stressful to the cat. Few cats tolerate a face mask for oxygen supplementation, but most will tolerate a 'flow-by' technique. A tracheostomy kit and surgeon should be readily available during the perianesthetic period.

SURGICAL TECHNIQUES

Arytenoid lateralization

Unilateral arytenoid lateralization is considered the surgical technique of choice for palliation of laryngeal paralysis in cats. The surgical technique is considered more challenging in cats than dogs due to the small size of the cat and the fragility of their laryngeal cartilages.[19,20] Generally, the technique is performed similarly in the cat and dog, with as many minor individual variations of technique as there are surgeons performing it. There is only one specific description of the surgical technique in cats[20] where it is performed in a similar manner to the dog. However, unlike some of the variations in techniques well described in the dog, the cricothyroid articulation was not disarticulated nor was the transverse arytenoid ligament transected in any of the ten cats in this retrospective study. Other surgeons also recommend leaving the cricothyroid articulation intact in cats to maintain stability of the cartilage 'chassis' and further comment that bilateral cricothyroid disruption leads to dorsoventral collapse of the rima glottides.[7] The author performs arytenoid lateralization in cats using a method identical with the technique she uses in dogs, including cricothyroid disarticulation, transection of the interarytenoid sesamoid band, and the use of two prosthetic sutures, a cricoarytenoid and thyroarytenoid suture.[28] Small gauge suture material (4/0 polypropylene) on a taper-cut cardiovascular needle is preferred by the author. Cutting needles should be avoided due to the risk of accidentally cutting through the small and delicate muscular process of the arytenoid cartilage.[19] The author prefers fine ophthalmic instruments for feline 'tie-back'. Very fine small curved mosquito forceps and cotton buds are useful for cricoarytenoid disarticulation.

The surgical technique used by the author is illustrated in a cadaver (Fig. 52-7) and described in Box 52-1.[28,29] The appearance of the larynx before (Fig. 52-8A) and after (Fig. 52-8B) left unilateral arytenoid lateralization by this technique in a cat with idiopathic laryngeal paralysis illustrates the effect of the 'tie-back' procedure on the rima glottidis area. To the author's knowledge, change in the rima glottidis area in experimental cats or cats with naturally occurring laryngeal paralysis treated by unilateral arytenoid lateralization has not been reported. A mean increase of nearly 250% was reported in dogs with naturally occurring laryngeal paralysis treated by unilateral arytenoid lateralization.[29]

Ventral laryngotomy

Ventral laryngotomy may be used for removal of laryngeal masses in cats,[24,27] and it has been reported for surgical excision of a laryngeal cyst.[10] Ventral laryngotomy is also used for treatment of laryngeal stenosis due to laryngeal webbing in the dog, but to the author's knowledge this indication has not yet been reported in the cat. Temporary tracheostomy is indicated for administration of anesthetic gases intraoperatively. Maintenance of the tracheostomy tube postoperatively is recommended.

The surgical technique of ventral laryngotomy is described in Box 52-2.[30] The author prefers 4/0 prolene on a taper-cut cardiovascular needle for simple continuous closure of the laryngotomy incision in the thyroid cartilage.

Laryngectomy

Complete laryngectomy and permanent tracheostomy has only been described in one cat for treatment of laryngeal adenocarcinoma.[23] Unfortunately, this cat survived only three days after surgery. To the author's knowledge, long-term survival following complete feline laryngectomy has not been reported.

POSTOPERATIVE CARE

Continuous monitoring, particularly in the early postoperative period, is essential following laryngeal surgery in any species and perhaps particularly in cats as they are prone to laryngospasm and may be more predisposed to laryngeal edema and laryngeal obstruction due to their small size.

Postoperative care following feline arytenoid lateralization should start with a smooth anesthetic recovery. Maintaining the endotracheal tube for control of the upper airway for as long as possible is paramount. Multimodal analgesic management, including administration of IV non-steroidal anti-inflammatory drugs when no contraindications (renal disease, hypotension) exist and microdose medetomidine (1 μg/kg IV) prior to anesthetic recovery is used by the author for feline upper respiratory surgical procedures with good results, in addition to narcotic analgesia. Continuing oxygen supplementation by face mask or flow-by technique following extubation also seems to be facilitated by the medetomidine administration. Frequent observation for signs of laryngeal edema or progressive respiratory distress is recommended. Temporary tracheostomy (see Chapter 46) may be required postoperatively in cats with progressive laryngeal edema or

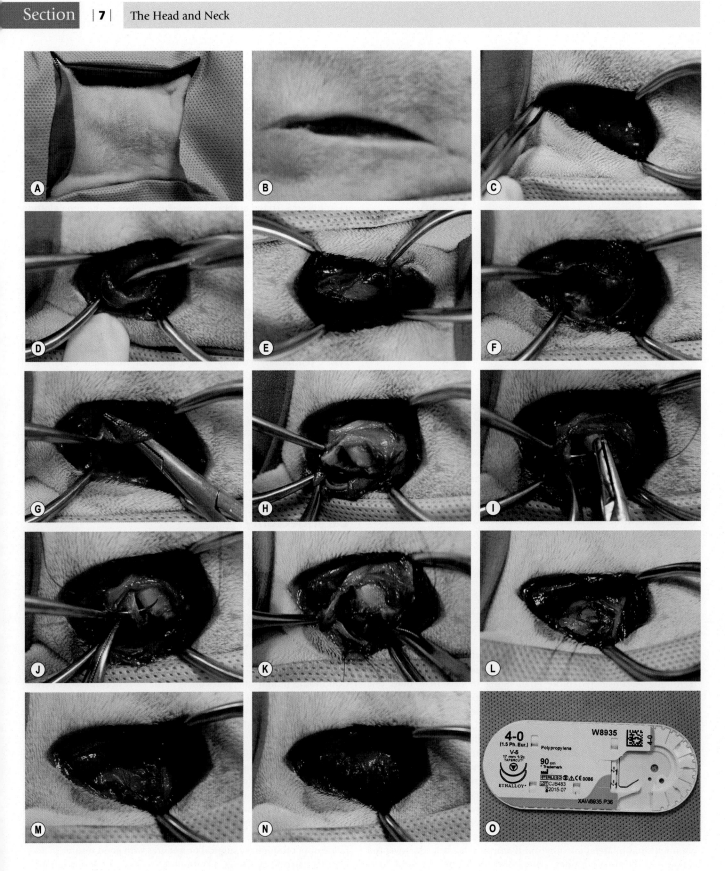

Box 52-1 **Arytenoid lateralization**

In cases of bilateral laryngeal paralysis either right or left arytenoid lateralization can be performed, based most commonly on the preference of the surgeon and their dominant hand. Right-handed surgeons generally find the left lateralization easier to perform, while left-handed surgeons tend to prefer the right. In cases of hemiparesis, the procedure should be performed on the affected side of the larynx.

The cat is positioned in lateral recumbency with a small roll under the neck at the level of the wings of the atlas. The forelimbs are pulled caudally and secured to the operating table. Care should be taken to avoid twisting the neck. A tape across the skull will help maintain straight positioning of the larynx. The surgical field is clipped and prepped before moving to the operating theatre to include the wing of the atlas dorsally, the ventral midline ventrally, the caudal edge of the mandibular body cranially, and 2–3 cm cranial to the point of the shoulder caudally. The surgical field is draped routinely for aseptic surgery and the ventral margin of the wing of the atlas is included in the field for orientation.

The wing of the atlas and the dorsal border of the thyroid cartilage of the larynx (Fig. 52-7A) are identified by palpation. A skin incision is made approximately 4 cm in length centered over the thyroid cartilage (Fig. 52-7B).

Using a combination of sharp and blunt dissection and maintaining careful hemostasis with electrocoagulation, the platysma muscle and subcutaneous tissue are dissected. In general this dissection will be ventral to the jugular vein. The jugular vein can be reflected either ventrally or dorsally as needed. The confluence of linguofacial and maxillary veins to the jugular vein is usually visible in the cranial part of the surgical field.

Dissection is continued to separate the sternocephalicus and sternohyoideus muscles, reflecting the former dorsally and the latter ventrally. Alternatively, if the separation of these muscles is indistinct, the dissection is continued deeper by separation of muscle in the direction of its fibers. In the cranial part of the surgical field, the mandibular salivary gland is sometimes visible (Fig. 52-7C).

The thyropharyngeus muscle is identified and incised at the midpoint of the dorsal edge of the thyroid cartilage (Fig. 52-7D). The incision is continued cranially and caudally using fine Metzenbaum scissors to expose the full length of the thyroid cartilage and intrinsic laryngeal muscles (Fig. 52-7E). In the dog, there is a membrane deep to the thyropharyngeus muscle that must be incised to expose the intrinsic laryngeal muscles. This structure is not apparent in the cat. Deep dissection cranial to the larynx must be avoided as perforation of the oropharyngeal mucosa may occur.

The cricothyroid joint is disarticulated by transection with Metzenbaum scissors. The thyroid cartilage is reflected laterally with baby Gelpi or Weitlaner self-retaining retractors or with a stay suture in

the thyroid cartilage (Fig. 52-7F). The muscular process of the arytenoid cartilage is identified. This is palpable as a small protuberance. The cranial laryngeal nerve is identified and avoided. The cricoarytenoideus dorsalis (CAD) muscle is identified, a fan-shaped muscle with the wide part dorsally and inserting on the muscular process. The arytenoideus lateralis (AL) muscle is identified. The CAD muscle is isolated caudally and the AL muscle cranially. A curved mosquito forceps is passed medial to these muscles (Fig. 52-7G). The muscles are transected, leaving a portion attached to the muscular process. This portion of muscle can be grasped with a mosquito forceps or fine rat-tooth forceps during cricoarytenoid disarticulation and placement of sutures. Direct handling of the cartilage of the muscular process is to be avoided.

The cricoarytenoid joint is disarticulated by gradual stretching with a fine curved mosquito forceps (Fig. 52-7H). Cotton buds are also useful in this maneuver to help break fibrous attachments. Some surgeons prefer sharp transection with fine Metzenbaum or iris scissors. The dissection is continued until the most medial edge of the articular face of the muscular process can be moved to the most lateral edge of the articular surface of the cricoid cartilage. In the 6 kg cat shown in Figure 52-7H, the articular face of the muscular process is an oval measuring 2.5 mm × 3 mm.

The interarytenoid sesamoid band can be transected blindly at this point. Many surgeons consider this step unnecessary. If undertaken, this is a common point of inadvertent penetration of the oropharynx.

The prosthetic suture(s) are pre-placed (Fig. 52-7K). The author prefers two prosthetic sutures of 3/0 or 4/0 prolene double-armed on a fine taper-cut needle (Fig. 52-7O). There are individual surgeon variations in suture placement. The author's personal preference is described.

The cricoarytenoid suture is preplaced first (Fig. 52-7L). The needle is passed from caudal to cranial and lateral to medial through the cricoid cartilage at the site of cricothyroid articulation. Taking care to avoid intralaryngeal nerve branches that may be crossing the field, the needle is passed from the articular surface of the muscular process to the lateral surface and back again (mattress suture) (Figs 52-7I,J). A mosquito is placed on the free ends of this suture and reflected caudally or dorsally during placement of the second suture.

The thyroarytenoid suture is pre-placed. The needle is passed from the lateral surface of the thyroid cartilage, then from the articular surface of the muscular process to its lateral surface and back again, and finally from the medial surface of the thyroid cartilage to exit laterally (horizontal mattress). The points of needle penetration are spaced in the muscular process as far from one another as possible, but well within the cartilage of the muscular process to avoid

---

Figure 52-7 Arytenoid lateralization surgical technique in a feline cadaver. **(A)** The cat is positioned in right lateral recumbency with a small roll under the neck. Palpable landmarks for the skin incision are the larynx and the wing on the atlas. The jugular vein is not visible in this cadaver, but is usually readily visible in the live patient by raising the vein with digital pressure at the thoracic inlet. **(B)** Skin incision. **(C)** The mandibular salivary gland is visible cranially in the surgical field. **(D)** Blunt dissection to the level of the thyropharyngeus muscle covering the lateral surface of the larynx. The mosquito forceps are medial to the dorsal edge of the thyroid cartilage and displacing it laterally to illustrate the point for division of the thyropharyngeus muscle. **(E)** Exposure of the left wing of the thyroid cartilage after longitudinal division of the thyropharyngeus muscle. **(F)** Lateral displacement of thyroid cartilage with baby Gelpi self-retaining retractor after cricothyroid disarticulation. **(G)** Isolation of arytenoideus transverses and cricoarytenoideus muscles with curved mosquito forceps passed beneath the muscles at the level of transection. **(H)** Using mosquito forceps on the remaining cricoarytenoideus dorsalis muscle attached to the muscular process for manipulation rather than handling the muscular process directly, the cricoarytenoid joint is disarticulated until the medial border of the articular face of the arytenoid cartilage can be lateralized to the lateral edge of the articular face of the cricoid cartilage. **(I)** Prolene (4/0) suture has already been passed through the cricoid cartilage caudally in this photograph. The first pass of a horizontal mattress suture through the articular face of the arytenoid cartilage is in progress. **(J)** Second pass of cricoarytenoid suture in horizontal mattress pattern through the articular surface of the arytenoid cartilage. **(K)** Pre-placed cricoarytenoid and thyroarytenoid sutures. **(L)** The cricoarytenoid suture is tied first, displacing the muscular process caudally. **(M)** The thyroarytenoid suture is tied. **(N)** Simple continuous appositional closure of the thyropharyngeus muscle. **(O)** The author's preferred suture material (prolene) and needle (V-5 17 mm 1/2 circular double-armed taper-cut) for feline arytenoid lateralization.

Box 52-1 Continued

breakage of the muscular process or cut-through by the mattress sutures.

The retractors or stay suture are removed, if still present, reflecting the thyroid cartilage laterally. The cricoarytenoid suture is tightened and tied first, observing caudal displacement of the muscular process. The thyroarytenoid suture is then tightened and tied (Fig. 52-7M). In some animals lateral displacement of the muscular process may be observed at this time, but may be obscured by the thyroid cartilage.

The wound is lavaged and the lavage fluid is removed by suction or with swabs. The endotracheal tube cuff should remain inflated prior to lavage as it can be inadvertently punctured with the needle in placement of the cricoarytenoid suture. If the oropharyngeal

mucosa has been inadvertently penetrated, the lavage fluid may be seen disappearing from the surgical field and may flow down the trachea if the endotracheal tube cuff is not inflated.

The cut edges of the thyropharyngeus muscle are reapposed with 4/0 monofilament absorbable suture material in a simple continuous pattern (Fig. 52-7N). The wound closure is continued routinely in layers.

At the completion of surgery, the cat is repositioned and the endotracheal tube removed for evaluation of the rima glottidis per os to confirm successful 'tie-back' (Fig. 52-8B) and to check for penetration of the oropharyngeal mucosa. The cat can be reintubated following inspection of the larynx if necessary.

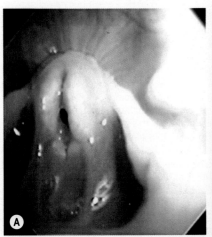 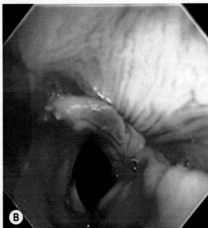

Figure 52-8 (A) Per os endoscopic view of the larynx of a cat with bilateral laryngeal paralysis. Note the erythema and edema of the laryngeal mucosa and narrow rima glottidis. **(B)** Per os endoscopic view of the same cat pictured in A following left unilateral arytenoid lateralization. Note the relative increase in size and altered shape of the rima glottidis after surgery.

Box 52-2 Ventral laryngotomy[30]

In most cases, the cat can be orotracheally intubated at induction of anesthesia, but temporary tracheostomy may be required intraoperatively to gain sufficient access and exposure to the laryngeal lumen. The surgeon and anesthetist must be prepared to change from orotracheal to tracheostomy intubation, thus a sterile cuffed endotracheal tube or tracheostomy tube and sterile anesthetic circuit tubing must be available.

The surgical site is clipped and prepared to include the caudal third of the mandibular bodies cranially, the shoulders caudally, and a sufficient margin laterally to avoid hair contamination of the field.

The cat is positioned in dorsal recumbency with a small roll under the neck at the level of the larynx. The head is secured to the surgery table by tape across the rostral mandible. The front limbs are positioned along the trunk and secured to the table. A vacuum positioning aid, trough, or sandbags can be used to maintain straight position on the operating table. Twisting of the neck or lateral deviation of the head or thorax is avoided to maintain normal orientation of the larynx and trachea. The surgical field is draped routinely for aseptic surgery.

The skin on the ventral midline is incised beginning 1 cm cranial to the palpable prominence of the thyroid cartilage and extending 1 cm caudal to the larynx. A temporary tracheostomy for intraoperative intubation can be performed at this point if required, either by extension of the primary skin incision to the level of tracheal ring 4–5 or by a separate skin incision on the ventral midline between tracheal rings 3 and 5. A separate skin incision for tracheostomy avoids the

presence of the temporary tracheostomy tube in the primary wound in cases where it must remain in situ postoperatively.

The subcutaneous tissue is dissected and the hyoid venous arch is identified, marking the cranial extent of the laryngotomy. The hyoid venous arch should not require ligation. The paired sternohyoideus muscles are separated to expose the ventral larynx. The laryngeal impar vein on the ventral surface of the larynx requires ligation or electrocoagulation if it is present.

The ventral cricothyroid ligament and the cricoid cartilage are identified. In most cases, the cricoid cartilage can be left intact, but the cricothyroid ligament needs to be divided on the midline. The ventral midline of the larynx is incised using a no. 11 or 15 scalpel blade, beginning at the caudal aspect of the thyroid cartilage. The laryngotomy incision is extended cranially with the scalpel blade or iris scissors until adequate exposure of the laryngeal lumen is obtained. Intralaryngeal dissection as appropriate for the clinical condition is continued.

The laryngeal lumen is lavaged prior to closure, ensuring presence of an inflated tracheal tube cuff prior to lavage. Lavage fluid is removed by suction.

The ventral laryngotomy is closed with 4/0 monofilament absorbable or non-absorbable suture material (personal preference of the author is 4/0 PDS-II or 4/0 prolene) on a fine needle in a simple continuous appositional pattern. The remainder of the wound is closed routinely in layers. Tracheostomy incisions are not routinely closed. If a tracheostomy tube was used, it is usually left in situ after surgery for a variable period of time as required.

respiratory distress. The cat should be maintained after surgery in an area where it can be monitored closely, with personnel and equipment for emergency tracheostomy nearby. Following arytenoid lateralization, the cat should be maintained on nil per os overnight to prevent aspiration of food or liquid in an animal not fully recovered from the effects of anesthesia. Maintenance IV fluid therapy is recommended until re-establishment of per os fluid intake. The author does not recommend change in the normal diet or feeding management of cats following arytenoid lateralization. Continued antibiotic administration should not be required postoperatively unless inadvertent penetration of the laryngeal mucosa intraoperatively occurred.

Postoperative management in an intensive care unit is recommended following ventral laryngotomy or laryngectomy in cats, with particular care required for the temporary or permanent tracheostomy present after surgery in these cases.

COMPLICATIONS AND PROGNOSIS

The most frequent complications following laryngeal surgery are airway obstruction and aspiration pneumonia. The incidence of complications in cats following laryngeal surgery appears to be higher than for the same procedures in dogs. In 14 cats with laryngeal paralysis treated by unilateral arytenoid lateralization, the postoperative complication rate was 50%.[19] Complications included pulmonary edema secondary to fluid overload, single episodes of dyspnea, mild dysphagia, coughing and gagging when eating, and loss of voice. In a review of 26 cats treated surgically by various techniques for laryngeal paralysis, 54% developed some type of postoperative complication while 15% developed aspiration pneumonia and died as a result.[20] In a retrospective study of tracheostomy in 23 cats including 13 with laryngeal masses, 40% of the cats studied had potentially life-threatening complications defined as total occlusion of the airway requiring immediate intervention or dislodgement of the tracheostomy tube.[22] In this study, cats with laryngeal masses were more likely to have occlusion of their tracheostomy tubes than cats without a laryngeal mass. All cats were considered at high risk of complications, but those with laryngeal masses were particularly predisposed. Excessive airway secretions secondary to the laryngeal mass were postulated to contribute to this high complication rate.

Other complications of arytenoid lateralization include fragmentation or avulsion of the muscular process either intraoperatively or postoperatively. Penetration of the oropharyngeal mucosa intraoperatively is usually inconsequential, although antimicrobial therapy is then warranted postoperatively. Wound complications such as edema, seroma or infection are rare.

The prognosis for cats with laryngeal lymphoma treated with multi-agent chemotherapy is favorable, with seven of eight cats in one study achieving complete remission with a median survival of 173 days.[31]

The prognosis in obstructive inflammatory laryngeal disease in cats reported to date is variable and the preferred method of treatment has not yet been determined. Long-term survival was reported in one cat managed by mass excision plus corticosteroid therapy.[27] Two of five cats in another report survived long term with medical therapy, although specific details of treatment of these surviving cats are difficult to extract from the report.[28]

REFERENCES

1. Reighard J, Jennings HS. Anatomy of the cat. 3rd ed. New York: Holt, Rinehart and Winston; 1934. p. 246–51.
2. Sebastiani AM, Fishbeck DW. Mammalian anatomy: the cat. Englewood: Morton Publishing Company; 1998. p. 108–9.
3. Hast MH. The larynx of roaring and non-roaring cats. J Anat 1989;163:117–21.
4. Hardie EM, Kolata RJ, Stone EA, et al. Laryngeal paralysis in three cats. J Am Vet Med Assoc 1981;179:879–82.
5. Weissengruber GE, Forstenpointner G, Peters G, et al. Hyoid apparatus and pharynx in the lion (*Panthera leo*), jaguar (*Panthera onca*), tiger (*Panthera tigris*), cheetah (*Acinonyx jubatus*) and domestic cat (*Felis silvestris* f. *catus*). J Anat 2002;201:195–209.
6. Busch DS, Noxon JO, Miller LD. Laryngeal paralysis and peripheral vestibular disease in a cat. J Am Anim Hosp Assoc 1992;28:82–6.
7. White RAS, Monnet E. The larynx. In: Brockman DJ, Holt DE, editors. BSAVA manual of canine and feline head, neck, and thoracic surgery. Quedgeley: British Small Animal Veterinary Association; 2005. p. 94–104.
8. Katada A, Nonaka S, Adachi M, et al. Functional electrical stimulation of laryngeal adductor muscle restores mobility of vocal fold and improves voice sounds in cats with unilateral laryngeal paralysis. Neurosci Res 2004;50:153–9.
9. Lascelles BDX, White RN. Tumours of the respiratory system and thoracic cavity. BSAVA manual of canine and feline oncology. 3rd ed. Quedgeley: British Small Animal Veterinary Association; 2011. p. 270–3.
10. Rudorf H, Lane JG, Brown PJ, Mackay A. Ultrasonographic diagnosis of a laryngeal cyst in a cat. J Small Anim Pract 1999;40:275–7.
11. Stadler K, Hartman S, Matheson J, O'Brien R. Computed tomographic imaging of dogs with primary laryngeal or tracheal airway obstruction. Vet Radiol Ultrasound 2011;52:377–84.
12. Dyson DH. Efficacy of lidocaine hydrochloride for laryngeal desensitization: a clinical comparison of techniques in the cat. J Am Vet Med Assoc 1988;192:1286–8.
13. Nelissen P, Corletto F, Aprea F, et al. Effect of three anesthetic induction protocols on laryngeal motion during laryngoscopy in normal cats. Vet Surg 2012;41:876–83.
14. Robinson EP, Johnston GR. Radiographic assessment of laryngeal reflexes in ketamine-anesthetized cats. Am J Vet Res 1986;47:1569–72.
15. Miller CJ, McKiernan BC, Pace J, Fettman MJ. The effects of doxapram hydrochloride (Dopram-V) on laryngeal function in healthy dogs. J Vet Intern Med 2002;16:524–8.
16. McKiernan BC. Possible laryngeal paralysis in a cat. Vet Med 2004;99:12–14.
17. Schachter S, Norris CR. Laryngeal paralysis in cats: 16 cases (1990–1999). J Am Vet Med Assoc 2000;216:1100–3.
18. LeCouteur RA. Feline neuromuscular disorders. Proceedings of the North American veterinary conference, Volume 20, Orlando, FL; 2006. p. 709–12.
19. Thunberg B, Lantz GC. Evaluation of unilateral arytenoid lateralization for the treatment of laryngeal paralysis in 14 cats. J Am Anim Hosp Assoc 2010;46:418–24.
20. Hardie RJ, Gunby J, Bjorling DE. Arytenoid lateralization for treatment of laryngeal paralysis in 10 cats. Vet Surg 2009;38:445–51.
21. Saik JE, Toll SL, Diters RW, et al. Canine and feline laryngeal neoplasia: a 10-year survey. J Am Anim Hosp Assoc 1986;22:359–65.
22. Guenther-Yenke CL, Rozanski EA. Tracheostomy in cats: 23 cases (1998–2006). J Feline Med Surg 2007;9:451–7.

23. Vasseur PB, Patnaik AK. Laryngeal adenocarcinoma in a cat. J Am Anim Hosp Assoc 1981;17:639–41.

24. Wheeldon EB, Amis TC. Laryngeal carcinoma in a cat. J Am Vet Med Assoc 1985;186:80–1.

25. Jakubiak MJ, Siedlecki CT, Zenger E, et al. Laryngeal, laryngotracheal, and tracheal masses in cats: 27 cases (1998–2003). J Am Anim Hosp Assoc 2005;41:310–16.

26. Harvey CE, O'Brien JA. Surgical treatment of miscellaneous laryngeal conditions in dogs and cats. J Am Anim Hosp Assoc 1982;18:557–62.

27. Tasker S, Foster DJ, Corcoran BM, et al. Obstructive inflammatory laryngeal disease in three cats. J Feline Med Surg 1999;1:53–9.

28. Costello MF, Keith D, Hendrick M, et al. Acute upper airway obstruction due to inflammatory laryngeal disease in 5 cats. J Vet Emerg Crit Care 2001;11:205–10.

29. Demetriou JD, Kirby BM. The effect of two modifications of unilateral arytenoids lateralization on rima glottides area in dogs. Vet Surg 2003;32:62–8.

30. Smith MM, Waldron DR. Atlas of Approaches for General Surgery of the Dog and Cat. Philadelphia: W B Saunders Company; 1993. p. 36–9, 44–7.

31. Taylor SS, Goodfellow MR, Browne WJ, et al. Feline extranodal lymphoma: response to chemotherapy and survival in 110 cats. J Small Anim Pract 2009;50: 584–92.

Chapter | 53 |

Thyroid and parathyroid

T. Sissener

Diseases of the thyroid and parathyroid glands are the most common indication for surgery in the neck of feline patients. Although they share a common anatomical location, the thyroid and parathyroid glands are functionally very different. The thyroid gland produces thyroxine, an important regulator of metabolic homeostasis. The parathyroid glands are responsible for calcium homeostasis.[1] Diseases of these glands can cause profound metabolic changes and surgery can be very rewarding in correctly selected patients. This chapter provides a comprehensive overview of thyroid and parathyroid surgical disease in cats with a particular focus on surgical management of feline hyperthyroidism.

SURGICAL ANATOMY

The thyroid glands are a paired set of adenomatous glands located in the neck at about the level of the fourth through eighth tracheal rings, lateral but adjacent to the trachea itself (Fig. 53-1). The right thyroid

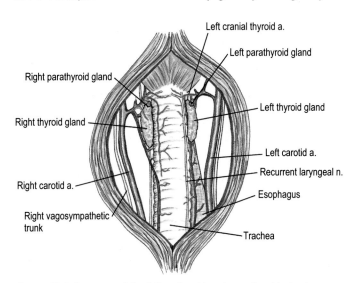

Right parathyroid gland

Right thyroid gland

Right carotid a.

Right vagosympathetic trunk

Left cranial thyroid a.

Left parathyroid gland

Left thyroid gland

Left carotid a.

Recurrent laryngeal n.

Esophagus

Trachea

Figure 53-1 Anatomy of the feline thyroid and parathyroid glands.

gland is normally located slightly cranial to the left gland. Closely associated with the thyroid glands are the much smaller and pale tan-colored parathyroid glands. Each side contains two parathyroid glands, one located at the cranial pole and outside the thyroid parenchyma (external parathyroid gland) and a second caudal parathyroid gland within the thyroid parenchyma itself (internal parathyroid gland). For this reason, the caudal internal parathyroid glands are more difficult to visualize during surgery.

The thyroid glands are encapsulated and ductless. The major blood supply to the thyroid glands is the cranial thyroid artery arising from the common carotid artery on each side. The artery enters the cranial pole and branches off to the parathyroid gland immediately or in some cases after traversing a short distance through the cranial pole of the thyroid gland. A caudal thyroid artery arising from the brachycephalic trunk is present in some but not all cats.[2] Venous drainage is through the cranial and caudal thyroid veins into the internal jugular vein.

The thyroid glands measure about 16 mm long, 4 mm wide, and 2 mm thick in the adult normal feline patient.[3] The parathyroid glands are typically about 1–2 mm in diameter with the cranial external parathyroid glands appearing well demarcated from adjacent thyroid tissue. There may be an isthmus of thyroid tissue connecting the right and left thyroid glands in some feline patients,[4] although this is more common in humans. Cats may also have ectopic thyroid tissue that can be located anywhere along the midline cervical area, thoracic inlet, or in some cases the thorax.[5] There has also been a report of cystic ectopic thyroid tissue in the tongue.[6] Studies have shown that 10–20% of hyperthyroid cats undergoing nuclear scintigraphy have ectopic hyperplastic thyroid tissue.[7,8] Failure to identify hyperplastic ectopic thyroid tissue preoperatively can be a cause of persistent hyperthyroidism after surgery. There may also be ectopic parathyroid tissue in up to 50% of cats that can be located in the peritracheal fascia, mediastinum, or pericardium.[2,7,9]

The left thyroid gland sits ventral to the esophagus and lateral to the trachea. This position partially separates the left thyroid from direct contact with the left common carotid artery. Medial and slightly dorsal to the left thyroid gland is the caudal laryngeal nerve which must be protected during dissection. On the right side, the recurrent laryngeal nerve is slightly dorsal to the right thyroid gland. The right common carotid artery and the right vagosympathetic trunk are

© 2014 Elsevier Ltd
DOI: 10.1016/B978-0-7020-4336-9.00053-6

located laterally. Care must be taken to preserve these structures during surgery. Bipolar electrocautery hemostasis is strongly recommended to ensure bleeding does not obscure the surgeon's view of these structures.

GENERAL CONSIDERATIONS

Diagnosis of thyroid and parathyroid disease is generally made with a combination of palpation, consistent clinical signs, blood tests, and ultrasound. Nuclear scintigraphy is also often utilized in hyperthyroid patients, although less frequently when radioactive iodine treatment is being planned. This is because the presence of ectopic thyroid tissue is less of a concern with this treatment modality. Since many of these patients are older and may have significant concurrent disease such as renal failure or cardiomyopathy, it is important to avoid stressful examination and blood collection. This may cause the cat to decompensate and experience a deterioration in clinical signs.

Physical examination is often rewarding. Palpation of the ventral cervical area of the neck is performed by running two fingers gently down either side of the trachea from the larynx to the manubrium while the neck is extended with the head in slight dorsal extension (Fig. 53-2). The examiner may feel a thyroid 'slip' or small mass that passes under the fingers on either side. In some cases, a thyroid slip may only be palpable unilaterally or the thyroid nodule(s) may be close to the thoracic inlet and not palpable.[2] A second palpation technique has also been described.[10] This is described as a semi-quantitative technique using a scale of 0 to 6. Cats with non-palpable lobes are scored as 0. A score of 1 is assigned to a lobe that is barely palpable and 6 to a lobe approximately 2.5 cm or greater in length. To palpate the right thyroid lobe, the cat's head is held with the clinician's left hand, the chin elevated to 45° from the horizontal and the head turned 45° to the left from the vertical. The tip of the right index finger is placed in the groove between the trachea and the right sternohyoideus muscle just below the larynx and run down the groove to the thoracic inlet. An enlarged lobe is typically felt as a 'pop'. If no

lobe is palpated on two runs, the cat's head is released and repositioned for a third try. If this is also negative, a final try using more finger contact (typically the flat part of the middle finger) is used. Comparison between this newer technique and the classic palpation technique has found good within- and between-examiner agreements for both, although due to familiarity the classic technique may be preferred.[11] Wetting the neck fur with water or clipping the area can also be helpful with either technique. Palpation of a nodule in this area is highly suggestive of a thyroid or parathyroid nodule, although there has also been a report of bilateral dermoid cysts presenting as enlarged thyroid glands in a cat.[12]

Signalment and clinical signs

Thyroid and parathyroid disease of cats tends to affect middle-aged and older patients. The reported age range is four to 22 years, but 95% of cats with hyperthyroidism are older than 10 years.[1] Juvenile hyperthyroidism has also been reported in an eight-month-old cat.[13] Clinical signs of hyperthyroidism are often slowly progressive and include weight loss, polyphagia, vomiting, polyuria, polydipsia, increased activity, restlessness, diarrhea, panting, and weakness. Cats may appear in thin body condition with an unkempt coat. Tachycardia, a gallop rhythm, or heart murmur may be appreciated on auscultation. Some cats may present with clinical signs of congestive heart failure as hyperthyroidism can induce a secondary cardiomyopathy (hypertrophic or dilative).[1] Respiratory distress, weakness, and cardiac arrhythmias may be present in these patients. Patients with larger cervical masses may have a cough, dysphagia, facial edema, and Horner syndrome.

A small subset of cats may present with apathetic hyperthyroidism where the clinical signs are depression, anorexia, and weakness. This is reported in less than 5% of cases[1] and is not typical.

Parathyroid disease in cats is much less common, but affected animals may present with clinical signs consistent with hypercalcemia. This is primarily polyuria and polydipsia, although lethargy, inappetence, vomiting, and weakness may also be observed. Cardiac changes are much less likely, although renal disease may be present in patients with chronic hypercalcemia.[1]

Biochemical and hematologic investigations

Screening tests for patients suspected of thyroid or parathyroid disease with hematology, biochemistry, and urinalysis is strongly recommended. Blood sampling from the jugular vein is not recommended, to avoid formation of a hematoma in the area.

Common abnormalities noted in cats with hyperthyroidism are mild erythrocytosis, high mean corpuscular volume, leukocytosis, lymphopenia, and eosinopenia. These changes are consistent with a stress response as a result of increased thyroid hormone levels. Blood biochemistry result may reveal elevated alanine aminotransferase (ALT), alkaline phosphatise (ALP), bilirubin, and lactate dehydrogenase (LDH). Interestingly, high serum liver enzyme levels do not seem to be associated with abnormalities in hepatic parenchyma and liver function, regardless of degree of increase. Serum liver enzyme activities were shown to return to normal after control of hyperthyroidism with ^{131}I therapy in one study.[14] Cats may also have renal dysfunction that is partially masked by the elevation of the renal glomerular filtration rate by hyperthyroidism. Azotemia, hyperphosphatemia, and hypokalemia may also be seen.[1,7]

Confirmation of hyperthyroidism is obtained by performing blood thyroid function tests (Fig. 53-3). High serum total thyroid hormone levels confirm hyperthyroidism. Measurement of resting total T_4 (TT_4) levels is preferred over T_3 levels. In cases where clinical signs are highly suggestive of hyperthyroidism but the TT_4 level is not elevated above

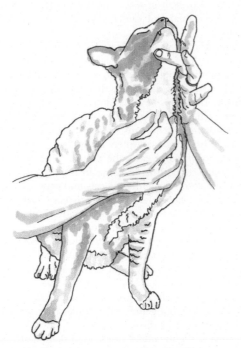

Figure 53-2 Palpation of cats to detect thyroid glands.

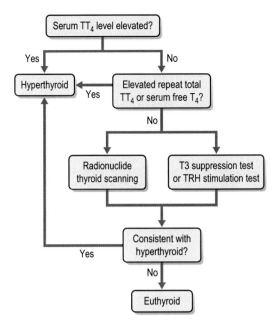

Figure 53-3 The diagnostic approach to feline hyperthyroidism.

normal, repeat total T$_4$ and free T$_4$ (fT$_4$) concentrations should be measured one to two weeks after the initial test. Serum fT$_4$ concentrations are more reliable than TT$_4$ in part because non-thyroidal illness has more of a suppressive effect on serum TT$_4$ than fT$_4$. Serum fT$_4$ is increased in many cats with occult hyperthyroidism and 'normal' TT$_4$ test results. If these tests are equivocal, radionuclide thyroid scanning is advised. The T$_3$ suppression test and thyroid releasing hormone stimulation test are also occasionally used in cats where TT$_4$ and fT$_4$ serum measurements are equivocal.[15] A recent study demonstrated a significantly higher risk of euthyroid geriatric cats becoming hyperthyroid if they had thyroid stimulating hormone (TSH) below the reference range. Cats that became hyperthyroid within 14 months also had higher ALP levels and higher prevalence of goiter than controls.[16]

An elevated ionized calcium level is the most common biochemical abnormality noted on cats with primary hyperparathyroidism. Isosthenuria may be seen on urinalysis. Azotemia may be occasionally noted. It is essential to rule out other causes of hypercalcemia, especially hypercalcemia of malignant disease. Thoracic and abdominal radiographs along with ultrasound of the abdomen and neck are essential. Parathyroid hormone or parathyroid hormone-related protein serum level tests of the radionuclide can also be utilized.[17]

Concurrent diseases

Concurrent diseases are often seen in hyperthyroid cats either as a result of increases in thyroid hormone or because the cat is older and more susceptible to other co-morbidities. Since they can have a profound impact on anesthesia and long-term prognosis, it is important to recognize these conditions before definitive treatment is undertaken.

Thyrotoxic cardiomyopathy may develop in cats with hyperthyroidism. This may either be hypertrophic or, less commonly, dilative cardiomyopathy. Tachycardia, pulse deficits, pounding heartbeat, a gallop rhythm, cardiac murmur, or muffled cardiac sounds secondary to pleural effusion may be noted on physical examination. Electrocardiographic abnormalities may also be noted, including arrhythmias, increased R-wave in lead II, and widened QRS complexes.[15] Thoracic radiographs may reveal pleural effusion, cardiomegaly, or pulmonary

edema. Echocardiogram may reveal thickening (hypertrophic) or dilation (dilative) changes to the atria, ventricles, and septum with decreased myocardial contractility. Hypertrophic thyrotoxic cardiomyopathy may be reversible once the cat is euthyroid, but dilative thyrotoxic cardiomyopathy is not.

Systemic hypertension is also common in cats with hyperthyroidism, but is commonly clinically silent. The hypertension results from the effects of increased β-adrenergic activity on heart rate, contractility, vasodilation, and activation of the renin–angiotensin–aldosterone system.[15] If hypertension does not resolve with treatment using anti-thyroid drugs, treatment with the calcium blocker amlodipine (0.13–0.3 mg/kg once daily) is recommended before surgery.

Renal insufficiency is a common condition in older cats. It may be masked by hyperthyroidism because of the increased glomerular filtration and renal perfusion that hyperthyroidism causes. Once the cat is treated for hyperthyroidism, these parameters decrease and the azotemia and clinical manifestations of renal disease may worsen or become apparent. Cats with azotemia noted before any treatment of hyperthyroidism should be placed on a trial therapy of methimazole or carbimazole to evaluate the extent of renal insufficiency before any definitive treatment is undertaken.

Gastrointestinal disorders are also common in cats with hyperthyroidism. Clinical signs including weight loss, anorexia, vomiting, and increased frequency of defecation are commonly noted. Since intestinal lymphoma and inflammatory bowel disease are also seen in older cats, care should be taken to palpate the abdomen carefully on physical examination. Any persistent gastrointestinal signs after treatment of hyperthyroidism warrant further investigation. A preoperative treatment period with carbimazole or methimazole can be useful in increasing the weight of the cat and resolving some of the gastrointestinal clinical signs before surgery.

Diagnostic imaging

Imaging can be very useful in the evaluation of patients with thyroid and parathyroid disease. The two primary modalities used are ultrasound and nuclear scintigraphy. Plain thoracic and abdominal radiographs are also helpful in the further evaluation of patients with hypercalcemia or those suspected of having malignant disease, to rule out metastatic disease or mediastinal masses.[18]

Ultrasound

Ultrasound imaging of the thyroid and parathyroid glands requires high frequency transducers in the 7.5–10 MHz range.[19] Transducers in this range allow resolution of smaller structures with better anatomical detail. In particular, this allows visualization of parathyroid adenomas that tend to be unilateral and can therefore help the surgeon plan the procedure. Ultrasound is also useful in evaluating unilateral versus bilateral thyroid disease, as well as the extent of any localized invasion that may be a result of thyroid or parathyroid adenocarcinoma.[20] Ultrasound of the thoracic inlet may also be helpful in localizing ectopic thyroid tissue. Thorough preoperative evaluation of patients will also often require echocardiography to evaluate underlying cardiac disease and ultrasonography of the urinary system to evaluate the kidneys and bladder. This can be performed with lower frequency transducers.

Nuclear scintigraphy

Hyperthyroid cats will have an increased uptake in the abnormal thyroid gland(s). Unilateral disease can be differentiated from bilateral disease and ectopic thyroid tissue can also be identified. Nuclear scintigraphy is not able to reliably distinguish between thyroid adeno-carcinoma and adenoma.[8] A comprehensive overview of nuclear scintigraphy is included in Chapter 8.

SURGICAL DISEASES OF THE THYROID GLANDS

The most common indication for surgery of the feline thyroid glands is removal of benign functional neoplastic thyroid tissue. Surgery to excise thyroid carcinoma is also performed, although carcinomas occur in only about 2–3% of patients with hyperthyroidism.[7,21] A thyroid cyst and thyroid cyst adenomas have also been reported in cats.[22] These cystic masses should be considered as differential diagnoses but are still relatively uncommon (Fig. 53-4). Surgical procedures to remove thyroid masses are usually elective and patients will often be higher risk anesthesia patients that benefit from preoperative stabilization and a thorough preoperative workup.

Hyperthyroidism

Hyperthyroidism is a condition resulting from excessive thyroid hormone levels produced by functional adenomatous or hyperplastic thyroid tissue. It is the most common endocrine disorder of cats.[21] The disease is bilateral in 70–90% of cats, resulting in enlargement of the thyroid glands on both sides.[1,7,23] Treatment options for cats with hyperthyroidism include the use of radioactive iodine, surgical thyroidectomy, and oral medication with methimazole and carbimazole. Selection of the appropriate treatment will depend on a variety of factors including age, concurrent diseases, availability of treatment options, and owner input.[24] Surgical thyroidectomy may not be the best option in all cats. Some cats may benefit from a more holistic treatment that balances the hyperthyroidism with treatment of concurrent underlying diseases such as renal failure and hyperaldosteronism.

Where available, radioactive iodine (^{131}I) is the treatment of choice for most cases of feline hyperthyroidism. Anesthesia is not required and a single dose of radioactive iodine will result in normal thyroid function in 95% of cats.[25] As the radioactive iodine is concentrated almost exclusively in hyperfunctional adenomatous hyperthyroid tissue, normal tissue and the parathyroid glands receive only a small radiation dose.[7,21,25] In addition, ectopic hyperplastic thyroid tissue is also treated regardless of the anatomic location. High-dose radioactive iodine therapy has also been used for the treatment of thyroid carcinomas.[26,27] A comprehensive overview of radioactive iodine therapy for feline hyperthyroidism is included in Chapter 8. The main limitations of radioactive iodine therapy are the availability of treatment facilities and costs.

Medical treatment of hyperthyroidism typically consists of oral medication with methimazole or carbimazole which block the synthesis of thyroid hormone.[28] Carbimazole is converted to methimazole after administration.[29] Side effects of methimazole include gastrointestinal upset, facial excoriation, neutropenia, and hepatic enzyme elevations.[30] Serious side effects such as agranulocytosis and thrombocytopenia have also been reported with methimazole but not carbimazole and therefore carbimazole is preferred when available.[1] Restoration of euthyroidism will lead to a drop in glomerular filtration rate of the kidneys. Treating azotemic hyperthyroid cats with an anti-thyroid drug until it can be determined whether correction of the hyperthyroid state will exacerbate the azotemia may be prudent.[31] Medical management is an important part of preparing a cat for definitive treatment with radioactive iodine or surgical thyroidectomy and can also be used for long-term treatment. However, one study reported a significantly lower survival time for cats treated with methimazole alone versus those treated with ^{131}I alone or methimazole followed by ^{131}I.[32] The main limitation of medical treatment is inability of the owner to orally dose the cat, although alternate options for medication delivery like transdermal patches have been developed.[33] A recent prescription diet for hyperthyroid cats has also been made available (Hill's Prescription Diet y/d, Hill's Pet Nutrition, Topeka, KS). The goal of the diet is to decrease thyroid hormone production by limiting iodine uptake without the use of additional anti-thyroid drugs. The diet also contains taurine and carnitine for cardiac health and lower phosphorous and sodium levels to support renal function.

Surgical thyroidectomy is a good treatment option in areas where accessibility to radioactive iodine treatment is limited and the owner wants to pursue treatment with curative intent. Thyroidectomy is also a good option in cats with poor tolerance to anti-thyroid drugs or in cats that are difficult to medicate. The surgical technique itself is well established and not particularly demanding, but concurrent diseases in many patients can increase anesthetic and surgical risks.

Other treatments, including percutaneous ultrasound-guided radio-frequency heat ablation, have been tried and have been shown to be effective transiently but not permanently.[34]

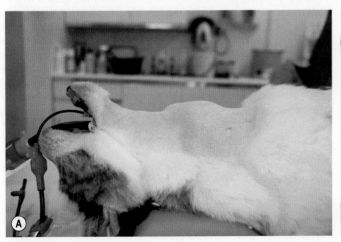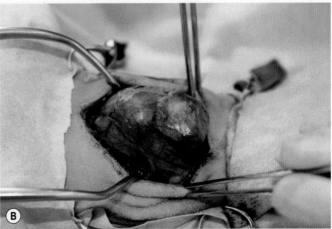

Figure 53-4 (A) An eight-year-old female neutered domestic short-hair cat with massive goiter. **(B)** Dysphagia was associated with a space occupying unilateral non-functional thyroid cyst which on histopathologic analysis was reported to be a cystic thyroid adenoma. *(Courtesy of Jon Hall.)*

Thyroid carcinomas

Similar to thyroid adenomas that are physiologically active and produce excess thyroxine, thyroid carcinomas can also be functional. In these cases, clinical signs and laboratory blood test results will often reflect similar physiologic changes. The definitive diagnosis of thyroid carcinoma requires histologic examination. Even with histology, thyroid carcinomas can be difficult to distinguish from adenoma. Ultimately, the determination is made on the basis of capsular and vascular invasion as well as evidence of metastatic spread.[1] Scintigraphy is unable to differentiate between thyroid adenomas and carcinomas, and in some cases non-functional carcinomas may not take up radioisotope.[1,8,35] The metastatic rate of feline carcinomas has been reported to be as high as 71%.[18] Primary thyroid carcinomas can also be found outside of the neck, presumably arising from ectopic thyroid tissue. An intrapericardial thyroid carcinoma has been reported in a cat with grossly normal appearing thyroid glands and normal serum thyroxine levels.[36]

The recommended treatment for feline thyroid carcinomas is surgical excision followed by radioactive iodine therapy.[37] Complete, histologically clean margin excision of the carcinoma can be curative if there is no evidence of metastatic spread. If microscopic tissue remains, recurrence is common and will often be seen within weeks of surgery.[1] High-dose radiation treatment is therefore recommended as an adjunct therapy and can result in survival times ranging from ten to 41 months.[26] Iatrogenic hypothyroidism can be a complication of the high-dose radioactive iodine treatment. This may contribute to development of azotemia in cats with underlying mild chronic kidney disease because it further reduces the glomerular filtration rate. Thyroxine supplementation in these cases may be required.[1,38]

SURGICAL DISEASES OF THE PARATHYROID GLANDS

In contrast to canine patients, primary disease or neoplasia of the feline parathyroid gland is rare.[39] The most common surgical problem with the parathyroid glands is iatrogenic hypoparathyroidism as a result of removal of the parathyroid glands during surgery to remove hyperplastic thyroid tissue. Primary hyperparathyroidism is sometimes encountered in feline patients, primarily as a cause of parathyroid adenoma. This results in clinical signs of hypercalcemia. The parathyroid glands are composed of chief cells that secrete parathyroid hormone, an important regulator of ionized calcium in the body. The effect of parathyroid hormone is to conserve calcium within the body and elevate serum calcium levels. A negative feedback loop and calcitonin produced from the parafollicular cells of the thyroid glands in response to hypercalcemia help maintain normal calcium levels.

Non-parathyroid malignant disease is the most common cause of hypercalcemia in cats.[40] It is therefore important to differentiate humoral hypercalcemia of malignancy from primary parathyroid disease. Humoral hypercalcemia is caused by parathyroid hormone-related protein (PTHrP) and not parathyroid hormone itself. Lymphosarcoma, lymphocytic leukemia, granulocytic leukemia, erythroleukemia, and squamous cell carcinoma have all been implicated in humoral hypercalcemia in cats.[39] Assays have been validated to assess both intact parathyroid hormone and parathyroid hormone-related protein in cats with humoral hypercalcemia.[17] These assays can be useful in the further investigation of cats with hyperthyroidism and differentiating parathyroid gland from non-parathyroid gland disease.

Chronic renal failure is commonly associated with increased secretion of parathyroid hormone and hyperplasia of the parathyroid glands leading to renal secondary hyperparathyroidism.[39] One study showed that hyperparathyroidism was present in 84% of cats with chronic renal failure.[41] Despite the high incidence of secondary hyperparathyroidism, hypercalcemia occurs in less than 10% of cats with chronic renal failure.[42] This type of hyperparathyroidism is not a disease of the parathyroid glands itself and therefore surgery is not indicated.

Parathyroid neoplasia

Parathyroid adenomas resulting in hypercalcemia have been reported in cats, either solitary or in conjunction with a thyroid adenoma.[22,43] It is important to distinguish between parathyroid adenoma and parathyroid gland hyperplasia that may affect all four glands. Parathyroid adenomas are typically solitary, unilateral, and often involve the external parathyroid gland.[1,44] The excess parathyroid hormone will suppress the other three parathyroid glands to the point that they can be difficult to locate during surgery. Ultrasonongraphically, one parathyroid gland will be prominent. Surgical excision of parathyroid adenomas is typically curative and the prognosis excellent as long as postoperative transient hypocalcemia is addressed. Primary or secondary parathyroid gland hyperplasia involves all four glands and surgical exploration or ultrasound will reveal symmetrical enlargement of all four parathyroid glands. Primary parathyroid gland hyperplasia involving all four glands may require resection of multiple parathyroid glands in some cases. It is important to rule out causes of secondary parathyroid gland hyperplasia before removing multiple parathyroid glands.

Parathyroid adenocarcinomas have also been reported and are similarly rare in the cat.[45] These can also be functional and secrete excess parathyroid hormone. The definitive diagnosis is made histologically and surgical excision is recommended. Due to the paucity of clinical data, the long-term prognosis is uncertain but may be fair to good if the carcinoma has remained encapsulated or can be removed with clean margins.[43]

PREOPERATIVE STABILIZATION

As most of the feline patients with hyperthyroidism are geriatric and many have other underlying conditions, preoperative stabilization to maximize the safety of anesthesia is important. Thyroidectomy is generally an elective procedure. A thorough evaluation of the patient is essential for a successful outcome. Discussion with the owner about the potential risks of anesthesia and surgery as well as the possible complications and other treatment options available should be performed.

Stabilization and medical management

Preoperative stabilization of the hyperthyroid cat with anti-thyroid drugs is preferred to minimize anesthetic and surgical complications.[1,46] The cat should preferably be made euthyroid by administration of methimazole or carbimazole for two to three weeks before surgery. A serum T_4 measurement preoperatively, confirming the cat is euthyroid, is preferable, but the blood sample should not be retrieved from the jugular vein to avoid the possibility of a hematoma in the neck that might impede surgery. Methimazole should be administered preoperatively to the cat the day of surgery.

If preoperative treatment with methimazole or carbimazole is not well tolerated, a β-adrenergic blocking agent such as propanolol or atenolol can be used. Atenolol (6.25–12.5 mg/cat once daily) may be preferred due to its once-daily dosing regime and cardioselective properties. Patients in congestive heart failure are first stabilized with diuretics and digitalis before use of beta-blockers.

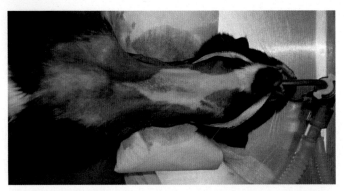

Figure 53-5 Positioning and preoperative preparation of a thyroidectomy patient. *(Courtesy of Jon Hall.)*

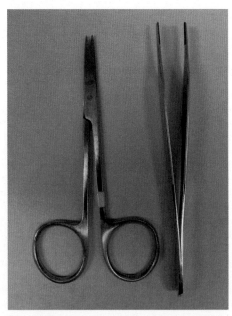

Figure 53-6 Iris scissors and Adson thumb forceps are useful instruments for performing thyroidectomy.

One study found that approximately 30% of hyperthyroid cats were hypokalemic preoperatively.[7] A preoperative electrolyte panel will reveal any hypokalemia and provide a baseline serum figure for ionized calcium. It is recommended that hypokalemic patients have intravenous supplementation with fluids containing added potassium chloride until normokalemia is achieved before surgery.

Stabilization of cats with primary hyperparathyroidism and resulting hypercalcemia usually consists of preoperative fluid diuresis. Furosemide can also be used to help lower calcium levels.[43]

Preparation for surgery

The cat should be fasted the night before surgery but should be left with access to clean water. The ventral half of the neck is clipped from the level of the ears caudal to 2 cm beyond the manubrium. This ensures that any necessary extension of the incision is not compromised by inadequate clipping. The cat is placed in dorsal recumbency with a small rolled-up towel as a bolster under the neck to slightly hyperextend the neck (Fig. 53-5).

Instrumentation should include a pair of blunt ended Gelpi retractors or an assistant with handheld retractors. Fine-tipped bipolar electrocautery forceps are essential to minimize hemorrhage and maintain visualization of the surgical field. A pair of iris or tenotomy scissors for fine dissection and non-traumatic thumb forceps are also recommended (Fig. 53-6).

Anesthesia

Acetylpromazine and an opioid such as hydromorphone, methadone, or buprenorphine are commonly used as premedication. This provides good sedation and the acetylpromazine some protection against arrhythmias. Some surgeons prefer to limit premedication and may only give buprenorphine. The induction agent commonly used is propofol, but etomidate can also be used in well sedated cats.

Anticholinergic agents such as atropine and glycopyrrolate are not used because the drug-induced tachycardia is counterproductive. Likewise, ketamine stimulates the sympathetic nervous system and is also generally avoided.[1]

Anesthesia should be maintained with isoflurane or sevoflurane after intubation. Halothane is avoided due to myocardial sensitization. Anesthetic monitoring equipment should include a blood pressure measurement capability, pulse oximetry, electrocardiogram, and an esophageal thermometer. It is important to keep hyperthyroid cats warm as they have little body fat. The rapid metabolic rate in hyperthyroid cats can increase the absorption, disruption, tissue uptake, and inactivation of anesthetic agents.[1]

SURGICAL TECHNIQUES

Thyroidectomy

There are four described methods for thyroidectomy (Box 53-1). In general, the intracapsular techniques are slightly more challenging and time consuming because they require peeling the thyroid parenchyma from the thyroid capsule. All four methods sacrifice the internal (caudal) parathyroid gland and the extracapsular technique sacrifices both parathyroid glands. If the cat is bilaterally affected, it is recommended that both thyroid glands be examined first before starting dissection, to determine on which side the external parathyroid may be easier to salvage. The external parathyroid glands are much smaller and pale tan colored in comparison to the darker thyroid glands (Fig. 53-7).

Care should be taken during dissection; manipulation and traction of the tissues around the external parathyroid may cause vasospasm, thrombosis, or damage to the vascular supply resulting in a greater likelihood of transient postoperative hypocalcemia. In cats with unilateral hypertrophic thyroid tissue, the contralateral gland may be very small or in some cases not visible. Staging bilaterally affected patients by separating the surgeries by three to four weeks has been advocated by some surgeons to avoid postoperative hypocalcemia. One study failed to demonstrate any difference in the incidence of hypocalcemia when an intracapsular technique was used, and the rate of hyperthyroid recurrence is high because of regrowth of microscopic or gross tissue that adheres and remains attached to the capsule.[1,47] Clinically significant hypocalcemia occurs in 6% or fewer cats when bilateral thyroidectomy is performed by an experienced surgeon.[1] As long as adequate support facilities are in place to effectively provide support and treatment of hypocalcemia should this complication occur, bilateral procedures are typically safe to be performed by experienced surgeons.

Parathyroid autotransplantation

Parathyroid autotransplantation is performed when parathyroid tissue has inadvertently been dissected free or lost its blood supply

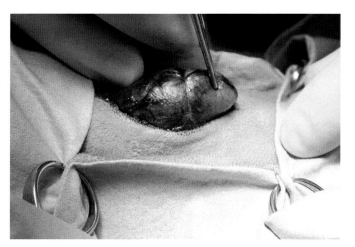

Figure 53-7 A thyroid adenoma is being removed using a modified extracapsular thyroidectomy technique in a 14-year-old cat. The forceps is pointing to the external parathyroid gland. Note the color difference between the darker thyroid gland and the paler parathyroid gland. *(Courtesy of Jon Hall.)*

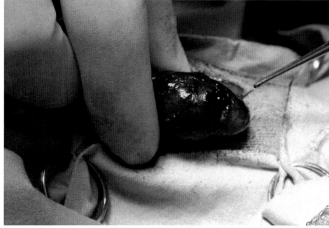

Figure 53-8 Modified extracapsular thyroidectomy is being performed in a 14-year old domestic short-haired cat. The capsule is being carefully dissected away from the parathyroid gland. *(Courtesy of Jon Hall.)*

Box 53-1 **Thyroidectomy**

The cat is positioned in dorsal recumbency with the head extended and care taken that the cat is straight and symmetrical on the table. A small rolled-up towel under the neck can serve to slightly bolster the neck upwards and contribute to better visualization. A ventral midline incision is made from the larynx to the manubrium. The sternohyoideus and sternothyroideus muscles are divided along the midline and held retracted with a self-retaining retractor during the exposure. The trachea can be visualized at this point and the paratracheal fascia lateral to the trachea can be bluntly dissected. Cotton-tipped swabs can be useful in gentle dissection of the area.

The thyroid glands are located and inspected. Adenomatous thyroid gland tissue is usually darker red or brown colored when compared to the typical tan appearance of a normal thyroid lobe. Unilateral patients may have an unaffected gland that is very atrophied, thin, and pale and hard to visualize. Following identification of the adenomatous thyroid tissue, the external parathyroid gland should be identified. It may lie at the cranial pole of the thyroid lobe, cranial to the entire lobe itself, or in rare cases over the middle or caudal part of the lobe. It is a discrete, spherical, pale tissue about 1–3 mm in diameter. Blood supply to the external parathyroid will be a branch of the cranial thyroid artery that may be visible where it enters the gland or it may arise from within the thyroid lobe.

At this point, the adenomatous thyroid tissue is removed by one of four techniques.

Modified extracapsular thyroidectomy

The modified extracapsular thyroidectomy removes all of the thyroid parenchyma and capsule while sparing the external parathyroid gland by use of fine-tipped bipolar electrocautery and accurate dissection around the periphery (Fig. 53-8 and Fig. 53-9A). The surgeon incises the capsule by use of a number 15 or 11 scalpel blade or iris scissors and continues the dissection carefully around the rim of the external parathyroid gland taking care to preserve the blood supply to the parathyroid. The cranial thyroid artery is ligated downstream to the bifurcation of the parathyroid vessel with fine 4/0 absorbable suture material. The thyroid can then be removed with ligation of the caudal thyroid artery in those cats where it is present. This is the technique preferred by the author.

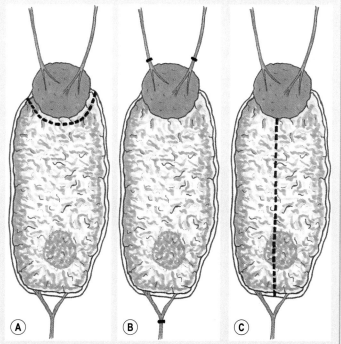

Figure 53-9 (A) Modified extracapsular thyroidectomy: careful removal of the thyroid adenoma while sparing the external parathyroid gland. **(B)** Extracapsular thyroidectomy: no effort is used to spare the external parathyroid gland. **(C)** Intracapsular thyroidectomy: the thyroid capsule and the external parathyroid gland are kept intact.

Extracapsular thyroidectomy

The extracapsular thyroidectomy technique involves removal of the whole thyroid gland with no attempt to spare the external parathyroid gland (Fig. 53-9B). The cranial and (if present) caudal thyroid artery are ligated.

Box 53-1 **Continued**

Intracapsular thyroidectomy

The intracapsular thyroidectomy technique is started by incising the thyroid capsule on the ventral surface. The thyroid parenchyma is gently teased away from the capsule by use of cotton tipped swabs and sharp dissection in some areas. The thyroid parenchyma including the internal parathyroid gland is removed but the whole thyroid capsule and external parathyroid gland are left intact (Fig. 53-9C). The cranial thyroid artery is ligated with 4/0 suture material distal to the branch that supplies the parathyroid gland. Despite meticulous dissection, this technique will often leave microscopic or gross adenomatous tissue behind and recurrence rate of hyperthyroidism is higher than with the other techniques.

Modified intracapsular thyroidectomy

After the thyroid parenchyma is removed as with the intracapsular technique above, the entire thyroid capsule is then also removed with the exception of a small cuff of tissue directly around the parathyroid gland.

Closure consists of apposing the sternohyoideus and sternothyroideus muscles along the midline with 3/0 absorbable suture such as poliglecaprone along with routine closure of the subcutaneous tissue and skin. It is recommended that the resected thyroid tissue be submitted for histopathologic analysis.

---

during surgery. A small incision producing a 'pocket' is made between muscular tissue in the adjacent area and the parathyroid gland placed within it. The incision is closed with a simple interrupted suture of non-absorbable suture material to mark the area. Studies show that serum calcium concentrations normalize after surgery much quicker in patients with autotransplantation than those where the parathyroid has been removed, but not as quickly as those that have had their parathyroid gland spared during surgery.[48]

Parathyroidectomy

Parathyroidectomy alone is performed in those few cases with primary hyperparathyroidism, typically due to a parathyroid adenoma. The adenomas typically affect the cranial external parathyroid glands. The adenoma is gently dissected out within its capsule with care to avoid damaging the cranial thyroid artery as much as possible. In those cases where the internal parathyroid gland is affected, a modified extracapsular or modified intracapsular technique (Box 53-1) can be performed.

POSTOPERATIVE CARE

Most cats are kept hospitalized 48 to 72 hours postoperatively to monitor recovery from anesthesia, provide analgesia, and provide postoperative supportive care. The ionized calcium levels should be measured at least once daily. The cat should be provided with a warm, comfortable cage to recover in. Postoperative analgesia is typically provided with buprenorphine. Non-steroidal anti-inflammatories are avoided unless there is absolute certainty that underlying renal compromise is not present.

COMPLICATIONS

Postoperative complications after thyroidectomy include hypocalcemia (hypoparathyroidism), laryngeal paralysis, Horner syndrome, recurrence of hyperthyroidism, and hypothyroidism.[1,2,7,9,23] Other less common complications can include swelling of the neck and laryngeal edema or spasm.[7]

Hypocalcemia is perhaps the most pressing complication postoperatively. If unilateral thyroidectomy is performed, hypocalcemia is unlikely. Daily monitoring of ionized calcium levels and comparison to preoperative levels is important. Clinical signs of hypocalcemia are typically noted two to five days after surgery and include muscle

Table 53-1 Treatment options for hypocalcemia following thyroidectomy or parathyroidectomy

Drug	Dose	Comments
Calcium gluconate 10%	Acutely: 0.25–1.5 mL/kg slowly IV to effect In fluids: 5–15 mg/kg/hour IV	Monitor serum ionized calcium levels regularly. Monitor heart rate during initial infusion
Calcium carbonate	Oral tablets 25–50 mg/kg/day or 15–20 mg/kg/meal	Typically 500 mg tablets that must be divided
1,25-Dihydroxyvitamin D3 (calcitriol)	20–30 ng/kg/day for three days then 5–15 ng/day	Quick onset, short half-life
Dihydrotachysterol	0.05 mg once daily for three days, then 0.025 mg once daily	Quick onset
Alfacalcidol	0.05 µg/kg orally once daily	Quick onset, short half-life

twitching, facial pruritis, spasms, panting, nervousness, and seizures. It is estimated that about 60% of cats with severe hypocalcemia demonstrate clinical signs.[1] Acute hypocalcemia is treated with intravenous 10% calcium gluconate (0.25–1.5 mL/kg) slowly intravenously over 10 to 20 minutes to effect. Intravenous calcium supplementation is then continued by placing 10 mL of 10% calcium gluconate in 250 mL lactated Ringer's solution and administered at 60 mL/kg per 24 hours.[1] Vitamin D supplementation and oral calcium can be started once the cat accepts oral medication. This can be gradually tapered over a four to ten week period by monitoring serum ionized calcium levels on an outpatient basis (Table 53-1). The goal is to maintain serum calcium levels in the low normal range to prevent clinical signs while stimulating growth and function of atrophied parathyroid tissue.

Laryngeal paralysis is typically a result of iatrogenic damage to the laryngeal nerves causing either neuropraxia or paresis of the nerves. The complication is avoided by careful and methodical dissection, with care regarding placement of retractors. In severe cases, postoperative recovery can be hampered by respiratory difficulty. One study reported the death of a cat within 72 hours of surgery that was thought to be caused by laryngeal edema from intubation or by bilateral recurrent laryngeal nerve damage.[7] Although a rarely reported complication, arytenoid lateralization may need to be performed in extreme cases (see Chapter 52).

Recurrence of hyperthyroidism is most likely the result of incomplete resection of hyperplastic thyroid tissue at the surgery site or ectopic hyperplastic thyroid tissue. Recurrence occurs within two to three years in 5–11% of cats after bilateral thyroidectomy.[1] When using the modified intracapsular or modified extracapsular techniques, recurrence of hyperthyroidism is more commonly due to ectopic tissue.[7] Nuclear scintigraphy is recommended and repeat surgery or radioactive iodine therapy considered. Some owners may elect to treat with anti-thyroid medication. Preoperative nuclear scintigraphy can be helpful in case selection; the optimal treatment for cats identified with ectopic hyperplastic thyroid tissue is radioactive iodine therapy, unless the ectopic tissue is accessible to surgical intervention.

Although transient hypothyroidism is observed in feline patients after thyroidectomy, it appears to rarely be a clinical concern. Most patients return to a euthyroid state, even those having undergone bilateral thyroidectomy. Thyroid supplementation has been suggested in some cases, particularly those that have received high doses of radioactive iodine after resection of thyroid carcinomas.[1,38]

PROGNOSIS

The prognosis after thyroidectomy to treat hyperthyroidism is generally good as long as the patient is evaluated properly preoperatively and precautions have been taken to address any postoperative complications. One study reported a mortality rate of 2% after modified intracapsular thyroidectomy.[7] Even though the majority of these patients are older and may be affected by multiple concurrent diseases that can all impact survival times, significant improvement in quality of life can be obtained by resolution of hyperthyroidism through thyroidectomy.

The prognosis after parathyroidectomy to treat parathyroid adenomas is thought to be generally good, with surgical excision typically resulting in resolution of clinical signs. Of the three reports of feline parathyroid adenocarcinomas in the literature, none were observed to have metastasized although one patient did develop chronic renal failure.[22] Prolonged hypercalcemia and secondary nephrocalcinosis or chronic interstitial nephritis were thought to be the likely causes in that case.

REFERENCES

1. Seguin B, Brownlee L. Thyroid and Parathyroid Glands. In: Tobias KM, Johnson SA, editors. Veterinary surgery small animal. St. Louis: Elsevier Saunders; 2003. p. 2043–8.
2. Anderson DM. The Thyroid and Parathyroid Glands. In: Brockman DJ, Holt DE, editors. BSAVA manual of canine and feline head, neck, and thoracic surgery. Quedgeley: British Small Animal Veterinary Association; 2005. p. 123–31.
3. Drost WT, Mattoon JS, Weisbrode SE. Use of helical computed tomography for measurement of thyroid glands in clinically normal cats. Am J Vet Res 2006;467–71.
4. Gilbert SG. The Digestive and Respiratory Systems. In: Gilbert SG, editor. Pictorial anatomy of the cat. Seattle: University of Washington Press; 1997; p. 40.
5. Lynn A, Dockins JM, Kuehn NF, et al. Caudal mediastinal thyroglossal duct cyst in a cat. J Small Anim Pract 2009;50: 147–50.
6. Reed TP, Brisson BA, Schutt LK. Cystic ectopic lingual thyroid tissue in a male cat. J Am Vet Med Assoc 2011;239:981–4.
7. Naan EC, Kirpensteijn J, Kooistra HS, Peeters ME. Results of thyroidectomy in 101 cats with hyperthyroidism. Vet Surg 2006;35:287–93.
8. Harvey AM, Hibbert A, Barrett EL, et al. Scintigraphic findings in 120 hyperthyroid cats. J Feline Med Surg 2009;11:96–106.
9. Welches CD, Scavelli TD, Matthiesen DT, Peterson ME. Occurrence of problems after three techniques of bilateral thyroidectomy in cats. Vet Surg 1989;18: 392–6.

10. Norsworthy GD, Adams VJ, McElhaney MR, Milios JA. Palpable thyroid and parathyroid nodules in asymptomatic cats. J Feline Med Surg 2002;4:145–51.
11. Paepe D, Smets P, van Hoek I, et al. Within- and between-examiner agreement for two thyroid palpation techniques in healthy and hyperthyroid cats. J Feline Med Surg 2008;10:558–65.
12. Tolbert K, Brown HM, Rakich PM, et al. Dermoid cysts presenting as enlarged thyroid glands in a cat. J Feline Med Sutg 2009;11:717–19.
13. Gordon JM, Ehrhart EJ, Sisson DD, Jones MA. Juvenile hyperthyroidism in a cat. J Am Anim Hospi Assoc 2003;39: 67–71.
14. Berent AC, Drobatz KJ, Ziemer L, et al. Liver function in cats with hyperthyroidism before and after ^{131}I therapy. J Vet Intern Medicine 2007;21: 1217–23.
15. Nelson RW, Couto CG. Disorders of the thyroid gland. In: Nelson RW, Couto CG, editors. Small animal internal medicine. St. Louis: Mosby; 2003. p. 691–728.
16. Wakeling J, Elliott J, Syme H. Evaluation of predictors for the diagnosis of hyperthyroidism in cats. J Vet Intern Medicine 2011;25:1057–65.
17. Bolliger AP, Graham PA, Richard V, et al. Detection of parathyroid hormone-related protein in cats with humoral hypercalcaemia of malignancy. Vet Clin Path 2002;31:3–8.
18. Turrel JM, Feldman EC, Nelson RW, Cain GR. Thyroid carcinoma causing hyperthyroidism in cats: 14 cases (1981–1986). J Am Anim Hosp Assoc 1988;193:359–64.

19. Wisner ER, Nyland TG. Ultrasonography of the thyroid and parathyroid glands. Vet Clin North Am Small Anim Pract 1998;28:973–91.
20. Wisner ER, Nyland TG. Ultrasonography of the thyroid and parathyroid glands. Vet Clin North Am Small Anim Pract 1998;28:973–91.
21. Mooney CT. Pathogenesis of feline hyperthyroidism. J Feline Med Surg 2002;4:167–9.
22. Phillips DE, Radlinsky MG, Fischer JR, Biller DS. Cystic thyroid and parathyroid lesions in cats. J Am Anim Hospi Assoc 2003;39:349–54.
23. Kaptein EM, Hays MT, Ferguson DC. Thyroid hormone metabolism. A comparative evaluation. Vet Clin North Am Small Anim Prac 1994;24: 431–63.
24. Flanders JA. Surgical options for the treatment of hyperthyroidism in the cat. J Feline Med Surg 1999;3:127–34.
25. Kintzer PP. Considerations in the treatment of feline hyperthyroidism. Vet Clin North Am Small Anim Pract 1994;24:577–85.
26. Hibbert A, Gruffydd-Jones T, Barrett EL, et al. Feline thyroid carcinoma: diagnosis and response to high-dose radioactice iodine treatment. J Feline Med Surg 2009;11:116–24.
27. Guptill L, Scott-Moncrieff CR, Janovitz EB, et al. Response to high-dose radioactive iodine administration in cats with thyroid carcinoma that had previously undergone surgery. J Am Vet Med Assoc 1995;207: 1055–8.
28. Mooney CT. Feline hyperthyroidism: diagnostics and therapeutics. Vet Clin

North Am Small Anim Pract 2001;31: 963–83.

29. Peterson ME, Aucoin DP. Comparison of the disposition of carbimazole and methimazole in clinically normal cats. Res Vet Sci 1993;54:351–3.

30. Trepanier LA. Pharmacologic management in feline hyperthyroidism. Vet Clin North Am Small Anim Pract 2007;37:775–88.

31. DiBartola SP, Broome MR, Stein BS, Nixon M. Effect of treatment of hyperthyroidism on renal function in cats. J Am Vet Med Assoc 1996;208:875–88.

32. Milner RJ, Channell CD, Levy JK, Schaer M. Survival times for cats with hyperthyroidism treated with ^{131}I, methimazole, or both: 167 cases (1996–2003). J Am Vet Med Assoc 2006;228:559–63.

33. Sartor LL, Trepanier LA, Kroll MM, et al. Efficacy and safety of transdermal methimazole in the treatment of cats with hyperthyroidism. J Vet Intern Med 2004;18:651–5.

34. Mallery KF, Pollard RE, Nelson RW, et al. Percutaneous ultrasound-guided radiofrequency ablation for treatment of hyperthyroidism in cats. J Am Vet Med Assoc 2003;223:1602–7.

35. Kintzer PP, Peterson ME. Nuclear medicine of the thyroid gland: Scintigraphy and radioiodine therapy. Vet Clin North Am Small Anim Prac 1994;24:587–605.

36. Knowles S, Uhl EW, Blas-Machado U, Butler AM. Intrapericardial ectopic thyroid carcinoma in a cat. J Vet Diagn Invest 2010;22:1010–13.

37. Waters CB, Scott-Moncrieff JC. Cancer of endocrine origin. In: Morrison WB, editor. Cancer in dogs and cats. Baltimore: Williams and Wilkins; 1998. p. 599.

38. Williams TL, Elliott J, Syme HM. Association of iatrogenic hypothyroidism with azotemia and reduced survival time in cats treated for hyperthyroidism. J Vet Intern Med 2010;24(5):1086–92.

39. Flanders JA. Parathyroid gland. In: Slatter D, editor. Textbook of small animal surgery. Philadelphia: Saunders; 1993. p. 1711–23.

40. Klausner JS, Bell FW, Hayden DW, et al. Hypercalcaemia in two cats with squamous cell carcinomas. J Am Vet Med Assoc 1990;196:103–5.

41. Barber PJ, Elliot J. Study of calcium homeostasis in feline hyperthyroidism. J Small Anim Pract 1996;37:575–9.

42. DiBartola SP, Rutgers HC, Zack PM, Tarr MJ. Clinicopathologic findings associated with chronic renal disease in cats: 74 cases (1973–1984). J Am Vet Med Assoc 1987;190:1196–200.

43. Kaplan E. Primary hyperparathyroidism and concurrent hyperthyroidism in a cat. Can Vet J 2002;43:117–19.

44. Bonczynski J. Primary hyperparathyroidism in dogs and cats. Clin Tech Small Anim Pract 2007;22: 70–4.

45. Cavana P, Vittone V, Capucchio MT, Farca AM. Parathyroid adenocarcinoma in a nephropathic Persian cat. J Fel Med Surg 2006;8:340–4.

46. Birchard SJ. Thyroidectomy in the cat. Clin Tech Small Anim Pract 2006;21: 29–33.

47. Flanders JA. Surgical options for treatment of hyperthyroidism in the cat. J Feline Med Surg 1999;1: 127–34.

48. Padgett SL, Tobias KM, Leathers CW, Wardrop KJ. Efficacy of parathyroid gland autotransplantation in maintaining serum calcium concentrations after bilateral thyroparathyroidectomy. J Am Anim Hosp Assoc 1998;34:219–24.

Chapter |54|

Nose

J.F. Ladlow

Diseases of the feline nose are relatively common and include neoplasia, rhinitis, foreign bodies, fungal infections, and polyps. Treatment protocols often include surgical techniques such as biopsies, rhinotomy or nasal planectomy. Complications of nasal procedures can be major but these can be minimized by careful preoperative diagnosis and planning.

SURGICAL ANATOMY

The nose consists of the nasal planum, the nasal cavities or fossae divided by the nasal septum, and the choanae that mark the start of the nasopharynx (Fig. 54-1). The nasal fossae are divided by a dorsal concha (the extension of an endoturbinate), a curved shelf of bone originating from the ethmoidal crest. The dorsal concha (previously nasoturbinate) separates the dorsal cavity into the dorsal meatus and the middle meatus. Ventrally, the ventral nasal concha (previously maxilloturbinate) extends from the conchal crest and divides into several delicate bony scrolls. The concha divides the nasal cavity into

the middle meatus and ventral meatus before forming the alar fold rostrally. Caudally, the ethmoturbinates extend from the midline ethmoidal plate to the cribriform plate; these ethmoid tubinates fill the presphenoid sinus and continue up into the frontal sinus. The ethmoturbinates can be divided into long, medially lying endoturbinates (usually seven in the cat) and smaller, more superficial ectoturbinates. The nasopharyngeal meatus is formed by the confluence of the caudal ends of the dorsal, middle, and ventral meatuses and runs to the choanae. The turbinates are covered by mucosa and act to direct the inspired air into the meatuses and humidify inspired air prior to passage to the lungs. They also act as a heat exchange mechanism and remove inhaled foreign material.

The nasal planum is pigmented and consists of tough, thickened keratinized squamous epithelium. The philtrum marks the midline and separates the two nares. The external nares are supported by the dorsolateral cartilage, ventrolateral cartilage, accessory cartilage, and cartilaginous septum. The dorsolateral cartilage is the largest of the nasal cartilages and merges with the ventral nasal concha (maxilloturbinate).

The olfactory receptors are located mainly on the ethmoturbinates and thus are in the caudodorsal section of the nasal cavity. The nasal mucosa is well vascularized and innervated. The blood supply originates from the maxillary artery that arborizes into the sphenopalatine and major palatine branches before continuing as the infraorbital artery. The sphenopalatine artery supplies the nasal conchae, and its terminal branches are known as the caudal lateral nasal arteries. Lymphatic drainage is to the retropharyngeal, parotid, and submandibular lymph nodes.

GENERAL CONSIDERATIONS

Clinical presentation

Clinical signs of nasal disease include sneezing, stertor, nasal discharge, epiphora, epistaxis, inappetence, dyspnea, and facial swelling or distortion (Fig. 54-2). The clinical signs are often non-specific and may be associated with a variety of underlying diseases such as

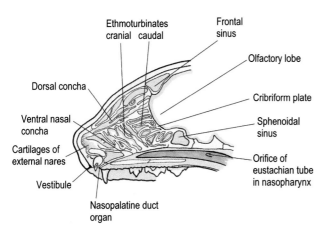

Figure 54-1 The nasal cavity of the cat, showing the position of the ethmoturbinates, nasoturbinates and maxilloturbinates.

© 2014 Elsevier Ltd
DOI: 10.1016/B978-0-7020-4336-9.00054-8

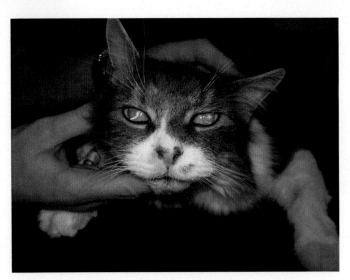

Figure 54-2 An eight-year-old female neutered domestic short-haired cat with a right-sided nasal discharge of five weeks' duration. A nasal carcinoma was diagnosed after rhinoscopy and biopsy.

infectious rhinitis, inflammatory rhinitis, tumors (such as lymphoma or adenocarcinoma), foreign bodies, hypertension, or trauma. Increased upper respiratory tract noise and dyspnea are more commonly seen with neoplasia than foreign bodies or rhinitis.[1]

Signalment may be helpful in prioritizing the differential diagnosis list; viral rhinitis is more common in older kittens while neoplasia is unusual in younger cats. A careful history is mandatory, including outdoor exposure, vaccination status, contact with other household or cattery cats, duration and progression of clinical signs, and response to previous treatments. Chronic post-viral rhinitis is seen in cats that have a history of cat flu. Cats with neoplasia tend to have a more acute history than those with rhinitis.

Clinical examination should include dental examination and careful auscultation of the larynx. Nasal airflow can be assessed by either holding cotton wool or thread in front of the nostrils or by looking for condensed water vapor on a microscope slide held in front of the nose. This should be assessed for both right and left nares. If epiphora is present, the patency of the nasolacrimal duct should be assessed with fluorescein dye. Facial deformity may be seen with neoplasia, fungal or mycobacterial disease whilst in oriental color point cats, nasal depigmentation may reflect increased temperature associated with chronic rhinitis. Depigmentation or ulceration of the nasal planum is commonly seen with nasal planum squamous cell carcinoma.

DIAGNOSTIC APPROACH

Although history and clinical signs can be helpful in prioritizing differential diagnoses, unfortunately there is considerable overlap between most of the underlying diseases. Thus a careful diagnostic approach is essential, involving blood profiles (and ideally feline leukemia virus (FeLV)/feline immunodeficiency virus (FIV) status), imaging (including rhinoscopy if available), and histology. It can be difficult to obtain a representative sample of tissue for biopsy unless a mass is directly visualized on rhinoscopy and thus a histopathology report of lymphoplasmacytic rhinitis in a cat with a rapid onset of progressive clinical signs warrants a repeat biopsy. It is also worth considering that in approximately 50% of cases of rhinitis in cats a diagnosis is not achieved after workup. In a retrospective study of 75

cats, the overall diagnostic yield was 36%. However, in 16 out of 23 cats that underwent nasal imaging, rhinoscopy and nasal biopsy, a specific etiological diagnosis was obtained, demonstrating that if nasal disease is to be investigated the investigation needs to be thorough.[2]

Diagnostic imaging

The nose can be imaged with radiography, computed tomography, or magnetic resonance imaging (MRI). For radiography, general anesthesia is essential for optimal views. A complete radiographic examination of the nose would include a lateral and dorsoventral skull and a dorsoventral intra-oral view; the latter being the most useful view. The dorsoventral intra-oral view gives good detail of the nasal chonchae and septum but requires non-screen film and thus cannot be performed with digital radiography. If digital radiography is being used, a ventro 30° rostral-dorsocaudal view can be used. In cases with suspected sinus involvement, though the lateral view is useful, a rostro-caudal sky-line or ventral 10° ventro-caudodorsal oblique sinus view is helpful, although in some cats, particularly brachycephalic breeds, this can be a very difficult view to achieve and perfect. Radiographic abnormalities include soft tissue opacity, loss of turbinate detail, lucent foci, displacement of midline structures, soft tissue opacity of the frontal sinus, and facial deformity. Unfortunately most of these changes can be seen in both rhinitis and neoplastic disease. In one study of 64 cats, rhinitis was more frequently associated with a normal radiographic appearance while neoplasia more frequently caused displacement of midline structures, unilateral soft tissue opacity, unilateral loss of turbinate detail, and evidence of bone invasion.[3] There was, however, considerable overlap between the two groups although none of the cats in the neoplastic group had normal radiographic changes. Computed tomography (CT) is better at localizing and determining the extent of nasal disease compared to radiography, but there is no difference in sensitivity of detection of the presence of nasal disease.[4]

Rhinoscopy

Rhinoscopy allows direct visualization of the nasal cavity and biopsy (at least the first sample) to be guided. Some diseases such as nasal hamartomas, fungal granulomas, and foreign bodies can be treated appropriately with this technique. Retrograde rhinoscopy is performed first using a fiberoptic bronchoscope to examine the nasopharynx and choanae so that hemorrhage does not obscure the view. Anterior rhinoscopy is then performed with a 2.7 mm or 0.9 mm diameter (for smaller cats) forward-viewing rigid endoscope (for details on equipment and technique, see Chapter 9). Isotonic fluid can be used during rhinoscopy to flush away blood contamination and aid hemostasis. In one study of 41 cats with chronic nasal disease, a mass was evident rhinoscopically in the 19 cats with neoplasia.[5]

Cytology, histology and culture

In feline nasal disease, cytologic analysis of samples from masses prepared by squash techniques can provide a relatively accurate diagnosis; agreement between cytologic and histologic diagnosis had a sensitivity of 0.94 and a specificity of 0.81 in one study of 30 cats.[6] With brush sampling, the results are far less reliable: one study of 12 cases had only a 25% agreement between cytology and histology.[7] The different results are probably due to the difficulty in locating a representative sample of tissue rather than superficial mucosa with the brush techniques as compared to the deeper sample obtained from a piece of abnormal tissue with the squash technique. Cytologic analysis will often yield a cell population suggestive of neutrophilic or suppurative rhinitis, indicating that chronic changes are not easily detected via cytology.[8] Even with biopsy and histology, incorrect diagnosis may occur as a result of the lesion being missed. Hence in an elderly cat with rapidly progressive clinical signs, repeat biopsy is indicated if a report of rhinitis is received, as neoplasia could still be present.

Sampling of nasal discharge is only of use where there is suspicion of infection with a *Cryptococcus* spp., as cryptococci can be easily recognized in the discharge as a round organism with a lucent halo on Romanowsky stains.[9]

For nasal planum squamous cell carcinomas, biopsy samples are required to confirm the diagnosis. Cytology in the form of exfoliative samples from the surface of the lesion is less invasive but often yields predominantly inflammatory cells that may mask the presence of neoplastic cells.

Culture of nasal samples is of use in neutrophilic suppurative inflammation as antibiotic therapy can be tailored accurately to the infection present. In other conditions, a positive culture result is often obtained with the usual infective agents including *Escherichia coli*, *Pseudomonas* spp., *Streptococcus* spp., *Staphylococcus* spp., *Pasteurella* spp., *Serratia* spp., *Klebsiella* spp., and *Proteus* spp.[7] Approximately half the cases will have mixed infections. These bacteria, however, are usually secondary invaders and whilst antibiotic treatment may temporarily improve the nasal discharge, it is unlikely to resolve the clinical signs in the long term.

SURGICAL DISEASES

The diseases in the nasal cavity that may benefit from or require surgical input include neoplasia (predominately for biopsies or planectomy), polyps, fungal rhinitis, nasal planum tumors, foreign bodies, and chronic sinusitis.

Nasal and paranasal sinus tumors

Nasal and paranasal sinus tumors constitute about 5% of tumors seen in the cat and are usually malignant.[10] They generally originate from epithelium (with a split of 35% adenocarcinoma, 35% squamous cell carcinoma, 20% adenomas and 10% from submucosal or minor salivary gland origin) or are malignant lymphoma (30% of all nasal tumors). B-cell lymphoma is more common than T-cell.[11] Other rarer tumors encountered in the nasal cavity include soft tissue sarcomas, chondrosarcoma, osteosarcoma, plasmacytoma, basal cell carcinoma, melanoma, and mastocytoma.[11]

Common clinical signs include nasal discharge, dyspnea, facial swelling, and epistaxis and these signs are not specific for neoplasia (Fig. 54-3). Seizures can be seen with olfactory neuroblastomas due to extension of the tumor into the brain.[11] Cats with carcinomas tend to present at an older age than cats with non-epithelial tumors (12.8 years versus 8.8 years), and males are more frequently affected than female, with a 60:40 ratio.[11] Routine staging should be performed to check for lymph node metastasis (though this is rare) or generalized disease, particularly affecting the kidney, in cats with nasal lymphoma.

Nasal planum tumors

The majority of tumors affecting the nasal planum are squamous cell carcinoma, although other rarer tumors, including basal cell carcinoma or mast cell tumor, can occur on the planum (Fig. 54-4). Fungal granulomas do occur over the maxillary bone but tend not to originate from the actual planum. Squamous cell carcinomas are associated with exposure to ultraviolet light and thus pale sparse hair cover may predispose a cat to this disease. As multiple sites can be affected, any

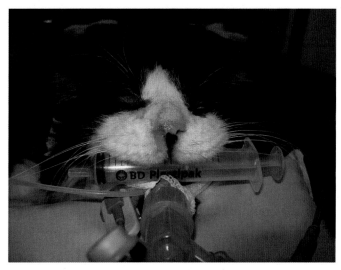

Figure 54-3 A nine-year-old male neutered domestic long-haired cat with a nasal lymphoma resulting in unilateral nasal discharge and distortion of the nose.

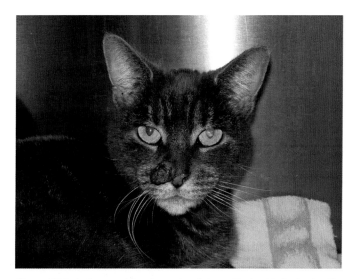

Figure 54-4 A six-year-old male neutered domestic short-haired cat with a soft tissue sarcoma originating from the right dorsal nasal planum.

cats with suspicious nasal lesions should have the other predilection sites inspected, such as the pinnae and eyelids. The typical history is one of a 'scratch' or superficial crusting lesion that fails to heal in an older cat. The tumors have often been present for weeks/months before veterinary advice is sought. In cats, the lesion usually originates from the external cornified part of the nasal planum (Fig. 54-5). Initial staging for nasal planum tumors consists of radiography of the skull and inflated thorax. For more extensive lesions, MRI or computed tomography (CT) are useful for surgical planning. Aspirates are taken of the local submandibular lymph nodes although usually the metastatic rate is low.

Superficial lesions (grade Tis and small T1a, see Table 54-1) can be treated with photodynamic therapy, strontium 90 brachytherapy, radiotherapy, hyperthermia, or cryosurgery.[12–17] More than one treatment may be required with both photodynamic therapy and strontium therapy, but the cosmetic results are relatively good[12,13,15] (Fig. 54-6). Deeper lesions over 5 mm are likely to recur with the more conservative therapies and surgical treatment in the form of nasal planum resection is advised.

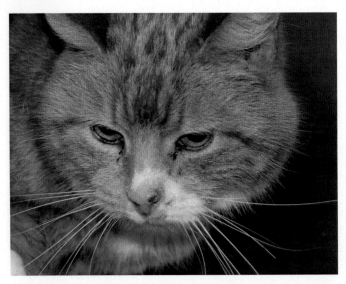

Figure 54-5 An early squamous cell carcinoma of the nasal planum in a 12-year-old male neutered domestic short-haired cat.

Table 54-1 World Health Organization staging of feline nasal squamous cell carcinoma	
Grade	**Description**
Tis	Carcinoma in situ Superficial ulcerative/crusting lesion not extending through the basement membrane
T1a	Larger lesion <1.5 cm, exophytic
T1b	Larger lesion >1.5 cm, superficial or minimally invasive
T2	Ulcerative or infiltrative lesion of 2 cm or larger
T3	Larger lesion 2–5 cm or with invasion of subcutis
T4	Invading muscle, bone or fascia

Nasal mesenchymal hamartoma/ inflammatory polyp

Nasal mesenchymal hamartomas are also known as inflammatory polyps but are distinct from nasopharyngeal polyps that originate from the bulla or Eustachian tube. Nasal mesenchymal hamartomas are firm or cystic as opposed to the firm pink masses that form nasopharyngeal polyps. Macroscopically, nasal mesenchymal hamartomas are formed of excessive mesenchymal tissue, mainly fibrous connective tissue and woven bone that is covered by ciliated columnar epithelium.[18] Hence the terminology nasal mesenchymal hamartoma is more appropriate than inflammatory polyp as the lesion is disorganized indigenous tissue.

Nasal mesenchymal hamartomas present in young cats, usually less than one year in age. Clinical signs include epistaxis, sneezing, stertorous breathing, and mild facial deformity while nasal discharge is unusual. Occasionally, polypoid tissue is seen protruding through the nares.[19] Although these lesions are benign they can be locally aggressive with radiographic features of loss of turbinates and soft tissue opacity within the nasal cavities (Fig. 54-7). Treatment consists of surgical excision, either via a rhinotomy (see below) or per-endoscopic removal. In one case series of five cats, three were treated

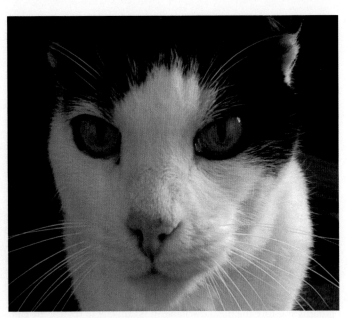

Figure 54-6 Appearance two years after photodynamic therapy (PDT) treatment of a nasal squamous cell carcinoma in an eight-year-old male neutered domestic short-haired cat.

endoscopically, of which one had recurrence but was cured by a second treatment. One cat had spontaneous resolution of clinical signs without treatment.[18]

Fungal rhinitis

Fungal infection in the nasal cavities of cats is rare, though over the last 20 years several case reports can be found in the literature.[20–26] Pre-existing nasal damage either due to a foreign body, lymphoplasmacytic rhinitis, feline rhinotracheitis virus or calicivirus, or neoplasia may compromise nasal defense mechanisms and allow fungal infections to take hold.[20,22] Clinical signs usually consist of a mucopurulent chronic nasal discharge with epistaxis, sneezing, stertor, and mandibular lymphadenopathy. In cats with cryptococcocis nasal deformity may be seen.

The fungal species most commonly identified are *Cryptococcus* spp. and *Aspergillus* spp., though *Penicillium* infection also occurs.[27] Disseminated aspergillosis is comparatively common and usually occurs in immunosuppressed cats[28] though FeLV/FIV infection has not been documented for the nasal cases.

Cryptococcus affects males and females equally, with an overrepresentation of younger cats (two to three years) and Siamese, Himalayan and Ragdoll breeds.[29] The nasal cavity is the most commonly affected site, with other predilection areas including the skin, especially over the nasal planum where ulcerated lesions may be seen, lungs, and lymph nodes. Cryptococcocis can be diagnosed using an immunoassay for the crytococcal polysaccharide capsular antigen (CALAS), cytologic examination, histopathology, or culture. Treatment of local disease is usually successful using azole anti-fungal drugs.[27]

In cases of aspergillosis, brachycephalic Persians and Himalayans are the most common breeds reported. This is the opposite of the canine cases that tend to be dolichocephalic breeds. There is no typical age group that is affected. Orbital involvement occurs in about one-third of cases with signs including exophthalmos, epiphora, anterior uveitis, resistance to retropulsion, and prolapse of the nictitating membrane.[24] Diagnosis is by imaging, rhinoscopy, and biopsy samples that are submitted for culture and histopathology (Fig. 54-8). Failure

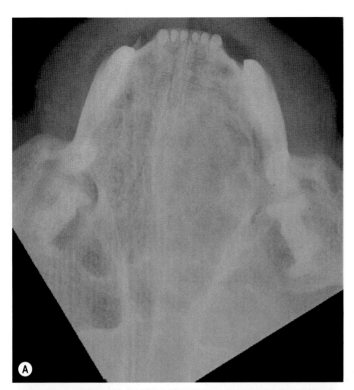

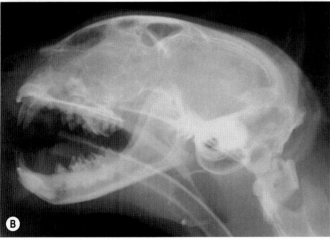

Figure 54-7 **(A)** An intra-oral dorsoventral view of the nasal cavity in a three-year-old male neutered cat demonstrating an expansile soft tissue opacity in the right nasal cavity with deviation of the vomer to the left. **(B)** A lateral skull radiograph shows increased opacity of the nasal cavity. The diagnosis in this case was nasal hamartoma (polyp).

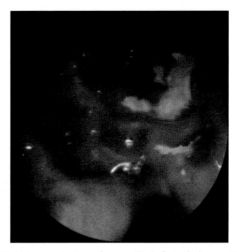

Figure 54-8 Rhinoscopic view of aspergillosis fungal plaque. *(Courtesy of Prue Neath.)*

Fungal infections of the subcutis of the nose

The skin overlying the nasal bones is a predilection site for fungal granulomas along with, to a lesser extent, other extremity sites such as digits and pinnae. These occur in cats of all ages though the incidence is more common in the middle-aged and elderly male cat.[31,32] There is usually a history of a chronic non-painful subcutaneous swelling, plaque, or non-healing wound that is non-responsive to antibiotic treatment (Fig. 54-8). The usual infective agents are *Alternaria* spp. though others are reported including *Mucor* spp., *Exophila* spp., *Ulocladium* spp.[31,33–35] Diagnosis involves cytologic analysis or biopsy of the swellings with histologic evidence of fungal hyphae along with fungal culture. In the case of alternariosis, the hyphae are hyaline and non-pigmented.

Treatment of alternariosis is most successful with surgical debridement (Fig. 54-9) followed by anti-fungal medication, but it can also be treated with protracted medication.[32] Recurrence is common. Successful treatment of the *Mucor* spp. case report involved five months of the second generation triazole, posaconazole.[33]

Foreign bodies

Nasal foreign bodies that have been reported in the cat include grass seeds, grass blades, air gun pellets, needles, stones, and canine teeth.[1,36,37] Clinical signs common to cats with nasal foreign bodies include nasal discharge and sneezing though facial distortion, cough, lethargy, and lymphadenopathy are also reported.[1] Foreign bodies may be retrieved by nasal flushing or rhinoscopy (Fig. 54-10). Occasionally, open rhinotomy approaches are required, particularly for larger foreign bodies such as teeth or air gun pellets.[36] If left in situ, foreign bodies will cause inflammation and a chronic rhinitis that may be difficult to resolve even after the foreign material has been removed.

Rhinitis

Chronic rhinitis is both a diagnostic and therapeutic challenge that is aided by classification of the inflammation by means of a biopsy. Clinical signs consist of a mucopurulent nasal discharge, often bilateral. Rhinitis can cause abnormal turbinate architecture or even destruction visible on endoscopy or advanced imaging.

In a retrospective study on rhinitis in cats, 20 cats had chronic non-specific rhinitis of over four weeks' duration. Of these 20 cats, acute

to culture fungal infections other than *Cryptococcus* spp. is common and histology reports of fungal hyphae, rhinoscopic findings of white-gray discharge/plaques or white-yellow fungal granulomas and turbinate destruction on imaging is diagnostic. Positive aspergillosis serology on ELISA is supportive of the diagnosis though false negative results occur.[20] Treatment protocols for aspergillosis include intranasal infusion of clotrimazole[21] or systemic anti-fungal agents such as itraconazole, fluconazole, and ketaconazole. There are too few cases in the literature to give an accurate prognosis on feline nasal aspergillosis though the cases treated with intranasal clotrimazole seemed to have resolution of the infection in about 50% of cases. Orbital involvement appears to be a negative prognostic indicator.[22,30]

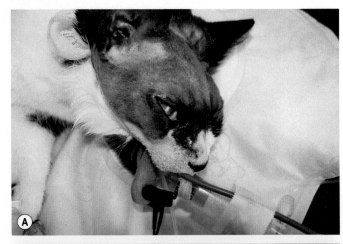

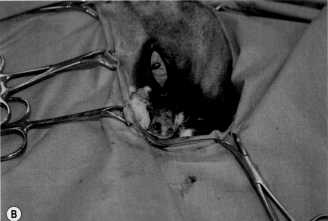

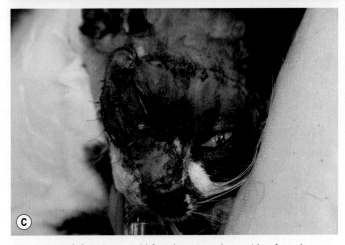

Figure 54-9 (A) A six-year-old female neutered cat with a fungal granuloma overlying the right nasal bone. **(B)** On surgical resection of the skin lesion, the underlying nasal bone was found to be eroded. **(C)** The skin defect was closed using a superficial temporal axial skin flap.

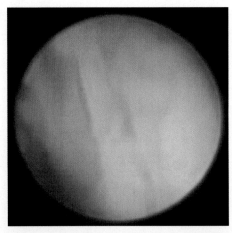

Figure 54-10 A rhinoscopic view of a grass blade nasal foreign body in a four-year-old female neutered domestic short-haired cat that presented with an abscess over the frontal sinus.

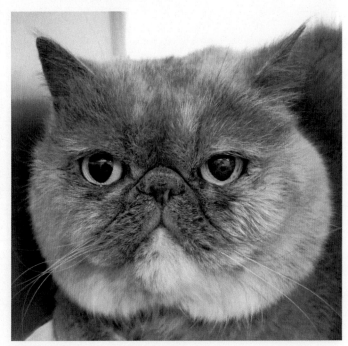

Figure 54-11 A five-year-old female neutered Persian with stenotic nares. This cat had no associated clinical signs.

neutrophilic inflammation was found in four cases, mixed lymphoplasmacytic and neutrophilic inflammation in 14 cases, and two cases had chronic lymphoplasmacytic inflammation.[7] Culture of the nasal discharge will usually yield bacterial growth, with the usual contaminants including *Escherichia coli*, *Pseudomonas* spp., *Streptococcus* spp., *Staphylococcus* spp., *Pasteurella* spp., *Serratia* spp., *Klebsiella* spp., and *Proteus* spp.[7] These bacteria are likely to be secondary infections as the likely etiology of many cases of feline rhinitis is viral, particularly

feline herpes virus (FHV-1) and feline coronavirus (FCV). *Chlamydophilia felis* and *Bordetella bronchiseptica* are also capable of causing a primary rhinitis.

In cases of feline rhinitis that have frontal sinus involvement and are refractory to medical treatment, it is possible that infection of the frontal sinus is producing a nidus of infection that is difficult to resolve. Surgical obliteration of the frontal sinus has been described to try and resolve any frontal sinus contribution to the rhinitis.[38,39] Results have only been reported in a limited number of cats and this procedure is not commonly performed, but out of six cats in one series, four cats had resolution of signs following surgery and two cats showed improvement.[39]

Stenotic nares

Some breeds of brachycephalic cat, particularly the Persian (Fig. 54-11) and Himalayan, have increased nasal resistance due to a combination of stenotic nares and incongruency between the size of the shortened nasal cavity and the nasal conchae. Clinical signs consist of upper respiratory tract noise, particularly stertor and occasional labored breathing.[40] The stenotic nares can be opened by a number of different techniques that reduce the size of the dorsolateral nasal cartilage. These include horizontal, lateral or vertical alaplasty, or punch resection alaplasty.[41]

GENERAL SURGICAL CONSIDERATIONS

Prior to performing any nasal procedures, the owners should be adequately prepared for postoperative complications and cosmetic alterations. Most nasal procedures, even biopsies, tend to result in a few days of hemorrhagic nasal discharge that can be profuse during sneezing episodes. Clipping of the face even before resection of tumors or surgical incisions can be disturbing to some owners. Preoperative photos of the likely immediate postoperative appearance can prepare owners and avoid the unfortunate scenario of tears on collection of their cat.

The nasal mucosa is friable with a tendency to marked hemorrhage when traumatized. Hematology profiles including coagulation profiles should thus be performed prior to planned procedures. In some surgeries such as rhinotomy and the combined nasal planectomy and premaxillectomy, there is the potential for rapid blood loss and blood products should be available even though transfusion is rarely required. Blood-typing is thus advisable (see Chapter 5). In middle-aged to elderly cats, biochemistry blood profiles are used primarily to screen for concurrent disease.

After induction maxillary nerve blocks, the introduction of local anesthetic such as bupivacaine or ropivacaine into the area of the infraorbital canal provides very useful intraoperative and initial postoperative analgesia (see Chapter 2). Local anesthetic spray can also be used in the nares prior to insertion of an endoscope or biopsy forceps as this is a very sensitive area and sneezing or movement during rhinoscopy can result in hemorrhage and an obscured view.

The pharynx should be packed with a mouth pack. This can be a swab or length of bandage to prevent aspiration of blood into the trachea and lungs. After completion of the surgery, the pharynx should be carefully inspected and suctioned if necessary after removal of the mouth pack. Recovery of the cat with the head down allows blood to run out of the nares and mouth rather than into the pharynx.

Useful surgical equipment includes an air powered burr that greatly aids rhinotomies, both ventral and dorsal. A Freer elevator is a good tool for elevation of periosteum and for checking the depth of osteotomies. Ice cold saline is used to flush the surgical site or pack exposed nasal cavity and aids hemostasis. An accurate set of weighing scales is required. Due to the potential for marked blood loss, swabs should be weighed during the procedure and, after the deduction of any fluids that were used, the increased weight in grams will give the blood loss in milliliters.

With rhinotomies and more aggressive nasal planectomies, the neck may be clipped for temporary carotid ligation whether this is planned as part of the procedure or as an emergency intervention after hemorrhage. After a ventral cervical midline incision, the carotid sheath is identified and the carotid artery is carefully isolated and occluded either with a bulldog clamp or a Rummel tourniquet. The advantage of using suture and Rummel tourniquet is that at the end of the procedure the tourniquet can be removed from the incision without needing to open the wound again. The carotid artery can be occluded for 40 minutes with no detrimental effects. In the cat, carotid ligation should be unilateral as the collateral vertebral blood supply is not as developed as in the dog and thus temporary bilateral carotid ligation

can lead to permanent blindness and neurologic deficits. Likewise, permanent carotid artery ligation is safe in the dog but this is not the case in the cat.[42]

Nasal surgery can lead to inappeteance postoperatively due to the lack of the sense of smell, obstruction of nasal airflow, and pain. In cats undergoing major procedures (rhinotomies, anti-fungal flushes, and nasal planectomy), it is worth placing an esophagostomy tube (see Chapters 6 and 12) at the end of surgery, particularly in sensitive or fussy cats. If cats do resume eating quickly then the feeding tube can be removed easily but for the reluctant cat it is a stress free way to supplement oral intake.

SURGICAL TECHNIQUES

Biopsies

It is prudent to warn owners that more than one biopsy may be required to obtain a diagnosis in nasal disease as it easy to miss lesions, particularly if blind biopsies are being taken.

Biopsy techniques include blind biopsies, rhinoscopically guided biopsies, nasal flushes, and trephination though the maxillary bone. As hemorrhage is likely in all these techniques, the pharynx should be packed as previously described (see above).

For blind biopsies, radiographs or advanced imaging should ideally be used to locate the approximate area of disease. A pair of crocodile or cup forceps is measured from the nares to the medial canthus of the eye and a piece of tape placed at this level to avoid damage to the cribriform plate. Multiple biopsies should be taken to try and maximize the chance of a diagnostic result. Blind biopsies can also be taken by using a stylet or 16 gauge catheter with an end that is cut obliquely and attached to a 10 mL syringe to apply negative pressure to the sample. Again, the stylet should be marked at the level of the medial canthus to prevent over-penetration.

With rhinoscopically guided biopsies, a sheath with a working channel will allow the passage of biopsy forceps alongside the scope so the tips of the forceps are visible. The area of suspicion should be biopsied first. The site of hemorrhage after the first biopsy can be flushed with cold isotonic fluids, thus allowing more guided biopsies to be taken. A pair of crocodile or cup forceps can also be passed parallel to the scope rather than through the biopsy channel in the scope, which allows bigger forceps to be used.

Nasal flushes rely on high-pressure saline being flushed through the nares with a 20 mL syringe whilst the other nostril is digitally occluded. The technique is repeated in each nostril two to three times to try and maximize tissue yield. This technique can yield large lumps of tissue if masses are present that will be located on a swab which is packing the pharynx. After the procedure, the pharynx should be checked and suctioned if necessary to remove debris. There is a risk of cerebral damage if the cribriform plate is damaged, though in one case series of 41 cases, of which 12 were cats, there was a 90% success rate of obtaining diagnostic material with no major adverse effects.[43]

If repeated nasal biopsies have failed to yield a diagnostic result, any mass lesion seen on imaging can be biopsied via trephination through the maxillary bone. In this case, a small area is clipped and prepped aseptically. After making a small skin incision, the bone is perforated with a Michel's trephine or K-wire of large enough diameter to allow crocodile forceps to be passed into the nasal cavity. This technique is rarely necessary but can be useful for tumors originating from the maxillary sinus.

In nasal planum squamous cell carcinomas, a superficial slice of the nasal planum taken using a scalpel blade often yields a diagnostic result. Alternative biopsy techniques include punch biopsies or incisional biopsies. Any postoperative hemorrhage is usually easily controlled with gentle pressure from surgical swabs.

Rhinotomy

The nasal cavity can be accessed from a dorsal or ventral approach. The ventral approach (Box 54-1) gives adequate exposure for exploration of the nasal cavity[44] and also gives a better cosmetic result with less chance of subcutaneous emphysema postoperatively.[45] The disadvantage of the ventral approach is that it involves working in the oral cavity, which can limit manipulation of instruments and require a pharyngostomy tube to be placed rather than an endotracheal tube. The dorsal approach (Box 54-2) gives good access to the nasal cavity but is more disfiguring, with a risk of postoperative subcutaneous emphysema.

Nasal planectomy

Nasal planectomy (Box 54-3) is the treatment of choice for squamous cell carcinomas of greater than 5 mm in depth that are likely to recur with the more conservative therapies. This surgery, though disfiguring, results in a good functional outcome and usually contented owners, with cats that are unconcerned (possibly unaware) of their appearance.

As the cosmetic appearance can be shocking, it is prudent to show the owners photos of cats that have undergone the procedure to prepare them fully for the postoperative appearance. Most owners, though initially distressed by the cosmetic appearance, will adjust to it easily. Occasionally owners find the postoperative appearance better than the preoperative tumor, particularly in the case of ulcerative tumors.

The excised tissue should always be submitted for histopathology examination. The pathologists are aided in their assessment of surgical margins if the cut edge of the tissue is marked with Indian ink. Alternatively, a few tiny samples from the wound bed can be submitted after excision of the tumor.

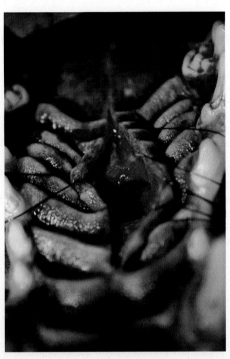

Figure 54-12 The use of stay sutures to increase exposure in a ventral rhinotomy.

Box 54-1 **Ventral rhinotomy**

The cat is placed in dorsal recumbency with the head secured in a level position with tape around the maxillary canines.

If the oral cavity is compromised by the presence of an endotracheal tube, a guarded pharyngostomy tube should be placed by making a small skin incision caudal to the hyoid apparatus onto the point of some large forceps such as Rochester carmalt that are then used to bring the tube into the pharynx. It is then retroflexed into the trachea. The pharynx is then packed with a swab.

The palate is then incised over the midline from the level of the canine teeth to the fourth premolars; any bleeding is stopped by swab pressure and sparing use of electrocoagulation. The mucoperiosteum is elevated to expose the palatine bone, taking care to avoid the major palatine artery which runs alongside the dental arcade from the carnassial tooth (see Fig. 56-1), and stay sutures are placed either side, at both the cranial and caudal ends of the incision, to maintain exposure (Fig. 54-12). If a large exposure is required, a hinged mucoperiosteal flap of palate is raised and retracted.

A burr is then used to gently burr through the palatine bone and access the nasal cavity/Unilateral or bilateral access can be obtained, depending on the extent of the nasal lesion. If a burr is not available, two holes can be made with K-wires and then connected with rongeurs which can be used to enlarge the cavity. Ice cold saline is used to decrease hemorrhage and flush the nasal cavity to allow the lesion to be visualized.

After removal of the mass or foreign body, the palatine mucoperiosteum is closed with a relatively long-lasting suture material such as polydiaxonone or glycomer 631 in a single layer using a simple interrupted suture.

Box 54-2 **Dorsal rhinotomy**

The cat is placed in sternal recumbency, with the nose positioned level on a sandbag. The pharynx is packed with a swab or bandage.

A midline incision is made from the medial canthus of the eye rostrally over the nasal bone. The skin and periosteum are elevated and retracted by stay sutures or Gelpi retractors placed in the tissues either side of the incision (Fig. 54-13A).

Hemorrhage is stopped by judicious use of bipolar electro-coagulation or swab pressure. A burr is used to gently burr through the nasal bone and access the nasal cavity (Fig. 54-13B). If a burr is not available, two holes can be made with K-wires and then connected with rongeurs, which can then be used to extend the cavity as necessary for exposure. Alternatively, an airsaw can be used to cut a rectangular flap of bone although this technique is difficult in cats due to the confined incisional area.

After removal of the abnormal tissue or foreign body the nasal cavity is flushed with ice cold saline and the periosteum closed with relatively long-lasting suture material such as polydioxanone or glycomer 631 and the mucosa and the skin is closed as a separate layer.

A small piece of sterile tube is sutured into the wound dorsally connecting the nasal cavity with the air to act as a drain for any subcutaneous air that accumulates. Alternatively, a small gap is left at the dorsal aspect of the incision though this can easily become occluded.

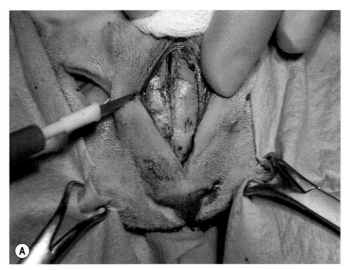

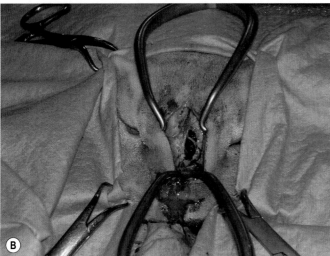

Figure 54-13 (A) A dorsal rhinotomy in a three-year-old male neutered cat. This is the same case as shown in Figure 54-7, and the expansile nature of the hamartoma can be seen affecting the nasal and frontal bones on the right. **(B)** Removal of the nasal bone with a burr revealed the hamartoma.

Anti-fungal flushing

A 1% solution of clotrimazole in propylene glycol has been described for intranasal flushing and is adapted from the canine technique.[12,13] The cat is placed in dorsal recumbency with the pharynx packed with swabs. A 14 French (Fr) Foley catheter is introduced into the right nares and advanced through the ventral meatus into the nasopharynx where inflation of the balloon prevents leakage of clotrimazole into the pharynx. Size 8 Fr Foley catheters with the tips cut off are then placed into each nare and inflated to prevent rostral leakage. Eight to 10 mL of clotrimazole solution is slowly and gently infused into each 8 Fr catheter until back-leakage occurs. The solution is left in situ for an hour, turning the cat into each lateral after 15 minutes and topping up with solution as the cat is turned.

If frontal sinus involvement is present, the frontal sinuses can be trephined (see below for detail) and debrided and 1% clotrimazole infused through the frontal sinuses into the nasal cavity after ensuring patency of drainage with saline. The ostium between the frontal and sphenoid cavities and the nasal cavity in cats is large, thus drainage should be rapid. Clotrimazole cream can be inserted into the frontal

Box 54-3 **Nasal planectomy**

The surgical clip is 1–2 cm from the planned surgical margins; whiskers are left in situ if possible. The skin is routinely aseptically prepared and the oral cavity prepped with a dilute povidone-iodine solution (Fig. 54-14A).

The cat is placed in ventral recumbency with the mouth slightly opened using a mouth gag. The drapes are placed in the mouth, covering the endotracheal tube and over the maxilla, but the commissures of the lips are exposed in case they are required during reconstruction.

The surgical margins are planned to extend to 1cm from the visible edge of the tumor if possible. If a 1 cm margin is not possible due to the size of lesion, a 0.5 cm margin will often result in clean surgical margins. After deciding on the surgical margins, the excision line is drawn on the skin with a sterile marker prior to the incision.

For small lesions, where removal of the nasal planum provides an adequate margin, the nasal planum and some of the underlying turbinates are sliced off using a scalpel with a number 10 or 15 blade starting dorsally with a 360° incision and angling ventrally to leave the lips in place. A small strip of skin is left in place at the rostral lip margins to aid reconstruction (Fig. 54-14B).

For larger tumors, or those situated more ventrally, the nasal planectomy should be combined with a premaxillectomy. After incising dorsally through the skin onto the maxillary bone, a full thickness labial incision is made perpendicular to the lip margin. The lips are very vascular and hemostasis is provided by the cautious use of electrosurgery, artery forceps, and ligation. Ice cold saline-soaked swabs are used to wrap the incised lip margins.

The incision is continued through the subcutis and nasolabial muscles to the maxillary bone. The rostral maxilla, nasal planum, turbinates, and palate are then removed with an oscillating saw. Swift removal followed by pressure applied with surgical swabs or ligation of the palatine arteries is the best way to control the hemorrhage.

Reconstruction

In cases where only the nasal planum has been resected, the skin can be sutured to the maxilla using simple interrupted rolling sutures or a purse-string suture. Simple interrupted rolling sutures are placed by anchoring the skin through holes made in the maxilla using K-wires and are more difficult to place than a purse string but give a good cosmetic appearance. The purse-string suture is faster and easier to perform but may result in more marked stenosis postsurgery. An absorbable suture of 2M or 1.5M monofilament suture such as polydioxanone is a good choice.

When the nasal planectomy has been combined with a premaxillectomy, unilateral or bilateral labial flaps are used to close the oral defect. The labio–gingival borders are incised as necessary to permit tension-free advancement, aiming for a palatobuccal recess of about 1 cm. Suturing the labial submucosa to the palatine bone using bone holes made with K-wires helps to prevent the formation of a rostral oronasal fistula, which can occur if the lip-palatine sutures break down (Fig. 54-15).

A three-layer closure of palatine periosteum/ bone tunnels to labial submucosa followed by oral mucosa medially and skin laterally is used.

sinuses at the end of the procedure for a longer lasting anti-fungal effect.[46]

The cat should be recovered with the head down to allow the anti-fungal solution to drain rostrally.

Sinus ablation

Frontal sinus ablation (Box 54-4) is advocated for treatment of chronic rhinitis with frontal sinus involvement. Obliteration of the frontal

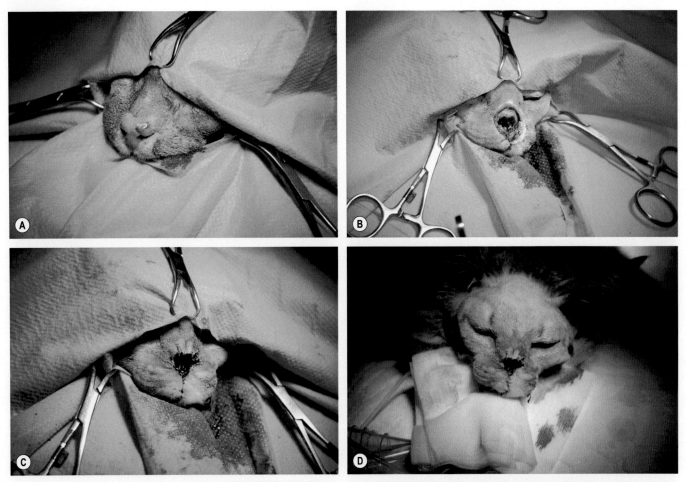

Figure 54-14 Nasal planectomy in a 12-year-old male neutered domestic short-haired cat. **(A)** The preoperative appearance. **(B)** Removal of the nasal planum using a 10 scalpel blade. **(C)** Reconstruction was performed using individual rolling sutures. **(D)** Immediate postoperative appearance.

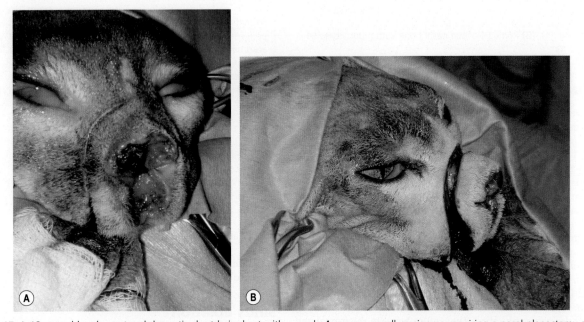

Figure 54-15 A 13-year-old male neutered domestic short-haired cat with a grade 4 squamous cell carcinoma requiring a nasal planectomy and maxillectomy. **(A)** The initial surgical incision is made after marking the margins on the skin with a sterile pen. **(B)** Appearance after incising through all the soft tissues. Hemorrhage is reduced by the use of ice cold saline.

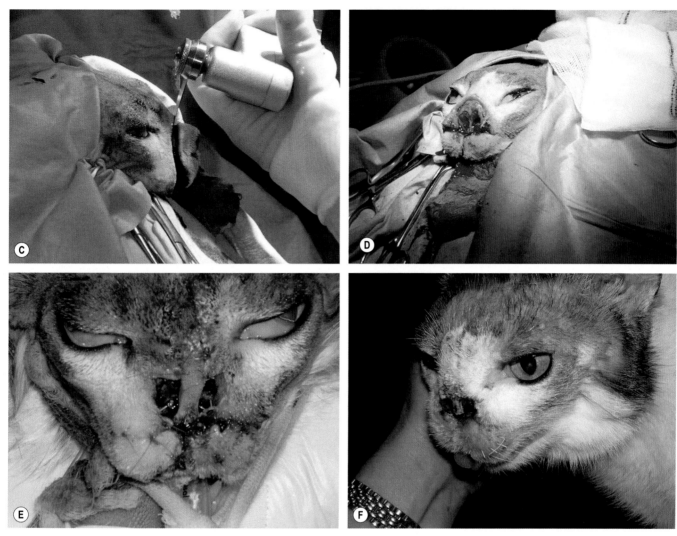

Figure 54-15, Continued (C) An oscillating saw is used to section through the nasal bone after the soft tissues have been incised. **(D)** Reconstruction is performed initially by incising along the gingival margin of the upper lips to advance the lip and recreate the philtrum. **(E)** Immediate postoperative appearance of the nasal planectomy and premaxillectomy. **(F)** The six week postoperative appearance. Clean surgical margins were obtained and no recurrence was noted at two years following surgery.

sinus with curettage of the ethmoid conchae removes the infection within the bony cavity and allows drainage to be re-established. Fat grafts can be used to encourage ablation of the sinuses.[31,32] Trephination and irrigation of the frontal sinuses without curettage produced an improvement in clinical signs in 20 cats but this was short term.[47]

Alaplasty

There are a number of techniques described for alaplasty (nares resection), including wedge resection (horizontal, vertical, and lateral) or punch biopsy. A horizontal wedge resection allows a deeper slice of tissue to be taken, which decreases the width of the alar fold (Box 54-5).

POSTOPERATIVE CARE

Although many cats will resume oral intake the day following surgery, the temporary disruption of the normal sense of smell combined with surgical stress, possible discomfort, and medications will result in

some cats being anorexic. Oral food that is initially offered should be soft and pungent.

Analgesia needs careful consideration. For the first 24 hours, once the local anesthetic nerve block has worn off, methadone is a good analgesic choice for planectomies and rhinotomies. An opiate with less sedative effects such as buprenorphine is then used with the addition of non-steroidal inflammatory drugs once food intake is reasonable.

A buster collar may be required and if so will need frequent cleaning. This is usually left in place for the first week though this depends on the temperament of the cat. Grooming will also need to be assisted in the first few weeks postsurgery. Immediately after nasal planectomy surgery the turbinates are exposed and bone is visible; however, a scab rapidly forms over the exposed tissue and granulation tissue usually covers the exposed bone within three weeks of surgery. In some cases, the nasal aperture will initially need gentle cleaning with damp cotton buds or swabs to remove food debris.

If a drain is placed in the wound during a rhinotomy, this can be removed after three to five days. If the drain becomes occluded and subcutaneous emphysema occurs this is usually self-resolving in seven

Box 54-4 Sinus ablation

The cat is initially positioned in dorsal recumbency and a piece of subcutaneous fat approximately 5 cm × 2 cm × 1 cm harvested from the ventral abdomen. The cat is then repositioned in sternal recumbency with its head elevated on a sandbag and stabilized with adhesive tape. A three-sided skin flap which hinges rostrally is made, starting at the midpoint between the base of the pinna and the lateral canthus of the eye, and then extending rostrally to the level of the lateral canthus and then connecting the two incisions dorsally across the temporal area (Fig. 54-16A).

The skin is elevated and retracted rostrally before a similarly positioned bone flap is created with an oscillating saw (Fig. 54-16B). The rostral side of the bone flap is scored with the saw to allow the bone flap to be hinged rostrally. Using surgical loupes or an operating microscope, the frontal sinuses are debrided and all the mucoperiosteal lining removed (Fig. 54-17). The ostium to the nasal cavity is checked for patency and increased in diameter, allowing the ethmoturbinates to be debrided. A piece of temporal muscle is then harvested and used to plug the ostium. The previously harvested fat graft is placed in the sinus prior to closure of the bone flap and the temporal fascia is resutured. The subcutaneous tissues and skin are closed routinely.

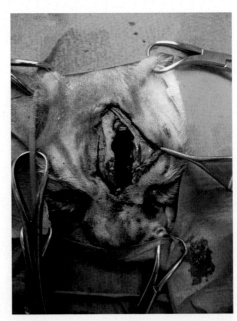

Figure 54-17 Unilateral sinus obliteration in a 13-year-old domestic short-haired cat that presented with chronic rhinitis refractory to medical treatment. MRI revealed sinus involvement.

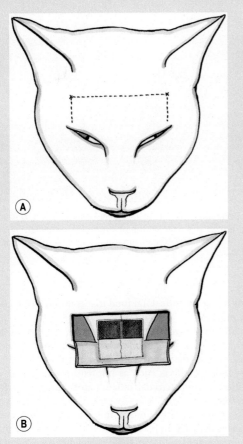

Figure 54-16 Sinus obliteration. **(A)** A three-sided rectangular flap of skin is made and hinged rostrally. **(B)** A smaller rectangular section of bone is cut and elevated to give access to the frontal sinuses.

COMPLICATIONS

With all nasal procedures some nasal hemorrhage is expected on recovery and for the following few days. Sneezing is common and can result in epistaxis. Anorexia is possible after planectomies and rhinotomies but in the author's cases has only ever been short term in duration.

Dorsal rhinotomies can produce subcutaneous emphysema in the first couple of weeks that is self-limiting and causes little morbidity. Dehiscence of ventral rhinotomies can result in an oronasal fistula but in a case series of 58 patients, including dogs and cats, only one incidence of an oronasal fistula was seen.[44] After both dorsal and ventral rhinotomies, a persistent nasal mucopurulent or serous discharge is common due to the altered architecture of the nasal conchae and resulting inflammation. With any facial surgery dehiscence is possible which may necessitate further surgery. There are a number of axial skin flaps that can be used for reconstruction and the local subdermal flaps are well vascularized (Fig. 54-19).

With nasal planectomies, dehiscence may be seen, usually of the premaxilla reconstruction, and this is usually only a cosmetic issue but the wound can be resutured if required. Nasal stenosis is sometimes apparent; the nasal orifice should be revised if this is causing a clinical problem. Mild nasal discharge may be noted after surgery due to the increased size of the nasal orifice and inflammation associated with exposure of the nasal turbinates. This is rarely a significant problem.

Recurrence of nasal planum squamous cell carcinomas may be seen if clean margins are not obtained. Radiotherapy in this area is often difficult after surgery due to the close proximity of the eyes and brain. If further surgical resection is possible this is often the best treatment.

Sinus curettage and obliteration can result in short duration subcutaneous emphysema. This is self-limiting and resolves in three to five days.

to ten days' time and there is little point in trying to remove the accumulated air prior to this time. Skin sutures, if present, are removed ten to 14 days postsurgery under sedation or general anesthesia, and the oral wounds after ventral rhinotomy are carefully checked at this stage to ensure adequate healing.

Box 54-5 **Alaplasty**

The cat is placed in sternal recumbency and the nostrils prepped with povidone-iodine.

Lateral wedge resection

An 11 blade is used to cut a wedge of tissue from the lateral cartilage (Fig. 54-18A). Hemorrhage is rapid but stops when the cut surfaces are re-apposed with a soft suture material such as polyglactin 10. Pressure is also applied by a sterile cotton bud. The sutures are left to fall out or removed two to three weeks postsurgery.

Punch resection technique

The lateral cartilage is stabilized with forceps and a 2 mm punch biopsy instrument used to remove a circular plug of tissue to the level of the alar fold (Fig. 54-18B). A 2–3 mm rim of tissue is left medially and laterally after the plug is sectioned. The tissue edges are then apposed with simple interrupted sutures.[34]

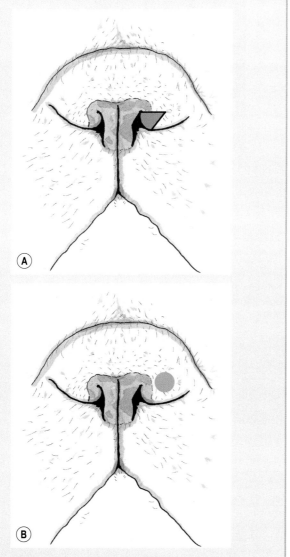

Figure 54-18 Stenotic nares correction. **(A)** Horizontal wedge technique. **(B)** Punch resection technique.

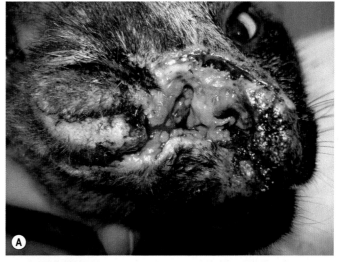

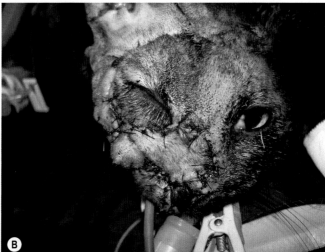

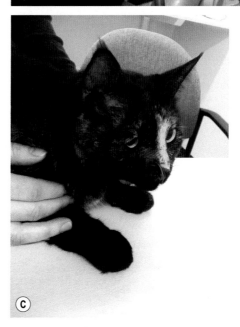

Figure 54-19 (A) Wound breakdown in a nine-year-old female neutered cat that had a chondrosarcoma removed from the maxillary bone. The superficial temporal axial pattern flap had distal necrosis. **(B)** The wound was reconstructed with a local subdermal rotation flap. **(C)** Six months postsurgery there is a good functional outcome with a reasonable cosmetic result.

PROGNOSIS

Nasal tumors

Both of the common nasal tumor types, lymphoma and carcinomas, can be treated effectively, albeit palliatively with radiotherapy, both orthovoltage and megavoltage; lymphomas are far more radiosensitive. There are few case series of non-lymphomatous nasal tumors in the literature but survival times are in the range of 315 days or 40% survival at one year for adenocarcinoma.[48,49] Lymphomas tend to have a better initial response to radiotherapy, with median survival times (when death from progression of the nasal tumor was analyzed) in the range of 530 days.[49,50] Similar survival times were obtained by using chemotherapy protocols but the inclusion of radiotherapy in the treatment protocol was pivotal for local disease control.[51] A variety of chemotherapeutic protocols are commonly used for nasal lymphoma (Box 54-6).

Little difference was noted in survival times of cats treated with either COP or Wisconsin–Madison (WM) in a study of 149 cats with lymphoma.[52] Surgical debulking of nasal tumors prior to radiotherapy or chemotherapy is not associated with improved survival times.[53]

Nasal planum squamous cell carcinomas

The one year survival rate after resection for nasal planum squamous cell carcinomas in cats is over 80% and disease free intervals postsurgery are reported as more than 500 days[54,55] (Fig. 54-20). There are fewer long-term reports following the more radical surgery[56] in cats but in the author's opinion and experience the results with combined nasal planectomy and premaxillectomy are very similar to those of nasal planectomy.

Fungal rhinitis

The prognosis for cats with aspergillosis rhinitis is guarded, with resolution of clinical signs in approximately half the cases treated. Orbital involvement appears to be a negative prognostic indicator.[14,22] Cryptococcosis is easier to treat. Cases that are localized to the nasal cavity were responsive to azole anti-fungal medication such as itraconazole, though therapy was often protracted (over a year) and relapse occurred in about one-third of cases.[18] In cases where the infection had invaded into the CNS additional treatment with amphotericin B with or without flucytosine was required.[20]

Box 54-6 **Chemotherapeutic agents commonly used for treatment of nasal lymphoma**

COP: vincristine, cyclophosphamide, prednisolone
Wisconsin–Madison (WM): vincristine, L-asparaginase, cyclophosphamide, prednisolone, doxorubicin, methotrexate
Prednisolone

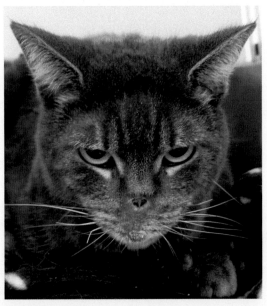

Figure 54-20 The long-term cosmetic appearance following a nasal planectomy. This cat had no obvious morbidity associated with the procedure

Sinus obliteration

There are few published clinical case series of sinus obliteration. In a series of six cats, three of the cat owners reported excellent results between 18 and 22 months postsurgery. Two cats were improved with only intermittent sneezing and discharge and one cat was lost to follow up.[30]

REFERENCES

1. Henderson SM, Bradley K, Day MJ, et al. Investigation of nasal disease in the cat- a retrospective study of 77 cases. J Feline Med Surg 2004;6:245–57.

2. Demko JL, Cohn LA. Chronic nasal discharge in cats: 75 cases (1993–2004). J Am Vet Med Assoc 2007;230:1032–7.

3. Lamb CR, Richbell S, Mantis P. Radiographic signs in cats with nasal disease. J Feline Med Surg 2003;5: 227–35.

4. Schoenborn WC, Wisner ER, Kass PP, Dale M. Retrospective assessment of computed tomographic imaging of feline sinonasal disease in 62 cats. Vet Radiol Ultrasound 2003;44(2):185–95.

5. Galler A, Shibly S, Bilek A, Hirt R. Chronic rhinitis in cats: A retrospective study. Schweiz Arch Tierheilkd 2012;154(5):209–16.

6. De Lorenzi D, Bertoncello D, Bottero E. Squash-preparation cytology from nasopharyngeal masses in the cat: cytological results and histological correlations in 30 cases. J Feline Med Surg 2008;10(1):55–60.

7. Michiels L, Day MJ. A retrospective study of non-specific rhinitis in 22 cats and the value of nasal cytology and histopathology. J Feline Med Surg 2003;5:279–85.

8. Cape L. Feline idiopathic chronic rhinosinusitis: a retrospective study of 30 cases. J Am Anim Hosp Assoc 1992;28:149–55.

9. Reed N, Gunn Moore D. Nasopharyngeal disease in cats. J Feline Med Surg 2012;14: 306–15.

10. Cox NR, Brawner WR, Powers RD, Wright JC. Tumors of the nose and paranasal sinuses in cats: 32 cases with comparison to a national database (1977–1987). J Am Anim Hosp Assoc 1991;27:339–47.

11. Mukaratirwa S, van der Linde-Sipman JS, Gruys E. Feline nasal and paranasal sinus tumours. Clinicopathological study, histomorphological description and diagnostic immunohistochemistry of 123 cases. J Feline Med Surg 2001;3:235–45.

12. Bexfield NH, Stell AJ, Gear RN, Dobson JM. Photodynamic therapy of superficial nasal planum squamous cell carcinomas in cats: 55 cases. J Vet Int Med 2008;22:1385–9.

13. Goodfellow M, Hayes A, Murphy S, Brearley M. A retrospective study of strontium 90 plesiotherapy for feline squamous cell carcinoma of the nasal planum. J Feline Med Surg 2006;8:169–76.

14. Grier RL, Brewer WG Jr, Theilen GH. Hyperthermic treatment of superficial tumours in cats and dogs. J Am Vet Med Assoc 1980;177:227–33.

15. Stell AJ, Dobson JM, Langmack K. Photodynamic therapy of feline superficial squamous cell carcinoma using topical 5-aminolaevulinic acid. J Small Anim Pract 2001;42:164–9.

16. Théon AP, Madewell BR, Shearn VI, Moulton JE. Prognostic factors associated with radiotherapy of squamous cell carcinoma of the nasal plane in cats. J Am Vet Med Assoc 1995;206:991–6.

17. Théon AP, VanVechten MK, Madewell BR. Intratumoral administration of carboplatin for treatment of squamous cell carcinomas of the nasal plane in cats. Am J Vet Res 1996;57:205–10.

18. Greci V, Mortellaro CM, Olivero D, et al. Inflammatory polyps of the nasal turbinates of cats: an argument for designation as feline mesenchymal nasal hamartoma. J Feline Med Surg 2011;13:213–19.

19. Chambers BA, Laksito MA, Fliegner RA, et al. Nasal vascular hamartoma in a domestic shorthair cat. Aust Vet Journal 2010;88:107–11.

20. Tomsa K, Glaus TM, Zimmer C, Greene CE. Fungal rhinitis and sinusitis in three cats. J Am Vet Med Assoc 2003;222:1380–4.

21. Furrow E, Groman RP. Intranasal infusion of clotrimazole for the treatment of nasal aspergillosis in two cats. J Am Vet Med Assoc 2009;235:1188–93.

22. Barachetti L, Mortellaro CM, Di Giancamillo M, et al. Bilateral orbital and nasal aspergillosis in a cat. Vet Ophthalmology 2009;12(3):176–82.

23. Peiffer RL, Belkin PV, Janke BH. Orbital cellulitis, sinusitis, and pneumonitis caused by Penicillium sp in a cat. J Am Vet Med Assoc 1980;176:449–551.

24. Wilkinson GT, Sutton RH, Grono LR. Aspergillus spp. infection associated with orbital cellulitis and sinusitis in a cat. J Small Anim Pract 1982;23:127–31.

25. Goodall SA, Lane JG, Warnock DW. The diagnosis and treatment of a case of nasal aspergillosis in a cat. J Small Anim Pract 1984;25:627–33.

26. Malik R, Wigney DI, Muir DB, et al. Cryptococcosis in cats:clinical and mycological assessment of 29 cases and evaluation of treatment using orally administered fluconazole. J Vet Mycology 1992;30(2):133–44.

27. Trivedi SR, Malik R, Meyer W, Sykes JE. Feline cryptococcosis: impact of current research on clinical management. J Feline Med Surg 2011;13(3):163–72.

28. Ossent P. Systemic aspergillosis and mucormycosis in 23 cats. Vet Rec 1987;120:330–3.

29. O'Brien CR, Krockenberger MB, Wigney DI, et al. Retrospective study of feline and canine cryptococcosis in Australia from 1981 to 2001:195 cases. Med Mycology 2004;42(5):449–60.

30. McLellan GJ, Aquino SM, Mason DR, et al. Use of posaconazole in the management of invasive orbital aspergillosis in a cat. J Am Anim Hosp Assoc 2006;42:302–7.

31. Miller RI. Nodular granulomatous fungal skin diseases of cats in the United Kingdom: a retrospective review. Vet Derm 2009;21:130–5.

32. Dye C, Johnson EM, Gruffydd-Jones TJ. Alternaeria species infection in nine domestic cats. J Feline Med Surg 2009;11(4):332–6.

33. Wray JD, Sparkes AH, Johnson EM. Infection of the subcutis of the nose in a cat caused by Mucor species: successful treatment using posaconazole. J Feline Med Surg 2008;10(5):523–7.

34. Bostock DE, Coloe PJ. Phaeohyphomycosis caused by Exophiala jeanselmei in a domestic cat. J Comp Path 1982;92:479–82.

35. Knights CB, Lee K, Rycroft AN, et al. Phaeohyphomycosis caused by Ulocladium species in a cat. Vet Rec 2008;162:415–17.

36. Planellas M, Roura X, García F, Pastor J. Chronic rhinitis secondary to the intrusion of a tooth into the nasal cavity of a cat. Vet Rec 2009;165:325–6.

37. Riley P. Nasopharyngeal grass foreign body in eight cats. J Am Vet Med Assoc 1993;202:299–300.

38. Anderson GI. The treatment of chronic sinusitis in six cats by ethmoid conchal curettage and autogenous fat graft sinus ablation. Vet Surg 1987;16(2):131–4.

39. Bright RM, Thacker L. Fate of autogenous fat implants in the frontal sinuses of cats. Am J Vet Res 1983;44(1):22–7.

40. Harvey CE. Surgical correction of stenotic nares in a cat. J Am Anim Hosp Assoc 1986;22:31–2.

41. Trostel CD, Frankel DJ. Punch resection alaplasty technique in dogs and cats with stenotic nares: 14 cases. J Am Anim Hosp Assoc 2010;46:5–11.

42. Holmes RL, Wolstencroft JH. Accessory sources of blood supply to the brain of the cat. J Physiol 1959;148:93–107.

43. Ashbaugh EA, McKiernan BC, Miller CJ, Powers B. Nasal hydropusion: A novel tumour biopsy technique. J Am Anim Hosp Assoc 2011;47:312–16.

44. Holmberg DL, Fries C, Cockshutt J, Van Pelt D. Ventral rhinotomy in the dog and cat. Vet Surg 1989;18(6):446–9.

45. Holmberg DL. Sequelae of ventral rhinotomy in dogs and acts with inflammatory and neoplastic nasal pathology: A retrospective study. Canadian Vet J 1996;36:483–5.

46. Sissener TR, Bacon NJ, Friend E, et al. Combined clotrimazole irrigation and depot therapy for canine nasal aspergillosis. J Small Anim Pract 2006;47(6):312–15.

47. Winstanley EW. Trephining frontal sinuses in the treatment of rhinitis and sinusitis in the cat. Vet Rec 1974;95:289.

48. Mellanby RJ, Herrtage ME, Dobson JM. Long-term outcome of eight cats with non-lymphoproliferative nasal tumours treated by megavoltage radiotherapy. J Feline Med Surg 2002;4:77–81.

49. Theon AP, Peaston AE, Madewell BR, Dungworth DL. Irradiation of non lymphoproliferative neoplasms of the nasal cavity and paranasal sinuses in 16 cats. J Am Vet Med Assoc 1994;204:78–83.

50. Haney SM, Beaver L, Turrel J, et al. Survival analysis of 97 cats with nasal lymphoma: A multi-institutional retrospective study (1986–2006). J Vet Int Med 2009;23:287–94.

51. Sfiligoi G, Théon AP, Kent MS. Response of nineteen cats with nasal lymphoma to radiation therapy and chemotherapy. Vet Rad Ultrasound 2007;48(4):388–93.

52. Taylor SS, Goodfellow MR, Browne WJ, et al. Feline extranodal lymphoma: response to chemotherapy and survival in 110 cats. J Small Anim Pract 2009;50:584–92.

53. Evans SM, Hendrick M. Radiotherapy of feline nasal tumours. Vet Radiol 1988;30(3):128–32.

54. Lana SE, Ogilvie GK, Withrow SJ, et al. Feline cutaneous squamous cell carcinoma of the nasal planum and pinnae: 61 cases. J Am Anim Hosp Assoc 1997;33:329–32.

55. Withrow SJ, Straw RC. 1990 Resection of the nasal planum in nine cats and five dogs. J Am Anim Hosp Assoc 1990;26:219–22.

56. Lascelles BD, Henderson RA, Seguin B, et al. Bilateral rostral maxillectomy and nasal planectomy for large rostral maxillofacial neoplasms in six dogs and one cat. J Am Anim Hosp Assoc 2004;40:137–46.

Chapter | 55 |

Mandibulectomy and maxillectomy

K.M. Pratschke, K.D. Smith

There are several indications for surgery of the maxilla and mandible in feline patients; this chapter will describe the indications and techniques of mandibulectomy and maxillectomy. There has traditionally been an assumption that cats do not tolerate such procedures well although this assumption has largely been based on opinion and anecdote with only limited documented information available for review. Indications for these procedures include oral neoplasia, non-neoplastic oral lesions, intractable infection, and traumatic injuries. The most commonly encountered oral tumors are squamous cell carcinoma (SCC) and fibrosarcoma, both of which are locally invasive and frequently invade bone. Maxillectomy and mandibulectomy allow resection of these tumors with wide margins,[1-4] and therefore provide potentially curative treatment. Traumatic injuries such as bite wounds, projectile injuries, and road traffic accidents may result in a degree of dysfunction that is not compatible with life, but which may be addressed via maxillectomy or mandibulectomy in a way that allows a good quality of life and normal or near normal function to be restored.

Fractures of the mandible and disorders of the temporomandibular joint including ankylosis and locking-jaw syndrome are common in the cat and these are covered in Chapter 26 of Feline Orthopedic Surgery and Musculoskeletal Disease.[5]

SURGICAL ANATOMY

The skull is a rigid structure made up of many bones, which articulates with the mandible at the two temporomandibular joints (Fig. 55-1). Maxillectomy may require removal of part or all of the maxilla, incisive, palatine, frontal, vomer, zygomatic, and lacrimal bones, so a thorough knowledge of regional anatomy is essential. The mandible is comprised of two hemimandibles firmly united rostrally at the mandibular symphysis (Fig. 55-2). The horizontal part is termed the body and the vertical part the ramus. The permanent dentition of the cat is coded 2(I3/3–C1/1–P3/2–M1/1), although in the experience of the authors use of this terminology is not consistent amongst veterinary surgeons. The premolars are numbered 2–4 on the upper arcade and 3–4 on the lower arcade.[6]

The lips in the cat are small and relatively immobile compared to dogs. They form a large rima oris with the upper and lower lips meeting at the commissure caudally. The lips consist of skin, muscle, and mucosa and contain numerous small scattered salivary glands. The cheeks form the buccal vestibule, which receives salivary secretions from the parotid, molar, and zygomatic salivary glands. The hard palate separates the oral and nasal cavities and is formed from the incisive, maxillary, and palatine bones. The oral aspect of the hard palate is covered by thick mucosa with transverse folds (rugae) that are continuous with the gingiva rostrally and laterally and the soft palate caudally. The floor of the oral cavity is supported by paired mylohyoideus muscles passing between the mandibular bodies. The ventral oral mucosa has two protuberances to either side of the lingual frenulum known as sublingual caruncles, marking the opening of the mandibular and sublingual salivary ducts.

The muscles of mastication attach mainly to the ramus of the mandible (Fig. 55-3). The temporalis muscle attaches to the coronoid process and the pterygoid muscles attach medially and caudally, ventral to the temporalis attachment. The masseter arises from the zygomatic process and attaches to the ventrolateral surface at the masseteric fossa. The digastricus attaches to the mandibular body.

Blood supply to the rostral skull and mandible is from branches of the maxillary artery. The inferior alveolar artery enters the mandible at the mandibular foramen then runs through the mandibular canal supplying teeth before branching to exit through the rostral, middle, and caudal mental foramina. The infraorbital artery, palatine arteries and external ophthalmic arteries branch from the maxillary artery medial to the rostral zygomatic arch. The infraorbital artery passes through the infraorbital canal to emerge at the infraorbital foramen, supplying the upper dental arcade, nose, and upper lip. The paired minor palatine arteries run ventrally and supply the soft and caudal hard palate. The paired major palatine arteries pass through the major palatine canals emerging at the major palatine foramen level with the caudal edge of the upper fourth premolar. Rostrally the sphenopalatine artery branches from the major palatine artery to pass through the palatine fissure to supply the interior of the rostral nasal cavity.

Lymphatic drainage is primarily to mandibular lymph nodes with regional drainage to both ipsilateral and contralateral retropharyngeal nodes, the cervical chain, and then the prescapular and anterior mediastinal nodes.

© 2014 Elsevier Ltd
DOI: 10.1016/B978-0-7020-4336-9.00055-X

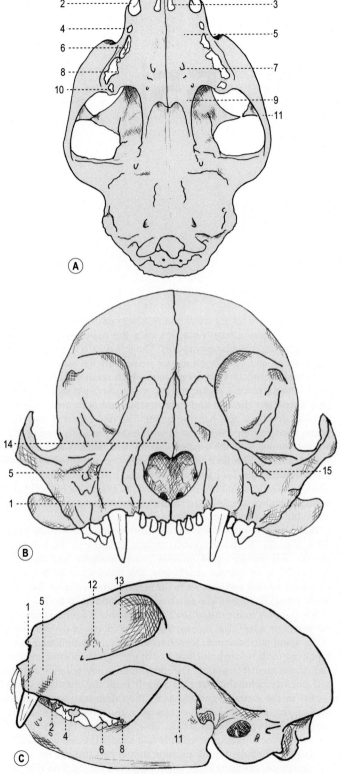

(A)

(B)

(C)

Figure 55-1 Three views of the feline skull are provided in this figure, lateral, ventrodorsal, and rostral. 1, Incisive bone; 2, canine tooth; 3, palatine fissure; 4, upper premolar 2; 5, maxilla; 6, upper premolar 3; 7, palatine foramen; 8, upper premolar 4; 9, palatine bone; 10, upper molar 1; 11, zygomatic arch; 12, lacrimal bone; 13, frontal bone; 14, nasal bone; 15, infraorbital foramen.

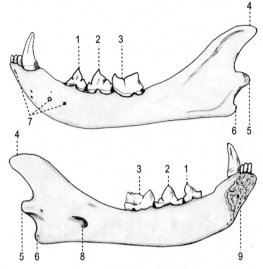

Figure 55-2 Two views of the feline mandible are provided in this figure, medial and lateral. 1, Premolar 3; 2, premolar 4; 3, molar 1; 4, coronoid process; 5, condylar process; 6, angular process; 7, mental foramina; 8, mandibular foramen; 9, mandibular symphysis.

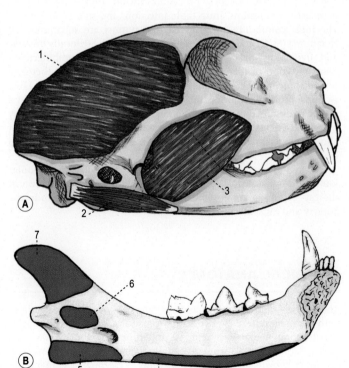

(A)

(B)

Figure 55-3 This picture illustrates the muscles of mastication on the lateral skull and the insertions on the medial mandible. 1, Temporalis; 2, digastricus; 3, masseter; 4, attachment of mylohyoideus; 5, attachment of digastricus; 6, attachment of medial pterygoid; 7, attachment of temporalis

GENERAL CONSIDERATIONS

Clinical presentation

Oral masses are often present for some time before the owner becomes aware of a problem and therefore may have reached an advanced stage of development. Clinical signs commonly encountered include ptyalism that may be hemorrhagic, weight loss, dysphagia, inappetence, and halitosis. Other signs can include epistaxis, exophthalmus, and tooth loss.

Diagnostic procedures

A minimum database of hematology, serum biochemistry, urinalysis, and feline leukemia virus (FeLV)/feline immunodeficiency virus (FIV) status should always be obtained prior to further diagnostic procedures, and a thorough examination of the oral cavity under general anesthesia is mandatory to fully assess the extent of disease. As the majority of feline oral masses are malignant, full staging is essential (see Chapter 14). Lymphatic spread is typically to the submandibular lymph nodes initially, then to the mediastinal and prescapular lymph nodes via the cervical chain.[7] Distant metastatic disease may be to the lungs, or other organs depending on the primary tumor type.

Diagnostic imaging is essential to assess the extent of the tumor and the invasion of local bone. Orthogonal radiographs of the skull as well as intraoral views may be used to assess invasion of bone via lysis or new bone production. However, radiographs may underestimate the extent of the tumor, as lysis is only evident once 40% of bone cortex has been destroyed.[8] Computed tomography combining plain and contrast images is very useful to assess maxillary masses that extend into the nasal cavity, and caudal mandibular masses,[9] and provides an enhanced level of detail over conventional radiography.[10,11]

In one study, just over half of cats and dogs with regional lymph node metastasis from oral tumors had submandibular lymph node enlargement,[12] although the likelihood of local lymphatic disease varies with tumor type. However, palpation of local and regional lymph nodes is not a sensitive test for lymph node metastasis and, as a minimum, fine needle aspiration for cytology should be performed. There is an argument, however, for performing either incisional or excisional biopsy in preference to aspiration as this is a more accurate way of staging local disease.[13,14] Tumor surface inflammation and necrosis mean that touch cytology preparations are often non-diagnostic or misleading and are therefore not recommended.

Biopsy is essential in determining the nature of an oral tumor. The biopsy tract should form part of the tissue that will be excised and should avoid normal peripheral tissues to prevent contamination. In humans, incisional biopsy of oral SCC results in transient release of tumor cells into the blood but there is no supporting evidence for biopsy-induced metastasis in small animals and the overall prognosis remains unaffected provided the biopsy tract has been correctly placed.[15]

SURGICAL DISEASES

Neoplastic diseases

Squamous cell carcinoma is the most common oral neoplasm in cats, comprising approximately 61–80% of all oral tumors.[16,17]

Development of oral SCC has been linked with environmental factors such as the use of flea collars, diet, and passive smoking.[18,19] Affected cats have a median age of 10–12 years and there is no sex predisposition. Grossly, the appearance is variable and may be proliferative or ulcerative, underlining the importance of biopsy for accurate diagnosis. Invasion of bone is common in feline oral SCC and is often aggressive with osteolysis, infection, and associated tooth loss.[20] Regional lymph node metastasis occurs in less than 25% of cases and distant metastasis is rare.[17] In the dog, the metastatic rate is site dependent, with rostral tumors having a lower metastatic potential than caudal or tonsilar SCCs.[21] There is currently no evidence that this is the case in the cat. A syndrome of paraneoplastic hypercalcemia has been described in two cats with SCC.[22]

Oral fibrosarcoma is the second most common oral neoplasm of cats, comprising approximately 13–17% of all oral tumors.[17] Affected cats have a median age of 10 years and there is no sex predisposition. Grossly, lesions characteristically appear firm and solid. These are locally aggressive tumors and bone involvement is common; however, the metastatic rate to regional and distant sites is low. In dogs the lungs are the most common site for metastasis,[23] but it is not clear if this is the case in the cat.[24]

Malignant melanoma is rare in cats, accounting for only 0.8% of feline oral tumors in a ten-year survey carried out in 1989; unfortunately, more recent data is not available.[16] Once again, it is locally aggressive although metastasis has not been reported in the cat. *Osteosarcoma* accounts for 2.4% of feline oral tumors and seems to be more commonly seen in the maxilla, although available numbers for analysis are low and the data is now quite old so its reliability is uncertain.[16] Although one study suggested that mandibular osteosarcoma in cats is associated with a good two-year survival rate,[24] two further studies concluded that axial osteosarcoma carried a poorer prognosis with shorter survival times when compared with feline appendicular osteosarcoma. Other tumor types reported include salivary gland adenocarcinoma, lymphoma, chondrosarcoma and osteoma, but these are more rare occurrences.[16,25]

Epulides and odontogenic tumors

Epulis is a clinical 'umbrella' term used to describe any one of a group of diseases characterized by grossly visible gingival proliferation; as such it does not constitute a histologic diagnosis.[26] In cats, epulides have been classified into four types: fibromatous, ossifying, acanthomatous, and giant cell. Fibromatous epulis was described as the third most common oral tumor in cats in the 1989 survey, representing 7.8% of all feline oral tumors.[16] However, a more recent study showed most fibromatous epulides also had acanthomatous and ossifying components so the true distribution is difficult to assess.[26] Lesions may be solitary or multiple, with multiple tumors being relatively common in cats under three years old.[26,27] Granulomas, which may be pyogenic or peripheral giant cell in nature, may resemble epulides grossly,[16,28] but peripheral giant cell epulis has been documented to show aggressive behavior such as rapid growth, ulceration, and osteolysis, which is not typical for most epulides.[26]

Odontogenic tumors or *ameloblastomas* are tumors of the epithelial cells of the dental lamina, and may resemble epulides clinically and histologically.[16] In dogs, fibromatous and ossifying epulides have been reclassified as peripheral odontogenic fibromas, but in cats it is still not clear whether they may be considered separate diseases.[16] Feline inductive odontogenic tumors, also known less correctly as feline inductive fibroameloblastoma, are unique to cats[29] and are most commonly seen in the rostral maxilla. They are described in young cats and may be locally invasive although metastasis has not been described. Amyloid-producing odontogenic tumors are rare in cats

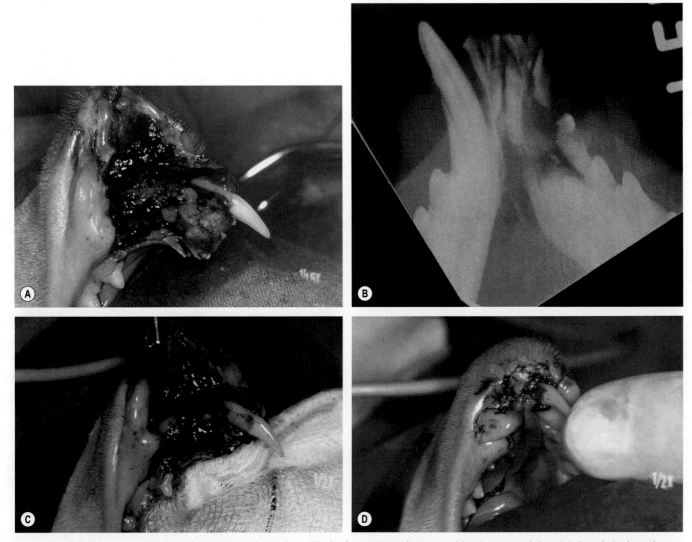

Figure 55-4 (A) Comminuted, open and contaminated rostral mandibular fracture in a three-year-old male neutered domestic long-haired cat that had been involved in a road traffic accident. **(B)** Intraoral radiograph shows comminution and loss of some of the incisors and rostral mandible. **(C)** The remaining rostral mandible and incisors were debrided. **(D)** Primary closure was possible.

and may be locally invasive but do not seem to metastasize.[30] Odontogenic cysts have been described in cats and may be maxillary or mandibular in nature.[31]

Other surgical conditions

Fractures of the mandible and maxilla may not always be amenable to repair, depending on location and severity. In some patients teeth may be absent, bone quality poor, periodontal disease may be severe, osteomyelitis may be present, or the fracture line may pass through an alveolus. In such cases partial mandibulectomy or maxillectomy may offer a superior prognosis to primary fracture repair, with a better quality of life and function (Fig. 55-4). To date, however, this treatment concept is only poorly documented in the available literature, and has been described in only a small case series in the dog[32] and not at all in cats. This means that unfortunately this aspect of orofacial surgery is currently based largely on individual experience and clinical anecdote rather than on widely available evidence. Partial maxillectomy has been reported in the management of oronasal fistula in the dog,[33] but there are no similar reports in the cat.

Cats with severe dental disease can have resorption of the tooth root socket, periapical infection, abscessation, and periosteal new bone. This must be differentiated from neoplasia and biopsy, with samples taken for culture and histopathologic analysis used to help in the differentiation. Removal of the offending tooth and debridement of the offending alveolus should be curative in such cases.

GENERAL PREOPERATIVE SURGICAL CONSIDERATIONS

Despite the increasing use and availability of radiation and chemotherapy, surgery offers a faster, cheaper, and sometimes more reliable method of therapy for most solid tumors. For many tumor types, aggressive surgical resection with appropriate margins remains the treatment of choice. When planning surgery the objectives of the treatment must be clearly defined, i.e., is surgery of curative intent, is it intended to debulk prior to adjunctive radiation, or is it solely palliative in nature?

Margins

Tumors may be surrounded by a pseudocapsule (a mix of normal and neoplastic cells) and/or a reactive zone (mainly inflammatory cells),[34] and these must be taken in to account with surgical planning and selection of appropriate margins. Removal of the tumor from within the pseudocapsule, an intracapsular resection, is rarely indicated but may be suitable when curetting a well-differentiated odontoma from the mandible. A marginal excision involves removal of the tumor by dissection in the reactive zone and is appropriate for some benign tumors but never for a malignant tumor.[35] Where the tumor is malignant and local infiltration is expected, wide excision is indicated. A benchmark of 10 mm is often used in veterinary medicine, based on recommendations for resection of oral SCCs in humans.[36,37] In reality, this margin has had little validation in veterinary medicine and may not be universally applicable, particularly for tumors that are considered less invasive or aggressive in nature.[34] More locally invasive and infiltrative tumors such as fibrosarcomas or feline squamous cell carcinomas, on the other hand, may require margins greater than 10 mm, and many surgeons will take 1.5–2 cm margins for oral sarcomas. This margin, however, is to a large extent arbitrary in nature, and its use has not been validated for clinical cases. Wide resection is typically achieved through partial mandibulectomy or maxillectomy whereas radical excision requires total hemimandibulectomy or rostral maxillectomy.[38]

Healing

Tissues of the oral cavity will heal readily due to good blood supply; however, basic principles of good surgical technique remain important and atraumatic tissue handling is essential. As most osteotomies will be performed with powered equipment, there is a tendency for irrigation with sterile saline during use to prevent thermal damage, although this is once again an approach that has not been clinically validated and is based largely on opinion rather than evidence. Oral tumor resections are considered clean-contaminated surgeries. In humans, such surgeries are considered to warrant prophylactic intravenous antibiosis.[39] Amoxicillin-clavulanate, some cephalosporins, and clindamycin have been suggested as the most appropriate for perioperative use in cats, based on the typical oral flora, but it should be borne in mind that this recommendation is now over 15 years old.[40]

Analgesia

Sensory nerve blocks of the infraorbital and inferior alveolar nerves[41] provide excellent analgesia and can prevent central sensitization, therefore they form a very useful part of a multimodal analgesic protocol (see Chapter 2). Blocking the infraorbital nerve will desensitize the upper dental arcade, the soft and hard palates ipsilaterally, and the muzzle. Blocking the inferior alveolar nerve will desensitize the lower dental arcade and chin.

SURGICAL TECHNIQUES

The patient is placed in lateral recumbency for most unilateral maxillectomy and mandibulectomy surgeries although for bilateral procedures dorsal or sternal recumbency may be preferable. The oropharynx is packed and hair is clipped on the affected side. The extent of the clip is dictated by the planned procedure, so for a partial hemimandibulectomy it may be adequate to clip ventral to the eye, whereas a maxillectomy involving partial orbitectomy may require a considerably wider clip. The planned reconstruction will also dictate the clip; for example, if the use of an omocervical flap (see Chapter 19) is anticipated then the clip must extend down the neck for the appropriate distance. The planned placement of a feeding tube at the end of the procedure will also require additional preoperative clipping. The mouth and skin are prepared aseptically; in people, chlorhexidine is considered most suitable for oral preparation,[42] but there are no similar studies in animals and povidone-iodine is commonly used for oral preparation. Following aseptic preparation and draping, the planned margins of the incision are outlined with a sterile skin marker.

Maxillectomy

Maxillectomy is performed at varying levels based on the location and extent of tissue to be removed and may be rostral, central, caudal, unilateral, or bilateral in differing combinations (Boxes 55-1 and 55-2; Fig. 55-5A,B).

Rostral maxillectomy may be performed unilaterally or bilaterally and involves excision of the incisive bone, rostral maxilla, the incisors, and canine teeth. A bilateral maxillectomy can be extended caudally to the level of the second premolar although this extent of maxillectomy has only been documented in dogs. A combined dorsal and intraoral approach has been described in dogs for maxillectomy for tumors involving tissues more caudal to the third premolar.[47] The results obtained in this study represented an improvement over previously reported studies, and the authors postulated this was due to the better exposure and access to the area afforded by the combined approach over the standard intraoral approach. There are currently no reports of this approach being used in a cat and it is likely that anatomic differences mean it will be both less applicable and less appropriate.

Given the 10 mm margins typically required around tumors, a unilateral rostral maxillectomy would rarely be suitable in cats. Where there has been extension of the tumor into the adjacent buccal or labial mucosa, reconstruction may not be possible using conventional techniques and consideration may need to be given to the use of novel techniques such as the temporal muscle flap (see Chapter 19).[46]

Mandibulectomy

Partial mandibulectomy techniques are described based on the area of mandible excised (Boxes 55-3 to 55-5; Fig. 55-5). Unilateral rostral mandibulectomy, although relatively commonly performed in dogs, is less suitable in the cat as proper application of the 10 mm margin around malignant tumors of the rostral mandible will usually incorporate the mandibular symphysis.[34] Bilateral rostral mandibulectomy foreshortens the mandible and has many similarities to the unilateral rostral mandibulectomy, although the mandibular body is transected bilaterally rostral to the third premolar.

Radical excision can be achieved by hemimandibulectomy and three-quarters mandibulectomy but there is only limited information available regarding how cats fare after this type of procedure, with the majority of clinical experience being related to dogs.

Mandibular rim excision, where only the dorsal cortex of the mandibular body is osteotomized and the ventral cortex is maintained has been described in dogs.[48] Although this has the advantage of maintaining mandibular integrity, the small size of the feline mandible is likely to preclude its use in cats for tumor resections other than for benign masses such as fibromatous or ossifying epulides.

POSTOPERATIVE CARE

Oropharyngeal swabs or packing should be removed and the oropharynx suctioned prior to extubation. Cats dislike having to open-mouth

Box 55-1 **Rostral maxillectomy** (Fig. 55-5A,B)

The cat is positioned in either ventral or lateral recumbency depending on the surgeon's preference. The oral mucosa and periosteum is incised at the level of the preplanned margin. If the margin crosses the major palatine artery, this should be identified and ligated prior to division. Although bone may be cut with an osteotome and mallet, the control offered by a powered saw is preferred by many surgeons although the precision of a small osteotomy and mallet may be useful for completion of osteotomy lines in areas that have limited access.

In the dog, various authors have recommended positioning the suture line over adjacent intact bone or leaving a flap of soft tissue to allow easier closure. Given the relatively small size of the feline skull, such flaps are rarely possible without compromising the surgical margins.

The maxillectomy line should extend dorsally to include the tooth roots; if they are inadvertently sectioned then any residual portions of root must be retrieved before closure. The nasal cavity is exposed following excision of the bone in a maxillectomy, and presurgical planning should include assessment regarding whether appropriate margins will require removal of nasal turbinates. This is a procedure

that may be associated with significant hemorrhage, so provision should be made for availability of blood products should they be required (see Chapter 5). Temporary carotid ligation prior to surgery has been used to control severe hemorrhage in the dog,[42] but this technique cannot be safely used in cats due to the risk of both morbidity and mortality.[43]

Closure of standard maxillectomy defects is achieved by raising a flap of vestibular mucosa-submucosa from the upper lip lateral to the defect. The incision is started parallel to the lateral edge of the defect then extended perpendicularly toward the lip margins. Dissection of the flap is continued until the defect can be closed without tension and without drawing the lip into the mouth to an extent that is likely to result in trauma from teeth. Synthetic absorbable sutures are used to attach the labial flap to the mucoperiosteum. Monofilament suture will cause less tissue drag during closure. A two-layer closure has been recommended to close submucosa and mucosa separately; however, in reality this may not always be possible in the cat where tissues are very thin.

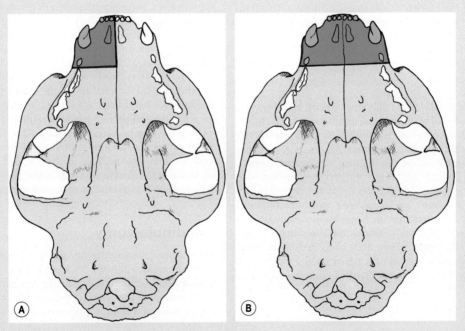

Figure 55-5 **(A)** Unilateral rostral maxillectomy; **(B)** bilateral rostral maxillectomy.

Box 55-2 **Central, caudal and hemimaxillectomy** (Fig. 55-6)

The cat is positioned in lateral recumbency. The caudal osteotomy required when performing caudal maxillectomy or hemimaxillectomy extends from the midline of the hard palate at the level of the upper molar to the rostral base of the zygomatic arch. This can be combined with resection of portions of the ventral orbit, zygomatic arch and ramus of the mandible as necessary (Fig. 55-10).

When performing central or caudal maxillectomy, transection of the infraorbital canal may be required. Ligation of the infraorbital vessels is not possible in advance so this cut should be the final one in the maxillectomy and suction should be used to identify, retrieve, and ligate the infraorbital and sphenopalatine arteries as rapidly and efficiently as possible.

Extension of the technique across the midline is limited by the availability of soft tissue for closure. If the defect cannot be closed with a labial flap as previously described in Box 55-1, then consideration should be given to the use of an axial pattern flap such as the caudal auricular, omocervical or superficial temporal,[44] possibly combined with a temporal muscle flap to provide additional soft tissue cover. Microvascular techniques may also be used to allow closure using a muscular (temporalis) or myocutaneous free flap[45] but access to the relevant equipment and expertise is likely to limit routine application of these techniques.

Box 55-2 **Continued**

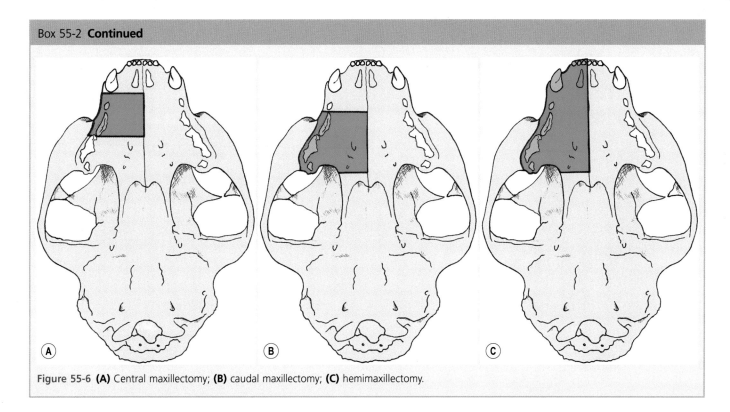

Figure 55-6 (A) Central maxillectomy; **(B)** caudal maxillectomy; **(C)** hemimaxillectomy.

Box 55-3 **Hemimandibulectomy** (Fig. 55-7)

With the patient in lateral recumbency, the oral mucosa and periosteum are incised at the level of the pre-planned margin. The symphysis is split to facilitate dissection and soft tissues elevated subperiosteally as much as surgical margins will permit.

To improve exposure caudally, the commissure of the lip may be incised full thickness toward the angle of the mandible. Following

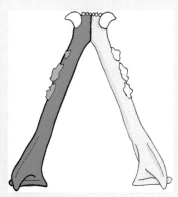

Figure 55-7 Hemimandibulectomy.

transection of the digastricus caudoventrally, the mandibular foramen is identified and the mandibular artery and vein ligated and transected as they enter the foramen. The vertical ramus is freed of its muscular attachments (pterygoid, masseter, and temporalis), with subperiosteal elevation of the muscles being a less traumatic option where possible.

The temporomandibular joint is incised and disarticulated, taking care to avoid the maxillary artery and its branches medially. Removal of the mandible is completed by dissection of remaining temporal muscle attachments from the coronoid process.

The exact method of closure is dependent on the extent of soft tissue resection, and as with the maxillectomy techniques there is no single description that will fit all cases. If labial and buccal mucosa remains, it may be apposed to sublingual mucosa using a synthetic absorbable suture in a simple continuous pattern or simple interrupted pattern depending on individual preference. If surgery requires removal of the labial mucosa rostrally, the skin may be sutured directly to the incisor gingiva. If the commissure was incised as part of surgery, it is closed in three layers, i.e., mucosa, muscularis, and skin (Fig. 55-11). Advancement of the commissure (commissurorrhaphy) to the level of the first premolar or canine teeth has been described in dogs to prevent the tongue hanging from the mouth; however, it is unknown whether a similar approach would be necessary or appropriate for cats.

breathe so if the nasal cavity has been entered and is therefore likely to be at least partially occluded from edema and blood clots the patient should be monitored carefully for dyspnea.

The patient should be carefully monitored for the first 12 hours following surgery in case of ongoing or recurring hmorrhage. Sedation may be indicated if the patient becomes distressed, particularly if this worsens respiratory function or causes recurrent hemorrhage.

Analgesia should be assessed regularly to ensure that appropriate levels are being provided; this will typically require a multimodal approach.

Intravenous fluid therapy is continued at maintenance levels, with electrolyte supplementation if required until normal oral feeding is restored. Although the majority of canine patients will readily eat with assistance within 24 hours of surgery, cats can be slower to eat.

Box 55-4 **Rostral mandibulectomy** (Fig. 55-8)

The cat is positioned in dorsal or lateral recumbency depending on the surgeon's preference.

Unilateral rostral mandibulectomy

The soft tissue incisions are determined by surgical margins and the oral mucosa and periosteum are incised at the level of the pre-planned margin. Care should be taken to ligate the middle mental blood vessels and to avoid the sublingual caruncle during dissection

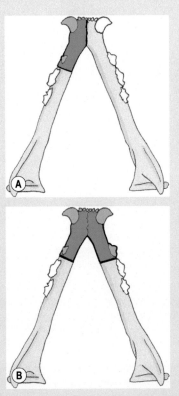

Figure 55-8 (A) Unilateral rostral mandibulectomy; **(B)** bilateral rostral mandibulectomy.

although this will sometimes not be possible if margins are to be maintained.

The mandible is osteotomized at the symphysis and at the body rostral to the third premolar using either an osteotome, air powered saw or drill, depending on individual preference.

The inferior alveolar artery should be ligated if possible, but in many cases hemorrhage from this vessel is best controlled through the application of pressure and use of a hemostatic agent such as bone wax in the mandibular canal.

The defect is reconstructed by raising a flap of labial mucosa-submucosa and suturing it to the sublingual mucosa and symphyseal gingiva.

In the dog, unilateral rostral mandibulectomy may be achieved without complete separation of the symphysis; however, this is unlikely to be feasible in the cat.

Stabilization of the remaining hemimandible with implants and grafts has been described but this is generally not considered necessary.

Bilateral rostral mandibulectomy

The cat is positioned in dorsal recumbency. The soft tissue incisions are determined by surgical margins and the oral mucosa and periosteum are incised at the level of the pre-planned margin. Care should be taken to ligate the middle mental blood vessels and to avoid the sublingual caruncle during dissection although this will sometimes not be possible if margins are to be maintained.

The mandible is osteotomized bilaterally at the body rostral to the third premolar using either an osteotome, air powered saw or drill, depending on individual preference.

The inferior alveolar artery should be ligated if possible, but in many cases hemorrhage from this vessel is best controlled through the application of pressure and use of a hemostatic agent such as bone wax in the mandibular canal.

Reconstruction can generally be achieved through suturing the labial mucosa to the sublingual mucosa without creating a labial flap. It is important to ensure the margin of the lip is positioned in an elevated position relative to the oral mucosa to prevent, or at least reduce, drooling.

Redundant skin may need to be resected from the chin to achieve a cosmetic closure. Where the lower lip has been resected to preserve surgical margins, skin may be sutured directly to the incisor gingiva.

Box 55-5 **Central and caudal mandibulectomy techniques** (Fig. 55-9)

Central (or segmental) mandibulectomy

This technique involves removal of part of the body of the mandible caudal to the second premolar. The oral mucosa and periosteum are incised at the level of the pre-planned margin, the osteotomy performed as described previously, and closure again achieved by raising a labial mucosa-submucosa flap.

It should be remembered that devitalization and death of the teeth rostral to the osteotomy will occur following full thickness segmental mandibulectomy. As malocclusion tends to occur after this procedure, and dogs will commonly 'grind' the molars in the caudal mandible after surgery, techniques for mandibular reconstruction have been described in the dog.[47] Similar techniques have not been described for cats and it is unknown whether they would be applicable or not.

Caudal mandibulectomy

Caudal mandibulectomy is not a commonly performed or required technique in veterinary surgery but may be indicated for caudally

located masses or management of traumatic injuries. The vertical ramus may be removed via an approach made over the zygomatic arch. Osteotomy of the zygomatic arch is described but is not always necessary.

An incision overlying the length of the arch is made and the temporal and masseter muscles are detached from the dorsal, ventral and medial aspects before the zygomatic arch is excised and wrapped in a blood-soaked swab. Dissection of the temporal and masseter muscles is continued to the vertical ramus taking care to preserve appropriate margins. The vertical ramus is osteotomized and removed, then the zygomatic arch may be re-attached at either end with orthopedic wire. Re-attachment of the masseter is achieved with synthetic non-absorbable suture looped around the zygomatic arch. Care should be taken to close dead space. This technique has been described via an oral approach,[33] but this is not in common clinical usage.

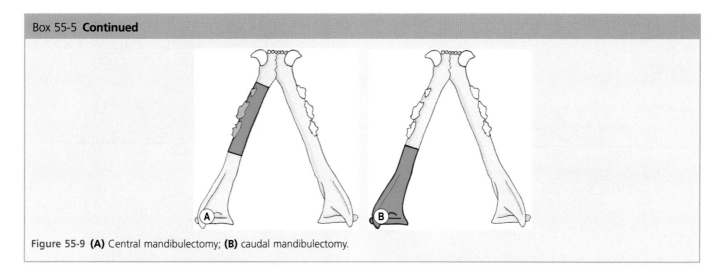

Figure 55-9 (A) Central mandibulectomy; **(B)** caudal mandibulectomy.

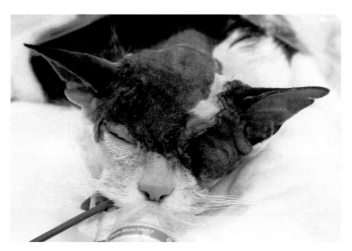

Figure 55-10 This cat had a maxillary fibrosarcoma that necessitated central maxillectomy combined with ocular exenteration and partial orbitectomy. The defect was reconstructed with an advancement flap from the dorsal head and neck.

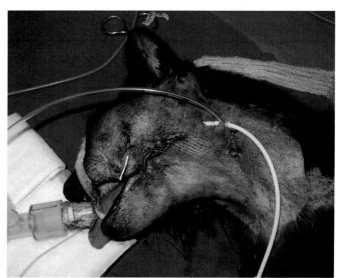

Figure 55-11 This cat had a mandibular squamous cell carcinoma for which hemimandibulectomy was performed incorporating a full thickness incision of the labial commissure to improve access. A local wound analgesia (soaker) catheter is in place as is an esophagostomy tube to enable provision of postoperative nutrition.

Dysphagia and/or inappetence is perceived to be fairly common following mandibulectomy and maxillectomy in cats and it may be worth thinking about placing either an esophagostomy or gastrostomy feeding tube at the time of surgery (see Chapter 12). Prehension and mastication may be affected by tension in the lips and a range of soft food should be offered, although foods that have a paste-like consistency should be avoided due to the potential for them to seep between sutures and cause local infection. Although there are no firm or clinically validated guidelines, water is usually offered six to 12 hours following surgery and eating should be encouraged with soft foods within 24 hours following surgery. Soft food should be continued for one month and chewing hard objects should be discouraged.

Excised tissue should always be sent for histologic evaluation to confirm both the histologic diagnosis and to evaluate surgical margins (Fig. 55-12), although it is important to remember that obtaining clear margins histologically may not prevent local recurrence of the tumor. For this reason, ongoing periodic monitoring is advisable[24] and oncologic re-evaluation should be considered every three to six months regardless of margins obtained.

COMPLICATIONS

As cats have minimal spacing between teeth, performing the osteotomy cuts required for either mandibulectomy or maxillectomy without causing tooth root damage is difficult. Any trauma to the tooth roots may result in death of the tooth requiring either vital pulpotomy or extraction at a later date.

In a retrospective case series of 42 cats undergoing mandibulectomy, postoperative complications were very common, in particular dysphagia and inappetence.[24] The majority of patients in this case series had either complete unilateral mandibulectomy or rostral bilateral mandibulectomy, and the authors reported an acute morbidity of 98%, with the more common complications including dysphagia, inappetence, ptyalism, mandibular drift, and tongue protrusion. Long-term morbidity was reported in 76%, predominantly related to dysphagia, inappetence, ptyalism, tongue protrusion, difficulty

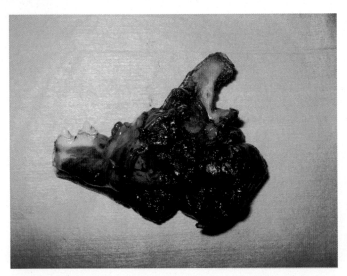

Figure 55-12 All tissues resected should be submitted for histology, including both bone and soft tissues. Information regarding margins in all involved tissues is essential to assess completeness of excision.

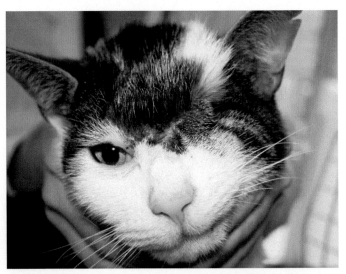

Figure 55-13 The postoperative appearance following even quite aggressive surgical procedures is often better than anticipated by owners, particularly once the hair coat has grown back. This is the cat seen immediately postoperatively in figure 55-10, and here at 12 months after surgery.

grooming, and dental malocclusion. Five cats were reported to never regain the ability to eat normally; however, two of these died only nine and 11 days after surgery and two more were euthanized at 37 and 68 days postsurgery. One of the five survived to 192 days when it was euthanized for local recurrence. All five had undergone relatively aggressive procedures, losing >50% of their mandible. An additional factor regarding assessment of postoperative complications in this series was that 12 of the 42 cats underwent adjunctive therapy including chemotherapy and radiation therapy, both of which could potentially play a role in inappetence. Although this issue was mentioned in the discussion it was not evaluated. It is important to give due consideration preoperatively to the potential for a feline patient to effectively lose the ability to eat voluntarily following an aggressive mandibulectomy procedure as some clients will not be willing to accept this type of complication.

Mandibular drift (medial movement of the remaining intact mandible) occurs if there has been disruption of the mandibular symphysis or body and may result in severe malocclusion in the cat. This was reported as a long-term complication in 37% of cats that had mandibulectomy in the retrospective study of 42 cats previously cited.[24] The same study reported ulceration of the hard palate by pressure from the lower canines following mandibulectomy in 18% of cases. Temporary interdental bonding has been suggested to prevent this but surgery to shorten or extract the canine teeth may ultimately be required.

Wound dehiscence is reportedly uncommon following mandibulectomy, being seen in only 12.5% of the 42 cats, although no information was provided regarding the severity and extent of dehiscence. Sublingual ranulae may occur several months after mandibulectomy but usually resolve spontaneously.[24]

There are only limited references within the veterinary literature to clinical cases where cats have undergone maxillectomy so it is difficult to be sure how much of what we know about the procedure in dogs might apply to cats. In dogs, dehiscence of the palate following maxillectomy has been reported in 7–33% of surgeries.[49,50] The vast majority occur caudal to the canine teeth and may be avoided by tension-free closure and careful surgical technique. In some cases it may be appropriate to pre-drill anchor holes for suture placement within bone on one side of the reconstruction if the use of soft tissue anchor points does not provide a sufficiently robust closure. Subcutaneous

emphysema may occur following maxillectomy but is usually mild and will resolve in five to six days. Medial deviation of the upper lip following rostral maxillectomy and upper canine tooth removal has been reported to render the lip susceptible to trauma from the lower canines in dogs; the two reported feline cases in the literature did not develop this complication. In one case series a single cat underwent left maxillectomy, with no postoperative complications recorded.[25] In another series reporting the outcome following bilateral rostral maxillectomy and nasal planectomy a single cat that underwent surgery was anorexic for six days postoperatively but was reported to have normal function and no complications at 66 months after surgery,[39] while three cats that underwent partial maxillectomy in a third series had no postoperative complications recorded.[3] Two case reports document unilateral maxillectomy, one in a four-month-old kitten and the other a two-year-old cat; in one report esophagostomy tube feeding was required for seven days postoperatively but follow up with the owners at seven months confirmed normal function.[45,51]

Although the numbers available for review are very limited it is interesting that maxillectomy seems to have a lesser risk of complications in cats and to have a far less profound effect on eating than does mandibulectomy.

Postoperative cosmetic appearance is generally much better than most owners imagine (Fig. 55-13), but concern regarding likely alterations in cosmetic appearance is a common reason for refusal of surgery. It can be valuable to have a library of pictures showing patients following surgery to demonstrate the good cosmetic outcomes that can be achieved in many cases, as well as to assist discussion of cases where the cosmetic change will be greater to help owners fully appreciate what they are agreeing to. Medial deviation of the upper lip is often the only sign of a rostral maxillectomy, while more caudal maxillectomies cause mild to moderate facial concavity. Unilateral canine tooth removal in rostral mandibulectomy often results in protrusion of the tongue from that side. Bilateral rostral mandibulectomy causes a more marked change in cosmetic appearance, with drooping of the lower jaw and difficulty maintaining the tongue within the mouth.

Despite complications, 83% of owners were satisfied with the outcome of surgery following mandibulectomy in Northup's case series of 42 cats, although a general observation that could be made is that owner satisfaction tended to also reflect survival times and outcome.[24]

PROGNOSIS

Tumor type, stage, and location are major determinants of prognosis where the primary disease is neoplastic. The prognosis for benign and non-neoplastic tumors is, on the whole, excellent. As a general caveat, there are only small numbers of cases reported and available for review, and there seem to be quite wide variations in outcome amongst these cases, so it is difficult to be certain of the accuracy of the numbers and percentages that are routinely quoted.

SCC carries a poor prognosis in the cat, with fewer than 10% of cats surviving to one year in one study,[8] although this was contradicted in a second, larger study, where 43% survival was identified at one year.[24] Overall, it does appear that SCC is associated with a significantly shorter survival time compared to fibrosarcomas and osteosarcomas,[24] although this is complicated by the fact that the majority of documented cases of feline SCC were already stage 3 at the time of diagnosis and treatment, meaning that they had already progressed to confirmed local invasion of bone and soft tissues including muscles, lymphatics, and nerves. There is a paucity of information regarding outcome in stage 1 SCC managed with early aggressive treatment, suggesting that many cases are not recognized at an earlier stage, although it is also possible that aggressive treatment is not being recommended until the disease has visibly progressed. There is a single case report of one cat that had maxillectomy for aggressive maxillary carcinoma (poorly differentiated) that was reported as alive and disease free at 27 months after surgery,[3] but this appears to be the exception rather than the rule. Wide excision of the primary tumor, removal of the submandibular lymph node and radiation may offer an improved prognosis for oral SCC,[24] but the potential adverse effects of more aggressive mandibulectomy procedures on eating function and quality of life must be considered. Clients should be made aware of this prior to surgery, and also of the fact that even with aggressive surgery followed by adjunctive therapy the prognosis remains guarded. Progression of local disease is the most common reason for euthanasia,[22,24,52] and this may well reflect the tendency towards less aggressive resections in cats. Caudal oral SCC is, as a rule, less amenable to therapy, resulting in a poorer prognosis.

Fibrosarcoma of the maxilla or mandible carries a better prognosis in the cat. Following mandibulectomy, a one-year survival of 67% was reported in Northup's series of 42 cats, regardless of local recurrence.[24] This is similar to the situation in dogs with soft tissue sarcoma, where the presence or absence of local recurrence has no influence on survival times or outcome. One report of a maxillary fibrosarcoma treated by unilateral premaxillectomy showed no recurrence within two years.[2]

Mandibular osteosarcomas were associated with 83% two-year survival following surgical resection in Northup's series.[24] Although specific information regarding the maxillary and mandibular osteosarcomas is not provided in two large studies of feline osteosarcoma, both concluded that overall axial osteosarcoma carried a poorer prognosis with shorter survival times when compared with appendicular osteosarcoma, which in cats generally has a much longer survival time reported postoperatively compared to the dog.[53,54]

In a recent report on seven cats with mandibular and maxillary osteoma, three were euthanized, one was treated by maxillectomy, one by mandibulectomy, and two with debulking. All four surviving cats were reported to have acceptable quality of life at one-year follow up.[25]

Fibromatous and acanthomatous epulides, although considered benign growths, may recur locally following marginal excision.[26] In the only report that documents cats with multiple epulides, 73% were reported to have local recurrence following surgical resection; however, the primary surgery in each case was actually limited to excisional biopsy and was not a curative intent procedure so this information should be interpreted with caution.[27]

REFERENCES

1. Emms SG, Harvey CE. Preliminary results of maxillectomy in the dog and cat. J Small Anim Pract 1986;27:291–306.

2. Salisbury SK, Richardson DC, Lantz GC. Partial maxillectomy and premaxillectomy in the treatment of oral neoplasia in the dog and cat. Vet Surg 1986;15:16–26.

3. Bradley RL, MacEwen EG, Loar AS. Mandibular resection for removal of oral tumors in 30 dogs and 6 cats. J Am Vet Med Assoc 1984;184(4):460–3.

4. Penwick RC, Nunamaker DM. Rostral mandibulectomy: A treatment for oral neoplasia in the dog and cat. J Am Anim Hosp Assoc 1987;23(1):19–25.

5. Voss K, Langley-Hobbs SJ, Grundemann S, Montavon PM. Mandible and maxilla. In: Montavon PM, Voss K, Langley-Hobbs SJ, editors. Feline orthopedic surgery and musculoskeletal disease. Edinburgh: Elsevier; 2009. p. 311–28.

6 Berman E, Davis J, Stara JF. A dental chart of the domestic cat (Felis catus L.). Lab Anim Care 1967;17(5):511–13.

7. Smith MM. Surgical approach for lymph node staging of oral and maxillofacial

neoplasms in dogs. J Am Anim Hosp Assoc 1995;31(6):514–18.

8. Reeves NCP, Turrel JM, Withrow SJ. Oral squamous-cell carcinoma in the cat. J Am Anim Hosp Assoc 1993;29(5):438–41.

9. Forrest LJ. The head: excluding the brain and orbit. Clin Tech Small Anim Pract 1999;14(3):170–6.

10. Van Camp S, Fisher P, Thrall DE. Dynamic CT measurement of contrast medium wash in kinetics in canine nasal tumors. Vet Radiol Ultrasound 2000;41(5):403–8.

11. Gendler A, Lewis JR, Reetz JA, Schwarz T.Computed tomographic features of oral squamous cell carcinoma in cats: 18 cases (2002–2008). J Am Vet Med Assoc 2010;236(3):319–25.

12. Herring ES, Smith MM, Robertson JL. Lymph node staging of oral and maxillofacial neoplasms in 31 dogs and cats. J Vet Dent 2002;19(3):122–6.

13. Williams LE, Packer RA. Association between lymph node size and metastasis in dogs with oral malignant melanoma:

100 cases (1987–2001). J Am Vet Med Assoc 2003;222(9):1234–6.

14. Gilson SD. Clinical management of the regional lymph node. Vet Clin North Am Small Anim Pract 1995;25(1):149–67.

15. Klopfleisch R, Sperling C, Kershaw O, Gruber AD. Does the taking of biopsies affect the metastatic potential of tumours? A systematic review of reports on veterinary and humans cases and animal models. Vet J 2011;190:e31–42.

16. Stebbins KE, Morse CC, Goldschmidt MH. Feline oral neoplasia: a ten-year survey. Vet Pathol 1989;26(2):121–8.

17. Liptak JM, Withrow SJ. Oral tumours. In: Withrow SJ, MacEwen EG, Editors. Small animal clinical oncology. Missouri: Saunders Elsevier; 2007. p. 455–75.

18. Bertone ER, Snyder LA, Moore AS. Environmental and lifestyle risk factors for oral squamous cell carcinoma in domestic cats. J Vet Int Med 2003;17(4):557–62.

19. Snyder LA, Bertone ER, Jakowski RM, et al. p53 expression and environmental tobacco smoke exposure in feline oral

squamous cell carcinoma. Vet Pathol 2004;41(3):209–14.

20. Martin CK, Tannehill-Gregg SH, Wolfe TD, Rosol TJ. Bone-invasive oral squamous cell carcinoma in cats: pathology and expression of parathyroid hormone-related protein. Vet Pathol 2011;48(1):302–12.

21. Theon AP, Rodriquez C, Madewell BR. Analysis of prognostic factors and patterns of failure in dogs with malignant oral tumors treated with megavoltage irradiation. J Am Vet Med Assoc 1997;210(6):778–84.

22. Hutson CA, Willauer CC, Walder EJ, et al. Treatment of mandibular squamous cell carcinoma in cats by use of mandibulectomy and radiotherapy: seven cases (1987–1989). J Am Vet Med Assoc 1992;201(5):777–81.

23. Kosovsky JK, Matthiesen DT, Marretta SM, Patnaik AK. Results of partial mandibulectomy for the treatment of oral tumors in 142 dogs. Vet Surg 1991;20(6):397–401.

24. Northrup NC, Selting KA, Rassnick KM, et al. Outcomes of cats with oral tumors treated with mandibulectomy: 42 cases. J Am Anim Hosp Assoc 2006;42(5):350–60.

25. Fiani N, Arzi B, Johnson EG, et al. Osteoma of the oral and maxillofacial regions in cats: 7 cases (1999–2009). J Am Vet Med Assoc 2011;238(11):1470–5.

26. de Bruijn ND, Kirpensteijn J, Neyens IJ, et al. A clinicopathological study of 52 feline epulides. Vet Pathol 2007;44(2):161–9.

27. Colgin LMA, Schulman FY, Dubielzig RR. Multiple epulides in 13 cats. Vet Pathol 2001;38(2):227–9.

28. Rothwell JT Valentine BA. Peripheral giant-cell granuloma in a cat. J Am Vet Med Assoc 1988;192(8):1105–6.

29. Gardner DG Dubielzig RR. Feline inductive odontogenic-tumor (inductive fibroameloblastoma) – a tumor unique to cats. J Oral Pathol Med 1995;24(4):185–90.

30. Bock P, Hach V, Baumgartner W. Oral masses in two cats. Vet Pathol 2011;48(4):906–10.

31. Gioso MA, Carvalho VGG. Maxillary dentigerous cyst in a cat. J Vet Dent 2003;20(1):28–30.

32. Lantz GC, Salisbury SK. partial mandibulectomy for treatment of mandibular fractures in dogs: 8 cases (1981–1984). J Am Vet Med Assoc 1987;191(2):243–5.

33. Salisbury SK Richardson DC. Partial maxillectomy for oronasal fistula repair in the dog. J Am Anim Hosp Assoc 1986;22(2):185–92.

34. Verstraete FJM, Mandibulectomy and maxillectomy. Vet Clin N Am Small Anim Pract 2005;35(4):1009–39.

35. Salisbury SK. Maxillectomy and mandibulectomy. In: Slatter DH, Editor. Textbook of small animal surgery. Philadelphia: WB Saunders; 2003. p. 561–72.

36. Batsakis JG. Surgical excision margins: A pathologist's perspective. Advan Anatom Pathol 1999;6(3):140–8.

37. McMahon J, O'Brien CJ, Pathak I, et al. Influence of condition of surgical margins on local recurrence and disease-specific survival in oral and oropharyngeal cancer. Br J Oral Maxillofac Surg 2003;41(4):224–31.

38. Lascelles BD, Henderson RA, Seguin B, et al. Bilateral rostral maxillectomy and nasal planectomy for large rostral maxillofacial neoplasms in six dogs and one cat. J Am Anim Hosp Assoc 2004;40(2):137–46.

39. Page CP, Bohnen JM, Fletcher JR, et al. Antimicrobial prophylaxis for surgical wounds. Guidelines for clinical care. Arch Surg 1993;128(1):79–88.

40. Harvey CE, Thornsberry C, Miller BR, Shofer FS. Antimicrobial susceptibility of subgingival bacterial flora in cats with gingivitis. J Vet Dent 1995;12(4):157–60.

41. Lemke KA, Dawson SD. Local and regional anesthesia. Vet Clin North Am Small Anim Pract 2000;30(4):839–57.

42. Summers AN, Larson DL, Edmiston CE, et al. Efficacy of preoperative decontamination of the oral cavity. Plast Reconstr Surg 2000;106(4):895–900; quiz 901.

43. Hedlund CS, Tangner CH, Elkins AD, et al. Temporary bilateral carotid-artery occlusion during surgical exploration of the nasal cavity of the dog. Vet Surg 1983;12(2):83–5.

44. De Ley G, Leusen I. Cerebrovascular reserve in the cat after acute bilateral carotid occlusion. Arch Int Physiol Biochim 1987;95(5):447–55.

45. Lester S, Pratschke K. Central hemimaxillectomy and reconstruction using a superficial temporal artery axial pattern flap in a domestic short hair cat. J Feline Med Surg 2003;5(4):241–4.

46. Cheung LK. An animal model for maxillary reconstruction using a temporalis muscle flap. J Oral Maxillofac Surg 1996;54(12):1439–45.

47. Lascelles BD, Thomson MJ, Dernell WS, et al. Combined dorsolateral and intraoral approach for the resection of tumors of the maxilla in the dog. J Am Anim Hosp Assoc 2003;39(3):294–305.

48. Arzi B. Verstraete FJM. Mandibular rim excision in seven dogs. Vet Surg 2010;39(2):226–31.

49. Harvey CE. Oral surgery. Radical resection of maxillary and mandibular lesions. Vet Clin North Am Small Anim Pract 1986;16(5):983–93.

50. Wallace J, Matthiesen DT, Patnaik AK. Hemimaxillectomy for the treatment of oral tumors in 69 dogs. Veterinary Surgery 1992;21(5):337–41.

51. Padgett SL, Tillson DM, Henry CJ, Buss MS. Gingival vascular hamartoma with associated paraneoplastic hyperglycemia in a kitten. J Am Vet Med Assoc 1997;210(7):914–15.

52. Bradney IW, Hobson HP, Stromberg PC, et al. Rostral mandibulectomy combined with intermandibular bone-graft in treatment of oral neoplasia. J Am Anim Hosp Assoc 1987;23(6):611–15.

53. Kessler M, Tassani-Prell M, von Bomhard D, Matis U. Osteosarcoma in cats: epidemiological, clinical and radiological findings in 78 animals (1990–1995). Tierarztl Prax 1997;25(3):275–83.

54. Heldmann E, Anderson MA, Wagner-Mann C. Feline osteosarcoma: 145 cases (1990–1995). J Am Anim Hosp Assoc 2000;36(6):518–21.

Chapter |56|

Palate

R.K. Sivacolundhu

Reconstruction of palatal defects in cats can be challenging and requires a detailed knowledge of local anatomy, as well as an understanding of the various options available to the surgeon.

SURGICAL ANATOMY

The secondary palate is a bony and soft tissue structure that separates the respiratory and digestive passages of the head.[1] The primary palate consists of the lips and premaxilla,[2] and conditions affecting these areas are covered in Chapters 49 and 55. The nasal cavity and nasopharynx lie dorsal to the secondary palate, while the oral cavity and oropharynx lie ventral to it. The bony hard palate lies rostrally and the membranous soft palate caudally.[1]

The hard palate is formed by fusion of the palatine, maxillary, and incisive bones on each side.[3] The soft palate extends caudally from the hard palate and this tends to be relatively short in the cat. There is a thin fold from its ventrolateral part that extends on each side to form the ventral wall of the tonsillar crypts.[1] The palate has mucosa both on the nasal and oral sides. The mucosa on the oral side of the hard palate is a tough, cornified squamous epithelium. While there are no muscles of the hard palate, the muscles of the soft palate consist of paired (intrinsic) palatine muscles, and paired (extrinsic) tensor and levator veli palatine muscles. There are many palatine glands that lie within the bulk of the soft palate, which have many openings throughout the surface of the soft palate.[1]

The maxillary artery is the main continuation of the external carotid artery. It supplies a branch to the mandible before extending rostrally to where it branches to become the minor palatine artery, major palatine artery and infraorbital artery.[3] The minor palatine arteries are the main blood supply to the soft palate, and the major palatine artery is the main blood supply to the hard palate.[1] The major palatine foramen is located medial to the fourth premolar tooth and there are one or more minor palatine foraminae located caudal to this.[3] The major palatine artery exits the skull through the major palatine foramen and courses rostrally along the ventral surface of the bony hard palate (Fig. 56-1). It supplies bone and soft tissues of the hard palate before reaching the midline palatine fissure where it anastomoses with the infraorbital artery.[3] The minor palatine artery(ies) exit the skull through the minor palatine foramen(ae) to supply the soft palate,

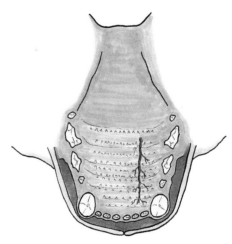

Figure 56-1 The major palatine artery exits the skull through the major palatine foramen and then courses rostrally. It is the main blood supply to the hard palate.

with contributions from the ascending pharyngeal artery and major palatine artery.[3] The arteries are dwarfed by the palatine plexus of veins, which mainly lie lateral to the paired slender palatine muscles.[1] Venous drainage of the hard palate is located in the submucosa covering the bony palate. Lymphatic drainage is usually via the medial retropharyngeal lymph nodes.[1]

The trigeminal nerve supplies the main sensory nerves to the palate. The major palatine branch of the maxillary division of the trigeminal nerve enters the palate through the major palatine foramen to supply sensory function to the hard palate, and the minor palatine branch enters through the minor palatine foramen to supply sensory function to the soft palate.[1,3] Branches of the glossopharyngeal and vagus nerves supply the muscles of the soft palate and pharynx.[1]

GENERAL CONSIDERATIONS

Diagnosis of congenital defects of the palate or oronasal fistulae is very easy and involves a simple physical examination. A sedation or general anesthetic may be required in animals that are difficult to

© 2014 Elsevier Ltd
DOI: 10.1016/B978-0-7020-4336-9.00056-1

examine. Animals may present with clinical signs of poor growth, nasal discharge, sneezing while eating, dyspnea, upper respiratory congestion, coughing, sneezing, or halitosis.[4,5] Middle ear disease associated with congenital palatine defects has been reported in a cat.[6] Neoplasia of the palate will often go unnoticed until a mass is interfering with deglutition, respiration, causes weight loss, local irritation, cessation of grooming, or ulcerates causing bleeding and/or halitosis due to superficial infection.[7] Palatal masses are often not painful.[7,8] Masses may be identified during routine dental procedures. Examination of the hard palate should be routine in any physical examination for amenable patients.

The majority of the hard and soft palate can be examined visually under a general anesthetic with the aid of a laryngoscope or other good light source. A more complete examination of the nasopharynx may be performed using a small flexible fiberoptic endoscope. Any masses seen should have a biopsy performed for histologic examination, and associated local lymph nodes should be aspirated to check for spread of disease. If histology is consistent with a malignancy, a computed tomographic scan (CT) is often worthwhile during the staging process to aid in identifying the extent of locoregional disease and thereby assisting in determining treatment options. If previous thoracic radiographs are clear for evidence of metastases, CT may aid in earlier detection of pulmonary metastases or local or thoracic lymphadenopathy. Staging tests performed will depend on the histologic diagnosis and expected biological behaviour of the mass, and will usually include a complete blood count, biochemical panel, and urinalysis. Other tests to consider may include abdominal ultrasonography, coagulation panel, other blood tests, or nuclear scintigraphy for primary bone tumors. For a detailed discussion of oral neoplasia readers are referred to Chapters 49 and 55.

Timing of surgery needs to be considered for correction of congenital clefts of the palate. While early surgery may cause interference with normal growth of the skull,[9,10] surgery is often performed before skeletal maturity without subsequent clinically apparent problems.[4] Animals may live with congenital defects of the palate for months prior to performing a surgical correction. Surgery should be performed sooner for animals that are not eating well or if their quality of life is otherwise significantly affected.[4] If early repair is performed, the reconstructed palate of a neonate grows rapidly, causing stretching and thinning of some repairs. This can result in oronasal fistulae, which can then be repaired after patients reach eight to ten months old.[2] Preoperative thoracic radiographs are performed since aspiration pneumonia is a possible complication of congenital palatine defects.[6] Otoscopic examination should be performed and skull radiographs considered, even in asymptomatic animals, due to the association of middle ear disease with congenital palatine defects.[6]

SURGICAL DISEASES

Defects in the hard and soft palates may be congenital or acquired. Congenital defects may include clefts of the hard and/or soft palate, and hypoplasia of the soft palate.[5] While congenital hard palate defects generally occur in the midline, defects in the soft palate may occur in the midline or as a unilateral (asymmetrical) or bilateral hypoplasia (Fig. 56-2).[5,11] While most cleft palates are believed to be inherited recessive or irregularly dominant traits, intrauterine infections and exposure to toxins at specific times during gestation may also result in a cleft palate.[12] Acquired defects occur as a result of trauma (Fig. 56-3), including surgery and/or radiation therapy, severe periodontal disease, tooth removals, resection of neoplasms, or severe chronic infections.[13] Siamese and Abyssinian cats may have a higher incidence of congenital palatal defects.[2,12,14]

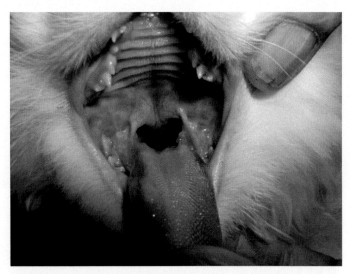

Figure 56-2 Congenital hypoplasia of the soft palate in a five-year-old cat, resulting in a 'uvula' *(Courtesy of Prue Neath.)*

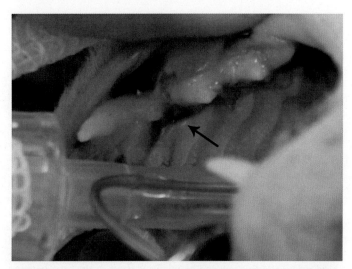

Figure 56-3 A small oronasal fistula (arrow) in a cat that occurred after a maxillary fracture along the dental arcade. The fistula healed without treatment. *(Courtesy of the University of Cambridge.)*

SURGICAL TECHNIQUES

Reconstruction of palatal defects can be challenging and requires a detailed knowledge of the local anatomy, as well as an understanding of the various options available to the surgeon.[13] This is particularly important in cases of large defects, or when radiation or previous surgeries have compromised local tissue.[15] The surgeon needs to work with the anatomical limitations, difficult access, and limited tissue available for local repair. Additionally, the repair must withstand the mechanical stresses induced during mastication and deglutition.[15] Consideration should be made as to whether to temporarily divert food with a feeding tube (see Chapter 12).

There are a number of general principles that should be followed when considering surgery on a patient with a palate defect (Box 56-1).[12]

Surgery of the hard and soft palate is generally performed with the animal in dorsal recumbency. A mouth gag is used to improve surgical access. A moistened swab may be used caudal to the soft palate to decrease risk of aspiration of blood. Wiping mucous membranes with 0.05% aqueous chlorhexidine is adequate for surgical preparation of the area.

Suture materials used are usually 4/0 or 5/0 absorbable monofilament suture material, depending on the size of the animal, type of repair and type of tissue being sutured.[13] Non-absorbable sutures have also been used. If knots are left on the epithelial surface, they will usually slough within three to four weeks regardless of the type of suture material being used.[16]

> ## Box 56-1 Surgical principles for repairing palatine defects
>
> - Make flaps large compared with the size of the defect to minimize tension
> - Preserve the vascular supply to flaps by elevating adequate underlying connective tissue. For the hard palate, the mucoperiosteum should be elevated as one layer, avoiding the major palatine artery, which exits the skull through the major palatine foramen medial to the fourth premolar tooth
> - Suture tissues to freshly incised epithelium, and make incisions with a scalpel blade rather than scissors to minimize crushing injuries
> - Arrange suture lines so that they are lying over connective tissue rather than over the defect, thereby preventing drying and contamination of the connective tissue side of the flap and decreasing the risk of dehiscence
> - Suture tissue gently and with large bites of tissue to minimize tension and interference with blood supply at the wound edges

There have been many techniques described to manage palatal defects, including local flaps[4,16–19] axial pattern flaps,[15,20] distant tissue using a rostral tongue flap,[21] auricular cartilage free grafts,[22] temporal muscle transfer,[23] free tissue (muscle) transfer with microvascular anastomosis,[24] and prosthetic appliances.[25,26] Due to the similarities in anatomy between dogs and cats, techniques that have previously been reported in dogs are likely to be applicable to cats although scientific reports are lacking.

Reconstruction of the hard palate

The more common or useful techniques for reconstruction of the hard palate include mucoperiosteal flaps, mucoperiosteal releasing incisions, local flaps from the soft palate, buccal mucosal flaps, double reposition flaps, auricular cartilage free grafts, temporal muscle transfer, and prosthetic appliances.[18,19,22,23,25–29]

Mucoperiosteal flaps and releasing incisions

Mucoperiosteal flaps are easy to perform (Box 56-2), being mindful of the location of the palatine artery. While a single overlapping mucoperiosteal flap may be used,[18] this may interfere with bone union in the case of a cleft palate.[2] Achieving a two-layer closure is preferable to allow a more anatomic closure and potentially allow bridging of the bone defect.[2]

Bipedicle flaps are most commonly used for closing cleft palate defects of the hard palate. Transposition flaps are useful for small defects anywhere on the palate and split palatal U-flap may be used to repair large caudal defects of the hard palate.[30]

Box 56-2 Mucoperiosteal flaps

Bipedicle

The cat is positioned in dorsal recumbency with the mouth held open with the use of a gag. Releasing incisions are made with a sharp scalpel blade in the hard palate mucosa longitudinally along the length of the defect, adjacent and medial to the dental arcade.[19] Incisions are also made 2–3 mm from the midline defect. Flap attachments are maintained rostrally and caudally. A hinged flap is created bilaterally by elevating the mucosa adjacent to the defect, hinging it across the defect and suturing it in the midline using simple interrupted sutures of 4/0 or 5/0 polydioxanone, thus reconstructing the nasal side of the defect. The bipedicled flaps may then be mobilized to reconstruct the oral side of the defect and are sutured primarily.[19] The large lateral defects with exposed palatine bone are left open and will rapidly epithelialize (Fig. 56-4).[2,13,19]

Transposition

A transposition flap may be elevated from the mucosa of the hard palate, usually with the base directed caudally.[13] The flap is simply transposed in to the defect and sutured primarily. If the palatine artery is preserved, a long thin flap may be elevated and rotated up to 180° to assist in closing large defects.[13,28]

Split palatal U-flap

The mucosa is incised 2–3 mm from the maxillary arcade, extending to the level of the first or second premolar teeth. The rostral extent of the incisions will depend on the size of the defect, and join in the midline to form a large U-shaped flap. A midline incision is created from the rostral extent of the defect to the rostral extent of the flap. Flaps are elevated and transposed caudally to cover the defect, being careful to avoid the palatine artery (Fig. 56-5).[30]

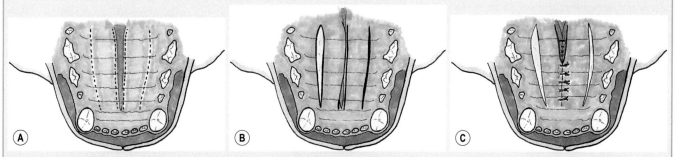

Figure 56-4 Bipedicle mucoperiosteal flap. **(A)** Incisions are created medially and laterally in the mucoperiosteum of the hard palate. **(B)** The bipedicle flaps are elevated, taking care to avoid the palatine artery. **(C)** Flaps are hinged and sutured to create the nasal mucosa, and the bipedicled flaps are sutured to reconstruct the oral mucosa. The donor site defects are left open and epithelialize rapidly.

Box 56-2 Continued

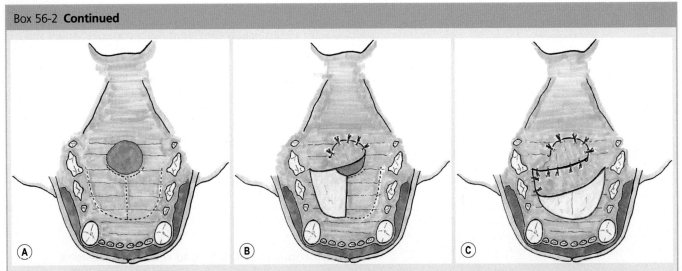

Figure 56-5 Split palatal U-flap. **(A)** The mucosa is incised 2–3 mm from the maxillary arcade, extending to the level of the first or second premolar teeth. The rostral extent of the incisions will depend on the size of the defect, and join in the midline to form a large U-shaped flap. A midline incision is created from the rostral extent of the defect to the rostral extent of the flap. **(B, C)** Flaps are elevated and transposed caudally to cover the defect, being careful to avoid the palatine artery. The large rostral defect is left open and heals rapidly via second intention healing.

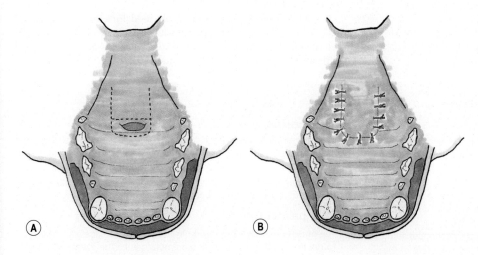

Figure 56-6 Soft palate advancement flap. **(A)** Flap incisions are extended caudally from the defect in to the soft palate, creating a partial-thickness advancement flap. **(B)** The flap is advanced and sutured primarily.

Local flaps from the soft palate

For large caudal defects of the hard palate, either hinged flaps or advancement flaps from the soft palate may be used.[13] For the hinged flap, an inverted U-incision is made in the soft palate caudal to the hard palate defect, and a flap elevated incorporating up to three quarters of the thickness of the soft palate elevated.[28] The flap is hinged cranially and sutured in to the defect. The donor site is only partially closed due to tension and will heal relatively quickly.[28] For the advancement flap, for caudal midline hard palate defects, incisions are extended caudally from the lateral extent of the defect. A split-thickness flap is elevated from the soft palate, and advanced over the defect due to the inherent elasticity of the tissue. The incisions and dissection extend far enough caudally to close the defect without tension (Fig. 56-6).[13,16]

Buccal mucosal flaps

Buccal mucosal flaps (Box 56-3) are very versatile flaps and often used in conjunction with maxillectomies. They are also very useful for closing oronasal fistulae associated with tooth removal.[13] Buccal mucosal transposition flaps based at the palatoglossal arches have been

described in dogs to reconstruct defects of the hard and soft palate.[12,17] If these flaps include the angularis oris artery and vein, they could be considered to be axial pattern flaps.[15] A similar technique is likely to be applicable in cats although studies have not been performed to show this. Random pattern buccal mucosal transposition flaps have been used in the dog to close large rostral hard palate defects.[13,27]

Combinations of hinged flaps in the hard palate and simple advancement flaps of the buccal mucosa are known as the double reposition flap and may be used to achieve a double-layer closure of defects (see Box 56-3).[29] Although single-layer closures may be more prone to dehiscence than double-layer closures, it is often adequate for repair in the absence of tension and if a good blood supply is maintained.[13]

Auricular cartilage free graft

Auricular cartilage provides a scaffold over which granulation tissue can form and subsequent epithelialization can occur and is useful for defects in the hard palate less than 8–10 mm in diameter (Box 56-4).[22] The exposed cartilage generally has epithelial coverage within four weeks. Premature detachment of the cartilage flap is a possible complication.[22]

Box 56-3 Buccal mucosal flaps

The cat is positioned in dorsal recumbency.

Simple advancement flap

Incisions are made in the mucosa and submucosa adjacent to the defect. Sufficient tissue is mobilized to allow a tension-free closure of the defect. The flap is sutured to freshly incised mucoperiosteum surrounding the defect using simple interrupted sutures.

Double reposition flap

A U-incision is placed in the hard palate adjacent to the defect while maintaining mucosal attachments at the base. It is hinged in to the defect and sutured primarily. A simple advancement flap of the buccal mucosa is then created and sutured in to the donor site of the hinged flap, thus creating a two-layer closure (Fig. 56-7).[29]

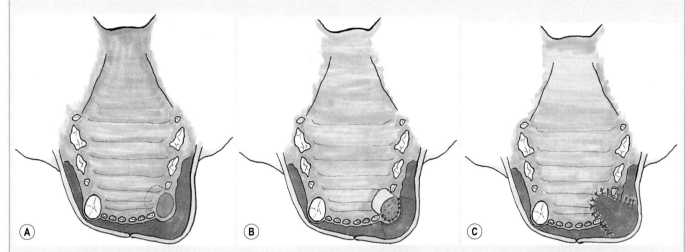

Figure 56-7 Double reposition flap. **(A)** A mucoperiosteal flap is created (dotted line) to hinge it in to the defect. **(B)** The hinged flap is sutured in to the defect and a buccal mucosal advancement flap is created in the adjacent tissue. **(C)** The buccal mucosal flap is used to cover the hinged flap and exposed palatine bone.

Box 56-4 Auricular cartilage free grafts

The cat is positioned in lateral recumbency for harvesting of the free graft, and then dorsal recumbency for the repair of the defect. A skin incision is made over the outer surface of the pinna and a round piece of cartilage excised that is slightly larger than the size of the defect in the palate. The rostral skin and surrounding cartilage is left intact. This does not affect the cosmetic appearance of the ear and closure is routine. Cartilage of the vertical canal has also been used for larger defects up to 8 mm × 10 mm in dimensions. Palatal mucosa is freed around the fistula margins for 2–3 mm to create a pocket for the graft. The auricular cartilage free graft, which is a few millimeters larger than the defect, is inserted into the pocket and secured with a single interrupted suture at the rostral and caudal ends.

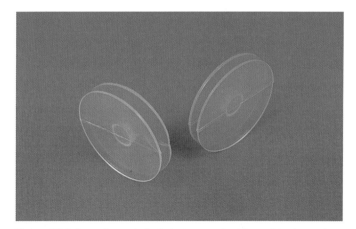

Figure 56-8 A nasal septal silastic button can be trimmed to size and used in palatine defects in the cat. *(Courtesy of Invotec International Inc., Jackson, Florida USA.)*

Temporal muscle transfer

Although temporal muscle transfer has not been reported clinically in cats, it has been described experimentally in association with maxillectomy in cats to reconstruct the defect.[23] This may prove to be a useful clinical technique in cats.

Prosthetic appliances

For oronasal fistulae refractory to surgical reconstruction, or for owners unwilling to go for repeated surgery, prosthetic appliances are an option.[25,26] Silastic buttons used for obturation of nasal septal perforations in humans may be used for 7–25 mm diameter defects in cats (Fig. 56-8).[26] The septal button is trimmed to the appropriate size and placed in the defect under general anesthesia. The button may

be maintained for over 12 months without the need for removal or cleaning, as long as food accumulation between the appliance and mucosa is minimal.[26]

Reconstruction of the soft palate

Methods of reconstruction of defects of the soft palate include soft palate mucosal flaps (Fig. 56-9) and releasing incisions (Box 56-5), buccal mucosal flaps, and pharyngeal wall flaps.[13] Soft palate mucosal flaps and releasing incisions are often used to reconstruct midline cleft palate defects.[13] Similar to releasing incisions in the hard palate mucoperiosteum, releasing incisions may be performed in the soft palate.

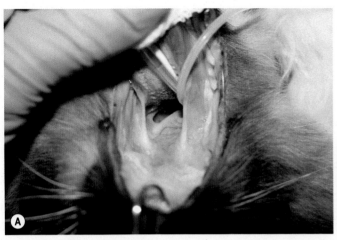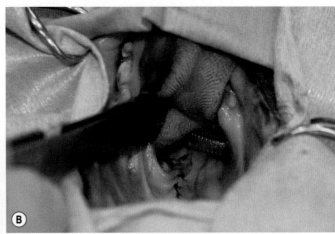

Figure 56-9 (A) Unilateral soft palate defect in a three-year-old female Birman. **(B)** The defect was repaired by incising the edges of the defect and closing the resulting ventral and dorsal flaps separately. A releasing incision was not required. *(Courtesy of Jane Ladlow.)*

Box 56-5 **Reconstruction of the soft palate**

The cat is positioned in dorsal recumbency.

Soft palate mucosal flaps and releasing incisions

Incisions are created in the nasal side and oral side of opposite sides of the defect, up to 5 mm from the edge of the defect.[4,13] Mucosal flaps are elevated from the nasal mucosa on one side and oral mucosa on the other. This requires gentle dissection and sharp scissors, particularly in the cat. The dissection creates two flaps, one based on the nasal side and the other on the oral side of the defect. The soft palate may then be approximated and sutured in two layers (Fig. 56-10). Simple interrupted sutures of a long-acting monofilament absorbable suture material such as polydioxanone are placed with knots on the nasal side and oral side of the nasal and oral mucosa, respectively.[2,4,13]

Buccal mucosal flap

An incision is made in the mucosa with the base at the palatoglossal arch, at the level of the caudal end of the hard palate. The length and width of the flap are determined by the size of the defect. A second mucosal incision is made with the dimensions of the defect in mind. The size of the flap should be larger than the size of the defect to allow for shortening of the flap as it is rotated. Bilateral flaps may be mobilized to allow for oral and nasal mucosal reconstruction. The existing soft palate and nasopharyngeal mucosa is incised to create edges for suturing to the flaps. If the flaps are reconstructing the caudal edge of the soft palate, the caudal edges of both flaps are sutured to each other. The donor sites are closed using a simple interrupted pattern (Fig. 56-11).[17] A vertical mattress suture may be used at the commissure of the lips to protect against dehiscence of the donor site during opening of the mouth.[15] If the angularis oris vessels are included in the flap, it is considered an axial pattern flap (see angularis oris axial pattern flap).[13,15] Use of the angularis oris mucosal axial pattern flap has not yet been reported in cats.

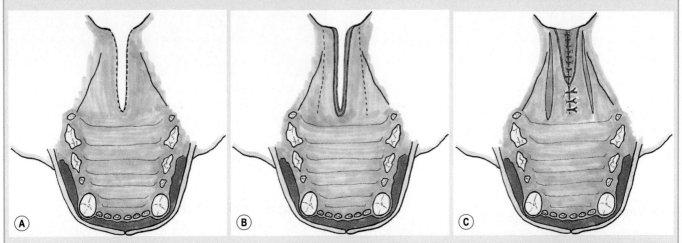

Figure 56-10 Soft palate mucosal flaps and releasing incisions. **(A)** Incisions are created in the nasal and oral side of opposite sides of the defect in the soft palate. **(B)** Two flaps are created, one based on the oral side of the defect and the other on the nasal side of the defect. **(C)** The soft palate is sutured in two layers with suture knots placed on the nasal and oral sides of the repair. Releasing incisions may be extended through the palatine muscles to decrease tension on the repair.

Box 56-5 **Continued**

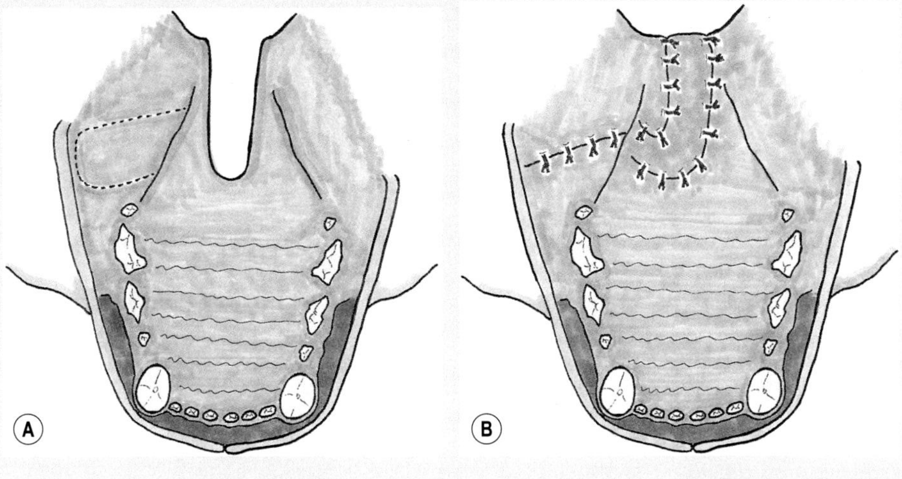

Figure 56-11 Buccal mucosal transposition flap for reconstruction of the soft palate. If the flap includes the angularis oris artery and vein, it is considered an angularis oris axial pattern flap. **(A)** A buccal mucosal transposition flap is created with the base at the palatoglossal arch. **(B)** It may be rotated and sutured to reconstruct large defects extending as far as the caudal edge of the soft palate. The donor site is closed using simple interrupted sutures.

To relieve tension on the subsequent repair, partial-thickness incisions are extended through the oropharyngeal mucosa and muscles of the soft palate, to the caudal edge of the soft palate.[2,13]

Buccal mucosal flaps for the soft palate

Buccal mucosal transposition flaps based at the palatoglossal arches have been used to reconstruct large defects of the soft palate in dogs.[17] It is likely that this technique is applicable to cats (see Box 56-5).

Pharyngeal wall flaps

Bilateral pharyngeal wall flaps and a caudally hinged hard palate mucoperiosteal flap have been used for reconstruction of a bilateral hypoplastic soft palate in a cat.[5] A flap of mucoperiosteum was created in the caudal hard palate, approximately 2 cm in length and extending from the left to right dental arcades. Care was taken to preserve the palatine arteries. The flap was hinged caudally to form the nasopharyngeal mucosa of the reconstructed soft palate. Bilateral pharyngeal wall flaps were then created with the bases extending from the caudal border of the last molar to the cranial border of the tonsillar crypt. The dimensions of each flap were such to allow suturing across the nasopharynx in an 'H-plasty' configuration over the mucoperiosteal flap.[5] Elevation of the flaps occurs deep to the submucosa to preserve the vascular supply.[8] The lateral edges of the mucoperiosteal flap were sutured to the donor defects in the pharyngeal walls. Donor sites in the hard palate and pharyngeal walls were left open.[5,13]

Axial pattern flaps

Axial pattern flaps may be used for reconstruction of the hard or soft palate. The angularis oris axial pattern flap, which has been reported in the dog, is the most versatile axial pattern flap for reconstruction of the palate.[15] A superficial cervical axial pattern skin flap has also been described for use in the palate, but requires use of a dermatome and a staged procedure.[20]

Angularis oris axial pattern flap

The use of the angularis oris buccal mucosal flap has not been reported in the cat but the technique for performing it in the dog is described (Box 56-6). Anecdotally in the author's and others' experiences,

Box 56-6 **The angularis oris pattern flap**

The cat is positioned in dorsal recumbency. The angularis oris artery is a branch of the facial artery that courses from near the cranial border of the masseter muscle to the ipsilateral commissure of the lips (Fig. 56-12). An incision is made through the skin over the artery from the commissure of the lips and extending caudally. The skin is reflected dorsally and ventrally to expose the angularis oris artery and vein. Transillumination has been used in dogs for vessels that are difficult to identify. A full thickness incision is made through the remaining cheek tissue dorsal and ventral to the angularis oris vessels, extending to the caudal extent of the buccal pouch. An island flap may be created by incising the buccal mucosa at the caudal extent of the buccal pouch, being careful not to traumatize the angularis oris vessels, which enter under the cranioventral border of the masseter muscle. The donor site is closed in two or three layers, including a large vertical mattress suture at the commissure of the lips to protect against dehiscence with movement of the jaw. The flap is rotated in to the defect and sutured primarily.[13,15]

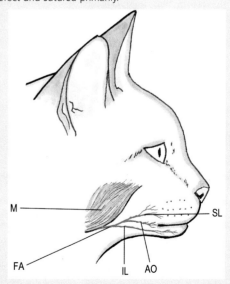

Figure 56-12 Diagram illustrating anatomy of the angularis oris artery in the cat. AO, angularis oris artery; FA, facial artery; IL, inferior labial artery; M, masseter muscle; SL, superior labial artery.

dyspnea is a possible complication in dogs following use of this flap. It is unclear how often this may occur, or if cats may have similar problems. It remains a very useful flap in the dog and may prove to be useful in the cat. In the dog it may reach the contralateral dental arcade, the distal gingival margin of the canine tooth, and the caudal soft palate.[15] Advantages of the flap include its highly vascular and robust character, high degree of mobility, and a surface of tough buccal mucosa.[15]

POSTOPERATIVE CARE

Intravenous fluids should be provided until the animal is eating and drinking, usually within 24 to 48 hours of surgery. Soft food is given for two to four weeks, and chewing on hard objects must be prevented. An Elizabethan collar should be used to prevent pawing at the mouth. Antibiotics are not required in most cases, although they may be used for cases of severe rhinitis. Healing should be evaluated two to four weeks after surgery.[31] Use of a feeding tube should be considered following major repairs (see Chapter 12).[13]

COMPLICATIONS AND PROGNOSIS

Clefts of the secondary palate can interfere with the ability to nurse, and some neonates die of malnutrition or aspiration pneumonia before other signs are recognized.[12] Clefts involving only the distal half of the soft palate are unlikely to result in significant clinical signs.[12] The prognosis for animals that have defects that are amenable to surgery, that are able to wait for surgery, and have no signs of aspiration pneumonia is excellent.[5,21] Even very young animals and animals with large defects can be successfully treated.[4,5] The main complication following surgical correction of a palatal defect is dehiscence of the repair leading to recurrence of clinical signs. Dehiscence may occur repeatedly.[22] Knowledge of the local anatomy and different techniques for reconstruction is vital in managing cases with large defects or dehiscence. A combination of techniques may be required.[5] Complications are minimized by adhering to basic principles of palate surgery, which include making flaps slightly larger than the defects to be reconstructed, maintaining vascularity to the flap, suturing flaps to freshly incised tissue edges, avoiding placement of suture lines over the defect, and gentle tissue handling (Box 56-1).[13]

REFERENCES

1. Evans HE. The digestive apparatus and abdomen. In: Evans HE, editor. Miller's anatomy of the dog. 3rd ed. Philadelphia: WB Saunders Co.; 1993. p. 385–462.

2. Nelson AW. Cleft palate. In: Slatter D, editor. Textbook of small animal surgery. 3rd ed. Philadelphia: Saunders Co.; 2003. p. 814–23.

3. Eubanks DL. Oral soft tissue anatomy in the dog and cat. J Vet Dent 2007;24(2): 126–9.

4. Griffiths LG, Sullivan M. Bilateral overlapping mucosal single-pedicle flaps for correction of soft palate defects. J Am Anim Hosp Assoc 2001;37(2): 183–6.

5. Headrick JF, McAnulty JF. Reconstruction of a bilateral hypoplastic soft palate in a cat. J Am Anim Hosp Assoc 2004;40(1): 86–90.

6. Gregory SP. Middle ear disease associated with congenital palatine defects in seven dogs and one cat. J Small Anim Pract 2000;41(9):398–401.

7. Northrup NC, Selting KA, Rassnick KM, et al. Outcomes of cats with oral tumors treated with mandibulectomy: 42 cases. J Am Anim Hosp Assoc 2006;42(5): 350–60.

8. Peterson NW, Buote NJ. Soft palate cyst in a cat. J Feline Med Surg 2011;13(8): 594–6.

9. Ishikawa Y, Goris RC, Nagaoka K. Use of a cortico-cancellous bone graft in the repair of a cleft palate in a dog. Vet Surg 1994;23(3):201–5.

10. Nguyen PN, Sullivan PK. Issues and controversies in the management of cleft palate. Clin Plast Surg 1993;20(4): 671–82.

11. Hammer DL, Sacks M. Surgical closure of cleft soft palate in a dog. J Am Vet Med Assoc 1971;158(3):342–5.

12. Pope ER, Constantinescu GM. Oral cavity. In: Bojrab MJ, editor. Current techniques in small animal surgery. 4th ed. Baltimore: Williams and Wilkins; 1998. p. 113–50.

13. Sivacolundhu RK. Use of local and axial pattern flaps for reconstruction of the hard and soft palate. Clin Tech Small Anim Pract 2007;22(2):61–9.

14. Noden DM, DeLahunta A. Craniofacial muscles and connective tissues. In: Noden DM, DeLahunta A, editors. Embryology of domestic animals. Baltimore: Williams and Wilkins; 1985. p. 156–95.

15. Bryant KJ, Moore K, McAnulty JF. Angularis oris axial pattern buccal flap for reconstruction of recurrent fistulae of the palate. Vet Surg 2003;32(2):113–19.

16. Harvey CE. Palate defects in dogs and cats. Complend Contin Educ Pract Vet 1987;9:404–18.

17. Sager M, Nefen S. Use of buccal mucosal flaps for the correction of congenital soft palate defects in three dogs. Vet Surg 1998;27(4):358–63.

18. Howard DR, Davis DG, Merkley DF, et al. Mucoperiosteal flap technique for cleft palate repair in dogs. J Am Vet Med Assoc 1974;165(4):352–4.

19. Knight G. Surgical closure of the cleft palate. Vet Rec 1958;(70):680–1.

20. Dundas JM, Fowler JD, Shmon CL, Clapson JB. Modification of the superficial cervical axial pattern skin flap for oral reconstruction. Vet Surg 2005;34(3): 206–13.

21. Robertson JJ, Dean PW. Repair of a traumatically induced oronasal fistula in a cat with a rostral tongue flap. Vet Surg 1987;16(2):164–6.

22. Cox CL, Hunt GB, Cadier MM. Repair of oronasal fistulae using auricular cartilage grafts in five cats. Vet Surg 2007;36(2): 164–9.

23. Cheung LK. An animal model for maxillary reconstruction using a temporalis muscle flap. J Oral Maxillofac Surg 1996;54(12):1439–45.

24. Degner DA, Lanz OI, Walshaw R. Myoperitoneal microvascular free flaps in dogs: an anatomical study and a clinical case report. Vet Surg 1996;25(6):463–70.

25. Coles BH, Underwood LC. Repair of the traumatic oronasal fistula in the cat with a prosthetic acrylic implant. Vet Rec 1988;122(15):359–60.

26. Smith MM, Rockhill AD. Prosthodontic appliance for repair of an oronasal fistula in a cat. J Am Vet Med Assoc 1996;208(9): 1410–12.

27. Banks TA, Straw RC. Multilobular osteochondrosarcoma of the hard palate in a dog. Aust Vet J 2004;82(7):409–12.

28. Beck JA, Strizek AA. Full-thickness resection of the hard palate for treatment of osteosarcoma in a dog. Aust Vet J 1999;77(3):163–5.

29. Ellison GW, Mulligan TW, Fagan DA. A double reposition flap technique for repair of recurrent oronasal fistulas in dogs. J Am Anim Hosp Assoc 1986;22: 803–8.

30. Beckman BW. Split palatal U-flap for repair of caudal palatal defects. J Vet Dent 2006;23(4):267–9.

31. Hedlund CS. Surgery of the oral cavity and oropharynx. In: Fossum TW, editor. Small animal surgery. 2nd ed. St. Louis: Mosby; 2002. p. 274–307.

Chapter |57|

Eyelids and orbit

C.E. Plummer

The feline eye exhibits a variety of diseases that are not seen or are uncommon in other species. There are a few specific indications for surgical procedures of the periocular structures and orbit and this chapter will focus on these. For further details of intraorbital and corneal surgery the reader is referred to specific ophthalmology texts and the current literature as these techniques often require specialized equipment and training.

SURGICAL ANATOMY

Eyelids

Eyelids are composed of several different tissue types. The outer layer of haired skin covers a tarsal plate and musculature, which control the movement and positions of the eyelids. The inner layer adjacent to the globe is the palpebral conjunctiva, a thin, vascular tissue resembling a mucous membrane. The eyelids function to protect and support the globe. This is achieved by three methods: (1) they act as an initial defense against external dangers due to the presence of an active blink reflex; (2) they remove dirt and debris from the surface of the eye; and (3) they contribute portions of the tear fluid and distribute it across the ocular surface.[1-5]

The skin of the eyelids is thinner and more pliable than in other parts of the integument to allow for ease of movement. The thin subcutaneous tissue attaches the skin to the deeper orbicularis oculi muscle, which controls eyelid closure. Additional subcutaneous muscles allow for elevation of the upper eyelid (*corrugators supercilii medialis* medially and *frontoauricularis* laterally and the *Müller muscle*) and elongation of the palpebral fissure (*retractor anguli oculi lateralis*).[1,3,4] Meibomian (or tarsal) glands are present along the margins of both the upper and lower eyelids and are responsible for producing the lipid fraction of the pre-ocular tear fluid. Their oily product exits through a series of openings that appear as little grey dots along the lid margin. Cilia, or eyelashes, are not normally present in the cat, although occasionally distichiasis, i.e., lashes that exit through the meibomian gland openings, are noted. Conjunctival goblet cells produce mucin, which is also a component of the tear fluid.

The eyelids are innervated by branches of the facial nerve (sympathetic fibers and motor function) and by branches of the trigeminal nerve (sensory function). The majority of the vascular supply to the eyelids originates at the lateral and medial canthi from branches of the superficial temporal, the external ethmoidal, and infraorbital arteries. Lymphatic drainage from the eyelids is primarily to the parotid and mandibular lymph nodes.[1,4]

Orbit

The feline orbit is relatively deep and, although it is not completely formed of bone, it provides considerable coverage and protection for the globe. The bones that compose the orbital walls in the cat include the sphenoid, maxillary, lacrimal, zygomatic, and frontal bones. The orbit is incomplete caudoventrally and laterally; the lateral aspect of the orbital rim is completed by the thick, fibrous orbital ligament, and the caudoventral and lateral walls of the orbit, which do not consist of bone, are bordered by the temporal, masseter, and pterygoid muscles. The small bony portion of the orbital floor in the cat consists of a thin shelf of maxillary bone, which holds the last molar teeth. A thick layer of fascial endorbita (periorbita) lines the inner bony and soft tissue margins of the orbit. The contents of the orbit include the globe with its muscular attachments, which originate at the orbit's apex and traverse the orbit to insert on the globe, anterior to its equator. These muscles consist of four bellies of the retractor bulbi muscle, which envelop the optic nerve along its path from the optic foramen to the posterior aspect of the globe, four rectus muscles, and two oblique muscles. The ventral oblique muscle is unique in that its origin is the medial orbital wall.

An extensive vascular supply is present in the orbit, most of which consists of various branches of the maxillary artery and their respective venous vessels which pass through the rostral alar foramen, the most ventrally situated foramen. The internal ophthalmic artery enters the orbit through the optic foramen with the optic nerve. The third, fourth, branches of the fifth, and the sixth cranial nerves, along with some autonomic fibers, enter the orbit through the orbital foramen and provide both sensory and motor innervation. The zygomatic salivary gland is small and lies close to the maxillary nerve near the ventral floor of the orbit. The nictitating membrane, or third eyelid,

DOI: 10.1016/B978-0-7020-4336-9.00057-3

inserts in the ventromedial orbit. Adipose tissue fills the remaining space of the orbit and acts as a cushion to support the globe.[1-3]

GENERAL CONSIDERATIONS

When evaluating a cat for eyelid or periorbital conditions the signalment, in particular the age and breed of the cat, is relevant. A full history should be obtained from the owner in relation to how long the problem has been present, vaccination history, and history of concurrent disease such as rhinitis, history of trauma, etc. A full investigation of eye problems should include an intraocular examination and evaluation of vision.[3,5]

Eyelid evaluation

Evaluation of the eyelids should begin with an appreciation of symmetry between the two eyes. Is the abnormality unilateral or does it affect both eyelids? Is the patient able to perform a complete blink when tactilely stimulated to do so (palpebral reflex)? Are swellings or ulcerations present? Mass lesions are often obvious, but many neoplastic lesions in cats will be tissue destructive rather than proliferative; squamous cell carcinoma is the classic example. Has the globe position deviated resulting in passive eyelid instability, as occurs with enophthalmos and secondary entropion? Secondary blepharospasm is common with painful disorders of the eyelids and this spastic trigeminal–facial nerve reflex may worsen the appearance of an eyelid defect. Prior to and as part of the planning for surgical approaches to eyelid abnormalities, a topical anesthetic should be applied to the eye in the conscious animal (prior to general anesthesia and sedation) in order to allow determination of the extent of the underlying structural problem. If the surgical plan is made without taking into account the aggravating effects of blepharospasm, an inappropriate repair may result.

The eyelids in the cat are tightly apposed to the globe and allow very little visualization of structures posterior to the corneoscleral limbus. Compared to the dog, there is little redundancy of eyelid tissue and facial skin, which makes blepharoplastic procedures more challenging.

For inflammatory and potentially neoplastic conditions, skin scrapings, fine needle aspirates or biopsies for histopathologic examination and microbiologic evaluation are usually indicated. If there is suspicion of systemic disease then virology or hematologic and biochemical analysis of blood may be necessary.

If a neoplastic condition is determined to be present, staging with thoracic and abdominal imaging and lymph node aspirates (see Chapter 14) may be indicated, depending upon the expected biologic behavior of the tumor.

Orbit evaluation

Evaluation of the orbit should begin with an external examination assessing globe position, symmetry, and globe mobility, followed by palpation of the orbital margins and retropulsion of the globe. If there is resistance to digital palpation and retropulsion, or the cat is unable to retract the globe, a retrobulbar space-occupying lesion is likely and imaging should be pursued to determine the character and the extent of the disease process. Inflammatory diseases of the orbit are often accompanied by pain when the extraocular muscles and globe are retracted, when the globe is retropulsed, or upon opening of the mouth. With cystic and neoplastic lesions, the retropulse reflex is impaired, but usually elicits no significant discomfort.

Diagnostic imaging

If surgical intervention in the orbit is anticipated, additional diagnostic procedures are recommended. B-scan ultrasonography of the orbit may provide useful information about the impact of the orbital disease on the globe and will often provide guidance for sampling of a lesion, but computed tomography (CT) and magnetic resonance imaging (MRI) are better options to delineate the extent and borders of the disease.[6,7] A study in a cat that compared orbital echography, skull radiography, CT, and MRI to assess a mass involving the orbit showed that MRI was the only technique that delineated the entire border of the tumor.[8]

Histopathology

Prior to surgical intervention, histopathologic evaluation of a biopsy specimen is advised to facilitate surgical and postoperative treatment planning. Depending upon the exact location of the lesion within the orbit, sampling may be performed posterior to the bony orbital rim or via the oral cavity. Since the ventral orbital floor is bordered only partially by bone, the soft tissue posterior to the last molar may be incised in order to access the ventral orbit. A scalpel blade is used to incise the mucosa and a hemostat is gently and bluntly introduced through the incision, through the pterygoid musculature and the periorbita into the orbit for blind sampling. Expansive lesions may extend into the oral cavity and may be grossly appreciable upon examination of the mouth. Care must be taken to avoid damaging the maxillary artery as it courses along the orbital floor.[1,2]

If a diagnosis of a malignant process in the orbit is determined, the patient should have thoracic and abdominal imaging and potentially aspirates of the regional lymph nodes performed for staging purposes (see Chapter 14).

SURGICAL DISEASES OF THE FELINE EYELIDS

Most eyelid disorders in cats will be the result of either congenital and developmental abnormalities or neoplastic diseases. Inflammatory conditions occur uncommonly and may be associated with infectious agents (*Demodex*, dermatophytoses, myiasis, FHV-1), autoimmune disorders (pemphigus, lupus, eosinophilic complex disease), or trauma and exposure to irritating compounds (drug reactions).[3]

Ankyloblepharon

Ankyloblepharon is fusion of the eyelids to one another. It is physiologic in the kitten until postnatal days 10–14.[4] If the eyelids remain closed beyond this time, this indicates either incomplete development of the eyelids and periocular structures or more likely viral conjunctivitis (infection acquired from the queen either during parturition or during the first few days following birth) that has resulted in conjunctival adhesions or symblepharon. When an infection is introduced to the conjunctival space beneath the fused eyelids, neonatal ophthalmia results, which requires manual (premature) opening of the palpebral fissure. Often these kittens will have gross swelling of their orbits and eyelids and may have purulent discharge exiting through a small rent in the palpebral fissure. If the lids are left apposed when such an infection is present, the ocular surface will be irreparably damaged and vision will be significantly impaired if not lost completely.

To open the lids, first topical anesthesia should be applied to the lid margins and then one side of a small scissor or a mosquito hemostat is placed through the rent in the fissure and gently advanced and

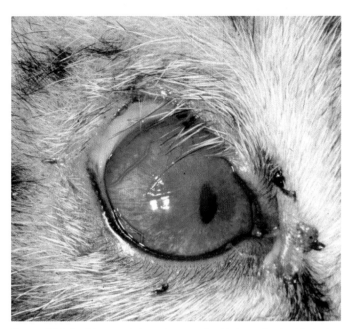

Figure 57-1 Eyelid agenesis in a nine-month-old domestic short-haired cat. The dorsotemporal eyelid margin is absent and trichasis is present. There is also keratitis, evidenced by corneal vascularization.

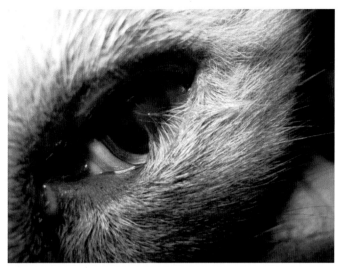

Figure 57-2 Lower lid lateral canthal entropion in an eight-month-old domestic short-haired cat.

elevated along the fused lid margins to break the adhesion. It is not recommended to cut the fissure since it is very easy to miss the line of fusion and cut the tiny lids themselves. Once the palpebral fissure is open, copious flushing should be performed to remove as much debris and infectious material as possible. Topical antibiotics and lubricants should be applied frequently thereafter (every four hours) because the blink reflex and tear production are usually underdeveloped at this young age. If there are corneal ulcerations present when the lids are opened, treatment with a topical antiviral medication, such as idoxuridine or cidofivir, should be started.

Eyelid agenesis

The incomplete formation of a portion of the eyelid is known as eyelid agenesis or coloboma (Fig. 57-1). It is usually associated with an absent eyelid margin.[3] The severity of this condition varies dramatically among affected individuals.[9] The majority of cases have absent lid tissue and margin along the temporal portion of the dorsal eyelid. Severe cases may have most of the upper lid missing, including the lateral canthus and portions of the lower lid as well. Mild cases may be managed medically with regular lubrication if minimal ocular irritation is present. Most cases, however, benefit from surgical reconstruction of the abnormal lids in order to provide greater coverage for the globe and to minimize discomfort from exposure and scarring that can impair vision. In many cases, ocular irritation will occur not only due to absent tissue and an impaired blink mechanism, but also as the result of trichiasis, in which hair from the face is deviated toward the cornea. Cats with eyelid agenesis often will have other ocular abnormalities including microphthalmia, cataract, retinal dysplasia, and keratoconjunctivitis sicca.[9] A thorough ophthalmic examination should be performed to determine the extent of this congenital disorder.

The surgical approach to this condition will vary depending upon the severity. In some cases, simple apposition of the normal margins will suffice; other cases will require sliding advancement grafts (see Boxes 57-4 and 57-5) or grafts of tissue from either the lower eyelid

or the commissure of the lip. Various surgical techniques have been employed.[1,10-14]

Entropion

Most cases of eyelid malposition in cats are because of entropion, i.e., the inversion of the eyelid margin rolling toward the globe.[3,15,16] Medial canthal entropion is almost universal in brachycephalic cats and is one of the causes of tear overflow and staining at the medial corners.[1,3] In these cases, if irritation is minimal and the face can be kept sufficiently clean, surgical repair is not always necessary. In cats that develop full lid or lateral entropion, surgical correction is indicated.[1,3,4,15] Most cats with entropion are only affected along the lower eyelid and occasionally at the lateral canthus (Fig. 57-2). Careful evaluation of the eyelid anatomy in affected cats is warranted since many cases have not only entropion, but also excessive length to their lower eyelid. In these cases shortening of the lower eyelid with a wedge resection may augment the repair.[16] Ectropion, or eversion of the eyelid, is exceedingly rare in cats, and typically only results from cicatrix formation.

Eyelid neoplasia

Since eyelid neoplasms in cats are usually malignant, it is fortunate that they are relatively uncommon, occurring with significantly less frequency than cutaneous neoplasms elsewhere on the body.[17,18] The prevalence of eyelid neoplasia increases with age in cats, but has not been found to correlate with breed or gender. The most common eyelid neoplasm in cats is squamous cell carcinoma. Other reported tumors include mastocytomas (Fig. 57-3), hemangiosarcomas and hemangiomas, fibrosarcomas, various neoplasms of glandular origin (adenomas, adenocarcinomas), basal cell carcinomas (Fig. 57-4), peripheral nerve sheath tumors, lymphomas, and others.[3,17,18] Squamous cell carcinomas usually appear as ulcerated lesions along the eyelid margin with a crusting surface (Fig. 57-5). White cats seem to have a predilection for the development of this tumor.[19] There is evidence for the role of actinic damage in the pathogenesis of this tumor.

Squamous cell carcinomas are amenable to various forms of treatment and wide surgical excision is often curative, although grafting procedures are usually necessary to fill the resultant defect of excision. Most other types of feline eyelid neoplasm are also amenable to

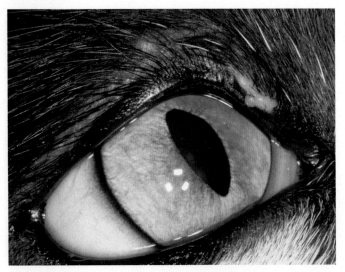

Figure 57-3 An 11-year-old domestic short-haired cat with an eyelid mast cell tumor.

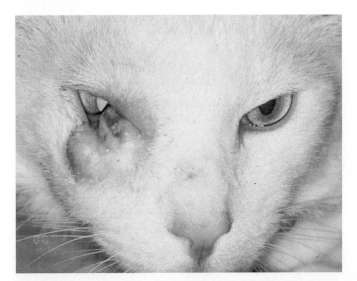

Figure 57-4 A 12-year-old domestic short-haired cat with an eyelid myxosarcoma.

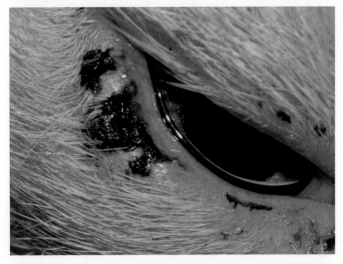

Figure 57-5 A nine-year-old domestic short-haired cat with an eyelid squamous cell carcinoma.

surgical excision, with variable recurrence rates.[1,3,17] Mast cell tumors of the eyelids in cats generally respond favorably to surgical excision. A recent retrospective study described results in 33 cats with periocular mast cell tumors, and reported that recurrences were rare and affected cats had a median survival time of 945 days.[20] Plesiotherapy with strontium-90 is another treatment option, either as a sole modality or in combination with surgical excision, that has excellent success rates.[20,21] However, extensive lesions or disseminated disease may be best approached with systemic chemotherapy rather than excision or local radiation in cats.[20] Cystic structures at the medial canthus that are benign and resemble apocrine hidrocystomas are occasionally noted in brachycephalic cats.[18,22] Recurrence is common following local excision of these lesions, according to the authors' experience and that of other veterinary ophthalmologists.[18]

SURGICAL DISEASES OF THE FELINE ORBIT

In the normal state, the feline eye rarely develops traumatic corneal ulcerations, exposure keratitis, and many of the other ocular conditions frequently diagnosed in other species. However, the feline orbit is relatively small, so when disease states occur, there is very little room for expansion or swelling. Early deviation (exophthalmos, strabismus, protrusion of the nictitans membrane) of the eye and the orbital contents is frequently accompanied by exposure keratitis, conjunctivitis, and chemosis. Brachycephalic individuals tend to have more shallow orbits and prominent globes, which may predispose them to even earlier exposure issues.

Orbital neoplasia

The most common disorders of the feline orbit are neoplastic proliferations. They tend to be malignant (90%) and usually of epithelial origin.[3] Squamous cell carcinomas are the most frequently reported orbital tumors in cats, followed by lymphoma (Fig. 57-6), fibrosarcoma and various bone tumors (Fig. 57-7).[23] At least fifteen different tumor types have been reported within the feline orbit.[23,24] Treatment strategies for each vary upon the extent of the lesion and the known or supposed biologic behavior of that type of tumor. Conservative surgical approaches to orbital neoplasms, which attempt to maintain the globe and vision, are usually associated with unacceptably high rates of tumor recurrence. Hence, the treatment of choice for orbital neoplasia is usually exenteration (see Box 57-7), which involves removal of the entire contents of the orbit including the globe. Orbitotomy techniques that spare the globe and seek to remove focal abnormalities within the orbit are rarely indicated in the cat and should be considered only in the case of small, well-defined lesions (preferably non-neoplastic or at least non-malignant). Advanced imaging of the head in cases of orbital neoplasia is strongly recommended because the incidence of concurrent orbital, nasal and sinus disease is high due to the close proximity of these spaces in cats.

Proptosis

Unfortunately, because of the rigid nature of the orbital support, when a traumatic insult is sustained and the globe suffers injury, the great amount of force necessary to affect the globe usually results in significant damage, which may be vision or globe threatening. Proptosis, or the capture of the eyelid margins behind the equator of the globe (Fig. 57-8), usually with anterior displacement of the globe, is often associated with significant facial and orbital trauma and fractures of the

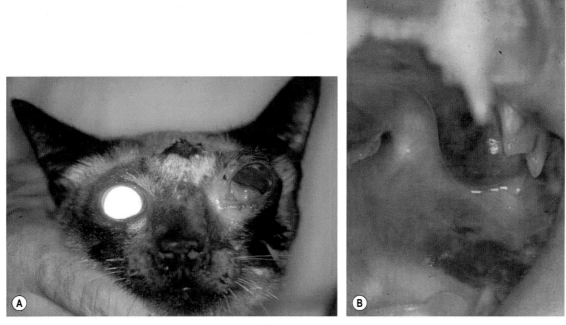

Figure 57-6 (A) A 12-year-old Siamese-cross with orbital lymphoma. **(B)** A bulging mass lesion and hemorrhage was noted posterior to the last upper maxillary molar upon oral examination of the cat.

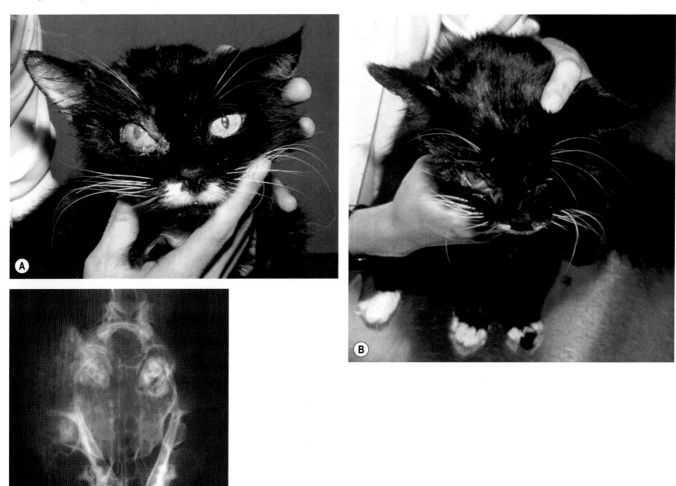

Figure 57-7 Osteosarcoma in a 14-year-old cat. **(A)** There is exophthalmos, dorsolateral strabismus and elevation of the third eyelid. **(B)** Viewed from above the anterior deviation of the globe can be better appreciated. **(C)** Radiograph shows extensive bony lysis of the orbit.

695

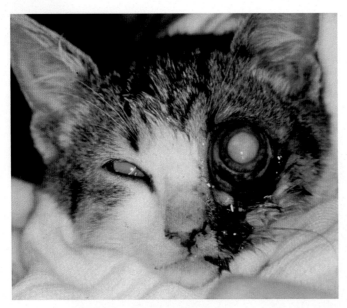

Figure 57-8 Traumatic proptosis in a kitten.

skull and mandible.[25] In most cases of traumatic proptosis in the cat, the affected globes are rendered non-visual and are so severely damaged that they require enucleation.[1] The contralateral eye may also be blinded by damage to the optic chiasm from the stretching forces placed upon the affected globe.[3] These cats are usually seriously injured and collapsed and should be triaged and treated first for shock, head-trauma, and concussive brain injury. If the globe can be salvaged, it should be kept well lubricated until the cat is stable enough to undergo anesthesia and a temporary tarsorrhaphy performed to provide for its protection.

Orbital inflammatory disorders

Orbital inflammatory disorders are fortunately uncommon in the cat. Orbital cellulitis and abscessation may be associated with trauma, foreign bodies, dental disease, extension of inflammatory nasal or sinus disease (especially if infectious), and rarely, immune-mediated inflammation.[3,26] Most of these conditions respond appropriately to medical therapy when the underlying etiology is recognized and treated. Surgical therapy is usually only indicated if it is necessary to establish drainage in the orbit (see above for details on accessing the retrobulbar space for diagnostics), to protect the globe if the function of the eyelids is impaired and the proper distribution of the tear film is not possible (temporary tarsorrhaphy), or to remove the eye if it has been irreparably damaged (enucleation). Most inflammatory orbital conditions that result in exophthalmos are associated with orbital, ocular, and oral pain and most patients have an inflammatory leukogram and may be febrile. The exception is the condition known as idiopathic sclerosing orbital disease or orbital pseudotumor.[26-28] This disorder has been diagnosed with increasing frequency of late and usually has an insidious onset. Clinical signs include exophthalmos, progressively decreasing ocular mobility, and exposure keratitis. The orbital tissues and eyelids become fixed in place by fibrous tissue. It begins in one eye but eventually progresses to involve both. Response to therapy (immunosuppressive therapy and radiation) is generally poor and enucleation is often necessary when the exposure keratitis progresses to ulceration and perforation.

PREPARATION FOR EYELID AND ORBITAL SURGERY

Due to the proximity of the lids to the sensitive ocular structures, preparation of the surgical site must differ somewhat from other sites on the body. Rather than cleaning and rinsing the eyelids with alcohol, chlorhexidine and other traditional sterilizing agents, which can be incredibly irritating and damaging to the corneal and conjunctival epithelia, it is recommended that a dilute (1:50) solution of povidine-iodine (solution, not scrub) be used to cleanse the site.[29] At least three scrubs of the skin with swabbing of the conjunctival fornices are recommended, followed by liberal rinsing of the site with normal saline.[1] Routine perioperative antibiotics (such as intravenous cefazolin) are useful to limit the incidence of peri- and postoperative infection.

Regional anesthesia is not a necessary adjunct to general anesthesia for eyelid procedures. And, in fact, the infusion of lidocaine or other injectable anesthetic agents may distort the anatomy of the eyelid and alter the results of the procedure. Once the surgical site has been prepared, care must be taken to ensure that the globe remains lubricated throughout the duration of the procedure. Artificial tear or broad-spectrum antibiotic (triple antibiotic combination) ointments can be applied sparingly. If these interfere with the surgical procedure, sterile saline may be used to repeatedly and frequently moisten the eye.

If an orbital procedure such as enucleation or exenteration is to be performed, a retrobulbar block may be considered. These blocks are more difficult to perform in cats than in other species due to limited retrobulbar space in the feline orbit. It can be difficult to achieve proper placement of the injection. There are several approaches to this block, but no matter which procedure is chosen, it is critical that the dose of local anesthetic be calculated carefully to avoid toxicity.[1,30,31] A 1.5–2.5 inch 22 gauge needle that has been bent to the approximate curve of the orbit wall can be inserted ventrolateral or dorsal to the globe through either the conjunctiva (for subconjunctival enucleations) or through the eyelid skin after cleaning and preparation (for transpalpebral enucleations) and advanced past the globe in a ventromedial direction towards the opposite temporomandibular joint until the base of the orbit is encountered. Regional retrobulbar and peribulbar anesthesia runs the risk of hemorrhage, globe perforation, intravascular or subarachnoid injection, and vagal reactions, but can significantly decrease the depth of general anesthesia necessary and decrease postoperative pain.[1,30,31]

SURGICAL TECHNIQUES AND MANAGEMENT OF EYELID DISEASE

Initial management of a developmental or neoplastic eyelid problem is in most cases surgical, with adjunctive medical support.[1] If a surgical procedure for the feline eyelid is to be performed, the surgeon should primarily consider the requisite functions of the eyelid and aim to restore or improve that function, not just the cosmetic appearance of the eye.

Tarsorrhaphy

A temporary tarsorrhaphy (Box 57-1) is the requisite surgical procedure for proptosed eyes that are salvageable and is also indicated when an orbital condition has resulted in exophthalmos and corneal exposure or if a facial paralysis has developed which impairs the animal's ability to blink and protect its globe.[1,2,25] The tarsorrhaphy should be left in place until the blink reflex returns and the orbital swelling has resolved; in most cases this will be a matter of two to four weeks. It is preferable to remove one tarsorrhapy suture at a time, rather than all at once, so that at least partial support for the globe is maintained for an extended time.

Simple lid mass resection

If a lesion to be removed involves less than one-third of the margin of the eyelid, simple full thickness resections are typically indicated (Box 57-2).

Modified Hotz–Celsus

The most commonly employed approach to entropion in the cat is to perform a modified Hotz–Celsus procedure (Box 57-3). The length and shape of the skin-orbicularis oculi incisions vary depending upon the amount and area of the entropion correction necessary (Fig. 57-11).

Combination Hotz-Celsus with lateral wedge resection

If lower lid entropion is accompanied by excessive lid length, the modified Hotz-Celsus procedure may be combined with a lid

---

Box 57-1 **Tarsorraphy**

The cat is positioned in sternal recumbency and the eye aseptically prepared for surgery. If the eyelid margins are caught behind the equator of the globe (e.g., with a proptosed eye), a lateral canthotomy will be necessary to release them. With blunt-tipped tenotomy, strabismus or Metzenbaum scissors, a 5–10 mm full thickness lateral canthotomy incision is made (perpendicular to the lateral canthus, as if extending the palpebral fissure laterally). The lids are then lifted from their inverted posture and repositioned in their normal anatomic position. The canthotomy incision is then closed with 4/0 or 5/0 non-absorbable suture with a figure-of-eight suture (Fig. 57-9A) at the margin of the lateral canthus, followed by interrupted sutures of the same material to close the remainder of the incision. Next, two or three horizontal mattress sutures are preplaced along and across the palpebral fissure with 4/0 non-absorbable suture material. These sutures should be placed only partial thickness through the eyelid; care should be taken not to go through the palpebral conjunctiva so that the suture does not contact the cornea when the fissure is closed. When there is tension on the lids, as in the case of a proptosis or extensive orbital swelling, stents should be employed to minimize damage to the eyelid skin and the potential for pull-through (Fig. 57-9B). Portions of sterilized rubber bands or intravenous tubing are useful for this purpose. The horizontal mattress sutures should be tightened slowly and the lids lifted over the exposed globe rather than the globe being pushed back into the orbit.

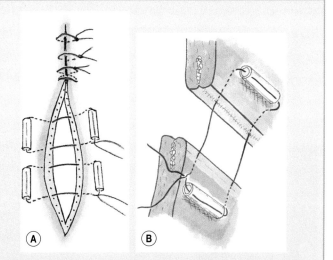

Figure 57-9 Temporary tarsorrhaphy. The lid fissure is closed with two or three horizontal mattress sutures, prevented from cutting into the skin by stents (e.g., infusion tubing). **(A)** If a canthotomy has been performed, it is closed with a figure-of eight suture at the margin and simple interrupted sutures for the length of the incision. **(B)** These sutures should be placed only partial thickness through the eyelid. Using 4/0 or 5/0 non-absorbable suture on a cutting or micropoint needle. (In the diagram the suture is shown loose and untied so the placement of the suture is clear. In the cat the suture will appose the eyelids – no suture should contact the cornea.)

Box 57-2 **Eyelid mass resection**

The cat is positioned in lateral recumbency and prepared for aseptic surgery. There are two options to consider.

Triangular wedge resection[1,4]

An incision is made with tenotomy scissors through the full thickness of the eyelid on either side of the defect or neoplasm so that the incisions intersect away from the lid margin (Fig. 57-10A).

The four-sided or 'house' technique[32]

Two parallel incisions are made on either side of the defect to be repaired or removed. These incisions should be perpendicular to the eyelid margin and palpebral fissure. Two additional incisions are then made to connect the initial cuts in an intersecting manner (as with the wedge). This procedure provides a larger surface area to distribute tension associated with wound apposition (Fig. 57-10B).

Closure

For either technique described above, the defect is then closed in two layers. The first a deep tarso-conjunctival layer with a simple continuous pattern of 5/0 to 6/0 absorbable suture. Care must be taken to ensure that the suture does not penetrate through the palpebral conjunctiva as corneal abrasions and ulcerations can result. The external layer is apposed with 5/0 non-absorbable suture in an interrupted pattern. The first suture placed in this repair is at the eyelid. This suture is the most critical for ensuring proper alignment and should be a figure-of-eight suture (Fig. 57-10C; a modification of the cruciate mattress suture). The remainder of the skin layer can be closed routinely with simple interrupted sutures (Fig. 57-10D,E).

Box 57-2 **Continued**

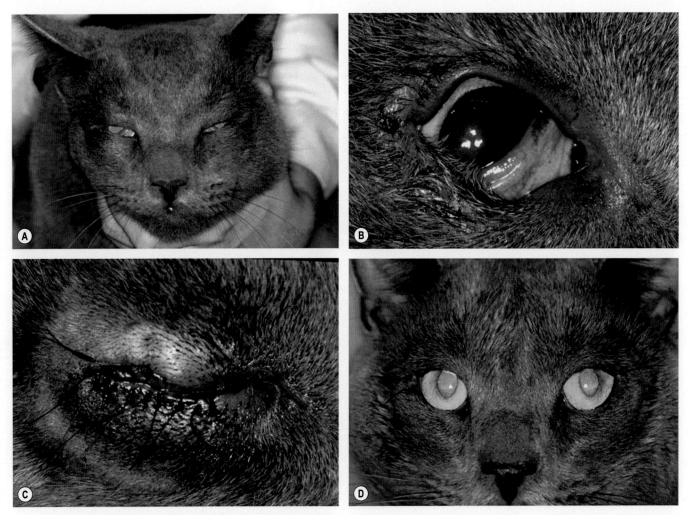

Figure 57-10 Simple lid resection. **(A)** A full-thickness wedge of tissue is removed. **(B)** A four-sided excision may decrease tension along the repaired incision line. **(C)** The first suture should be placed to appose the eyelid margin. A figure-of-eight suture, which is essentially a modified cruciate mattress suture, will accomplish this nicely. **(D)** The deep layer should not penetrate through the palpebral conjunctiva. **(E)** Final appearance.

Figure 57-11 (A) Bilateral lower eyelid entropion in an un-neutered male cat. **(B)** Trichiasis has occurred as a result of the lid inversion. **(C)** Immediate postoperative appearance after correction of the entropion with Hotz–Celsus. **(D)** Postoperative appearance at suture removal.

shortening procedure.[16] The excessive length of the lower lid is estimated or measured with Jameson calipers. If the patient is only unilaterally affected with entropion, it can be helpful to measure the length of the lower lid of the non-affected eye for comparison. When the surgeon has determined how much to shorten the eyelid length, a full-thickness wedge resection is performed (see Box 57-2) in the lateral lower eyelid. The eyelid margin is then apposed with a

figure-of-eight suture of 5/0 non-absorbable material. The modified Hotz-Celsus (see Box 57-3) is then performed as usual.

Sliding skin graft

The sliding skin graft, or H-plasty, is employed when a traumatic or surgical defect involves greater than one-third of the eyelid margin

Box 57-3 **Modified Hotz–Celsus** (Fig. 57-12)

The cat is placed in lateral recumbency and prepared for aseptic surgery. A lid plate is placed behind the eyelid to prevent full thickness incisions through the eyelid and damage to the globe. The initial incision is made 1–2 mm from the eyelid margin (usually where the skin pigmentation stops and the skin hair begins) through the skin into the orbicularis oculi muscle. The length of this incision will depend upon the length of the lid that is affected by inversion. A second elliptical incision that joins to the ends of the first incision is made ventral (or proximal) to the first; the width is dependent upon the amount of tissue that needs to be removed to evert the eyelid into its normal position. The delineated segment of skin with a small amount of underlying muscle is removed with tenotomy scissors. The orbicularis muscle in cats may be difficult to discern; as long as the skin is excised fully, a sufficient amount of adjacent muscle should accompany it. The resultant defect is then closed with 5/0 non-absorbable suture in a simple interrupted pattern. Closure of the incision should begin in its center and split the distance between sutures until it is completely closed and sutures are 1–2 mm apart. The suture knots should be directed away from the globe or the near tags cut short and the far tags left longer to facilitate removal. As the incision heals, wound contraction will result in an additional 0.5–1 mm eversion.

The Hotz–Celsus procedure can be modified further for medial entropion (Fig. 57-12D), such as is common in brachycephalic animals. A triangular incision is made at the medial canthus in the lower eyelid wherein the tip of the triangle is opposite the lower lacrimal punctum. This incision should not be deeper than the orbicularis muscle or damage to the nasolacrimal puncta and canaliculus can occur. Closure is routine with a simple interrupted 5/0 non-absorbable repair.

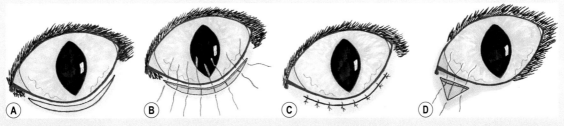

Figure 57-12 Modified Hotz–Celsus. **(A)** An elliptical incision delineates the tissue to be removed. **(B)** The skin and a small portion of the underlying orbicularis oculi muscle is excised. One suture is initially placed in the center of the surgical eyelid wound and then the subsequent sutures placed. **(C)** Final appearance of Hotz-Celsus repaired with simple interrupted sutures. **(D)** Modification of the Hotz-Celsus for focal medial canthal entropion.

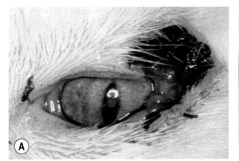
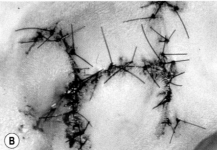
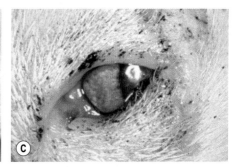

Figure 57-13 **(A)** Squamous cell carcinoma affecting the eyelid at the lateral canthus. **(B)** Immediate postoperative appearance after excision of the neoplasm and repair of the resultant defect with two sliding skin advancement grafts, one in the upper lid and one in the lower lid. **(C)** Postoperative appearance. The palpebral fissure is shortened, but the lids are functional and there was complete excision of the tumor.

(Box 57-4).[1,4] This procedure is appropriate for both upper and lower eyelid repairs (Fig. 57-13).

Roberts–Bistner procedure and modifications

Although there are innumerable surgical approaches to the correction of eyelid agenesis in the cat, the most common is the Roberts–Bistner procedure (Box 57-5), or a modification thereof. This procedure involves transplanting a myocutaneous pedicle from the lower eyelid beneath the margin into the upper lid defect (Fig. 57-15).[11] The donor area on the nictitans is left to heal by second intention. The base of the conjunctival pedicle is transected three to four weeks following the initial surgery. This can usually be accomplished with topical anesthesia alone, negating the need for a second episode of general anesthesia.

Lip-to-lid resection

The lip-to-lid procedure (Box 57-6) is useful for grafting of large defects in the lower eyelid following resection of neoplastic lesions[33,34] (Fig. 57-17).

ORBITAL SURGERY

Because there is limited peribulbar space in the feline orbit, surgical procedures are more difficult to perform than in other species.[1,3]

Box 57-4 The sliding skin graft

After full thickness excision of the lesion, two slightly diverging incisions are made with a scalpel blade in the eyelid, that are approximately twice as long as the height of the defect (Fig. 57-14A). Two equal sized triangles of skin are removed at the proximal tips of both incisions to accommodate the shifting of the graft into the defect. After liberal dissection to separate the skin graft from its underlying subcutaneous attachments, the graft is advanced into the defect, which will collapse the triangles (Fig. 57-14B). The graft should be advanced 0.5–1 mm beyond the normal margin of the

eyelid to compensate for postoperative shrinkage and secured with 5/0 non-absorbable simple interrupted sutures (Fig. 57-14C). The sliding skin graft should be lined on its underside with mucosa, either adjacent conjunctiva that can be recruited or free grafts of conjunctiva from elsewhere or free grafts of buccal mucosa. This lining should be attached to the posterior aspect of the skin flap with 6/0 absorbable suture in a simple continuous pattern so that the knots are either buried or exposed on the skin side. A temporary tarsorrhaphy is helpful if there is tension on the advancement graft.

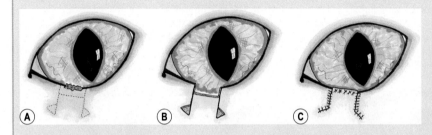

Figure 57-14 Sliding advancement graft. **(A)** The margins of the graft to be advanced are determined by the size of the lesion. **(B)** Two triangular pieces of skin are removed at either side of the graft's base to prevent dog-ears. **(C)** Once advanced, the graft is sutured in place and the triangles closed.

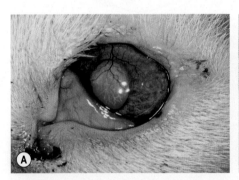
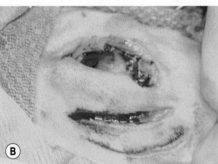
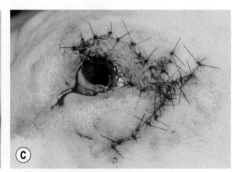

Figure 57-15 (A) Eyelid agenesis in the cat. Note the trichiasis and the extensive corneal vascularization. **(B)** Intraoperative appearance of eye during harvesting of myocutaneous graft during Roberts-Bistner repair of eyelid agenesis. **(C)** Immediate postoperative appearance.

Box 57-5 The Robert–Bistner procedure

The recipient bed is first prepared by dividing the lid skin that is present from the palpebral conjunctiva with either a scalpel blade or a pair of Westcott scissors (Fig. 57-16A). A scalpel blade is then used to make an initial incision in the skin 2–3 mm ventral to the lower eyelid margin that is slightly longer than the length of the upper lid defect (Fig. 57-16B). A second parallel incision should provide a pedicle that is 1.0 mm wider than the height of the upper lid defect. This pedicle is elevated with scissors and should include skin and orbicularis oculi

musculature. It is then rotated into the upper lid defect and sutured in place with 5/0 simple interrupted non-absorbable sutures (Fig. 57-16C). The donor bed is reapposed similarly. If there is sufficient conjunctiva separated from the recipient bed during preparation of the site, it should be used to cover the posterior aspect of the graft and sutured to the new lid margin with 6/0 absorbable suture in a simple continuous pattern with the knots either buried or exposed on the skin surface.

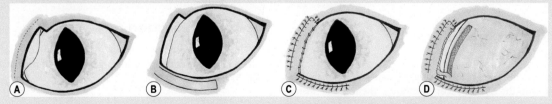

Figure 57-16 Myocutaneous graft repair of eyelid agenesis. **(A)** The recipient bed is prepared by dissecting the underlying conjunctiva away from the eyelid skin. **(B)** A pedicle of skin and orbicularis oculi muscle is harvested from the lower eyelid. **(C)** The skin graft is sutured in place in the recipient bed. **(D)** The Dziezyc–Millichamp modification harvests a pedicle of conjunctiva from the anterior face of the third eyelid to line the posterior surface of the skin graft. The conjunctival pedicle is left attached at its base laterally. The conjunctival defect on the third eyelid will be left to heal by second intention.

Box 57-5 **Continued**

Modifications

Modification of this technique utilizes conjunctiva from other sources if there is not enough available from the recipient bed. The Dziezyc–Millichamp modification proceeds as above, but the conjunctiva used to line the posterior surface of the skin graft is recruited from the anterior face of the nictitating membrane (Fig. 57-16D).[20] A pedicle graft of conjunctiva with its base at the lateral aspect of the nictitans is prepared with scissors then rotated 180° and apposed to the posterior surface of the skin graft and secured in place with 6/0 to 7/0 absorbable suture in a simple continuous pattern.

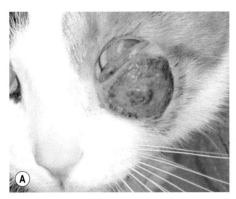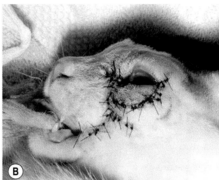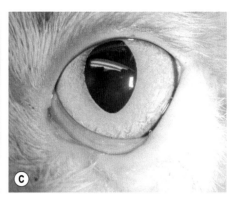

Figure 57-17 **(A)** Basal cell carcinoma of the lower eyelid. **(B)** Immediate postoperative appearance following excision of the neoplasm and repair of the resultant defect with a lip-to-lid graft. **(C)** Postoperative appearance of eyelid margin following lip-to-lid repair. Mild ectropion is present.

Box 57-6 **Lip-to-lid** (Fig. 57-18)

For this procedure it is helpful to draw the proposed incisions with a marking pen before committing to the cuts. The lesion to be removed should be excised from the lower lid full thickness in its entirety with tenotomy or Metzenbaum scissors. Two parallel incisions are made through the lip at a 45° angle to the commissure of the lip beneath the lower eyelid. Once enough oral mucosa has been exposed and elevated with the lip graft so that when placed into the recipient bed the missing conjunctiva is replaced, the oral mucosa should be carefully split so that it remains within the oral cavity while the skin graft from above continues to be harvested for transfer. The rostral aspect of the lip graft incision is continued so that it connects with the medial aspect of the eyelid defect. The graft is carefully undermined and rotated into the position of the former eyelid margin. The oral mucosal defect is apposed with 4/0 absorbable suture in a simple continuous pattern. The graft is initially sutured in place by apposing its oral mucosa to the remaining conjunctival edges with 6/0 buried simple interrupted absorbable sutures. The cutaneous surface of the graft is sutured in a simple interrupted pattern with 5/0 non-absorbable material. The cutaneous donor bed is closed similarly to repair the defect in the lip.

A modification of this technique that places the lateral commissure of the lip in place of the lateral canthus to correct eyelid agenesis has been described.[14]

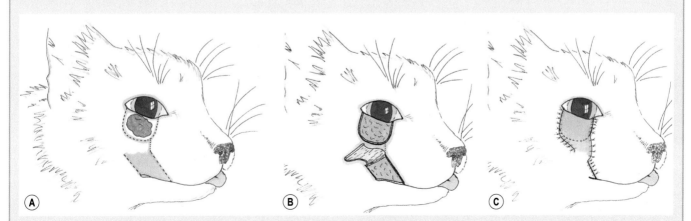

Figure 57-18 Lip-to-lid resection. **(A)** The tissues to be excised and transposed are delineated. **(B)** A section of lip with oral mucosa is elevated. The oral mucosa is split, when enough has been harvested with the skin graft, to replace the conjunctival defect to be created with the lid excision. Once the eyelid defect has been created, the incisions between the lip and the lid defects are connected. **(C)** The lid graft is rotated into position and sutured in place. The remaining oral mucosa is reapposed.

Enucleation

Enucleation or removal of the globe, the eyelid margins, and the nictitating membrane and its associated gland, is indicated in many different situations (Box 57-7).

There are two main approaches to removal of the globe, the subconjunctival technique and the transpalpebral technique[1] (Box 57-8). The transpalpebral technique is recommended in cases of ocular neoplasia or intraocular or ocular surface infections in order to decrease the chances of extension of disease into adjacent tissues.[35] In all other instances, the choice of which procedure to perform is surgeon preference, although the subconjunctival technique is reported by most surgeons to be more rapid and associated with less intra and postoperative hemorrhage.[1] Also, the subconjunctival technique may be preferable in cats as a matter of course since tissues are often easier to identify with this approach.[36] In cases of refractory glaucoma wherein the globe has become enlarged, limiting the already limited space in the orbit, it may be helpful to place a small gauge needle (30 or 25 gauge) into the anterior chamber at the corneoscleral limbus to remove a small amount of aqueous humor to make the globe smaller and facilitate manipulation of the globe within the orbit. If this is done, the globe may become somewhat flaccid which can make

---

Box 57-7 **Indications for enucleation**

- Intraocular tumors are present that are not amenable to local excision and are still confined within the globe, especially if they have resulted in secondary glaucoma
- Intraocular infections have destroyed the globe and are potential sources of systemic infection
- Proptosis of the globe has occurred with extensive damage to the globe, rupture of multiple extraocular muscles or severing of the optic nerve
- Intraocular inflammation has destroyed the globe, resulted in blindness and pain
- Glaucoma is uncontrolled with medical therapy, especially if buphthalmos is causing problems with corneal exposure
- Extensive trauma to the globe or corneal defects that do not have the possibility of successful repair
- Congenital defects, such as microphthalmia when sight is not present, result in chronic problems like conjunctivitis and keratitis

---

Box 57-8 **Enucleation**

The cat is positioned in lateral recumbency and prepared for aseptic surgery.

Subconjunctival enucleation (Figs 57-19A,B,C)

With blunt-tipped tenotomy, strabismus or Metzenbaum scissors, a 5–10 mm full thickness lateral canthotomy incision is made (perpendicular to the lateral canthus, as if extending the palpebral fissure laterally). This will facilitate exposure of the globe. The nictitating membrane may be removed at this time or following removal of the globe. The nictitating membrane is grasped and retracted with forceps to allow visualization of its deep extent. Two small hemostats are clamped at its base from either side and then it, along with the gland at its base, is excised with Mayo scissors. Next the bulbar conjunctiva in incised 3–5 mm posterior to the limbus with curved tenotomy, strabismus or blunt-tipped Metzenbaum scissors. This incision is extended 360° around the globe. Blunt dissection is then performed underneath the bulbar conjunctiva posterior to this incision until the insertions of the extraocular muscles are identified. The transection of these muscles is facilitated by introduction of a small muscle hook to elevate the muscle from the sclera. The tendinous insertions of all four rectus muscles are cut, followed by transection of the oblique and retractor bulbi muscle insertions. The globe should at this time be mobile and may displace forward slightly. There should be sufficient room to maneuver a small curved hemostat behind the globe to clamp the optic nerve and its adjacent vasculature. With curved Metzenbaum or enucleation scissors, the optic nerve is severed anterior to the hemostat. If there is not enough room for both instruments behind the globe, which is often the case in cats, then the nerve should be clamped for a moment, then the hemostat removed followed by transection of the nerve with the scissor. In most cases, it is not necessary to place a ligature on the stump of the nerve and blood vessels. The globe is removed and the orbit inspected. Bleeding vessels that can be identified may be addressed with ligatures or point cautery. Direct pressure with a surgical sponge may stop or slow diffuse oozing.

Next, 4–6 mm of the eyelid margins, including the lateral and medial canthi are removed with scissors and any remaining conjunctiva within the orbit is removed at this time.

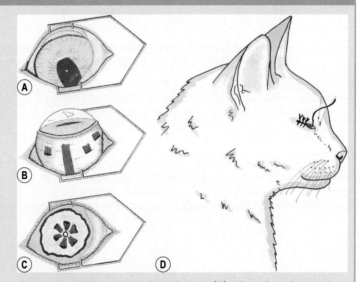

Figure 57-19 Subconjunctival enucleation. **(A)** A lateral canthotomy is performed to facilitate exposure. **(B)** A 360° incision in the conjunctiva is made. Blunt dissection underneath the conjunctiva will expose the insertions of the extraocular muscles which are transected. **(C)** Once the muscular attachments of the globe have been severed, the optic nerve is clamped, then transected and the globe is removed. **(D)** The margins of the eyelids are removed prior to a two-layer closure.

Transpalpebral enucleation

The palpebral fissure is sutured closed with 4/0 to 5/0 non-absorbable suture in a simple continuous pattern (Fig. 57-20A). If the tags of suture are left long on either side of the fissure, they can be grasped with hemostats to facilitate exposure of the surgical site. The eyelid skin is then incised circumferentially with a scalpel blade approximately 4–6 mm from the margins (to avoid the base of the glands in the lid margin). Care must be taken to incise the skin

---

Box 57-8 **Continued**

and subcutaneous tissues alone, without penetrating through the palpebral conjunctiva. Once the submucosa of the conjunctiva is reached and identified, blunt dissection with curved tenotomy, strabismus or Metzenbaum scissors will continue posteriorly above the conjunctiva until the fornices are passed and the sclera can be visualized. The extraocular muscles are identified and transected (Fig. 57-20B). Once all the extraocular muscles are transected, the optic nerve is clamped, transected and the globe is removed (Fig. 57-20C).

Enucleation closure (Figs 57-19D and 57-20D)

If a silicone implant (see Chapter 10) is to be placed within the empty orbit, it should be prepared by soaking in betadine solution followed by roughening or scarification by several incisions with a scalpel blade to roughen its surface and improve its orbital retention. The implant will then be placed within the orbit and a mesh of suture placed across the orbit from the dorsal to ventral orbital rims to facilitate its positioning. A simple continuous pattern of 3/0 to 4/0 absorbable suture will span the orbit over the implant with bites taken along the orbital rims through the periorbita. If no implant is to be placed, this meshwork may still be placed in an attempt to minimize the depression of skin into the empty orbit that results from loss of orbital contents. A standard two-layer closure of the remaining subcutaneous tissue and skin over the orbit is then performed. The subcutaneous tissues should be apposed with 4/0 to 5/0 absorbable suture in a simple continuous pattern. The skin may then be apposed with either 4/0 to 5/0 non-absorbable interrupted sutures or 4/0 to 5/0 absorbable suture in an intradermal pattern. If skin sutures are to be removed, they should remain in place for at least 10-14 days following surgery.

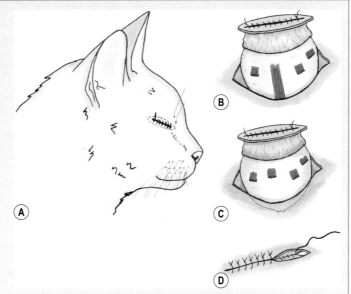

Figure 57-20 Transpalpebral enucleation. **(A)** The eyelids are sutured closed prior to the initial incision and an elliptical incision is made around the closed palpebral fissure. **(B)** Blunt dissection of the subcutaneous layers is performed until the insertions of the extraocular muscles are identified and transected at their origins. Care must be taken to avoid entering the conjunctival space surrounding the ocular surface when performing this dissection. **(C)** Once all the extraocular muscles are transected the optic nerve is clamped, then transected and the globe is removed. **(D)** Closure is in two layers.

Box 57-9 **Exenteration**

The cat is positioned in lateral recumbency for surgery and prepared aseptically. The palpebral fissure is sutured closed with 4/0 to 5/0 non-absorbable suture in a simple continuous pattern. If the tags of suture are left long on either side of the fissure, they can be grasped with hemostats to facilitate exposure of the surgical site. The eyelid skin is then incised circumferentially with a scalpel blade approximately 4–6 mm from the margins (to avoid the base of the glands in the lid margin). Care must be taken to incise the skin and subcutaneous tissues alone, without penetrating through the palpebral conjunctiva. Once the submucosa of the conjunctiva is reached and identified, blunt dissection with curved tenotomy, strabismus or Metzenbaum scissors

will continue posteriorly above the conjunctiva until the fornices are passed and the sclera can be visualized. The initial incision is extended caudally through the orbicularis oculi muscles of the eyelids and the orbital fascia toward the orbital rim. The extraocular muscles are incised as close to their origins as possible and the optic nerve is clamped and severed as in a routine enucleation. A periosteal elevator may be used to remove the periorbita from the orbital bones and the orbital lacrimal gland from the dorsal orbit. Once the globe and its associated tissues are removed, remaining connective tissue and fat within the orbit may be excised if necessary. Closure is as in a routine enucleation.

delineation of its margins more difficult during the procedure, so care should be taken not to unwittingly damage the globe during its dissection. It is imperative to avoid excessive traction on the globe during enucleation in the cat. The retrobulbar optic nerve (from the posterior globe to the optic chiasm) is relatively short and traction on the diseased globe during its removal may damage the optic chiasm and the opposite optic nerve, rendering the patient blind.[1,3]

Exenteration

Exenteration (Box 57-9) involves the removal of not only the globe, but also the extraocular muscles and periorbita. This technique is usually indicated when there is orbital neoplasia (Fig. 57-21). The orbital depression that results from exenteration is more marked that that following enucleation alone. In cases of exenteration which

require removal of more skin that the eyelid margins alone and there is insufficient skin left to close the orbital defect, a caudal-auricular axial pattern flap may be used (see Chapter 19).[37]

POSTOPERATIVE CARE

Eyelid surgery

The most important part of the postoperative care of patients that have undergone some form of blepharoplasty is diligent attention to preventing self-trauma and dehiscence of the suture line. The importance of this for the success of the procedure should be stringently stressed to the caretaker. Rigid Elizabethan collars are the most common

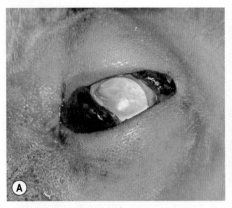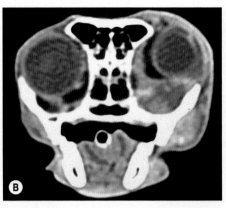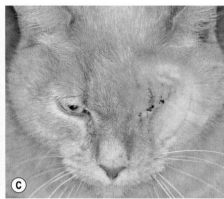

Figure 57-21 (A) A 12-year-old domestic short-haired cat with exophthalmos, chemosis and conjunctival hyperemia resultant from an undifferentiated orbital sarcoma. Note the dilated pupil which suggests damage to the optic nerve and the dull, lackluster appearance of the cornea, an indication that the ability to blink has been compromised. **(B)** Computed tomographic scan shows a mass in the ventral orbit causing exophthalmos. **(C)** Postoperative appearance two weeks following exenteration.

means to limit the patient's ability to disturb the surgical site. Topical lubricants and broad-spectrum antibiotics are usually employed to minimize the likelihood of irritation to the ocular surface and infection of the surgical site. Systemic antibiotics following surgery are not usually necessary if appropriate perioperative antibiotics are used unless an infectious process is present at the time surgery is performed. If the patient is systemically able to tolerate non-steroidal anti-inflammatory agents, such as meloxicam, these are helpful to minimize pain and tissue swelling. Skin sutures should be left in place for at least ten to 14 days, preferably longer, as premature removal of sutures can result in dehiscence and lid defects and may necessitate additional surgery.

Orbital surgery

If proper sterile and careful surgical technique is employed in orbital procedures, the postoperative recovery of the patient is usually uneventful. If preoperative retrobulbar anesthesia is administered (see Chapter 2), the requisite postoperative analgesia will be minimized. If they are not contraindicated by a systemic condition, non-steroidal anti-inflammatory agents administered systemically usually significantly improve patients' postoperative comfort. Systemically administered antibiotics are usually unnecessary if perioperative antibiotics are given, unless there is concern because an infectious process necessitated the orbital surgery or removal of the globe. Postoperative

swelling may be decreased with prompt and repeated (as long as it is tolerated) application of a cold compress to the surgical site.

COMPLICATIONS AND PROGNOSIS

Eyelids

Complications of eyelid surgery may include suture dehiscence, infection, recurrence of the original problem, trichiasis, corneal ulceration, swelling, and discomfort. Cats latently infected with FHV-1 may suffer from recrudescent disease (conjunctivitis, corneal ulcers, upper respiratory signs) initiated by the stress of general anesthesia, hospitalization, and treatment.

Orbit

The most common complications following enucleation and exenteration are hemorrhage and infection.[1,2,35,36] In globe sparing procedures, damage to the globe, persistent displacement or deviation of the globe, exposure keratitis, corneal ulcerations that may progress or be slow to heal, keratoconjunctivitis, blindness, and recurrence or progression of the primary disease process (tumor recurrence, recrudescence of infection, etc.) are possible. Prognosis is highly dependent upon the etiology of the disorder.

REFERENCES

1. Gelatt KN, Gelatt JP. Small animal ophthalmic surgery. Oxford: Butterworth-Heinemann; 2001. p. 46–124.

2. Spiess BM. Diseases and surgery of the canine orbit. In: Gelatt KN, editor. Veterinary ophthalmology. Ames: Blackwell; 2007. p. 539–62.

3. Stiles J, Townsend WM. Feline ophthalmology. In: Gelatt KN, editor. Veterinary ophthalmology. Ames: Blackwell; 2007. p. 1095–164.

4. Stades FC, Gelatt KN. Diseases and surgery of the canine eyelid. In: Gelatt KN, editor. Veterinary ophthalmology. Ames: Blackwell; 2007. p. 563–617.

5. Ollivier FJ, Plummer CE, Barrie KP. Ophthalmic examination techniques. In: Gelatt KN, editor. Veterinary ophthalmology. Ames: Blackwell; 2007. p. 438–83.

6. Calia C, Kirschner SE, Baer KE, Stefanacci JD. The use of computed tomography scan for the evaluation of orbital diseases in cats and dogs. Vet Comp Ophthalmol 1994;4:24–7.

7. Grahn BH, Stewart WA, Towner RA, Noseworthy MD. Magnetic resonance imaging of the canine and feline eye, orbit, and optic nerves and its clinical application. Cn Vet J 1993;34:418–24.

8. Ramsey D, Gerding PA, Losonsky JM, et al. Comparative value of diagnostic imaging techniques in a cat with exophthalmos. Vet Comp Ophthalmol 1994;4:198–202.

9. Belhorn RW, Barnett KC, Henkind P. Ocular colobomas in domestic cats. J Am Vet Med Assoc 1971;159:1015–21.

10. Roberts SR, Bistner SI. Surgical correction of eyelid agenesis. Mod Vet Pract 1968;49:40–3.

11. Dziezyc J, Millichamp NJ. Surgical correction of eyelid agenesis in a cat. J Am Anim Hosp Assoc 1989;25:513–16.

12. Wolfer J. Correction of eyelid coloboma in four cats using subdermal collagen and

a modified stades technique. Vet Ophthalmol 2002;4:269–72.

13. Esson D. A modification of the mustarde technique for the surgical repair of a large feline eyelid coloboma. Vet Ophthalmol 2001;4:159–60.

14. Whittaker CJ, Wilkie DA, Simpson DJ, et al. Lip commissure to eyelid transposition for the repair of feline eyelid agenesis. Vet Ophthalmol 2010;13:173–8.

15. Williams DL, Kim JY. Feline entropion: a case series of 50 affected animals (2003–2008). Vet Ophthalmol 2009;12:221–6.

16. Read RA, Broun HC. Entropion correction in dogs and cats using a combination Hotz-Celsus and lateral wedge resection: results in 311 eyes. Vet Ophthalmol 2007;10:6–11.

17. McLaughlin SA, Whitely RD, Gilger BC, et al. Eyelid neoplasia in cats: a review of demographic data (1979–1989). J Am Anim Hosp Assoc 1993;29:63–7.

18. Newkirk KM, Rohrbach BW. A retrospective study of eyelid tumors from 43 cats. Vet Pathol 2009;46:916–27.

19. Dorn CR, Taylor DO, Schneider R. Sunlight exposure and risk of developing cutaneous and oral squamous cell carcinoma in white cats. Journal of the National Cancer Institute 1971;46:1073–8.

20. Montgomery KW, van der Woerdt A, Aquino SM, et al. Periocular cutaneous mast cell tumors in cats: evaluation of surgical excision (33 cases). Vet Ophthalmol 2010;13:26–30.

21. Turrel JM, Farrelly J, Page RL, et al. Evaluation of strontium 90 irradiation in treatment of cutaneous mast cell tumors in cats: 35 cases (1992–2002). J Am Vet Med Assoc 2006;228:898–901.

22. Cantaloube B, Raymond-Letron I, Regnier A. Multiple eyelid apocrine hidrocystomas in two persian cats. Vet Ophthalmol 2004;7:121–5.

23. Gilger BC, McLaughlin SA, Whitley RD, Wright JC. Orbital neoplasms in cats: 21 cases (1974–1990). J Am Vet Med Assoc 1992;201:1083–6.

24. Attali-Soussay K, Jegou JP, Clerc B. Retrobulbar tumors in dogs and cats: 25 cases. Veterinary Ophthalmology 2001;4:19–27.

25. Gilger BC, Hamilton HL, Wilkie DA, et al. Traumatic ocular proptoses in dogs and cats: 84 cases (1980–1993). J Am Anim Hosp Assoc 1995;206:1186–90.

26. Van der Woerdt A. Orbital inflammatory disease and psuedotumor in dogs and cats. Vet Clin North Am Small Anim Pract 2008;38:389–401.

27. Billson FM, Miller-Michau T, Mould JR, Davidson MG. Idiopathic sclerosing orbital pseudotumor in 7 cats. Vet Ophthalmol 2006;9:45–52.

28. Bell CM, Schwarz T, Dubielzig RR. Diagnostic features of feline restrictive orbital myofibroblastic sarcoma. Vet Pathol 2010. [Epub ahead of print]

29. Apt L, Isenberg S, Yoshimori R, Paez JH. Chemical preparation of the eye in ophthalmic surgery. III. Effect of povidone-iodine on the conjunctiva. Arch Ophthalmol 1984;102(5):728–9.

30. Ahmad S, Ahmad A, Benzon HT. Clinical experience with the peribulbar block for ophthalmic surgery. Region Anesthes 1993;18:184–8.

31. Skarda RT, Tranquilli WJ. Local and regional anesthetic and analgesic techniques: cats. In: Tranquilli WJ, Thurmon JC, Grimm KA, editors. Lumb and Jones veterinary anesthesia and analgesia. 4th ed. Ames: Blackwell; 2007. p. 595–603.

32. Peiffer RL. Four-sided excision of canine eyelid neoplasms. Journal of Canine Practice 1979;6:35–8.

33. Pavletic MM. Mucocutaneous subdermal plexus flap from the lip for lower eyelid restoration in the dog. J Am Vet Med Assoc 1982;180:921–6.

34. Hunt GB. Use of the lip-to-lid flap for replacement of the lower eyelid in five cats. Vet Surg 2006;35:284–6.

35. Wolf E. Enucleation of the globe. In: Bojrab M, editor. Current techniques in small animal surgery. Philadelphia: Lea & Febiger; 1990. p. 119–23.

36. Kuhns E. Enucleation of the eye by subconjunctival ablation. Vet Med Small Anim Clin 1976;71:1433–40.

37. Stiles J, Townsend W, Willis M, et al. Use of a caudal auricular axial pattern flap in three cats and one dog following orbital exenteration. Vet Ophthalmol 2003;6:121–6.

Chapter |58|

Neurocranium

B.P. Meij

Intracranial tumors are relatively common in cats. Due to availability of advanced imaging techniques like computed tomography (CT) and magnetic resonance imaging (MRI), a confirmed diagnosis of intracranial neoplasia is being made possible in an increasing number of affected patients. Furthermore, developments in the field of veterinary neurology, anesthesia, emergency and critical care, neurosurgery, and radiotherapy have resulted in an improved prognosis following treatment. However, the biggest challenge for the veterinary surgeon is early diagnosis of feline intracranial neoplasia, when clinical signs may be non-specific, which would improve the outcome of neurosurgery and radiation therapy.

This chapter will cover surgical therapy of brain tumors, and other operable neurocranial diseases in cats.

SURGICAL ANATOMY

The skull and brain

The feline skull is somewhat more accessible than the canine skull due to less overlying muscle and a thinner calvarium. Also, the increased mobility of the skull in relation to the cervical spine facilitates the caudal approach because it is possible to position and stabilize the cat's skull in hyperflexion. The function of the feline skull is to protect the brain. The brain can be divided into three large regions: cerebrum, cerebellum, and brainstem.[1] The cerebrum consists of the paired cerebral hemispheres that are separated by a longitudinal fissure. The cerebral hemispheres are composed of cerebral cortex (gray matter) and underlying white matter. Each cerebral hemisphere contains a lateral ventricle that communicates with the third ventricle through an interventricular foramen. The olfactory nerve originates from the rostral extensions of the cerebrum, the olfactory bulbs. The other cranial nerves originate from the brainstem. The cerebellum is separated from the cerebrum by a transverse fissure that holds the tentorium. The brainstem occupies the middle and caudal fossae of the floor of the cranial vault and is continuous with the spinal cord. It contains the third and fourth ventricle. The thalamus, subthalamus, hypothalamus, and epithalamus are components of the brainstem. The hypothalamus is connected to the hypophysis, which resides in the pituitary fossa bordered rostrally by the tuberculum sphenoidalis and caudally by the dorsum sellae. The third ventricle runs deep into the posterior lobe (Fig. 58-1) of the pituitary gland. The pituitary gland is composed of the anterior lobe and a neurointermediate lobe. In the cat, the pars intermedia is a prominent layer, which can be visualized by immunohistochemical staining (Fig. 58-1).

Vascular supply

The major venous sinuses into which the veins of the brain drain are the basilar, paired transverse, confluens, and dorsal sagittal sinuses. The locations of these sinuses are generally used as landmarks for the various surgical approaches to the brain and care should be taken to avoid them. The middle meningeal artery and its rostral and caudal branches supply the dura and the adjacent portions of the skull. The ethmoidal artery reaches the dura after passing through the ethmoidal foramen and runs between the cribriform plate and olfactory bulb. The internal carotid arteries and the basilar artery give rise through the caudal communicating arteries to the arterial cerebral circle (of Willis) at the base of the brain with the hypophysis at its center (Fig. 58-2). Arterial branches sprouting from the circle constitute the arterial supply to the brain. Rostral, middle, and caudal cerebral arteries originate from the circle and run between the gyri in the sulci. Also, the cerebellum receives blood from the circle by way of the rostral cerebellar artery. The anterior lobe of the hypophysis has no direct arterial supply but receives blood from the median eminence through long portal veins. The neurointermediate lobe receives a direct arterial supply from the fused caudal intercarotid arteries and the caudal hypophyseal artery. These run partly in the rostral intercavernous sinus and perforate the dura to connect directly to the neural lobe.[2]

GENERAL CONSIDERATIONS

Brain and the mass effect

Cats with signs attributable to a suspected intracranial mass may present in several ways and the clinical signs may represent different underlying causes (Box 58-1).

© 2014 Elsevier Ltd
DOI: 10.1016/B978-0-7020-4336-9.00058-5

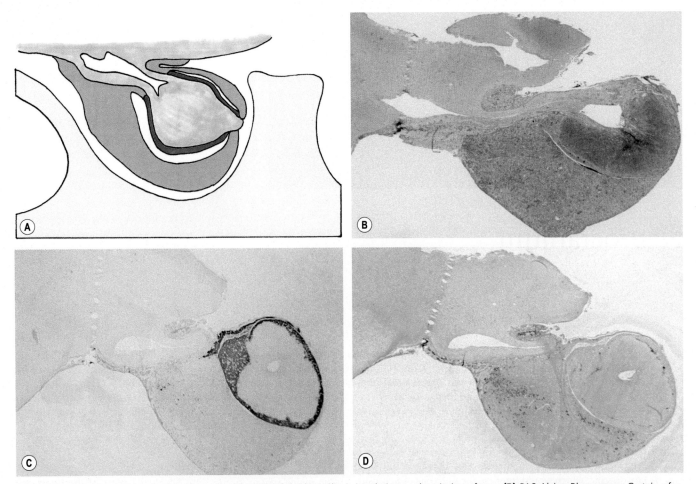

Figure 58-1 (A) Schematic sagittal median representation of the hypophysis in relation to the pituitary fossa. **(B)** PAS-Alcian Blue-orange G stain of a sagittal section of the cat pituitary. The third ventricle runs deep into the posterior lobe (blue), which is surrounded by a thin rim of pars intermedia. Sections of the cat pituitary stained with an antibody against **(C)** α-melanocyte stimulating hormone and **(D)** adrenocorticotropin, which illustrates that in the cat the anterior lobe extends upwards around the pituitary stalk. *(Courtesy of Professor A. Rijnberk and Dr H.S. Kooistra.)*

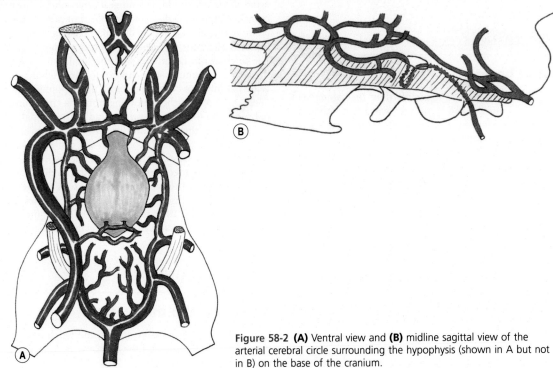

Figure 58-2 (A) Ventral view and **(B)** midline sagittal view of the arterial cerebral circle surrounding the hypophysis (shown in A but not in B) on the base of the cranium.

1. Primary mass effects due to the intracranial tumor
2. Secondary effects of a mass in the bony calvarium that is affecting adjacent 'normal' brain tissue
3. An endocrine disorder due to an endocrine-active tumor, e.g., pituitary adenoma
4. A combination of the above

Clinical signs

The cat with an intracranial tumor is a diagnostic challenge since the mass effects can initially be absent or very subtle and clinical signs vary from mild depression to secondary epilepsy.[3-5] Also, pituitary adenomas in cats manifest themselves by endocrinologic syndromes (diabetes mellitus, acromegaly, and/or Cushing's syndrome) that may delay the diagnosis of a large intracranial pituitary mass.[6] For further details on clinical signs in pituitary adenomas with endocrine syndromes, please see Chapter 35 and the sections below (Cushing's disease and acromegaly).

Historical findings in cats with intracranial tumors (other than functional pituitary adenomas) include subtle to overt altered behavior (e.g., hiding, personality changes, lethargy, poor appetite, disorientation, and aggressive behavior), seizures, impaired vision, weakness (para-, hemi- or tetraparesis), and altered consciousness (e.g., depressed, obtunded, stuporous, or comatose).[7,8] The severity of clinical signs depends on the tumor location, size, invasiveness, and growth rate. For example, tumors close to the cerebellum will cause an ataxic gait whereas tumors close to the optic chiasm will impair vision. Behavioral changes (rather than seizures) are often the first and most common findings in cats with brain tumors. In a study of 61 cats with intracranial neoplasia, only 23% had a history of seizures.[8] In another study of 125 cats with recurrent seizures, primary epilepsy was compared with secondary epilepsy in relation to signalment, history, ictal pattern, clinical and neurologic findings. Seizure etiology was classified as primary in 47 (38%) and secondary in 78 (62%) cats. Secondary epilepsy was caused by intracranial neoplasia in only 16 of 78 cats.[9]

Abnormal clinical findings associated with brain neoplasia include weight loss despite normal appetite, decreased and no appetite, decreased thirst, and bradycardia. Neurologic abnormalities include seizures, circling, locomotor disturbances, visual deficits, hearing loss, altered states of consciousness, and head pressing. Acute post-retinal blindness may be the sole neurologic deficit.[10] Neurologic signs alone may be enough for neuroanatomic localization of the tumor. Characteristic neurologic signs of focal intracranial lesions affecting the forebrain (seizures), cerebral cortex (head pressing), thalamus (personality changes, visual deficits), brainstem (cranial nerve deficits), vestibular systems (nystagmus), and cerebellum (ataxia, intention tremor) may help neurolocalization, but precise pinpointing to a specific region is often difficult since neurologic examination in cats may be hampered by their unwillingness to cooperate, absence of cranial nerve deficits and overlap of neurologic signs.

Diagnostic procedures

When an intracranial mass is suspected, the imaging tool of choice is MRI in most instances since mineralization and invasion into bone by brain tumors are rare. However, when MRI is not available contrast-enhanced CT is also a valuable diagnostic tool since brain tumors usually damage the blood–brain barrier, resulting in enhancement of tumor tissue adjacent to unaffected brain tissue. In cases of skull trauma, CT is a better diagnostic procedure than MRI since it gives more information on position of the skull fracture fragments. In cases of brain abscess, MRI or contrast-enhanced CT is diagnostic.

Radiography

Skull radiography is not a valuable diagnostic tool for differentiation or localization of primary intracranial neoplasia, since mineralization and invasion into bone are rare.[5] Exceptions are hyperostosis adjacent to the meningioma with invasion of the calvarium causing erosion or complete calvarial disruption,[11] invasion of the calvarium and brain by local extension (e.g., with skull osteosarcomas, nasal adenocarcinomas, and squamous cell carcinomas of the middle ear), and calcification or mineralization of an intracranial neoplasm (e.g., with meningioma).

Advanced imaging

As definite therapy (surgery, chemotherapy, radiotherapy) requires knowledge of the precise anatomic location and size of the intracranial neoplasm, preoperative CT or MRI is necessary. In rare instances a brain biopsy under image guidance (e.g., free-hand, CT-guided, frame-aided or frameless stereotactic neuronavigation using CT or MRI data) is indicated to determine the histologic type and best treatment option. Cats with suspected metastatic intracranial neoplasia should have further imaging such as thoracic and abdominal CT to identify the primary tumor, to stage the tumor, and check for metastases elsewhere.

MRI is an excellent diagnostic tool for detection of intracranial tumors in cats and it provides important information to aid in the diagnosis of tumor type.[12,13] MRI of the feline cranium has been performed using a low-field open magnet (0.2 Tesla) or a high-field closed magnet (1.5 Tesla).[12] Transverse spin echo T1-weighted, proton density-weighted, and T2-weighted images are usually acquired before contrast injection. Transverse spin echo and gradient echo T1-weighted images can be acquired after intravenous contrast injection (gadolinium dimeglumine, 0.1 mmol/kg).

MRI and contrast-enhanced CT[14,15] are the methods of choice for pituitary imaging as they can confirm the diagnosis of a pituitary tumor (Fig. 58-3). When pituitary surgery is a treatment option, CT is preferred to low-field MRI because of better resolution with modern CT scanners and the ability to precisely define the surgical landmarks.[16] Contrast-enhanced MRI[16,17] and CT[18,19] reveal the pituitary dimensions (height, width, length) and allow for calculation of the pituitary height/brain area (P/B) ratio.[20] However, it must be emphasized that the reference range for non-enlarged (P/B ≤0.31) versus enlarged (P/B >0.31) pituitaries was established for canines, and it is the author's experience that this is somewhat different for felines. The upper normal P/B ratio for the cat is most likely higher and in the range of 0.40, but this still needs to be established. Dynamic CT also allows for visualization of the neurointermediate lobe (NIL), and analysis of its enhancement, the so called 'pituitary flush'. Distortion or displacement of the flush gives insight into lateralization (left/right) or dorsal/ventral localization of the adenoma.[18]

Cerebrospinal fluid analysis

Cerebrospinal fluid (CSF) analysis is rarely diagnostic for intracranial neoplasia but may be performed for purposes of differential diagnosis. The most common CSF abnormality associated with brain tumors is increased protein concentration; however, normal CSF does not preclude neoplasia.

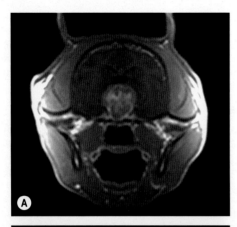

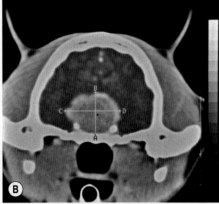

Figure 58-3 **(A)** Transverse T1-weighted MR image in a 10-year-old male European short-hair cat with post-retinal blindness, aggressiveness and hypersensitive behavior shows a large pituitary mass with a diameter of 17 mm. **(B)** Contrast-enhanced transverse CT image in a 14-year-old castrated male domestic short-haired cat presented with mild clinical signs of hyperadrenocorticism and central blindness shows a very large pituitary tumor (A–B = 13.6 mm; C–D = 17.9 mm). CT is superior to MRI for imaging the tumor mass in relation to bony landmarks.

SURGICAL DISEASES

Trauma

Trauma to the feline calvarium occurs frequently and is mainly caused by motor vehicle accidents, penetrating bites or gunshot wounds, falls, and kicks.[5] Severe trauma is generally necessary to cause significant brain injury due to the protective musculature and calvarium. More than 50% of head trauma patients have associated injuries including thoracic trauma (pulmonary edema, pneumothorax, contusion) and fractures (spine, pelvis, long bones, mandible, maxilla).[5] Diagnostic imaging of head trauma patients should include thoracic radiographs to assess for thoracic abnormalities.

The cat's state of consciousness is usually altered to some degree (depressed, obtunded, stuporous, or comatose). Cats with head trauma should be carefully examined and both a general and neurologic examination should be frequently repeated to assess ongoing pulmonary and myocardial changes and intracranial damage. Ischemia and hemorrhage in damaged brain disrupts cell-membrane integrity by release of free radicals. Electrolyte disturbances in the damaged brain can cause brain edema, which increases ischemia and hypoxia. Both brain edema and accumulation of blood increase intracranial pressure, decrease perfusion pressure, increase hypoxia and cause further ischemia.

Medical treatment should be the first line of treatment in head trauma patients and is directed at reversing brain edema, hypoxia, ischemia, and increased intracranial pressure and preventing infection. Stuporous or comatose cats presented with head trauma should be initially treated with appropriate fluid therapy to maintain systolic blood pressure. The cat should be placed in an oxygen-rich environment (e.g., oxygen cage, nasal oxygen) and efficacy of oxygen supplementation can be monitored with arterial blood gas analysis, arterial blood pressure measurements through arterial catheterization, electrocardiography, capnography, and pulsoximetry. Mannitol (20%) in a dosage of 0.5–1.5 g/kg IV over 20 minutes (limited to three boluses per 24 hours) is administered to decrease intracranial pressure. Furosemide (2.2–4.4 mg/kg IV) is synergistic in reducing intracranial pressure. Methylprednisolone sodium succinate (30 mg/kg IV, repeat after six hours) given within 12 hours after trauma is thought to help restore membrane integrity by removing free oxygen radicals from the damaged brain area.[5] Seizures can be controlled with anticonvulsants (diazepam 0.5 mg/kg bolus IV, repeat if necessary; phenobarbital 2–5 mg/kg as a bolus IV, to effect). If the cat has an open wound or open skull fracture, cephalozin (20 mg/kg IV, repeat every eight hours) is started and continued orally for ten days.

When the cat is hemodynamically stable and medical treatment has been initiated, CT or MRI is performed to localize the lesion. Skull radiographs are not helpful in assessing intracranial trauma. CT is preferable because it is quicker and better for imaging fractures and associated acute hemorrhage than MRI.

If the lesion is located in an area amenable to surgical decompression (i.e., through craniotomy) and is removable (e.g., hematoma and fracture fragment) then surgical intervention should be considered (see Box 58-2). Depressed skull fractures can be carefully reduced; skull fragments are removed when they are embedded in brain parenchyma. Underlying dura, arachnoid, and brain parenchyma are examined for hemorrhage. If an epidural, subdural, or subarachnoid hematoma is seen, the hematoma is gently lifted with a brain spatula and controllable suction. Small dural and arachnoid vessels are cauterized with bipolar cautery and pieces of thrombin gel foam are used to enhance coagulation. After hematoma removal the surgical field is gently irrigated with warmed sterile saline (NaCl 0.9%) solution. Dural tears are not closed and fracture fragments are not replaced.

Brain abscess

Brain abscesses are extremely rare in cats and it was only recently that the first well documented case was described, suspected to be secondary to a bite wound.[21] A nine-year-old male castrated European short-hair cat was presented with a six-day history of progressive depression and ataxic gait. Neurologic examination revealed depression, absent menace in the left eye, absent pupillary light reflex in the right eye, anisocoria, circling to the right, and delayed proprioception in all limbs. MRI showed a space-occupying right temporal lobe lesion adjacent to a small defect in the temporal bone suggestive of a meningoencephalitis with concurrent abscess formation (Fig. 58-4). The site was surgically approached by a rostrotentorial craniectomy. A cerebral abscess was found and debrided. *Propionibacteria* spp. was cultured from the purulent fluid. Histopathologic examination of the removed tissue demonstrated a subacute to chronic purulent encephalitis with extensive necrosis of brain tissue. Neurologic signs resolved completely within two weeks and full recovery was observed four weeks after surgery.

Neoplasia

The incidence of intracranial neoplasia in cats is approximately 3.5 per 100 000.[6] The most common primary brain tumor is meningioma.

Primary brain tumors other than meningiomas, such as gliomas (astrocytoma, oligodendroglioma), choroid plexus tumors, or ependymoma are rare in cats.

The therapeutic options available for cats are rapidly expanding, co-existent with advances in the veterinary fields of anesthesia and analgesia. In academia or specialized veterinary institutions the treatment options include neurosurgery, with total or subtotal resection of brain tumors, primary or adjuvant radiotherapy by linear accelerator or intralesional radiation therapy, or medical therapy with chemotherapeutic drugs or hormonal agents.

Meningiomas

Meningiomas are mesenchymal tumors that arise from the dura mater, arachnoid (most commonly), or pia mater. Feline meningiomas are generally solitary but multiple meningiomas have been reported.[22–24] Meningiomas are most commonly located over the cerebral hemispheres but may also originate in other locations, e.g., rostral to the pituitary fossa in the area of the optic chiasm (Fig. 58-5). Meningiomas grow slowly, accounting for the insidious onset of clinical signs, usually starting with behavioral changes. The average age of cats with meningioma is 12 years (range five to 17 years). A gender predilection has not been identified, although some reports suggest a higher incidence in male cats. All breeds of cats appear to be affected by meningiomas. Diagnosis is confirmed with MRI: meningiomas typically show hyperintensity of the mass lesion on T1-weighted pre- and post-contrast sequences (Fig. 58-6).[3] The dural tail sign seen on MRI is also very specific for meningioma.[25] However, absence of hyperintensity and the dural tail sign in some cases and the overlap in the MRI appearance between different types of primary brain tumors often precludes a definite diagnosis of meningioma on the basis of imaging alone.

Meningiomas, particularly those located over the cerebral convexities or in the frontal lobes of the cerebrum, may often be completely removed by surgery (see Box 58-2). Final diagnosis is based on histology with hematoxylin and eosin staining.[13] Immunohistochemistry for vimentin, CD34, and E-cadherin is proposed to support a diagnosis of meningioma in surgical or postmortem samples.[26] Studies have also shown that expression of metalloproteinase-2, progesterone receptor, and Ki67 holds some prognostic value in feline meningiomas.[27,28]

Surgical removal of solitary meningioma in cats results in excellent long-term survival and is the first choice of treatment. In a series of ten cats, one cat died immediately after surgery, and three cats died of concurrent disease unrelated to cerebral neoplasia two to 30 months after surgery.[29] In another study, four cats that had surgical removal of solitary meningioma had a mean survival time of 485 days, with two cats surviving more than two years after surgery.[30] A report of 17 cats with meningioma treated by surgical removal indicated that three died in the immediate postoperative period, three cats died with tumor recurrence at three months, nine months, and 72 months after surgery, and the remaining 11 cats survived without tumor recurrence for 18 to 47 months (median 27 months) postoperatively.[31] The results of craniotomy in 42 cats with meningioma indicated a median survival

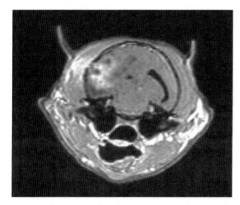

Figure 58-4 Transverse T1-weighted image in a nine-year-old male castrated European short-hair cat with a history of depression and ataxic gait. A space-occupying, contrast enhancing lesion is present in the right temporal musculature and right temporal cerebral lobe. A midline shift with compression and displacement of the right and lateral ventricle is apparent. After craniectomy and dural incision a yellow viscous discharge was found, confirming the diagnosis of cerebral abscess.

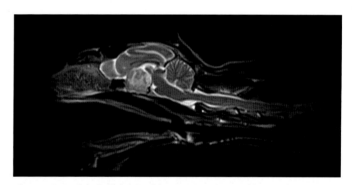

Figure 58-5 High-field (1.5 Tesla) MRI in a 10-year-old male European short-hair cat with post-retinal blindness, aggressiveness and hypersensitive behavior. Sagittal T2-weighted gadolinium-enhanced MR image shows a large hyperintense intracranial mass in the planum sphenoidalis with extension into the pituitary fossa.

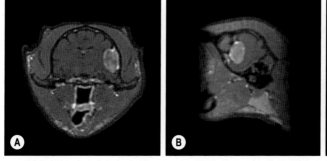
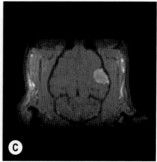

Figure 58-6 (A) Transverse, **(B)** parasagittal, and **(C)** dorsal T1-post contrast (gadolinium) T1-weighted MR images in a 12-year-old cat with a history of seizures. A hyperintense extra-axial intracranial mass was found. The dural tail sign is visible on the transverse image at the upper margin of the tumor close to the skull bone (A). Surgery and histopathology confirmed the diagnosis of meningioma.

of 26 months (range three days to 54 months) and the overall survival was 71% at 6 months, 66% at one year, and 50% at two years.[32] In a report on surgical removal of tentorial meningiomas in six cats, one cat died immediately postoperatively and five cats survived with a median survival of 20 months (range six to 30 months) but all died or were euthanized because of tumor regrowth.[33]

In contrast, there is a significant morbidity and mortality associated with the surgical removal of neoplasia other than meningiomas, especially when these are located in the caudal fossa and brainstem. In addition to providing a tissue diagnosis of tumor type, partial removal of a brain neoplasm may relieve signs of cerebral dysfunction and, in turn, may render an animal a better candidate for other forms of therapy. Cytoreduction lessens the volume of tumor available for therapy using other treatment regimes, such as radiation therapy. Surgical biopsy or cytoreduction must be approached with care, as seeding of a tumor to previously uninvolved tissue is a risk.

Pituitary gland adenomas

Pituitary adenomas are considered benign tumors although in humans they have been reported to invade surrounding tissues such as the dura mater, the cavernous sinus, and the sphenoid sinus.[34] Due to their extension and infiltration of regional structures, these invasive adenomas have a high rate of recurrence after surgical resection in humans.

Pituitary adenomas in cats show a greater diversity in cell characteristics than their canine counterparts. In addition to corticotroph (ACTH cell) adenomas, causing pituitary-dependent hyperadrenocorticism or Cushing's disease,[2,4] and somatotroph (GH cell) adenomas causing acromegaly,[35] a melanotroph (α-MSH cell) adenoma[36] and double (ACTH and GH cell) adenomas[37,38] have also been described in cats. Prolactin (PRL) cell adenomas (prolactinomas) have not been described in cats. Endocrinologically non-functioning pituitary tumors occur in older cats and comprise 9% of the feline intracranial neoplasia that leads to neurologic signs due to tumor mass effect on the brain.[7]

Cushing's disease

Cortisol is the main glucocorticoid released by the adrenal glands in cats. Thus endogenous glucocorticoid excess is essentially hyperadrenocorticism. Prolonged exposure to inappropriately elevated plasma concentrations of free cortisol leads to a variety of signs consistent with Cushing's syndrome. In cats, pituitary-dependent hyperadrenocorticism is a rare disease of middle-aged and older animals[39] and the disease is the result of excessive ACTH secretion by a pituitary adenoma. The pituitary lesions producing the excess of ACTH range from small hyperplastic cell nests of corticotroph (or melanotroph) cells to adenomas and large tumors. Pituitary adenomas may extend and infiltrate into surrounding tissues such as cavernous sinus, dura mater, brain tissue, third ventricle and rarely, sphenoid bone. These are called invasive adenomas, whereas only the exceptional tumors associated with extracranial metastasis are called carcinomas. Corticotroph adenomas may co-occur with somatotroph adenomas in the cat and these are called double adenomas.[37,38]

Many clinical signs can be related to the actions of excessive glucocorticoids, i.e., increased gluconeogenesis, lipogenesis and protein catabolism. The cardinal physical features are central obesity and atrophy of muscles and thinning of skin. In addition, polyuria and polydipsia and polyphagia are often dominant features. Depending on the duration of the glucocorticoid excess the changes may range from cessation of shedding, no regrowth of clipped hair, some thinning of the coat, to alopecia and a thin and wrinkled skin (Fig. 58-7A). The skin thinning and the immune suppression make the animals prone to skin lesions and skin infections (Fig. 58-8). The polyuria is known to be due to both impaired osmoregulation of vasopressin

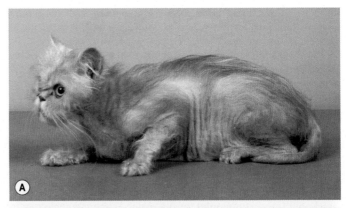
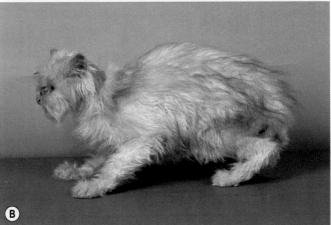

Figure 58-7 (A) Lateral view of a six-year-old Persian cat with pituitary-dependent hyperadrenocorticism showing alopecia and a thin and wrinkled skin with folds. The urinary corticoid/creatinine ratio was 73 × 10⁻⁶ which is above the upper limit of the reference range (42 × 10⁻⁶). **(B)** At four months after trans-sphenoidal hypophysectomy the hair coat had regrown on the abdomen and flank of the cat and the UCCR was 1.3 × 10⁻⁶.

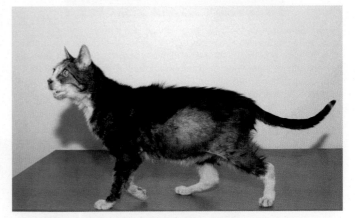

Figure 58-8 A 17-year-old castrated male cat, referred because of problems controlling its diabetes mellitus. In addition to polyuria, polydispia, and weight loss, there was alopecia and muscular weakness in the hind legs. Basal UCCRs on two consecutive days (73 × 10⁻⁶ and 88 × 10⁻⁶) were above the upper limit of the reference range (42 × 10⁻⁶). After three oral doses of 0.1 mg dexamethasone per kg body weight the UCCR decreased to 9 × 10⁻⁶ indicating pituitary-dependent hyperadrenocorticism. CT revealed the pituitary to be moderately enlarged (height 4.2 mm, width 4.0 mm) with displacement of the neurohypophyseal flush.

release and interference of the glucocorticoid excess with the action of vasopressin. In cats, the cutaneous manifestations are initially less pronounced than in the dog. Furthermore, glucocorticoid excess gives rise less readily to polyuria/polydipsia in cats, and it may become obvious only when diabetes mellitus develops.

Cats are susceptible to the diabetogenic effects of glucocorticoids. In the majority of the described cases of feline hyperadrenocorticism the disease was associated with diabetes mellitus and the suspicion of hyperadrenocorticism has often arisen specifically because of insulin resistance encountered in the treatment of diabetes mellitus.[39] Endogenous glucocorticoid excess increases blood pressure. In cats with hyperadrenocorticism decreased thyroxine (T_4) concentrations can be found, as a consequence of altered transport, distribution, and metabolism of thyroxine, rather than hyposecretion. Clinical neurologic manifestations of the disease are only observed when the pituitary tumor develops to be large enough to cause a mass effect.[40] These neurologic abnormalities are often vague, including lethargy, inappetence, and mental dullness.

The tests for diagnosis of hyperadrenocorticism are described in Chapter 35. Resistance to glucocorticoid feedback is significantly correlated with the size of the pituitary gland. Large tumors tend to be more resistant to the suppressive effect of dexamethasone due to their size, and they often release ACTH precursors like pro-opiomelanocortin (POMC). There is also a report of a cat with a melanotroph pars intermedia adenoma with extremely elevated plasma concentrations of α-MSH and no evidence for ACTH-dependent hyperadrenocorticism.[36]

Diagnostic imaging may help to complete the picture of the physical and hormonal changes that can be associated with hyperadrenocorticism (see Chapter 35).[35] Ultrasonography of the adrenal glands and CT or MRI of the pituitary (see above) and adrenal glands are the imaging techniques now most frequently used, especially in the search for the location and the characterization of the source of the hormone excess. This visualization is imperative in institutions where hypophysectomy or pituitary irradiation is an option for treatment. For hypophysectomy the surgical landmarks in relation to the pituitary tumor are best visualized with contrast-enhanced CT (Fig. 58-9) and for pituitary irradiation using a linear accelerator the exact pituitary zones for intense radiation need to be outlined with MRI or CT.

Spontaneous recovery of pituitary-dependent hyperadrenocorticism is rare and life expectancy in severe cases is usually less than one year if the disease is left untreated. Death may ensue as a result of complications such as heart failure, thromboembolism, or diabetes mellitus. In mild cases with apparently little progression, the course of the disease may be followed for some time with measurements of urine cortisol/creatinine ratio (UCCR), although the usefulness of UCCR is debatable due to a high rate of false positives. To minimize the risk for false positives repeated urine samples are needed that are collected in a stress-free environment. The treatment of pituitary-dependent hyperadrenocorticism should ideally be directed at the elimination of the stimulus for the augmented production of cortisol, i.e., the pituitary lesion causing the excessive ACTH secretion. In the last decade experience has been gained with a microsurgical technique for trans-sphenoidal hypophysectomy (see Box 58-3) in the treatment of cats with pituitary-dependent hyperadrenocorticism.[41] With appropriate short-term and long-term substitution therapies, pituitary surgery is an effective treatment. It can only be performed in specialized institutions with intensive perioperative care and where imaging techniques such as CT and MRI enable assessment of localization and size of the pituitary gland prior to surgery. In a study of seven cats that underwent hypophysectomy for Cushing's disease, two cats died within four weeks after surgery of non-related disease. In the five remaining cats, hyperadrenocorticism went into clinical and biochemical remission (follow-up periods six to 46 months). Hyperadrenocorticism recurred

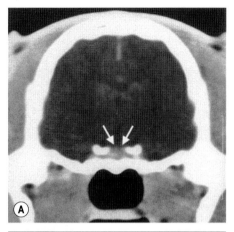

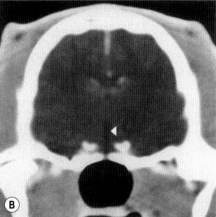

Figure 58-9 **(A)** Contrast-enhanced transverse CT images through the pituitary fossa in a seven-year-old European short-hair cat with Cushing's disease. The urinary corticoid/creatinine ratio was 77×10^{-6} (reference range 8×10^{-6} to 42×10^{-6}). The pituitary (arrows) is not enlarged and is 3.5 mm high, 4.7 mm wide, and the pituitary height/brain area ratio is 0.36. **(B)** At three months after trans-sphenoidal hypophysectomy, the UCCR was 2.3×10^{-6} and there was complete remission of signs of hyperadrenocorticism. There is no contrast enhancement in the pituitary fossa, and the third ventricle is indicated (arrowhead).

after 19 months in one cat. In two of four cats that had concurrent diabetes mellitus, insulin treatment could be discontinued at one and five months after hypophysectomy.[41] Prognosis after hypophysectomy for Cushing's disease in cats is determined by co-existing disease, and thorough presurgical screening is imperative. The main advantage for long-term survival, compared to approaches at the adrenal level, is in the prevention of neurologic problems that may occur as a result of an expanding pituitary tumor.

Radiation therapy for pituitary macroadenomas may lead to some decrease in the tumor mass and peritumoral edema, but concurrent adrenocortical suppression treatment is needed. Radiation therapy does not usually reduce the hypersecretion of ACTH sufficiently so additional therapy at the adrenal level is required.[42–47]

Treatment of adrenal-dependent disease is described in Chapter 35 and in the literature.[42–47]

Acromegaly

In cats, chronic hypersecretion of growth hormone (GH) by a functional pituitary adenoma causes acromegaly.[35] The clinical signs are dominated by concurrent insulin-resistant diabetes mellitus. Although acromegaly is being recognized in cats with increasing frequency, there

Table 58-1 Signalment, imaging data, and insulin requirements in three diabetic cats with acromegaly treated by hypophysectomy

Parameter	Cat 1	Cat 2	Cat 3
Breed	DS	DS	DS
Gender	MC	MC	FC
Age (years)	11	10	10
Body weight (kg)	7.2	9.4	4.3
CT pituitary height (mm)	4.5	13.3	5.2
CT pituitary width (mm)	4.2	13.4	8.3
CT pituitary length (mm)	4.7	14.0	4.0
CT pituitary height/brain area (P/B)[a]	0.50	1.41	0.60
Insulin demand (total IU/day) before HX	100	200	17
Insulin demand four weeks after HX	0	0	0

DS, Domestic short-haired cat; FC, female castrated; HX, hypophysectomy; MC, male castrated.

[a]Reference P/B for cats: P/B <0.40.

Table 58-2 Basal plasma hormone concentrations in three diabetic cats with acromegaly treated by hypophysectomy

Hormones	Values			Reference values
	Cat 1	Cat 2	Cat 3	
Thyroxine (nmol/L [μg/dL])	22 (1.7)	11 (0.8)	11(0.8)	15–45 (1.2–3.5)
Cortisol (nmol/L [μg/dL])	211 (7.3)	203 (7.0)	NA	12–263 (0.4–9.5)
ACTH (ng/L)	26	21	21	15–358
α-MSH (ng/L)	257	82	NA	29–503
GH (μg/L)	51	>100	>50	0.8–7.2
GH (μg/L) one year after HX	2.4	3.1	1.9	0.8–7.2
IGF-1 (μg/L)	3871	2497	1136	39–590
IGF-1 (μg/L) one year after HX	113	34	76	39–590

Basal plasma concentrations of cortisol, ACTH, α-MSH, GH, and IGF-1 before HX are means calculated from two values. The data are presented in SI units (and traditional units in brackets). HX, hypophysectomy; NA, not available. Reference values for ACTH, α-MSH, and cortisol,[51] and GH and IGF-1.[52]

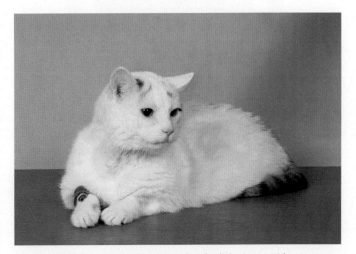

Figure 58-10 An 11-year-old castrated male diabetic cat with acromegaly showing increased body weight and a dull hair coat. Plasma concentration of GH was 51 μg/L (reference range 0.8–7.2 μg/L) and of IGF-1 3871 μg/L (reference range 39–590 μg/L).

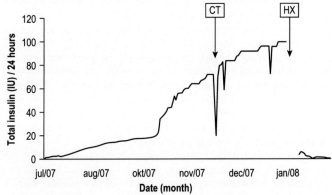

Figure 58-11 Insulin requirements over a six-month period in a diabetic cat with acromegaly treated by trans-sphenoidal hypophysectomy (HX). CT indicates when computed tomography was performed. At three weeks after surgery the cat no longer required insulin treatment.

have been few reports of experience with treatment. Usually, treatment of the diabetes is aimed at regulation of glucose levels with insulin medication, but as long as the primary cause remains untreated insulin requirements usually increase over time and can become extremely high. Successful treatment of acromegaly in a diabetic cat by pituitary surgery has been reported recently.[48]

Affected cats are usually male and castrated and approximately ten years old (Table 58-1). They present with insulin-resistant diabetes mellitus, ravenous appetite, coarse facial features, a dull hair coat, and sometimes increased interdental spacing, a combination of features that is well-described in feline acromegaly (Fig. 58-10). The ravenous appetite and the combined anabolic actions of hyperinsulinaemia (in the initial stages) and the excess GH, lead to an increase in body weight. In a 24-hour glucose curve, the plasma glucose concentrations are elevated and insulin requirements progressively increase, indicating insulin resistance (Fig. 58-11). In general practice, acromegaly is

confirmed by measuring elevated plasma concentrations of insulin-like growth factor-1 (IGF-1); GH measurements are restricted to institutions that have access to a reliable GH assay (Table 58-2).[49,50] The pituitary–adrenocortical system can be further investigated by measuring plasma concentrations of α-MSH, ACTH, and cortisol. The basal plasma concentrations of α-MSH, ACTH, and cortisol are usually in the reference range (see Table 58-2), but acromegaly and Cushing's disease may occur simultaneously in diabetic cats due to double adenomas.[37,38] The plasma total thyroxine concentration can be within the reference range (Table 58-1) or can be decreased due to compression and atrophy of the unaffected pituitary gland by a large adenoma (secondary hypothyroidism).

Pituitary imaging (see above) supports the diagnosis of a pituitary adenoma (Figs 58-9 and 58-12A), and in cats with acromegaly the palatum molle may be thickened, which may be evident on a sagittal reconstruction of the CT images (Fig. 58-12B). This may also be noted

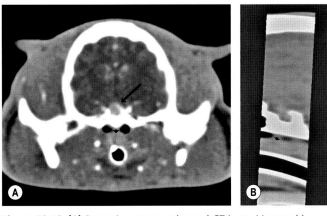

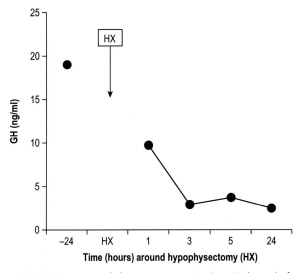

Figure 58-12 **(A)** Dynamic contrast-enhanced CT in an 11-year-old castrated male cat with acromegaly. The pituitary is enlarged, measuring 4.5 mm in height, 4.2 mm in width, and 4.7 mm in length. The pituitary flush is displaced to the right and dorsal side of the gland (arrow) indicative of a pituitary adenoma on the left and ventral side. **(B)** Sagittal reconstruction shows the thickened palatum molle (arrowhead) between the tracheal tube and sphenoid bone.

Figure 58-13 Plasma growth hormone concentrations 24 hours before and one, three, five and 24 hours after hypophysectomy (HX) in a diabetic cat with acromegaly.

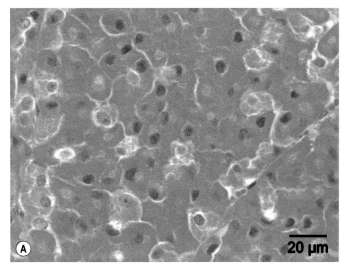

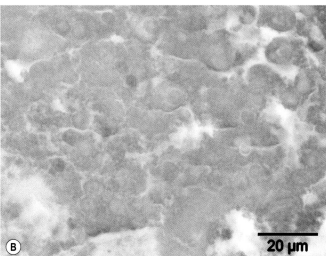

Figure 58-14 Somatotroph pituitary adenoma in a cat with acromegaly. **(A)** Adenomatous nodule comprised of acidophilic cells with uniform nuclei and low mitotic index; hematoxylin and eosin staining. **(B)** Positive immunocytochemical staining of the adenomatous tissue for growth hormone.

during the approach for trans-sphenoidal hypophysectomy:[48] the soft palate is thicker than normal and the mucoperiosteum covers the sphenoid bone in thick folds. During hypophysectomy (see Box 58-3) the pituitary is carefully examined and, when possible, non-affected pituitary tissue (normal specimen) and adenomatous pituitary tissue (tumor specimen) is collected separately for routine histopathology and immunocytochemistry. When the pituitary adenoma is successfully removed, plasma GH concentrations show a rapid decline within five hours after hypophysectomy (Fig. 58-13). Microscopic examination of hematoxylin and eosin (H&E) stained sections of specimens may show uniform adenomatous nodules of acidophilic cells with infiltrative growth pattern in pre-existent pituitary tissue (Fig. 58-14A). Additional immunohistochemical staining for ACTH, α-MSH, and GH is needed to confirm the cell type of the pituitary adenoma. In a typical pituitary GH cell (somatotroph), adenoma nodules stain positive for GH (Fig. 58-14B) whereas cells in the pre-existent pituitary tissue stain sporadically positive for GH and ACTH.

Recovery from surgery is rapid in acromegalic cats; the cats will start to eat and drink within 1 or 2 days after surgery or they may be force-fed through an esophageal tube. The insulin demand rapidly decreases from presurgical values to zero values within four weeks after surgery (see Table 58-1 and Fig. 58-11).[48] The explanation for this dramatic response (more than a 90% decrease in the first week after hypophysectomy) may be the immediate decrease in GH levels, which is evident from the five-hour postoperative GH profile (Fig. 58-13). The elevated GH and IGF-1 levels apparently cause no permanent irreversible damage to the insulin responsiveness of pancreatic endocrine and peripheral tissues. This is in sharp contrast with insulin-resistant diabetes mellitus caused by Cushing's disease in dogs, which is usually irreversible.

Medication after surgery consists of desmopressin, cortisone acetate, and thyroxine as described previously.[2,15] Polydipsia further resolves at home. Basal UCCRs, measured in two consecutive morning urine samples collected at home at six months after surgery, are usually below the reference range (8×10^{-6} to 42×10^{-6}).[53] At one year after surgery, remission of acromegaly should be confirmed by normalization of plasma concentrations of GH and IGF-1 (Table 58-2). However,

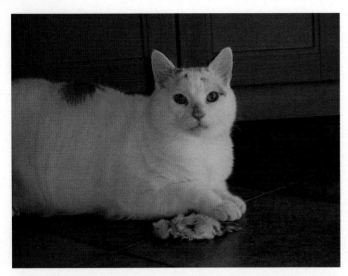

Figure 58-15 The same cat as in Figure 58-10 at one year after hypophysectomy no longer requires insulin medication. The cat had resumed its normal behavior at home and had developed a healthy full hair coat. Plasma concentration of growth hormone was 2.4 μg/L (reference range 0.8–7.2 μg/L) and of IGF-1 113 μg/L (reference range 39–590 μg/L).

the appetite of the cat may remain high, leading to a gain in body weight (Fig. 58-15). This increased food intake may lead to obesity, which in turn causes peripheral insulin resistance and ultimately may lead to diabetes mellitus. The exact reasons for this are unclear but it has been hypothesized that the central hypothalamic regulation of food intake has been disturbed by the enlarged pituitary.

Cryohypophysectomy has been reported in two cats. In one cat this resulted in diminished insulin resistance, but GH and IGF-1 data were not available.[54] The cat showed neurologic deterioration and blindness after cryohypophysectomy that was later attributed by the authors to enrofloxacin medication.[55] In the other cat, cryohypophysectomy led to persistent insulin resistance and no significant lowering of plasma IGF-1 concentrations.[56]

The most frequently reported treatment for feline acromegaly has been radiation therapy. In five cases cobalt 60 (gamma) radiation lowered the insulin requirement transiently and reduced the size of the pituitary tumor.[35,57] In one cat in which linear accelerator (high-energy X-ray) radiation was used, insulin resistance was reduced but the plasma IGF-1 concentration remained elevated and acromegaly continued as an active disease process.[58] Beta radiation reduced the insulin requirement only slightly in one cat but linear accelerator radiation reduced the insulin dose in another cat by half.[59] Radiation therapy is variably successful, primarily because of the partial and delayed effect of radiation necrosis.[35,57,58,60] In a recent study, including 14 cats with acromegaly, hypofractionated radiotherapy improved diabetic control in 13 of 14 cats and complete resolution of diabetes mellitus was achieved in six cats.[61] However, in eight cats in which IGF-1 concentrations were also measured after radiotherapy, changes in the concentration of IGF-1 did not reflect the clinical improvement in glycemic control. In six cats, IGF-1 concentrations remained within the range considered diagnostic for acromegaly.[61]

Medical treatment with the somatostatin analog octreotide[35] and a dopamine agonist[62] has not been successful in reducing the insulin requirements in cats with acromegaly. In one cat treated with the somatostatin analog octreotide, plasma GH concentration was normalized,[4] but in four others octreotide had little or no effect on serum GH levels.[35] A pre-entry test with a single intravenous injection of octreotide was introduced recently to evaluate the potential effectiveness of octreotide treatment in acromegalic cats.[38] Those responding favorably might be candidates for long-acting release (LAR) octreotide treatment. The recently introduced GH-receptor antagonist pegvisomant has been reported to be effective, safe, and well tolerated in humans with acromegaly.[63] However, as long as there are no species-specific antagonists, this approach is not an option for dogs and cats.

Non-functioning pituitary adenoma

The non-endocrine manifestations of pituitary adenomas result from pressure by the tumor on adjacent structures in the brain. In addition, such cats may have anterior pituitary failure. Large pituitary masses can cause partial or complete anterior pituitary hormone deficiency. In principle, deficiency of all six major hormones (LH, FSH, GH, TSH, ACTH, and PRL) can occur. The interpretation of results of suprapituitary stimulation tests may pose problems when there is also hormone excess that may affect the secretion of other pituitary hormones.[4] The pituitary enlargement may also have consequences for posterior lobe function. The following hormone deficiencies may occur. In the adult cat, GH deficiency is not easily recognized as a pathologic syndrome, although longstanding GH deficiency may lead to less activity, muscle atrophy, and skin atrophy with alopecia. Total or partial TSH deficiency is often part of hypopituitarism and results in hypothyroidism. Secondary adrenocortical failure may occur late in the development of large pituitary tumors. The resulting cortisol deficiency may contribute to the gradual deterioration of the animal and a relatively trivial illness or anesthesia may precipitate vascular collapse. Gonadotropin deficiency in female cats may remain unnoticed because of the naturally long interestrous intervals. In male cats the continuing decrease in gonadotropin secretion results in testicular atrophy. The testes are very small and soft and the unchanged epididymis is more easily delineated than it normally is. Posterior pituitary failure is unusual in anterior pituitary disease that remains restricted to the pituitary fossa, but more common when the suprasellar extension of larger tumors compresses the hypothalamus and causes regression of the supra-optic and paraventricular nuclei with vasopressin deficiency and diabetes insipidus.

Continued suprasellar expansion of the tumor exerts pressure on the diaphragma sellae mater, the hypothalamus and, if the expansion is sufficiently rostral, the optic chiasm. Lateral suprasellar extension of pituitary tumors may impair oculomotor nerve function.[64] The expanding tumor can be expected to cause headache and visual field defects in the cat, but because of the lack of an autoanamnesis, the veterinarian must initially often rely on rather vague and non-specific symptoms. These include lethargy, a tendency to seek seclusion, and a decrease in appetite. The suspicion of a mass effect from a pituitary tumor may be supported by the owner's description of the animal's tendency to lower its head to avoid being patted. In cats this may also lead to increased aggressiveness towards the owner and strangers and is probably due to headache. Progressive enlargement of the mass may give rise to severe neurologic abnormalities such as pacing, head pressing, and circling. There may be continuous vocalization (howling). Seizures usually do not occur. Very large pituitary tumors may cause pressure on the optic chiasm to such an extent that visual disturbances are noticed by the owner.[40] Physical examination can reveal a variety of signs, including dullness, one or more of the above neurologic signs, weight loss due to increasing anorexia, and occasionally mydriasis with or without anisocoria. Papillary edema is occasionally found on ophthalmoscopic examination.

The mass effects may also have a very sudden character. The syndrome in humans and dogs known as pituitary apoplexy is characterized by the peracute occurrence of headache, vomiting, visual impairment, and loss of consciousness.[65] It is caused by either hemorrhage or infarction within a pituitary tumor or a non-tumorous pituitary gland. This syndrome has now been described in dogs but not in cats. The three most severe canine cases were presented in an emergency situation with sudden-onset collapse, and severe depression; in two of these dogs there was loss of vision with bilateral mydriasis. In four dogs there was a large corticotroph adenoma with hemorrhage. In the one dog without pituitary tumor the hemorrhage was most likely part of the hemorrhagic diathesis due to idiopathic thrombocytopenia.[65]

Indications of low basal functions of peripheral endocrine glands, i.e., a low plasma concentration of thyroxine and a low urinary corticoid excretion, may support the suspicion of anterior pituitary failure. However, the diagnosis of partial or total hypopituitarism should be made by demonstrating the deficiencies of pituitary hormones. This can be accomplished by stimulation tests with hypophysiotropic hormones such as GHRH, GnRH, CRH, and TRH. Measurement of the respective pituitary hormones (GH, LH, ACTH, PRL, and TSH) permits assessment of pituitary reserve capacity.[4]

Contrast-enhanced helical CT and MRI provide imaging of the pituitary with high spatial and contrast resolution, allowing the identification of pituitary enlargement and its relationship to surrounding structures and bony anatomic landmarks for surgical intervention (Fig. 58-16).[14] Dynamic helical CT and MRI allow visualization of the posterior lobe. Inability to visualize the posterior lobe in very large pituitary tumors may indicate hypopituitarism and vasopressin insufficiency (Fig. 58-17).[18]

Anterior pituitary failure can be treated by substituting for the deficient hormone production by the target glands. Since gonadal hormones are not essential, treatment amounts to oral administration of thyroxine (10–15 µg/kg twice daily) and cortisone (0.25–0.5 mg/kg twice daily). The owners usually report that this treatment brings about some improvement in alertness and also in appetite if the animal had been anorectic. Especially when by virtue of its size the tumor has already had neurologic effects, the improvement, if any, will be only temporary. Immediate corticosteroid administration is indicated in cases suspected of pituitary apoplexy; in such a crisis the dose should be four to five times the long-term substitution dose.

In principle, there are three options to reduce the size of the pituitary tumor: medical therapy, hypophysectomy, and radiation therapy. Most experience with medical treatment has been gained in dogs with pituitary-dependent hyperadrenocorticism. Dopaminergic drugs such as bromocriptine did not effectively decrease cortisol production,[66] but in a recent study using the dopamine D2 receptor agonist cabergoline better results were obtained. Cabergoline has a higher affinity for the D2 receptor and has a longer half-life than bromocriptine. Despite the fact that D2 receptors are only moderately expressed in tumorous and non-tumorous dog pituitaries,[67] 17 out of 40 dogs responded to cabergoline with decreased cortisol production and decreased tumor size. Among the non-responders there were many dogs with large pituitary tumors.[68] Whether this medical strategy is an option in cats with non-functioning pituitary adenomas remains to be investigated.

Hypophysectomy (see Box 58-3) is used successfully in the treatment of pituitary-dependent hyperadrenocorticism[41] and acromegaly,[48] and with increasing experience the technique also allows the removal of non-functioning pituitary tumors up to 1–2 cm in diameter. Total or subtotal removal of large and giant pituitary tumors with mass effect gives immediate relief, resolution of neurologic signs, and return of appetite. The cat can resume a normal life for many months

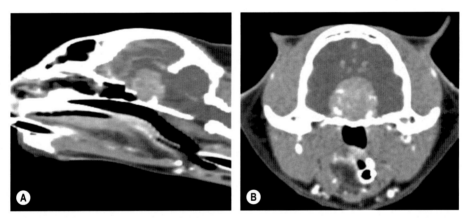

Figure 58-16 (A) Sagittal and **(B)** transverse contrast-enhanced CT of the skull in a four-year-old female castrated domestic short-haired cat with depression and anorexia. A large pituitary mass was detected measuring 16.5 mm in height, 18.8 mm in width, and 19.6 mm in length. The pituitary height/brain area ratio was 1.90.

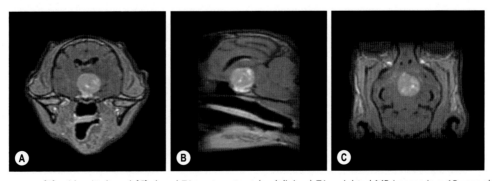

Figure 58-17 (A) Transverse, **(B)** midsagittal, and **(C)** dorsal T1-post contrast (gadolinium) T1-weighted MR images in a 13-year-old male castrated domestic short-haired cat with a history of depression, circling, and ataxic gait. A hyperintense pituitary mass was found.

to years after surgery. In cases with return of the pituitary mass a repeat trans-sphenoidal pituitary debulking is an option to control the tumor growth over time.

Radiation therapy (see Chapter 15) is indicated in cats when a pituitary tumor is causing neurologic abnormalities.[69] It reduces the size of the tumor and thereby the neurologic manifestations. For cats a median survival time of 17.4 months has been reported.[60] Radiation therapy does not cause a prompt reduction in pituitary hypersecretion, and cats with pituitary-dependent hyperadrenocorticism or acromegaly may require continued medical treatment. Cats with a macrotumor and diabetes mellitus may not require insulin treatment after the completion of a series of fractionated radiation therapy treatments.[70] Acute side effects of radiation treatment include local skin changes (erythema, hair loss, leukotrichia), pharyngeal mucositis, and mild otitis externa. The risk of late side effects (hearing impairment, brain necrosis/fibrosis) depends on the volume of brain tissue treated, and the daily and the total dose of radiation administered.[69] Recently, brachytherapy, or interstitial radiation therapy has been introduced in domestic animals; by intralesional injection of radioactive holmium-166 microspheres for treatment of giant pituitary adenomas, tumor shrinkage is accomplished.[71] Whether this works for large non-functioning pituitary adenomas in cats remains to be investigated.

SURGICAL TECHNIQUES

Craniotomy and craniectomy

Craniotomy in the cat requires specific medical and anesthetic management with respect to intracranial pressure and blood flow, antibiotics, anticonvulsants, and diuretics. Proper anesthetic management (see Chapter 2) includes arterial catheterization, appropriate induction and maintenance agents, and modest hyperventilation (end-tidal carbon dioxide approximately 28–32 mmHg). Arterial catheterization is used to constantly monitor arterial blood pressure and end-tidal capnography is used for continuous monitoring of carbon dioxide. Periodic arterial blood sampling for carbon dioxide levels aids anesthetic monitoring. Modest hyperventilation using a mechanical ventilator reduces arterial carbon dioxide, decreases cerebral blood flow, and lowers intracranial pressure.[5] Autologous blood donation before surgery is considered safe for cats undergoing craniectomy for resection of meningioma.[72]

The craniotomy/craniectomy procedure is described in Box 58-2. The term craniectomy is used when the bone flap that is created during craniotomy is not replaced. The most common approaches to the feline calvarium[5] are: (1) rostrotentorial transparietal or

---

Box 58-2 Craniotomy and craniectomy

Most craniotomies are performed with the cat in sternal recumbency. A head stand, a vacuum cushion and/or surgical tape is used to stabilize the head (Fig. 58-19). In general, craniotomy starts with a skin incision (Fig. 58-20A) and detachment of the temporal muscle mass from the skull (Fig. 58-20B). Bipolar electro-coagulation is used for hemostasis. The outline of the craniotomy is marked with a sterile pencil or with the electrical or air-powered burr. Usually three (triangular craniotomy) or four (rectangular craniotomy) holes are burred, stopping short of the dura mater. The burr holes are connected with grooves that are carefully deepened until a paper-thin inner cortical lamina separates the burr from the dura mater. Hemorrhage from venous sinuses within the bone itself is plugged with bone wax. Using fine neurosurgical probes and Kerrison punches the remaining inner cortical bone layer on the bottom of the grooves is broken away or removed with the punches, thereby isolating the craniotomy flap from the feline skull (Fig. 58-20C).

The bone flap is carefully lifted with a periosteal elevator or pediatric brain spatula by detaching the dura mater from the inside of the bone flap (Fig. 58-20D). Care is taken not to damage the middle meningeal artery. The bone flap is removed and stored in sterile solution but is usually not replaced (craniectomy). From this moment on it is important to use some sort of magnification, either an operating loupe (3–4× magnification) or an operating microscope (10× magnification). Before incising the dura mater, stay sutures (e.g., 6-0 polydioxanone) are strategically placed in the exposed dura mater to allow lateral reflection of the dura after incision. By lifting the dura mater with the sutures, the dura mater can be carefully incised with an arachnoid knife.

With a meningioma the tumor usually arises from the dura itself and then the dura mater needs to be circumferentially excised together with the tumor. In gliomas the dura mater can be preserved and used for closure after tumor extraction. With peripheral brain tumors, the tumor margins are carefully explored with neurosurgical probes. Small vessels leading to the tumor can be cauterized with bipolar electrocautery. Diffuse hemorrhage can be controlled with thrombin gel foam. Suction devices with a controllable degree of suction are used to remove neoplastic tissue. Suction should be used with care since normal brain parenchyma has a weak consistency and is easily damaged or sucked away when the tip of the suction device locks on unaffected brain tissue. To prevent this, a small 1 cm × 1 cm piece of gauze may be placed on the tip of the suction device to protect the brain tissue. In this way the suction device can also be used as a dull dissector between tumor and normal brain tissue.

With meningiomas there is usually a sharp border between tumor and normal brain parenchyma and the tumor may roll out of the calvarium (Fig. 58-20E). Meningioma tissue has a firmer consistency than brain tissue and it may help to put a retraction suture through the center of the tumor. Other primary brain tumors are less firm and debulking is done based on abnormal color (gray, glassy-like, dark) and consistency (necrotic, hemorrhagic, mucoid, cystic compartments) and available imaging during surgery. It is essential for the veterinary neurosurgeon to develop some sort of comparative instinct between intraoperative real time dimensions (sizes and volume) and comparative values measured preoperatively from the imaging data set. This way the neurosurgeon can safely assess when it is time to stop the debulking procedure as the borders between normal and tumor tissue become less well defined.

After tumor removal there may be a significant impression left on the brain (e.g., in meningioma) or a defect where part of the brain has been removed (e.g., in glioma) and this cavity is filled up with thrombin gel foam. For limited craniotomies the bone flap is not usually replaced. In an extensive craniotomy (bilateral rostrotentorial craniectomy combined with frontal sinus craniectomy), a gamma-irradiated calvarial allograft has been described to repair the calvarial defect in a cat with a psammomatous meningioma.[73] When the dura mater cannot be sutured a fascial transplant (from the temporal muscle) can be sutured to the dura mater to close the calvarium. After osteotomy of the zygomatic arch, the bone continuity is restored with cerclage wire or monofilament sutures. The temporal muscle is reflected over the craniotomy opening and re-attached to its insertion on the midline (Fig. 58-20F). The wound is closed in a routine manner. The surgical specimen is sent for histopathology (Fig. 58-20G).

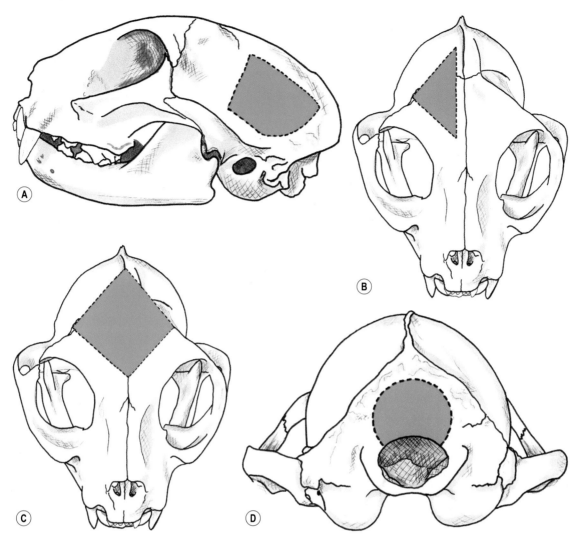

Figure 58-18 Schematic outline of the feline skull for **(A)** rostrotentorial craniotomy, **(B)** unilateral transfrontal sinus craniotomy, **(C)** bilateral transfrontal sinus craniotomy, and **(D)** suboccipital craniotomy.

transtemporal craniotomy (Fig. 58-18A) with or without osteotomy of the zygomatic arch; (2) unilateral (Fig. 58-18B) or bilateral (Fig. 58-18C) transfrontal sinus craniotomy; (3) caudotentorial craniotomy; or (4) suboccipital craniotomy (Fig. 58-18D). Craniotomy approaches can be combined or modified to improve exposure to various aspects of the cerebral hemispheres and cerebellum.[74]

Trans-sphenoidal hypophysectomy

Trans-sphenoidal hypophysectomy is indicated for tumors in the pituitary fossa and parasellar region (Fig. 58-21). The protocol described in Box 58-3 has been used successfully for hypophysectomy in cats with pituitary adenomas by the author.[41] After premedication with medetomidine (0.1 mg/kg IM), anesthesia is induced with propofol (5 mg/kg IV). The trachea is intubated, and inhalation anesthesia is maintained in a semiclosed system with a mixture of isoflurane, nitrous oxide, and oxygen. Analgesia is provided by sufentanil administered by an IV pump at a rate of 2.5 µg/kg/hour. Electrocardiography, capnography, pulsoximetry, and invasive or non-invasive measurement of blood pressure are used to monitor the cat during surgery. Amoxicillin and clavulanic acid (20 mg/kg IV) and hydrocortisone (1 mg/kg IV) are administered before surgery. During surgery the cat

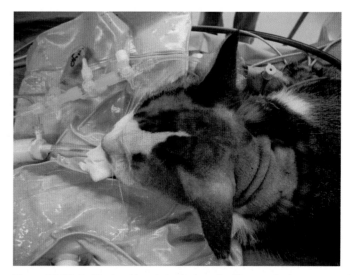

Figure 58-19 Positioning (dorsal view) of a cat with a cerebral meningioma for left-sided rostrotentorial craniotomy. The head is supported by a vacuum cushion.

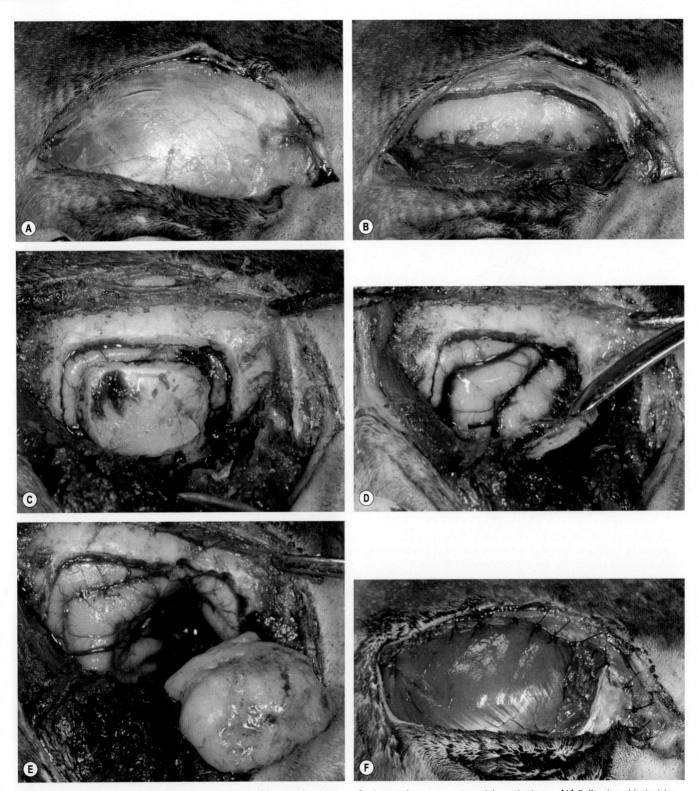

Figure 58-20 Rostrotentorial craniotomy in a 12-year-old cat with a history of seizures due to an extra-axial meningioma. **(A)** Following skin incision, **(B)** the temporal muscle is detached from the calvarium. **(C)** The bone flap is isolated with an electrical burr and punches and **(D)** removed. **(E)** The meningioma is removed. **(F)** The temporal muscle is re-attached.

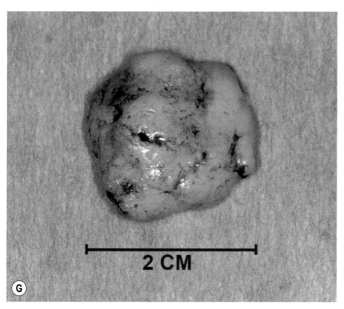

Figure 50-20, Continued **(G)** The surgical specimen is sent for histopathology.

receives lactated Ringer's solution (50 ml/kg IV). Trans-sphenoidal hypophysectomy is performed as described previously for dogs but with some modifications adapted to the feline species.[2,15,75,76]

Immediately after removal of the pituitary gland, treatment is started with hydrocortisone (1 mg/kg IV) every six hours, and desmopressin, one drop into the conjunctival sac every eight hours.[76] After surgery, the antidote atipamezole (0.25 mg/kg IV) is administered. Postoperative analgesia is achieved with buprenorphine (0.3 μg/kg IV) every eight hours. Amoxicillin and clavulanic acid are continued at a dose rate of 20 mg/kg IV every 12 hours. The cat has to recover in an intensive care unit. Fluid administration consists of a combined IV infusion of a 0.45% NaCl and 2.5% glucose solution supplemented with 10 mEq KCl/500 mL. The infusion rate (50 mL/kg/24 hours) is guided by central venous pressure measurements (reference ranges, 0–5 cm saline pressure) through a jugular infusion line. Plasma sodium and potassium concentrations and osmolality are measured before and immediately after surgery and at 8, 24, and 48 hours after surgery. Drinking is allowed as soon as the cat is awake. The Schirmer tear test (STT) is performed on the first day after surgery. When the cat resumes drinking and eating, oral substitution therapy is started by administering cortisone acetate, 1 mg/kg every 12 hours and thyroxine, 10–15 μg/kg every 12 hours. Once at home the dose of cortisone acetate is gradually lowered (in cats with Cushing's disease) over

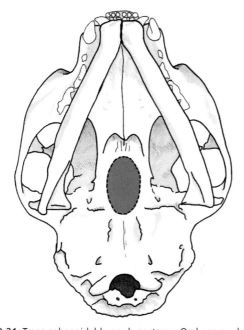

Figure 58-21 Trans-sphenoidal hypophysectomy. Oral approach to the brain.

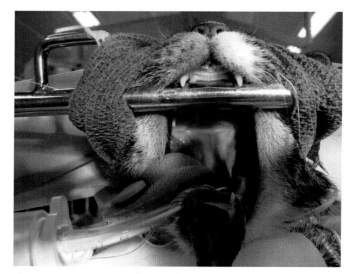

Figure 58-22 Positioning of the cat for trans-sphenoidal hypophysectomy. The upper jaw is fixed to a metal bar attached to the side of the operating table and the neck is supported.

Box 58-3 **Trans-sphenoidal hypophysectomy**

The cat is placed in sternal recumbency and the upper jaw is fixed to a padded metal bar attached to the side of the operating table (Fig. 58-22). The head and neck are supported by a vacuum cushion and care is taken not to hyperextend the neck, for which the cat is particularly vulnerable (risk of brainstem necrosis). The head is fixed with elastic bandage and tape to the metal bar and the lower jaw is gently reflected downwards with elastic bandage. The cuffed tracheal tube is taped beneath the tongue to the lower jaw and reflected laterally out of the surgical field. The surgeon is positioned in front of the operating table, facing the cat. The table is tilted at a 40° angle, which gives the

surgeon an unobstructed view of the oropharynx almost perpendicular to the plane of the sphenoid bone. The mouth and surgical field are irrigated with 10% povidone-iodine solution. The cuff of the tracheal tube is re-checked for adequate pressure. Following draping, the surgical field is bordered by the metal bar behind the feline teeth dorsally, the commissure of the lips laterally, and the base of the tongue ventrally. A gauze sponge is placed in the oropharynx to prevent blood or irrigation solution from leaking into the larynx.

Orientation is obtained by identifying the pterygoid hamular processes. The soft palate is incised in the midline with an electrical

Box 58-3 **Continued**

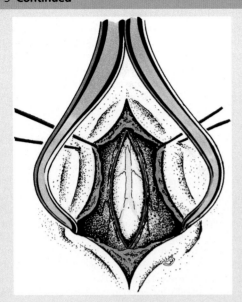

Figure 58-23 Anatomy of the trans-sphenoidal approach. The mucoperiosteum has been incised in the midline and is reflected laterally to expose the sphenoid bone. The bones and their sutures are indicated.

surgical knife over a distance of 1–2 cm between the hamular processes. The palatine mucosa is retracted with a small Gelpi retractor and two stay sutures, exposing the pterygoid bones and their caudoventral angles, and the pterygoid hamular processes, which can be palpated with a small probe. The slit-like orifices of the Eustachian tubes are identified at the base of the pterygoid bones at the level of the hamular processes. A small piece of gauze is placed in the caudal nasopharynx. The mucoperiosteum is incised in the midline using electrosurgery and reflected laterally using a periosteal elevator, thereby exposing the outer cortical lamina of the sphenoid bone. The basisphenoid and the presphenoid bones and their fissures are identified (Fig. 58-23). The position of the burr slot is determined by correlating the location of the pituitary fossa and pituitary gland to the caudal edge of the pterygoid hamuli with sequential, contrast-enhanced CT images that are available in the operating room. The shape of the outer cortical lamina of the sphenoid bone, visible on the transverse CT images and in the surgical field, is also helpful in determining the correct location for burring. In the cat, on the midline from rostral to caudal, a prominent ridge in the presphenoid bone is visible which flattens in the basisphenoid bone and turns into a groove in the direction of the occipitosphenoid bone. Access to the pituitary fossa is obtained with an air-powered burr and bone punches. Between burring episodes, the surgical field is flushed with 0.9% sodium chloride solution for cooling and removal of bone debris. Burring progresses from the outer cortical table of the sphenoid bone, through the middle cancellous bone, to the inner cortical table. The latter, forming the bottom of the burr slot, is identified when the red cancellous layer is replaced by a white inner cortical table.

The sphenoid bone in cats at the level of the pituitary fossa is usually not thicker than 5 mm. In the cat, the rostral part of the solid sphenoid bone continues into an air-filled sinus and in the burring process this may be opened (Fig. 58-24). In pituitary macroadenomas with rostral extension, this air-filled sinus may actually facilitate tumor debulking since the thin layer of bone on the bottom of the sinus is easily removed exposing the rostral extension of the tumor mass. Hemorrhage from the cancellous bone is controlled with bone wax. Burring is discontinued when the pituitary tumor becomes visible through the paper-thin inner cortical layer bordered by the blue cavernous sinuses

laterally. At this point a 3.3× operating loupe is essential to provide magnification. With a small 90° angled, ball-tipped hook an opening is created in the bone by breaking away the paper-thin flakes of the inner cortical lamina. A 1 mm 40° up-biting and a 3 mm (flatfoot) 40° up-biting Kerrison bone punch is used to enlarge the opening created in the inner cortical lamina of the sphenoid bone.

The size of the opening that is necessary for pituitary tumor removal is defined by the pituitary tumor dimensions. In pituitary adenomas with a diameter of 10 mm the opening can be extended rostrally into the air-filled sphenoid sinus (Fig. 58-24). The color of the pituitary is usually normal (pinkish-white oval structure) in non-enlarged pituitaries and gray, brown or dark blue in enlarged pituitaries. In enlarged pituitaries the cavernous sinuses are usually displaced laterally and are not visible through the burr hole. The dura mater is incised in a cruciate pattern with a no. 11 surgical knife or an arachnoid neurosurgical knife. Immediately following incision, the pituitary tissue starts to protrude through the dural opening. The pituitary tumor margins are carefully explored on the left and right lateral margins and on the upper surface of the tumor. On the caudal side the separation between the pituitary and the dorsum sellae can be explored with the probe. The pituitary tumor is detached from the fossa circumferentially using a small 90° angled ball-tipped probe, except for the caudal attachment to the dorsum sellae which will be preserved as long as possible since it contains the caudal hypophyseal artery to the neurointermediate lobe. Extraction of the pituitary tumor is done with fine surgical neurosurgical grasping forceps and controlled suction, which will break the pituitary stalk from the hypothalamus. Pituitary tumor fragments are collected separately (tumor adenoma specimen, non-affected specimen, neurointermediate lobe specimen) in formalin for histology and immunocytochemistry (Fig. 58-24).

Severance of the caudal attachment of the pituitary to the base of the dorsum sellae will usually cause a small arterial hemorrhage that can be best dealt with in the final phase of pituitary tumor extraction. The stump containing the artery that is attached to the base of the dorsum sellae can easily be cauterized with bipolar electrocautery. Incision of the dura mater and detachment of the pituitary is followed by leakage of cerebrospinal fluid (CSF) from the chiasmatic cistern. After removal of the pituitary, the CSF emerging from the infundibular recess can be seen to ebb and flow with respiratory movements of the cat. The hypophyseal fossa is inspected for completeness of hypophysectomy and using a small swab of thrombin gel foam and limited suction with a 2 mm suction cannula any remaining pituitary tumor fragments are removed. The edges of the incised dura mater retract in a ring bordering the opening of the inner cortical lamina of the sphenoid bone. The infundibular recess, which gives access to the third ventricle, is sometimes visible in the rostral half of the ventral hypothalamic surface. The base of the dorsum sellae marked by the caudal border of the pituitary fossa is carefully explored with the ball-tipped probe for pituitary remnants. The intact half-moon shaped cavernous sinuses are observed laterally. Completeness of hypophysectomy is assessed by the surgeon during surgery by the following criteria: (1) unobstructed view of the hypothalamus and the opening to the third ventricle, and (2) absence of pituitary remnants on careful exploration of the hypophyseal fossa and the dorsum sellae with a ball-tipped probe.

The opening to the pituitary fossa is filled with a piece of absorbable gelatin sponge to prevent oozing of blood and CSF. The gauze in the caudal nasopharynx is removed. The burr slot in the sphenoid bone is filled with bone wax and the mucoperiosteum is closed when possible. The soft palate incision is closed using two separate layers of polyglactin 910 sutures. The mucosal layer facing the nasopharynx is closed with a simple continuous suture pattern and the mucosal layer facing the oropharynx with simple interrupted sutures. The gauze in the caudal oropharynx is removed.

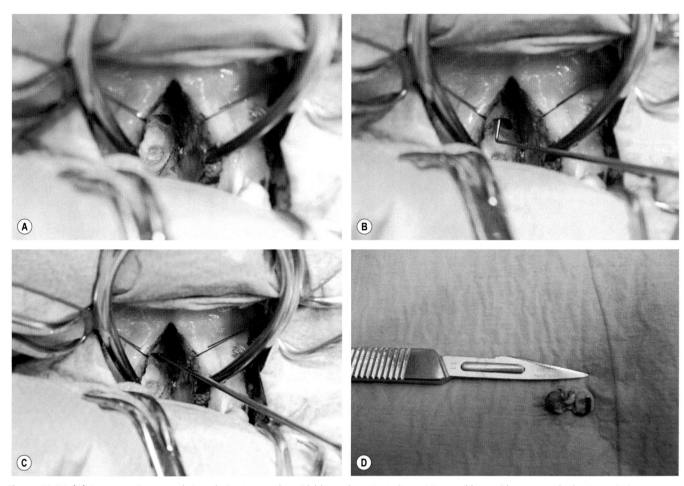

Figure 58-24 (A) Intraoperative ventral view during trans-sphenoidal hypophysectomy in an 11-year-old cat with acromegaly due to a pituitary adenoma. **(B, C)** The soft palate is retracted and the pituitary tumor is visible through the trans-sphenoidal slot. The air-filled sphenoid sinus has been opened rostral to the pituitary and is explored with a probe. **(D)** After hypophysectomy, the surgical specimen is sent for histology and immunocytochemistry.

a period of four weeks to 0.25 mg/kg, every 12 hours. Desmopressin is discontinued at two weeks after surgery. Antibiotic treatment is continued for 14 days postoperatively and consists of oral administration of amoxicillin and clavulanic acid, 12.5 mg/kg every 12 hours. Drinking behavior is monitored by the owner for at least four weeks after surgery by recording daily water intake. If there is persistent polyuria after discontinuation of desmopressin, this treatment is resumed. Follow up for remission is by hormone measurements (UCCR in Cushing's disease and plasma GH and IGF-1 measurements in acromegaly (Table 58-2)) and imaging (Fig. 58-25).

POSTOPERATIVE CARE

After surgery of the neurocranium, cats should recover in a padded cage (Fig. 58-26) in an intensive care unit and be given analgesics, anticonvulsants, corticosteroids, diuretics, antibiotics, and oxygen

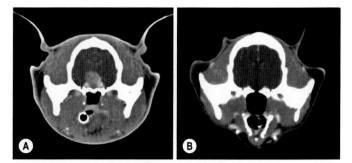

Figure 58-25 Transverse contrast-enhanced CT of a 10-year-old male castrated domestic short-haired cat with diabetes mellitus and acromegaly (plasma growth hormone (GH) >100 µg/L) due to a pituitary adenoma **(A)** before and **(B)** 3 months after trans-sphenoidal hypophysectomy. At three weeks after surgery the cat no longer required insulin treatment, at three months after hypophysectomy no pituitary remnants were visible on CT, and at one year after surgery plasma growth hormone was 3.1 µg/L (reference range 0.8–7.2 µg/L).

supplementation based on the indication for surgery (intracranial neoplasia, pituitary adenoma with endocrine syndrome, cranial trauma).[5] In addition, monitoring during the first days after surgery should include serial general and neurologic examinations, blood hematology (e.g., packed cell volume), electrolytes (e.g., sodium, potassium, osmolality), blood gas analyses, arterial and venous pressure measurements, and urine output. For postoperative care after trans-sphenoidal hypophysectomy, please see above.

Discharge from the hospital depends on the patient's status and owner compliance. Cats need to be scheduled for routine follow-up examinations by neurologists, endocrinologists and/or neurosurgeons at various intervals depending upon their condition and tumor type. In cases of cranial trauma and resection of meningioma or pituitary adenomas, re-evaluation with imaging is proposed but no sooner than three months after surgery with CT or MRI. Anticonvulsant therapy and adjuvant therapy (e.g., chemotherapy and radiotherapy) are re-evaluated.

COMPLICATIONS

The most common complications associated with craniotomy, craniectomy, brain parenchymal resection, and cranial trauma include uncontrollable brain swelling, brain herniation (Fig. 58-27), increased cranial pressure, seizures, hemorrhage, and infection. In case of incomplete resection of cranial neoplasia, recurrence of the mass effect may occur in the long term.

The most common complications after hypophysectomy include hypothalamic damage and hemorrhage, brainstem necrosis, postoperative coma and apnea, electrolyte (sodium and potassium) disturbances, infection, purulent rhinitis, nasal stridor, dehiscence of the soft palate (Fig. 58-28), and aspiration pneumonia. In the long term the most common complication is recurrence of the endocrine syndrome (acromegaly or Cushing's disease) or pituitary mass regrowth.

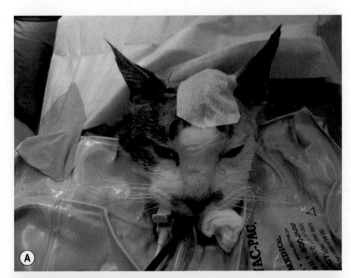

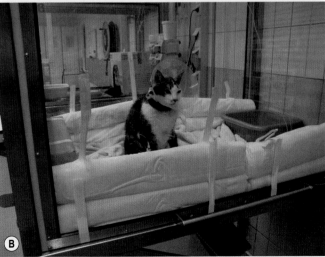

Figure 58-26 (A) Postoperative view after left-sided craniotomy for an extra-axial meningioma. **(B)** Recovery of the cat in a padded cage on the intensive care unit.

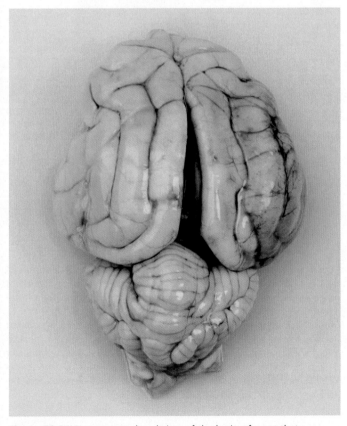

Figure 58-27 Postmortem dorsal view of the brain of a cat that underwent right-sided rostrotentorial craniotomy for a large meningioma. The tumor was completely resected and the bone flap was not replaced. In the intensive care unit the cat's neurologic condition rapidly worsened on the second day after surgery with coma and death. The brain shows an elevated area of cerebral swelling and herniation at the level of the craniotomy site.

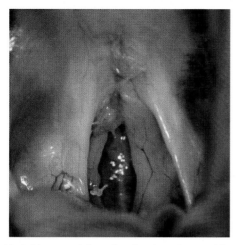

Figure 58-28 Dehiscence of the soft palate in a six-year-old Russian blue at three weeks after trans-sphenoidal hypophysectomy for Cushing's disease. Top is rostral.

PROGNOSIS

Unfavorable prognosticators for intracranial disease and surgical resection include severe neurologic deficits at initial presentation, rapidly progressive disease course, presence of irregular borders on brain imaging, technical inability to provide surgery with or without radiotherapy, co-morbidity in old cats due to co-existent diseases like renal dysfunction or diabetes mellitus.[7,8] The prognosis for cats with non-meningioma intracranial neoplasia is usually unfavorable.[7,8] The prognosis for cats with resectable meningiomas (e.g., clean margins on imaging and histology, absence of invasive behavior, single versus multiple locations) is excellent.[24,31,32] Local regrowth of feline meningiomas (like anaplastic meningiomas) after surgical resection occurs in approximately 20% to 30% of cases.[24,31,32]

Prognosis after hypophysectomy for Cushing's disease in cats is determined by co-existing disease and thorough presurgical screening is imperative. Recent experiences with hypophysectomy as primary treatment for feline acromegaly caused by pituitary somatotroph adenoma are very promising.[48] Diabetes mellitus is completely reversible after surgery (Table 58-1).

REFERENCES

1. Done SH, Goody C, Evans SA, Stickland NC. Veterinary anatomy volume 3. The Dog & Cat. 2nd ed. London: Mosby; 2009.

2. Meij BP. Hypophysectomy as a treatment for canine and feline Cushing's disease. Vet Clin North Am Small Anim Pract 2001;31:1015–41.

3. Lorenz MD, Coates JR, Kent M. Stupor or coma. In: Lorenz MD, Coates JR, Kent M, editors. Handbook of veterinary neurology. 5th ed. St. Louis: Elsevier Saunders; 2011. p. 346–83.

4. Seim HB III. Surgery of the Brain. In: Fossum TW, editor. Small animal surgery. 3rd ed. St. Louis: Mosby Elsevier; 2007. p. 1379–401.

5. LeCouteur RA, Withrow SJ. Tumours of the nervous system. In: Withrow SJ, Vail DM, editors. Small animal oncology. 4th ed. St. Louis: Saunders Elsevier; 2007. p. 659–85.

6. Meij BP, Kooistra HS, Rijnberk A. Hypothalamus-pituitary system. In: Rijnberk A, Kooistra HS, editors. Clinical endocrinology of dogs and cats. Hannover: Schlütersche; 2010. p. 13–54.

7. Troxel MT, Vite CH, Van Winkle TJ, et al. Feline intracranial neoplasia: retrospective review of 160 cases (1985–2001). J Vet Intern Med 2003;17:850–9.

8. Tomek A, Cizinauskas S, Doherr M, et al. Intracranial neoplasia in 61 cats: localisation, tumour types and seizure patterns. J Feline Med Surg 2006;8: 243–53.

9. Pákozdy A, Leschnik M, Sarchahi AA, et al. Clinical comparison of primary versus secondary epilepsy in 125 cats. J Feline Med Surg 2010;12:910–16.

10. Seruca C, Ródenas S, Leiva M, et al. Acute postretinal blindness: ophthalmologic, neurologic, and magnetic resonance imaging findings in dogs and cats (seven cases). Vet Ophthalmol 2010;13:307–14.

11. Gutierrez-Quintana R, Gunn-Moore DA, Lamm CG, Penderis J. Feline intracranial meningioma with skull erosion and tumour extension into an area of skull hyperostosis. J Feline Med Surg 2011;13: 296–9.

12. Troxel MT, Vite CH, Massicotte C, et al. Magnetic resonance imaging features of feline intracranial neoplasia: retrospective analysis of 46 cats. J Vet Intern Med 2004;18:176–89.

13. Mattoon JS, Wisner ER. What's under the cat's hat: feline intracranial neoplasia and magnetic resonance imaging. J Vet Intern Med 2004;18:139–40.

14. Van der Vlugt-Meijer RH, Voorhout G, Meij BP. Imaging of the pituitary gland in dogs with pituitary-dependent hyperadrenocorticism. Mol Cell Endocrinol 2002;197:81–7.

15. Meij BP, Voorhout G, Rijnberk A. Progress in transsphenoidal hypophysectomy for treatment of pituitary-dependent hyperadrenocorticism in dogs and cats. Mol Cell Endocrinol 2002;197:89–96.

16. Auriemma E, Barthez PY, van der Vlugt-Meijer RH, et al. Computed tomography and low-field magnetic resonance imaging of the pituitary gland in dogs with pituitary-dependent hyperadrenocorticism: 11 cases (2001–2003). J Am Vet Med Assoc 2009;235:409–14.

17. Van der Vlugt-Meijer RH, Meij BP, Voorhout G. Thin-slice three-dimensional gradient-echo magnetic resonance imaging of the pituitary gland in healthy dogs. Am J Vet Res 2006;67:1865–72.

18. Van der Vlugt-Meijer RH, Meij BP, van den Ingh TS, et al. Dynamic computed tomography of the pituitary gland in dogs with pituitary-dependent hyperadrenocorticism. J Vet Intern Med 2003;17:773–80.

19. Van der Vlugt-Meijer RH, Meij BP, Voorhout G. Dynamic helical computed tomography of the pituitary gland in healthy dogs. Vet Radiol Ultrasound 2007;48:118–24.

20. Kooistra HS, Voorhout G, Mol JA, Rijnberk A. Correlation between impairment of glucocorticoid feedback and the size of the pituitary gland in dogs with pituitary-dependent hyperadrenocorticism. J Endocrinol 1997;152:387–94.

21. Wouters EGH, Beukers M, Theyse LF. Surgical treatment of a cerebral brain abscess in a cat. Vet Comp Orthop Traumatol 2011;24:72–5.

22. Forterre F, Tomek A, Konar M, et al. Multiple meningiomas: clinical, radiological, surgical, and pathological findings with outcome in four cats. J Feline Med Surg 2007;9:36–43.

23. Tomek A, Forterre E, Konar M, et al. Intracranial meningiomas associated with cervical syringohydromyelia in a cat. Schweiz Arch Tierheilkd 2008;150:123–8.

24. Nafe LA. Meningiomas in cats: a retrospective clinical study of 36 cases. J Am Vet Med Assoc 1979;174:1224–7.

25. Graham JP, Newell SM, Voges AK, et al. The dural tail sign in the diagnosis of meningiomas. Vet Radiol Ultrasound 1998;39:297–302.

26. Ramos-Vara JA, Miller MA, Gilbreath E, Patterson JS. Immunohistochemical detection of CD34, E-cadherin, claudin-1, glucose transporter 1, laminin, and protein gene product 9.5 in 28 canine and 8 feline meningiomas. Vet Pathol 2010;47:725–37.

27. Mandara MT, Pavone S, Mandrioli L, et al. Matrix metalloproteinase-2 and matrix metalloproteinase-9 expression in canine and feline meningioma. Vet Pathol 2009;46:836–45.

28. Adamo PF, Cantile C, Steinberg H. Evaluation of progesterone and estrogen receptor expression in 15 meningiomas of dogs and cats. Am J Vet Res 2003;64: 1310–18.

29. Lawson DC, Burk RL, Prata RG. Cerebral meningioma in the cat: Diagnosis and surgical treatment of ten cases. J Am Anim Hosp Assoc 1984;20:333–42.

30. Niebauer GW, Dayrell-Hart BL, Speciale J. Evaluation of craniotomy in dogs and cats. J Am Vet Med Assoc 1991;198:89–95.

31. Gallagher JG, Berg J, Knowles KE, et al. Prognosis after surgical excision of cerebral meningiomas in cats: 17 cases (1986–1992). J Am Vet Med Assoc 1993;203:1437–40.

32. Gordon LE, Thacher C, Matthiesen DT, Joseph RJ. Results of craniotomy for the treatment of cerebral meningioma in 42 cats. Vet Surg 1994;23:94–100.

33. Forterre F, Fritsch G, Kaiser S, et al. Surgical approach for tentorial meningiomas in cats: a review of six cases. J Feline Med Surg 2006;8:227–33.

34. Meij BP, Lopes MB, Ellegala DB, et al. The long-term significance of microscopic dural invasion in 354 patients with pituitary adenomas treated with transsphenoidal surgery. J Neurosurg 2002;96:195–208.

35. Peterson ME, Taylor RS, Greco DS, et al. Acromegaly in 14 cats. J Vet Int Med 1990;4:192–201.

36. Meij BP, van der Vlugt-Meijer RH, van den Ingh TS, et al. Melanotroph pituitary adenoma in a cat with diabetes mellitus. Vet Path 2005;42:92–7.

37. Meij BP, van der Vlugt-Meijer RH, van den Ingh TS, Rijnberk A. Somatotroph and corticotroph pituitary adenoma (double adenoma) in a cat with diabetes mellitus and hyperadrenocorticism. J Comp Path 2004;130:209–15.

38. Slingerland LI, Voorhout G, Rijnberk A, Kooistra HS. Growth hormone excess and the effect of octreotide in cats with diabetes mellitus. Dom Anim Endocrinol 2008;35:352–61.

39. Galac S, Reusch CE, Kooistra HS, et al. Adrenals. In: Rijnberk A, Kooistra HS, editors. Clinical endocrinology of dogs and cats. Hannover: Schlütersche; 2010. p. 93–154.

40. Fracassi F, Mandrioli L, Diana A, et al. Pituitary macroadenoma in a cat with diabetes mellitus, hypercortisolism and neurological signs. J Vet Med A Physiol Pathol Clin Med 2007;54:359–63.

41. Meij BP, Voorhout G, Van Den Ingh TS, Rijnberk A. Transsphenoidal hypophysectomy for treatment of pituitary-dependent hyperadrenocorticism in 7 cats. Vet Surg 2001;30:72–86.

42. Duesberg CA, Nelson RW, Feldman EC, et al. Adrenalectomy for treatment of hyperadrenocorticism in cats: 10 cases (1988–1992). J Am Vet Med Assoc 1995;207:1066–70.

43. Watson PJ, Herrtage ME. Hyperadrenocorticism in six cats. J Small Anim Pract 1998;39:175–84.

44. Daley CA, Zerbe CA, Schick RO, Powers RD. Use of metyrapone to treat pituitary-dependent hyperadrenocorticism in a cat with large cutaneous wounds. J Am Vet Med Assoc 1993;202:956–60.

45. Moore LE, Biller DS, Olsen DE. Hyperadrenocorticism treated with metyrapone followed by bilateral adrenalectomy in a cat. J Am Vet Med Assoc 2000;217:691–4.

46. Skelly BJ, Petrus D, Nicholls PK. Use of trilostane for the treatment of pituitary-dependent hyperadrenocorticism in a cat. J Small Anim Pract 2003;44:269–72.

47. Neiger R, Witt AL, Noble A, German AJ. Trilostane therapy for treatment of pituitary-dependent hyperadrenocorticism in 5 cats. J Vet Intern Med 2004;18: 160–4.

48. Meij BP, Auriemma E, Grinwis G, et al. Successful treatment of acromegaly in a diabetic cat with transsphenoidal hypophysectomy. J Feline Med Surg 2010;12:406–10.

49. Berg RI, Nelson RW, Feldman EC, et al. Serum insulin-like growth factor-I concentration in cats with diabetes mellitus and acromegaly. J Vet Intern Med 2007;21:892–8.

50. Niessen SJ, Petrie G, Gaudiano F, et al. Feline acromegaly: an underdiagnosed endocrinopathy? J Vet Intern Med 2007;21:899–905.

51. Javadi S, Slingerland LI, van de Beek MG, et al. Plasma renin activity and plasma concentrations of aldosterone, cortisol, adrenocorticotropic hormone, and alpha-melanocyte-stimulating hormone in healthy cats. J Vet Intern Med 2004;18: 625–31.

52. Norman EJ, Mooney CT. Diagnosis and management of diabetes mellitus in five cats with somatotrophic abnormalities. J Feline Med Surg 2000;2:183–90.

53. de Lange MS, Galac S, Trip MR, Kooistra HS. High urinary corticoid/creatinine ratios in cats with hyperthyroidism. J Vet Intern Med 2004;18:152–5.

54. Abrams-Ogg ACG, Holmberg DL, Stewart WA, Claffey FP. Acromegaly in a cat: diagnosis by magnetic resonance imaging and treatment by cryohypophysectomy. Can Vet J 1993;34:682–5.

55. Abrams-Ogg ACG, Holmberg DL, Quinn RF, et al. Blindness now attributed to enrofloxacin therapy in a previously reported case of a cat with acromegaly treated by cryohypophysectomy. Can Vet J 2002;43:53–4.

56. Blois SL, Holmberg DL. Cryohypophysectomy used in the treatment of a case of feline acromegaly. J Small Anim Pract 2008;49:596–600.

57. Goossens MM, Feldman EC, Nelson RW, et al. Cobalt 60 irradiation of pituitary gland tumors in three cats with acromegaly. J Am Vet Med Assoc 1998;213:374–6.

58. Littler RM, Polton GA, Brearley MJ. Resolution of diabetes mellitus but not acromegaly in a cat with a pituitary macroadenoma treated with hypofractionated radiation. J Small Anim Pract 2006;47:392–5.

59. Kaser-Hotz B, Rohrer CR, Stankeova S, et al. Radiotherapy of pituitary tumours in five cats. J Small Anim Pract 2002;43: 303–7.

60. Mayer MN, Greco DS, LaRue SM. Outcomes of pituitary tumor irradiation in cats. J Vet Int Med 2006;20:1151–4.

61. Dunning MD, Lowrie CS, Bexfield NH, et al. Exogenous insulin treatment after hypofractionated radiotherapy in cats with diabetes mellitus and acromegaly. J Vet Intern Med 2009;23:243–9.

62. Abraham LA, Helmond SE, Mitten RW, et al. Treatment of an acromegalic cat with the dopamine agonist L-deprenyl. Austr Vet J 2002;80:479–83.

63. Higham C, Chung TT, Lawrance J, et al. Long term experience of pegvisomant therapy as a treatment for acromegaly. Clin Endocrinol (Oxf) 2009;71: 86–91.

64. Allgoewer I, Grevel V, Philipp K, et al. Somatotropic pituitary adenoma with lesions of the oculomotor nerve in a cat. Tierärztl Prax Ausg K Kleintiere Heimtiere 1998;26:267–72.

65. Bertolini G, Rossetti E, Caldin M. Pituitary apoplexy-like disease in 4 dogs. J Vet Intern Med 2007;21:1251–7.

66. Rijnberk A, Mol JA, Kwant MM, Croughs RJ. Effects of bromocriptine on corticotrophin, melanotrophin and corticosteroid secretion in dogs with pituitary-dependent hyperadrenocorticism. J Endocrinol 1988;118:271–7.

67. De Bruin C, Hanson JM, Meij BP, et al. Expression and functional analysis of dopamine receptor subtype 2 and somatostatin receptor subtypes in canine Cushing's disease. Endocrinology 2008;149:4357–66.

68. Castillo VA, Gómez NV, Lalia JC, et al. Cushing's disease in dogs: Cabergoline treatment. Res Vet Sci 2008;85:26–34.

69. Mayer MN, Treuil PL. Radiation therapy for pituitary tumors in the dog and cat. Can Vet J 2007;48:316–18.

70. Brearley MJ, Polton GA, Littler RM, Niessen SJ. Coarse fractionated radiation therapy for pituitary tumours in cats: a retrospective study of 12 cases. Vet Comp Oncol 2006;4:209–17.

71. Van de Bovenkamp CG, Meij BP, Stassen QE, et al. Administration of radioactive holmium-166 microsphere in domestic animals with inoperable tumors. Tijdschr Diergeneeskd 2009;134:532–3.

72. Fusco JV, Hohenhaus AE, Aiken SW, et al. Autologous blood collection and transfusion in cats undergoing partial craniectomy. J Am Vet Med Assoc 2000;216:1584–8.

73. O'Brien CS, Bagley RS, Hicks DG, et al. Gamma-irradiated calvarium allograft cranioplasty in a cat following brain tumor removal. J Am Anim Hosp Assoc 2010;46:268–73.

74. Forterre F, Jaggy A, Rohrbach H, et al. Modified temporal approach for a rostro-temporal basal meningioma in a cat. J Feline Med Surg 2009;11:510–13.

75. Meij BP, Voorhout G, Van den Ingh TS, et al. Transsphenoidal hypophysectomy in beagle dogs: evaluation of a microsurgical technique. Vet Surg 1997;26:295–309.

76. Meij BP. Treatment protocols. Pituitary. Hypophysectomy. In: Rijnberk A, Kooistra HS, editors. Clinical endocrinology of dogs and cats. 2nd ed. Hannover: Schlütersche; 2010. p. 315–16.

Index

Printed in the United States
By Bookmasters